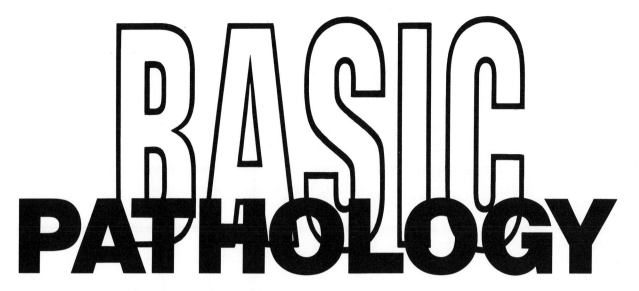

# BASIC PATHOLOGY

**FOURTH EDITION**

## STANLEY L. ROBBINS, M.D.
Visiting Professor of Pathology, Harvard Medical School
Senior Pathologist, Brigham and Women's Hospital
Boston, Massachusetts

## VINAY KUMAR, M.D.
Charles T. Ashworth Professor of Pathology, Department of Pathology
University of Texas, Southwestern Medical School
Dallas, Texas

1987
**W. B. SAUNDERS COMPANY**

Philadelphia   London   Toronto   Sydney   Tokyo   Hong Kong

W. B. Saunders Company:    West Washington Square
                           Philadelphia, PA 19105

**Library of Congress Cataloging-in-Publication Data**

Robbins, Stanley L. (Stanley Leonard), 1915–

Basic pathology.

Includes bibliographies and index.

1. Pathology.    I. Kumar, Vinay.    II. Title.
   [DNLM: 1. Pathology.    QZ 4 R636b]

RB111.R6    1987    616.07    86–21984

ISBN 0–7216–1814–6

Listed here is the latest translated edition of this book together with the language of the translation and the publisher.

Spanish (*1st Edition*)—NEISA, Mexico City, D.F., Mexico

Spanish (*3rd Edition*)—Nueva Editorial Interamericana S.A. de C.V., Mexico City, Mexico

*Editor*:  Dean Manke
*Developmental Editor*:  Kathleen McCullough
*Designer*:  W. B. Saunders Staff
*Production Manager*:  Bob Butler
*Manuscript Editor*:  Linda Mills
*Illustration Coordinator*:  Walter Verbitski
*Indexer*:  Angela Holt

Basic Pathology                                                    ISBN 0–7216–1814–6

Last digit is the print number:    9   8   7   6   5   4   3   2   1

To
JEREMY AND JOSEPH
AND TO
AMBIKA AND ROHIT
WITH LOVE

# Preface

The preface of the previous edition of this text began with the words, "It is a pleasure to write. . . ." It is an even greater pleasure to write the preface for this edition of *Basic Pathology*. We are grateful and encouraged by the acceptance of its forebears and hope that the present edition will be up to their standards. Indeed, if time, effort, and dedication to the task have any meaning, this edition will surpass the previous ones.

Our goals remain substantially unaltered:

To present a balanced and accurate picture of the central body of knowledge of pathology in as clear, dynamic, accurate, and readable a manner as possible.

To accord space to subjects in proportion to their clinical or biologic significance, providing rounded, reasonably complete discussions of the more important.

To maintain the book's "slimness" by selectivity and judicious omission rather than by sketchy telegraphic brevity.

To relate lesions and dysfunctions to the diseases they produce, never losing sight of the meaning of the word "dis-ease."

Above all, to be meticulous about clarity, readability, and the quality of the language.

Even though the goals remain as before, this edition differs greatly from its predecessor. Entire chapters have been rewritten, and all have been extensively revised. No single line from the previous edition has been retained without rigorous appraisal. Several new contributors have added their expertise. A chapter on disorders of the oral cavity and teeth has been added. With particular pride we point to the large number of new illustrations, especially the introduction of drawings, diagrams, flow charts, and additional tables and outlines to support and augment the writing. We strongly subscribe to the old saying, "a single picture is worth a thousand words," but only if the image is crystal clear, interpretable, representative, and photogenic. It goes without saying that a strenuous effort was made to incorporate the best and latest information available. New diseases and revised concepts of old diseases are found throughout, as, for example, the current state of knowledge about the Acquired Immunodeficiency Syndrome (AIDS) and the explosion of information about oncogenes and their roles in the causation of cancer. A liberal number of references on points or subjects of interest are included to provide source material to those wanting to know more, and all the chapter bibliographies have been extensively revised, sometimes to the point of total replacement. Significant contributions in the 1985 and 1986 literature were incorporated up to the moment the book "went to press" because they are key to understanding advances in the field.

The format of the book is basically the same as in the previous edition. The first portion deals with the basic mechanisms and principles of general pathology, detailing to the extent of our current knowledge "the machinery that turns the wheels" and the terminology. Although the reasonably well-established concepts are emphasized, emerging trends are flagged when they seem promising. Pains have been taken to differentiate the known from the half-known and the unknown, to foster critical awareness of the many fields left to conquer.

The second portion of the text covers systemic pathology, sequentially considering the organs and systems of the body. In each chapter the more important diseases are considered in reasonable detail as dynamic processes from their origins to their ultimate consequences on the tissues and organs and on the patient as a whole. Individual entities are always taken up in the whole and not dismembered into component parts discussed in several chapters. No attempt is made at encyclopedic coverage; marginal disorders are either treated briefly or entirely omitted. Better to know 90% well, than 100% half-well. Only time and reader response will tell us whether our judgments were sound.

We hope we have succeeded in presenting the broad dimensions of pathology in an understandable and enjoyable manner. Learning can be and should be satisfying, stimulating, and, yes, even fun. The extent to which we have encouraged the reader to want to know more is a measure of our success.

# Acknowledgments

The completion of a text not only brings an appreciated respite from many, many months of demanding effort, it also provides a welcome opportunity to acknowledge in writing the many kind souls who helped along the way. First among them are our personal editorial assistants: Ms. Sandra Jeffries, Ms. Deborah Scott, and Ms. Malorye Allison. To Sandra, the book was her "baby," on which she lavished endless care, labor, and love. She helped in the literature search, typed manuscript, edited it, and in general organized the endless detail. Her standards of excellence never permitted her to falter in her pursuit of perfection. Deborah and Malorye likewise never settled for anything less than the very best. To all of them we are indebted not only for all of their contributions but also for setting the example that nothing but the best effort would suffice. Less deeply involved in secretarial, literature search, and editorial capacities were Marcia Diefendorf, Eileen Fonferko, and Beverly Shackelford. Their help was willingly and expertly given, often at times of great pressure and need, and so we are all the more grateful. To these valued helpmates an awareness that their labors did not go unnoticed and our grateful thanks.

Particularly deserving of our thanks are our medical artist-illustrators, Ms. Marcia Williams and Mr. Michael Schenk. Their deft and elegant drawings grace many pages of this text and add welcome amplification and clarification to the writing. From long hours of working with them we learned that, demanding and laborious as the rendering of a drawing may be, it is child's play compared to the capturing of a complex concept in a comprehensible visual image. We hope only that the reader will receive as much pleasure from these contributions as the authors received from working with their creators.

We owe much to the contributors who have so unmistakably enhanced the quality of this text with their expertise. Dr. Ramzi Cotran, our close friend, colleague, and fellow author, graciously took time from a very busy schedule to revise the chapters on disease at the cellular level and the kidney and its collecting system. Dr. Maximilian Buja was kind enough to re-do the chapters on blood vessels and the heart, areas in which he is an acknowledged expert. Dr. L. Eversole assumed the difficult task of preparing a new chapter on the teeth and oral cavity, and Dr. James Morris revised in a superb fashion the chapter on the nervous system. Their contributions are deeply appreciated not only for their authority and excellence but also for their being provided on time.

Many colleague-friends helped in innumerable ways—providing choice illustrations, guiding us to excellent slides for photography, providing valuable suggestions, and offering helpful critiques. Among them are Drs. R. Ehrmann, J. Godleski, F. Lichtenberg, G. Pincus, M. Warhol, and W. Welch (at Boston) and Drs. D. Burns, J. Hernandez, R. McKenna, F. Silva, A. Weinberg, and C. White III (at Dallas); others are acknowledged with their illustrations. Although the individual contributions may not loom large in the overall perspective of the entire text, they were greatly needed from time to time and so the more valuable; collectively they have added a great deal to the quality of the finished product. Special mention should be made of past and present Pathology House Officers of the Brigham and Women's Hospital for their many kindnesses, such as an illustration from their personal collections or the preparation of a photomicrograph. With apologies they are not named individually for fear of egregious omissions.

Thanks should also be extended to W. B. Saunders and in particular Linda Mills and Kathleen McCullough of the editorial department. Although there are always endless details involved in the production and printing of a text that could constitute points of irritation and frustration, we are happy to acknowledge that none disturbed the team effort, leaving no doubt in our minds about W. B. Saunders' desire to produce the best possible text.

Finally, but no less deeply felt, some personal debts of obligation. Writing is a lonely business that inevitably excludes others for long periods of time. To our wives, Elly Robbins and Raminder Kumar, and to our children and grandchildren our apologies for our protracted and repeated absences, and our thanks for their patience. Each of us wishes also to acknowledge the pleasure it has been having the other for a co-author. It is not that we always thought alike, but that we were always willing to acknowledge the worth of the other's thoughts.

# Contents

I

# 1

# Cell Injury and Adaptation

RAMZI S. COTRAN, M.D.*

Acknowledging that the whole is greater than the sum of its parts, every human is ultimately a fiendishly complicated and clever aggregation of cells.

*F. B. Mallory Professor of Pathology, Harvard Medical School; Chairman, Department of Pathology, Brigham and Women's Hospital, Boston.

The health of the individual has its origin in healthy cells. Disease, on the other hand, reflects dysfunction of a significant number of cells. It is necessary then to begin our consideration of pathology with an examination of disease at the cellular and subcellular levels.

The normal cell is a restless, pulsating microcosm constantly modifying its structure and function in response to changing demands and stresses. Until these stresses become too severe, the cell tends to maintain a relatively narrow range of structure and function, designated as "normal." Just as the individual must adapt to the constantly changing demands and stresses of life, so must the cell. Within limits, cellular adaptation achieves an altered but steady state, preserving the health of the cell despite continued stress. However, if the limits of adaptive capability are exceeded, injury or even cell death results. In response to progressive levels of stress, then, the cell may (1) adapt, (2) be reversibly injured, or (3) die (Fig. 1–1). We can draw an analogy to a stately tree exposed to a wind storm. Up to a point the tree bends and yields to the stresses of the wind forces but rapidly resumes its erectness when the stresses abate. The windswept conformation of the tree on the shoreline is a beautiful example of an adaptive, altered, but steady state permitting continued survival and growth. More severe wind may break branches and strip leaves, but such injury is compatible with recovery and survival. A hurricane, however, may be more than the tree can withstand and leave it an uprooted victim of stresses too great for survival.

*The normal cell, the adapted cell, the injured cell, and the irreversibly injured or dead cell are hazily delimited states along a continuum of function and structure.* In response to moderate stress the cell might pass through a succession of stages of adaptation and injury, only to die eventually. More severe stress might induce direct injury and, of course, intense injury might kill immediately. One cannot assume that all stressed or injured cells pass through every stage of reaction. Whether a specific form of stress induces adaptation, injury, or cell death depends not only on the nature and severity of the stress but also on many variables relating to the cells themselves, such as particular vulnerability, differ-

3

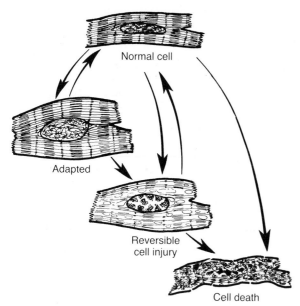

Figure 1–1. The relationships among normal, adapted, reversibly injured, and dead myocardial cells. The cellular adaptation depicted here is hypertrophy, and the type of cellular injury is ischemic.

and molecular biological techniques. The time lag required to produce the visible changes of cellular adaptation, injury, or death varies with the discriminatory ability of the methods used to detect these changes. With histochemical or ultrastructural techniques, changes can be seen in minutes or hours, but it may be much longer before they become evident with the light microscope or on gross examination of the tissue. Despite sophisticated methods of morphologic and biochemical investigation, the boundary lines between these stages are still difficult to define, and there are no clear benchmarks by which the severely stressed but still normal cell can be distinguished from the cell that has been taxed to the point of injury. Similarly, there are no certain measurements by which the injured but still viable cell can be differentiated from one that is fatally injured.

The following sections consider first the broad categories of stresses and noxious influences that induce cellular injury, death, and adaptation; then each of these three states will be taken up individually.

# CAUSES OF CELLULAR INJURY, DEATH, AND ADAPTATION

The stresses that induce altered morphologic states in the cell range from the gross physical violence of a crushing blow to the subtle dislocations involved in the absence of a single enzyme, as occurs in many genetic conditions. The broad categories of adverse influences known to affect cellular functions include (1) hypoxia, (2) chemicals and drugs, (3) physical agents, (4) microbiologic agents, (5) immune mechanisms, (6) genetic defects, (7) nutritional imbalances, and (8) aging.

## HYPOXIA

Hypoxia, an extremely important and common cause of cell injury and cell death, impinges on aerobic oxidative respiration. Loss of blood supply, which may occur when the arterial flow or the venous drainage is impeded by vascular disease or luminal clots, is the most common cause of hypoxia. Another frequent cause is inadequate oxygenation of the blood owing to cardiorespiratory failure. Loss of the oxygen-carrying *capacity* of the blood, as in anemia or carbon monoxide poisoning (producing a stable carbon monoxyhemoglobin that blocks oxygen carriage), is a third, less frequent basis for oxygen deprivation. Depending on the severity of the hypoxic state, cells may adapt, undergo injury, or die. For example, if the femoral artery is narrowed, the skeletal muscle cells of the leg may shrink in size (atrophy). This reduction in cell mass achieves a balance between metabolic needs and the available oxygen supply.

entiation, blood supply, nutrition, and previous state of the cell.

In many instances there are ready explanations for particular cell vulnerabilities. Carbon tetrachloride, inhaled or ingested, is metabolized in the liver, and free radicals (discussed later), which are far more toxic than the parent compound, are released there. Thus, liver cells bear the brunt of this form of injury. Cardiac muscle cells have a high rate of metabolism and thus are very susceptible to hypoxia. Sometimes the site of attack or delivery of the stressful influence determines the particular cells affected. For example, the pulmonary parenchyma is attacked directly by inhaled toxic gases. Despite these obvious explanations there are many instances in which stressful agents induce changes in mysterious sites. We only partly know why, for example, the polio virus, which usually enters the body through the gastrointestinal tract, attacks principally anterior horn ganglion cells in the spinal cord or why a toxic level of lead absorbed into the bloodstream exerts its effect principally on the hematopoietic system, the central nervous system, and the kidneys. Nonetheless, it is important to know the major targets of the various forms of stress in order to make an educated guess at the etiology of the cellular change from the selective sites of involvement. Thus, the child with an anemia and manifestations of diffuse central nervous system involvement may well be a victim of lead poisoning.

All stresses and noxious influences exert their effects first at the molecular level. The molecular and functional changes always precede the morphologic alterations and are now being elucidated by cellular

More severe hypoxia would, of course, induce cell injury or cell death.

## CHEMICALS (INCLUDING DRUGS)

Chemicals and drugs are important causes of cell adaptation, injury, and death. Virtually any chemical agent or drug may be implicated. Even an innocuous substance such as glucose, if sufficiently concentrated, may so derange the osmotic environment of the cell that it causes injury or cell death. Agents commonly known as poisons may cause severe cell damage and possibly death of the whole organism. Many of these chemicals and drugs effect their changes by acting on some vital function of the cell, such as membrane permeability, osmotic homeostasis, or the integrity of an enzyme or cofactor. As mentioned earlier, the individual agent usually has specific targets within the body, affecting some cells and sparing others. In some cases this selectivity reflects the cell populations involved in the absorption, transport, and metabolism of the agent. Barbiturates evoke changes in liver cells because it is these cells that are involved in the degradation of such drugs. When mercuric chloride is ingested it is absorbed from the stomach and excreted through the kidneys and colon. Thus it exerts its principal effects on these organs. However, we do not always have satisfactory explanations for the selective points of attack of the many chemicals and drugs that induce cellular changes.

## PHYSICAL AGENTS

Trauma, extremes of heat or cold, sudden changes in atmospheric pressure, radiant energy, and electrical energy all have wide-ranging effects on cells. *Mechanical trauma* may cause subtle but significant dislocations of the intracellular organization of organelles or, at the other extreme, may destroy the cell by completely disrupting it.

Cold and heat are evident causes of stress, cell injury and even cell death. *Low temperature* acts in a number of ways. At first it induces vasoconstriction and impairs the blood supply to cells. Injury to the vasomotor control, with marked vasodilatation, stagnation of blood flow, and sometimes intravascular coagulation, may follow. When the temperature becomes sufficiently low, intracellular water crystallizes. Damaging *high temperatures* may of course incinerate tissues, but long before this point is reached increased temperature causes injury by inducing hypermetabolism, exceeding the capacity of the available blood supply. Hypermetabolism also leads to the accumulation of acid metabolites, which lowers the pH of the cell to critical levels.

*Sudden changes in atmospheric pressure* also may lead to impairment of the blood supply to cells. Deep sea divers or tunnel diggers, when working under increased atmospheric pressure, have higher levels of atmospheric gases dissolved in their blood. If such individuals return to normal pressure too quickly the dissolved gases come out of solution rapidly and form air bubbles within the circulation. Oxygen is readily redissolved, but nitrogen is less soluble and may persist as small bubbles that become trapped in the microcirculation, blocking blood flow and ultimately causing hypoxic injury to cells. This disorder is called "caisson disease."

The damaging effects of *radiant energy* were all too vividly illustrated by the atomic bombs dropped on Japan (p. 279). Less grotesque exposure to radiant energy may also be injurious, either because of direct ionization of chemical compounds contained within the cell or because of ionization of cellular water, producing free "hot" radicals that secondarily interact with intracellular constituents (p. 9). Radiant energy also induces varying mutations that may injure or even kill cells.

*Electrical energy* generates heat when it passes through the body and may thus produce burns. More importantly, however, it may interfere with neural conduction pathways and often causes death from cardiac arrhythmias. The extent of damage induced by electrical current depends on its voltage and amperage, the tissue resistance (hence the generation of heat), and the pathway followed by the current from its point of entrance in the body to its point of exit.

## MICROBIOLOGIC AGENTS

A host of living agents, ranging in size from the submicroscopic viruses to grossly visible nematodes, may attack humans and cause cell injury, cell death, or death of the individual. Here it is possible to discuss only a few generalizations about how these living forms affect cells. *Viruses* and *rickettsias* are obligate intracellular parasites—that is, they can survive only within living cells. The interaction between viruses and host cells takes many forms. Many viruses parasitize cells apparently without affecting them; these have been termed "passenger viruses." Those that induce cellular changes fall into two broad categories: (1) agents capable of causing cell death (cytolytic) and (2) agents that stimulate cell replication and possibly cause tumors (oncogenic). The mechanisms by which some viruses cause cell injury are discussed on page 11, and the issue of viral oncogenesis is reviewed in the chapter on neoplasia (p. 204).

*Bacteria* are almost as unpredictable in their effects as viruses.[1] Some are harmless commensals, and some even contribute to human survival. The *Escherichia coli* flora of the gut, for example, constitutes a valuable source of vitamin K. However, even *E. coli* may cause disease in infants, who have little or no immunity to these otherwise innocuous organisms, or in debilitated or immunodeficient adults. Similarly, many individuals harbor potentially pathogenic bacteria in the oropharynx but develop a significant clinical infection only when rendered vulnerable. The administration of broad-spectrum antibiotics may destroy the normal coliform flora of the gut and permit swallowed staphylococci to multiply wildly within the intestinal tract. A staphylococcal enteritis then ensues, which can lead to bacteremia and death. In contrast, other bacteria, such as the agents causing syphilis, gonorrhea, or plague, almost always cause disease if the organism gains a portal of entry.

How bacteria evoke cellular injury and disease is imperfectly understood. Some organisms liberate exotoxins capable of causing cell injury at a distance from the site of implantation of the bacteria. Other agents elaborate endotoxins that are released only on disintegration of the organisms. In addition, some bacteria may damage cells by elaborating a variety of enzymes such as lecithinase (*Clostridium perfringens*), capable of destroying cell membranes, or hemolysins (beta-hemolytic streptococci), which lyse red cells. Another potential mechanism of bacterial injury is the development of hypersensitivity to the agent, leading to damaging immunologic reactions.

We know little about how *fungi, protozoa,* and *helminths* cause cell damage and disease. Some, such as the Histoplasma, Coccidioides, and Blastomyces, induce sensitization reactions; but others, such as the Actinomyces, do not. How protozoa induce cell injury is sometimes remarkably clear and at other times obscure. Amebiasis is caused by a protozoan that elaborates powerful cytopathic enzymes and so destroys tissues wherever it implants. The plasmodia of malaria invade and eventually destroy red cells by releasing toxic metabolites as well as malarial pigment derived from hemoglobin. The causative agent of toxoplasmosis, however, is an obligate intracellular protozoan that causes considerable tissue damage by obscure mechanisms in its sites of localization. Helminthic infections have their own specific sites of localization and induce cell injury for the most part by obscure means. The agent of trichinosis preferentially invades striated muscle (cardiac and skeletal) and eventually destroys parasitized cells. The trichina worm may usurp the energy supplies of the cell, or possibly its metabolic end products are toxic, but these explanations are speculative. Filariasis is characterized by intense fibrosis at sites of localization, but we do not understand precisely why such inflammatory fibrosis evolves.

## IMMUNE MECHANISMS

Immune reactions have come to be recognized as not uncommon causes of cell damage and disease. The trigger antigen may be exogenous in origin, as for example the resin of poison ivy, or it may be endogenous (e.g., cellular antigens). The latter evoke so-called autoimmune diseases. The effect of immune reactions on cells is discussed in Chapter 5, page 136.

## GENETIC DERANGEMENTS

Critical to the cell's homeostasis is its normal genetic apparatus. Mutations, whatever their origin, may have no recognizable effect, may deprive the cell of a single enzyme (*inborn errors of metabolism*), or may be so severe that they are incompatible with cell survival. The mutation may appear during gametogenesis, in the early zygote, or in adult cells (a somatic mutation). Indeed, as will be discussed, somatic mutations may underlie the origins of cancerous transformation of cells. As is well known, some genetic abnormalities are transmitted as familial traits, such as sickle cell anemia. More is said about genetic derangements in Chapter 4, page 84.

## NUTRITIONAL IMBALANCES

It is sad to report that deficiencies in nutrition not only are important causes of cell injury today but threaten to become devastating problems in the future. Protein-calorie deficiencies (which scourge many developing nations) are the most obvious examples. Avitaminoses also are rampant in deprived populations and are not uncommon even in industrialized nations having relatively high standards of living. Ironically, excesses in nutrition, privileged only to upper economic groups, are important causes of morbidity and mortality. Excess calories and diets rich in animal fats are now strongly implicated in the development of atherosclerosis. Obesity alone leads to an increased vulnerability to certain disorders. Unfortunately, both obesity and atherosclerosis have become virtually epidemic in some countries, such as the United States. All of these disorders are obviously associated with cell injury and cell death.

## AGING

The mechanisms of cellular adaptations and injury in aging cells are discussed on page 12.

## PATHOGENESIS

The problem of unraveling the biochemical sequence of events responsible for cell injury has proved to be immensely complex. Injury to cells may have many causes, and there is probably no common final pathway of cell death. The many macromolecules, enzymes, biochemical systems, and organelles

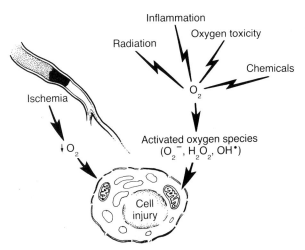

**Figure 1–2.** The critical role of oxygen in cell injury. Ischemia causes cell injury by reducing cellular oxygen supplies, whereas other stimuli, such as radiation, induce damage via toxic activated oxygen species (p. 9).

within the cell are so closely interdependent that it is difficult to differentiate the primary target of injury from the secondary ripple effects. The "point of no return," i.e., the point at which irreversible damage and cell death occur, is still largely undetermined.

With certain injurious agents, the mechanisms and loci of attack are well defined. Cyanide represents an intracellular asphyxiant in that it inactivates cytochrome oxidase. Certain anaerobic bacteria, such as *Clostridium perfringens*, elaborate phospholipases, which attack phospholipids in cell membranes. Other isolated examples exist, but the modes of action of many injurious agents are largely unknown. Recent work, however, suggests a central role for *oxygen* in cell injury (Fig. 1–2). Lack of oxygen clearly underlies the pathogenesis of cell injury in ischemia, but it also is becoming abundantly clear that *partially reduced activated oxygen species* are important mediators of cell death in many pathological conditions.[2–4] As we shall see, these free radical species cause lipid peroxidation and other deleterious effects on cell structure. In the following account we shall concentrate on hypoxic injury, some forms of chemical injury, and injury induced by viruses as model systems of cell injury.

## ISCHEMIC AND HYPOXIC INJURY

**Sequence of Events.** The sequence of morphologic changes following acute hypoxic injury has been studied extensively in humans, in experimental animals, and in culture systems,[5] and reasonable schemes concerning the mechanisms underlying these changes have emerged (Fig. 1–3).

*The first point of attack of hypoxia is the cell's aerobic respiration, i.e., oxidative phosphorylation by mitochondria.* The generation of ATP thus slows down or stops. This loss of ATP has widespread effects on many systems within the cell. In particular, the activity of the ouabain-sensitive ATPase of the cell membrane is decreased, causing failure of the active membrane "sodium pump," accumulation of sodium intracellularly, and diffusion of potassium out of the cell. The net gain of solute is accompanied by an iso-osmotic gain of water, producing *acute cellular swelling.*

The decrease in cellular ATP and associated increase in AMP also stimulate the enzyme phosphofructokinase, which results in an increased rate of anaerobic glycolysis to maintain the cell's energy sources by generating ATP from glycogen. Glycogen is thus rapidly depleted, a phenomenon that can be appreciated histologically if tissues are stained for glycogen (such as with the periodic acid–Schiff stain [PAS]). Glycolysis results in the accumulation of lactic acid and inorganic phosphates from the hydrolysis of phosphate esters. *This reduces the intracellular pH.*

The next phenomenon to occur is *detachment of ribosomes from the granular endoplasmic reticulum and dissociation of polysomes into monosomes.* If hypoxia continues, other alterations take place and, again, are reflections of increased membrane permeability and diminished mitochondrial function. *Blebs* may form at the cell surface. "Myelin" figures (concentric laminations), derived from plasma as well as organellar membranes, are seen within the cytoplasm or extracellularly. At this time the mitochondria appear either normal, or slightly swollen, or actually condensed; the endoplasmic reticulum is dilated; and the entire cell is markedly swollen.

*All the above disturbances are reversible* if oxygenation is restored. However, if ischemia persists, irreversible injury ensues. Irreversible injury is associated morphologically with severe vacuolization of the mitochondria, including their cristae; extensive damage to plasma membranes; swelling of lysosomes; and—particularly if the ischemic zone is reperfused—massive *calcium influx* into the cell. *Amorphous densities develop in the mitochondrial matrix.* In the myocardium, these are early indications of irreversible injury and can be seen as soon as 30 to 40 minutes after ischemia. There is continued loss of proteins, essential coenzymes, and ribonucleic acids from the hyperpermeable membranes. The cells may also leak metabolites, which are vital for the reconstitution of ATP, thus further depleting net intracellular high-energy phosphates.

The falling pH leads to injury to the lysosomal membranes, followed by leakage of their enzymes into the cytoplasm, activation of acid hydrolases, and enzymatic digestion of cell components, evidenced by loss of ribonucleoprotein, deoxyribonucleoprotein, and glycogen.

Following cell death, cell components are progressively degraded, and there is leakage of cellular

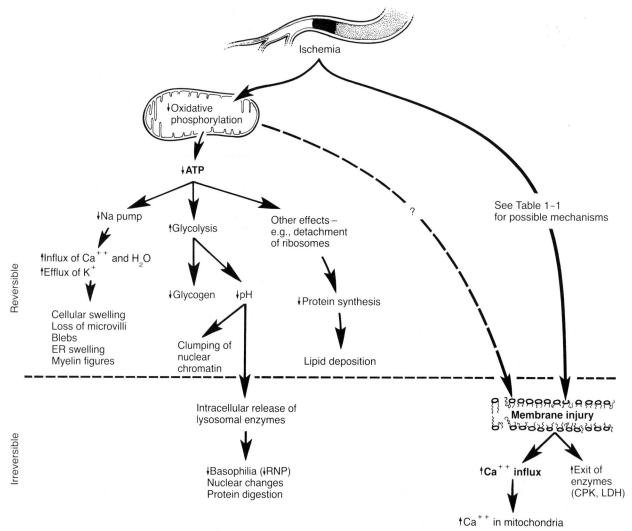

**Figure 1–3.** Postulated sequence of events in ischemic injury. Note that although reduced oxidative phosphorylation and ATP levels have a central role, ischemia causes direct membrane damage by currently uncertain mechanisms, listed in Table 1–1 (p. 9).

enzymes into the extracellular space and, conversely, entry of extracellular macromolecules from the interstitial space into the dead cells. Finally, the dead cell may become replaced by large masses composed of phospholipids, in the form of "myelin figures." These are then either phagocytosed by other cells or degraded further into fatty acids. *Calcification* of such fatty acid residues may occur with the formation of calcium soaps.

At this point in the story, we should note that leakage of intracellular enzymes across the abnormally permeable plasma membrane and into the serum provides important clinical indicators of cell death. Cardiac muscle, for example, contains glutamic-oxaloacetic transaminase (GOT), pyruvic transaminases, lactic dehydrogenase (LDH), and creatine kinase (CK). Elevated serum levels of such enzymes, and particularly the isoenzymes specific for heart

muscle (e.g., CK-MB), are valuable clinical criteria of myocardial infarction, a locus of ischemic cell death in heart muscle.

**MECHANISMS OF IRREVERSIBLE INJURY.** The sequence of events for hypoxia was described as a continuum from its initiation to ultimate digestion of the lethally injured cell by lysosomal enzymes. But at what point did the cell actually die? *And what are the critical events for irreversible injury?* Two phenomena consistently characterize irreversibility. The first is the *inability to reverse mitochondrial dysfunction* (lack of oxidative phosphorylation and ATP generation) upon reperfusion or reoxygenation, and the second is the development of *profound disturbances in membrane function.*[6, 7]

It would be reasonable to consider that progressive depletion of ATP in itself at some critical juncture constitutes a lethal event, but the evidence on this

Table 1–1. POSSIBLE CAUSES OF
MEMBRANE DAMAGE IN
IRREVERSIBLE ISCHEMIC INJURY

1. Depletion of cellular ATP
2. Loss of membrane phospholipids (decreased synthesis or
   increased degradation)
3. Lipid breakdown products (free fatty acids; lysophospholipids)
4. Toxic oxygen species
5. Cytoskeletal alterations
6. Rupture of lysosomes

issue is conflicting. Although numerous alterations in mitochondrial structure and function are found in ischemic tissues, it has been possible experimentally to dissociate these changes as well as ATP depletion from the inevitability of cell death.[8]

*A great deal of evidence favors cell membrane damage as a central factor in the pathogenesis of irreversible cell injury.*[9] As should be well known, the cell membrane consists of a lipid-protein mosaic made up of a bimolecular layer of phospholipids and globular proteins embedded within the lipid bilayer. An intact plasma membrane is essential to the maintenance of normal cell permeability and volume. Loss of volume regulation, increased permeability to extracellular molecules such as inulin, and demonstrable plasma membrane ultrastructural defects occur in the earliest stages of irreversible injury.

The biochemical basis of this membrane damage is now under intensive study. The potential causes of membrane damage are listed in Table 1–1. Each one of these has been implicated at one time or another as the final pathway of lethal injury, and all may play a role. Activated oxygen species, for example, appear to be important in reperfusion injury that follows temporary ischemia.[10] In liver ischemia, net loss of membrane phospholipid, possibly by activation of phospholipases, has been shown to be associated with irreversible damage.[6]

Whatever the mechanism(s), the resultant membrane damage causes further influx of calcium from the extracellular space, where it is present in high concentrations ($>10^{-3}$ M). When, in addition, the ischemic tissue is reperfused to some extent, as may occur *in vivo*, the scene is set for a massive influx of calcium. Farber has argued that this calcium influx may be the "coup de grâce" that determines irreversible injury, not only after ischemia but also in toxic injury.[6] Calcium is taken up avidly by mitochondria after reoxygenation and permanently poisons them, inhibits cellular enzymes, denatures proteins, and causes the cytologic alterations characteristic of coagulative necrosis.

It is evident that the precise molecular events that initiate irreversible anoxic cell injury are still incompletely understood. Indeed, it may well be that several mechanisms, acting at more than one locus,

underlie cell death. *For now it must suffice that hypoxia affects oxidative phosphorylation and hence the synthesis of vital ATP supplies, that membrane damage is critical to the development of lethal cell injury, and that calcium ions may under some conditions be important mediators of the biochemical alterations leading to cell death.*

## FREE RADICAL MEDIATION OF CELL INJURY

It can be deduced from our discussion of hypoxic cell injury that any agent that can cause direct damage to the cell membrane or to the membranes of critical cell organelles can trigger a sequence of events that, in the end, may mimic those occurring in hypoxia. Some chemicals cause membrane injury *directly*. For example, in *mercuric chloride poisoning*, mercury binds to the sulfhydryl groups of the cell membrane and other proteins, causing increased membrane permeability and inhibition of ATPase-dependent transport. Most other toxic chemicals, however, are not biologically active but must be converted to reactive toxic metabolites by specific target cells. Although these metabolites might cause membrane damage and cell injury by *direct covalent binding* to membrane protein and lipids, by far the most important mechanisms of membrane injury involve the formation of *reactive free radicals* and subsequent *lipid peroxidation*.[4, 11] Free radical injury, particularly by activated oxygen species, is emerging as a final common pathway of cell injury in such varied processes as chemical and radiation injury, oxygen and other gaseous toxicity, cellular aging, microbial killing by phagocytic cells, inflammatory damage, tumor destruction by macrophages, and others.

What is a free radical? In most atoms, the electron orbitals are filled with paired electrons spinning in opposite directions, thus canceling each other's physicochemical reactivity. A free radical is a chemical species that has a single unpaired electron in an outer orbital. In such a state the radical is extremely reactive and unstable and enters into reactions in cells with inorganic or organic chemicals—proteins, lipids, carbohydrates—particularly with key molecules in membranes and nucleic acids. Moreover, free radicals initiate autocatalytic reactions whereby molecules with which they react are themselves converted into free radicals to thus propagate the chain of damage.

Radicals may be initiated within cells by the absorption of radiant energy (e.g., ultraviolet light, x-rays) or in the reduction-oxidation (redox) reactions that occur during normal physiologic processes, or they may be derived from the enzymatic metabolism of exogenous chemicals. Radiant energy may lyse water to release such radicals as OH· (hydroxyl ion) and H·. Another free radical is superoxide $O_2^-$, which is derived by reduction of molecular oxygen. Normally oxygen is reduced to water, but in some reactions, particularly those involving xanthine oxidase (other enzymes may also be implicated), $O_2^-$ may be formed. Fortunately, its formation is rare in normal oxidation-reduction reactions. Some metals such as iron, called transitional because they change valency states, can accept or donate free electrons during transit and thereby catalyze free radical formation ($Fe^{++} + H_2O_2 \rightarrow Fe^{+++} + OH\cdot + OH^-$). Certain exogenous chemicals such as $CCl_4$ can also be converted into free radicals, as will be discussed below.

The effects of these reactive species are wide-ranging. Free radicals in the presence of oxygen may cause peroxidation of lipids within organellar membranes to damage endoplasmic reticulum, mitochondria, and other microsomal components. Lipid peroxidation is the process by which fats become rancid when inadequately refrigerated and exposed to air. Peroxidation of lipids may also occur in living cells. Polyunsaturated lipids, such as those in membranes, possess double bonds between some of the carbon atoms, which weaken the carbon-hydrogen bonds of these carbon atoms. Such bonds are vulnerable to attack by oxygen-derived free radicals. The lipid-radical interactions yield peroxides, which are themselves unstable and reactive, and an autocatalytic chain reaction ensues, resulting in extensive membrane, organellar, and cellular damage. Cross-linking of proteins (the most labile amino acids are methionine, histidine, cystine, and lysine) may also occur and raise havoc throughout the cell, in particular inactivating enzymes, especially sulfhydryl enzymes. Interactions with nucleic acids induce mutations in the genetic code, which, if not repaired, induce cellular derangements. Much more could be said about this large and complex subject, but it will suffice for our purposes to cite a few specific examples of free radical injury.

**CARBON TETRACHLORIDE–INDUCED INJURY.** One of the best characterized models of free radical injury is that produced in the liver by $CCl_4$ poisoning.[7] This halogenated hydrocarbon is used widely in the dry-cleaning industry. Its toxic effect is not due to the $CCl_4$ molecule but to conversion of the molecule to the toxic free radical $CCl_3\cdot$ in the smooth endoplasmic reticulum (SER) by the mixed-function (P-450) oxidase system of enzymes involved in the metabolism of lipid-soluble drugs and other compounds. The free radicals produced locally cause autooxidation of the polyenoic fatty acids present within the membrane phospholipids. There, oxidative decomposition of the lipid is initiated, and organic peroxides are formed after reacting with oxygen (lipid peroxidation). This *reaction is autocatalytic* in that new radicals are formed from the peroxide radicals themselves. Thus, rapid breakdown of the structure and function of the endoplasmic reticulum is due to decomposition of the lipid. *It is no surprise, therefore, that $CCl_4$-*

*induced liver cell injury is both severe and extremely rapid in onset.* Within less than 30 minutes there is a decline in hepatic protein synthesis of both plasma proteins and endogenous protein enzymes, and within 2 hours, swelling of SER and dissociation of ribosomes from the rough endoplasmic reticulum (Fig. 1–4).

Accumulation of lipid then ensues, due to the inability of cells to synthesize lipoprotein from triglycerides and "lipid acceptor protein." Mitochondrial injury occurs after injury to the endoplasmic reticulum, and this is followed by progressive swelling of the cells due to increased permeability of the plasma membrane. Plasma membrane damage is thought to be caused by relatively stable fatty aldehydes, which are produced by lipid peroxidation in the SER but are able to act at distant sites.[11] This is followed by massive influx of calcium and cell death.

**OTHER FORMS OF FREE RADICAL INJURY.** Radiation is another example of free radical injury, mediated by radiolysis of water, producing free radicals such as $OH\cdot$, $H\cdot$, and $HOO\cdot$. These radicals may then interact with membranes, nucleic acids, or other key elements within the cell. Autocatalytic reactions are initiated, which may ultimately result in the induction of mutations or the death of the cell.

It has long been known that the lung and other tissues are subject to injury when exposed to high concentrations of $O_2$. Free radical formation is believed to underlie the pulmonary changes of *"oxygen toxicity."* Analogous changes may underlie the ocular injuries (retrolental fibroplasia) in newborns placed in incubators having excessive levels of oxygen. Oxygen-derived reactive species, derived largely from leukocytes, are also important mediators of cell injury in various other types of inflammation.[12]

The accumulation of injury caused by free radicals over the years may be responsible for certain aspects of *aging and the aging of cells.* Lipofuscin, a pigment described in more detail on page 21, accumulates in a variety of tissues (particularly the heart, liver, and brain) as a function of age. The pigment represents complexes of lipid and protein that are derived from the lipid peroxidation of polyunsaturated lipids of subcellular membranes.[13] Conceivably over the span of years, free radicals derived either from physiologic redox reactions or from long exposure to exogenous environmental agents cause the cumulative peroxidation of membrane lipids and the accumulation of lipofuscin. Alternatively, with aging there maybe progressive loss of some of the protective mechanisms, as will now be discussed.

Once free radicals are formed, how does the body get rid of them? They may spontaneously decay. Superoxide, for example, is unstable and decays spontaneously into oxygen and hydrogen peroxide. The rate of such decay is significantly increased by the catalytic action of *superoxide dismutases* found in many cell types. A number of other enzymes—glutathione synthetase, glutathione peroxi-

Figure 1–4. Rat liver cell after carbon tetrachloride intoxication, showing well-developed swelling of endoplasmic reticulum and shedding of ribosomes. Mitochondria at this stage are unaltered. (From Robbins, S. L., Cotran, R. S., and Kumar, V.: Pathologic Basis of Disease. 3rd ed. Philadelphia, W. B. Saunders Co., 1984. Courtesy of Dr. O. Iseri.)

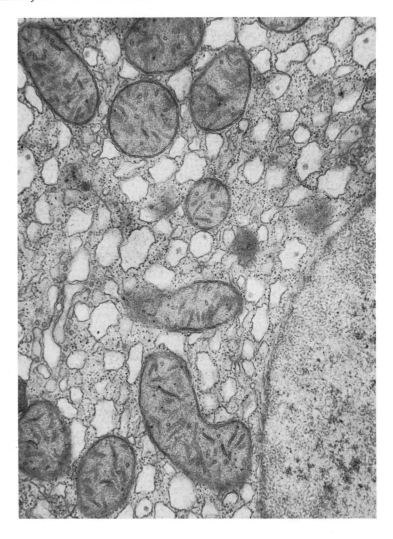

dase, glucose-6-phosphate dehydrogenase, and catalase—also provide defense against free radicals. From an evolutionary point of view such enzymes may have evolved to protect cells from free radical injury. The dismutases catalyze the scavenging of superoxides by forming $H_2O_2$, which is then decomposed to $O_2$ and $H_2O$ by catalases.[12] Some dismutases contain both copper and zinc; others, manganese; and still others, iron. The metals participate in this scavenging by accepting or donating an electron. Alternatively, endogenous or exogenous antioxidants—e.g., vitamin E; sulfhydryls such as cysteine or glutathione and ceruloplasmin—may either block the initiation of free radicals or inactivate them. In summary, the net potential for free radical injury flows from the balance between their initiation and their being scavenged. Thus, cells are more or less vulnerable to free radical injury depending on the presence and quantity of defensive enzymes and antioxidants that serve as protective mechanisms.

Although free radicals are discussed here mainly in the context of their damaging effects on tissues, it should be pointed out that free radicals such as

superoxide are also utilized by phagocytic cells to kill ingested microbes (p. 35). This, then is one of several examples whereby a given reaction can be beneficial or harmful to the integrity of the organism, depending on the context.

## VIRUS-INDUCED CELL INJURY

As stated earlier, the viruses that induce cellular changes are of two types: (1) *cytolytic* or *cytopathic* viruses, which cause various degrees of cell injury and cell death, and (2) *oncogenic* viruses, which stimulate host cell replication and may produce tumors. Here we are concerned with the cytopathic effects of viruses and some of the mechanisms by which cell injury occurs.

Viruses are thought to cause cell injury by one of two general mechanisms.[14] The first is the direct cytopathic effect, in which rapidly replicating virus particles interfere with some aspect of cell metabolism and thus cause cellular damage. The second mechanism involves the induction of an immunological response against viral or virus-altered cell antigens and the destruction of the cell by either antibody or cell-mediated reactions. The damage to hepatocytes caused by hepatitis B virus, for example, seems to be mediated by cytolysis induced by T lymphocytes (see p. 574).

Most cytopathic viruses have a high degree of specificity for certain cell types (viral tropism), caused in part by the presence of membrane receptors on host cells, which interact with specific viral structures. The interactions between viruses and receptors allow the virus to attach to, and then enter and injure, the host cell and thus are major determinants of virulence. In such viral infections as poliomyelitis, adenovirus infection, and influenza, specific viral polypeptides are responsible for these interactions; in the case of reovirus a single surface protein, the sigma 1 polypeptide, accounts for the specificity of this agent for certain cells of the central nervous system.[15] Following attachment, viruses without envelopes enter the cell by phagocytosis of the intact virion, whereas viruses with envelopes gain entrance by fusion of the viral envelope with the plasma membrane of the host. Following entry into the cell, active replication of the viruses ensues.

The nature of the cell response to viral replication depends to a large extent on the specific viral agent and the species of the host cells. *Cell lysis*, apparently due to major depression of cellular metabolism caused by explosive viral replication, is one end of the spectrum. Cytolytic viruses use cellular ATP, ribosomes, transfer RNA, enzymes, and other biosynthetic processes of the host cell to replicate, and in so doing subvert the cell's metabolism. Many viruses *alter macromolecular synthesis* by host cells, and the viral components that mediate these effects are now beginning to be unraveled. For example, the polio virus is known to inhibit the formation of active complexes that initiate protein synthesis.[15] Some viruses, including the pox virus and reoviruses, cause *cytoskeletal alterations*, such as disruption of vimentin intermediate filaments, and organizational changes in microtubules. Several common respiratory viruses cause additions or deletions in the number of microtubules in cilia of epithelial cells, thus interfering with ciliary motion and with clearance of particles from respiratory passages.[16] Cells sometimes respond to infection with the measles or herpes virus by the *formation of syncytial or multinucleate giant cells*, caused by cell-to-cell fusion. This fusion appears to require the insertion of viral glycoproteins into host surface membranes and a viral effect on the cytoskeleton. *Inclusion bodies* either in the nucleus or cytoplasm, or both, are found in infections with herpes viruses, measles, and rabies (Fig. 1–5). They often contain virus particles and cellular membranous or fibrillar material. But recall that cell death is one end of the spectrum of viral interactions with cells; the

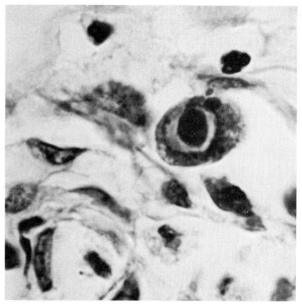

**Figure 1–5.** Large basophilic intranuclear inclusion of the cytomegalovirus (a herpesvirus). The inclusion is set off by a cleared halo in an enlarged nucleus, typical of this viral infection.

other end is cell replication caused by oncogenic viruses.

## CELLULAR AGING

Aging has many dimensions and can be characterized in many ways.[17] Shakespeare probably did it best in his elegant description of the Seven Ages of Man. It begins at the moment of conception, involves the differentiation and maturation of the organism and its cells, at some variable point of time leads to the progressive loss of functional capacity characteristic of senescence, and ends in death. We discuss cellular aging here because it could represent the progressive accumulation over the years of alterations in structure and function that may lead to cell death or at least diminished capacity of the cell to respond to injury. In the context of cell aging, a question arises—are the changes of cell senescence the consequence of genetic programs inherent in cells or are they the consequence of the accumulation over time of repeated cell injuries? These two possibilities are by no means mutually exclusive, and it is highly likely that both contribute. The notion that each cell has a limited, genetically determined replicative life span has come from the tissue culture studies of Hayflick and others, who pointed to the fact that when fibroblasts are grown in vitro, they undergo some $50 \pm 10$ doublings and then stop replicating.[18]

In contrast to the controversial concept of inherent limited replication, other workers contend that cells are potentially immortal but mitotic errors produce cells that are committed to die and these eventually replace the immortal cells. Thus senescence and cell death are the consequence of progressive acquisition during the life span of the cell of inappropriate genetic information hampering normal cell function. It is here that environmental influences may play a role. There is agreement that changes occurring in postreplicating cells are important in cell aging.[19] Morphologically, senescent cells in culture become larger, are occasionally multinucleate, develop vacuoles of various sizes, and are more prone to injury than nonsenescent cells. In vivo in the central nervous system, cell loss eventually occurs in some of the neuronal cells of the cerebellum. In some neurons there is also a characteristic "neurofibrillary" degeneration that occurs in aging brains and is more pronounced in patients with senile dementia and Alzheimer's disease. Since a number of environmental agents to which aging individuals are increasingly exposed (such as ultraviolet light, chemicals, x-rays and food products) are capable of causing both somatic mutations and changes in a variety of cytoplasmic constituents, it is thought that these postreplicative changes in aging cells are caused by repeated environmental injury. One evidence for this scenario is the cellular accumulation of lipofuscin pigment, the yellow-brown wear and tear pigment that is the final breakdown product of autophagic vacuoles (p. 21). The biochemical composition of lipofuscin suggests that it is derived through lipid peroxidation, perhaps from repeated free radical injury induced by environmental factors.

Much more might be said about the mechanisms responsible for the cellular alterations that occur in cell aging, but it suffices here to say that according to present best evidence, some of these mechanisms are probably merely an extension of those involved in the maturation and differentiation of cells and others are due to environmental influences that may well interact with these mechanisms.

Against this background of the agents and their mediators that cause cell injury, we can now turn to their morphologic effects on cells.

## MORPHOLOGY OF CELL INJURY

### ULTRASTRUCTURAL CHANGES

We can now examine the morphologic changes in reversibly and lethally injured cells, and we shall begin with the ultrastructural changes (Fig. 1–6).

*Changes ascribable to alterations in the plasma membrane* are seen early in cell injury, reflecting the disturbances in ion and volume regulation induced by loss of ATP. These include cell swelling, formation of cytoplasmic blebs, blunting and distortion of microvilli, creation of myelin figures, and deterioration and loosening of intercellular attachments. These changes can occur rapidly and are readily reversible. In later stages of irreversible injury, breaks are seen in both the membranes enclosing the cell and those of the organelles.

*Mitochondrial* changes occur extremely rapidly after ischemic injury but are delayed in some forms of chemical injury. Early after ischemia, the mito-

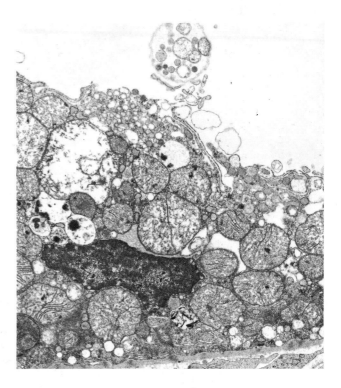

Figure 1–6. Proximal tubular cell showing irreversible ischemic injury. Note the markedly swollen mitochondria containing amorphous densities, disrupted cell membranes, and a dense pyknotic nucleus. (From Robbins, S. L., Cotran, R. S., and Kumar, V.: Pathologic Basis of Disease. 3rd ed. Philadelphia, W. B. Saunders Co., 1984, p. 7.)

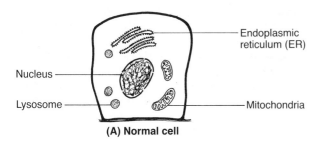

**(A) Normal cell**

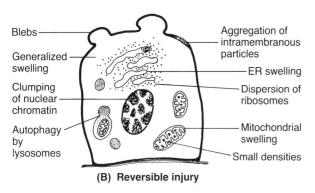

**(B) Reversible injury**

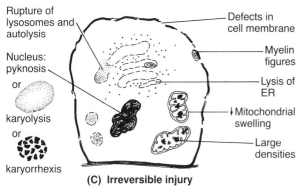

**(C) Irreversible injury**

Figure 1–7. Schematic representation of the ultrastructural changes in reversible (*B*) and irreversible (*C*) cell injury (see text).

chondria appear condensed. However, this is quickly followed by *swelling of mitochondria* due to the ionic shifts that occur in the mitochondrial inner compartment. Characteristic *amorphous densities* appear as early as 30 minutes after ischemia in the myocardium, where they correlate with the onset of irreversibility. These densities consist of lipids or lipid-protein complexes, but with reperfusion and in chemical injury dense granules appear that are rich in *calcium*. With irreversible injury comes increased swelling of mitochondria, and, finally, there is outright rupture of the mitochondrial membranes, followed by calcification.

Dilatation of the *endoplasmic reticulum* occurs early after injury, probably owing to changes in ion and water movement. This is followed by detachment of ribosomes and disaggregation of polysomes, with a decrease of protein synthesis. These responses are also reversible, but with further injury there is pro-

gressive fragmentation of the endoplasmic reticulum and formation of myelin figures.

Changes in the *lysosomes* generally appear late. In the stages of reversible injury, lysosomes may be clear and often swollen, but there is no evidence of leakage of lysosomal enzymes. *After* the onset of lethal injury, lysosomes rupture and eventually may disappear as recognizable structures from the disfigured carcass of the dead cell. A summary of these ultrastructural changes is given in Figure 1–7.

## LIGHT MICROSCOPIC PATTERNS

### Reversible Injury

In classic pathology, the morphologic changes resulting from nonlethal injury to cells were termed degenerations, but today they are more simply designated *reversible injuries*. Two patterns can be recognized under the light microscope: *cellular swelling* and *fatty change*. Cellular swelling appears whenever cells are incapable of maintaining ionic and fluid homeostasis. *Fatty change*, under some circumstances, may be another indicator of reversible cell injury. It is a less universal reaction, principally encountered in cells involved in and dependent on fat metabolism, such as the hepatocyte and myocardial cell. Since it is a form of intracellular accumulation, it is described later in this chapter.

**Cellular swelling** is the first manifestation of almost all forms of injury to cells, resulting from a shift of extracellular water into the cell caused by mechanisms described earlier. It is a difficult morphologic change to appreciate with the light microscope; it may be more apparent at the level of the whole organ. When it affects all cells in an organ, it causes some pallor, increased turgor, and increase in weight of the organ. Microscopically, enlargement of cells is most often discernible by compression of the microvasculature of the organ as, for example, the hepatic sinusoids and the capillary network within the renal cortex.

If water continues to accumulate within cells, small clear vacuoles appear within the cytoplasm. These vacuoles presumably represent distended and pinched-off or sequestered segments of the endoplasmic reticulum. This pattern of nonlethal injury is sometimes called **"hydropic change"** or **"vacuolar degeneration"** (Fig. 1–8). Swelling of cells is reversible and is usually without significant functional effect.

### Cell Death—Necrosis

Cells can be recognized as dead with the light microscope only after they have undergone the sequence of changes referred to as necrosis.[20] *Necrosis may be defined as the morphologic changes caused by the progressive degradative action of enzymes on the lethally injured cell.* The formalin-fixed cells studied in histology are dead, but all enzymic action

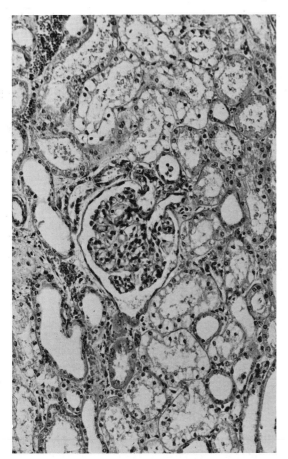

Figure 1–8. Cellular swelling of renal tubular epithelial cells seen in the center field above and below the glomerulus. The cleared, vacuolated cells contain dark displaced nuclei, suggesting that the swelling has been followed by death of the cells.

is stopped at once by the fixative and so the cells are not necrotic. Two essentially concurrent processes bring about the changes of necrosis: (1) enzymic digestion of the cell and (2) denaturation of proteins. The catalytic enzymes are derived either from the lysosomes of the dead cells, in which case the enzymic digestion is referred to as *autolysis*, or from the lysosomes of immigrant leukocytes, termed *heterolysis*. Depending on whether enzymic digestion or denaturation of proteins is ascendent, two quite distinctive patterns of cell necrosis develop. In the former, the progressive catalysis of cell structures leads to so-called *liquefactive necrosis*, whereas in the latter, *coagulative necrosis* develops. Both of these processes require hours to develop and so there would be no detectable changes in cells if, for example, a myocardial infarct caused sudden death. The only telling evidence might be occlusion of a coronary artery.

**The hallmarks of cell death are found in the nucleus**. In well-advanced but reversible injury the chromatin often becomes clumped against the nuclear membrane. With death of the cell further nuclear changes

appear in the form of one of three patterns (Fig. 1–7C). The basophilia of the chromatin may fade (**karyolysis**), a change that presumably reflects the activation of the DNAses as the pH of the cell drops. A second pattern is **pyknosis**, characterized by nuclear shrinkage and increased basophilia. Here the DNA apparently condenses into a solid, shrunken basophilic mass. In the third possible pattern, known as **karyorrhexis**, the pyknotic or partially pyknotic nucleus undergoes fragmentation. With the passage of time (a day or two), in one way or another the nucleus in the necrotic cell totally disappears. Meanwhile, the cytoplasm has become transformed into an acidophilic, granular opaque mass. This acidophilia represents an affinity for acid dyes (eosinophilia), resulting in part from denaturation of cytoplasmic proteins, which exposes basic groups, and in part from activation of acid ribonuclease, which destroys the normally basophilic cytoplasmic RNA. In this manner, the necrotic cell becomes converted into an acidophilic anucleate carcass.

Once the cell has died and has undergone the early alterations described above, one of three distinctive sequences ensues. The mass of necrotic cells may undergo **coagulative necrosis, liquefactive necrosis**, or, in special circumstances, **caseous necrosis** (Fig. 1–9).

**Coagulative necrosis** implies preservation of the basic outline of the coagulated cell for a span of at least some days. Presumably the injury or the subsequent increasing intracellular acidosis denatures not only structural proteins but also enzymic proteins and so blocks the proteolysis of the cell. For a time, then, the general morphologic shape of the cell is remarkably preserved. **The process of coagulative necrosis is characteristic of hypoxic death of cells in all tissues save the brain**. The myocardial infarct is a prime example. Here, acidophilic, coagulated, anucleate cells persist for weeks (Fig. 1–10). Ultimately, the necrotic myocardial cells are removed by fragmentation and phagocytosis of the cellular debris by scavenger white cells or by the action of proteolytic lysosomal enzymes brought in by the immigrant white cells.

**Liquefactive necrosis** resulting from autolysis or het-

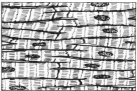

Normal cells

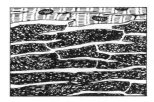
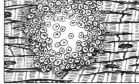

Coagulative necrosis            Liquefactive necrosis

Figure 1–9. Schematic representation of coagulative and liquefactive necrosis in myocardium (see Figs. 1–10 and 1–11).

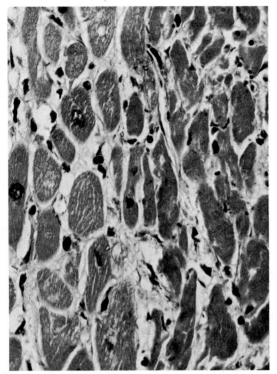

Figure 1–10. Myocardium, with preserved normal fibers on the left. The right half of the figure reveals coagulative necrosis of the fibers, with loss of nuclei and clumping of the cytoplasm but with preservation of basic outlines of the cells.

erolysis is mainly characteristic of focal bacterial infections, since bacteria constitute powerful stimuli to the accumulation of white cells (Fig. 1–11). For obscure reasons, hypoxic death of cells within the central nervous system evokes liquefactive necrosis, yet hypoxic death of heart muscle cells, liver cells, kidney cells, and, in fact, most other cells in the body is followed by coagulative necrosis. Whatever the pathogenesis, liquefaction essentially digests the dead carcasses of cells and often leaves a tissue defect filled with immigrant leukocytes, creating an abscess.

**Caseous necrosis**, a distinctive form of coagulative necrosis, is encountered most often in foci of tuberculous infection. The term "caseous" is derived from the gross appearance (i.e., white and cheesy) of the areas of necrosis. Histologically, the necrotic focus appears as an amorphous granular debris seemingly composed of fragmented, coagulated cells with a distinctive inflammatory enclosing border known as a granulomatous reaction (p. 47). It is important to be able to recognize this morphologic pattern because it is evoked by only a limited number of agents. Among these, tuberculosis is preeminent, as is discussed in greater detail on page 437.

*Apoptosis* is an unusual distinctive morphologic pattern of cell death (derived from Greek for "dropping off").[21] It usually involves single cells, or clusters of cells, and appears on H and E sections as a round or oval mass of intensely eosinophilic cytoplasm, often with pyknotic nuclear fragments. One example is the acidophilic *Councilman body* seen in the liver in toxic or viral hepatitis, but apoptosis also occurs in a variety of other pathologic and physiologic conditions. It is thought that the alterations initially involve rapid condensation and fragmentation of nuclear chromatin, probably through activation of an endogenous endonuclease.[22] The precise mechanisms of cell injury in apoptosis are still unclear, as are their relationship to the mechanism of necrosis.

*Enzymic fat necrosis* is a term that is well fixed in medical parlance but does not in reality denote a specific pattern of necrosis. Rather, it is descriptive of *focal areas of destruction of fat resulting from abnormal release of activated pancreatic enzymes into the substance of the pancreas and the peritoneal cavity.* This occurs in the uncommon but calamitous abdominal emergency known as "acute pancreatic necrosis." In this condition, discussed more completely on page 603, activated pancreatic enzymes escape from acinar cells and ducts; the activated enzymes liquefy fat cell membranes, and the activated lipases split the triglyceride esters contained within fat cells. *The released fatty acids combine with calcium to produce grossly visible chalky white areas,* which enable the surgeon and the pathologist to identify this disease on inspection of involved fat depots.

*Fibrinoid necrosis* is another somewhat inappropriate but nonetheless useful term. It is most often applied in those immunologic injuries to arteries and arterioles that are characterized by the accumulation of pink-staining homogeneous masses of fibrin, immunoglobulins, and other plasma proteins within the walls of affected vessels. Indeed, the vessels may become necrotic, and it is the combination of cell

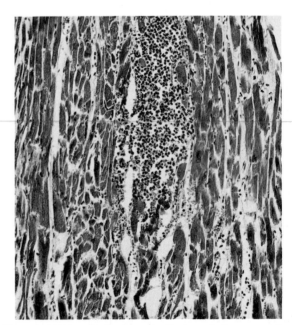

Figure 1–11. Liquefactive necrosis of a focus in the myocardium caused by bacterial seeding. The focus is filled with white cells, creating a myocardial abscess.

death and deposition of fibrin-like material that gives rise to the term *fibrinoid necrosis*. It is in reality not a pattern of cell death but rather a distinctive pattern of tissue reaction to certain forms of injury.

*Gangrenous necrosis* is generally applied to a limb, usually the lower limb, which has lost its blood supply and has subsequently been attacked by bacteria. Thus the initial hypoxic coagulative necrosis is modified by the liquefactive action of enzymes derived from the bacteria and such white cells as may have gained access to the necrotic tissue. When the coagulative pattern predominates, it is referred to as *dry gangrene*. If the bacterial invasion has introduced significant liquefaction, it is termed *wet gangrene*.

Ultimately, in the living patient, most necrotic cells and their debris disappear. Even coagulated cells are eventually removed by a combined process of enzymic digestion and fragmentation, with phagocytosis of the particulate debris by scavenger leukocytes. If necrotic cells and cellular debris are not promptly destroyed and reabsorbed, they tend to attract calcium salts and other minerals and become calcified. This phenomenon, so-called *dystrophic calcification*, is considered on page 25.

## INTRACELLULAR ACCUMULATIONS

This section deals with an assortment of intracellular accumulations that may or may not impair the normal function of the cell. In general, intracellular accumulations imply either (1) presentation to the cell of excessive amounts of some normal metabolite, (2) accumulation of some abnormal nonmetabolizable product, or (3) excessive intracellular synthesis of some product. Intracellular accumulation of glycogen in diabetic patients who have prolonged high blood glucose levels is an example of the first mechanism. The second pathway might involve the intracellular accumulation of some abnormal product resulting from an inborn error of metabolism. The third instance is exemplified by excessive synthesis of a pigment, such as melanin, encountered in certain disease states, such as adrenal insufficiency. Some of these intracellular accumulations are apparently without functional effect, but others overload the cell and cause cell injury and dysfunction. All are important, however, because they may provide morphologic evidence of the underlying causation of the disease.

### LIPIDS

#### Fatty Change

Fatty change refers to any abnormal accumulation of fat within parenchymal cells. Several pathogenetic mechanisms underlie fatty change, but in all cases *the appearance of fat vacuoles within cells, whether small or large, represents an absolute increase in intracellular lipids.* It does not represent so-called unmasking of the normal fat content of cells. Fatty change is sometimes preceded by cellular swelling. Although it is by itself an indicator of nonlethal injury, fatty change is sometimes the harbinger of cell death and, in many situations, is encountered in cells adjacent to those that have died and undergone necrosis.

The genesis of fatty change of the liver has largely been unraveled and will be considered here in some detail. Under normal conditions lipids are transported to the liver from adipose tissue and from the diet. From adipose tissue, lipids are released and transported in only one form—free fatty acids (FFA). Dietary lipids, on the other hand, are transported either as chylomicra (lipid particles consisting of triglyceride, phospholipid, and protein) or as free fatty acids. Some fatty acids are synthesized from acetate within the liver proper. Whatever their origin, most fatty acids in the liver are esterified to triglycerides; some are converted to cholesterol, incorporated into phospholipids, or oxidized in mitochondria into ketone bodies.

*In order to be secreted by the liver, intracellular triglycerides must be complexed with specific apoprotein molecules called "lipid acceptor proteins" to form lipoproteins* (p. 287). Excess accumulation of triglycerides, causing a fatty liver, results from the following six defects, sometimes acting in combination (Fig. 1–12): (1) *Excessive entry of free fatty acids into the liver.* In starvation, for example, adipose depots are mobilized, and more fatty acids are brought to the liver, where they are synthesized into triglycerides.

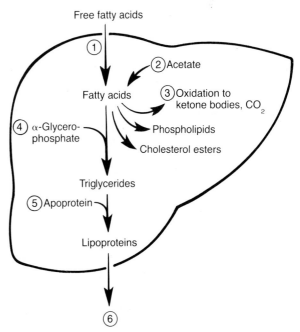

**Figure 1–12.** Lipid metabolism in liver cells. The numbers refer to possible abnormalities leading to fatty liver, as indicated in the text.

Corticosteroids also produce lipid mobilization from adipose tissue. (2) *Enhanced fatty acid synthesis from acetate.* (3) *Decreased fatty acid oxidation.* Both (2) and (3) lead to increased esterification of fatty acids to triglycerides. (4) *Increased esterification of fatty acids to triglycerides, owing to an increase in alpha glycerophosphate, the carbohydrate backbone involved in such esterification.* This is thought to be one effect of alcohol excess. (5) *Decreased apoprotein synthesis.* As stressed earlier, this protein is necessary for the conversion of triglycerides to lipoproteins, the only form in which lipid is excreted from the liver. This mechanism has been well established as the cause of fatty accumulation caused by carbon tetrachloride and by malnutrition. (6) *Impaired lipoprotein secretion from the liver.* This seems to be involved in an experimental model of fatty liver induced by the administration of orotic acid. *Alcohol*, at least in industrialized countries, is perhaps the most common cause of fatty liver.[23] Alcohol is a hepatotoxin that alters mitochondrial and microsomal functions. At present it appears that fatty change and the hepatotoxic effects of alcohol can be attributed to its oxidation by liver enzymes to acetylaldehyde (p. 267). Increased free fatty acid mobilization, diminished triglyceride utilization, decreased fatty acid oxidation, increased esterification, a block in lipoprotein excretion, as well as direct damage to the endoplasmic reticulum by free radicals produced by ethanol metabolism have all been implicated.

Mild fatty change has no effect on cellular function. More severe fatty change may impair liver function, but unless some vital intracellular process is irreversibly damaged (such as in carbon tetrachloride poisoning), fatty change per se is reversible. The fatty liver in the alcoholic, for example, may become enormously enlarged and may indeed be associated with functional deficit and, by a complex process to be described later (p. 584), may lead to a progressive form of fibrosis of the liver termed *cirrhosis*. However, in the alcoholic who has not yet developed cirrhosis and who wisely adopts an alcohol-free balanced diet, it is quite remarkable to observe the return of the enlarged fatty liver to normal size, structure, and function.

Fatty change is most often seen in the liver and heart, but it may occur in other organs.

**LIVER.** In the liver, mild fatty change may not affect the gross appearance. With progressive accumulation, the organ enlarges and becomes increasingly yellow until, in extreme instances, the liver may weigh 3 to 6 kg and be transformed into a bright yellow, soft, greasy organ. Fatty change begins with the development of minute, membrane-bounded inclusions (liposomes) closely applied to the endoplasmic reticulum and probably derived from it. It is first manifested under the light microscope by the appearance of small fat vacuoles in the cytoplasm around the nucleus. As the process progresses, the

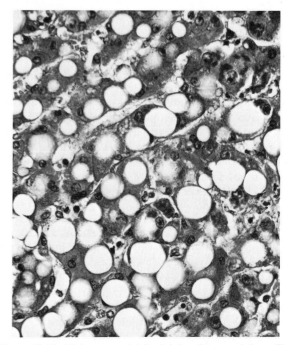

**Figure 1–13.** High-power detail of fatty change of liver. The variability in size of vacuoles is evident. In some cells, the well-preserved nucleus is squeezed into the displaced rim of cytoplasm about the fat vacuole.

vacuoles coalesce to create cleared spaces that displace the nucleus to the periphery of the cell (Fig. 1–13).

**HEART.** Lipid, as neutral fat, is quite frequently found in heart muscle in the form of small droplets. It occurs in two patterns. In one, prolonged moderate hypoxia such as that produced by profound anemia causes intracellular deposits of fat, which create grossly apparent bands of yellowed myocardium alternating with bands of darker, red-brown, uninvolved myocardium (tigered effect). In the other pattern of fatty change produced by more profound hypoxia or some forms of myocarditis (e.g., diphtheritic), the myocardial cells are uniformly affected. The mechanism by which the diphtheria bacillus causes a fatty heart is apparently the production of an exotoxin that interferes with the metabolism of carnitine, a cofactor for the oxidation of long-chain fatty acids.

### Other Lipid Accumulations

As detailed previously, the overload of parenchymal liver cells by triglycerides is termed "fatty change." By quite different mechanisms, *phagocytic cells may become overloaded with lipid (triglycerides and cholesterol).* Scavenger macrophages, wherever in contact with the lipid debris of necrotic cells, may become stuffed with lipid because of their phagocytic activities. Macrophages at the margin of an inflammatory focus may become so filled with minute vacuoles of lipids as to impart a foaminess to their cytoplasm (*foam cells*).

Intracellular accumulations of cholesterol and choles-terol esters are also prominent in certain diseases. The most important is atherosclerosis, in which smooth mus-cle cells and macrophages within the intimal layer of the aorta and large arteries are filled with lipid. Such cells appear foamy, and aggregates of them in the intima produce the cholesterol-laden atheromas characteristic of this serious disorder. Many of these fat-laden cells rupture, releasing the lipids into the ground substance of the intima. The mechanisms of lipid accumulation in these cells in atherosclerosis are discussed in Chapter 10. The extracellular cholesterol esters may crystallize in the shape of long needles, producing quite distinctive clefts in tissue sections.

Intracellular accumulations of cholesterol and cho-lesterol esters within macrophages are also character-istic of acquired and hereditary hyperlipidemic states. Usually, these lesions are found in the subepithelial connective tissue of the skin and in tendons, produc-ing tumorous masses known as *xanthomas*.

*Fatty ingrowth* (or stromal infiltration of fat) refers to the accumulation of adipose tissue within the stromal connective tissue of parenchyma.

Fatty ingrowth is most commonly encountered in the heart and pancreas, where adult adipose cells appear within the connective tissue stroma. In the heart, there is an increase of subepicardial fat that extends in continuity as finger-like projections between the muscle bundles. These insinuations may extend throughout the thickness of the myocardium to appear beneath the endocardium as small yellow deposits. The adult fat cells separate but do not damage the adjacent myocardial cells. In the pancreas, the fat is found in the connective tissue septa of the pancreatic lobules. The glandular tissue may be-come so dispersed as to be almost invisible on gross inspection.

As far as is known, stromal infiltration of fat rarely affects cardiac or pancreatic function.

## PROTEINS

Protein accumulations may be encountered in cells either because excesses are presented to the cells or because the cells synthesize excessive amounts. Nor-mally, trace amounts of albumin, filtered through the glomerulus, are reabsorbed in the proximal convo-luted tubules. Any disorder producing heavy protein-uria leads to pinocytotic reabsorption of the protein. When these pinocytotic vesicles in the epithelial cells fuse with lysosomes, hyaline cytoplasmic droplets, which appear pink in hematoxylin and eosin stains, are formed. If the proteinuria abates, the protein droplets are metabolized and disappear. Accumula-tions of immunoglobulins synthesized in the cisternae of the rough endoplasmic reticulum of plasma cells may create rounded, acidophilic *Russell bodies*.

## GLYCOGEN

Excessive intracellular deposits of glycogen are seen in patients with an abnormality in either glucose or glycogen metabolism. Whatever the clinical set-ting, the glycogen masses appear as clear vacuoles within the cytoplasm that are PAS positive.

Diabetes mellitus is the prime example of a disor-der of glucose metabolism. In this disease, glycogen is found in the epithelial cells of the distal portions of the proximal convoluted tubules and sometimes in the descending loop of Henle, as well as within liver cells, beta cells of the islets of Langerhans, and heart muscle cells.

The intracellular glycogen produces marked vacuoli-zation of the cytoplasm to the point at which the cells appear to be entirely cleared. For obscure reasons, glycogen deposition in hepatocytes appears by light mi-croscopy within nuclei, which thus become swollen and clear, giving the nucleus a ground-glass appearance. Such glycogen accumulation has no clinical significance.

Glycogen also accumulates within the cells in a group of closely related disorders, all genetic, collec-tively referred to as the *glycogen storage diseases*, or *glycogenoses*. In these disorders, either there is a lack of one or several of the enzymes that metabolize normal glycogen, or some abnormal form of glycogen is synthesized and cannot be metabolized. In the various syndromes (discussed in Chapter 4), the intracellular accumulations affect mainly myocardial muscle, skeletal muscle, and hepatic and renal cells. In all instances the glycogen appears as clear, intra-cytoplasmic vacuoles. These diseases represent in-stances in which massive stockpiling of substances within cells causes secondary injury and cell death.[24]

## COMPLEX LIPIDS AND CARBOHYDRATES

Intracellular accumulations of a variety of abnormal metabolites characterize a growing list of inborn errors of metabolism collectively referred to as the "storage diseases" (p. 110). These abnormal products collect within cells throughout the body, principally those in the reticuloendothelial system. The abnor-mal products range from the complex lipids (in Gaucher's, Tay-Sachs, and Niemann-Pick diseases) to complex carbohydrates (in Hurler's and Hunter's syndromes) to other, more exotic products, such as glycolipids and mucolipids. In all of these rare con-ditions, the precise identification of the stored prod-uct requires specific biochemical or enzymic analysis.

## PIGMENTS

Pigments of either exogenous or endogenous origin may accumulate within cells. Although most are relatively innocuous, they often provide clues to the existence and nature of an underlying disorder.

## Exogenous Pigments

Accumulations of exogenous carbon dust in the macrophages of the alveoli and the lymphatic channels blacken the tissues of the lungs (*anthracosis*). It is a universal indication of the air pollution to which the coal miner and the urban dweller are exposed. When these macrophages drain to the regional lymph nodes, they similarly blacken them. In coal miners, heavy pulmonary accumulations may give rise to so called "*coal-worker's pneumoconiosis*" (CWP). However, CWP does not interfere or at worst interferes only mildly with respiratory function, except in extreme instances, when it may become transformed into "*progressive massive fibrosis*" of the lungs, a disabling pneumoconiosis (p. 256). Those living in iron mining communities may develop a rust-like discoloration of the lung (*siderosis*). Here again, the pigmentation does not seem to be associated with damage but implies heavy air pollution. In some of these mining areas, however, the iron dust is associated with silica dust (*siderosilicosis*), and the silica evokes a serious fibrosing reaction, described later in the consideration of *silicosis* (p. 257)..

Tattooing may cause dermal pigmentation of an innocuous but sometimes embarrassing nature. The tattoo pigment has the distressing property of persisting in situ throughout life in dermal macrophages, creating difficulties if one wishes to marry Mary when the seductive adornment is titled Alice.

## Endogenous Pigments

Five forms of pigment are of endogenous origin. Among these, hemosiderin, hematin, and bilirubin are hemoglobin-derived; lipofuscin and melanin are not. Each is considered below.

*Hemosiderin* is a golden-yellow to brown, granular or crystalline, iron-containing pigment readily visible with the light microscope. Its derivation is discussed in detail on page 353, so it suffices for now to state that the individual granules of hemosiderin comprise aggregates of ferritin micelles, which can only be seen with the electron microscope. Ferritin is composed of a protein known as apoferritin complexed to iron to create dense particles (6.1 nm in radius) arranged in tetrads. Ferritin is present in many cell types normally. When there is an excess of iron either locally or systemically, the ferritin aggregates into iron-containing granules of hemosiderin. Helpful in differentiating hemosiderin from other pigments such as lipofuscin or melanin, which do not contain iron, is the Prussian blue histochemical reaction. The colorless potassium ferrocyanide reacts with the ferric ions to produce the insoluble blue ferric ferrocyanide, confirming the iron content of the hemosiderin pigment. Hemosiderin pigmentation of cells and tissues

may occur as a local process or systemically throughout the body.

*Local excesses of iron* may be produced by internal hemorrhages (within tissues or closed body cavities) or by long-standing vascular congestion that presumably leads to minute hemorrhages. The common bruise following an injury provides an excellent example of the local formation of hemosiderin. The color changes that occur in the bruise reflect the transformation of the hemoglobin. The bruise begins with the blue-red color of erythrocytes, which accumulate at the site of hemorrhage. These are phagocytized by macrophages, which break down the hemoglobin to produce at first biliverdin (yellow-green), then bilirubin (green-brown), and eventually, from the contained iron, hemosiderin (golden yellow). The lung in long-standing heart failure is a prime example of protracted congestion leading to the appearance of hemosiderin in phagocytic mononuclear cells in the alveoli. These pigmented macrophages thus are often called "heart failure cells"

*Systemic hemosiderosis* is encountered whenever there is iron overload in the body. Depending upon the amount and cause of the iron excess, the pigment is first deposited in mononuclear phagocytes throughout the body, but the iron and pigment may then be recycled to parenchymal cells, such as those in the liver, kidneys, endocrine glands, pancreas, and other organs. More intensive pigment deposition in parenchymal organs is characteristic of *hemochromatosis*, the most extreme example of systemic iron overload (p. 594), with its cell and organ injury.

In most instances, the intracellular accumulation of hemosiderin pigment does not damage the cell and so does not impair either cell or organ function. Indeed, the iron contained within this pigment can be mobilized and hemosiderin will therefore disappear in time if the cause for the excess iron abates. As is well known, a black and blue bruise eventually disappears.

*Hematin* is a relatively uncommon hemoglobin-derived pigment of uncertain composition. It is seen following massive hemolysis of red cells, such as may occur with a transfusion reaction or in the parasitic destruction of erythrocytes in malaria. This pigment is also golden yellow but is virtually confined to the reticuloendothelial cells in the body. Despite its content of iron, hematin fails to react with the Prussian blue method, presumably because the iron is still tightly bound to heme and therefore un-ionized.

*Bilirubin*, the normal yellow-brown-green pigment of bile, is also derived from hemoglobin but does not contain iron. As you know, it is largely derived from the heme pigment of hemoglobin released by the breakdown of obsolete red cells in the mononuclear-phagocyte or reticuloendothelial system. Promptly bound to albumin, the bilirubin is transported through the blood to the liver cells, where it is eventually conjugated into a diglucuronide and secreted into the bile. Further details on the synthesis and normal metabolism of this pigment can be found on page 564. For our present purposes, it suffices to say that the normal plasma contains from 0.4 to 1.0 mg of total bile pigments per 100 ml. At these levels, the pigment cannot be identified within cells or tissues. Increased plasma levels of bilirubin (hyperbilirubinemia) can be caused by a variety of disorders that derange the normal metabolism of bilirubin—e.g., increased breakdown of red cells (hemolytic jaundice); intrahepatic disorders that damage liver cells, thus impairing the conjugation and excretion of bilirubin (intrahepatic cholestasis); and diseases that block the outflow of bile (extrahepatic or posthepatic cholestasis). With hyperbilirubinemia, the tissues and fluids of the body become bile-stained, and it is the yellowing of the skin and sclerae that produces clinically apparent *jaundice*.

The bilirubin is visible within cells morphologically only when the jaundice is well marked. It appears as a green-brown to black, amorphous, globular, intracytoplasmic deposit. Most often hepatocytes are affected, but in severe jaundice bilirubin also may be observed in renal tubular epithelial cells and dermal macrophages.

*Lipofuscin* is an insoluble pigment also known as lipochrome, ceroid, and "wear-and-tear" or aging pigment. Its importance lies in its being the "telltale" sign of free radical injury and lipid peroxidation. In tissue sections it appears as a yellow-brown, finely granular intracytoplasmic pigment. Lipofuscin is seen in cells undergoing slow, regressive changes such as in the atrophy accompanying advanced age and chronic injury, it is particularly prominent in the liver and heart of aging patients or patients with severe malnutrition, and it is usually accompanied by organ shrinkage (*brown atrophy*).

Lipofuscin represents the indigestible residues of autophagic vacuoles formed during aging or atrophy. The pigment appears to be composed of polymers of lipids and phospholipids complexed with protein, suggesting *that it is derived through lipid peroxidation of polyunsaturated lipids of subcellular membranes* and is consistent with the theory that free radical formation causes the progressive deterioration of cell membranes in aging (see p. 12). The high rate of lipofuscin formation in relatively young people who die of inanition results from lack of dietary antioxidants that help prevent auto-oxidation.

*Melanin* (derived from the Greek work *melas*, meaning black) is an endogenous, non-hemoglobin-derived, brown-black pigment formed when the enzyme tyrosinase catalyzes the oxidation of tyrosine to dihydroxyphenylalanine (DOPA). At the ultrastructural level, DOPA is aggregated or polymerized in the Golgi apparatus and incorporated there into small membrane-bound organelles known as melanosomes. It is these melanosomes, or aggregates of them, that constitute the pigment granules visible with the light microscope.

Melanocytes are normally present in the skin, hair follicles, uveal tract, retinal pigmented epithelium, inner ear, leptomeninges, ovary, adrenal medulla, bladder, and substantia nigra of the brain. In the skin, melanocytes comprise dendritic cells in the dermoepidermal junction. These cells apparently connect through their dendrites with the basal cells of the epidermis and through some incredible process inject minute granules of melanin (melanosomes) into the basal cells. In this manner we acquire the color of our skin. Phagocytic cells in the dermis can accumulate melanin either from nearby melanocytes or from basal epidermal cells to thus be transformed into melanophores. Aggregates of these melanophores create freckles which darken, as is well known, after exposure to sunlight because of the actinic stimulation of melanin synthesis in melanocytes.

In humans, melanin synthesis is under adrenal and pituitary control. Adrenal steroids suppress and pituitary adrenocorticotropic hormone (ACTH) stimulates its synthesis. Excess melanin synthesis is thus encountered in adrenal insufficiency (with its compensatory hypersecretion of ACTH) and in some hyperpituitary states.

*Albinos* suffer from a hereditary lack of tyrosinase. Thus they are unable to synthesize melanin and are extremely vulnerable to sunlight. Lacking the protective pigment mantle in the skin against the actinic activity of sunlight, as well as the light-shielding action of the pigment in the eye, they are prone to develop sunburn and skin cancers and have extreme visual sensitivity to light.

For all practical purposes melanin is the only endogenous *brown-black* pigment. The only other is homogentisic acid, a black pigment that occurs in patients with alkaptonuria, a rare metabolic disease. Here the pigment is deposited in the skin, connective tissue, and cartilage, and the pigmentation is known as "ochronosis."

# SUBCELLULAR ALTERATIONS

To this point in the chapter the focus has been on the cell as a unit. However, certain conditions are associated with rather distinctive alterations in cell organelles or cytoskeleton. Some of these alterations coexist with those described for acute lethal injury; others represent more chronic forms of cell injury, and others still are adaptive responses that involve specific cellular organelles. Here we shall touch on only some of the more common or interesting of these reactions.

## MEMBRANES AND MEMBRANE SKELETON

We have seen how ischemic or toxic injury causes reversible and irreversible membrane damage, the latter characterized by permanent loss of membrane permeability. There are, however, many other defects in the molecular structure of the plasma membrane and its associated components. Some of these are genetic in origin, involving the number or the affinity of membrane receptors such as occurs in familial hypercholesterolemia (p. 105); others relate to acquired antibodies to such receptors, e.g., the thyrotropin receptor in primary hyperthyroidism (p. 681); and still others are defects in the *membrane skeleton*, i.e., the filamentous meshwork of proteins lining the inner membrane surface of certain cells, particularly erythrocytes.[25] These proteins consist of *spectrin, actin, protein 4.1,* and *ankyrin,* and their interactions determine the structural stability of the cell membrane. It has been shown that membrane-skeletal flaws may account for some important red cell disorders (p. 353). For example, in some patients with *hereditary spherocytosis,* in which the red cells are spheroid rather than discoid (and more prone to fragmentation), the defect in red cell shape is caused by abnormal spectrin molecules that are incapable of binding protein 4.1 and thus unable to maintain the stability of the red cell membrane.[26] Spectrin-like molecules have now been found to occur in a variety of other cell types (e.g., endothelium), and it is possible that defects in such molecules may be involved in specific disorders.[27]

## LYSOSOMES: HETEROPHAGY AND AUTOPHAGY

As is well known, lysosomes are membrane-bound cytoplasmic bodies, 0.2 to 0.8 μm in diameter, which contain a variety of hydrolytic enzymes. Lysosomes are involved in the breakdown of phagocytosed material in one of two ways (Fig. 1–14).

**HETEROPHAGOCYTOSIS.** In this phenomenon materials from the external environment are taken up through the process of *endocytosis.* Uptake of particulate matter is known as *phagocytosis,* and that of soluble smaller macromolecules as *pinocytosis.* Heterophagy is most common in the "professional" phagocytes, such as neutrophils and macrophages, but also occurs in other cell types. Examples of heterophagocytosis include the uptake and digestion of bacteria by neutrophilic leukocytes, the removal of necrotic cells by macrophages, and the reabsorption by the pinocytotic vesicles of the proximal convoluted tubules (heteropinocytosis) of protein that may filter across the renal glomerulus. Fusion of the phagocytic vacuole with a lysosome then occurs, possibly with digestion of the engulfed material.

**AUTOPHAGOCYTOSIS.** In many instances, individual cell organelles, such as mitochondria or endoplasmic reticulum, suffer focal injury and must then be digested if the cell's normal function is to be preserved. The lysosomes involved in such autodigestion are called *autolysosomes* and the process is called *auto-*

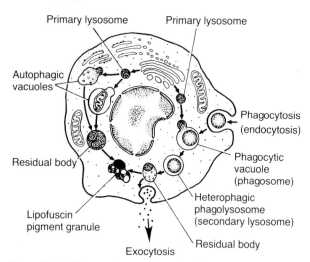

**Figure 1–14.** Schematic representation of lysosomal breakdown of phagocytosed material. Autophagy is depicted on the left side of the cell, and heterophagy is seen on the right. (From Robbins, S. L., Cotran, R. S., and Kumar, V.: Pathologic Basis of Disease. 3rd ed. Philadelphia, W. B. Saunders Co., 1984, p. 26.)

*phagy.* Autophagy is particularly pronounced in cells undergoing atrophy.

The enzymes in the lysosomes are capable of breaking down most proteins and carbohydrates, but some lipids remain undigested. Lysosomes with undigested debris may persist within cells as *residual bodies* or may be extruded. *Lipofuscin pigment* granules, discussed earlier, represent undigested material that results from intracellular lipid peroxidation. Certain indigestible pigments, such as carbon particles inhaled from the atmosphere or pigment inoculated in tattoos, can persist in phagolysosomes of macrophages for decades.

Lysosomes are also wastebaskets in which cells sequester abnormal substances when these cannot be adequately metabolized. Hereditary *lysosomal storage disorders,* marked by deficiencies of enzymes that degrade mucopolysaccharides, cause abnormal amounts of these compounds to be sequestered in the lysosomes of cells all over the body, particularly neurons, leading to severe abnormalities.

## INDUCTION (HYPERTROPHY) OF SMOOTH ENDOPLASMIC RETICULUM

It is known that protracted human use of barbiturates leads to a state of increased tolerance, so that repeated identical doses lead to progressively shorter time spans of sleep. The patients have thus "adapted" to the medication. The basis of this adaptation has been traced to induction of increased volume (hypertrophy) of the smooth endoplasmic reticulum (SER) of hepatocytes.[28] Barbiturates are detoxified in the liver by oxidative demethylation, which involves the P-450–centered mixed-function oxidase system found in the smooth endoplasmic reticulum (SER). The barbiturates stimulate (*induce*) the synthesis of more enzymes as well as more SER. In this manner, the cell is better able to detoxify the drugs and so adapt to its altered environment. The mixed-function oxidase system of the SER is also involved in the metabolism of other exogenous compounds—carcinogenic hydrocarbons, steroids, carbon tetrachloride, alcohol, insecticides, and others. Thus hepatic cells that have already undergone inductive changes metabolize all of these products more rapidly.

## MITOCHONDRIA

We have seen that mitochondrial dysfunction plays an important role in acute cell injury. In addition, however, various alterations in the number, size, and shape of mitochondria occur in some pathologic conditions. For example, in cell hypertrophy and atrophy there is an increase and decrease, respectively, in the number of mitochondria in cells. Mitochondria may assume an extremely large and abnormal shape (megamitochondria). These can be seen in the liver in alcoholic liver disease and in certain nutritional deficiencies, in skeletal muscle fibers in some myopathies, and in other cells in which there is alteration in mitochondrial growth and replication. In addition, large and highly pleomorphic mitochondria are seen commonly in tumor cells.

## CYTOSKELETON

Abnormalities of the cytoskeleton underlie a variety of pathological states. The *cytoskeleton* consists of microtubules (20 to 25 nm in diameter), thin actin filaments (6 to 8 nm), thick myosin filaments (15 nm), and various classes of intermediate filaments (10 nm).[29] Several other nonpolymerized and nonfilamentous forms of contractile proteins also exist. Cytoskeletal abnormalities may be reflected by defects in cell function, such as cell locomotion and intracellular organelle movements, or in some instances by intracellular accumulations of fibrillar material. Only a few examples will be cited.

Functioning myofilaments and microtubules are essential for various stages of leukocyte migration and phagocytosis, and functional deficiencies of the cytoskeleton appear to underlie certain defects in leukocyte movement toward an injurious stimulus (chemotaxis, p. 36) or the ability of such cells to perform phagocytosis adequately. For example, a defect of microtubule polymerization in the *Chédiak-Higashi syndrome* causes delayed or decreased fusion of lysosomes with phagosomes in leukocytes and thus impairs phagocytosis (p. 36). Some drugs, such as cytochalasin B, inhibit microfilament function and thus affect phagocytosis. Defects in the organization of lowly microtubules can destroy a man by inhibiting sperm motility to cause male sterility and by immobilizing the cilia of respiratory epithelium, causing interference with the ability of such epithelium to clear inhaled bacteria, leading to often fatal lung infections (the immotile cilia syndrome).

Two common histologic entities have recently been traced to accumulations of *intermediate filaments*. One is the *Mallory body*, or "alcoholic hyaline," an eosinophilic intracytoplasmic inclusion in liver cells that is highly characteristic of alcoholic liver disease. Such inclusions are now known to be composed largely of intermediate filaments of predominantly *prekeratin* composition, suggesting that a cytoskeletal defect with loss of intracellular organization may be a mechanism of cell injury in alcoholic liver disease.[30] Another is the *neurofibrillary tangle* found in the brains of patients with Alzheimer's disease, an important cause of presenile dementia. Tangles are now thought to contain cross-linked neuronal intermediate filaments, and it is believed that such cross-linking may interfere with the dynamics of neuronal cytoskeleton and the maintenance of axons and dendrites.[31]

Undoubtedly the burgeoning field of "cytoskeletal pathology" will soon uncover many more instances in which abnormalities of the cytoskeleton contribute to the expression of disease.

# CELLULAR ADAPTATION

Just as animals, including humans, have adapted to environmental changes in the evolution of their species, so do cells adapt to changes in their microenvironment. The normal cell does not exist in a rigidly fixed functional and morphologic state. Rather it traverses a fluid range of structure and function reflecting the changing demands of life. Organelles become senescent and are replaced by more or fewer new ones to adapt to the metabolic demands. When stresses or noxious influences impinge upon the cell, it will, to the extent possible, adapt and achieve an altered steady state, permitting it to survive within its changed environment. As before, there is continuing turnover of the cells' substructure with adjustment of the number of organelles to meet the level of stress. A new but altered equilibrium is achieved. We have just begun to understand the many facets and manifestations of cellular adaptation. One example of adaptation—induction of SER—has already been described (p. 22). There follow some additional examples.

## ATROPHY

*Shrinkage in the size of the cell by loss of cell substance is known as atrophy.* It represents a form of adaptive response. When a sufficient number of cells are involved, the entire tissue or organ diminishes in size or becomes atrophic (Fig. 1–15).

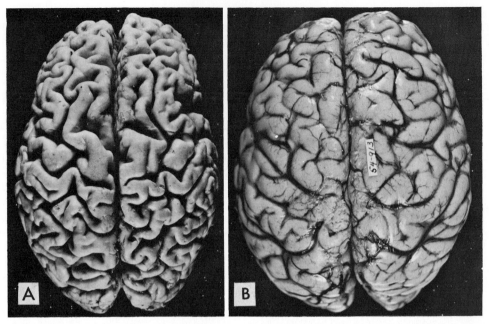

**Figure 1–15.** *A,* Physiologic atrophy of the brain in an 82-year-old male. The meninges have been stripped. *B,* Normal brain of a 35-year-old male. (From Robbins, S. L., Cotran, R. S., and Kumar, V.: Pathologic Basis of Disease. Philadelphia, W. B. Saunders Co., 1984, p. 30.)

The apparent causes of atrophy are (1) decreased workload, (2) loss of innervation, (3) diminished blood supply, (4) inadequate nutrition, and (5) loss of endocrine stimulation. The fundamental cellular change is identical in all, representing a retreat by the cell to a smaller size at which survival is still possible. The cell contains fewer mitochondria and myofilaments and less endoplasmic reticulum.

The biochemical mechanisms of atrophy are not very well understood. There is a finely regulated balance between protein synthesis and degradation in normal cells, and either decreased synthesis, increased catabolism, or both may cause atrophy. Hormones, particularly insulin, thyroid hormones, glucocorticoids, and prostaglandins, influence such protein turnover.[32] Thus only slight increases of degradation over a long period of time may result in atrophy, as seems to occur in some muscle dystrophies. The concentration of hydrolytic proteases within the cell increases in atrophy; however, these enzymes are not simply released into the cytoplasm, since this might lead to uncontrolled cellular destruction. Rather, they are incorporated into autophagic vacuoles. Thus in many situations atrophy is accompanied by a marked increase in the number of *autophagic vacuoles.*

## HYPERTROPHY

*Hypertrophy refers to an increase in the size of cells and, with such change, an increase in the size of the organ.* Hypertrophy can be caused by increased functional demand or by specific hormonal stimulation and may occur under both physiologic and pathologic conditions. The physiologic growth of the uterus during pregnancy involves both hypertrophy and hyperplasia. The cellular hypertrophy is stimulated by estrogenic hormones through smooth muscle estrogen receptors, which allow for interactions of the hormones with nuclear DNA, eventually resulting in increased synthesis of smooth muscle proteins and increase in cell size. This is then physiologic hypertrophy effected by hormonal stimulation. Hypertrophy as an adaptive response is exemplified by muscular enlargement. The striated muscle cells in both the heart and skeletal muscle are most capable of hypertrophy, perhaps because they cannot adapt to increased metabolic demands by mitotic division and the formation of more cells to share the work (Fig. 1–16).

The environmental change that produces hypertrophy of striated muscle appears mainly to be increased workload. In the heart a stimulus is high blood pressure; in skeletal muscles, heavy work. There is a synthesis of more enzymes and filaments, achieving a balance between the demand and the cell's functional capacity. The greater number of myofilaments permits an increased workload with a level of metabolic activity per unit volume of cell not different from that borne by the normal cell. Thus the draft horse readily pulls the load that would break the back of a pony. A decrease in protein degradation, with a normal or slightly increased amount of protein synthesis, may also cause hypertrophy. Intracellular enzymes, including proteases, are responsible for such protein degradation, and thus any alterations in these intracellular enzymes may affect cellular pro-

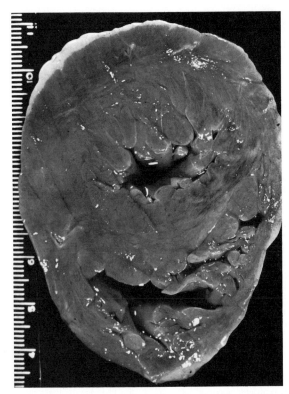

Figure 1–16. A cross section of a heart with marked left ventricular hypertrophy. The left ventricular wall is over 2 cm in thickness (normal, 1 to 1.5 cm). On the right side of the interventricular septum, the mottled, dark area is a focus of fresh ischemic necrosis (myocardial infarct).

tein mass. Whatever the exact mechanism of hypertrophy, however, it eventually reaches a limit beyond which enlargement of muscle mass is no longer able to compensate for the increased burden, and cardiac failure, for example, ensues. At this stage a number of "degenerative" changes occur in the myocardial fibers, of which the most important are lysis and loss of myofibrillar contractile elements. The limiting factors for continued hypertrophy and the causes of regressive changes are incompletely understood; they may be due to limitation of the vascular supply to the enlarged fibers, to diminished oxidative capabilities of mitochondria, or to alterations in protein synthesis and degradation.

# CALCIFICATION

Pathologic calcification is a common process that implies the abnormal deposition of calcium salts, together with smaller amounts of iron, magnesium, and other mineral salts. When the deposition occurs in dead or dying tissues, it is known as *dystrophic calcification; it may occur despite normal serum levels of calcium and in the absence of derangements in calcium metabolism.* In contrast, the deposition of calcium salts in normal tissues is known as *metastatic calcification, and it almost always reflects some de-rangement in calcium metabolism, leading to hypercalcemia.*

## DYSTROPHIC CALCIFICATION

This alteration is encountered in areas of coagulation, in caseous and liquefactive necrosis, and in foci of enzymic necrosis of fat whenever the necrotic tissue persists for a long period of time. It commonly develops in damaged heart valves, hampering their function (Fig. 1–17). Calcification is almost inevitable in the atheromas of advanced atherosclerosis, which, as will be seen, are focal intimal injuries in the aorta and larger arteries that are characterized by the accumulation of lipids (p. 292).

Whatever the site of deposition, the calcium salts appear macroscopically as fine, white granules or clumps, often felt as gritty deposits. Sometimes, a tuberculous lymph node is virtually converted to stone. Histologically, calcification can be **intracellular** or **extracellular** basophilic deposits, or **both**. In time, **heterotopic bone** may be formed in the focus of calcification.

The pathogenesis of dystrophic calcification involves *initiation* and *propagation* leading ultimately to the formation of crystalline calcium phosphate. Initiation in *extracellular* sites occurs in membrane-bound *vesicles*, about 200 nm in diameter; in cartilage and bone they are known as *matrix vesicles*, whereas in pathologic calcification they seem to be derived from degenerating or aging cells. It is thought that

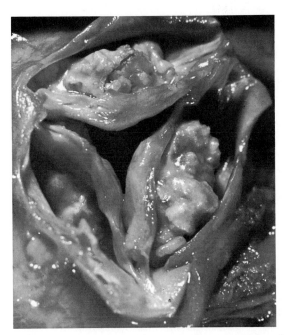

Figure 1–17. A view looking down onto the unopened aortic valve in a heart with healed (old) rheumatic aortic endocarditis. The semilunar cusps are thickened and fibrotic. Behind each leaflet are seen irregular masses of piled-up dystrophic calcification.

calcium is concentrated in these vesicles by its affinity to acidic phospholipids, and phosphates accumulate as a result of the action of membrane-bound phosphatases.[33] Initiation of *intracellular* calcification occurs in the *mitochondria* of dead or dying cells that accumulate calcium, as described earlier. Propagation of crystal formation then occurs, dependent on the concentration of $Ca^{++}$ and $PO_4$ in the extracellular spaces, the presence of mineral inhibitors, and the presence of collagen. The latter appears to increase the rate of crystal proliferation.

Although dystrophic calcification may be simply a "telltale" sign of previous cell injury, it is often a cause of organ dysfunction. Such is the case in calcific valvular disease and atherosclerosis, as will become clear in the further discussion of these diseases.

## METASTATIC CALCIFICATION

*This alteration may occur in normal tissues whenever there is hypercalcemia.* Hypercalcemia also accentuates dystrophic calcification. The causes of hypercalcemia include hyperparathyroidism; vitamin D intoxication; systemic sarcoidosis; milk-alkali syndrome; hyperthyroidism; idiopathic hypercalcemia of infancy; Addison's disease (adrenocortical insufficiency); increased bone catabolism associated with multiple myeloma, metastatic cancer, and leukemia; and decreased bone formation as occurs in immobilization. Hypercalcemia also arises in some instances of advanced renal failure with phosphate retention, leading to secondary hyperparathyroidism.

Metastatic calcification may occur widely throughout the body but principally affects the interstitial tissues of the blood vessels, kidneys, lungs, and gastric mucosa. In all these sites, the calcium salts morphologically resemble those described in dystrophic calcification. Metastatic calcification appears to begin also in mitochondria except in kidney tubules, where it develops in the basement membranes, probably in relation to extracellular vesicles budding from the epithelial cells. On occasion, massive involvement of the lungs produces remarkable x-ray films and respiratory deficits. Massive deposits in the kidney (nephrocalcinosis) may in time cause renal damage.

## HYALINE CHANGE

Hyaline deposits may occur within cells, between cells, and, more widely, as hyalinization of tissues, and so it is necessary that the term "hyaline" be clarified. *"Hyaline" is a descriptive adjective for any homogeneous, glassy, pink-appearing substance in routine tissue sections.* The term is applied to a variety of histologic changes solely in a descriptive sense: (1) Dense collagenous fibrous scars may assume a homogeneous pink hyaline appearance.

(2) Thickening and reduplication of basement membranes, as in arterioles in long-standing hypertension, give rise to what is termed hyaline arteriolosclerosis. (3) The abnormal extracellular proteinaceous deposits in amyloidosis (p. 168) appear hyaline with the light microscope. (4) The droplets of reabsorbed protein encountered in the renal tubular epithelial cells in clinical states associated with excessive proteinuria have a hyaline, glassy, pink appearance in routine tissue sections. (5) Certain viral infections are marked by the appearance of hyaline viral inclusions within involved cells. (6) In chronic alchoholism, particularly when it has led to cirrhosis of the liver, the hepatocytes may develop cytoplasmic hyaline deposits, usually referred to as alcoholic hyalin, which is described more fully on page 586. It must be apparent that the term "hyaline" is applied to a heterogeneous group of anatomic changes merely in an attempt to categorize their appearance in stained tissue sections.

## References

1. Mäkelä, P. F., et al.: Evasion of host defenses (group report). *In* Smith, J. J., et al. (eds.): The Molecular Basis of Microbial Pathogenicity. Berlin, Dahlem Konferenzen, 1980, pp. 175–198.
2. Weiss, S. J., and LoBuglio, A. F.: Phagocyte-generated oxygen metabolites and cellular injury. Lab. Invest. 47:5, 1982.
3. Freeman, B. A., and Crapo, J. D.: Biology of disease: Free radicals and tissue injury. Lab. Invest. 47:412, 1982.
4. DiGuiseppi, J., and Fridovich, I.: The toxicity of molecular oxygen. Crit. Rev. Toxicol. 12:315, 1984.
5. Cowley, R. A., and Trump, B. F.: Pathophysiology of Shock, Anoxia, and Ischemia. Baltimore, Williams & Wilkins Co., 1981.
6. Farber, J. L.: Membrane injury and calcium homeostasis in the pathogenesis of coagulative necrosis. Lab. Invest. 47:114, 1982.
7. Smuckler, E. A., and James, J. L.: Irreversible cell injury. Pharmacol. Rev. 36:778, 1984.
8. Lemasters, J. J., et al.: Cell surface charges and enzyme release during hypoxia and reoxygenation in the isolated, perfused rat liver. J. Cell Biol. 97:778, 1984.
9. Matthys, E., et al.: Lipid alterations induced by renal ischemia: Pathogenetic factor in membrane damage. Kidney Int. 26:153, 1984.
10. McCord, J. M.: Oxygen-derived free radicals in postischemic tissue injury. N. Engl. J. Med. 312:159, 1985.
11. Comporti, M.: Lipid peroxidation and cellular damage in toxic liver injury. Lab. Invest. 53:599, 1985.
12. Fligiel, S. E. G., et al.: Evidence for a role of hydroxyl radical in immune-complex-induced vasculitis. Am. J. Pathol. 115:375, 1984.
13. Farber, E., et al.: Cell suicide and cell death. *In* Aldrige, W. N. (ed.): Mechanisms of Toxicity. London, Macmillan & Co., 1971, pp. 163–170.
14. Johnson, T. C.: Virus-host interactions: General concepts and defense mechanisms. *In* Youmans, G. P., et al. (eds.): The Biologic and Clinical Basis of Infectious Diseases. 3rd ed. Philadelphia, W. B. Saunders Co., 1985, pp. 35–44.
15. Sharpe, A. H., and Fields, B. N.: Pathogenesis of viral infections: Basic concepts derived from the reovirus model. N. Eng. J. Med. 312:486, 1985.
16. Notkin, A. C.: Molecular biology and viral pathogenesis—Clinical spinoff. N. Engl. J. Med. 312:507, 1985.
17. Smith, J. R., and Lincoln, D. W.: Aging of cells in culture. Int. Rev. Cytol. 89:151, 1984.

18. Hayflick, L.: The biology of human aging. Adv. Pathobiol. 7:21, 1980.

19. Martin, G. M.: Cellular aging (parts I and II). Am. J. Pathol. 89:484, 1977.

20. Majno, G., et al.: Cellular death and necrosis: Chemical, physical, and morphologic changes in rat liver. Virchows Arch. 333:421, 1960.

21. Searle, J., et al.: Necrosis and apoptosis: Distinct modes of cell death with fundamentally different significance. Pathol. Annu. 17:229, 1982.

22. Wyllie, A. H., et al.: Chromatin cleavage in apoptosis: Associated with condensed chromatin morphology and dependence on macromolecular synthesis. J. Pathol. 142:67, 1984.

23. Lieber, C. S.: Metabolism and metabolic effects of alcohol. Med. Clin. North Am. 68:3, 1984.

24. Stanbury, J. B.: The Metabolic Basis of Inherited Disease. 5th ed. New York, McGraw-Hill Book Co., 1983.

25. Marchesi, V. T.: The cytoskeletal system of red blood cells. Hosp. Prac. 20:113, 120, 125, 1985.

26. Shohet, S. B., and Lux, S. E.: The erythrocyte membrane skeleton: Pathophysiology. Hosp. Prac. 19:89, 1984.

27. Bennett, V., et al.: Ankyrin and synapsin: Spectrin antibody proteins associated with cell membrane. J. Cell Biol. 29:157, 1985.

28. Jones, A. L., and Fawcett, D. W.: Hypertrophy of the agranular endoplasmic reticulum in hamster liver induced by phenobarbital. J. Histochem. Cytochem. 14:215, 1966.

29. Gabbiani, G., and Kocher, O.: Cytocontractile and cytoskeletal elements in pathologic processes: Pathogenetic role and diagnostic value. Arch. Pathol. Lab. Med. 107:662, 1983.

30. French, S. W.: Present understanding of the development of Mallory's body. Arch. Pathol. Lab. Med. 107:445, 1983.

31. Selkoe, D. J., et al.: Paired helical filaments in human neurons: Relationship to neurofilaments. Ann. N. Y. Acad. Sci. 455:583, 1985.

32. Goldberg, A. L., et al.: Hormonal regulation of protein degradation and synthesis in skeletal muscle. Fed. Proc. 39:31, 1980.

33. Kim, K. M.: Pathological calcification. In Trump, B., and Arsila, A. (eds.): Pathobiology of Cell Membranes. Vol. 3. New York, Academic Press, 1983.

# 2

# Inflammation and Repair

Humans could not long survive in their sometimes hostile environment without the protective responses of inflammation and repair. Infections would run amok, burns would not heal, and wounds would remain festering, open sores. *Inflammation is the reaction of living tissues to all forms of injury. It involves vascular, neurologic, humoral, and cellular responses at the site of injury.* The inflammatory process destroys, dilutes, or contains the injurious agent and paves the way for repair of the damaged site. In the course of achieving its desirable ends, the inflammatory reaction often evokes prominent clinical manifestations, such as pain, as any patient with acute appendicitis will attest (note: inflammatory involvement of an organ or tissue is designated by the suffix "-itis"). *Repair is the process by which lost or destroyed cells are replaced by vital cells*, sometimes by regeneration of the native parenchymal cells but more often by fibroblastic scar-forming cells. Thus the inflammatory-reparative processes contain and neutralize the injury and restore the morphologic continuity of tissues, although not always their specialized function, as will be evident later. In some instances the inflammatory-reparative processes may be harmful. An overreactive inflammatory response (hypersensitivity) to a bee sting may indeed cause death. Similarly, scarring, such as sometimes follows bacteria-induced inflammatory reactions in the pericardial sac, may so encase the heart in dense fibrous tissue that it forever impairs cardiac function. Notwithstanding such possible untoward consequences, the inflammatory and reparative responses are fundamental to the survival of the organism.

Although inflammation and repair are two somewhat distinct processes, they are closely interwoven in the response of tissues to injury. Inflammation dominates the early events and repair assumes major importance later. Nevertheless, repair begins early in the inflammatory response, although it reaches completion only after active inflammation has subsided. If the injury is slight and the inflammatory response neutralizes it before there is much tissue damage, there may be little to be repaired. Such injuries may be completely reconstituted by regeneration of parenchymal cells, or at most there is only slight scarring. When the offending agent has caused considerable loss of cells, repair with substantial scar formation may become dominant. Because of the complexity of the many concurrent events in the inflammatory-reparative process, the discussion that follows will be somewhat artificially divided into separate considerations of inflammation and repair.

# Inflammation

## ACUTE INFLAMMATION

Acute inflammation comprises the immediate and early response to an injurious agent. It is of relatively short duration lasting for hours or days. As mentioned earlier, inflammation is basically a defensive reaction in the host. Since the two major defensive components, antibodies and leukocytes, are normally carried in the bloodstream, it is not surprising that vascular phenomena play a major role in the inflammatory process. Simple logic suggests that introduction of an injurious agent into the tissues should have two major effects: marshalling of defensive elements in the immediate vicinity of the offending agent, and emigration of the "combat troops" from the vasculature into the "battlefield," the tissues. Therefore, acute inflammation has three major components: (1) *alterations in vascular caliber that lead to an increase in blood flow,* (2) *structural changes in the microvasculature that permit the plasma proteins and leukocytes to leave the circulation,* and (3) *aggregation of the leukocytes in the focus of injury.* The protein-rich fluid and white cells that accumulate in the extravascular space as a result of an inflammatory reaction constitute an *exudate.*

The events in the acute inflammatory process are largely mediated by the production and release of a variety of chemical mediators. Despite the diversity of the injurious influences and the tissues involved in inflammation, similar chemical mediators are released; hence *the immediate inflammatory response is virtually stereotyped.* Thus microbiologic infections; injuries caused by heat, cold, or radiant energy; electrical or chemical injury; and mechanical trauma evoke similar immediate inflammatory reactions. Although the basic nature of the inflammatory process is stereotyped, its intensity and extent depend on the severity of the injury and the reactive capability of the host. Acute inflammation may remain confined to the site of injury and evoke only local signs and symptoms (to be described later as the cardinal signs of inflammation) or may be extensive and induce systemic signs and symptoms as well as involve secondary lines of defense, such as lymphoid tissue.

## VASCULAR CHANGES

The vascular response at a site of injury is fundamental to the acute inflammatory reaction. Without an adequate blood supply, tissues cannot mount an inflammatory reaction. The vascular changes can be segregated into alterations in blood flow and alterations in permeability.

### *Alterations in Blood Flow*

Directly after an injury, arteriolar dilatation, possibly preceded by a fleeting interval of vasoconstric-

tion, occurs at the local site. Precapillary sphincters open, leading to increased flow in previously functioning capillaries, as well as opening of inactive capillary beds. Concomitantly, the postcapillary venules dilate and fill with the rapidly flowing blood (Fig. 2–1). Thus, the microvasculature at the site of injury becomes dilated and filled with blood (*congestion*). Except in the case of very mild injury, the initial surge of blood flow (*hyperemia*) is followed by slowing of the bloodstream, changes in intravascular pressure, and alterations in the orientation of the formed elements with respect to the vessel walls. Stagnation of flow is the consequence of several events. As hyperemia develops, the venules and capillaries become abnormally permeable, resulting in the escape of plasma water. The viscosity of the blood is thus increased, leading to both packing (sludging) of the red cells and increased frictional resistance to flow. Therefore the outflow of blood from the local site is impeded, contributing to the stasis and stagnation. Decreased outflow, coupled with the increased inflow of blood from the arterioles, leads to elevation of hydrostatic pressure in the capillaries and venules (important to our later consideration of exudate formation). In the slowly moving blood, clumps of red cells assume a major central position and the leukocytes, principally neutrophils, assume a more peripheral orientation (margination) (Fig. 2–2).

The time relationships of these vascular changes

NORMAL

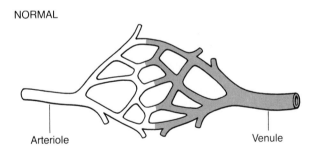

INFLAMED

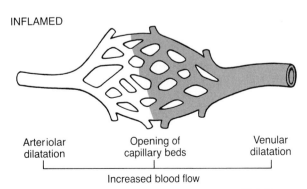

**Figure 2–1.** Alterations in blood flow associated with inflammation.

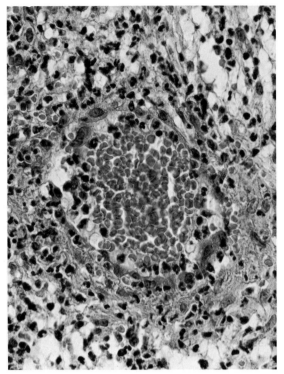

Figure 2–2. A dilated, congested venule with peripheral orientation (margination) of neutrophils. Many neutrophils have emigrated into the perivascular edematous tissue.

depend to some extent on the severity of the injury. Arteriolar dilatation becomes evident within a few minutes of the injury. Slowing and stagnation are apparent within 10 to 30 minutes.

### Alterations in Vascular Permeability—Exudation

*Increased vascular permeability with the escape of plasma proteins and white cells is known as exudation and is a major feature of all acute inflammatory reactions.* The mechanisms leading to increased permeability in acute inflammation are best discussed in the context of the normal structure of the microvasculature.

Omitting much detail, we may state that the microcirculation consists essentially of continuous channels of branching and anastomosing endothelium-lined tubes. The endothelial cell layer is enclosed within a continuous basement membrane. Although lacking in liver sinusoids and very thin in the lungs, in most tissues the basement membrane is sufficiently well developed to be seen on electron microscopy. Often it splits to enfold pericytes. The endothelial cell itself has been likened to a fried egg in appearance, with the central thick portion enclosing the nucleus, from which a thin attenuated cytoplasmic sheet extends out in all directions. The endothelial lining of all venules and most of the capillaries in the body is of the so-called *continuous* type, i.e., an unbroken cytoplasmic layer with tightly closed intercellular junctions.

Movement of fluid normally occurs out of and back into the microvasculature. Such movement, according to *Starling's law*, is regulated largely by the balance of intravascular hydrostatic pressure and opposing effects of colloid osmotic pressure exerted by plasma proteins. At the arteriolar end of the capillaries, high hydrostatic pressure forces fluids out into the interstitial tissue spaces by ultrafiltration (Fig. 2–3). This leads to an increased intravascular concentration of plasma proteins and a resulting increase in colloid osmotic pressure, which draws fluid in at the venular ends of capillaries. Such an exchange normally leads to a slight net efflux of fluid, which is drained from the tissue spaces by lymphatics. Normally capillaries allow free movement of water, salts, and solutes up to a molecular weight of 10,000 daltons. Movement of plasma proteins with molecular weights higher than 10,000 daltons is increasingly restricted as the size of the protein molecule increases.

With this brief overview of the normal capillary structure and fluid exchange, it is now possible to consider the development of exudation and edema (tissue swelling) at inflammatory sites. As already stated, an *exudate is an inflammatory extravascular fluid having a high specific gravity* (above 1.020) which often contains 2 to 4 gm per cent of protein, as well as white cells that have emigrated. It accumulates as a result of increased vascular permeability (which allows large plasma protein molecules to escape), the elevation in intravascular hydrostatic pressure brought about by increased local blood flow (Fig. 2–3), and a complex series of white cell events (to be described) leading to their emigration. In contrast, *transudate is a fluid that finds its way into the tissue spaces exclusively as a result of increased intravascular hydrostatic pressure.* The specific gravity of transudates is generally less than 1.012, a reflection of their low protein content. Formation of transudates is discussed later in Chapter 3. It should be remembered, however, that in mild injuries there is only a slight increase in vascular permeability, and as a result exudates are formed predominantly owing to the increase in hydrostatic pressure. The protein content of such an exudate may be only slightly greater than that of a transudate.

**PATTERNS OF INCREASED VASCULAR PERMEABILITY.** The timing and rate of development of exudation and edema at the site of acute inflammation vary with the severity of the injury. When the skin of the guinea pig is exposed to graded severities of thermal injury, three temporal patterns of exudation can be identified.[1] Mild injuries induce an *immediate transient permeability response*, which begins within one to two minutes following the application of heat and phases out within 15 to 30 minutes. Although it is rare, the reaction may persist for as long as an hour. As we shall see, this immediate response appears to be mediated largely by histamine and bradykinin. Electron micrographs of the inflammatory sites indicate that endothelial cells in small venules appear contracted, creating interendothelial gaps that are 0.5 to 1.0 μm wide. It is through these gaps that the leakage of plasma proteins occurs. The contraction of endothelial cells is believed to result from the action of histamine on these cells. Of note, there is no effect on the capillaries at this stage. This pattern of inflammatory exudation is encountered in very mild clinical inflammatory reactions.

Slightly more severe injuries induce a so-called *delayed prolonged response*. Here the increase in permeability is delayed for a period ranging from 30 minutes to 10 hours and reaches a peak, depending on the time of onset, between four and 24 hours after the injury. Sunburn, commonly experienced after the sunbathers return from the beach, is an example of the delayed-prolonged response. It appears that the delayed wave of increased permeability involves leakage from both venules and capillaries through interendothelial cell gaps. However, in contrast to the immediate-transient response, the intercellular gaps are believed to result from injury to the endothelium followed by passive retraction, rather than histamine-mediated contraction described earlier.[1]

Severe levels of injury induce an *immediate prolonged reaction*. Here the increase in permeability rises to an early peak, as in the immediate response, but remains at a high plateau at least as long as in the delayed pattern. Presumably here the more intense levels of heat have caused not only the death of endothelial cells but also their immediate disruption, causing abnormal leakage involving arterioles, capillaries, and venules. It should be emphasized that although these three patterns of permeability response can be identified clearly in the experimental model and may also occur in humans, in all likelihood clinically significant injuries produce the immediate prolonged reaction.

## WHITE CELL EVENTS

The massing of white cells, principally neutrophils and monocytes, at a site of injury may well constitute the most important aspect of the inflammatory reaction. White cells are capable of engulfing foreign particulate matter, including bacteria and the debris of necrotic cells, and their lysosomal enzymes contribute in a number of ways to the defensive response. As we shall see, several leukocyte products

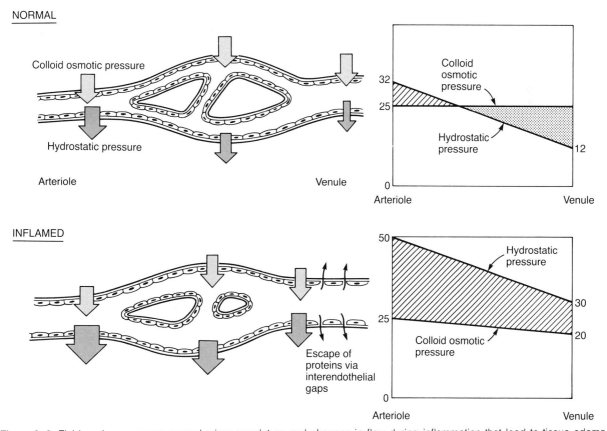

**Figure 2–3.** Fluid exchange across normal microvasculature and changes in flow during inflammation that lead to tissue edema. Note that both an increase in the hydrostatic pressure and vascular permeability contribute to the formation of inflammatory exudate. Strength of forces is scaled to size of arrows. (Modified from Wright, G.: An Introduction to Pathology. 3rd ed. London, Longmans Greens and Company, 1958.)

are by themselves pro-inflammatory, thus serving to "fuel the fire" and in some cases contribute significantly to tissue damage. The lymphocyte plays very little, if any, role in the acute phases of inflammation but principally contributes to the reactions in chronic long-standing inflammatory processes and in those of immunologic origin. Lymphocytes will be considered later in the discussion of chronic inflammation (p. 41). We can consider the sequence by which white cells aggregate and act at the inflammatory site under the following headings: (1) margination and pavementing, (2) emigration, (3) chemotaxis, and (4) phagocytosis.[2]

### Margination and Pavementing

In the inflammatory focus, the onset of stagnation in the microcirculation induces red cell clumping to form aggregates larger than individual leukocytes. According to physical flow laws, these red cell masses assume a central location within the axial stream and the white cells are displaced to the periphery (*margination*). Thus leukocytes come to occupy positions in contact with the endothelial surfaces. At first they slowly tumble or roll along the endothelial surface in the sluggish margins of the stream, but soon the cells appear to stick to and *pavement* the endothelial surfaces (Fig. 2–2).

The question of why leukocytes stick to the endothelium is still unanswered. Although several mechanisms, such as alterations in the surface charge of the leukocytes or elaboration of adhesive chemicals by injured endothelial cells, have been entertained, best documented is the role of factors that are chemotactic for leukocytes (p. 33). For example, leukotriene B$_4$, a product of arachidonic acid metabolism, and C5a (a complement component) have been shown to both increase leukocyte adhesion to endothelial cells and serve as chemoattractants for leukocytes.

*Pavementing* requires the presence of divalent cations such as Ca$^{++}$ and Mg$^{++}$, but their precise role remains mysterious. It is of interest that the administration of large doses of adrenal steroids reduces or totally blocks the phenomenon of pavementing. Glucocorticoids may act by inhibiting the synthesis of arachidonic acid from membrane phospholipids, thereby affecting the production of leukotriene B$_4$ (p. 39). This action of steroids may in part account for their well-known inhibitory effect on the inflammatory response. The patient on long-term adrenal steroid therapy is especially susceptible to uncontrolled bacterial infections.

### Emigration

As the term implies, emigration refers to the process by which motile white cells migrate out of blood vessels. Although all leukocytes are more or less motile, the most active are the neutrophils and monocytes; the most sluggish are the lymphocytes.

The principal sites of emigration of white cells are the interendothelial junctions. Although widening of the intercellular cell junctions (brought about by vasoactive amines) facilitates white cell emigration, leukocytes are known to be able to insert themselves through unaltered, apparently closed interendothelial cell junctions. During their migration across the vessel wall, leukocytes arrest temporarily under the basement membrane, but after a short period in this location they traverse it to enter the interstitial space. A second phenomenon has also been noted; on occasion a spurt of red cells may burst through the vessel wall behind an exiting white cell. This red cell movement, called diapedesis ("to walk between"), is believed to be passive and to result from hydrostatic pressure squeezing the thin envelope through a small defect. Thus red cell diapedesis is a passive phenomenon, whereas white cell emigration is an active, energy-dependent process.

The first cells to appear in perivascular spaces are the neutrophils, usually followed by monocytes (once outside the vascular compartment, monocytes are referred to as macrophages or histiocytes). There are some exceptions to this general sequence. Certain organisms, such as the tubercle and typhoid bacilli, evoke a predominantly mononuclear reaction from the outset. Similarly, viral infections and many immune reactions are characterized principally by the accumulation of lymphocytes. Despite these exceptions, most acute inflammations are marked by large numbers of neutrophils (Fig. 2–4). Several influences determine the sequence of appearance of the various white cell types in the inflammatory focus. The neutrophils appear first, owing in large part to their greater mobility and to the fact that they are present in greater number in the circulation. Furthermore, factors that act on neutrophils are activated early during the inflammatory response. Because of their short half-life the extravasated neutrophils do not survive for more than 24 to 48 hours. Monocytes begin to replace neutrophils by 48 hours, partly because the factors causing their recruitment are far more sustained, and partly because their life span ranges from weeks to months.

### Chemotaxis

After leaving the blood vessels, the leukocytes move in the general direction of the site of the injury. Such directional migration of white cells is mediated by diffusible chemical attractants and is hence called *chemotaxis*. Chemotaxis can be graphically documented in vitro in the Boyden chamber. A micropore membrane permeable to migrating cells separates an upper compartment containing the cell suspension from the lower compartment containing the test chemotactic solution. The number of cells that have migrated through the filter in a given time is a measure of the chemotactic effectiveness of the solution in the lower compartment. Most observations

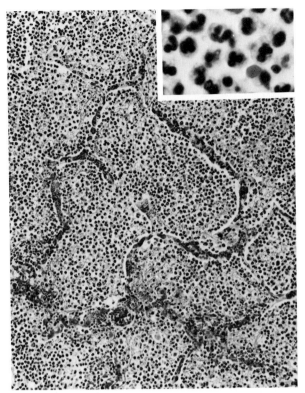

Figure 2–4. Photomicrograph of an acutely inflamed lung (pneumonia) showing emigration of inflammatory cells into the alveoli. Most of the cells in the exudate are neutrophils (*inset*) (Courtesy of Dr. Charles L. White III, Department of Pathology, Southwestern Medical School, Dallas, TX.)

relating to chemotaxis and chemotactic factors have been obtained by this technique.

Almost all classes of leukocytes are affected by chemotactic factors to a variable degree. Neutrophils and monocytes are the most reactive to chemotactic stimuli, whereas lymphocytes in general react poorly. Some chemotactic factors affect both neutrophils and monocytes; others are selective in their action on various white cells. Chemotactic factors may be endogenous, derived from plasma proteins (complement components), or exogenous—e.g., bacterial products.

*The most important chemotactic factors for neutrophils* are (1) *C5a*, a component of the complement system, (2) *leukotriene B$_4$*, a product of arachidonic acid metabolism, and (3) *bacterial products*. The first two are detailed later in this chapter. Chemotactic factors can be isolated from a variety of bacteria, including *Staphylococcus aureus* and *Escherichia coli*. The best studied chemotactic factors of bacterial origin are peptides with N-formyl-methionine–terminal amino acids. Synthetic oligopeptides such as formyl-methionyleucylphenylalanine (f-MLP), which resemble naturally occurring bacterial chemotactic factors, have been used extensively in the study of chemotaxis.

*Chemotactic agents acting on monocytes and mac-rophages* include C5a, leukotriene B$_4$, bacterial factors, fractions from neutrophils, lymphokines generated by exposure of sensitized lymphocytes to antigens, and fibronectin fragments. It is worth noting that neutrophils, possibly through the basic peptides in their lysosomal granules, play an important role in the formation of chemotactic agents for macrophages. Herein may lie the explanation for the fact that neutrophils emigrate first and provide a continuing stimulus for monocyte emigration. Chemotactic factors also act on eosinophils. In certain types of hypersensitivity reactions (Type 1), the inflammatory exudate is very rich in eosinophils, which are attracted by the release of eosinophil chemotactic factors of anaphylaxis (ECF-A) from mast cells (p. 137) and certain products of arachidonic acid metabolism such as prostaglandin D$_2$.

Although the mechanisms by which chemotactic factors interact with the leukocytes and signal them to move are not fully understood, the following are established[3]:

○ the initial interaction between chemotactic factors and leukocytes is receptor-mediated; cell surface receptors for C5a, leukotriene B$_4$, and f-MLP are present on human neutrophils and monocytes

○ the binding of chemotactic factors to their cell surface receptors leads to a net influx of calcium, which plays a key role in the ensuing locomotion

○ leukocytes can "sense" the concentration gradient of chemotactic factors, allowing them to align their advancing edge (head) toward the source of the factor (Fig. 2–5)

○ the ameboid movement necessary for locomotion is mediated by the microfilaments actin and myosin, present in the cytosol

○ the ability to move in a specific direction requires the participation of microtubules. Disruption of microtubules by the drug colchicine leads to haphazard, nondirectional movements.

### Phagocytosis

Phagocytosis can be resolved into three distinct but interrelated steps: (1) attachment of the particle to the surface of the phagocyte; (2) engulfment; and (3) killing and degradation of the ingested microbe or particle.

ATTACHMENT AND RECOGNITION. Although phagocytic cells can attach to inert particles and bacteria without any specific recognition process, it has long been known that phagocytosis of microorganisms is greatly facilitated if they are coated with *opsonins* in serum (e.g., IgG, C3) (Fig. 2–6). The cell surfaces of neutrophils and macrophages have receptors for the Fc portion of the immunoglobulin IgG and the third component of complement (C3b). When a microorganism is coated with IgG antibodies present in the serum, the Fc portion of the immunoglobulin molecule provides a site for attachment to the surface of the phagocyte. Similarly, the presence of C3b recep-

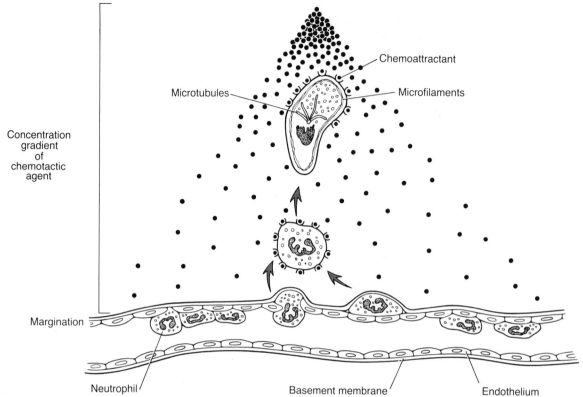

**Figure 2–5.** Schematic diagram depicting margination and emigration of neutrophils in response to a chemotactic agent. The chemoattractant binds to cell surface receptors on neutrophils. For simplicity the leukocytes within blood vessels are shown without the receptors.

tors on the phagocyte favors attachment and phagocytosis if C3b is fixed to the surface of the microorganism. As we shall see, C3b may be generated either by the antibody-dependent or the alternate pathway of complement activation (p. 38). Receptor-mediated attachment of opsonized bacteria has been called the recognition step of phagocytosis.

**ENGULFMENT.** After the opsonized bacterium is attached to the surface, the phagocytic cell then appears to flow partially around the particle, to create, in effect, a deep pocket. The mouth of such an invagination is pulled shut through formation of microfilaments in the surrounding cytoplasm, which act like a purse-string suture. The particle is now enclosed in a membrane-bound cytoplasmic vesicle known as a phagosome.[4] Even as the phagosome is forming, before it is fully enclosed, the cytoplasmic granules of the neutrophils fuse with the phagosome and discharge their contents into it, a process called degranulation (Fig. 2–6). The two types of granules in the neutrophil cytoplasm are (1) *azurophil (primary) granules*, which are lysosomes that contain acid hydrolases, neutral proteases, cationic proteins, myeloperoxidase, and lysozyme; and (2) *specific (secondary) granules*, which contain lysozyme and lactoferrin but no hydrolases or peroxidase. Macrophages also contain azurophil granules. The process of degranulation pours into the phagosome a battery of powerful enzymes, which constitute the cell's weaponry against the trapped microorganism. During degranulation enzymes as well as reactive oxygen metabolites (discussed later) also leak into the extracellular environment because some granules discharge their contents before the phagosome is completely closed (a process called "regurgitation during feeding"). Since some of the chemicals within the granules can act as mediators, they help to promote the inflammatory response (p. 41). Unfortunately, lysosomal enzymes and oxygen-derived free radicals can also attack normal tissue cells in the vicinity. This then is the price that the body pays for defending itself against invasion.[5]

Engulfment is an energy-dependent process that requires the presence of $Ca^{++}$ and $Mg^{++}$. There is little doubt that microfilaments are involved in exerting the forces necessary to produce invagination, closure, and degranulation. In this process they are assisted by microtubules, which are made up of the noncontractile protein tubulin. Profound metabolic changes occur in the cell following phagocytosis, including increased glycolysis, oxygen consumption ("the oxygen burst"), and increased glucose utilization by the hexose monophosphate shunt. It should be noted that the increase in oxygen consumption has nothing to do with increased energy production via mitochondrial respiration, but rather its purpose is to produce powerful antimicrobial agents, as will be discussed in the next section. The ability to respire anaerobically via glycolysis is crucial to neutrophils, since they must function in the center of inflammatory foci under hypoxic conditions.

**KILLING AND DEGRADATION.** Once a microorganism has been engulfed, what is its fate? Although most are readily destroyed by the phagocyte, some particularly virulent organisms may destroy the leukocyte. On the other hand, certain organisms, such as the acid-fast bacilli causing tuberculosis and leprosy, can survive within viable phagocytes. Transport of such infected white cells through the lymphatics to the lymph nodes can result in spread of the infection. The factors that determine whether engulfed bacteria will be killed within their membrane-bound prisons or will survive are poorly understood. However, we do know of a variety of microbicidal mechanisms within the phagocytic cells, which are classified as oxygen-dependent or oxygen-independent.

*Oxygen-Dependent Mechanisms* (Fig. 2–6). Contact between the neutrophil and the particulate stim-

ulus leads to rapid activation of a membrane enzyme called NADPH oxidase. This enzyme oxidizes NADPH to $NADP^+ + H^+$ and in the process reduces oxygen to the superoxide anion $O_2^-$. In the phagosome most of the $O_2^-$ is converted into $H_2O_2$ by spontaneous dismutation:[6]

$$2\ O_2^- + 2\ H^+ \rightarrow H_2O_2 + O_2$$

Although both $O_2^-$ and $H_2O_2$ (the immediate products of the respiratory burst) can kill bacteria, they are only weakly microbicidal. Instead they provide starting materials for powerful and more important microbicidal oxidants. In the presence of the enzyme myeloperoxidase (present normally in the neutrophil granules), $H_2O_2$ reacts with a halide ion—e.g., chloride ($Cl^-$) to form hypochlorite. This is the well-known and powerful antimicrobial agent also used in chlorinating drinking water and swimming pools. In other reactions, the superoxide anion $O_2^-$ acts as a precursor for potent free radicals such as OH:

$$O_2^- + H_2O_2 \rightarrow OH\cdot + OH^- + O_2$$

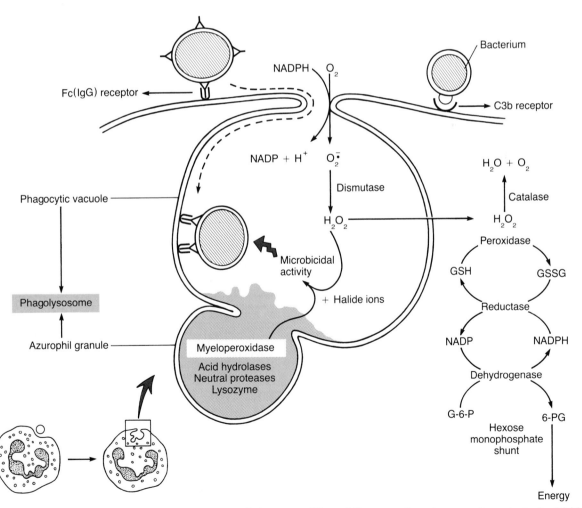

**Figure 2–6.** Schematic diagram of bacterial phagocytosis by neutrophils and the generation of oxygen-dependent microbicidal mechanisms within the phagolysosome.

The $H_2O_2$-halide-myeloperoxidase system is considered to be the major antimicrobial system within the neutrophil. Since the $H_2O_2$ produced within the phagosome can diffuse into the cytoplasm, the cell must protect itself from its toxic action. Most of the $H_2O_2$ is broken down by catalase into $H_2O$ and oxygen, and some of it is destroyed by the action of glutathione peroxidase. It may be noted in Figure 2–6 that two of the reactions discussed make $NADP^+$ available for the hexose monophosphate shunt, which therefore becomes greatly stimulated.

*Oxygen-Independent Mechanisms.* These include the following lysosomal agents: arginine-rich cationic proteins (phagocytin), enzymes such as lysozyme and elastase, and lactoferrin, an iron-binding protein. All of these have some antimicrobial activity. The low pH within the phagosomes (3.4 to 4.0) resulting from accelerated glycolysis may also be bactericidal. However, the lysosomal enzymes generally are more important for the digestion and degradation of killed microorganisms than for direct killing.

Although this discussion of phagocytosis applies in a general way to both macrophages and neutrophils, there are some differences between these two cell types. For example, although monocytes contain myeloperoxidase, once they enter tissues and transform into macrophages, they lose this enzyme. They can, however, like neutrophils generate $H_2O_2$ and other microbicidal free radicals. As we shall see later (p. 144), macrophage functions, including phagocytosis, can be markedly stimulated by lymphocyte products called lymphokines. As scavengers, macrophages are much more effective than neutrophils.

### Defects in Leukocyte Function

From the preceding discussion it is obvious that leukocytes play a cardinal role in host defense. Not surprisingly, therefore, defects in leukocyte function, both genetic and acquired, lead to an increased vulnerability to infections. Impairments of virtually every phase of leukocyte function—from adherence to vascular endothelium to microbicidal activity—have been described. Although individually rare, these disorders underscore the importance of the complex series of events that must occur *in vivo* following invasion by microorganisms. Only the most important of the leukocyte defects are briefly noted here. Details may be found in a recent review.[7]

1. DEFECTS IN CHEMOTAXIS. These can be classified into two major categories: (a) Intrinsic cellular defects—e.g., Chédiak-Higashi syndrome and diabetes mellitus (p. 59). In Chédiak-Higashi syndrome, an autosomal recessive disorder, there are multiple abnormalities including disordered assembly of microtubules, which impairs locomotion. (b) Extrinsic—e.g., defective generation of chemotactic factors such as complement deficiency states.

2. DEFECTS IN PHAGOCYTOSIS. These may also be intrinsic (e.g., neutrophil "actin dysfunction," dia-

betes mellitus) or extrinsic to the leukocytes. The latter include deficiencies of immunoglobulins or complement and the resultant failure of opsonization.

3. DEFECTS IN MICROBICIDAL ACTIVITY. This is illustrated by a childhood disease called chronic granulomatous disease (CGD), a condition in which there is a deficiency of NADPH oxidase. As a result, engulfment of bacteria is not followed by activation of oxygen-dependent killing mechanisms. The defective killing of bacteria by CGD neutrophils is somewhat selective. Many bacteria produce $H_2O_2$ during their own metabolism. Neutrophils of CGD patients can harness this $H_2O_2$ to produce bactericidal compounds, since the myeloperoxidase-halide system is normal. However, certain bacteria such as *S. aureus* possess catalase, which inactivates $H_2O_2$ and thus prevents its utilization by the neutrophils. Against such bacteria the CGD neutrophils are defenseless. In contrast, a measure of resistance is present against catalase-negative bacteria such as pneumococci.

4. MIXED DEFECTS. In some diseases, exemplified by diabetes mellitus (p. 59) and Chédiak-Higashi syndrome, several defects are present. The latter is characterized by neutropenia, decreased chemotaxis, defective degranulation, and delayed microbial killing. Neutrophils and other leukocytes have giant granules which can be readily appreciated in peripheral blood smears. The molecular basis of this genetic disorder is unknown but abnormal microtubule function is suspected.

**SUMMARY OF THE ACUTE INFLAMMATORY RESPONSE.** At this point it would be profitable to review the events in acute inflammation discussed so far. The vascular phenomena are characterized by increased blood flow to the injured area, resulting mainly from arteriolar dilatation and opening of capillary beds. Increased vascular permeability results in the collection of protein-rich extravascular fluid, which forms the exudate. Plasma proteins leave the vessels, either through widened interendothelial cell junctions of the venules or by direct endothelial cell injury. The leukocytes, predominantly neutrophils, also leave the microvasculature through the interendothelial cell route and migrate to the site of injury under the influence of chemotactic agents. Phagocytosis of the offending agent follows, which may lead to the death of the microorganism. With this overview we can proceed to a discussion of the mediators that bring about these phenomena.

## MEDIATORS OF ACUTE INFLAMMATION

### Neurogenic Mechanisms

In the very early phases of the reaction to injury, neurogenic mechanisms participate. Recall that following injury there is a very fleeting phase of arteriolar vasoconstriction, followed soon by dilatation of the arterioles leading into the inflammatory focus. Insights into these events are provided by the "triple response of Lewis."[8] When the skin is heavily stroked by a dull instrument, such as the tip of a pencil or a ruler edge, a *dull red line* corresponding to the line of pressure appears in approximately 1 minute. Soon a *bright red halo* or *flare* surrounds the stroke mark. Thereafter, the third component appears—the *edematous wheal (swelling)* along the line of the original stroke mark. Lewis showed that the second component of this triple response—the flare—could be blocked by prior anesthesia or interruption of the nervous pathways into the area. He concluded that this event was mediated by neurogenic vasodilatation of arterioles. Presumably this occurs through an antidromic axon reflex arc involving the vasomotor innervation of the arterioles. The first and third components of the triple response were not affected by blocking the nervous pathways, and Lewis attributed these to the release in injured tissues of an "H substance," which he later designated as histamine. The transient phase of vasoconstriction in the usual injury is, then, neurogenic in origin, but soon the antidromic reflex inhibits the vasoconstrictive impulses and contributes to the vasodilatation. Even without neural connections, however, the major aspects of the acute inflammatory response would take place, because, as we shall see, the principle mediators are chemical.

### Chemical Mediators

Chemicals derived from either plasma or the tissues are the major link between the occurrence of injury and the onset of the phenomena that constitute inflammation. Several general comments can be made about chemical mediators. Since the basic pattern of acute inflammation is stereotyped, regardless of the tissue or the causative agent, it follows that essentially similar chemical mediators widely distributed in the body are likely to be involved in most forms of inflammation. Several mediators can interact with each other, thus providing biologic mechanisms for amplifying the mediator actions. Furthermore, like all processes in the body, inflammation must be controlled. One mechanism of effecting control is the rapid local inactivation of the chemical mediator by enzyme systems or antagonists. Imperfections in the control systems can lead to serious consequences, including occurrence of disease, as exemplified by alpha-1-antitrypsin deficiency (p. 419) and hereditary angioedema.

So many chemical mediators have been identified that we are confronted with an embarrassment of riches. Identification of those that are significant in humans is a difficult task at present. All mediators (some with greater proof of their relevance than others) can be categorized as falling into one of the following groups:

○ vasoactive amines—histamine and serotonin
○ plasma proteases—the kinin system, the comple-

ment system, and the coagulation-fibrinolytic system
○ arachidonic acid (AA) metabolites—the prostaglandins and leukotrienes
○ products of leukocytes—lysosomal enzymes and lymphokines
○ miscellaneous—oxygen-derived free radicals, platelet activating factor (PAF-acether)

**VASOACTIVE AMINES.** Histamine is widely distributed in tissues, the richest source being the mast cells that are normally present in the connective tissue adjacent to blood vessels. It is also found in blood basophils and platelets. Preformed histamine is present in mast cell granules and is released by mast cell degranulation in response to a variety of stimuli: (1) physical injury such as trauma or heat, (2) immunologic reactions involving binding of IgE antibodies to mast cells (p. 137), (3) fragments of complement called anaphylatoxins, and (4) cationic lysosomal proteins derived from neutrophils. In humans, histamine causes dilatation of the arterioles and increases vascular permeability of the venules. It is considered to be the principal mediator of the immediate phase of increased vascular permeability, causing venular endothelial contraction and widening of the interendothelial cell junctions (p. 31). Histamine acts by binding to H-1-type histamine receptors present on the vascular endothelium. It is important to note that antihistamine drugs can inhibit only the early phase of increased vascular permeability and that histamine has no role in the delayed sustained phase of increased permeability.

Soon after its release from mast cells, histamine is inactivated by histaminase. In addition to its role in vascular phenomena, histamine has been reported to be specifically chemotactic for eosinophils. Although serotonin (5-hydroxytryptamine) induces effects similar to histamine in rodents, its role as a mediator in humans is not established.

**PLASMA PROTEASES.** A variety of phenomena in the inflammatory response are mediated by three interrelated plasma-derived factors—kinins, complement, and the clotting system (Fig. 2–7).

*The Kinin System.* This system, when activated, leads to the formation of bradykinin. Like histamine, bradykinin causes arteriolar dilatation, increased permeability of venules, and extravascular smooth muscle contraction. Unlike histamine, it is not chemotactic for leukocytes but causes pain when injected into the skin. Like histamine, it acts on endothelial cells to increase the gaps between cells. It is rapidly inactivated by kininases present in plasma and tissues, and its role is limited to the early phase of increased vascular permeability. Bradykinin is a polypeptide that (unlike histamine) is derived from plasma where it is present in a precursor form called *high-molecular-weight kininogen (HMWK)*. This precursor glycoprotein is cleaved by a proteolytic enzyme *kallikrein*, which must be activated from its own precursor, prekallikrein, by activated factor XII

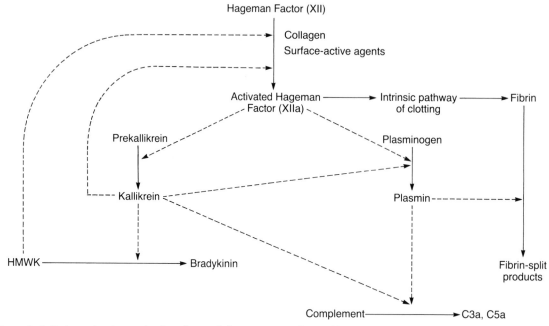

**Figure 2–7.** Pathway for the production of some inflammatory mediators. Note the interactions between various mediators.

of the clotting system (Hageman factor), which results from contact of factor XII with the injured tissues, especially collagen and vascular basement membrane. Figure 2–7 illustrates the close interaction between the clotting and the kinin-generating systems and also the amplifying effect of kallikrein on the activation of Hageman factor.

**The Complement System.** The complement system consists of a series of plasma proteins that play an important role in both immunity and inflammation. Complement components present as inactive forms in plasma are numbered C1 through C9. Although it is not our intention to go into the detailed sequence of the activation of the "complement cascade," a brief review of the salient features will be helpful to our discussion.[9] The most critical step in the elaboration of the biologic functions of complement is the activation of the third component, C3 (Fig. 2–8). All other complement components can be grouped into functional units in relation to their interaction with C3. Cleavage of C3 can occur by the so-called *classical pathway*, which is triggered by fixation of C1 to antibody (IgM or IgG) combined with antigen, or by the *alternate pathway*. The alternate pathway, which does not require activation by antigen-antibody complexes, can be triggered by bacterial polysaccharides such as endotoxins and human IgA. It involves the participation of a distinct set of serum components called the properdin system (properdin [P], factors B and D). Whichever pathway is involved in the cleavage of C3, there is a single amplification mechanism composed of the alternate pathway proteins, which promote further conversion of C3 to C3b. Once C3b is generated, it utilizes a common final *effector* sequence involving C5 through C9, which leads to

the generation of several biologically active factors and lysis of antibody-coated cells. The recognition in recent years of the alternate pathway has strengthened the belief that complement proteins generate important mediators of inflammation, both in immunologic and in nonimmunologic settings. Complement-derived factors affect a variety of phenomena in acute inflammation as follows:

1. VASCULAR PHENOMENA. C3a and C5a (also called anaphylatoxins), which are the split products of the corresponding complement components increase vascular permeability and cause vasodilatation by releasing histamine from mast cells. C5a also activates the lipoxygenase pathway of arachidonic acid metabolism in neutrophils and monocytes, causing further synthesis and release of inflammatory mediators.

2. CHEMOTAXIS. As mentioned previously (p. 32),

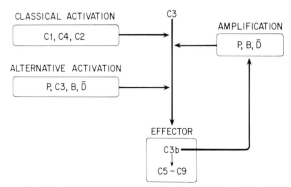

**Figure 2–8.** Pathways of complement activation. (From Fearon, D. T., and Austen, K. F.: *In* McCarty, D. J., and Hollander, J. L. [eds.]: Arthritis and Allied Conditions. 10th ed. Philadelphia, Lea & Febiger, 1985.)

C5a, a split product of C5, causes adhesion of neutrophils to the endothelium and is chemotactic for monocytes and neutrophils.

3. PHAGOCYTOSIS. C3b, when fixed to the bacterial cell wall (p. 33), acts as an opsonin and favors phagocytosis by neutrophils and macrophages, which bear cell surface receptors for C3b.

Among the complement components, C3 and C5 are undoubtedly the most important mediators. Their significance is further enhanced by the fact that, in addition to the mechanisms discussed above, C3 and C5 can be activated by several proteolytic enzymes present within the inflammatory exudate. These include plasmin and lysosomal enzymes released from neutrophils (see discussion later in this chapter). Thus, the chemotactic effect of complement and the complement-activating effects of neutrophils can set up a self-perpetuating cycle of neutrophil emigration.

*The Clotting System.* As mentioned earlier, Hageman factor (XII) is activated during inflammation as a consequence of tissue injury. This event is of singular importance, since it sets into motion several reactions that intercalate with the activation of complement and the kinin systems (Fig. 2–7). Most of these have been discussed earlier; it is worth pointing out, however, that plasmin itself can act on Hageman factor, producing subunits that are powerful activators of prekallikrein.

### ARACHIDONIC ACID METABOLITES—THE PROSTAGLANDINS AND LEUKOTRIENES.

It is now widely recognized that products derived from the metabolism of arachidonic acid are ubiquitous in mammalian tissues. They affect a variety of biologic processes, including inflammation and hemostasis, and play important physiologic roles in the renal, cardiovascular, and pulmonary systems, to name a few. Here we will briefly review some of the important pathways in arachidonic acid metabolism and the role of its metabolites in inflammation. Detailed reviews of this subject are available.[10, 11]

Arachidonic acid (AA) is a polyunsaturated fatty acid that is present in large amounts in phospholipids of the cell membrane. In order for it to be utilized by the cell to generate mediators, AA must be released from membrane phospholipids by activation of cellular phospholipases. During inflammation, lysosomes of neutrophils are believed to be an important source of phospholipases. Other chemical mediators such as C5a can also activate phospholipases and trigger the AA cascade. Arachidonic acid metabolism proceeds along one of two major pathways (Fig. 2–9), named after the enzymes that initiate the reactions:

(1) *The cyclooxygenase pathway.* This leads initially to the formation of a cyclic endoperoxide, prostaglandin $G_2$ (PG$G_2$), which in turn is converted into prostaglandin $H_2$ (PG$H_2$) by a peroxidase. PG$H_2$, itself highly unstable, is a precursor of the biologically active end products of the cyclooxygenase pathway. These include PG$E_2$, PG$D_2$, PG$F_{2\alpha}$, PG$I_2$ (prostacy-

clin), and TX$A_2$ (thromboxane), each of which is derived from PG$H_2$ by the action of a specific enzyme. Some of these enzymes have restricted tissue distribution. For example, platelets contain the enzyme thromboxane synthetase, and hence TX$A_2$ is the major product of PG$H_2$ in these cells. TX$A_2$ is a potent platelet aggregating agent and vasoconstrictor, itself unstable and rapidly converted to its inactive form TX$B_2$. Vascular endothelium, on the other hand, lacks thromboxane synthetase but possesses prostacyclin synthetase, which leads to the formation of prostacyclin (PG$I_2$) and its stable end product PG$F_{1\alpha}$. Prostacyclin is a vasodilator and a potent inhibitor of platelet aggregation. The opposing roles of TX$A_2$ and PG$I_2$ in hemostasis are further discussed on page 68. PG$D_2$ is the major metabolite of the cyclooxygenase pathway in mast cells; along with PG$E_2$ and PG$F_2$ (which are more widely distributed) it causes vasodilatation and potentiates edema formation. It should be noted that aspirin and nonsteroidal anti-inflammatory agents such as indomethacin inhibit cyclooxygenase and thus inhibit prostaglandin synthesis. Lipooxygenase is not affected by these anti-inflammatory agents.

(2) *Lipoxygenase pathway.* The importance of this pathway in generating powerful pro-inflammatory substances is now well established.[12, 13] The initial reaction along this pathway is the addition of a hydroperoxy group to AA at 5-, 12-, or 15-carbon positions of AA by enzymes called 5-, 12-, or 15-lipoxygenases, respectively. 5-Lipoxygenase is the predominant enzyme in neutrophils, and the metabolites derived by its actions are the best characterized. Our discussion will therefore be limited to the 5-lipoxygenase pathway. The 5-hydroperoxy derivative of AA, called 5-HPETE, is quite unstable and is either reduced to 5-HETE (which is chemotactic for neutrophils) or converted into a family of compounds collectively called *leukotrienes.* The first leukotriene generated from 5-HPETE is called leukotriene $A_4$ (LT$A_4$), which in turn gives rise to leukotriene $B_4$ (LT$B_4$) by enzymatic hydrolysis or to leukotriene $C_4$ (LT$C_4$) by addition of glutathione. LT$C_4$ is converted to leukotriene $D_4$ (LT$D_4$) and finally to leukotriene $E_4$ (LT$E_4$). LT$B_4$ is a potent chemotactic agent and causes aggregation of neutrophils. LT$C_4$ and LT$D_4$ collectively account for the biologic activity previously known as slow-reacting-substance of anaphylaxis (p. 137). They cause vasconstriction, bronchospasm, and increased vascular permeability.

As may be surmised from the preceding discussion, AA metabolites affect various facets of inflammation. These are summarized below:

1. VASCULAR PHENOMENA. Prostaglandin $E_2$ and prostacyclin are potent *vasodilators.* Their effect is predominantly on arterioles and, unlike histamine, vasodilatation is slow in onset and lasts for several hours. PG$D_2$, a product of mast cells, also causes vasodilation and may therefore be an important mediator at the sites where mast cells are triggered (p.

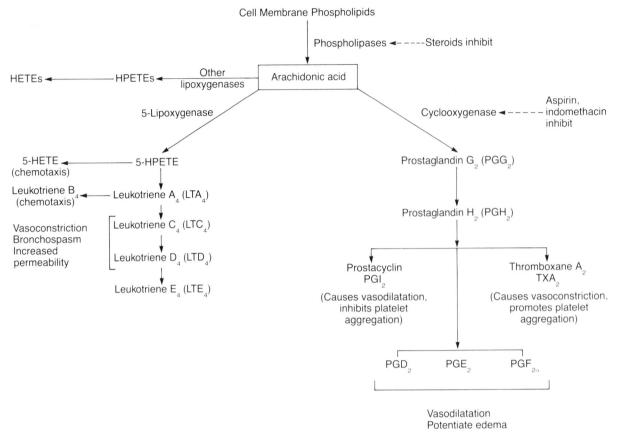

Figure 2–9. Generation of arachidonic acid metabolites and their role in inflammation.

137). $PGE_2$ and prostacyclin do not themselves affect vascular permeability but potentiate edema formation by increasing the permeability-increasing effect of other mediators such as histamine. This may result from their ability to increase blood flow into the inflamed area. As might be expected, increased blood flow would not only potentiate edema formation but also favor the influx of leukocytes into an area of inflammation. Whereas products of the cyclooxygenase pathway act predominantly as vasodilators, $LTC_4$ and $LTD_4$ generated by the 5-lipoxygenase pathway are extremely potent at increasing vascular permeability. Their effects, like those of histamine, are exerted on venules, but their potency is approximately 1000 times greater than histamine's. They also cause vasoconstriction and bronchospasm.

2. CHEMOTAXIS. $LTB_4$ is a powerful chemoattractant of neutrophils and monocytes. It also causes adhesion of neutrophils to the vascular endothelium, leading to the formation of conspicuous aggregates within the microvasculature. Its potency as a chemotactic agent is comparable to that of C5a, although it does not induce the same degree of generalized neutrophil activation (e.g., production of other mediators and free radicals). 5-HETE, another product of the lipoxygenase pathway, is also chemotactic, although not as powerful as $LTB_4$.

3. PAIN. $PGE_2$ produces pain and more importantly potentiates the pain-inducing effects of bradykinin. Prostaglandin $E_2$ may also be involved in the causation of fever.

*In summary, prostaglandins and leukotrienes can mediate virtually every step of acute inflammation.* Although the effects of the AA metabolites have been investigated most extensively in vitro, there is mounting evidence for their role in vivo.[10, 13] Prostaglandins and leukotrienes can be found in inflammatory exudates, and agents that suppress cyclooxygenase (aspirin, indomethacin) also suppresss inflammation in vivo. Glucocorticoids, which are powerful anti-inflammatory agents, may act at least in part by inducing the synthesis of a protein (called lipomodulin or macrocortin) that inhibits phospholipase $A_2$. Recall that phospholipases are required for the generation of AA from the phospholipids of the cell. Thus glucocorticoids, by blocking the synthesis of AA, may effectively prevent the subsequent generation of prostaglandins and leukotrienes.[14]

**MISCELLANEOUS MEDIATORS.** A host of other inflammatory mediators have been proposed. The activities ascribed to them can be readily demonstrated in vitro, but relative to the other mediators their roles in vivo are less well characterized. Important in this category are *oxygen-derived free radicals* and *PAF-acether.*

As noted previously, reactive oxygen metabolites generated within phagocytic cells during phagocytosis may leak into the extracellular milieu. It is suggested that these highly toxic free radicals increase vascular permeability by causing damage to capillary endothelium. In addition, superoxide and hydroxyl ions may also cause nonenzymatic peroxidation of AA resulting in generation of chemotactic lipids. While these reactions may indeed contribute to inflammation[15] and the accompanying tissue damage, it must be recalled that serum, tissue fluids, and most cells possess fairly effective, antioxidant mechanisms (p. 10) and therefore the damage inflicted in vivo by reactive oxygen intermediates may not be as great as one would suspect from in vitro experiments.

*PAF-acether* is the newest addition to the family of lipid mediators. Its biologic effects have been known for years as platelet-activating factor (PAF) because it causes platelet aggregation after being released from mast cells. Only recently, however, has it been chemically characterized and rechristened PAF-acether. In addition to mast cells, several other cell types including neutrophils and macrophages can synthesize PAF-acether. It increases vascular permeability, causes increased leukocyte adhesion, and stimulates both neutrophils and macrophages. It is not clear whether its effects are mediated directly or by the stimulation of AA metabolism in leukocytes. These and other questions relating to its role in vivo await further clarification.[16]

**LEUKOCYTE PRODUCTS.** Lysosomal contents of neutrophils, when released, provide several mediators of acute inflammation. Enzymes and other proteins are released from neutrophils by several mechanisms: following death of neutrophils, by leakage during the formation of the phagocytic vacuole (p. 34), and by reverse endocytosis. In the latter process, attempted phagocytosis of immune complexes attached to flat surfaces leads to exocytosis (expulsion) of lysosomal enzymes into the medium. The effects of many of these sustances have been discussed earlier in this section and will be mentioned briefly here. *Neutral proteases* including enzymes such as elastase, collagenase, and cathepsin can mediate tissue injury by degrading elastin, collagen, and other tissue proteins. Proteases may cleave C3 and C5 directly to generate anaphylatoxins. Kallikrein released from the lysosomes promotes the generation of bradykinin. Cationic proteins include several biologically active factors that (a) increase vascular permeability by causing mast cell degranulation, (b) possess chemotactic activity for monocytes, and (c) immobilize neutrophils at the site of inflammation. Neutrophils are also a source of phospholipase required for arachidonic acid

synthesis. Furthermore, *stimulation of the neutrophil surface even in the absence of phagocytosis can trigger the arachidonic acid cascade and subsequent release of its mediators.*

Monocytes and macrophages, like neutrophils, contain many biologically active pro-inflammatory substances in their lysosomes. Their release may be important not only in acute but also in chronic inflammation. Lymphocytes that have been sensitized to antigens release a variety of biologically active products called lymphokines (p. 144), which include factors that mediate the accumulation and activation of macrophages at sites of inflammation. They are important in chronic inflammation.

A summary of the mediators of inflammation is presented in Table 2–1.

# CHRONIC INFLAMMATION

To this point, the inflammatory process has been described in terms of the immediate reaction to injury, which gives rise to acute inflammation. Acute reactions are seen when the stimulus to inflammation is transient, as in physical trauma, burns (whether caused by excess heat or by chemicals), and microbiologic infections that are rapidly eradicated by the defensive forces of the body. *The acute response is characterized principally by the vascular and exudative changes already discussed.* The white cells that participate in the acute reaction are principally neutrophils and macrophages. In contrast with acute inflammation, *chronic inflammation results from injurious stimuli that are persistent, often for weeks or*

**Table 2–1.** SUMMARY OF MEDIATORS IN INFLAMMATION

| Event | Mediator or Mechanism |
|---|---|
| Vasodilatation | Histamine |
| | Bradykinin |
| | Prostaglandins—$PGI_2$, $PGE_2$, $PGD_2$, $PGF_{2\alpha}$ |
| Increased vascular permeability | Histamine |
| | Bradykinin |
| | C3a and C5a (anaphylatoxins) |
| | Leukotriene $C_4$, $D_4$, $E_4$ |
| | PAF-acether |
| | Oxygen metabolites |
| Margination | $LTB_4$ |
| | C5a |
| Chemotaxis | $LTB_4$ |
| | C5a |
| | Bacterial products |
| | Neutrophil cationic proteins |
| | Lymphokines |
| Fever | Endogenous pyrogen—IL-1 |
| | $PGE_2$ |
| Pain | $PGE_2$ |
| | Bradykinin |

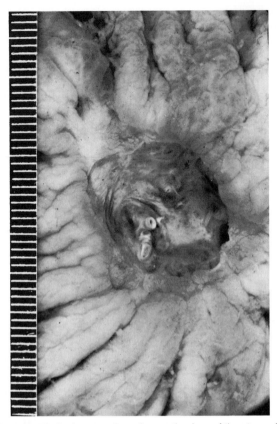

Figure 2–10. A close-up view of a peptic ulcer of the stomach. The crater is surrounded by the rugal folds of the gastric mucosa. An eroded artery, which caused the fatal hemorrhage, protrudes from the floor of the ulcer.

*months, leading to mononuclear cell infiltration and proliferation of fibroblasts.* The latter is a manifestation of repair which proceeds concomitantly. The accumulated white cells are chiefly macrophages and lymphocytes and sometimes plasma cells. Thus the leukocytic exudate in chronic inflammation is called mononuclear to distinguish it from the polymorphonuclear exudation of acute inflammation.

Chronic inflammation may arise in one of two ways. It may follow acute inflammation, or the response may be chronic almost from the onset. Acute to chronic transition occurs when the acute inflammatory response cannot be resolved, due either to the persistence of the injurious agent or to some interference in the normal process of healing. For example, bacterial infection of the lung may begin as a focus of acute inflammation (pneumonia), but its failure to resolve may lead to extensive tissue destruction and formation of a cavity in which the inflammation continues to smolder, leading eventually to a chronic lung abscess. An example of chronic inflammation with persisting acute inflammation is the peptic ulcer of the duodenum or stomach. *An ulcer is a local excavation of the surface of an organ or tissue resulting from the sloughing of inflammatory necrotic tissue* (Fig. 2–10). Peptic ulcers may persist for years. The base of the ulcer is often covered by a

layer of acute exudate composed of fibrin and enmeshed neutrophils. Deep to this layer large numbers of lymphocytes and macrophages, and some plasma cells, are found. Deeper yet there may be dense fibrosis indicative of the chronicity of the ulcer crater. Thus, in the same lesion we see an acute neutrophilic exudate as well as unmistakable evidence of chronic inflammation.

There are some settings in which chronic inflammation is initiated as a primary process. Often the injurious agents are of low toxicity in comparison with those leading to acute inflammation. Three major groups can be identified:

(1) *Persistent infections* by certain intracellular micro-organisms, such as tubercle bacilli, *Treponema pallidum* (causative organism of syphilis), and certain fungi. These organisms are of low toxicity and evoke an immunologic reaction called delayed hypersensitivity (p. 143). The inflammatory response often takes a specific pattern called a granulomatous reaction, which will be discussed later in this chapter.

(2) *Prolonged exposure to nondegradable inanimate material*; this includes silica particles, which after being inhaled for a prolonged period set up a chronic inflammatory response in the lungs called *silicosis* (p. 257). Silica may act as both a chemical and a mechanical irritant. On the other hand, large foreign bodies such as splinters and sutures may provoke chronic inflammation, mainly by physical or mechanical irritation. The response in these cases is aptly termed *foreign body reaction* and often includes *giant cells* formed by fusion of macrophages.

(3) Under certain conditions, immune reactions are set up against the individual's own tissues, leading to *autoimmune diseases* (see p. 148). In these diseases, autoantigens evoke a self-perpetuating immunologic reaction that results in several chronic inflammatory diseases, such as rheumatoid arthritis.

Some inflammations are difficult to categorize as either acute or chronic because there is no sharp line, either clinically or morphologically, that divides them. Arbitrarily it is said that when an inflammation lasts longer than 4 to 6 weeks, it is chronic. However, since much depends on the effectiveness of the host response and the nature of the injury, time limits are without meaning. The differentiation of acute from chronic inflammation can be best made on the basis of the morphologic pattern of the reaction.

### Chronic Inflammatory Cells

As mentioned earlier, chronic inflammation is characterized by the presence of mononuclear cells, which include macrophages, lymphocytes, and plasma cells (Fig. 2–11). Although repair often accompanies chronic inflammation, and fibroblasts and collagen are frequently intermingled with chronic inflammatory cells, the processes involved in repair will be discussed separately in a later section. We

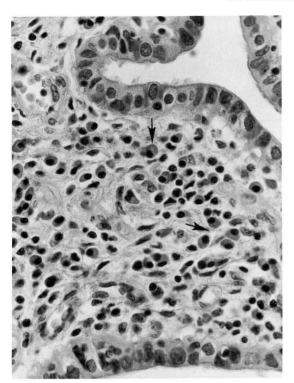

Figure 2–11. Chronic inflammation of the fallopian tube. The subepithelial connective tissue is infiltrated with mononuclear white cells, principally plasma cells marked by eccentric nuclei (see arrows).

will begin our discussion with a brief review of the biology of macrophages.

Traditionally macrophages have been considered scavengers, but they are now known to play several other important functions in inflammation and immunity.[17, 18] Tissue macrophages are but one component of the *mononuclear phagocyte system (MPS)*, previously known as reticuloendothelial system (RES). The MPS consists of closely related cells of bone marrow origin (whose members include blood monocytes) and tissue macrophages. The latter are diffusely scattered in the connective tissues or clustered in organs such as the liver (Kupffer cells), spleen and lymph nodes (sinus histiocytes), and lungs (alveolar macrophages). All arise from a common precursor in the bone marrow, which gives rise to blood monocytes. From the blood, monocytes migrate into various tissues and transform into macrophages. The half-life of blood monocytes is about one day, whereas the life span of tissue macrophages is several months. In addition to phagocytosis, already discussed, macrophages possess several other features that are important in their role as inflammatory cells. *Mononuclear phagocytes have the property of being "activated,"* a process that results in an increase in cell size, increased levels of lysosomal enzymes, more active metabolism, and most importantly greater ability to phagocytose and kill ingested microbes. Macrophage activation is a complex multistep process, occurring in response to external stimuli,

that must be presented in an orderly sequence.[19] Activation signals include lymphokines (such as γ-interferon) secreted by sensitized T lymphocytes, bacterial endotoxins, and contact with fibronectin-coated surfaces and a variety of chemicals, some of which are generated during acute inflammation. Following activation, the *macrophages secrete a wide variety of biologically active products*, many of which are intimately related to their role in inflammation and repair. Over 50 bioactive products of macrophages have been identified! These can be grouped into the following major categories (Table 2–2):

(a) *Enzymes*: both neutral and acid proteases. Several neutral proteases such as elastase and collagenase were previously mentioned as mediators of tissue damage in inflammation. Others, such as plasminogen activator, trigger the production of plasmin and greatly amplify the generation of pro-inflammatory substances (Fig. 2–7).

(b) *Plasma proteins*: these include complement proteins and coagulation proteins such as tissue factor and factors V, VII, IX, and X.

(c) *Reactive metabolites of oxygen.*

(d) *Lipid mediators* including products of AA metabolism and PAF-acether.

(e) *Factors regulating proliferation and functions of other cells*: these include *interferon*; *growth factors* for fibroblasts, endothelial cells, and primitive myeloid cells; and *interleukin-1*, a molecule with wide-ranging effects such as production of fever (endogenous pyrogen), activation of T and B lymphocytes, stimulation of collagenase production by fibroblasts, and secretion of acute phase reactants by the liver, to name a few.[20]

It should be noted that although this impressive arsenal of mediators, enzymes, and factors makes macrophages powerful allies in the body's defense against unwanted invaders, the very same weaponry can also induce considerable tissue damage when macrophages are inappropriately activated, as may occur in autoimmune diseases.

Returning to the presence of macrophages at sites

**Table 2–2.** PRODUCTS RELEASED BY MACROPHAGES

1. *Enzymes*
     Neutral proteases
       Elastase
       Collagenase
       Plasminogen activator
     Acid hydrolases
       Phosphatases
       Lipases
2. *Plasma proteins*
     Complement components (e.g., C1 to C5, properdin)
     Coagulation factors (e.g., factors V, VII, tissue factor)
3. *Reactive metabolites of oxygen*
4. *Lipid mediators of inflammation*
5. *Factors regulating function of other cells*
     Interferons, angiogenesis factors, and interleukin-1, for example

of chronic inflammation, it must be obvious that they are derived from blood monocytes that emigrate from the blood vessels under the influence of chemotactic factors. The steady release of lymphocyte-derived factors (p. 144) is an important mechanism by which macrophages continue to accumulate at the site of chronic inflammation. Once in the tissues, macrophages have the ability to survive for long periods, outliving neutrophils, which may have been the earliest cells to arrive. Macrophages also have a limited capacity to divide. Fusion of macrophages can lead to formation of large cells having multiple nuclei, called giant cells. Lymphocytes are also seen in most forms of chronic inflammation. As we shall discuss in Chapter 5, lymphocytes are involved in both cell-mediated and humoral immune responses. Many stimuli that evoke chronic inflammation, such as mycobacteria, are also antigenic and therefore capable of stimulating immune responses. It is easy to understand the presence of lymphocytes and antibody-secreting plasma cells in such cases. For reasons not entirely clear, lymphocytes can also be seen in apparently nonimmunologic chronic inflammations such as those induced by foreign bodies. It is very likely that in all inflammations there is release of cellular antigens which, in effect, provide an immunologic component to the response. Eosinophils, which are seen in some cases of chronic inflammation, are characteristic of inflammatory responses induced by parasites.

# MORPHOLOGIC PATTERNS OF ACUTE AND CHRONIC INFLAMMATION

The immediate response to all forms of injury is virtually stereotyped, as described earlier. However, within the first few days, several influences relating to the injurious agent begin to condition and modify the course and morphologic expression of the inflammatory response. These influences include the intensity of the injury, nature of the causative agent, and in some instances location of the inflammation.

Exudation and consequent edema or swelling is one of the characteristic features of the inflammatory response. It is virtually always present in the acute inflammatory reaction but may also persist into the chronic stages. In very mild injuries, it may be so slight as to escape detection. The nature and amount of exudate depend on the intensity of the injury and the specific injurious agent.

## Serous Inflammation

In general, mild injuries tend to evoke a protein-poor *serous inflammatory reaction*. An example of a serous reaction is the skin blister that follows a mild burn. In the course of a few days, the serous exudate is slowly resorbed and the inflammatory state subsides.

## Fibrinous Inflammation

With more severe injuries and the resulting greater vascular permeability, larger molecules pass the vascular barrier. A fibrinous inflammatory exudate develops when the vascular leaks are large enough to permit the passage of fibrinogen molecules. Acute rheumatic carditis classically evokes a fibrous pericarditis (Fig. 2–12). In the same way, ischemic necrosis of a portion of the myocardium (myocardial infarct) often causes a fibrinous pericarditis in the overlying epicardium. Histologically, fibrin appears as an eosinophilic meshwork of threads or sometimes as an amorphous coagulum (Fig. 2–13). Fibrinous exudates may be removed by fibrinolysis, followed by removal of other debris by macrophages. This process, called *resolution*, may restore normal tissue structure. However, when the fibrin is not removed, it may stimulate the ingrowth of fibroblasts and blood vessels and thus lead to scarring. Conversion of the fibrinous exudate to scar tissue (termed *organization*) within the pericardial sac will lead either to opaque fibrous thickening of the pericardium and epicardium in the area of exudation or, more often, to the development of fibrous strands that bridge the pericardial space. It is evident, then, that fibrinous exudation may have more serious consequences than serous exudation.

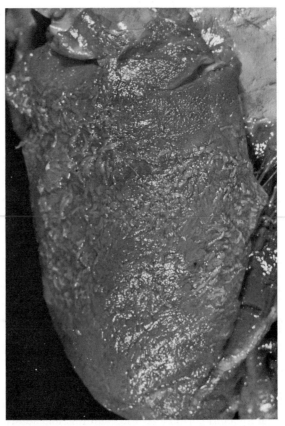

Figure 2–12. View of the epicardial surface of the heart, heavily layered with a shaggy fibrinous exudate—the so-called bread and butter pericarditis.

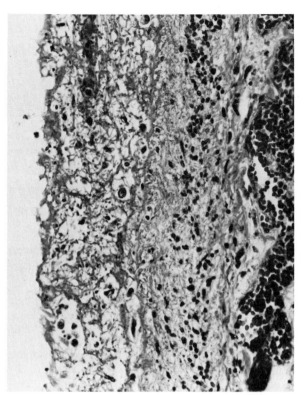

Figure 2–13. Fibrinous inflammation of the pleura. A meshwork of fibrin strands on the left is seen overlying the congested and inflamed pleura. (Courtesy of Dr. Charles L. White III, Department of Pathology, Southwestern Medical School, Dallas, TX.)

## Purulent or Suppurative Inflammation

This pattern is characterized by liquifactive necrosis associated with emigration of large numbers of neutrophils. Such an exudate, also called *pus*, is caused by certain bacteria, and is discussed next.

*Localized suppurative infections* are caused by a great variety of bacteria that are collectively referred to as pyogens (pus-producers). *Pus may be defined as an inflammatory exudate rich in proteins that contains viable leukocytes admixed with cell debris derived from necrotic native and immigrant white cells.* Included among the pyogens are staphylococci, many gram-negative bacilli (*E. coli, Klebsiella pneumoniae, Proteus* strains, and *Pseudomonas aeruginosa*), the meningococci, gonococci, and pneumococci. Infections with these agents induce local collections of pus at the site of implantation. Staphylococci are perhaps the most frequent cause of localized suppurative or pyogenic infections. When implanted beneath the skin or in a solid organ, the pyogens produce an *abcess*—a localized collection of pus. Pyogenic infections of the skin range from the simple hair follicle infection (*folliculitis*) to the *furuncle* (which involves suppuration of subcutaneous tissue, also called a "boil"), to the multiple deep-seated abscesses known as *carbuncles*. The gram-negative rods, on the other hand, are more often the cause of suppurative urinary tract infections, such as those that involve the urinary

bladder (*cystitis*) or the kidney (*pyelonephritis*). The favorite site of attack of the gonococcus is the genital tract (male or female), whereas the meningococcus implants on the oronasopharyngeal mucosa, whence it spreads to the meninges (*suppurative meningitis*). All the pyogens, wherever they become implanted, are capable of invading blood vessels to produce bacteremia, with the potential seeding of any or all of the other organs and tissues in the body. In this fashion, a neglected staphylococcal or gonococcal infection, for example, may give rise to bacterial implantation of the heart valves (*infective endocarditis*), or to meningitis or a brain abscess. In the course of progression of any infection, the regional lymph nodes or the entire lymphoid system of the body may become involved, as will be discussed more fully later.

A subgroup of suppurative infections is the *spreading suppurative infection* classically caused by the streptococci, particularly those of the beta-hemolytic Lancefield group A. Infections with these organisms tend to trek rapidly through large areas of tissue, such as an entire forearm, one side of the face, or even large tracts of the abdominal wall. Characteristic of such spreading infection is brawny edema and fiery red hyperemia of the inflammatory area known as *cellulitis* (also referred to as a *phlegmon*). Instead of producing focal abscesses filled with thick purulent exudate, the streptococci tend to evoke a watery suppurative reaction distributed throughout the cleavage planes and tissue spaces. This morphologic pattern reflects the bacterial elaboration of large amounts of hyaluronidases that break down polysaccharide ground substance, fibrinolysins that digest fibrin barriers, and lecithinases that destroy cell membranes. As might be anticipated, in this type of spreading infection, the lymphatics are particularly prone to secondary involvement (*lymphangitis*). In these infections one can sometimes observe subcutaneous red streaks extending proximally from areas of injury toward the regional lymph nodes. The regional nodes undergo striking inflammatory reactive hyperplasia, and too often the organisms invade the bloodstream, producing bacteremia. Sometimes a streptococcal infection remains fairly superficial and affects only the skin, superficial subcutaneous tissues, and skin lymphatics in a pattern known as *erysipelas*.

The other, less virulent Lancefield groups of streptococci tend to produce focal suppurative reactions in the pattern of the pyogens already mentioned. It should be noted that the immunologic reactions to the streptococcal infections may themselves be responsible for very serious poststreptococcal systemic diseases, such as rheumatic fever (p. 328) and glomerulonephritis (p. 468).

Some inflammatory reactions are characterized by mixed patterns of exudation—for example, *serofibrinous*. An injury may evoke a serous reaction at the outset, with subsequent transformation to the fibrinous pattern.

## Membranous (Pseudomembranous) Inflammation

This term is given to those inflammatory reactions on the surface of mucous membranes that are characterized by the formation of a superficial membranous layer of exudate containing the causative agents, precipitated fibrin, necrotic native cells, and inflammatory white cells. Membranous inflammation is most frequently encountered in the oropharynx, trachea, bronchi, and gastrointestinal tract. Diphtheria, now fortunately rare, is a classic example of membranous inflammation of the pharynx and respiratory passages. In diphtheria, the causative organism, *Corynebacterium diphtheriae*, establishes itself superficially on the surface of the mucous membranes of the pharyngeal region or the trachea and major bronchi. Here it causes necrosis and desquamation of the epithelium by its powerful exotoxin, and it also leads to the formation of a fibrin-rich inflammatory exudate. The necrotic mucosal cells and the fibrin meshwork with entrapped leukocytes constitute the gray-white membrane that is attached to the submucosal tissues. Should it become loosened and be inhaled, it may cause asphyxiation, particularly in young children. Diphtheritic infections, however, have other serious implications, resulting from the absorption into the bloodstream of the exotoxin elaborated by the organism, which often causes severe injury to the myocardial cells.

A much more common form of pseudomembranous inflammation is seen in the colon and sometimes the lower small intestines and is caused by *Clostridium difficile*. It is described on page 547, but briefly, *C. difficile* is a minor commensal in the gut that proliferates in those receiving broad-spectrum antibiotics destroying the competitive normal flora. The inflammation and necrosis of the bowel mucosa results from the action of an enterotoxin. Similar lesions can also be caused (although less frequently) by staphylococci, invasive shigellae, and *C. perfringens*. Whatever the causative agent, the common denominator is necrosis and inflammation of the mucosa caused by powerful exotoxins, leading to formation of a membrane-like structure, as described previously.

## Histiocytic Inflammatory Reactions

*Diffuse involvement of the mononuclear phagocyte system and focal histiocytic aggregations* are characteristics of the *Salmonella* infections. Within this group, typhoid fever, produced by *Salmonella typhi*, is most serious (p. 546). The other organisms tend to produce less threatening febrile illness, often with gastrointestinal manifestations. In these diseases, there is widespread involvement of the lymph nodes, as well as of the spleen and liver. In all sites, the macrophages are hypertrophied. These often undergo proliferation to produce focal aggregations of macrophages (histiocytes). In the gastrointestinal tract, typhoid fever induces hyperplasia and enlargement of

Peyer's patches, often with ulceration of the overlying mucosa. Diffuse involvement of the MPS is also caused by *Histoplasma capsulatum*, a common fungal infection in the midwestern United States.

## Interstitial and Perivascular Inflammations

Perivascular accumulations (cuffing) and interstitial infiltrations of mononuclear leukocytes are seen in viral, rickettsial, and syphilitic infections. Lymphocytes and macrophages—and, to a lesser extent, plasma cells—are involved principally. Rarely, in extremely acute viral infections, there may be a polymorphonuclear leukocytic reaction. Thus, the various viral agents that cause encephalitis (p. 730) tend to evoke mononuclear cuffing about the small vessels of the brain substance (Fig. 2–14). Poliomyelitis is similarly characterized by mononuclear interstitial and perivascular infiltrates. In addition, viral myocarditis is characterized by intercellular edema and infiltrations of mononuclear white cells (Fig. 2–15). The response to rickettsial infections is virtually the same except that there is often proliferation of the endothelial cells as well as a perivascular reaction. Actual parasitization of the endothelial cells by the rickettsial organisms appears to lead to the proliferative reaction in these cells. There is often necrosis and rupture of the walls of the small blood vessels as a result of this involvement. *Typhus fever*, for ex-

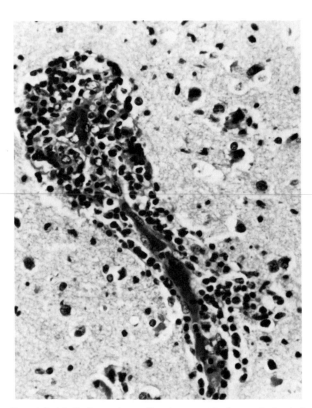

Figure 2–14. Perivascular cuffing by mononuclear cells in viral encephalitis. (Courtesy of Dr. Charles L. White III, Department of Pathology, Southwestern Medical School, Dallas, TX.)

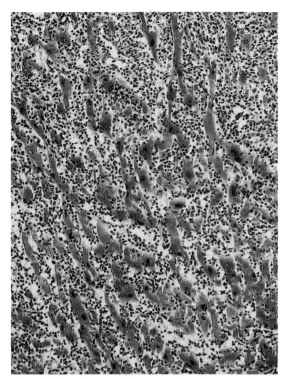

**Figure 2–15.** Viral myocarditis. The myocardial cells are widely separated by edema and an infiltration of mononuclear white cells.

ample, produces striking vascular and perivascular reactions in the brain and any other tissue affected. *Rocky Mountain spotted fever* causes a similar reaction, not only in the brain but also in the small vessels of the skin, hence the skin rash. Syphilis, too, induces perivascular cuffing, largely by plasma cells (p. 626).

We still do not understand such a predictable mononuclear infiltrate. Possibly immunologic mechanisms are involved, thus evoking immunologically competent cells, i.e., lymphocytes, plasma cells, and macrophages.

### Granulomatous Inflammation

This is a distinctive morphologic pattern of inflammatory reaction encountered in relatively few diseases. Tuberculosis is the archetype of the granulomatous diseases, but sarcoidosis, cat-scratch disease, lymphogranuloma inguinale, leprosy, brucellosis, syphilis, some of the mycotic infections, berylliosis, and reactions to irritant lipids are also included. Recognition of the granulomatous pattern in a lymph node biopsy, for example, is of great importance because of the limited number of possible conditions causing it, some of which are extremely threatening. *A granuloma consists of a microscopic aggregation of histiocytes (macrophages) that have been transformed into epithelial-like cells and are therefore designated epithelioid cells, surrounded by a collar of mononuclear leukocytes, principally lym-*

*phocytes and occasionally plasma cells* (Fig. 2–16). In the usual hematoxylin and eosin preparations the epithelioid cells have a pale pink granular cytoplasm with indistinct cell boundaries, often appearing to merge into one another. The nucleus is less dense than that of a lymphocyte (vesicular), is oval or elongated, and may show folding of the nuclear membrane.

Older granulomas develop an enclosing rim of fibroblasts and connective tissue. Frequently, but not invariably, *large giant cells* are found in the periphery or sometimes in the center of granulomas. These giant cells may achieve diameters of 40 to 50 μm. They comprise a large mass of cytoplasm containing numerous (20 or more) small nuclei. Two types of giant cells are encountered. The *Langhans type* is said to be characteristic of tuberculosis but in reality may be found in any of the granulomatous reactions. The nuclei in this form tend to be arranged about the periphery of the cell, sometimes encircling the cytoplasm and at other times producing horseshoe patterns. The individual nuclei are quite small and have a diameter that is only a very small fraction of the diameter of the entire cell. *The foreign body–type giant cell* differs in that the numerous nuclei are scattered throughout the cytoplasm in no distinctive pattern. Both forms of giant cells are believed to arise from fusion of macrophages. Although some observers rely heavily on the finding of giant cells, *the identification of a granulomatous reaction actually rests on the recognition of epithelioid cells.*

The formation of granulomas in most instances is a reflection of the buildup of cell-mediated immunity (delayed hypersensitivity, p. 143) to the causative agent. Specifically sensitized T lymphocytes liberate several soluble factors (lymphokines), some of which attract, immobilize, and activate more macrophages. Simultaneously, the macrophages undergo epithelioid cell transformation (Fig. 2–16). The exact mechanism of transformation is not clear. We do know

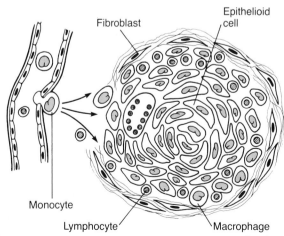

**Figure 2–16.** A schematic illustration of a granuloma. The large cell with multiple nuclei is a giant cell.

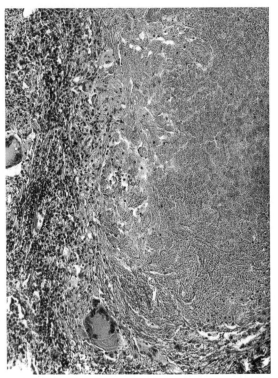

Figure 2–17. Caseous necrosis (upper right) in a tuberculous granuloma (a caseating tubercle). In the necrotic focus, all cell detail is obliterated by granular debris. The enclosing wall contains several large multinucleate giant cells of the Langhans type, with peripheral orientation of the nuclei.

that epithelioid cells are poorly phagocytic, and under the electron microscope they show prominent endoplasmic reticulum, vacuoles, and Golgi apparatus. These morphologic features suggest that epithelioid cells represent a stage of macrophage differentiation with predominantly secretory functions.

Although all the disorders previously mentioned are characterized by granuloma formation, certain variations in the granulomatous pattern are encountered among the various diseases. *The granuloma of tuberculosis classically has central caseous necrosis, as is discussed in greater detail on page 439* (Fig. 2–17). The fusion of many caseating granulomas may give rise to extensive macroscopic lesions of caseous necrosis involving large areas of the lung. The same caseating lesion is produced in all tissues affected. In contrast, *sarcoidosis almost never produces central necrosis, and so the sarcoid granuloma is often called a "hard tubercle,"* whereas the tuberculous granuloma is often referred to as a "soft tubercle." Syphilis produces gummatous necrosis in the center of its granuloma. Gummatous necrosis tends to have a rubbery consistency, firmer than the soft, cheesy texture of the tuberculous reaction. Berylliosis may cause central necrosis, but classically polymorphonuclear leukocytes are present in the necrotic center, a distinctly unusual finding in tuberculosis. Some of the differential features are outlined in Table 2–3.

# ROLE OF LYMPHATICS, LYMPHOID TISSUE, AND MONONUCLEAR-PHAGOCYTE SYSTEM

Lymphatics are almost as omnipresent as capillaries. In tissues terminal lymphatics are blind-ending, thin-walled tubes. All are lined with continuous epithelium having loose cell junctions and basement membranes in the larger channels. One function of lymphatics is to drain the small amount of low-protein tissue fluid that is normally formed by ultrafiltration of the blood (p. 30). In an inflammatory response, there is increased regional lymphatic flow of a fluid having a higher than usual protein content and containing increased numbers of leukocytes. These vessels drain off the fluid and cellular exudate from the area of reaction. Regrettably, lymphatic drainage also provides channels for the dissemination of the injurious agent. Inflammatory involvement of lymphatic channels (*lymphangitis*) and the regional filtering lymph nodes (*reactive lymphadenitis*) may develop. Reactive lymphadenitis is associated with a variety of changes, prominent among which are enlargements of the lymphoid follicles and increases in the number of histiocytes lining the sinuses. Often there is phagocytosis of cell debris by the phagocytic cells of the sinuses and follicles. Occasionally polymorphonuclear cells and particulate debris can be identified in the sinuses. If significant numbers of viable bacteria drain to the node, they may set up secondary sites of necrosis, which leads to the destruction of the lymph node and accumulation of exudate in these sites.

*Nevertheless, the regional lymph nodes constitute important secondary lines of defense, which, in general, tend to screen off the infection from the remainder of the body.* As would be expected, if these secondary lines of defense are overwhelmed, the inflammatory reaction may extend through the body. This dissemination is encountered only in severe inflammatory reactions and usually implies drainage of the infection through the blood as well as through the entire lymphatic system. With microbiologic infections that involve the bloodstream, cells of MPS, particularly Kupffer cells of the liver and splenic macrophages, constitute the main line of defense. When infections become generalized, tender lymphadenopathy appears, accompanied by hepatomegaly and splenomegaly. For this reason, the astute clinician always palpates for enlargement of the lymph nodes, liver, and spleen in febrile patients suspected of having a disseminated microbiologic infection.

# CLINICAL MANIFESTATIONS OF ACUTE AND CHRONIC INFLAMMATION

From what has already been said, and indeed as everyone knows from personal experience, inflam-

**Table 2–3.** MAJOR GRANULOMATOUS INFLAMMATIONS*

| Disease | Cause | Tissue Reaction |
| --- | --- | --- |
| Tuberculosis | *Mycobacterium tuberculosis* | Noncaseating tubercle (*granuloma prototype*): A focus of epithelioid cells, rimmed by fibroblasts, lymphocytes, histiocytes, occasional Langhans' giant cell. Caseating tubercle: Central amorphous granular debris, loss of all cellular detail. |
| Sarcoidosis | Unknown | Noncaseating granuloma: Giant cell (Langhans' and foreign body types); asteroids in giant cells; occasional Schaumann's body (concentric calcific concretion). |
| Certain fungal infections | | Granuloma usually larger than single tubercle with central granular debris; often contains causal organism and recognizable neutrophils. |
| | *Histoplasma capsulatum* | Organism is yeast-like, round to oval, budding, 2 to 4 μm; usually intracellular. |
| | *Cryptococcus neoformans* | Organism is yeast-like, sometimes budding; 5 to10 μm; large, clear capsule. |
| | *Blastomyces dermatitidis* | Organism is yeast-like, budding; 5 to 15 μm; thick, doubly refractile capsule. |
| | *Coccidioides immitis* | Organism appears as spherical (30–80 μm) cyst containing endospores of 3 to 5 μm each. |
| Syphilis | *Treponema pallidum* | Gumma: Microscopic to grossly visible lesion, enclosing wall of histiocytes, fibroblasts, and lymphocytes; plasma cell infiltrate; center cells are necrotic without loss of cellular outline. |
| Cat-scratch disease | Unknown | Rounded or stellate granuloma containing central granular debris and recognizable neutrophils; giant cells uncommon. |
| Berylliosis (chronic) | Beryllium | Fibrosing granuloma resembling noncaseating lesions of sarcoidosis. Asteroids and Schaumann's bodies may be present. |
| Lymphogranuloma inguinale (venereum) | Chlamydiae | Granulomatous enclosing rim composed mostly of macrophages and reticuloendothelial cells about a microabscess containing viable and necrotic neutrophils. |

*Modified from Robbins, S. L., Cotran, R. S., and Kumar, V.: Pathologic Basis of Disease. 3rd ed. Philadelphia, W. B. Saunders Co., 1984, p.65.

mations are painful and cause other local manifestations. Some (streptococcal tonsillitis is a good example) also evoke systemic signs and symptoms, such as fever, malaise, and loss of appetite. It is our purpose here to correlate the inflammatory changes already described with the resultant clinical findings.

The local manifestations of acute inflammation and active chronic inflammation have long been known as the *cardinal signs of inflammation—i.e., rubor (redness), calor (heat), tumor (swelling), dolor (pain) and functio laesa (loss of function)*. The pathophysiology of some of these cardinal signs is readily evident. The local heat and redness result from the increased blood flow in the microcirculation at the site of injury. The swelling is obviously the consequence of exudation, with its increase of interstitial fluid. Pain is less easily explained. It has been attributed simplistically to pressure on nerve endings resulting from exudation. Although this explanation may be valid, there is reason to believe that chemical mediators such as bradykinin and prostaglandins are also involved. The loss of function may be explained on mechanistic grounds. A painful infection in or

about the elbow joint might lead to voluntary immobilization of the joint; but such an explanation would hardly suffice for the loss of liver function seen in diffuse hepatitis. Conceivably, the hyperemia of inflammation raises the temperature in the microenvironment of the cells, impairing enzyme function; or the increased metabolic activity of an inflammatory focus might lower the pH and interfere with function in that way. These suggestions are, however, hypothetical. We simply do not understand functio laesa.

*The cardinal signs classically are evoked by all significant acute inflammations.* They may also be present with active chronic inflammations, those in which cellular necrosis is still present in the chronic inflammatory focus. As the flame of the inflammatory focus burns out, the cardinal signs fade and disappear. First the redness and local heat abate, then the pain, but the swelling and loss of function may persist for some time, even in those chronic inflammatory responses that smolder for months. Eventually all the cardinal signs disappear, leaving perhaps only some induration (increased consistency) as a sign of the proliferative fibroplasia of chronic inflammation.

Systemic manifestations, all too familar to anyone who has suffered from a severe sore throat or a respiratory infection, may be evoked by acute or chronic inflammation. *Fever* is one of the most prominent systemic manifestations, particularly in inflammatory states associated with spread of organisms into the bloodstream. Bacteremia usually induces a high fever (102° to 104° F) characterized by dramatic swings in temperature producing so-called spikes on the temperature chart. Usually these patients have violent shaking chills, which may indeed rattle the bed. The origin of fever is uncertain. Although it may in part be caused by release of bacterial endotoxins, in addition interleukin-1 (IL-1), previously described as endogenous pyrogen released from leukocytes, is an important mediator of hyperpyrexia. It is believed that IL-1 initiates fever by inducing the synthesis of $PGE_2$ in the anterior hypothalamus. Antipyretic agents such as aspirin reduce fever by suppressing the synthesis of $PGE_2$ without affecting IL-1 production.[20]

*Leukocytosis (increase in the number of circulating white cells) is another characteristic of significant acute and chronic inflammations.* In acute appendicitis, for example, the white cell count may rise to 25,000 leukocytes (mostly neutrophils) per $mm^3$ of blood. Indeed, some inflammatory states evoke extreme elevations of the white count to levels above 50,000 per $mm^3$ of blood. Such extreme elevations are sometimes called *leukemoid reactions* because they approach the white cell count encountered in leukemia. Granulocytosis results from both an increase in the release of neutrophils from the postmitotic pool in the bone marrow and increased for-

mation of neutrophils.[21] During inflammation macrophages and activated T cells secrete colony-stimulating factor, which promotes differentiation of granulocytes from their precursors in the bone marrow. With increased granulocytopoiesis some immature neutrophils escape from the marrow into the circulation. The appearance of many "juvenile" forms of neutrophils in the peripheral blood smear is described as "shift to the left."

Not all inflammatory states evoke a neutrophilic leukocytosis. Infectious mononucleosis, whooping cough, mumps, rubella, and undulant fever characteristically produce a lymphocytosis instead. Allergic inflammatory reactions (hay fever, bronchial asthma, and systemic angiitides) and parasitic infections typically elicit an eosinophilia. Moreover, the white cell count in the circulating blood actually drops in certain inflammatory states. Infections caused by viruses, rickettsiae and protozoa, and the salmonelloses, as well as overwhelming bacterial infections, may be marked by leukopenia rather than leukocytosis.

A number of other ill-defined and inconstant systemic manifestations may appear in patients with febrile inflammatory states—e.g., headache, listlessness, malaise, loss of appetite, and general disability. One would suspect the formation of humoral substances as the underlying basis for these nonspecific complaints, but none has been identified. Despite our lack of understanding of their origins, malaise, debility, and the other manifestations of general ill health are clinically significant, since they are responsible for much of the suffering of the patient with inflammatory disease.

# Repair

In the inflammatory-reparative reaction, repair begins soon after the injury, while the acute inflammatory reaction is still in full swing. But it cannot be completed until the injurious agent has been destroyed or neutralized. *Repair consists of the replacement of dead cells by viable cells.* These new cells may be derived either from the parenchyma or from the connective tissue stroma of the injured tissue. It is hardly necessary to point out that in the evolutionary process mammals lost the capacity to regenerate total structures, such as a limb, as many of the simpler aquatic and amphibious animals can. Indeed, the regenerative capacity of humans is quite limited. Only some of their cells are capable of regeneration and then only under specific conditions. Repair of destroyed cells therefore usually involves some connective tissue proliferation with the formation of a fibrous scar. Although the anatomic continuity of the tissue may be restored thereby, such repair is obviously imperfect, since it replaces functioning parenchymal cells with nonspecialized connective tissue.

Scarring thus diminishes the reserve of the organ or tissue involved.

Morphologic descriptions of parenchymal regeneration will be presented first, then connective tissue scarring will be described, followed by a discussion of our present understanding of the mechanisms and forces that govern repair.

## PARENCHYMAL REGENERATION

Replacement of destroyed parenchymal cells by proliferation of reserve cells can occur only in those tissues in which the cells retain the capacity to replicate. Other factors also influence the regenerative process, but let us first consider the ability of cells to divide. *The cells of the body have been divided into three groups, based on their regenerative capacity: labile, stable, and permanent.* The first two groups are able to proliferate throughout life, whereas permanent cells cannot reproduce themselves. Obviously, injury that destroys permanent cells can never be repaired by proliferation of the preserved parenchymal elements.

*Labile cells* continue to multiply throughout life to replace those shed or destroyed by normal physiologic processes. These include the cells of all epithelial surfaces, as well as lymphoid and hematopoietic cells. Included among the epithelial surfaces are the epidermis; the linings of the oral cavity, gastrointestinal tract, respiratory tract, and the male and female genital tracts; and the linings of ducts. In all these sites the surface cells exfoliate throughout life and are replaced by continued proliferation of reserve elements. Indeed, the lining of the small intestine is totally replaced every few days; the regenerative capacity of such cells obviously is enormous. The cells of the bone marrow and the lymphoid structures, including the spleen, are also labile cells. In these tissues, there is constant replacement of cells that have a life span ranging from a few days to possibly years.

*Stable cells* retain the latent capacity to regenerate, but under normal circumstances do not actively replicate because they have a survival time measured in terms of years and possibly equal to the life of the organism. The parenchymal cells of all glands in the body, including the liver, pancreas, salivary and endocrine glands, kidney tubular cells, and glands of the skin, are stable cells. For example, mitotic figures are rare to the point of being virtually nonexistent in normal adult liver, yet the liver has the capacity to regenerate large excised portions. It is possible to remove 80% of the liver in an experimental animal and find, in about a week, a liver of essentially normal weight. Humans too have a remarkable capacity to regenerate excised liver, as has been documented in patients who have had hepatectomies for primary liver cell cancer.

The mesenchymal cells of the body and their derivatives also fall into the category of stable cells. It is well known that fibroblasts and the more primitive mesenchymal cells retain great regenerative capacity. Moreover, many of these mesenchymal cells have the further ability to differentiate along a number of lines, thus making possible the replacement of specialized mesenchymal elements. Injuries involving bone are often accompanied by differentiation of mesenchymal cells into chondroblasts or osteoblasts. In adipose tissue, these same mesenchymal cells may become repositories for the storage of lipids and in this way be transformed into fat cells.

Endothelial and smooth muscle cells are also stable cells. Adult vascular endothelium has a low rate of turnover. However, endothelial cell injury such as that caused by trauma is followed by regeneration. Smooth muscle cell replication can be seen under hormonal influences—for example, in the myometrium and also following vascular injury in large blood vessels.

*Permanent cells* comprise neurons and skeletal and cardiac muscle cells. Destruction of a neuron, whether it is in the central nervous system or in one of the ganglia, represents a permanent loss. However, this statement does not refer to the ability of the nerve cell to replace its severed axon process. If the cell body of the neuron is not destroyed, the cell may regrow any of its extended processes. New axons grow at the rate of three to four millimeters per day, but in such regrowth, they must follow the preexisting pathway of the degenerating axon, or the regrowth becomes tangled and disoriented and, therefore, nonfunctional. The disoriented growing axon process may give rise to a mass of tangled fibers, sometimes termed an *amputation* or *traumatic neuroma*. It is for this reason that coaptation of severed nerves is of importance in surgical repair; it provides an appropriate "road map" for the regenerating axon fibers. With regard to the striated muscles, there is some evidence that cardiac and skeletal muscle cells can regenerate.[22] However, if such a capacity exists, it is of little significance in repair, since loss of muscle is always replaced by scar tissue. Scarring almost inevitably follows myocardial infarction, and one does not encounter in the margins of the infarct replicative activity in the still vital myocardial cells (Fig. 2–18).

*The perfection of parenchymal repair of an injury depends on more than the ability of cells to regenerate. Preservation of the stromal architecture or framework of the injured tissue is also necessary.* In injury to the liver, for example, if the supporting reticular framework is preserved, there is orderly regeneration of liver cells and the normal lobular

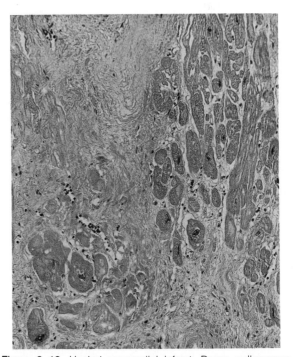

**Figure 2–18.** Healed myocardial infarct. Dense collagenous scar has replaced most of the myocardial fibers in the area of ischemic necrosis.

architecture and function are restored. Such is the case in mild viral hepatitis; however, in severe hepatitis (acute massive necrosis of the liver) there is massive liver cell injury accompanied by collapse or destruction of the stromal elements. If the individual survives, regeneration of the liver is disorderly and may lead to scar formation. Functional recovery is not perfect in such instances. Similarly, if the kidney is exposed to a toxic agent that destroys renal tubular cells but does not affect the tubular basement membranes or the underlying stroma, regeneration of tubular cells may completely restore normal structure and function. If, on the other hand, the stromal framework of the tubules is lost, as with a renal infarct, perfect reconstruction is not possible, and scarring ensues. Thus the perfection of repair depends to a considerable extent on the survival of the basic framework of the tissue. When this is lost, regeneration may restore mass but not complete function.

## REPAIR BY CONNECTIVE TISSUE

*Proliferation of fibroblasts and capillary buds and the subsequent laying down of collagen to produce a scar is the usual consequence of most tissue damage.* The only exceptions have already been cited. Connective tissue scarring is a ubiquitous and efficient method of repair but, as has been indicated, it necessitates a loss of specialized parenchymal function (Fig. 2–19). *Connective tissue repair is traditionally considered as either primary union (e.g., that which takes place when surgical wound margins are nicely coapted by sutures) or secondary union (e.g., that which occurs when the loss of tissue prevents such coaptation).* In the former instance, there is little or no loss of substance; exudate and necrotic debris are minimal and the repair occurs quite promptly. When there has been a significant loss of tissue, as in an open wound, and there is a considerable amount of exudate or necrotic debris to be removed, the healing takes place more slowly. In either case the tissue defect, large or small, is initially filled up with highly vascularized connective tissue called *granulation tissue*. The term "granulation tissue" (not to be confused with granulomatous inflammation, p. 47), is derived from its gross appearance, which is pink, soft, and granular. *Microscopically, it consists of newly formed small blood vessels embedded in loose (edematous) ground substance containing fibroblasts and inflammatory cells* (Fig. 2–20). Formation of granulation tissue begins early in the process of healing. It may be recalled that macrophages begin to accumulate at sites of inflammation within 48 hours and start scavenging the dead tissue, including dead and dying neutrophils. Although macrophages form the major leukocytic component of granulation tissue, there is a varying admixture of other inflammatory cells including lymphocytes, eo-

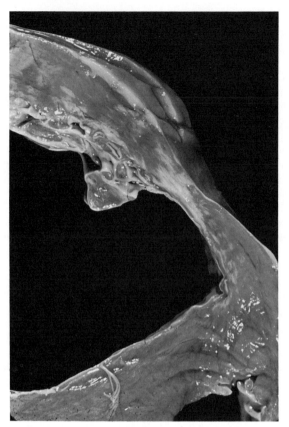

Figure 2–19. The pale areas within the thinned-out cross section of the heart are fibrous scar resulting from the replacement of myocardial fibers by scar tissue.

sinophils, mast cells, and some persisting neutrophils. Capillaries enter the area by budding from the undamaged blood vessels at the edges of the wound. It is noteworthy that macrophages secrete factors that promote neovascularization (angiogenesis). Initially the capillary buds are solid nubbins of endothelial cells that rapidly develop a lumen, into which blood flows. The newly formed blood vessels are leaky, allowing seepage of proteins and leukocytes into extravascular space. Therefore, young granulation tissue is edematous and soft. Presumably the leakiness of capillaries allows escape of nutrients to fibroblasts which must gear up to produce ground substance and collagen. Fibroblasts, like capillaries, migrate into the wound bed under the influence of chemotactic factors (to be described later). In newly formed granulation tissue the normal "skinny" spindle-shaped fibroblasts become plump, acquire increased amounts of rough endoplasmic reticulum, and can be mistaken for macrophages on cursory examination. As granulation tissue matures, inflammatory cells decrease in number, fibroblasts lay down collagen, and the capillaries become much less prominent. What emerges is an avascular, relatively acellular scar, with inactive spindle-shaped fibroblasts tucked in between collagen fibers. With this back-

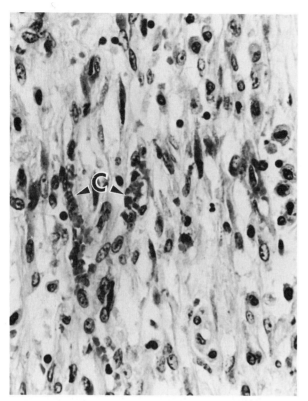

Figure 2–20. Granulation tissue containing spindle-shaped fibroblasts, mononuclear inflammatory cells, and capillaries (C) embedded in loose ground substance. (Courtesy of Dr. Charles L. White III, Department of Pathology, Southwestern Medical School, Dallas, TX.)

ground on the formation of granulation tissue we can now discuss the two forms of repair.

### Healing by Primary Union ("First Intention Healing")

Within the *first postoperative day* after the wound has been coapted by sutures, the line of incision promptly fills with blood clots. The surface of this clot dries, creating a crust or scab that seals the wound. The usual acute inflammatory reaction ensues in the margins of the wound, and a significant polymorphonuclear infiltrate is present.

During the *second day*, two separate activities begin concurrently: reepithelialization of the surface and fibrous bridging of the subepithelial cleft. Both depend heavily on the fibrin mesh-work in the blood clot, since it provides a structural scaffold along which the epithelial cells, fibroblasts, and capillary buds migrate. Small tongue-like processes of cells protrude beneath the surface crust, toward the midline from the epithelial margins. Within 48 hours these spurs connect to complete the epithelial covering of the wound. At first, the surface epithelium is only a single layer of cells in the midportion of the incision. Soon thereafter, progressive proliferation gives rise to the many-layered differentiated squamous epithe-

lium characteristic of the normal epidermis. Damaged hair follicles, sweat glands, and sebaceous glands may similarly regenerate. However, adnexal structures that have been totally destroyed cannot be replaced. During the second day, the fibroblasts at the margin of the incision hypertrophy and develop increased basophilia of their cytoplasm.

By the *third postoperative day* the acute inflammatory response begins to subside, and the neutrophils are largely replaced by macrophages, which débride the wound margins of destroyed cells as well as bits and pieces of fibrin.

By *day five* the incisional space is usually filled with a highly vascularized, loose granulation tissue. Scattered collagen fibrils may now be present.

By the *end of the first week*, then, the wound is covered with an epidermis of approximately normal thickness, and the subepithelial cleft is bridged by a vascularized connective tissue beginning to lay down collagen fibrils.

During the *second week* there is continued proliferation of fibroblasts and vessels and the progressive accumulation of collagen. By now the fibrin scaffold has entirely disappeared. The scar is still bright red owing to the increased vascularization and, as will be seen (p. 56), it has not yet attained significant tensile strength. Indeed, most of the tensile strength of a recent wound is attributable to the coapting surgical sutures and to the epithelial bridge. However, the inflammatory reaction has now almost completely abated, leaving only a few scattered macrophages and perhaps a sparse infiltrate of lymphocytes.

By the end of the second week the basic structure of the scar is already established and a long process (which will achieve blanching of the scar by compression of the vascular channels, accumulation of collagen, and steady increase in the tensile strength of the wound) is under way. As will be discussed later, however, even well-healed surgical scars may never regain the tensile strength, extensibility, and elasticity of normal, unwounded skin.[23]

### Healing by Secondary Union ("Second Intention Healing")

This is a more prolonged process because of the need to remove all dead tissue and necrotic debris and to fill in the tissue defect with vital cells. The base and margins of the defect are first layered with granulation tissue. Fibroblastic proliferation and capillary budding begin while the acute and sometimes chronic inflammatory reaction is still active in the center of the wound. As the leukocytes remove the exudate and debris the wound "granulates" in from its margins. At the same time, in surface wounds the epithelial margins migrate and proliferate, but only insofar as the underlying granulation tissue provides a base upon which they may grow. To some extent, the advancing epithelial cells grow downward over the edges and indeed a small mass of buried epithelium may be found in the newly formed granulation tissue.

A second remarkable phenomenon—*wound contraction*—aids in the repair of large defects, at least those on the surface of the body. It has been shown that a defect of about 40 cm² in the skin of a rabbit becomes reduced over the course of six weeks to 5 to 10% of its original size, largely by contraction. Remarkably, *all wounds halve their size at about the same rate.* Similar contraction may occur in deep wounds, but it has been less well studied. The mechanism of wound contraction appears to involve contraction of fibroblasts within the granulation tissue.[24] Indeed, myofilaments have been identified within these cells, justifying their designation as *myofibroblasts.*[25] By shortening, these multipotential mesenchymal cells are able to reduce significantly the size of the defect that must be filled eventually by granulation tissue and covered with epithelium.

*In review, then, healing by second intention differs in important ways from healing by first intention. Invariably, large tissue defects have more necrotic cells and exudate that must be cleared. Ingrowth of granulation tissue plays a far more prominent role in second intention healing. Moreover, this granulation tissue almost always has a more intense suffusion of neutrophils and macrophages because of the stronger inflammatory reaction elicited by the larger lesion. And, finally, wound contraction occurs only when there are large defects, since there is no significant loss of tissue in wounds that heal by first intention. As a consequence of these features, healing by second intention almost invariably results in the production of more scar and greater loss of specialized function. Thus, in large skin wounds there may be permanent loss of skin appendages (hair, sweat, and sebaceous glands) in the scarred area. Obviously first intention healing proceeds to completion more rapidly than the more complicated healing by second intention.*

Two aberrations may occur in wound healing, whether the process is by first or second intention. The accumulation of excessive amounts of collagen may give rise to a protruding, tumorous scar known as a *keloid.* Keloid formation appears to be an individual predisposition and, for reasons unknown, this aberration is somewhat more common in blacks. We still do not know the mechanisms involved in keloid formation. The other deviation in wound healing is the formation of excessive amounts of granulation tissue, which protrudes above the level of the surrounding skin and in fact blocks reepithelialization. This has been called *exuberant granulation* or, with more literary fervor, *"proud flesh."* Excessive granulations must be removed by cautery or surgical excision to permit restoration of the continuity of the epithelium.

Although the focus of much of the preceding discussion has been repair of skin wounds, the same basic characteristics of repair apply to the healing of defects in other organs and tissues of the body. Thus, repair of an abscess in the lung or an infarct in the kidney pursues the same course as that of an open wound on the surface of the body. The necrotic tissue and inflammatory debris must be removed. Similarly, the cell loss must be replaced, to the extent possible, by marginal regeneration of parenchymal cells, followed by ingrowth of vascularized connective tissue which, over the course of months, becomes progressively more collagenous. Thus, as was emphasized earlier, healing of most wounds represents a combination of parenchymal regeneration and connective tissue scarring, although in the individual instance one phenomenon may be predominant.

## BONE REPAIR

Repair of a bone injury is essentially another instance of connective tissue healing. It differs from soft tissue repair insofar as formation of the specialized calcified tissue of bone involves the activity of osteoblasts and osteoclasts. Bone-forming cells are derived from the periosteum and endosteum in the area of injury or, possibly, from the metaplastic transformation of primitive mesenchymal cells or fibroblasts in the adjacent connective tissues. Repair of a bone may be so perfect that it cannot be visualized at a later date by x-rays or even histologic examination.

Repair of a fracture may be taken as a model of the processes of bone healing.[26] Bone, with its contained marrow, is a highly vascularized tissue. When fractured, there is considerable hemorrhage into the site. A clot fills the region between the two fractured ends, as well as any space created by tearing of adjacent tissues, such as the periosteum and endosteum. Formation of granulation tissue within the meshwork of blood clot ensues just as has been described in the healing of soft tissue. By the second or third day, rapidly proliferating chondroblasts and osteoblasts, looking very much like plump fibroblasts, appear in the areas proximate to the injured periosteum and endosteum.

Toward the end of the first week islands of cartilage appear in the granulation tissue that has replaced the clot. The combination of fibroblastic tissue and islands of cartilage forms a fairly firm but still yielding fusiform sleeve that bridges the fracture site. This bridging tissue is known as a *soft tissue* or *provisional callus (procallus).* By the end of the first week some calcium is deposited in the cartilaginous matrix, further hardening the provisional callus and splinting the fractured ends of the bone. About this time, the osteoblasts of periosteal and endosteal origin begin to lay down osteoid, the protein matrix of bone. Eventually the procallus becomes traversed by a maze of osteoid trabeculae laid down in a haphazard pattern. Progressive calcification of the osteoid trabeculae ensues. In this manner, the provisional callus is replaced ultimately by *bony callus*. The fracture is now rigidly united, but there is excess bone within the marrow space and encircling the external aspect of the fracture site. This stage of repair might be reached in four to six weeks, depending upon a number of conditions, which will be mentioned later in this chapter. The excess bone within the marrow space, as well as around the fracture, is slowly remodeled (i.e., resorbed by osteoclasts), while at the same time neo-osteogenesis and increased calcification within the normal bone contours further strengthen and reinforce the trabeculae. Stress—or more precisely, direction of thrust of weight bearing—appears to guide the pattern of remodeling. Ultimately, the marrow cavity is restored to its original dimensions, and the bone marrow regrows to its prefracture stage of development. Additional details of this remarkable reconstitution of original structure may be found in the excellent discussion by Ham and McCormack.[27]

*Many factors are important in this healing process in bone. Primary among them is adequate immobilization.* It should be apparent that if the fractured ends are not firmly immobilized, *hard* tissue, such as the calcified osteoid trabeculae, cannot be formed. Instead, collagenized fibrous tissue may replace the soft tissue callus, which will block all possibility of later bony repair. In the same way, interposition of nearby soft tissues between the fractured ends will likewise block the formation of the new bone bridge between the two fractured ends.

*If hemorrhage is excessive, a large provisional callus is formed, which requires more time to be replaced.* At the same time, the excess hemorrhage leads to the formation of a larger bony callus that must eventually be remodeled and removed.

*Infection of a fracture site is a serious complication.* Bacteria introduced into the fresh blood clot literally run amok. The infection not only causes secondary tissue damage but also inhibits callus formation.

*Proper reduction of the fracture greatly speeds repair.* Proper alignment reduces the distance between the fractured ends and permits rapid union. It is remarkable to observe at a much later date a fracture that could not be realigned—the repair may be slowed but, as long as other complications do not exist, it proceeds nonetheless. The bony union will in time be sufficiently strong to bear weight, and the remodeling may eventually create a straight shaft, although it may be shortened owing to the loss in length created by the initial bowing. Obviously, miracles do not happen, and if the malalignment is marked, deformity or nonunion may result. An additional consideration in bone repair is the metabolic environment. Involved here are an adequate blood supply, nutrition (particularly vitamin C and calcium), and normal levels of hormones (particularly estrogens), which appear to influence osteoblastic activity. Of these factors, the blood supply is most critical. A fracture that destroys the arterial supply, or multiple fractures that create devascularized bone fragments, greatly retard and sometimes block bone healing for months or years. Despite all these limiting qualifications, the repair of bone injury is one of the most remarkable demonstrations of the reparative capacity of the body.

## COLLAGENIZATION AND WOUND STRENGTH

Scarring is an inevitable consequence of all repair save for the ideal situation in which an entirely parenchymal injury permits perfect regeneration and reconstitution of the original architecture. Fibroblasts are the work horses of scar formation, and collagen is their essential product that ultimately provides the tensile strength in the healing of soft tissue wounds. Knowledge of collagen structure and its biosynthesis has advanced our understanding of wound healing as well as inherited disorders of collagen structure (p. 117). Here we will briefly survey the biology of collagen; details can be found in recent reviews.[28–30]

Collagen is the single most abundant protein in mammals. Recent advances into its detailed structure and synthesis indicate that collagen constitutes a family of genetically and structurally distinct molecules. Over eight different kinds of collagens having distinctive tissue distribution have been identified. Types I, II, and III are interstitial in location and have fibrillar structure, whereas type IV and V are amorphous (nonfibrillar) materials found in interstitial tissues and basement membranes (Table 2–4). Types VI, VII, and VIII are neither abundant, nor have they been fully characterized.[28]

The basic unit of collagen is the rod-shaped collagen molecule, 300 nm long and 1.5 nm in diameter. Each molecule is made up of three polypeptide chains (α-chains), each of which is coiled into a left-handed helix, and the three helical chains are twisted around each other into a right-handed supercoil (Fig. 2–21). Several genetically and biochemically distinct α chains have been recognized. Their nomenclature is somewhat confusing but can be understood by using the composition of type I collagen as an example. Type I collagen contains two types of chains—designated α1 and α2. To these abbreviations is added the type of collagen in parentheses, e.g., α1(I). Since there are two α1 chains and one α2 chain in type I

α 1
α 1
α 2

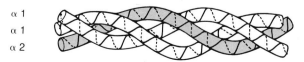

Figure 2–21. Schematic diagram showing the collagen triple helix. Note two α1 chains and one α2 chain characteristic of type I collagen.

**Table 2–4. TYPES OF COLLAGEN**

| Type | Molecular Formula | Characteristics |
|---|---|---|
| I | [α1 (I)$_2$α2] | Predominant structural collagen of the body; most abundant in skin, tendon, ligament, and cornea. Constitutes 80 to 85% of dermal and bone collagen. Chemically characterized by two types of α chains, both relatively low in hydroxylysine. |
| II | [α1 (II)]$_3$ | Found in cartilage, vitreous humor, and nucleus pulposus; not present in skin. Rich in hydroxylysine and heavily glycosylated. |
| III | [α1 (III)]$_3$ | Abundant in blood vessels and uterus; in skin it forms 10 to 20% of total collagen. Rich in hydroxyproline and contains interchain disulfide bonds. |
| IV | Unknown Contains α1 (IV) and α2 (IV) chains | Found in basement membranes. Very rich in hydroxylysine; almost fully glycosylated. |
| V | Unknown Contains α1 (V), α2 (V), and possibly α3 (V) | Found in basement membranes. Widespread in small amounts. Prominent in placenta. |

collagen, its molecular formula is [α1(I)$_2$α2]. The structure, tissue distribution, and some distinctive features of five collagen types are summarized in Table 2–4. It should be noted that as compared with other proteins, collagens contain large amounts of hydroxyproline and hydroxylysine, which serve important roles in the maintainance of the structure and strength of collagen. This will become apparent as we review the steps in collagen synthesis.

As with all other proteins, biosynthesis of collagen precursors occurs on ribosomes. The newly formed procollagen molecules undergo post-translational modifications in the cisternae of endoplasmic reticulum before being secreted by the Golgi apparatus. The posttranslational modifications include hydroxylation of the proline (representing about 10% of the amino acids in an α chain) and lysine residues. The hydroxylation reaction, which requires vitamin C as a cofactor, is followed by glycosylation of hydroxylysyl residues. Inter- and intrachain disulfide bonds are then introduced, which along with hydroxylation of lysine facilitate the formation of the triple helix. The helical procollagen molecule is still soluble, due to the presence of noncollagen sequences at the N- and C-terminals. Solubility allows the completed procollagen molecule to be transported to the Golgi apparatus for eventual secretion from the fibroblast. Once outside the cell, soluble procollagen is rapidly converted into insoluble collagen by enzymes (procolla-

gen peptidases) that cleave the N- and C-terminal noncollagen peptides. Collagen molecules then spontaneously aggregate into mature fibrils, which lack the tensile strength of mature collagen. *Oxidation of lysyl and hydroxylysyl residues by the extracellular copper-containing enzyme lysyl oxidase follows, leading to formation of cross-linkages. This last step is crucial to the development of structural stability in mature collagen.*

In addition to their role in collagen synthesis, the fibroblasts are also involved in the formation of other extracellular connective tissue components. These include elastic fibers and an amorphous sol-gel matrix containing various glycosaminoglycans (GAG), linked covalently to proteins (*proteoglycans*), and several glycoproteins such as *fibronectin*. This glycoprotein, which modulates cell-matrix interactions during healing, will be discussed in a later section. Here we will offer some brief comments about elastin, an important noncollagen intercellular fiber.[29] As is evident from the name, elastic fibers provide "elastic recoil," rather than structural strength. Thus their function is complimentary to that of collagen. Elastic fibers contain two protein components: *elastin*, which is amorphous, and *microfibrils*, which are fibrillar glycosylated polypeptides. Like collagen, elastin is rich in the amino acid lysine, which is involved in the formation of interchain cross-linkages, a process catalyzed by the enzyme lysyl oxidase. Thus genetic or acquired disorders that impair the formation of cross-linkages affect the structural stability as well as elasticity of the connective tissue, leading in some cases to disastrous consequences such as dissecting aneurysms of the aorta (p. 302)

With this overview of connective tissue synthesis and breakdown we can now examine the factors that affect the strength of a cutaneous wound such as an operative incision.

The acquisition of tensile strength follows a sigmoid curve.[31] The first phase has been described as the catabolic period, when there may actually be destruction of collagen. The second (anabolic, proliferative, or collagen) phase generally begins on day five. Thereafter there is a progressive increase in tensile strength up to day 100, during which 70 to 90% of the strength of unwounded skin is achieved. This is followed by a virtual plateau, which is maintained for years and perhaps for the life of the patient. When the plateau phase is more closely investigated, we find that the total collagen content of a wound stabilizes while collagen is still actively synthesized. Clearly, collagen is removed at the same time that more is added (collagen remodeling). This dynamic state is achieved by collagenases derived from inflammatory cells and fibroblasts, which break down mature collagen. Thus, lysis of collagen is an important controlling factor. Another interesting observation emerges from the study of the collagen content of wounds. Biochemical analysis reveals that the collagen content of wounds returns to normal levels far more rapidly than recovery of wound strength. Indeed, collagen content of the wound reaches normal levels by 60 to 70 days, at a time when the wound has recovered only 25 to 35% of its strength. Thus, strength in wounds is not simply a function of the amount of collagen. It is likely that the type of collagen formed and the extent of cross-linking also affect the strength of wound. In the adult skin 80 to 85% of the dermal collagen is type I, which has high tensile strength, whereas collagen deposited early in wound healing is of type III, which is the predominant form in embryonic skin. With passage of time there is a gradual shift in the ratio of types I and III to that more characteristic of adult skin. Concomitantly, there may be greater cross-linkage as well.

Since wounds require 100 days to regain 70 to 90% of the tensile strength of unwounded skin, how is it possible to discharge patients from the hospital within the first postoperative week? The answer lies in the art and skill of the surgeon and in the use of sutures. Carefully sutured wounds have approximately 70% of the strength of unwounded skin immediately following surgery.[32] If sutures are removed at the end of the first week, wound strength is only at approximately the five to 10% level![31] It should be amply evident now that the study of wound repair has wide-ranging ramifications, particularly for the postoperative patient.

# MECHANISMS INVOLVED IN REPAIR

Even the simple forms of repair, such as healing of surgical wounds, are finely orchestrated phenomena. Consider the numerous actors and their roles: epithelial cells must proliferate, migrate to cover the defect, and cease to divide once the gap is bridged. Underneath the epithelium, inflammatory cells accumulate, the sleepy fibroblasts are aroused and coaxed to migrate into the wound, where they secrete matrix components, and then revert to their "siesta" when the wound is healed. Surely the epithelium, endothelium, and fibroblasts must receive coordinated and sequential cues to perform their flawless acts. What are these signals? The answers are not clear and much research continues, since the understanding of growth control has implications extending into the realm of cancer biology, as we shall see. Here we will consider only three aspects of the wide array of regulatory factors that affect the healing of wounds: cell-cell interactions, cell-matrix interactions, and stimulatory hormones or growth factors.

## Cell-Cell Interactions

As mentioned earlier, reepithelization of surgical wounds begins within 24 hours of injury and the gap is usually covered by 48 hours. During regeneration of liver after partial hepatectomy, the liver cells burst into mitoses but cease to divide when normal liver substance is restored. What signals the cells to stop dividing? Answers to these questions have been sought by investigating the growth behavior of cells in vitro. When certain normal cells are lightly seeded in Petri dishes, they proliferate, migrate, and eventually form confluent monolayers. At this point cells cease to divide, a phenomenon called *contact inhibition*. It is proposed that cells are inhibited from proliferation by interchange of signals or substances at contact points. As will be discussed later (p. 198), growth of normal cells in tissue cultures is also regulated by cell density (*density-dependent inhibition*). Could it be that when normal cells reach confluence or acquire certain densities, there is a down-regulation of receptors for growth factors? Whatever the mechanisms, they must be important in vivo or else humans would be covered with tumors at sites of healing wounds!

## Cell-Matrix Interactions

Much evidence has accumulated to indicate that the orderly movement and proliferation of cells within a healing wound is influenced not only by signals derived from other cells but also from the extracellular matrix.[33, 34] The extracellular matrix is an organized complex of collagens, glycosaminoglycans, proteoglycans, and glycoproteins. Of these, much attention has focused on the *fibronectins*, which are a family of adhesive high-molecular-weight glycoproteins. Fibronectin is associated with cell surfaces, basement membranes, and pericellular matrices. It is produced by fibroblasts, endothelial cells, and monocytes, among others. An immunologically and structurally similar fibronectin is also found in the plasma. During wound healing fibronectin concentration in the wound bed is higher than in the adjacent tissue. It is believed that early in the process of healing, plasma fibronectin coats the fibrin scaffold within the clot (p. 53). Since fibronectin is highly adhesive, it facilitates the migration of epithelium and inflammatory cells along the fibrin meshwork. Not only does fibronectin provide anchorage to various cell types, it also participates actively in cellular influx. Intact fibronectin and its fragments are chemotactic for monocytes and, more importantly, for fibroblasts. Experimental evidence suggests that migration of endothelial cells and their organization into capillaries is also facilitated by fibronectin. In addition, it stimulates the release of fibroblast growth factors from monocytes. The fibroblasts that migrate into the wound themselves secrete large amounts of fibronectin and shortly thereafter type III collagen. In addition, other matrix components such as proteoglycans are codeposited with fibronectin. All these observations suggest that fibronectin plays a central role in the organization of granulation tissue. As wound healing progresses, the synthesis of fibronectin and type III collagen declines, and the fibroblasts turn to the secretion of type I collagen.

### Growth Factors

Thus far we have discussed the regeneration, migration, and organization of cells in the wound. But what triggers these cells to divide? Theoretically, one of two mechanisms may be involved: (1) loss of factors that normally inhibit cell division; (2) release of growth-stimulating factors. At one time, the concept that proliferation occurred because of reduced levels of growth inhibitory substances called *chalones* was popular. It was proposed that chalones were products of differentiated cells, and with loss of cells (as would occur in wounding) the local concentration of chalones might fall. This in turn would be expected to release cells from the antimitotic effect of the chalone. Although the chalone concept is still alive, it does not have many followers.

Much more interest and excitement surrounds the discovery of a variety of growth-stimulatory factors.[35-37] The list of growth factors is ever increasing. Some of the better characterized factors include epidermal growth factor (EGF), nerve growth factor (NGF), platelet-derived growth factor (PDGF), macrophage-derived growth factor (MDGF), and fibroblast growth factor (FGF). All of these are polypeptides with hormone-like structure. In tissue culture a variety of cell types have been shown to divide in response to these growth factors. Thus the targets of EGF action include not only several types of epithelial cells but also fibroblasts, glial cells, and kidney cells. The ability to respond to PDGF, however, seems to be limited to connective tissue cells such as fibroblasts and smooth muscle cells. MDGF acts on fibroblasts and endothelial cells. In all cases the responsive cells possess specific cell-surface receptors for the growth factors.

It is not difficult to visualize how these factors may be relevant in wound healing. Platelets are present quite early at the site of an injury, due to their involvement in hemostasis. PDGF is a growth factor for fibroblasts and also chemotactic for leukocytes. Influx and activation of macrophages would yield MDGF, which stimulates both angiogenesis and fibroplasia. Although most of the actions of growth factors have been investigated in vitro, it is very likely that they are also relevant in vivo. Furthermore, their role in vivo may not be restricted to wound healing but could also affect pathologic processes such as atherosclerosis (p. 293) and oncogenesis (p. 210).

*To summarize, repair is accomplished by proliferation of epithelial, parenchymal, and connective tissue cells under the influence of stimulatory hormones or growth factors. The proliferating cells migrate into the wound in an orderly fashion dictated by transmission of poorly defined signals between cells themselves and modulatory influences of the extracellular matrix. Unlike neoplastic proliferations, to be discussed later (p. 185), cell growth associated with repair is regulated, and it ceases when healing is completed.*

# OVERVIEW OF THE INFLAMMATORY-REPARATIVE RESPONSE

At this point, a backward look may help to interrelate the multitude of changes occurring simultaneously or sequentially in the inflammatory-reparative response. Figure 2–22 offers an overview of the possible pathways. This schema reemphasizes certain important concepts. Not all injuries result in permanent damage; some are resolved with almost perfect repair. More often, the injury and inflammatory response result in residual scarring. Although it is functionally imperfect, the scarring provides a permanent patch that permits the residual parenchyma more or less to continue functioning. Sometimes, however, the scar itself is so large or so situated that it may cause permanent dysfunction, as for example in a healed myocardial infarct. In this case, the fibrous tissue not only represents a loss of preexisting contractile muscle but also constitutes a permanent burden to the overworked residual muscle.

# FACTORS MODIFYING THE QUALITY AND ADEQUACY OF THE INFLAMMATORY-REPARATIVE RESPONSE

The quality and adequacy of the inflammatory reaction and reparative response are determined by factors relating to both the injurious agent and to the host. The outcome of an injury is determined by the balance achieved between the defensive, healing capability of the host and the destructive influence of the injurious agent. Much has already been said about the impact of the intensity, duration, and nature of the injury. Here we are primarily concerned with the host factors, which are equally important in this equation. Only the more important ones will be discussed, under the headings of systemic and local influences.

### Systemic Influences

At one time "prevailing wisdom" about the effects of *age* held that the elderly heal more slowly and less adequately than the young.[38] Yet there is little valid documentation of this view. In one study there was no difference between tensile strength values of the healing wounds of two age groups of rats, one young (eight months old) and the other old (20 months). However, the thickness of the scar was greater in the

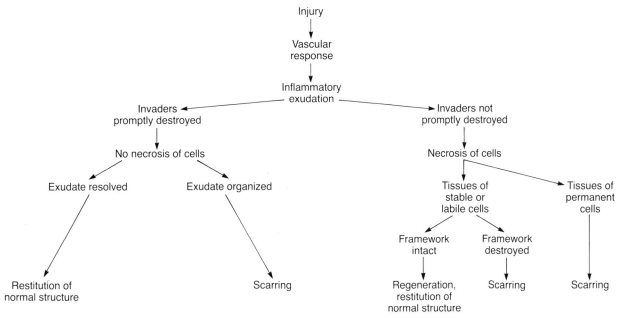

Injury
↓
Vascular response
↓
Inflammatory exudation

Invaders promptly destroyed ← Inflammatory exudation → Invaders not promptly destroyed

No necrosis of cells

Necrosis of cells

Exudate resolved     Exudate organized

Tissues of stable or labile cells     Tissues of permanent cells

Framework intact     Framework destroyed

Restitution of normal structure     Scarring

Regeneration, restitution of normal structure     Scarring     Scarring

Figure 2–22. Pathways of reparative response.

younger animals.[39] In another study no significant differences were found in the adequacy of repair among various age groups of rats. Thus there is little to support the view that age per se has any effect on wound healing. Co-existent atherosclerosis or malnutrition may, however, retard healing, as is discussed below.

The *nutrition* of the patient is of unchallenged importance. Both experimental and clinical observations indicate that severe protein depletion impairs wound healing. Although the protein-deficient patient can derive most of the tissue building blocks for wound repair by mobilization of body tissues, methionine and cystine may be in inadequate supply for the sulfation of the mucopolysaccharides that form the ground substance. Vitamin C plays an important role in collagen formation; it catalyzes the hydroxylation of lysine and proline by activation of inactive enzymes prolyl and lysyl hydroxylase. Deficiencies of ascorbic acid lead to defective collagen formation since hydroxylation is necessary for the formation of stable helical configuration. Underhydroxylated collagen undergoes increased intracellular degradation, and that which is secreted cannot form fibrils. Since cross-linkage also depends upon hydroxylation of lysine, any collagen formed is very fragile. In vitamin C deficiency, therefore, the rate of wound healing and the tensile strength of wounds is markedly impaired. Zinc may be another substance required for adequate wound healing. Zinc levels in tissues may fall after burns, and wound healing is delayed in patients with zinc deficiency. The importance of zinc lies in the fact that several enzymes required for DNA and RNA synthesis are zinc dependent.[40]

*Derangements in the blood* may have a profound effect on the inflammatory-reparative response. No one would deny that a deficiency of circulating granulocytes (granulocytopenia), or defects in leukocyte functions, predispose the patient to bacterial infections and render the leukocytic exudation inadequate to control bacterial invasion. The loss of neutrophils also impairs lysosomal proteolysis of dead cells and exudate, hampering repair. In bleeding disorders, excessive hemorrhage into the wound provides a rich substrate for the growth of itinerant bacteria. Moreover, the clot with its hemoglobin must be removed before repair can be completed.

*Diabetes mellitus* is a particularly important predisposing factor in microbiologic infections.[41] Diabetic patients tend to develop significant clinical infections more frequently than controls. They are particularly likely to develop tuberculosis, skin infections, infections of the urinary tract, and mycotic infections. It is not that these patients are more vulnerable to bacterial invasion but rather that they are less able to control the invasion once it is established. The nature of this susceptibility to infection is still incompletely understood. Diabetics are prone to develop generalized arterial disease and so may suffer from inadequate blood supply to the area of injury. Sometimes they are dehydrated and have serious electrolyte disturbances. Because the skin of a diabetic patient contains high levels of glucose, survival of implanted bacteria is favored. The neutrophils of diabetic patients have diminished chemotaxis and decreased phagocytic capacity and are inefficient in intracellular killing of bacteria.[42] All of these abnormalities hamper the inflammatory response and render the diabetic patient vulnerable to serious infections.

*Hormones,* particularly the adrenal steroids, have a depressant effect on the inflammatory and reparative reactions. Glucocorticosteroids have a variety of effects on the inflammatory response.[41] In experimental animals, high levels of cortisol prevent vasodilatation and increased vascular permeability of the acute inflammatory response. Corticosteroids also interfere with chemotaxis and adhesion of leukocytes to endothelium, leading therefore to greatly reduced leukocyte infiltration. Intracellular killing of tubercle bacilli by rabbit macrophages is impaired by cortisol treatment. Generation of prostaglandins and leukotrienes from stimulated phagocytic cells is decreased. The mechanism of action of steroids on the generation of lipid mediators is believed to involve inhibition of phospholipase $A_2$, which is the enzyme necessary for the synthesis of arachidonic acid (p. 39).

In the experimental animal pretreated with cortisol, fibroplasia is inhibited, new collagen formation is retarded, and neovascularization is slowed. Again, the mechanisms are not established. There is evidence that the steroids impair formation of the mucopolysaccharide ground substance so important in the formation of mature collagen. Thus steroids seem to suppress virtually every step of the inflammatory-reparative response.

It should be obvious, therefore, that it is unwise to administer glucocorticoids to patients with infections or wounds unless other disorders absolutely dictate the need for such treatment. On the other side of the coin, steroids are sometimes used to suppress inflammations associated with eye infections, chronic bursitis, or chronic inflammatory involvement of joints. In these cases, continued inflammation can lead to serious derangement in functions.

### Local Influences

*Adequacy of local blood supply* may well be the single most important influence in determining the quality and adequacy of the inflammatory-reparative response. Arterial disease, which reduces blood flow, and venous disorders, which retard drainage, seriously hamper the response to injury. For this reason, even a trivial injury to the toe in an aged individual with advanced atherosclerosis of the arteries in the lower leg may culminate weeks or months later in an amputation of the leg. Varicose veins of the leg result in hampered venous efflux, cause chronic edema of the lower leg, and restrict adequate arterial inflow. Secondarily infected ulcerations (well recognized by the designation "varicose ulcers") are common following injuries to the legs of these patients.

*Infection* of "clean wounds," whatever its cause, is a serious hindrance to repair. The more intense inflammatory reaction and copious exudation tend to separate tissue edges, build up pressure within the inflammatory site, and contribute to destruction of both native and immigrant white cells, thus enlarging the initial tissue injury. Healing by first intention may perforce be transformed into healing by second intention, with its more protracted course.

*Foreign bodies* are fairly obvious stimuli to inflammation and impediments to healing. Indeed, they must be removed by enzymic action (if they are biodegradable), by sequestration within multinucleate giant cells, or by extrusion from the wound, either spontaneously or with the aid of surgery. Repair cannot be completed until one of these resolutions has been achieved. It must be remembered that sutures represent foreign bodies. Meticulous coaptation of wound margins permits primary union and not only reduces the amount of inflammation but also greatly facilitates and speeds repair. On the other hand, as we have seen, sutures constitute stimuli to inflammation and, when on the skin surface, invite bacterial contamination of the suture tracts. The use of just enough and not too many sutures is not only a surgical science but also an art.

*Immobilization of wounds* is of primary importance in fractures. It may also be beneficial in large soft tissue injuries in which movement may induce secondary hemorrhages and dislocation of tissue approximation.

*Location of the injury* may significantly alter the end result. It is apparent that perfect reconstruction of tissues is possible only when the site of injury involves stable and labile cells. All destruction of permanent cells must result in irrevocable loss of specialized function. The functional loss may be unimportant when there is a large reserve, although to some extent the reserve is thereby diminished. Thus, the location of an injury impinges on the adequacy and quality of the end result. The location of the response also has other implications. Inflammations may arise within natural body cavities or tissue spaces, such as the peritoneal, pleural, and pericardial spaces, or in loose connective tissue. Although inflammatory exudate may readily fill the spaces, if resolution follows, virtually normal structure and function are restored. Similarly, resolution of inflammatory exudate within the pulmonary alveoli may leave no permanent damage if the pulmonary parenchyma has not been destroyed. At some later date, the lungs might appear entirely normal. By contrast, bacterial invasion of the liver or kidney with the production of an abscess might be repaired by marginal parenchymal regeneration but almost inevitably involves some scarring.

In closing, it is hardly necessary to point out that an understanding of the basic mechanisms and principles of inflammation and repair is fundamental to the proper treatment of the innumerable injuries encountered in everyday medicine. Stated in another way, clinical treatment of tissue injury consists, in essence, of the attempt to modify favorably by judicious interventions the physiologic and pathologic processes of the inflammatory and reparative response. A century ago "laudable pus" was a common expression that implied recognition of the important role of the inflammatory reaction in the body's defense. Often the pus is indeed laudable.

## References

1. Hurley, J. V.: Acute inflammation. 2nd ed. New York, Churchill Livingstone, 1983, p. 38.
2. Wade, B. H., and Mandell, G. L.: Polymorphonuclear leukocytes: Dedicated professional phagocytes. Am. J. Med. 74:686, 1983.
3. Palmbald, J.: The role of granulocytes in inflammation. Scand. J. Rheumatol. 13:163, 1984.
4. Aggeler, J., and Werb, Z.: Ultrastructural aspects of phagocytosis by macrophages. In Weissmann, G. (ed.): Advances in Inflammation Research. Vol. 8. New York, Raven Press, 1984, p. 35.
5. Korchak, H. M., et al.: Neutrophil stimulation: Receptor, membrane and metabolic events. Fed. Proc. 43:2749, 1984.
6. Babior, B. M.: The respiratory burst of phagocytes. J. Clin. Invest. 73:599, 1984.
7. Quie, P. G., and Hetherington, S. V.: Patients with disorders of phagocytic cell function. Ped. Infect. Dis. 3:272, 1984.
8. Lewis, T.: The Blood Vessels of the Human Skin and Their Responses. London, Shaw, 1927.
9. Cooper, N. R.: The complement system. In Stites, D. P., et al. (eds.): Basic and Clinical Immunology. 5th ed. Los Altos, Lange Medical Publications, 1984, p. 119.
10. Ford-Hutchinson, A. W.: Leukotrienes: Their formation and role as inflammatory mediators. Fed. Proc. 44:25, 1985.
11. Demers, L. M.: Prostaglandins in human disease. Clin. Lab. Med. 4:889, 1984.
12. Malmsten, C.L.: Leukotrienes: Mediators of inflammation and immediate hypersensitivity reactions. C.R.C. Crit. Rev. Immunol. 4:307, 1984.
13. Stenson, W. F., and Parker, C. W.: Leukotrienes. Adv. Int. Med. 30:175, 1984.
14. Flower, R. J., et al.: Macrocortin and the mechanism of action of the glucocorticoids. In Otterness, I., et al. (eds.): Advances in Inflammation Research. Vol. 7. New York, Raven Press, 1984, p. 61.
15. Flohe, L., Giertz, H., and Beckman, R.: Free radical scavengers as anti-inflammatory drugs? In Bonta, I. L., et al. (eds.): The Pharmacology of Inflammation. Amsterdam, Elsevier, 1985, p. 255.
16. Benveniste, J.: PAF-Acetheter (Platelet activating factor). Adv. Prostaglandin Thromboxane Leukotriene Res. 13:11, 1985.
17. Lasser, A.: The mononuclear phagocyte system. Hum. Pathol. 14:108, 1983.
18. Allison, A. C.: Role of macrophage activation in the pathogenesis of chronic inflammation and its pharmacologic control. Adv. Inflam. Res. 1:201, 1984.
19. Werb, Z.: Macrophages. In Stites, D. P., et al. (eds.): Basic and Clinical Immunology. 5th ed. Los Altos, Lange Medical Publications, 1984, p. 104.
20. Dinarello, C. A., and Mier, J. W.: Interleukins. Annu. Rev. Med. 37:173, 1986.
21. Boggs, D. R., and Winkelstein, A.: White Cell Manual. 4th ed. Philadelphia, F. A. Davis Co., 1983, p. 34.
22. Hay, E. D.: Skeletal muscle regeneration. N. Engl. J. Med. 284:1033, 1971.
23. Dunphy, J. E.: The healing of wounds. Can. J. Surg. 10:281, 1967.
24. Ryan, G. B., and Majno, G.: Acute inflammation, a review. Am. J. Pathol. 86:185, 1977.
25. Gabbiani, G., et al.: Granulation tissue as a contractile organ: A study of structure and function. J. Exp. Med. 135:719, 1972.
26. Byers, P. D., et al.: The healing of bone and articular cartilage. In Glynn, L. E., et al. (eds.): Handbook of Inflammation. Vol. 3. Amsterdam, Elsevier, 1981, p. 343.
27. Ham, A. W., and McCormack, D. H.: Histology. 8th ed. Philadelphia, J. B. Lippincott, 1979, p. 377.
28. Prockop, D. J., and Kivirikko, K. I.: Heritable diseases of collagen. N. Engl. J. Med. 311:376, 1984.
29. Bole, G. G.: Rheumatic diseases. In Sodeman, W. A., and Sodeman, T. M. (eds.): Sodeman's Pathologic Physiology, Mechanisms of Disease. 7th ed. Philadelphia, W. B. Saunders Co., p. 485, 1985.
30. Nimni, M. E.: Collagen, structure, function, and metabolism in normal and fibrotic tissues. Semin. Arth. Rheum. 13:1, 1983.
31. Peacock, E. E.: Wound Repair. 3rd ed. Philadelphia, W. B. Saunders Co., 1984, p. 102.
32. Lichtenstein, I. L., et al.: The dynamics of wound healing. Surg. Gynecol. Obstet. 130:685, 1970.
33. Grinnell, F.: Fibronectin and wound healing. J. Cell. Biochem. 26:107, 1984.
34. Wagner, B. M.: Wound healing revisited: Fibronectin and company. Hum. Pathol. 16:1081, 1985.
35. Gospodarowicz, D.: Growth factors and their actions in vivo and in vitro. J. Pathol. 141:201, 1983.
36. James, R.: Polypeptide growth factors. Ann Rev. Biochem. 53:259, 1984.
37. Bowen-Pope, D. F., and Ross, R.: Platelet-derived growth factor. Clin. Endocrinol. Metab. 13:191, 1984.
38. Dingman, R. O.: Factors of clinical significance affecting wound healing. Laryngoscope 83:1540, 1973.
39. Sussman, M. D.: Aging of connective tissue: Physical properties of healing wounds in young and old rats. Am. J. Physiol. 224:1167, 1973.
40. Editorial: A radical approach to zinc. Lancet 1:191, 1978.
41. Leme, J. G.: The endocrine and nervous system in inflammation: Pharmacologic considerations. In Glynn, L. E., et al. (eds.): Handbook of Inflammations. New York, Elsevier, 1985, p. 195.
42. Nolan, C. M., et al.: Further characterization of the impaired bactericidal function of granulocytes in patients with poorly controlled diabetes. Diabetes 27:889, 1978.

# 3
# Fluid and Hemodynamic Derangements

Survival of cells and tissues is exquisitely dependent on the oxygen contained within a normal blood supply. What may be less apparent is their dependence on a normal fluid balance. Approximately 60% of a person's lean body weight is water. This is divided between the intracellular compartment (40%) and the extracellular compartment (interstitial fluid, 15%; plasma water, 5%). Derangements in either blood supply or fluid balance cause some of the most commonly encountered disorders in medical practice: edema, congestion, hemorrhage, shock, and the three interrelated conditions—thrombosis, embolism, and infarction. Not only are these disorders common; they are major causes of mortality. Pulmonary edema is often the terminal event in most forms of heart disease. Hemorrhage and shock are virtually daily problems in the emergency room of any large hospital. Thrombosis, embolism, and infarction underlie three of the most important disorders in industrialized nations: myocardial infarction, pulmonary embolism, and cerebrovascular accidents (strokes). This chapter, then, deals with the predominating mechanisms of morbidity and mortality.

## EDEMA

The term *edema* refers to the accumulation of abnormal amounts of fluid in the intercellular tissue spaces or body cavities. It may occur as a generalized or a localized disorder. The term *anasarca* is used when the edema is severe and generalized, producing marked swelling of the subcutaneous tissues. Edematous collections in the various serous cavities of the body are given the special designations *hydrothorax*, *hydropericardium*, and *hydroperitoneum* (more commonly called *ascites*). The fluid of noninflammatory edema, such as develops in hydrodynamic derangements, is a transudate, low in protein and other colloids, with a specific gravity usually below 1.012. Inflammatory collections of fluid are rich in proteins (see p. 30) and therefore have a higher specific gravity—usually over 1.020.

Edema is the result of an increase in the forces tending to move fluids from the intravascular compartment into the interstitial fluid. The normal interchange of fluid, as proposed by Starling, is regulated by the hydrostatic and osmotic pressures within and without the vascular compartment. As indicated in Figure 3–1, intravascular hydrostatic pressure and interstitial colloid osmotic pressure tend to move fluid outward through the capillary wall, whereas interstitial fluid pressure and intravascular colloid osmotic pressure tend to move fluid inward. Since the hydrostatic and osmotic forces exerted by the interstitial fluid are relatively small and remain unchanged between the arteriolar and venular ends of the capillary, they do not play a major role in the regulation of extracellular fluid volume. *The opposing effects of intravascular hydrostatic pressure and plasma colloid osmotic pressure are the major factors to be considered in the pathogenesis of edema.* At the arteriolar end of the capillary bed, the hydrostatic pressure is about 35 mm Hg. At the venular end it falls to 12 to 15 mm Hg. The colloid osmotic pressure of the plasma is 20 to 25 mm Hg, rising slightly at

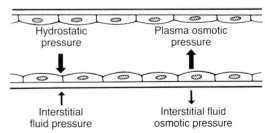

**Figure 3–1.** Factors affecting the flow of fluid across capillary wall.

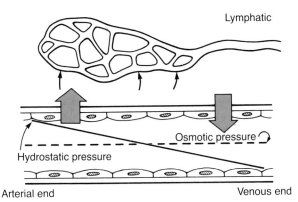

**Figure 3–2.** Normal formation and drainage of interstitial fluid.

Lymphatic

Osmotic pressure

Hydrostatic pressure

Arterial end     Venous end

**Table 3–1. CAUSES OF EDEMA**

| Primary Cause | Clinical Examples | |
|---|---|---|
| | *Localized Edema* | *Generalized Edema* |
| 1. Increased hydrostatic pressure | Venous obstruction Thrombosis External compression— e.g., tumors | Congestive heart failure |
| 2. Reduced colloid osmotic pressure of plasma— hypoalbuminemia | None | (a) Excessive loss of albumin— e.g., renal disease (b) Decreased synthesis of albumin— e.g., diffuse liver disease |
| 3. Lymphatic obstruction | Neoplastic or inflammatory obstruction | None |
| 4. Sodium retention | None | Renal disease with salt retention |

the venular end as fluid escapes (Fig. 3–2). Thus fluid leaves at the arteriolar end of the capillary bed and returns at the venular end. Not all of the fluid in the interstitial spaces returns to the venules; some is drained off through the lymphatics, to be returned to the bloodstream only indirectly.

From this brief review of the formation and drainage of interstitial fluid we can deduce that edema will occur when there is:
○ *an increase in intravascular hydrostatic pressure*
○ *a fall in colloid osmotic pressure of the plasma*
○ *an impairment in the flow of lymph.*

These constitute the important *primary causes* of noninflammatory edema. To this list must be added *renal retention of salt and water*, which may be a primary disturbance when there is kidney disease or may be a secondary event contributing to edema of other causes. Table 3–1 lists the primary causes of edema and the associated clinical conditions. Not included in this table is inflammatory edema, which,

as already discussed (p. 30), results from an increase in vascular permeability brought about by the action of chemical mediators.

*Increased hydrostatic pressure* may result from an impaired venous outflow, most frequently encountered in the lower extremities, secondary to the development of obstructive thromboses. The resulting edema is localized to the legs. A generalized increase in venous pressure and systemic edema occurs when there is congestive heart failure (p. 314) affecting right ventricular function. Although increased venous hydrostatic pressure is an important factor, the pathogenesis of cardiac edema is far more complex (Fig. 3–3). Congestive heart failure is associated with reduced cardiac output and reduced renal

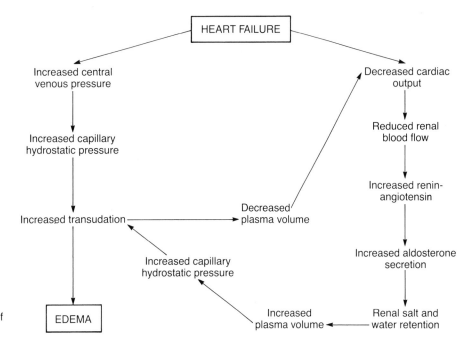

**Figure 3–3.** Pathogenesis of edema in heart failure.

HEART FAILURE

Increased central venous pressure

Increased capillary hydrostatic pressure

Increased transudation

EDEMA

Decreased plasma volume

Increased capillary hydrostatic pressure

Increased plasma volume

Decreased cardiac output

Reduced renal blood flow

Increased renin-angiotensin

Increased aldosterone secretion

Renal salt and water retention

blood flow. Through a series of complex regulatory mechanisms, a reduction in renal perfusion or perfusion pressure triggers the renin-angiotensin-aldosterone axis, resulting in renal retention of $Na^+$ and water (*secondary aldosteronism*). Expansion of the intravascular volume resulting from this sequence of events does not improve renal perfusion, since the failing heart is unable to increase cardiac output. With the extra fluid load (which the heart is unable to handle) there is further increase in venous pressure and edema formation. Thus a vicious circle of fluid retention and worsening edema sets in. Not surprisingly, therefore, restriction of salt intake and administration of diuretics and aldosterone antagonists reduce the edema of congestive heart failure.

*Reduced osmotic pressure of the plasma* results from excessive loss or reduced synthesis of serum albumin. The most important cause of increased loss of albumin is certain diseases of the kidney in which the glomerular basement membrane is abnormally permeable to albumin. The resulting *nephrotic syndrome* (p. 464) is characterized by generalized edema. Reduced synthesis of serum proteins occurs with diffuse diseases of the liver, such as cirrhosis (p. 582), or in association with malnutrition (p. 236). In all these instances, movement of fluid from the intravascular to the interstitial compartment leads to a contraction of plasma volume. Predictably, a reduction in renal perfusion follows, and secondary aldosteronism sets in. However, the retained salt and water cannot correct the deficit in plasma volume, since the primary defect of too little serum proteins persists. Once again, we see that the edema initiated by one mechanism gets complicated by secondary salt and fluid retention.

*Lymphatic obstruction* is another primary cause of edema. Impaired lymphatic drainage and consequent lymphedema is usually localized and may result from inflammatory or neoplastic obstruction. Filariasis, a parasitic infection, often causes massive fibrosis of the lymph nodes and lymphatic channels in the inguinal region. The resulting edema of the external genitalia and the lower limbs is so extreme, it is called *elephantiasis*. Cancer of the breast is sometimes treated by removal or irradiation of the entire breast along with all or most of the lymph nodes in the axilla. Consequently, postoperative edema of the arm often follows such therapy and can be a troublesome clinical problem.

*Sodium retention* along with obligate water retention has already been mentioned as a contributing factor in several forms of edema. Salt retention may be a primary cause of edema when there is acute reduction in renal function, as may be encountered in poststreptococcal glomerulonephritis (p. 468) or in acute renal failure (p. 476). The retained salt and water cause expansion of intravascular fluid volume and lead secondarily to increased hydrostatic pressure and, consequently, edema.

**MORPHOLOGY.** The morphologic changes of edema are much more evident grossly than microscopically. Although any organ or tissue in the body may be involved, edema is encountered most often in three sites: the subcutaneous tissues, usually in the lower extremities; the lungs; and the brain.

**Subcutaneous edema of the lower parts of the body is a prominent manifestation of cardiac failure, particularly failure of the right ventricle.** Although right ventricular failure obviously affects the entire systemic venous return to the heart, edema is most prominent in the lower extremities because they are subject to the highest hydrostatic pressures. If the patient is confined to bed, sacral edema may become evident. **Since the distribution of the edema is influenced by gravity, it is termed "dependent."**

Edema produced by **renal dysfunction** results from proteinuria and sodium retention. It tends to be generalized and more severe than cardiac edema, affecting all parts of the body equally. However, it may manifest itself initially in those tissues that have a loose connective tissue matrix, such as the eyelids (**periorbital edema**). Such generalized edema merits the designation anasarca. Finger pressure over edematous subcutaneous tissue will squeeze out the fluid and produce pitted depressions, hence the common clinical term **pitting edema.** Incision of edematous subcutaneous tissues will disclose an increased oozing of interstitial fluid, but it is usually slight and difficult to appreciate.

Microscopically, it may be extremely difficult to detect the increase of interstitial fluid in the subcutaneous connective tissue. Occasionally, a fine granular precipitate (a residuum of the trace amounts of protein in the edema fluid) is seen between the separated connective tissue fibers and cells. Dilatation of lymphatics may be present.

The **lungs**, composed of a loose, honeycombed tissue, are particularly susceptible to edema. **Pulmonary edema** is a prominent manifestation of left ventricular failure (Fig. 3–4). It may also be encountered in renal failure, in the so-called adult respiratory distress syndrome (p. 410), in infections of the lung and hypersensitivity reactions. The changes are described more fully in the consideration of congestive heart failure on page 313.

Edema of the **brain** is encountered in a variety of clinical circumstances, such as brain trauma, meningitis, encephalitis, hypertensive crises, and any form of obstruction to the venous outflow of the brain. This condition is described on page 726.

**Solid organs**, such as the liver and kidneys, may be involved when edema is systemic in distribution. Such involvement is evidenced only by a slight increase in size and weight, and possibly by some pallor. The capsule may be tense. The changes are rarely sufficiently well marked to be clearly identified by inspection, and the scales provide the most reliable indication.

**CLINICAL CORRELATION.** Edema may give rise to minor clinical problems, or it can be lethal. Edema of the subcutaneous tissues in cardiac or renal failure

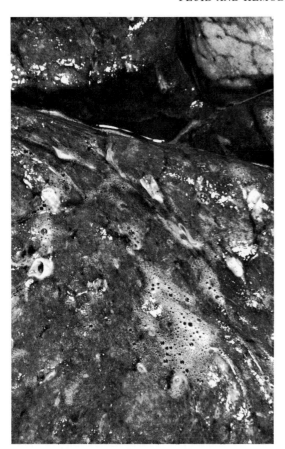

Figure 3–4. Pulmonary edema. A close-up view of the transected surface of a very wet lung, from which frothy edema fluid exudes.

is important chiefly because it indicates underlying disease, but it sometimes impairs healing of wounds or infections. Since edema of the lungs (pulmonary edema) impairs normal ventilatory function, it may be lethal. The fluid first collects within the alveolar walls around the capillaries, producing an "alveolo-capillary block" in oxygen diffusion. The impact on ventilatory function may seem disproportionate to the relatively small amounts of fluid required to produce such a block. In the later stages, when the fluid collects within the alveolar spaces, it creates a favorable soil for bacterial infection, termed *hypostatic pneumonia*. Edema of the brain can be a serious clinical problem and possibly cause death if it is sufficiently marked. The increased mass of brain substance may cause herniation of the cerebellar tonsils into the foramen magnum or may cause shearing stresses on the blood supply to the brain stem. Both conditions secondarily impinge upon medullary centers to cause death.

## HYPEREMIA OR CONGESTION

These synonyms refer to a local increased volume of blood caused by dilatation of the small vessels.

*Active hyperemia* results from an augmented arterial inflow, such as occurs in the muscles during exercise, at sites of inflammation, and in the pleasing neuro-vascular dilatation termed blushing. *Passive congestion* results from diminished venous outflow such as follows cardiac failure or obstructive venous disease. Thus, in cardiac failure the appearance of edema is almost always accompanied by passive congestion, giving rise to the more appropriate designation *congestion and edema. Chronic passive congestion of the lungs is one of the most reliable postmortem indicators of left ventricular cardiac failure.* When congestion is encountered in the lower extremities, the legs are abnormally cool and either pale, owing to the predominance of edema, or dusky blue-gray, owing to the venous congestion accompanying the edema.

## HEMORRHAGE

Hemorrhage obviously implies rupture of a blood vessel. Rupture of a large artery or vein is almost always caused by some form of injury, such as trauma, atherosclerosis, or inflammatory or neoplastic erosion of the vessel wall. Rupture of a large artery in the brain is a frequent cause of death in hypertensive patients (Fig. 3–5). An increased tendency to hemorrhage is encountered in a wide variety of clinical disorders known collectively as the *hemorrhagic diatheses*. These are discussed in Chapter 12.

Hemorrhages may be external and exsanguinating. When the blood is trapped within the tissues of the body, the accumulation is referred to as a *hematoma*. Rupture of the aorta, for example, in a dissecting or atherosclerotic aneurysm, may cause a massive retroperitoneal hematoma with sufficient loss of blood to cause death. When the blood accumulates in one of the body cavities it is referred to as *hemothorax, hemopericardium, hemoperitoneum,* or *hemarthrosis*. Minute hemorrhages into the skin, mucous membranes, or serosal surfaces are known as *petechiae*. Slightly larger hemorrhages are designated *purpura*. A large (over 1 to 2 cm in diameter) subcutaneous hematoma, an example of which is the common bruise, is called an *ecchymosis*. The released hemoglobin is converted into bilirubin and eventually into hemosiderin. Patients sustaining a large hemorrhage, such as massive gastrointestinal bleeding, a pulmonary hemorrhage or infarct (p. 77), or a hematoma, sometimes become jaundiced owing to the breakdown of red cells and subsequent release of bilirubin.

The significance of hemorrhage depends on the volume of blood loss, the rate of loss, and the site of hemorrhage. Sudden losses of up to 20% of the blood volume or slow losses of even larger amounts may have little clinical significance. Larger or more acute losses may induce hemorrhagic (hypovolemic) shock (p. 79). The site of the hemorrhage is, of course,

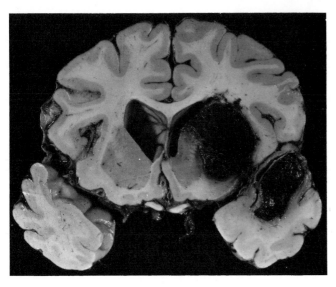

Figure 3–5. A fatal intracerebral hemorrhage in a 65-year-old hypertensive male.

important; a hemorrhage that would be trivial in the subcutaneous tissues may cause death when located in the brain stem. Repeated external hemorrhages (i.e., those in which the blood is shed—as from the skin, gastrointestinal tract, or female genital tract) represent losses of not only blood volume but also valuable iron. Usually the small but repeated volume losses are rapidly corrected by movement of water from the interstitial spaces into the vascular compartment, but the chronic loss of iron may lead to an iron deficiency anemia. In contrast, when the red cells are retained, as occurs with hemorrhages into the body cavities, joints, or tissues, the iron can be recaptured for synthesis of hemoglobin.

## THROMBOSIS

The formation of a clotted mass of blood in the noninterrupted cardiovascular system is known as *thrombosis*, and the mass itself is termed a *thrombus*. Blood clotting, when it plugs a severed vessel, may be life-saving; when it occludes a functioning vessel supplying a vital structure, it may be life-threatening. In addition, some part or all of the thrombus may break loose to create an *embolus* that flows downstream to lodge at a distant site. Thrombosis and embolism are, then, closely interrelated, as is indicated by the commonly used term *thromboembolism*. The potential consequence of both thrombosis and embolism is ischemic necrosis of cells and tissue, known as *infarction*. Thromboembolic infarctions of the heart, lungs, and brain are dominating causes of morbidity and mortality in industrialized nations and account collectively for more deaths than those caused by all forms of cancer and infectious disease together. Here we consider the subject of thrombosis, and in later sections, embolism and infarction.

**PATHOGENESIS.** The development of a thrombus is best viewed as the consequence of inappropriate activation of the process of normal hemostasis. We should briefly review, then, normal hemostasis.

*Normal Hemostasis.* When a vessel is severed, it almost immediately contracts owing to reflex neurogenic mechanisms, possibly augmented by such humoral factors as certain prostaglandin derivatives. Such vascular contraction is most evident in vessels having well-defined muscular walls, but it also occurs in the sphincteric mechanisms situated at the junction of meta-arterioles and capillaries, thereby shutting off capillary beds. Soon, however, the vascular spasm abates and bleeding would resume were it not for activation of the platelet and coagulation systems. We can dissect the ensuing process of hemostasis by considering the three major contributors to it: (1) *endothelial cell injury*, (2) *platelets*, and (3) *the coagulation system.*[1, 2]

*Endothelial cells*, once considered inert barriers between platelets, clotting factors, and the subendothelial tissues, are now known to be active in modulating several aspects of the hemostasis-coagulation sequence. On the one hand they possess antiplatelet and anticoagulant properties; on the other hand they exert procoagulant functions (Fig. 3–6). Once clots are formed, endothelial cells also participate in fibrinolysis, as will be discussed later. Only some properties of the "schizophrenic" endothelial cells are summarized here. For details the reader is referred to a recent review.[1] Consider first those aspects of the endothelium that oppose clotting. *Intact endothelium insulates the blood platelets and coagulation proteins from the highly thrombogenic subendothelial components, principally collagen.* Platelets flowing in the bloodstream do not adhere to the endothelium. This "antiplatelet" function seems intrinsic to their plasma membrane and is not dependent upon the production of prostacyclin (PGI$_2$). On the other hand, once platelets are "activated" (following focal endothelial injury), they are inhibited from adhering to the surrounding uninjured endothelial cells by the action of prostacyclin. The latter, which belongs to the family of prostaglandins (p. 39), is also a powerful inhibitor of platelet aggregation and a potent vasodilator. $PGI_2$ synthesis in endothelial cells is stimulated by thrombin and other undefined serum factors produced during coagulation. Another mechanism by which endothelial cells inhibit platelet aggregation is by enzymatic degradation of ADP, a powerful platelet-aggregating agent that, as we shall discuss, is released from activated platelets.

In addition to their antiplatelet activities, endothelial cells also express powerful anticoagulant functions. These are mediated primarily by two cell-surface molecules: *a heparin-like substance* and the protein *thrombomodulin* (Fig. 3–6). The heparin-like substance, presumably heparan sulfate, acts indirectly. It greatly facilitates the actions of naturally occurring anticoagulant protein antithrombin III, which inactivates thrombin and several other coagulation factors including factor Xa. These *anticoagulant actions of antithrombin III are accelerated approximately 2000 times after it binds to heparan sulfate on the endothelial cells*. Thrombomodulin, the other anticoagulant moiety present on the endothelial cell surface, also acts indirectly. It accelerates the activation of yet another naturally occurring anticoagu-

lant called protein C. *Activated protein C inhibits clotting by proteolytic cleavage of factors V and VIII. However, protein C itself has to be activated by thrombin, and this reaction proceeds very slowly unless thrombin is first bound to thrombomodulin* (Fig. 3–6). It is interesting to note that the procoagulant activity of thrombin (clotting of fibrinogen, activation of factor V) is markedly reduced after binding to thrombomodulin. *Thus thrombin-thrombomodulin complex formed on the endothelial cells inhibits clotting at two different levels—it favors anticoagulation by activating protein C, and it reduces the clot-promoting activity of thrombin.*

While on one hand endothelial cells oppose blood clotting and thrombosis, on the other hand they are prohemostatic, affecting both platelets and coagulation proteins. As mentioned earlier, endothelial injury leads to the first step in hemostasis, i.e., adhesion of platelets to subendothelial collagen. However, the role of endothelium in the adhesion of platelets to the vessel wall is not merely to "move themselves out of the way." Endothelial cells synthesize and secrete von Willebrand's factor (a component of factor VIII complex), which is essential for the adhesion of platelets to collagen and other surfaces. Tissue factor released from endothelial cells that have been injured or perturbed (for example, by exposure to endotoxin

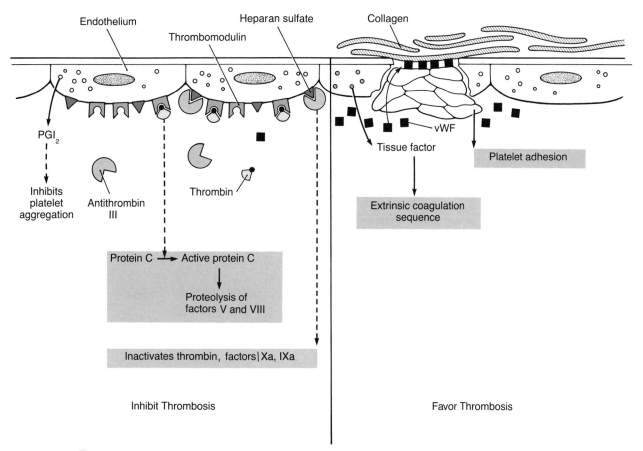

**Figure 3–6.** A schematic illustration of the procoagulant and anticoagulant activities of endothelial cells.

or sublethal injury) activates the extrinsic clotting pathway. Recent investigations have revealed that endothelial cells can bind to activated forms of factors IX and X,[3] and cell-bound factors seem to be more active than their counterparts in solution. This may be one mechanism by which the coagulation process remains localized to the vicinity of injured endothelium.

*In summary, intact endothelial cells, although multifunctional, predominantly serve to inhibit platelet adherence and initiation of blood clotting. Conversely, injury to endothelial cells represents a loss of anticlotting mechanisms and thus contributes to hemostasis and, as will be seen, to thrombosis.*

*Platelets,* as must already be evident, play a key role in normal hemostasis. Once viewed as banal or anucleate fragments of megakaryocytes, they are now recognized as extremely important and complex elements of the blood. In their circulating form, they appear as relatively smooth discs enclosed within a typical plasma membrane, itself coated by a glycocalyx. Within the platelets there is an open canalicular system representing deep invaginations of the plasma membrane; an elaborate complex of microtubules and microfilaments, the latter composed of the contractile proteins actin and myosin; and mitochondria, lysosomes, and two specific types of granules.[4] *Alpha granules* contain fibrinogen, fibronectin, factors V and VIII, platelet factor 4 (a heparin-neutralizing polypeptide), and platelet-derived growth factor (PDGF). The other form of granules are the *electron-dense bodies* that are the storage sites for a nonmetabolic pool of adenine nucleotides (ADP, ATP), ionized calcium, histamine, serotonin (5-HT), and epinephrine.

Injury to a vessel exposes a number of elements in the vascular wall to platelets—subendothelial collagen, capillary basal lamina, fibroblasts, and smooth muscle cells. Although all are capable of causing platelet adhesion, collagen is the most powerful stimulus. On contact with collagen, for example, platelets undergo a number of changes, which can be listed as *adhesion, release reaction (or secretion), and aggregation.* Together these phenomena are referred to as "platelet activation" (Fig. 3–7).

Despite intensive study, the precise changes that impart stickiness are still mysterious. This much is known—factor VIII, von Willebrand factor (vWF), is definitely involved. According to one widely accepted view, von Willebrand's factor acts as a "glue" between platelet surface and collagen. Specific receptors for vWF have been found on platelets, and vWF can bind to collagen. In patients with inherited deficiency of vWF (von Willebrand's disease, p. 399) platelet adhesion to collagen and other surfaces is impaired. Adhesion of platelets to subendothelial collagen is followed soon by *secretion*—or the so-called *release reaction*—during which ADP, serotonin, and various other platelet contents are released. Secretion of ADP is a particularly important event since ADP

causes *platelet aggregation* (platelets adhering to other platelets) and it also augments the release of ADP from other platelets. Thus an autocatalytic reaction is set into motion and leads to the buildup of an enlarging platelet aggregate. Initially, platelet aggregation is reversible, and the breach in the vessel wall is sealed by a "temporary hemostatic plug." Soon, however, under the influence of thrombin, thromboxane $A_2$ (discussed later), and increasing amounts of ADP, platelets contract and a mass of irreversibly aggregated platelets ("viscous metamorphosis") is produced. It will be recalled (p. 39) that $TXA_2$ is a prostaglandin that is synthesized by the platelets and, like prostacyclin, is a product of the cyclooxygenase pathway of arachidonic acid metabolism (p. 39). However, prostacyclin and $TXA_2$ have opposing actions—prostacyclin inhibits platelet aggregation and is a vasodilator, whereas $TXA_2$ is a powerful aggregator and vasconstrictor. *The interplay of prostacyclin and $TXA_2$ constitutes a finely balanced mechanism for modulation of human platelet function, which, in the normal state, prevents intravascular platelet aggregation and clotting, but following endothelial injury favors the formation of hemostatic plug.*

The buildup of a platelet mass at a site of vascular injury serves many functions. It alone may suffice as a hemostatic plug to control bleeding in small vessels. The aggregated platelets make available platelet fac-

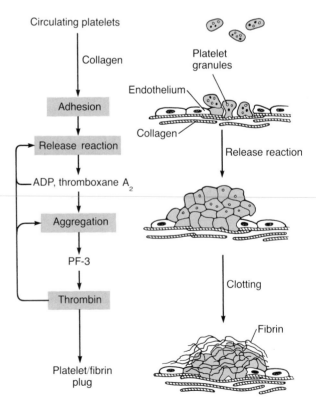

**Figure 3–7.** Platelet functions in hemostasis. (Modified from Taussig, M. J.: Processes in Pathology. 2nd ed. Oxford, Blackwell Scientific, 1984, p. 627).

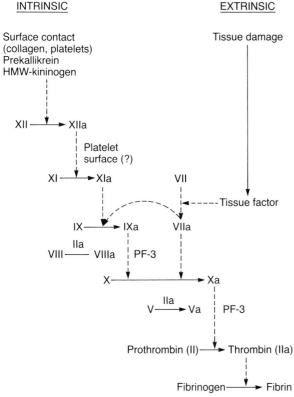

**Figure 3–8.** The coagulation cascade.

of an *enzyme* (activated coagulation factor) a *substrate* (proenzyme form of coagulation factor), and a *cofactor* (reaction accelerator). These components are assembled on a *phospholipid surface* and held together by *calcium ions*. Thus clotting tends to remain localized to sites where such an assembly can occur, e.g., on the surface of activated platelets. One of the key reactions in blood clotting, conversion of factor X to Xa, is illustrated in Figure 3–9.

It has been customary to divide the blood coagulation scheme into an *extrinsic* and *intrinsic* pathway, both of which converge at the point where factor X is activated (Fig. 3–8). However, it is now clear that such a division is probably an artifact of in vitro testing methods and that there are several interconnections between the so-called intrinsic and extrinsic pathways. An important example of such "crosstalk" between pathways is the demonstration that the conversion of factor IX to IXa is brought about not only by the "contact-activated" factors of the intrinsic pathway but also by factor VII, the initiator of the extrinsic pathway (Fig. 3–8). The fact that patients with congenital deficiencies of the contact-activated factors (such as factor XII, prekallikrein, and high-molecular-weight kininogen) do not have any bleeding disorders has cast serious doubts on the in vivo significance of these factors in hemostasis.[2, 5]

Once the coagulation cascade has been activated, it must be contained to the local site of vascular injury lest clotting involve the entire vascular tree.

tor 3 for the coagulation sequence. *Platelet factor 3 (unlike most other platelet constituents) is not a secreted product but rather a phospholipid complex that is activated or in some manner exposed on the platelet surface.* This phenomenon is of singular importance, since virtually every step in the coagulation sequence discussed below requires a phospholipid surface (see Fig. 3–9). The platelet surface therefore serves as a haven for the accumulation of thrombin, which itself is a potent inducer of platelet aggregation. Thus a feedback loop is built into the platelet system, augmenting the buildup of a hemostatic plug while contributing to the clotting sequence. Fibrin, the end product of coagulation, serves to cement the aggregated platelets. The events described thus far are summarized in Figure 3–7.

*Coagulation system,* the third component of the hemostatic process, is a major contributor to thrombus formation. It is not our intention to delve into the details of the clotting sequence[2] but to highlight certain general principles and newer concepts with relevance to hemostasis and thrombogenesis.

○ The coagulation sequence comprises, in essence, a series of transformations of proenzymes to activated enzymes culminating in the formation of thrombin, which converts the soluble plasma protein fibrinogen to the insoluble fibrous protein fibrin (Fig. 3–8).

○ Each reaction in the coagulation pathway results from the assembly of a reaction complex composed

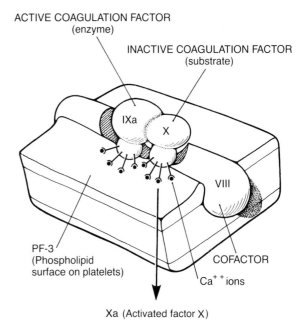

**Figure 3–9.** A schematic illustration of the conversion of factor X to factor Xa. The reaction complex consisting of an enzyme (factor IXa), a substrate (factor X), and a reaction accelerator (factor VIII) are assembled on the surface of platelets. Ca++ ions hold the assembled components together and are essential for the reaction. (Modified from Mann, K. G.: Clin. Lab. Med. 4:217, 1984.)

The most powerful control is the *fibrinolytic system.* Plasminogen normally present in plasma can be converted to plasmin by a tissue plasminogen activator (t-PA) present in most tissue cells, including endothelial cells. Urokinase or u-PA is a similar but chemically distinct activator of plasminogen extracted initially from human urine. Other PAs of exogenous origin (e.g., streptokinase) have also been identified. Another endogenous mechanism of plasminogen to plasmin conversion involves factor XII. Thus activated factor XII not only can initiate clotting and eventual fibrin formation but can also set into motion mechanisms leading to fibrinolysis. As fibrin is split by plasmin, its products (fibrin split products) themselves inhibit platelet aggregation and coagulation. Besides splitting fibrin, *plasmin* can also degrade fibrinogen and factors VIII and V. Normal human plasma also contains several protease inhibitors that can neutralize several of the clotting factors. Of principal importance is antithrombin III; it inhibits thrombin and factor Xa and, at slower rates, factors XIIa, XIa, and IXa. The facilitation of antithrombin III action by heparin-like substances was discussed earlier (p. 67). Protein C is another important naturally occurring anticoagulant. Its activation by thrombin-thrombomodulin complex on endothelial cells has already been described (p. 67). In this intricate system of checks and balances there are also inhibitors of plasmin, including alpha$_2$-macroglobulin and an alpha$_2$-plasmin inhibitor. There are other controlling mechanisms as well. The flow of blood past a nonocclusive clot serves as a controlling influence, since it dilutes activated factors at the local site and also carries them to the liver, where some (in particular, factors IX, X, and XI) are removed. Although still other controlling mechanisms might be mentioned, suffice it to say that clotting, once initiated, does not run rampant throughout the vascular tree. The significance of control mechanisms is highlighted by recurrent thromboembolism in patients with inherited deficiencies of antithrombin III or protein C.[6] With this overview of normal hemostasis, attention can be turned to its participation in the formation of thrombi.

***Thrombogenesis.*** The influences that predispose to thrombus formation are: (1) endothelial injury, (2) stasis or turbulence of blood flow, and (3) hypercoagulability of the blood.

*Endothelial injury* is the dominant influence in thrombogenesis, and the only one which by and of itself may lead to thrombus formation. This is amply documented by the frequency with which thrombi appear on ulcerated plaques in severely atherosclerotic arteries, particularly in the aorta; at sites of traumatic or inflammatory injury to vessels; and within the cardiac chambers when there has been injury to the endocardium, as may occur with myocardial infarction or in any form of myocarditis. The injury may be subtler in nature—hemodynamic stresses of hypertension, bacterial toxins, or endo-

toxins—and such adverse influences as homocystinuria, hypercholesterolemia, and products absorbed from cigarette smoke may also represent potential causes of endothelial injury.[7] Overt in many of these situations and perhaps covert in others is endothelial damage and exposure of subendothelial collagen (as well as other platelet activators), adherence of platelets (Fig. 3–10), release of tissue factor, and local depletion of prostacyclin and plasminogen activator. However, it should be stressed that the endothelial injury may be subtle and not detectable even under the electron microscope.

*Stasis and turbulence* (with its pockets of stasis) constitute major thrombogenic influences.[8] In normal laminar blood flow, all of the formed elements are separated from the endothelial surface by a clear plasmatic zone. Stasis and turbulence (1) disrupt laminar flow and permit platelets to come into contact with the endothelium; (2) prevent dilution of activated clotting factors to subcritical concentrations; (3) retard the inflow of clotting factors inhibitors; (4) permit the buildup of platelet aggregates and nascent fibrin either in the sluggish stream or in the pockets of stasis; (5) promote endothelial cell hypoxia and injury, predisposing to platelet and fibrin deposition as well as reducing release of t-PA[9]; and (6) the turbulence provides an additional mechanism for endothelial injury. *Stasis plays a dominant role in venous flow because of the low velocity of blood flow in veins.* Hume and associates have documented the

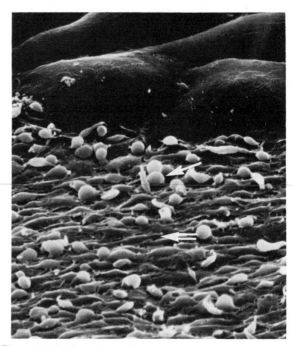

**Figure 3–10.** Scanning electron micrograph of an area of experimental endothelial denudation with only a few intact endothelial cells seen above. Numerous platelets are adherent to the subendothelium. Discoid and rounded platelets (arrow) are seen on top of an earlier layer of tightly adherent, elongated, flattened platelets (double arrow). (Courtesy of Dr. C. Haudenschild, Mallory Institute of Pathology.)

origin of venous thrombi in the sinuses behind the valve cusps in the deep veins of the lower leg.[10] A similar phenomenon probably occurs in the auricular appendages of the heart when there is atrial fibrillation or massive dilatation of the atria, as for example with mitral stenosis. Stasis and turbulence undoubtedly contribute to the development of thrombi within aneurysmal dilatations, which are already favored sites for thrombosis because of the underlying vascular disease and endothelial injury, e.g., atherosclerosis leading to aneurysm formation.

*Hypercoagulability* can be defined as an alteration of the blood or specifically the clotting mechanism that in some way predisposes to thrombosis. This can be documented easily in the test tube and can be established fairly clearly in the laboratory animal, but it has proved to be an elusive phenomenon to confirm in humans. Yet there can be no doubt of the existence of a thrombotic diathesis in many clinical settings—with the nephrotic syndrome, following severe trauma or burns, in disseminated cancer, in later pregnancy, with cardiac failure, and particularly with the long-term use of oral contraceptives.[11] In some of these settings, for example with cardiac failure or following trauma, other influences such as stasis or vascular injury may be the most important mechanism. But the frequency of thrombosis in patients having disseminated cancer and in late pregnancy (discussed more completely on p. 73), and the increased frequency of both venous and arterial thromboses in females who have used oral contraceptives, point to hypercoagulability as the predisposing mechanism. However, in most of these instances it has been difficult to define the precise basis for hypercoagulability. In users of oral contraceptives an increase in concentrations of plasma fibrinogen, prothrombin, and factors VII, VIII, and X can be demonstrated, as can a decrease in fibrinolytic activity; yet it has not been possible to prove a cause-and-effect relationship between the abnormalities in laboratory tests and increased thromboses.[11] In patients with disseminated cancer, secretion of thrombogenic factors or absorption of procoagulant products from necrotic tumor cells has been proposed as the basis for the tendency toward thrombosis.[12] Scattered reports call attention to increased numbers of platelets and increased platelet stickiness in one or another clinical setting, particularly in hyperlipidemia. In summary, despite suggestive clinical and some laboratory evidence, the role of a hypercoagulable state in thrombogenesis is hypothetical at best. The only exceptions to this generalization are the inherited deficiencies of antithrombin III and protein C already mentioned.

**MORPHOLOGY OF THROMBI.** Thrombi may develop anywhere in the cardiovascular system: in the chambers of the heart, arteries, veins, or capillaries. All are essentially intravascular clots, the composition, size, and shape of which are dictated by their site of origin. Those arising in the arterial side of the circulation (including the heart) differ somewhat from those arising in the venous side. Arterial or cardiac thrombi usually begin at a site of endothelial injury, or turbulence, either from some lesion or because a vessel bifurcates or branches. Classically the arterial thrombus is a dry, friable, tangled gray mass that on transection usually discloses darker gray lines of aggregated platelets interspersed between paler layers of coagulated fibrin. These lamellations are known as the **lines of Zahn.** Because they are largely composed of platelets and fibrin, **arterial thrombi are known as white or conglutination thrombi.** When arterial thrombi arise in the capacious chambers of the heart or in the aorta, they are usually applied to one wall of the underlying structure and thus are termed **mural thrombi** (Fig. 3–11). Mural thrombi also develop in abnormal dilatations of arteries (aneurysms). In arteries smaller than the aorta the thrombus usually builds up rapidly until it completely obstructs the lumen, producing a so-called **occlusive thrombus.** Any artery may be affected, but the most common and most important sites of involvement in order of frequency are as follows: coronary, cerebral, femoral, iliac, popliteal, and mesenteric arteries. **The term "thrombus," unless otherwise designated, implies the occlusive type.**

Venous thrombosis, also known as **phlebothrombosis,** is almost invariably occlusive. In fact, the thrombus often creates a long cast of the lumen of the vein. In the slower-moving blood of the veins, the coagulation simulates that in a test tube. Thus, these thrombi have a much

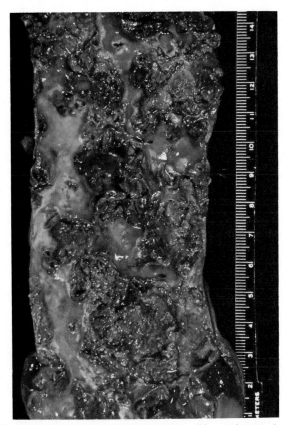

Figure 3–11. Numerous friable mural thrombi superimposed on advanced atherosclerotic lesions of the aorta.

richer admixture of erythrocytes and are therefore known as **red, coagulative,** or **stasis thrombi.** On transection laminations are not well developed, but tangled strands of fibrin can usually be seen. **Phlebothrombosis most commonly affects the veins of the lower extremities (90%) in approximately the following order of frequency: deep calf, femoral, popliteal, and iliac veins.** Less commonly, venous thrombi may develop in the periprostatic plexus, or the ovarian and periuterine veins.[10] Rarely, they occur in the portal vein or its radicles or in the dural sinuses.

Coagulation thrombi can be readily confused with postmortem clots at autopsy. The postmortem clot forms a cast of the vessel, but it is rubbery and gelatinous. The dependent portions of the clot where the red cells have settled by gravity tend to resemble dark red "currant jelly." The supernatant, free of red cells, has a yellow "chicken fat" appearance. Characteristically the postmortem clot is not attached to the underlying wall. In contrast, coagulation thrombi are more firm, almost always have a point of attachment, and on transection disclose barely visible tangled strands of pale gray fibrin.

Arterial and venous thrombi vary enormously in size. They range from small, irregular, roughly spherical masses to enormously elongated, snake-like structures that are formed when a long tail builds up behind the occluding head. In the arterial circulation the tail builds up retrograde to the direction of flow. On the venous side the tail extends in the direction of the blood flow, i.e., toward the heart. Often such propagations extend to the next major vascular branch.

A small or large area of attachment to the underlying vessel or heart wall is characteristic of all thromboses. Frequently the attachment is most firm at the point of origin, and the propagating tail may or may not be attached. It is this loosely attached tail which, in veins, is most likely to fragment to create an embolus. On the arterial side of the circulation, embolization usually implies detachment of the entire or almost the entire thrombus.

In special circumstances thrombi may be deposited on the heart valves. Blood-borne infections may attack heart valves (**bacterial** or **infective endocarditis),** creating ideal sites for the development of thrombotic masses. These masses, laden with microorganisms, are referred to as vegetations. Less commonly, noninfective, **verrucous endocarditis** may appear in patients who have systemic lupus erythematosus (p. 155). Vegetations may also develop on underlying **nonbacterial (thrombotic) endocarditis** in older patients with terminal cancers or other chronic ailments, and sometimes in young patients with nonfatal disorders. In these conditions hypercoagulability of the blood, subtle endothelial injuries, or both are invoked as the causative mechanisms.

If a patient survives the immediate effects of vascular obstruction, what happens to the thrombus over the course of days and weeks? One of the following sequences evolves: (1) the thrombus may propagate and eventually cause obstruction of some critical vessel, (2) it may embolize, (3) it may be removed by fibrinolytic activity, or (4) it may undergo organization and become recanalized—that is, incorporated within the vessel wall. The first two eventualities need no further comment here. There is evidence that fibrinolytic removal may occur. By angiography, pulmonary thromboemboli have been observed to shrink rapidly and even be totally lysed soon after their development.[13, 14] Such a happy outcome is most likely within the first day or two, presumably because as the thrombus ages and the fibrin undergoes continued polymerization, it is more resistant to proteolysis. It is relevant in this connection to note that infusion of fibrinolytic agents within hours of the acute event is being actively pursued as a modality in the management of coronary thrombosis. Initial results of thrombolytic therapy with streptokinase and more recently with genetically engineered tissue plasminogen activator are promising[15] and additional clinical trials are currently under way.

When a thrombus persists in situ for a few days, it is likely to become **organized.** This term refers to the ingrowth of subendothelial smooth muscle cells and mesenchymal cells into the fibrinous thrombus. In time the thrombus becomes populated with these spindle cells, and capillary channels are formed. Simultaneously the surface of the thrombus becomes covered with a layer of apparent endothelial cells. The capillary channels may anastomose to create thoroughfares from one end of the thrombus to the other through which blood may flow, reestablishing to some extent the continuity of the lumen of the original vessel. This process is known as **recanalization** of the thrombus (Fig. 3–12). In this manner the thrombus is converted into a vascularized subendothelial mass of connective tissue and eventually incorporated into the wall of the vessel. With the passage of time and the contraction of the mesenchymal cells, only a fibrous lump or thickening may remain to mark the site. Occasionally, instead of becoming organized, the center of the thrombus undergoes enzymic digestion to produce so-called **puriform (resembling pus) softening.** This action presumably reflects the release of lysosomal enzymes derived from the trapped leukocytes and platelets. This sequence is particularly likely in large thrombi within aneurysmal dilatations or within mural thrombi in the cardiac chambers. If a bacteremia occurs, such puriform debris is an ideal culture medium, which may convert the thrombus into a septic mass of pus.

**CLINICAL CORRELATION.** Thrombi are of critical importance for two reasons: (1) *they cause obstruction of arteries and veins* and (2) *they provide possible sources of emboli.* As generalizations, although venous thrombi may cause erythema and edema in dependent parts, they are of far graver consequence because thrombi usually arising in the deep veins of the legs are responsible for one of the major causes of death in the United States—namely, pulmonary embolization and infarction (p. 407).[16] In contrast, although arterial thrombi may of course embolize, much more important is their obstructive role in myocardial infarction, when the coronary arteries are involved, and in encephalomalacia (a form of stroke), when the arteries in the brain are involved.

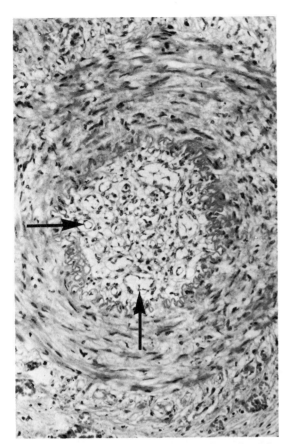

Figure 3–12. A completely organized and recanalized thromboembolus within an artery. The newly formed connective tissue is perforated by numerous vascular channels, several of which are marked by arrows.

As pointed out earlier, most venous thrombi are occlusive. As noted, the portal vein and its tributaries, the periovarian and periprostatic plexuses, are infrequent sites of involvement; *the great preponderance of venous thrombi arise in either the superficial or the deep veins of the leg.* Superficial thrombi usually occur in the saphenous system, particularly when there are varicosities. Such thrombi may cause local swelling, pain, tenderness, and erythema along the course of the involved vein, but only rarely do they embolize. However, the local edema and impaired venous drainage predispose the skin to infections from slight trauma and to the development of *varicose ulcers.* It is the deep thrombi in the veins of the calf muscles and in the popliteal, femoral, and iliac veins that tend to embolize. They may also cause edema of the foot and ankle and produce pain and tenderness on compression of the calf muscles (by either squeezing the calf muscles or forced dorsiflexion of the foot), known as Homan's sign. However, in *approximately half of the patients such thrombi are entirely asymptomatic* and can be documented only by using such sophisticated diagnostic techniques as radiolabeled fibrinogen assay, plethysmography, contrast venograms, and ultrasonic velocity measurements. The venous obstruction is soon com-

pensated for by the opening of collateral bypass channels of drainage. The most serious aspect of venous thrombosis in the deep veins of the leg, as mentioned, is its potential for causing pulmonary embolization and infarction.

It is necessary to digress for a moment to clarify the commonly used clinical term *"thrombophlebitis." This designation is often applied to phlebothrombosis* because the pain, tenderness, and erythema sometimes encountered at the local site are vaguely ascribed to a chronic inflammatory reaction in the wall of the involved vein, hence the term "thrombophlebitis." Morphologic studies, however, rarely disclose significant inflammatory changes in such vessels, and the pain, tenderness, and erythema are more reasonably attributed to local vascular stasis, edema, and distention of the affected vessel. Thus, *there is no valid distinction between phlebothrombosis and thrombophlebitis.*

Certain clinical settings are particularly associated with venous thrombosis, but advanced age, bed rest, and immobilization increase the hazard. The reduced physical activity in older age lessens the milking action of the muscles in the lower leg and so slows the venous return. Immobilization and bed rest carry the same implications. The specific clinical settings in which venous thrombosis is most likely to occur have already been mentioned in the discussion of thrombogenesis but for emphasis are repeated here. They include cardiac failure, severe trauma or burns, postoperative and postpartum states, the nephrotic syndrome, disseminated cancer (and in fact, all serious illnesses), and the use of oral contraceptives. Cardiac failure is an obvious cause of sluggish venous circulation. Trauma, surgery, and burns usually imply reduced physical activity, injury to vessels, release of procoagulant substances from tissues, and reduced t-PA activity.[7] In a series of 125 injured and burned patients, Sevitt encountered the following: 65% of all patients had venous thrombi; of those with thrombi, 74% had involvement of the veins of the calf, 70% had pelvic or thigh vein thrombi, and 37% had popliteal vein involvement.[17] Many factors act in concert to predispose to thrombosis in the puerperal and postpartum states. During delivery there is trauma to vessels and the potential for the entrance of amniotic fluid, bearing platelet-aggregating and possibly procoagulant factors into the pelvic veins (p. 76). But, in addition, there is a distinct hazard of venous thrombosis in the third trimester of pregnancy, as well as in the postdelivery period, giving rise to the designation "milk leg" or "phlegmasia alba dolens" (painful white leg). The basis for such predisposition is not entirely clear but has been attributed to hypercoagulability as well as to some inhibition of fibrinolysis.

Predisposition to venous thrombosis in any of the veins of the body in patients with cancer, particularly with abdominal neoplasms (such as carcinoma of the pancreas), was first noted by Trousseau and so is referred to as *Trousseau's sign*. Frequently the thrombi develop at one site only to disappear and reappear elsewhere, giving rise to the pattern known as *"migratory thrombophlebitis."* The basis for such a thrombotic diathesis probably involves a number of influences, including age, surgical procedures, confinement to bed, and, in addition, development of hypercoagulability due to release of procoagulant material from tumor cells.[12] Thus there are many possible mechanisms leading to a thrombotic diathesis in cancer.

Despite some persisting controversies, *it is generally accepted that women who use oral contraceptives are at an increased risk of developing thrombosis and its attendant complications such as embolism.* This subject is discussed in greater detail on p. 266; suffice it to say that the risk is highest in women between 35 and 45 years of age, and concomitant cigarette smoking compounds the hazards of thrombotic disease considerably.

*Arterial thrombi are particularly likely to develop in patients with myocardial infarction, rheumatic heart disease, florid atherosclerosis, and aneurysmal dilatations of the aorta or other major arteries.*[18] Myocardial infarction usually is associated with damage to the adjacent endocardium, providing a site for the origin of a mural thrombus, usually within the left ventricle (Fig. 3–13). Stasis and turbulence within the affected cardiac chamber are usually also present because of dyskinetic contraction of the myocardium or the development of cardiac irregularities. Advanced age, bed rest, and impaired circulation compound the problem. Rheumatic heart disease often leads to marked stenosis of the mitral valve and, along with it, stasis within the markedly dilated left atrium and atrial appendage. Concomitantly there may be cardiac arrhythmias augmenting the stasis. Florid atherosclerosis underlying the dominant causes of mortality in industrialized nations—i.e., myocardial infarction and stroke—is a prime initiator of thromboses for what must now be obvious reasons. But, in addition to all of the serious obstructive consequences, thrombi in the aorta and in the cardiac chambers often yield fragments that embolize to such sites as (1) the brain, (2) the kidney, (3) the legs, and (4) the spleen. Other tissues or organs may also be affected, but the brain, kidneys, and spleen constitute prime targets because of their large blood flow volume. The iliac, femoral, and more distal arteries of the lower legs represent the "ends of the line" of the aortic flow.

Although many high-risk clinical disorders have been cited, it should emphasized that thrombosis may occur in any clinical setting and sometimes arises in otherwise healthy, active young individuals, particularly those whose work involves long periods of standing or sitting. Therefore, no individual is immune, and ultimately thrombosis is an unpredictable, puzzling disorder of quixotic nature.

## MICROCIRCULATORY THROMBOSIS—DISSEMINATED INTRAVASCULAR COAGULATION (DIC)

In many disease states, minute thrombi form in widely dispersed sites within the microcirculation, principally in capillaries and venules. The thrombi are largely made up of aggregated platelets admixed with some fibrin. They are rarely visible on gross inspection but in the aggregate can cause circulatory insufficiency, principally in the lungs, brain, heart, and kidneys. DIC is not a primary disorder; rather, it is a complication of some underlying disease which, in some manner, activates the processes involved in blood clotting.[19] Paradoxically, the innumerable small thrombi may lead to a hemorrhagic diathesis. The bleeding tendency is probably attributable to the rapid consumption of platelets, prothrombin, fibrinogen, and factors V, VIII, and X; hence DIC is sometimes also referred to as *defibrination syndrome* or *consumption coagulopathy*. The clinical settings in which DIC is encountered are extremely diverse and are discussed in greater detail on page 395. It suffices for here that this complex clotting disorder may, on the one hand, cause clinical manifestations by occlusion of the microcirculation in one or more organs or, on the other hand, lead to a serious hemorrhagic diathesis.

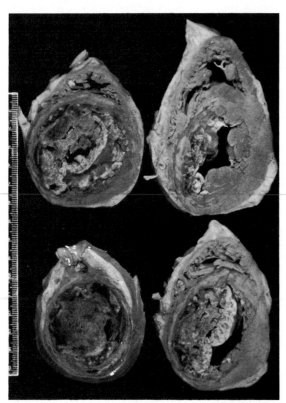

Figure 3–13. Multiple transections of the ventricles of a heart with a recent myocardial infarction. The left ventricle is virtually filled with thrombus, particularly toward the apex of the heart.

# EMBOLISM

*Embolism refers to occlusion of some part of the cardiovascular system by the impaction of some mass (embolus) transported to the site through the bloodstream.* The great majority of emboli represent some part or the whole of a dislodged thrombus, hence the commonly used term *thromboembolism.* Much less commonly, embolization is produced by droplets of fat, undissolved air or gas bubbles, atherosclerotic debris (cholesterol emboli), tumor fragments, bits of bone marrow, or any other substance that gains entry to the bloodstream (such as a bullet). Collectively, the unusual forms of embolism account for less than 1% of all instances, and so, unless otherwise indicated, embolism is considered to be thrombotic in origin.

Embolism may occur within either the venous or the arterial system. **In approximately 95% of instances, venous emboli arise from thrombi** within the veins of the leg in the locations previously mentioned (p. 72). Much more rarely they arise in pelvic veins, the right heart, or elsewhere. They drain through progressively larger channels, usually pass through the right heart, and become lodged in the pulmonary circulation (Fig. 3–14). Regrettably, not one but many emboli may become

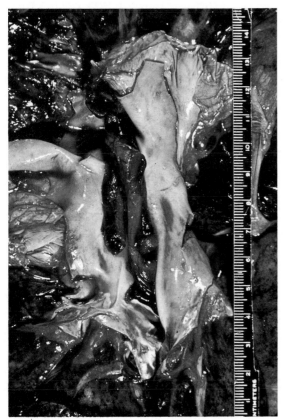

Figure 3–14. The opened major pulmonary arteries in the root of the lung. A large, coiled embolus having the diameter of one of the large veins in the leg was the cause of the sudden death of this patient.

dislodged, often at recurrent intervals. Thus, the patient who has had one pulmonary embolus is at high risk of having more. Indeed, at times the pulmonary circulation is peppered by a shower of small fragments. Rarely, a large, snake-like mass may become coiled upon itself and lodge in one of the valvular orifices of the right side of the heart. Alternatively, it may impinge on the bifurcation of the main pulmonary artery and sit astride the two major subdivisions, thus creating a **saddle embolus.** The size of the vessel occluded obviously depends on the size of the mass. Very infrequently, when congenital malformations of the heart produce right-to-left shunts, venous emboli may enter the left heart chambers and thus gain access to the arterial system. This phenomenon is known as **paradoxical embolism.**

Pulmonary embolism is the most serious form of thromboembolic disease. It is an extremely common clinical problem that is discussed in greater detail on page 407. Here we wish to discuss it only as an archetype, albeit the most important, of embolic disease. Meticulous dissection of the lungs reveals evidence of pulmonary embolism in up to 64% of autopsies.[20] Many of these emboli were small, produced no clinical symptoms and were of little significance. Nonetheless, past surveys have disclosed that pulmonary embolism is the prime or contributing cause of death in about 15% of hospitalized patients[21] and one of the most common causes of death among hospitalized patients in the United States.[16] Not all pulmonary emboli are fatal. Much depends on the size of the occluded vessel and the status of the patient's cardiovascular system. Large emboli (which obstruct more than 50% of pulmonary vascular flow) are often fatal because they cause either mechanical obstruction and massive strain on the right side of the heart (acute cor pulmonale) or sudden, severe hypoxemia. Reflex vascular and bronchiolar constriction worsens the respiratory deficit.[22] Death may be literally instantaneous, before ischemic changes can evolve in the lung parenchyma. Smaller emboli pass into the smaller branches of the pulmonary arterial system to cause either pulmonary hemorrhage or pulmonary infarction (p. 408). In younger patients with good cardiac function, the bronchial circulation may be sufficient to maintain the vitality of the lung tissue even though the pulmonary arterial supply is cut off. Intra-alveolar hemorrhage then results from collateral flow into the ischemic, weakened capillaries deprived of much of their blood supply. With less effective cardiac circulation, the bronchial supply may not suffice and infarction develops. It is estimated that overall only 10% of pulmonary emboli result in infarction.

It is remarkable that in those who survive pulmonary embolism, resolution of pulmonary vascular obstruction begins rapidly owing to activation of fibrinolysis and apparent fragmentation of the clot. Normal blood flow as evidenced by pulmonary angiography may be restored in 10 to 14 days.

*Arterial emboli* most commonly arise from intracardiac mural thrombi. Less often they take origin from mural thrombi in an aortic aneurysm or from those overlying atherosclerotic plaques in the aorta or some other large artery. Infrequently arterial emboli arise from fragmentation of a vegetation on a heart valve (discussed in more detail on p. 337). Occlusive thrombi in arteries of medium to small size rarely embolize, since they are usually firmly lodged at their sites of origin. In contrast to venous emboli, arterial masses usually follow a shorter pathway, since they travel through vessels of progressively diminishing caliber. The site of lodgement depends to a considerable extent on the point of origin of the thromboembolus and the volume of blood flow through an organ or tissue. The consequences of such emboli are somewhat dependent on the richness of the vascular supply of the affected tissue, its vulnerability to ischemia, and the caliber of the vessel occluded. These considerations are dealt with on page 78.

## FAT EMBOLISM

Minute globules of fat can often be demonstrated in the circulation following fractures of the shafts of long bones (which have fatty marrows) and rarely with soft tissue trauma and burns. Presumably the microglobules are released by injury to marrow or adipose tissue and gain access to the circulation by rupture of the marrow vascular sinusoids or venules. It should be emphasized that whereas *traumatic fat embolism can be demonstrated anatomically in approximately 90% of individuals sustaining severe skeletal injuries, only about 1% of these individuals manifest clinical signs or symptoms known as fat embolism syndrome.* It is characterized by pulmonary insufficiency (resembling the acute respiratory distress syndrome, p. 410), neurologic symptoms, anemia, and thrombocytopenia. Typically the symptoms appear after a latent period of 24 to 72 hours after injury. There is sudden onset of tachypnea, dyspnea, and tachycardia. Neurologic symptoms include irritability and restlessness, which progress to delirium or coma. Petechial skin rash is common. The fat embolism syndrome is fatal in about 10% of cases.[23, 24]

The pathogenesis of this symptom complex is not entirely clear but is believed to involve both mechanical obstruction and chemical injury. It is proposed that microaggregates of neutral fat cause occlusion of pulmonary or cerebral microvasculature, and the free fatty acids released from fat globules result in toxic injury to the vascular endothelium.[23, 24] The petechial skin rash is related to rapid onset of thrombocytopenia. Presumably myriads of fat globules are coated with platelets, thus depleting circulating platelets.

The microscopic demonstration of fat microglobules in tissues or organs requires special techniques using frozen sections and fat stains because the emboli are dissolved out of the blood by the usual solvents employed in paraffin embedding of tissues. Sometimes the microemboli can be identified in the gross specimen by gentle pressure on fresh tissue slices immersed in saline, which releases the droplets and permits them to float to the surface.

## CAISSON DISEASE

A particular form of gas embolism, known as *caisson disease* or *decompression sickness*, may appear in deep sea and scuba divers, in underwater construction workers, and in individuals in unpressurized aircraft that ascend rapidly to high altitudes. As deep sea divers descend to greater depths, air pressure is increased within the diving suit and helmet to compensate for the water pressure. The gases within the pressurized air are dissolved in the blood, tissue fluid, and fat. If the diver then ascends to the surface too rapidly, the dissolved oxygen, carbon dioxide, and nitrogen may come out of solution in the form of minute bubbles. Although the first two gases are rapidly solubilized, the nitrogen is of low solubility and persists as minute bubbles. Essentially the same sequence transpires with ascent from normal atmospheric pressures to the rarefied atmosphere of high altitudes.

The formation of minute gas bubbles within the skeletal muscles and supporting tissues in and about joints creates what is known as *"the bends."* Emboli may induce foci of necrosis in the brain, highly vascularized bones, the heart, or other tissues or organs. In the lungs, edema, hemorrhages, and focal atelectasis or emphysema may appear, sometimes leading to sudden respiratory distress, called *"the chokes."* Treatment of gas embolism consists of placing the individual in a compression chamber where the barometric pressure may be raised. This speeds the solution of the gas bubbles and permits slow decompression of the individual. However, when this condition is unrecognized, or when such therapy is not available, serious medical consequences may occur, as is still evident among native sponge and pearl divers in many locales around the world.

## AMNIOTIC FLUID EMBOLISM (AMNIOTIC FLUID INFUSION)

This disorder of mysterious origin occurs in about one in 50,000 to 80,000 deliveries. As the other major causes of maternal mortality—pulmonary thromboembolism, hemorrhage, and toxemia—decrease in incidence, amniotic embolism is assuming increased importance because it is often fatal, totally unpredictable, and largely unpreventable.[25] Typically it appears in older, multiparous patients who have a tumultuous labor, and it is characterized by sudden dyspnea, cyanosis, collapse, hemorrhage, and often convulsions followed by coma. Despite emergency therapy, which can only be supportive, 85 to 90% of these patients die.[26] The classic findings in the pulmonary arterioles and capillaries at autopsy comprise epithelial squames from fetal skin; lanugo hairs; fat from vernix caseosa; and mucin, presumed to be from the fetal gastrointestinal tract. Extensive fibrin thrombi, indicative of disseminated intravascular coagulation (DIC) (p. 397), are found in the small vessels of uterus, lung, kidney, thyroid, and myocardium.

The pathogenesis of amniotic fluid embolism is still unclear. There is little doubt that the symptom complex is triggered by infusions of amniotic fluid into the blood. Such entry may occur through endocervical veins, the uteroplacental site, or lacerations of the uterus or cervix. At one time it was thought that particulate matter within the amniotic fluid (e.g., epithelial squames, vernix caseosa) was responsible for pulmonary vascular obstruction. Recently attention has turned to the possibility that vasoactive substances within the amniotic fluid such as prostaglandins may be the cause of pulmonary vasconstriction. Additionally, one or more thrombogenic factors within the amniotic fluid induce intravascular coagulation, leading in effect to DIC and its attendant complications such as hemorrhages and acute renal failure. Present therapy is directed toward countering shock, hypoxemia, and controlling DIC.

## INFARCTION

*An infarct is an area of ischemic necrosis within a tissue or organ produced by occlusion of either its arterial supply or its venous drainage.* Nearly all infarcts result from thrombotic or embolic occlusion, but sometimes infarction may be caused by other mechanisms, such as ballooning of an atheroma secondary to hemorrhage within a plaque. Other uncommon causes include twisting of the vessels to the ovary or a loop of bowel, compression of the blood supply of a loop of bowel in a hernial sac, or trapping of a viscus under a peritoneal adhesion. In these last-mentioned situations the veins alone or both the veins and arteries may be blocked, but often the final occlusive episode is thrombotic closure of the already narrowed vessel. However, vascular occlusion does not always produce infarction, as will become clear later.

*Nearly 99% of infarcts are caused by thromboembolic events and almost all are the result of arterial occlusions.* Emboli arising in the heart or major arteries must impact in arteries. Similarly, venous thromboemboli lodge in the pulmonary arterial system and so cause arterial infarcts. Although venous thrombosis may cause infarction of some tissue or organ, more often it merely induces venous obstruction. Usually bypass channels develop, providing some outflow from the area, which in turn permits some improvement in the arterial inflow. Infarcts caused by venous thrombosis are more likely in organs having a single venous outflow channel, such as the testis and ovary.

**Infarcts are crudely divided into two types—white (anemic) and red (hemorrhagic).** This differentiation is quite arbitrary and is based merely upon the amount of hemorrhage that occurs in the area of infarction at the moment of vascular occlusion. This in turn depends on the solidity of the tissue involved and on the type of vascular compromise (venous or arterial). Most infarcts in solid organs result from arterial occlusion and are white or pale. The solidity of the tissue limits the amount of hemorrhage into the area of ischemic necrosis. **The heart, spleen, and kidneys exemplify solid, compact organs that develop white or pale infarcts. In contrast, the lung usually suffers hemorrhagic or red infarction** (Fig. 3–15). This loose, spongy organ permits blood to collect in the infarct from the anastomotic capillary circulation in the margins of the necrotic area. Hemorrhagic infarction is also encountered in those organs in which the venous outflow is limited to the obstructed vessel and in which bypass channels cannot develop. The ovary and the testis are the best examples of such. The entire ovarian blood supply and outflow pass through the mesovarium, and the testicular venous drainage traverses the spermatic cord. A twist in either of these organs may occlude only the thin-walled venous outflow tract. Similarly, hemorrhagic venous infarction may be encountered in loops of the intestine or in the brain (from bilateral occlusion of the jugular vein). Another uncommon mech-

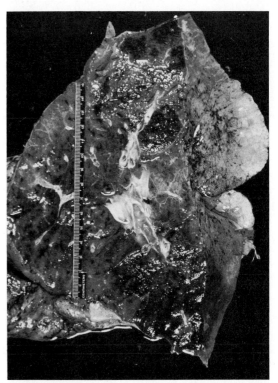

Figure 3–15. The transected surface of a lung, showing several dark hemorrhagic infarcts most evident at the apex and lower right. The infarction is recent and poorly demarcated from the adjacent, preserved lung substance.

anism for hemorrhagic infarction of the brain deserves passing mention. An arterial embolus may impact in a large artery such as the middle cerebral and induce a large area of nonhemorrhagic infarction. Subsequently, the embolus may shatter and the small fragments may move onward into smaller vessels, permitting "reflow" and hemorrhage into the primary area of ischemia.

All infarcts, red and white, tend to be wedge-shaped, with the occluded vessel at the apex and the periphery of the organ forming the base. Sometimes the margins are quite irregular, reflecting the pattern of vascular supply from adjacent vessels. When the base is a serosal surface, there is often a covering fibrinous exudate. At the outset, all infarcts are poorly defined and slightly hemorrhagic. In solid organs in which the lesions have relatively little hemorrhage, the contained red cells are laked and the released hemoglobin either diffuses out or is transformed to hemosiderin. **Thus, in the course of approximately 48 hours, infarcts in solid organs become progressively more pale and more sharply delimited** (Fig. 3–16). In spongy organs, such as the lungs, too many red cells are present to permit the lesion ever to become pale. The infarct is at first spongy and cyanotic (red-blue). Over the course of a few days, it becomes more firm and brown, reflecting the development of hemosiderin pigment. The margins of both types of infarcts, in the course of a few days, become progres-sively better defined. The delimitation is produced by the hypermia accompanying the acute inflammatory response from the surrounding vital substance.

The dominant histologic characteristic of infarction is ischemic coagulative necrosis of affected cells (p. 15). It should be noted, however, that if the patient dies imme-diately after having sustained the infarction, insufficient time may have elapsed to permit the enzymic alteration in cells that follow cell death. Thus, for example, in sudden death after myocardial infarction both light and electron microscopy may disclose no demonstrable cytologic or histologic changes in the heart. The dynamic sequence and time required for the appearance of changes following cell death have been described in Chapter 1, to which reference should be made for an understanding of this important consideration. In hemorrhagic or red infarcts, the suffusion of red cells often seems to obliterate the native underlying architecture. In this connection, the pulmonary hemorrhage is distinguished from an infarct by preservation of the native structure. Only the alveolar spaces are filled with red cells; the alveolar walls, blood vessels and stroma are preserved.

Most infarcts are ultimately replaced by scar tissue, which often contains hemosiderin granules as residua of the broken-down red cells. The time required for repair of an infarct depends on many factors, particularly on the size of the lesion, the adequacy of the still preserved blood supply supporting the fibroproliferative response, and the availability of the nutrients required for the prolif-eration of fibroblasts and blood vessels.

When an infarct is produced by an infected embolus (**septic embolus**), as may occur with a fragment of a bacterial vegetation from a heart valve, or when organ-isms of bacteremic origin seed the area of devitalized tissue, the infarct virtually is converted to an abscess.

**FACTORS CONDITIONING THE DEVELOPMENT OF AN INFARCT.** Occlusion of an artery or vein may have little or no effect on the involved tissue, or it may cause death of the tissue, and indeed of the individ-ual. *The major determinants include (1) the nature of the vascular supply, (2) the rate of development of the occlusion, (3) the vulnerability of the tissue to hypoxia, and (4) the oxygen-carrying capacity of the blood.*

*Nature of Vascular Supply.* The availability of an *alternative or newly acquired source of blood supply* is perhaps the most important factor in determining whether occlusion of a vessel will cause damage.

As was indicated previously, blockage of a small radicle of the pulmonary arterial tree may be without effect in a young person having a normal bronchial circulation. The same applies to the liver, with its double blood supply of hepatic artery and portal vein. In the young, healthy individual, occlusion of one point in the circle of Willis may be without effect if the patient's vessels are not narrowed by preexistent disease. Infarction or gangrene of the hand or forearm is almost never encountered, because of the double arterial supply through the radial and ulnar arteries, with their numerous interconnections. Such could

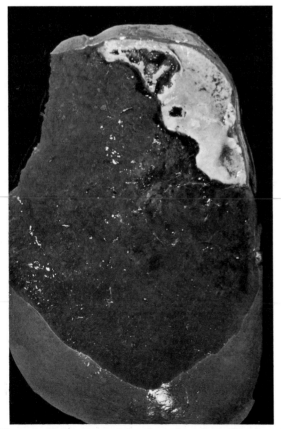

**Figure 3–16.** The transected surface of a spleen with a 1-week-old pale, sharply demarcated infarct.

occur only if both major arteries were simultaneously occluded.

Newly acquired *collateral circulation* may be equally effective in preventing infarction. The coronary arterial supply to the myocardium is an excellent case in point. Small anastomoses normally exist between the three major coronary trunks—i.e., the left anterior descending, the left circumflex, and the right coronary arteries. If one of these trunks is slowly narrowed, as by an atheroma, these anastomoses may enlarge sufficiently to prevent infarction, even though the major coronary artery is eventually occluded.

*Rate of Development of Occlusion.* Slowly developing occlusions are less likely to cause infarction since they provide an opportunity for alternative pathways of flow and anastomotic bypass channels to develop.

*Vulnerability of Tissue to Hypoxia.* The susceptibility of the tissue to hypoxia influences the likelihood of infarction. Neurons of the nervous system undergo irreversible damage when deprived of their blood supply for 3 to 4 minutes. Myocardial cells, although hardier than neurons, are also quite sensitive to anoxia. In contrast, the fibroblasts within the myocardium are unaffected and are quite resistant to hypoxia. The epithelial cells of the proximal renal tubules are much more vulnerable to hypoxia than are the other segments of the nephron.

*Oxygen-Carrying Capacity of Blood. The oxygen level of the blood* will obviously be of significance in determining the effect of vascular occlusion or narrowing. The anemic or cyanotic patient tolerates arterial insufficiency less well than does the normal patient. Occlusion of a small vessel might lead to an infarction in those so handicapped, whereas it would be without effect at normal levels of oxygen transport. In this way, cardiac decompensation with its circulatory stasis and possibly reduced levels of oxygen saturation of the blood contribute to, and indeed may be critical in, determining whether the patient with a pulmonary arterial occlusion will develop only a pulmonary hemorrhage or an infarction.

CLINICAL CORRELATION. Infarction of tissues underlies some of the most frequent as well as most serious clinical disorders. The two most common forms of infarction are myocardial and pulmonary. The primary cause of death today in the United States and in other industrialized nations is coronary heart disease, and the great preponderance of these deaths result from myocardial infarction. Less awesome, but still gravely significant, is pulmonary infarction. Infarction of the brain (encephalomalacia) (p. 734) is another very common "infarct killer." Infarction of the small or large intestine happily is not a common disease, but when it does occur, it is frequently fatal. Less grave, but nonetheless productive of clinical signs and symptoms and possibly of serious disease, are renal and splenic infarcts.

Infarctions tend to have a special gravity because they are most common in patients least able to withstand them. Thus infarcts tend to occur in aged individuals with advanced atherosclerosis or cardiac decompensation. The postoperative and postdelivery periods are also times of increased vulnerability. The anemic or cyanotic patient is often fragile and poorly prepared for further insult. The triad of thrombosis, embolism, and infarction therefore resembles the proverbial vultures always hovering over the heads of those least able to withstand the attack.

# SHOCK

Shock, often loosely called "vascular collapse," is traditionally viewed as a perfusion deficit, *a state in which the supply of blood to the tissues is inadequate to meet the metabolic demands.* It initially causes reversible hypoxic injury, but if it is sufficiently prolonged, cells and tissues suffer irreversible injury, which leads eventually to death. This definition stresses hemodynamic failure and is quite appropriate for some forms of shock (e.g., that induced by massive hemorrhage or extensive myocardial infarction). However, it is inadequate for shock induced by overwhelming sepsis (Table 3–2). The latter, as we shall see, is a multifactorial disorder in which toxic cellular injury and consequent inability to use available substrate is as important as failure of perfusion.[27]

Shock may be precipitated by any massive insult to the body, such as profuse hemorrhage, severe trauma or burns, extensive myocardial infarction, massive pulmonary embolism, or uncontrolled bacterial sepsis. All these various causes of shock can be grouped under a mechanistic classification presented in Table 3–2. A review of this table will indicate that the mechanisms underlying cardiogenic and hypovolemic shock are fairly obvious. As might be ex-

**Table 3–2. CLASSIFICATION OF SHOCK**

| Type of Shock | Clinical Examples | Principal Mechanisms |
| --- | --- | --- |
| *Cardiogenic* | Myocardial infarction Rupture of heart Arrhythmias Cardiac tamponade Pulmonary embolism | Failure of myocardial pump due to intrinsic myocardial damage or extrinsic pressure or obstruction to outflow |
| *Hypovolemic* | Hemorrhage Fluid loss—e.g., vomiting, diarrhea, burns | Inadequate blood or plasma volume |
| *Septic* | Overwhelming bacterial infections: gram-negative septicemia ("endotoxic shock") or gram-positive septicemia | Peripheral vasodilatation and pooling of blood; cell membrane injury, endothelial cell injury with disseminated intravascular coagulation |
| *Neurogenic* | Anesthesia, spinal cord injury | Peripheral vasodilatation with pooling of blood |

pected, they are *associated with low cardiac output, hypotension, impaired tissue perfusion, and cellular hypoxia*. The basis of septic shock is much more complex and still imperfectly understood.[28] The majority of cases of septic shock are caused by endotoxin-producing gram-negative bacilli—*Escherichia coli, Klebsiella pneumoniae*, Proteus species, *Pseudomonas aeruginosa*—and hence the term *endotoxic shock*. However, gram-positive cocci such as pneumococci and streptococci may produce a similar syndrome. In contrast to hypovolemic and cardiogenic shock, the *cardiac output in septic shock is not low at the outset*. However, the total peripheral resistance is inappropriately low, owing to arteriolar vasodilatation. This results principally from release of vasoactive mediators such as complement components, kinins, and platelet products (Fig. 3–17; see also Chapter 2) but direct toxic injury to the vessels may also be involved. As a consequence, veins (the so-called capacitance vessels) become engorged with blood, producing peripheral pooling. *Thus a state of relative hypovolemia and impaired perfusion results from a disproportion between circulating blood volume and the expanded volume of the circulating bed.* Sequestration of large volumes of blood in the capacitance vessels impairs venous return and leads eventually to low cardiac output. Endotoxins or other bacterial toxins play havoc on many other fronts: *Endothelial injury* leads to activation of both the

intrinsic and extrinsic clotting pathways, leading to *disseminated intravascular coagulation*, which further aggravates tissue hypoxia. Activation of *complement* generates many factors, including those that increase vascular permeability and attract neutrophils. The latter serve as reservoirs of additional toxic and vasoactive moieties (p. 41). More recently, endotoxin-mediated activation of the mononuclear phagocyte system and the consequent release of interleukin 1 (IL-1) from macrophages has received much attention.[29] As indicated in Figure 3–17, IL-1 affects several organ systems including endocrine pancreas, muscle, and hypothalamus. We mentioned earlier that bacterial toxins also cause direct injury to cells and tissues. Thus even the cells that are well perfused fail to extract adequate oxygen from the blood. This results in a subnormal arteriovenous oxygen difference often noted in septic shock. *To summarize, septic shock is associated with distributive defects (peripheral pooling), endotoxin-mediated activation of the inflammatory-immune response, and direct toxic injury to cells and tissues.*

**STAGES OF SHOCK.** Shock is a progressive disorder that, if uncorrected, may lead to death. Unless the insult is massive and rapidly lethal (e.g., a massive hemorrhage from a ruptured aortic aneurysm or an extensive infarct affecting the left ventricle), shock tends to evolve through three stages (Fig. 3–18): (I) an initial *nonprogressive phase* during which reflex

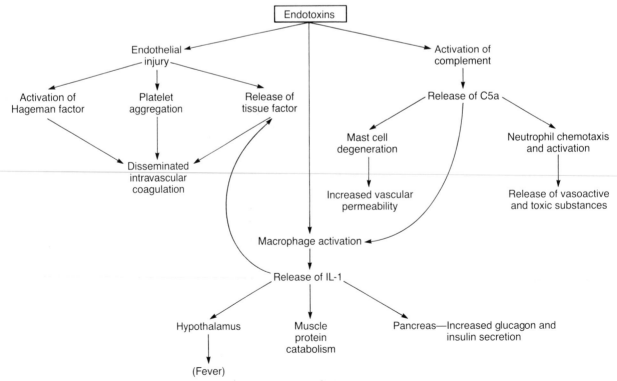

Figure 3–17. Role of endotoxins in the pathogenesis of septic shock.

compensatory mechanisms are activated and perfusion of vital organs is preserved; (II) *a progressive stage* characterized by tissue hypoperfusion and onset of an ever-widening circle of circulatory and metabolic imbalances, and finally, (III) an *irreversible stage* that sets in after the body has incurred cellular and tissue injury so severe that even if therapy corrects the hemodynamic defects, survival is not possible. Admittedly, these stages are somewhat arbitrary, but a brief discussion of this sequence will serve to integrate the sequential pathophysiologic and clinical alterations in shock.

During "early shock" (say, following blood loss), a *variety of neurohumoral mechanisms come into play to maintain cardiac output and blood pressure.* These include the baroreceptor reflexes, release of catecholamines, activation of the renin-angiotensin axis, antidiuretic hormone release, and generalized sympathetic stimulation.[30] The effect of all these is to produce *tachycardia, peripheral vasoconstriction, and conservation of fluid by the kidney.* The vasoconstrictor response is responsible for the coolness and pallor of skin. Since the coronary and cerebral vessels are less affected by the sympathetic response, their caliber is not significantly affected and thus oxygen continues to be delivered to these vital organs. Obviously, therapeutic maneuvers have the best chance of success at this stage. Uncorrected, shock passes imperceptibly to the progressive phase, during which the vital organs begin to experience significant hypoxia. With persistent oxygen deficit there is impair-

ment of intracellular aerobic respiration, followed by anaerobic glycolysis and excessive production of lactate, which often induces metabolic *lactic acidosis.* The lowering of pH in the tissues obtunds the vasomotor response; arterioles dilate and blood begins to pool in the microcirculation. Peripheral pooling not only worsens the cardiac output, it also favors anoxic injury to endothelial cells, thereby setting the stage for *disseminated intravascular coagulation.* Release of thromboxane $A_2$, a potent platelet aggregator, has also been implicated in the occlusion of microvasculature.[31] With widespread tissue hypoxia, the function of vital organs begins to deteriorate; often *the patient is confused and the urinary output begins to fall.*

At some point in the downward spiral there is transition from the reversible to the irreversible stage. Widespread cell injury allows leakage of lysosomal enzymes that further aggravate the shock state. *The ischemic pancreas liberates a myocardial depressant factor (MDF),* worsening the already poor cardiac performance. Endotoxic shock may be superimposed on hypovolemic or cardiogenic shock if the ischemic intestinal mucosa allows intestinal flora to enter the circulation. By this stage *the patient has complete renal shutdown due to acute tubular necrosis.* In closing, one may ask when does shock become irreversible? Some would argue that if the initiating cause is removed, shock is reversible at any stage. The issue is moot, but one fact is not: death from shock, despite the heroic measures afforded by modern intensive care units, is still an everyday affair.

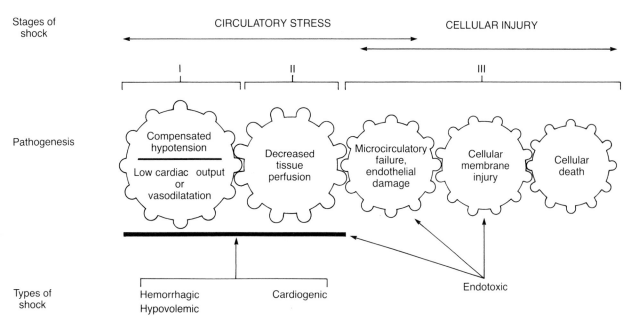

**Figure 3–18.** Pathogenesis and stages of shock. Stage I is nonprogressive, stage II is progressive, and stage III is irreversible. Note that endotoxic shock is multifactorial; it is associated with vasodilatation, decreased tissue perfusion, endothelial damage, and direct cellular injury. (Modified from Wyngaarden, J. B., and Smith, L. H., Jr.: Cecil Textbook of Medicine. 17th ed. Philadelphia, W. B. Saunders Co., 1985, p. 212.)

**MORPHOLOGY.** The cellular and tissue changes induced by shock are essentially those of hypoxic injury; only their distribution is somewhat distinctive. These were detailed earlier in Chapter 1.

Although cellular changes may appear in any tissue, they are particularly evident in the brain, heart, lungs, kidneys, adrenals, and gastrointestinal tract.

The **brain** may develop so-called ischemic encephalopathy, discussed on page 733.

The **heart** may disclose a variety of changes. Extensive lesions such as myocardial infarction or myocardial disease may, of course, be present. In addition, subendocardial hemorrhages and necrosis or "zonal lesions" sometimes appear in all forms of shock. The term "zonal lesions" refers to apparent hypercontraction of a myocyte, inducing shortening and scalloping of the sarcomere, fragmentation of the Z band, distortion of the myofilaments, and displacement of the mitochondria away from the intercalated disc. Subendocardial hemorrhages and zonal lesions are not diagnostic of shock and may be seen following administration of catecholamines or after prolonged use of the heart-lung bypass pump in cardiac surgery.

The **kidneys** may be severely affected in shock, and so oliguria, anuria, and electrolyte disturbances constitute major clinical problems. The renal changes are referred to as **acute tubular necrosis**, but since similar changes may be encountered in other settings, they are described in detail on page 476.

The **lungs** are seldom affected in pure hypovolemic shock because they are resistant to hypoxic injury. But when the vascular collapse is caused by bacterial sepsis or trauma, changes may appear that in essence consist of severe edema. The pulmonary lesions are now referred to as the "adult respiratory distress syndrome" or "diffuse alveolar damage." Since these anatomic changes may be caused by a variety of clinical derangements, they are described on page 412.

The **adrenal** alterations encountered in shock comprise in essence those common to all forms of stress and so might be referred to as **"the stress response."** Early there is focal depletion of lipids in the cortical cells beginning in the zona reticularis and then spreading progressively outward into the zona fasciculata. This loss of corticolipids implies not adrenal exhaustion but rather reversion of the relatively inactive vacuolated cells to metabolically active cells that utilize stored lipids for the synthesis of steroids. Isolated cell necroses may develop, creating apparent lumina or "pseudotubules."

The **gastrointestinal tract** may suffer patchy mucosal hemorrhages and necroses, referred to as "hemorrhagic enteropathy" (p. 526) (Fig. 3–19).

The **liver** may sometimes develop fatty change and, with severe perfusion deficits, central necrosis.

Virtually all of these organ changes may revert to normal if the patient survives. However, loss of neurons from the brain and of myocytes from the heart is, of course, irreversible. Moreover, persistent pulmonary septal edema may be converted into septal fibrosis, which is

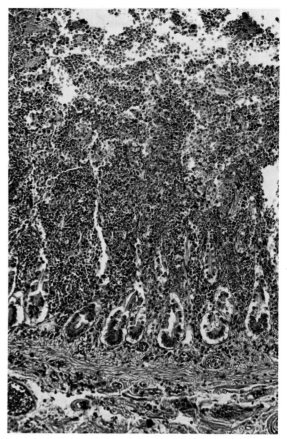

Figure 3–19. Hemorrhagic enteropathy in the colon. The superficial mucosa is entirely obscured by the extensive hemorrhage; only the bases of the colonic glands are visible. The submucosa is unaffected.

irreversible. However, most patients suffering shock of such severity as to produce irreversible changes succumb before these alterations become well developed.

**CLINICAL COURSE.** The clinical manifestations depend upon the precipitating insult. In hypovolemic and cardiogenic shock, *the patient presents with hypotension; an ashen gray pallor; cool, clammy skin; weak, thready pulse; and rapid cardiac and respiratory rates. With uncontrolled sepsis, however, the skin may be warm and indeed flushed owing to peripheral vasodilation.* The course of the patient in shock is beset with a sequence of hazards and pitfalls. The initial threat to life stems from the underlying catastrophe that precipitated the shock, such as the myocardial infarct, severe hemorrhage, or uncontrolled bacterial infection. However, the cardiac, cerebral, and pulmonary changes secondary to the shock state materially worsen the problem. Soon electrolyte disturbances and metabolic acidosis make their unwanted contributions. If all of these grave problems are survived, *the patient enters a second phase dominated by renal insufficiency* as is detailed on page 477. This may appear any time from the second to the sixth day and is marked by a progressive fall in urine output. Without going into detail, serious fluid and electrolyte imbalances now appear. If these can be managed with appropriate therapy, return of renal function is heralded by a "urinary flood tide." During this diuretic phase there is an increased vulnerability to microbiologic infections.

It is evident that the postshock course of the patient does not lack for threats to life. The prognosis varies with the origin of shock and its duration. For example, 80% of young, otherwise healthy patients with hypovolemic shock survive with appropriate management, whereas cardiogenic shock associated with extensive myocardial infarction, and gram-negative shock carry a mortality of 70 to 80%, even with the best care currently available.

## References

1. Jaffe, E. A.: Physiologic function of normal endothelial cells. Ann. N. Y. Acad. Sci. *454*:297, 1985.
2. Lammie, B., and Griffin, J. H.: Formation of the fibrin clot: The balance of procoagulant and inhibitory factors. Clin. Hematol. *14*:281, 1985.
3. Naworth, P., Kisiel, W., and Stern, D.: The role of endothelium in the hemostatic balance of hemostasis. Clin. Hematol. *14*:531, 1985.
4. Holmsen, H.: Platelet metabolism and activation. Semin. Hematol. *22*:219, 1985.
5. Bennett, J. S.: Blood coagulation and coagulation tests. Med. Clin. North Am. *68*:557, 1984.
6. Brandt, J. T.: The role of natural coagulation inhibitors in hemostasis. Clin. Lab. Med. *4*:245, 1984.
7. Shattil, S. J.: Diagnosis and treatment of recurrent venous thromboembolism. Med. Clin. North Am. *68*:577, 1984.
8. Fry, D. L.: Hemodynamic injury. *In* Chandler, A. B., et al. (eds.): The Thrombotic Process in Atherogenesis. New York, Plenum Press, 1978, p. 353.
9. Hamer, J. D., et al.: The $pO_2$ in venous valve pockets: Its possible bearing on thrombogenesis. Br. J. Surg. *68*:166, 1981.
10. Hume, M., et al.: Venous Thrombosis in Pulmonary Embolism. Cambridge, Harvard University Press, 1970, p. 25.
11. Beller, F. K., and Ebert, C. A.: Effects of oral contraceptives on blood coagulation. A review. Obstet. Gynecol. Surv. *40*:425, 1985.
12. Al-Mondhiry, H.: Tumor interaction with hemostasis: The rationale for use of platelet inhibitors and anti-coagulants in treatment of cancer. Am. J. Hematol. *16*:193, 1984.
13. Sabiston, D. C.: Pulmonary embolism. Surg. Gynecol. Obstet. *126*:1075, 1976.
14. Editorial: What happens to blood clots in the lungs? Lancet *1*:194, 1978.
15. Relman, A.: Intravenous thrombolysis in acute myocardial infarction: A progress report. N. Engl. J. Med. *312*:915, 1985.
16. Sharma, G. V. R. K., and Sasahara, A. A.: Diagnosis and treatment of pulmonary embolism. Med. Clin. North Am. *63*:239, 1979.
17. Sevitt, S.: Venous thrombosis and pulmonary embolism. Am. J. Med. *33*:703, 1962.
18. Schwartz, C. J., et al.: Clinical and pathological aspects of arterial thrombosis and thromboembolism. Adv. Exp. Med. Biol. *104*:111, 1978.
19. Lerner, R. G.: The defibrination syndrome. Med. Clin. North Am. *60*:871, 1976.
20. Frieman, D. G., et al.: Frequency of pulmonary thromboembolism in man. N. Engl. J. Med. *272*:1278, 1975.
21. McGlynn, J. T., Jr., et al.: Pulmonary embolism. J.A.C.E.P. *8*:532, 1979.
22. Sabiston, D. C.: Pathophysiology, diagnosis and management of pulmonary embolism. Am. J. Surg. *138*:384, 1979.
23. Peltier, L. F.: Fat embolism. Clin. Orthoped. *187*:3, 1984.
24. Seroto, M. L.: Fat embolism syndrome. West. J. Med. *141*:501, 1984.
25. Price, T. M., et al.: Amniotic fluid embolism. Three case reports with a review of the literature. Obstet. Gynecol. Surv. *40*:462, 1985.
26. Morgan, M.: Amniotic fluid embolism. Anaesthesia *34*:20, 1979.
27. Mizock, B.: Septic shock—A metabolic perspective. Arch. Int. Med. *144*:579, 1984.
28. Schwartz, R. A., and Cerra, F. B.: Shock: A practical approach. Urol. Clin. North Am. *10*:89, 1983.
29. Filkins, J. P.: Monokines and metabolic pathophysiology of shock. Fed. Proc. *44*:300, 1985.
30. Bond, R. F., and Johnson, G.: Vascular adrenergic interactions during hemorrhagic shock. Fed. Proc. *44*:281, 1985.
31. Lefer, A. M.: Eicosanoids as mediators of ischemia and shock. Fed. Proc. *44*:275, 1985.

# 4

# Genetic Diseases

From time immemorial every lover has intuitively known what science now stands on the threshold of proving—his loved one is truly unique. Even seemingly identical, monozygotic female twins probably have biochemical differences as a result of random inactivation of one of the X chromosomes. Within the past decade, remarkable advances have allowed deep penetrations into the mysteries of the genetic code and have disclosed seemingly endless genotypic and biochemical variations among individuals.[1] Recall that until as recently as 1956, when Tjio and Levan established the correct human chromosome count as 46, it was believed that humans possessed 48 chromosomes. Much of the recent progress in medical genetics has resulted from application of recombinant DNA techniques. It is possible, for example, to excise human genes and insert them into bacterial plasmids or phages, which are utilized as "cloning vectors." Under appropriate conditions, the human gene that has recombined with the DNA of the cloning vector can be replicated, transcribed, and translated. This technique has opened up new possibilities to analyze human genetic material, piece by piece. Several genes that cause serious disease have been characterized by these techniques. The origin of sickle cell anemia has been traced to the subtlest of mutations, the substitution of one purine base in the DNA sequence for another, resulting in the incorporation of valine rather than glutamic acid into the beta hemoglobin chains. More than 100 hemoglobin variants have subsequently been identified, arising from similar point mutations.

We are at the threshold of major medical applications of the burgeoning field of genetic engineering. It is now possible to produce a variety of ultrapure biologically active molecules by inserting cloned genes into bacterial plasmids. Examples of such products in current use include insulin, growth hormone, interferons, and interleukin 2 (an immunomodulator). The list continues to grow.[2] Current techniques also allow induction of site-localized mutations of DNA in vitro, making possible the repair or creation of mutations, the conversion of a gene of one species to the same gene of another, and the creation of genes for peptide analogs. Indeed, writers of science fiction may have to search for other professions!

Traditionally, the diseases of humans have been segregated into three categories: (1) those that are basically genetically determined, (2) those that are almost entirely environmentally determined, and (3) those to which both "nature" and "nurture" contribute. Advances in knowledge, however, have tended to blur these distinctions. At one time microbiologic infections were cited as examples of disorders arising wholly from environmental influences, but it is now clear that to some extent heredity conditions the immune response and the susceptibility to microbiologic infections. Despite these uncertainties, there is a large and ever-growing list of disorders referred to as "genetic diseases," whose prevalence is not generally appreciated.

Surveys indicate that as many as 20% of the pediatric inpatients in university hospital populations suffer from disorders of genetic origin. These data express only the tip of the iceberg. Chromosome aberrations have been identified in up to 50% of spontaneous abortuses during the first trimester. Only those mutations compatible with independent existence constitute the reservoir of genetic disease in the population at large. Many more abortuses must have had gene mutations.

It is beyond the scope of this book to review normal human genetics. It is necessary, however, to clarify several commonly used terms—*hereditary, familial,* and *congenital.* Hereditary disorders, by definition, are derived from one's parents, are transmitted in the gametes through the generations, and therefore are familial. The term *congenital* simply implies "born with." It should be noted that some congenital diseases are not genetic, as for example congenital syphilis. On the other hand, not all genetic diseases are congenital; patients with hereditary Huntington's chorea, for example, begin to manifest their condition only after the third or fourth decade of life.

*Genetic disorders fall into three major categories:* (1) *diseases with multifactorial (polygenic) inheritance,* (2) *those related to mutant genes of large effect, and* (3) *those arising in chromosomal aberrations.* The first category includes some of the most common disorders of humans, such as hypertension and diabetes mellitus. Multifactorial or polygenic inheritance implies that usually both genetic and environmental influences condition the expression of a phenotypic characteristic or disease. The genetic component involves the additive result of multiple genes of small effect; the environmental contribution may be small or large, and in some cases is required for expression of the phenotypic attribute. The second category, sometimes referred to as "mendelian disorders," includes many relatively rare conditions such as the "storage" diseases and inborn errors of metabolism, all resulting from single gene mutations of large effect. Most of these conditions are hereditary and familial. The third category includes disorders that have been shown to be the consequence of numerical or structural abnormalities in the chromosomes.

Each of these three categories will be discussed separately in the material to follow.

# DISORDERS WITH MULTIFACTORIAL (POLYGENIC) INHERITANCE

Multifactorial inheritance (also called polygenic) is involved in many of the physiologic characteristics of humans (e.g., height, weight, blood pressure, and hair color). *It may be defined as a physiologic or pathologic trait governed by the additive effect of two or more genes of small effect but conditioned by environmental, nongenetic influences.* Even monozygous twins reared separately may achieve different heights because of nutritional or other environmental influences. When surveyed in a large population, phenotypic attributes governed by multifactorial inheritance fall on a continuous or Gaussian distribution (Fig. 4–1). Presumably there is some threshold effect so that a disorder becomes manifest only when a certain number of effector genes as well as conditioning environmental influences are involved. The threshold effect also explains why parents of a child with a polygenic disorder may themselves be normal. Once the threshold value is exceeded, the severity of the disease is directly proportional to the number and the degree of influence of the pathologic genes.

Multifactorial disorders run in families, since family members share many of their genes as well as environmental influences. The risk of a disorder's being expressed depends to a large extent on the relationship of the family member to the proband. However, as pointed out, all multifactorial disorders involve environmental influences, and so risk factors are, at best, approximations. The concordance rate of a disease in monozygous twins is significantly less than 100% when multifactorial inheritance is involved. However, the chance of concordance in monozygous twins is much higher than that between first-degree relatives (siblings, parents, and offspring). For most multifactorial disorders, the first-degree relatives of the affected individual have a 5 to 10% risk of developing the disease. Since the second-degree relatives (uncles, aunts) share only one fourth of their genes with the proband, their risk of developing the disease is only in the range of 0.5 to 1%.

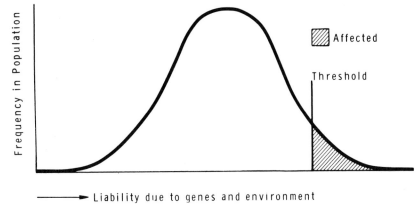

Figure 4–1. Multifactorial inheritance. The continuous distribution of the liability to develop a multifactorial disease is determined by many genes and the environment. A threshold of liability indicates the limit beyond which disease is expressed. (From Elsas, L. J., and Priest, J. H.: Medical Genetics. *In* Sodeman, W. A., and Sodeman, T. M. [eds.]: Pathologic Physiology: Mechanisms of Disease. 7th ed. Philadelphia, W. B. Saunders Co., 1985, p. 61.)

It is extremely difficult to establish multifactorial inheritance for any disease—much more difficult than for disorders related to mutant genes of large effect or those arising in chromosomal aberrations. Ascribing a disease to multifactorial inheritance must be based on familial clusterings and the exclusion of mendelian and chromosomal modes of transmission. This form of inheritance is believed to underlie such common diseases as diabetes mellitus, hypertension, gout, schizophrenia, manic depression, and certain forms of congenital heart disease, as well as some skeletal abnormalities. Hypertension provides an excellent example of multifactorial inheritance. There is good evidence that the level of blood pressure of an individual, at least in some part, is under genetic control, apparently governed by multiple genes of small effect. The pressure levels of the population at large fall along a continuous Gaussian curve of distribution. At some arbitrary level of blood pressure, hypertension is said to exist, since pressures above this level are associated with a significant disadvantage to the individual. Hypertension is described in Chapter 14. Here we will discuss diabetes mellitus, a common multifactorial disorder that affects multiple organ systems.

# DIABETES MELLITUS

Diabetes mellitus is a chronic disorder affecting carbohydrate, fat, and protein metabolism. *A defective or deficient insulin secretory response, which translates into impaired carbohydrate (glucose) use, is a characteristic feature of diabetes mellitus, as is the resulting hyperglycemia.* To this brief characterization the following qualifications must be added: (1) *Idiopathic (genetic) diabetes mellitus* must be distinguished from *secondary diabetes*, that is, hyperglycemia resulting from destruction of pancreatic islets by inflammation, surgery, tumors, or iron overload (hemochromatosis) or from endocrinopathies (e.g., Cushing's syndrome, acromegaly, and pheochromocytoma). The pathogenesis and clinical consequences of secondary diabetes differ from those of idiopathic diabetes. (2) Even "idiopathic diabetes mellitus" represents a heterogeneous group of disorders having hyperglycemia as a common feature. These can be basically divided into two variants, which differ from each other in their patterns of inheritance, insulin responses, and origins. *One variant, called insulin-dependent diabetes mellitus (IDDM), "Type I," "juvenile-onset," and "ketosis-prone diabetes," is seen in about 10% of all idiopathic diabetics. The remaining 90% of patients have the other variant, designated non–insulin-dependent diabetes mellitus (NIDDM).* This form of the disease often appears in adult life and so is sometimes referred to as "adult-onset or Type II diabetes." (3) Although heredity undoubtedly plays an important role in the development of both of these variants, environmental influ-

ences that "stress" the insulin-carbohydrate axis (e.g., viral infections, obesity, pregnancy) play a significant role in the expression of diabetes mellitus. (4) Most important, *the long-term effects of idiopathic diabetes mellitus are manifest principally in the vascular system, in the forms of atherosclerosis and small vessel disease (microangiopathy).* These vascular sequelae have devastating consequences, which spare no organ in the body.

**CLASSIFICATION.** Until recently, several classifications of diabetes have existed, based on differing criteria; some use clinical features, others etiology, and some the presumed natural history of diabetes. This led to confusion in terminology and, more importantly, to a lack of uniformity in the reporting of results by various investigators. In an attempt to overcome these problems, the National Diabetes Data Group of the National Institutes of Health has developed a classification incorporating all currently available information (Table 4–1).[3] Not included in this table but discussed in detail in the paper cited are criteria for diagnosis, a clinical procedure for classification, standards for evaluating obesity, and a wealth of other useful information.

**INCIDENCE.** With an annual death toll of about 35,000, diabetes mellitus is the seventh leading cause of death in the United States. The exact prevalence of diabetes is difficult to estimate since there are no "genetic markers" and identification is therefore based on the presence of symptoms. Given these limitations, it is estimated that the prevalence of diabetes is 1 to 2% in the adult population.

**INHERITANCE.** It has long been known that diabetes mellitus is at least in part a genetic familial disorder. However, the precise mode of inheritance of the gene or genes for susceptibility remains unknown. Part of the problem stems from the fact that until recently it was assumed that idiopathic diabetes mellitus was a homogeneous entity, and therefore attempts were made to find a single pattern of inheritance that would fit all cases. It is now agreed that IDDM and NIDDM exhibit substantial genetic differences. Evidence in support of such a conclusion derives from studies of identical twins and of histocompatibility antigens.

Among identical twins, the concordance rate (i.e., both twins affected) of IDDM is approximately 50%, whereas with NIDDM the rate is over 90%.[4] It is clear from this study that genetic factors are of greater importance in the genesis of NIDDM than in that of IDDM. Since discordance between identical twins is as frequent as concordance in IDDM, environmental factors must play a large role in its development. The question is, do environmental factors alone govern the occurrence of IDDM or, alternatively, do genetic factors act in concert with some environmental agent? The answer to this question is provided by the study of HLA types in diabetes mellitus. As will be discussed in another chapter (p. 133), HLA refers to a polymorphic gene complex that codes for certain cell-surface antigens found on leukocytes and other tissue cells. In Caucasoid populations there is a strong positive association between IDDM and HLA-DR3 and -DR4 antigens. Individuals who are HLA-DR3–positive have a fivefold greater risk of developing IDDM, as compared with those who are HLA-DR3–negative. The relative risk with HLA-DR4 is approximately 6.8. It is noteworthy that the relative risk in DR3/DR4 heterozygotes is more than additive (approximately 14.3) suggesting that there are two distinct susceptibility genes linked to the HLA-DR region.[5] Since genes that regulate the normal immune response (Ir genes) also map within the HLA-D region, these studies raise the possibility that the diabetogenic genes may function by regulating the immune response to potentially damaging environmental (microbiologic) agents. *No association with*

*HLA is seen in NIDDM,* which not only confirms the impression from twin studies that NIDDM is distinct from IDDM but also suggests that the susceptibility genes for NIDDM are not linked to the HLA region of the genome.

Despite all the collective evidence supporting some role for genetic factors in both IDDM and NIDDM, the specific inheritance patterns of both variants of the disease are still unknown. Virtually every mode of transmission has been invoked, including autosomal recessive, autosomal dominant, and multifactorial (polygenic). Although minor subsets may differ, *currently favored is the view that both IDDM and NIDDM are multifactorial disorders*, a proposal that best fits the wide variation in severity of both forms of the disease and provides for a role for environmental factors.

**Table 4–1.** CLASSIFICATION OF DIABETES MELLITUS AND OTHER CATEGORIES OF GLUCOSE INTOLERANCE*

| Class | Former Terminology | Associated Factors | Clinical Characteristics |
|---|---|---|---|
| *Clinical Classes* | | | |
| *Diabetes Mellitus (DM)* | | | |
| Insulin-dependent type (IDDM)—Type I | Juvenile diabetes Ketosis-prone diabetes Brittle diabetes | Associated with certain HLA types and presence of autoimmune reactions. Both genetic and environmental (viral) factors involved in etiology. | Absolute lack of insulin and dependent upon injected insulin to prevent ketosis and preserve life. In most cases onset in youth, but may occur at any age. |
| Non-insulin-dependent types (NIDDM)—Type II 1. Obese NIDDM 2. Nonobese NIDDM | Adult-onset DM Maturity-onset DM Ketosis-resistant DM | Probably multiple origins. Both genetic and environmental factors involved. Obesity is suspected as an etiologic factor and used for subclassification. No HLA linkage. | Serum insulin levels normal, elevated, or low. In most cases onset after age 40, but can occur at any age. About 60% of subjects are obese. |
| Other types, include DM associated with other identifiable causes | Secondary DM | (1) Pancreatic disease, (2) hormonal diseases (e.g., Cushing's), (3) drug-induced, (4) insulin receptor abnormalities, (5) certain genetic syndromes. | Diabetes mellitus and associated clinical features. |
| *Impaired Glucose Tolerance (IGT)* | Asymptomatic DM Chemical diabetes Latent diabetes | Glucose intolerance mild; may be due to normal variation in a population. In some cases represents a stage in development of NIDDM or IDDM. Majority remain in this class for years or return to normal glucose tolerance. | Glucose tolerance test (GTT) shows values between normal and diabetic. Some suggestion of increased risk for arterial disease but clinically significant renal and retinal lesions absent. |
| *Gestational Diabetes (GDM)* | Gestational diabetes | Glucose intolerance that has its onset and recognition during pregnancy. Complex metabolic and hormonal factors involved, including insulin resistance. Diabetics who become pregnant are not included. Associated with increased perinatal complications and with increased risk for progression to diabetes in 5 to 10 years after childbirth. | |
| *Statistical Risk Classes* | | | |
| *Previous Abnormality of Glucose Tolerance (PrevAGT)* | Latent diabetes Prediabetes | Persons who have normal glucose tolerance now but have previously demonstrated diabetic hyperglycemia or IGT either spontaneously or in response to an identifiable stimulus. Individuals with GDM who return to normal form a subclass of PrevAGT. It is likely that the risk of these patients' developing DM is higher. | |
| *Potential Abnormality of Glucose Tolerance (PotAGT)* | Prediabetes | Individuals who have never exhibited abnormal glucose tolerance but have a substantially increased risk for development of diabetes (e.g., monozygotic twin, sibling, or offspring of a known diabetic). | |

*Modified from National Diabetes Data Group: Classification and diagnosis of diabetes mellitus and other categories of glucose intolerance. Diabetes 28:1039, 1979.

**ENVIRONMENTAL INFLUENCES.** A number of constitutional and environmental factors *(diabetogenic influences)* predispose to diabetes mellitus and significantly affect its incidence in those who are genetically predisposed. Most important among them is *obesity.* Approximately 80% of patients with NIDDM are obese and, conversely, about 60% of markedly overweight individuals have some form of carbohydrate intolerance demonstrable by glucose tolerance tests. Frequently weight loss corrects the carbohydrate metabolic abnormality in the nondiabetic and significantly ameliorates the carbohydrate intolerance in the diabetic.

*Pregnancy* is another major diabetogenic influence; its effect is attributed to the appearance of an increased resistance to insulin or some diminished effectiveness of insulin. Overt diabetes so precipitated may revert to a subclinical stage following delivery (PrevAGT, Table 4–1), but the diabetogenic tendency grows stronger with increasing parity. *All forms of stress, including trauma, infections, hypoxia, and hyperthermia,* may unmask diabetes in those harboring the hereditary trait. It is a well-recognized clinical phenomenon that the insulin requirements of the diabetic mount significantly during periods of stress, particularly with infections. Stress may produce its effects through the release of catecholamines, which induce glycogenolysis and lipolysis. The glycogenolysis further burdens beta cells and the free fatty acids exert an insulin antagonism. Thus, although the diabetic state is inherited as a genetic trait, the expression of this genotype is conditioned by environmental influences.

### PATHOGENESIS

*Normal Insulin Metabolism.* The chemical structure, biosynthesis, and secretory pathways of insulin are understood in elegant detail. It is not our purpose to delve into the depths of insulin physiology, but some aspects of insulin release and action are described briefly to facilitate discussion of the pathogenesis of diabetes mellitus. Insulin is synthesized within the beta cells of the pancreas from proinsulin and is stored within membrane-bound granules derived from the Golgi complex. Its release from the beta cells occurs as a biphasic process involving two pools of insulin. A rise in the blood glucose levels, for example, calls forth an immediate release of insulin, presumably that stored in the beta-cell granules. If the secretory stimulus persists, a delayed and protracted response follows, which involves active synthesis of insulin. Among the many substances known to trigger insulin release, glucose is the most important.

Glucose initiates both synthesis and release of insulin. Other agents, however, including gut hormones, certain amino acids (principally leucine and arginine), and sulfonylureas do not initiate insulin synthesis. The "gut" hormones probably initiate release of insulin following a meal, in anticipation of the absorption of glucose. The precise steps and signals involved in insulin release are still not clear, but they are of considerable interest because, as we shall see, one of the factors believed to be important in the causation of NIDDM involves defective transmission of the insulinogenic signal.

Insulin is a major anabolic hormone. It is necessary for: (1) transmembrane transport of glucose and amino acids, (2) glycogen formation in liver and skeletal muscles, (3) glucose conversion to triglycerides, (4) nucleic acid synthesis, and (5) protein synthesis. Its prime metabolic function is to increase the rate of glucose transport into certain cells in the body. These are the striated muscle cells (including myocardial cells), fibroblasts, and fat cells, representing collectively about two thirds of the entire body weight.

How insulin interacts with its target cells is not entirely clear. The process begins with binding to a cell surface receptor (Fig. 4–2). Since the amount of insulin bound to the cells is affected by the availability of receptors, their number and function are important in regulating the action of insulin. Receptor-bound insulin triggers the formation of a series of "second

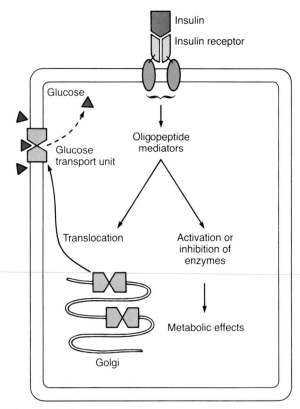

**Figure 4–2.** Schematic model of insulin action on an insulin-responsive cell. Insulin induces the formation of intracellular oligopeptides that affect the function of several enzymes involved in metabolic pathways and cause translocation of glucose transport units from the Golgi apparatus to the plasma membrane. (Modified from Truglia, J. A., et al.: Insulin resistance: Receptor and post-binding deficits in human obesity and non-insulin-dependent diabetes mellitus. Am. J. Med. 79(Suppl. 2B):13, 1985.)

messengers," which are released from the inner aspect of the cell membrane into the cytosol. The second messengers, believed to be oligopeptides,[6] serve to activate (or inactivate) insulin-sensitive enzymes in the mitochondria, endoplasmic reticulum, nucleus, and other intracellular locations. One of the important early effects of insulin that is mediated by second messengers involves translocation of glucose transport units from the Golgi apparatus to the plasma membrane, thus facilitating cellular uptake of glucose (Fig. 4–2).[7]

With this brief characterization of normal insulin secretion and action, we can review the metabolic consequences of insulin lack.

***Metabolic Derangements in Diabetes Mellitus.*** All diabetics, regardless of their genetic and environmental backgrounds and the age of onset of their disease, have in common a relative or absolute lack of insulin or inadequate insulin function. Thus, they suffer from an inability to utilize glucose adequately, since transfer of glucose from blood into muscles and adipose tissue is insulin dependent. Concomitantly, there is stimulation of glycogenolysis, which is normally inhibited by insulin. Both derangements lead to *an accumulation of glucose in the blood (hyperglycemia) to the point where the renal threshold for glucose reabsorption is exceeded and glycosuria results.* The major source of energy becomes fatty acids, mobilized from triglycerides stored within fat depots. In the liver, fatty acids are oxidized to ketone bodies (acetoacetic acid, acetone and β-hydroxybutyric acid), which are used by muscle, heart, kidney, and brain. In IDDM, and much less often in NIDDM, *the rate of formation of ketone bodies may exceed the rate of their utilization, and hence ketosis along with metabolic acidosis may result.* Since tissues appear to be starving for glucose, proteins from both the diet and tissues are used for gluconeogenesis. Thus, anabolic processes, such as the synthesis of glycogen, triglycerides, and proteins, are sacrificed to catabolic activities, including glycogenolysis, gluconeogenesis, and the mobilization of fats. As a result, the diabetic state, which begins as an insulin defect, fans out in ever-widening circles. Although there is considerable overlap in the metabolic alterations in the two major variants of diabetes mellitus, in NIDDM metabolic disturbances are less severe and ketoacidosis is rare.

With this background it is possible to list three major categories of etiologic factors that may result in diabetes mellitus (Fig. 4–3).

○ Abnormalities in pancreatic beta cells, ranging from loss of beta cells to a failure of intact beta cells to release insulin.

○ Abnormalities in plasma, such as circulating anti-insulin antibodies.

○ Abnormalities in the action of insulin on its target cells: reduced levels of insulin receptors or failure of bound insulin to generate second messengers (postreceptor defects).

Abnormalities in plasma are rarely the primary

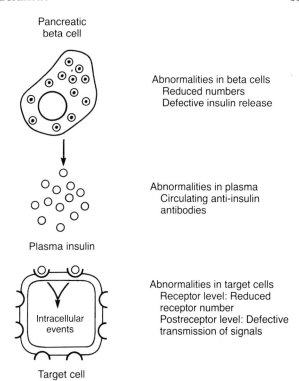

Figure 4–3. Etiologic factors in diabetes mellitus.

cause of diabetes mellitus, but the other two factors are of significance in the pathogenesis of diabetes mellitus. The accumulating evidence strongly suggests that IDDM and NIDDM have different origins and different derangements in insulin kinetics. Each of the variants, therefore, requires separate consideration.

***Insulin-dependent (Type I) Diabetes.*** This form of diabetes results from a severe, absolute lack of insulin. The plasma insulin level is low due to a reduction in the beta-cell mass, which is characteristic in this pattern of the disease. These patients require exogenous insulin for survival; hence the term insulin-dependent.

What causes the loss of beta cells? Three interlocking mechanisms are thought to be responsible: *environmental insult, genetic vulnerability,* and *autoimmunity.*[8] Although no definite environmental agent has been identified, viruses as a cause of diabetes mellitus have been suspected for many years. Several investigators have noted seasonal variation in the diagnosis of new cases; these seasonal trends often correspond to the prevalence of common viral infections in the community.[9] The viral infections implicated include mumps, measles, Coxsackie B, cytomegalovirus, rubella, and infectious mononucleosis,[10] and more recently slow viruses tropic for beta cells have been included.[11] This circumstantial evidence has been strengthened by a report that documented the isolation of Coxsackie B4 virus from the pancreas of a child with acute onset diabetic ketoacidosis.[12] Inoculation of mice with the human isolate produced beta-cell damage and hyperglycemia, supporting an etiologic role for the virus.

If viruses are involved in the origin of IDDM, the question arises, do they act directly on beta cells to cause their destruction? It is widely believed that in most cases direct destruction of the islets by the viruses is not the major cause of beta cell loss in IDDM. It is considered much more likely that viruses or other undefined environmental agents either initiate or unmask destructive autoimmune reactions in genetically predisposed individuals. As already mentioned, IDDM is associated with certain HLA types. Possibly, then, *the associated HLA-linked immune response genes in such individuals render them vulnerable to beta cell–damaging viral infections and at the same time predispose them to the induction of an autoimmune reaction once antigens are released from damaged beta cells. Alternatively, viral infection of the beta cells may merely lead to terminal decompensation of the insulin-secreting cells, whose mass has been gradually eroded over the preceding years by autoimmune reactions initiated by genetically determined abnormalities in immunoregulation*[13] (Fig. 4–4).

A role for autoimmunity in the pathogenesis of IDDM is supported by several morphologic, clinical, and experimental observations. Lymphocytic infiltration of the islets, often intense ("insulitis"), is frequently observed in cases of recent onset.[14] Up to 90% of patients have islet cell antibodies (ICAs) when tested within one year of diagnosis.[15] After one year the percentage of ICA-positive patients drops to 20 to 25%, possibly because loss of a majority of beta cells reduces antigen stimulation and the formation of ICAs. Furthermore, recent studies indicate that asymptomatic individuals who have a higher than normal risk of developing IDDM (monozygotic twin or first-degree relative of a patient) develop ICA months to years prior to the clinical onset of IDDM.[13] Evidence for cell-mediated autoimmunity against islet cells has also been found.[16] Of interest, in approximately one fifth of the cases of IDDM, other endocrine disorders suspected to be of autoimmune origin are also present. These include Addison's disease, hypothyroidism, and Graves' disease, suggesting that IDDM may be but one manifestation of a broad derangement in anti-self reactivity. *To summarize, there is overwhelming evidence implicating immunologically mediated injury as the cause of beta cell loss in IDDM.*[16A] Quite logically, therefore, drug-induced immunosuppression is currently being evaluated for the treatment of this form of diabetes.[17]

We should not close this discussion of IDDM without reference to the controversy regarding the role of glucagon excess in the pathogenesis of diabetes mellitus. Unger and associates have suggested that diabetes mellitus (both IDDM and NIDDM) is a bihormonal disorder characterized by both a lack of insulin and an excess of glucagon.[18] Several observations support such a contention: (1) Metabolic properties of glucagon qualify it as a potential diabetogenic hormone. Glucagon is known to inhibit glycogen storage, promote glycogenolysis, stimulate lipolysis, and favor ketogenesis. (2) Plasma glucagon levels are usually elevated in both forms of diabetes, especially in ketoacidosis. (3) Correction of hyperglucagonemia reduces or corrects diabetic abnormalities.[19] Nevertheless, the possible role of glucagon as an essential comediator is not universally accepted.[20] For example, diabetes mellitus can occur in the total absence of glucagon following pancreatectomy.[21] Moreover, it is pointed out that glucagon excess may be a consequence of low insulin levels rather than a primary abnormality. A balanced review of this controversy concludes that *although excess glucagon contributes to the metabolic abnormalities in diabetes mellitus, there is no evidence that it is an essential co-mediator.*[22]

***Non–insulin-dependent (Type II) Diabetes.*** This form of diabetes is associated with both a derangement in insulin secretion that is delayed or, in some cases, insufficient relative to the glucose load and an inability of peripheral tissues to respond to insulin (insulin resistance). It should be noted, however, that unlike IDDM, the lack of insulin is not severe and hence *insulin resistance is believed to play a major role in the pathogenesis of NIDDM.* In the following discussion each of these two factors will be considered separately, beginning with the role of insulin deficiency in NIDDM.

As previously noted, glucose-induced secretion of insulin occurs in two phases: an initial rapid phase followed by a delayed response. Loss of the first phase of insulin secretion (the glucose response) is seen in NIDDM, often at an early stage of the

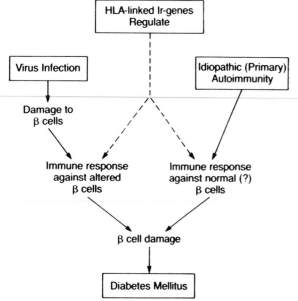

**Figure 4–4.** A simplified schema to show pathways of β-cell destruction leading to insulin-dependent (Type I) diabetes mellitus.

disease, when glucose levels are only slightly elevated.[23] The second phase of insulin secretion is normal and the peak plasma insulin may actually be higher than in controls. Despite the loss of the early response to glucose, the acute response to other secretagogues such as arginine and isoproterenol remains normal. This suggests a specific abnormality of the glucose receptor in the beta cells rather than an inadequacy of insulin synthesis or storage. *Do patients with NIDDM also have some deficiency of insulin?* The answer to this question is complicated by the frequent occurrence of obesity in patients with NIDDM. Obesity, even in the absence of diabetes, is characterized by insulin resistance and hyperinsulinemia. Since most patients with NIDDM are obese, their plasma insulin levels are "elevated." However, when obese NIDDM patients are compared with weight-matched nondiabetics, it appears that the insulin levels of obese diabetics (although well above those of lean nondiabetics) are below those observed in obese nondiabetics, suggesting a state of relative insulin deficiency. Furthermore, in patients with moderately severe NIDDM (fasting plasma glucose levels of 200 to 300 mg/dl) it is possible to demonstrate an absolute deficiency of insulin. We can conclude, therefore, that *most patients with Type II diabetes have a relative or absolute deficiency of insulin. However, this insulin deficiency is milder than that of Type I diabetes and is not an early feature of this variant of diabetes.*

The pathogenesis of the insulin deficiency in NIDDM is not entirely clear. Unlike IDDM, there is no evidence for viral or immunologic injury to the islet cells. According to one view, all the somatic cells of diabetics, including pancreatic beta cells, are genetically vulnerable to injury, leading to accelerated cell turnover and premature aging.[24] This theory not only attempts to explain premature islet cell failure but suggests that accelerated atherosclerosis and microangiopathy result from the increased vulnerability of endothelial cells and pericytes.

Since in most patients with NIDDM insulin deficiency is not of sufficient magnitude to explain the metabolic disturbances, it is logical to suspect some impairment in insulin action. Indeed in recent years an impressive body of data has accumulated that implicates insulin resistance as a major factor in the pathogenesis of NIDDM.[7, 25] Insulin resistance is a complex phenomenon, not restricted to the diabetic syndrome. In both obesity and pregnancy (even in the absence of diabetes) the insulin sensitivity of tissues decreases, but the pancreas compensates by pouring out excessive amounts of insulin (accounting for the hyperinsulinemia noted in obese individuals). Thus, if there were a defect in insulin production, obesity would unmask it and precipitate diabetes. Clearly, obesity is an important diabetogenic influence, and, not surprisingly, approximately 80% of NIDDM patients are obese. In many obese diabetics, especially early in the course of the disease, impaired

glucose tolerance can be reversed by weight loss. Although obesity is emphasized as a factor in insulin resistance, the latter is also encountered in nonobese patients with Type II diabetes.

*What is the cellular basis for insulin resistance?* Since binding to cell surface receptors is essential for insulin action, much attention is focused on the number of receptors available for insulin binding and the postbinding events. A decrease in the number of insulin receptors has been noted in cells obtained from obese as well as nonobese NIDDM patients. Although a reduction in receptor concentration on the target cells contributes to impaired insulin action, the full extent of insulin resistance in NIDDM cannot be explained solely on the basis of reduced receptor availability. It is now widely believed that the major cause of insulin resistance in NIDDM is a failure of cell-bound insulin to generate intracellular signals. The molecular basis of these "postreceptor" defects is under investigation.

*To summarize, NIDDM may be viewed as a complex, multifactorial disorder involving both impaired insulin release and end-organ insensitivity. Insulin resistance could produce excessive stress on beta cells, which may fail in the face of sustained need for a state of hyperinsulinism. Possibly, pancreatic beta cells in NIDDM are genetically vulnerable to such stress. Thus, insulin resistance might initiate the chain of events that in time leads to a deficient or deranged insulin secretory response. The jigsaw puzzle is still incomplete, but each year sees a few more pieces fitted into place.*

**MORPHOLOGY.** The diabetic at death may have many morphologic changes suggestive of the diagnosis and a few virtually diagnostic findings, or there may be no lesions that might not also be found in age-matched nondiabetics. This variability is poorly understood, but two factors are probably significant: (1) the duration of the disease and (2) the severity of the disease. The duration of diabetes strongly influences the development of anatomic changes. Generally the diabetic with disease of 10 to 15 years' duration develops dermal, renal, and retinal microangiopathy, as well as atherosclerosis more severe than that found in age-matched controls. The severity of the metabolic derangement also correlates with the likelihood of morphologic changes. In the presentation that follows, attention will be focused on those morphologic changes that are most characteristic of diabetes.

***Basement Membrane Thickening (BMT) and Microangiopathy.*** Thickening of basement membrane is characteristic of diabetes mellitus. When it affects capillaries, it is referred to as microangiopathy. This microvascular alteration is most evident in the capillaries of the skin, skeletal muscle, retina, renal glomeruli, and renal medulla. However, BMT is also seen in such nonvascular structures as renal tubules, Bowman's capsule, peripheral nerves, placenta, and possibly other sites.[24] The normal basal lamina consists of a relatively uniform layer of extracellular material separating parenchymal or endothelial cells from the surrounding connective tissue stroma. In diabetes this single layer is widened and sometimes replaced by concentric layers of hyaline material composed predominantly of type IV collagen.[26] Such laminar thickening causes narrowing of the lumina of affected capillaries. It should be noted that indistinguishable microangiopathy can be found in aged nondiabetic patients, but rarely to the extent seen in patients with long-standing diabetes.

*Pancreas.* Changes in the pancreas are inconstant and only rarely of diagnostic value. Distinctive changes are more commonly associated with IDDM than with NIDDM.[14] Indeed, the pancreas may appear virtually normal in individuals with NIDDM unless precise quantitation of the islet cell mass is attempted. When present, the changes include one or more of the following: (1) reduction in the size and number of islets, (2) increase in the size and number of islets, (3) beta-cell degranulation, (4) glycogen accumulation within beta cells, (5) amyloid replacement of islets, and (6) leukocytic infiltration of the islets.[27] **Reduction in the size and number of islets** is most commonly seen in IDDM, particularly with rapidly advancing disease. Most of the islets are so small as to escape detection in routinely stained sections. Subtle reduction in the islet cell mass can be demonstrated in NIDDM as well, but this requires special morphometric studies. An **increase in the number and size of islets** is especially characteristic of nondiabetic newborns of diabetic mothers. It is proposed that in this situation the fetal islets undergo hyperplasia in response to the maternal hyperglycemia. Hyperplasia may also be seen early in patients with IDDM, presumably as a compensatory response of the beta cells to injury. **Beta-cell degranulation** implies depletion of stored insulin and is most commonly seen in IDDM. **Glycogen accumulation** appears as small or large, clear cytoplasmic vacuoles within beta cells that show a positive PAS reaction. This change is usually considered to be reversible and a reflection of poor control and long periods of hyperglycemia prior to death. **Amyloid replacement** of islets appears as deposits of pink, amorphous material beginning in and around capillaries and between cells. At advanced stages the islets may be virtually obliterated (Fig. 4–5). This change is often seen in long-standing cases of NIDDM. Similar lesions may be found in elderly nondiabetics.

**Two types of leukocytic infiltration are found in the islets,** principally in Type I diabetes. The most common pattern is a heavy lymphocytic infiltration within and about the islets, a picture referred to as "insulitis." As discussed earlier, this suggests an immunologic reaction. Eosinophilic infiltrates associated with severe regressive and necrotic changes in beta cells may also be found, particularly in diabetic infants who fail to survive the immediate postnatal period. Only these inflammatory reactions and total depletion of beta-cell granules are diagnostic of diabetes mellitus.

*Vascular System.* Diabetes exacts a heavy toll of the vascular system. Whatever the age at onset, **in the course of 10 to 15 years of the disease, most diabetics**

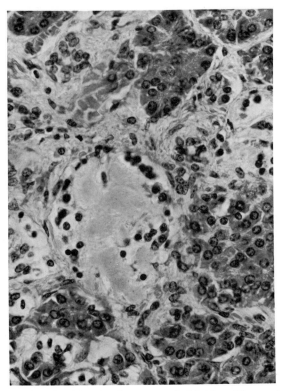

Figure 4–5. Amyloidosis of a pancreatic islet in a 65-year-old male with diabetes of 25 years' duration.

**have developed significant vascular abnormalities.** Indeed, about 80% of diabetics die of some form of cardiovascular (including renal vascular) disease, compared with 40 to 50% of nondiabetics. Vessels of all sizes are affected, from the aorta down to the smallest arterioles and capillaries.

The aorta and large- and medium-sized arteries suffer from accelerated severe **atherosclerosis.** Since atherosclerosis is a disease common to both diabetics and nondiabetics, it will be discussed in greater detail on page 286.

**Myocardial infarction, caused by atherosclerosis of the coronary arteries, is the most common cause of death in diabetics.** Significantly, it is almost as common in the diabetic female as it is in the diabetic male. In contrast, myocardial infarction is uncommon in nondiabetic females of reproductive age (p. 320). Gangrene of the lower extremities, as a result of advanced vascular disease, is about 100 times more common in diabetics than in the general population. The larger renal arteries are also subject to severe atherosclerosis. However, the most damaging effect of diabetes on the kidneys is exerted at the level of the glomeruli and the microcirculation. This is the subject of a later discussion.

The bases of accelerated atherosclerosis are not well understood, and in all likelihood multiple factors are involved.[28] About one third of NIDDM patients and over half of those with IDDM have elevated blood lipid levels known to predispose to atherosclerosis. But the remainder also have an increased predisposition to atherosclerosis, and so other mechanisms must also be involved. Qualitative changes in the lipoproteins brought about by excessive nonenzymatic glycosylation (described later) may affect their turnover and tissue deposition. Low levels of high-density lipoproteins (HDL) have been demonstrated in NIDDM.[29] Since HDL has been suggested as a "protective molecule" against atherosclerosis (p. 288), this could contribute to increased susceptibility to atherosclerosis. Hyperglycemia may itself be injurious to the intima, and deranged arterial wall metabolism may therefore set the stage for atherosclerosis. Finally, since platelets are intimately involved in the pathogenesis of atherosclerosis (p. 293), one cannot ignore the possible role of the reported platelet abnormalities in diabetes mellitus.[30] In addition to all these factors, diabetics tend to have an increased incidence of hypertension, which is a well-known risk factor for atherosclerosis (p. 288).

**Hyaline arteriolosclerosis,** the vascular lesion associated with hypertension (p. 483), is both more prevalent and more severe in diabetics than in nondiabetics. However, it is not specific for diabetes and may be seen in elderly nondiabetics without hypertension. It takes the form of an amorphous, hyaline thickening of the wall of the arterioles, which causes narrowing of the lumen (Fig. 4–6). Not surprisingly, in the diabetic it is related not only to the duration of the disease but also to the level of the blood pressure. The cause and nature of this vascular change are still uncertain. Although at one time it was attributed to hypertension, so common among diabetics, it can also be seen in diabetics who do not have hypertension. It has been proposed that the hyaline material

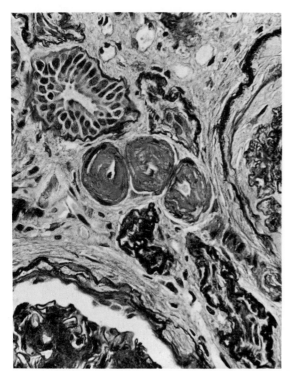

**Figure 4–6.** Hyaline arteriosclerosis. Note a markedly thickened, tortuous afferent arteriole (cut in three planes). The amorphous nature of the thickened vascular wall is evident.

comprises deposits of plasma proteins. Presumably these penetrate into the abnormally permeable walls of the arterioles by a process termed insudation.[31] This concept relates the arteriolosclerosis to the exudative lesions of the glomerulus, described later.

***Kidneys.*** The kidneys are prime targets of diabetes. In fact, renal failure is second only to myocardial infarction as a cause of death from this disease. **Four types of lesions, collectively termed "diabetic nephropathy," are encountered: (1) glomerular lesions; (2) renal vascular lesions, principally arteriolosclerosis; (3) pyelonephritis, including necrotizing papillitis; and (4) glycogen and fatty changes in the tubular epithelium.**

A variety of forms of glomerular involvement may be present: diffuse glomerulosclerosis, nodular glomerulosclerosis (Kimmelstiel-Wilson lesion), "fibrin caps," and "capsular drops." The last two are sometimes called exudative lesions. The sclerotic lesions of the glomeruli destroy renal function and constitute potentially fatal forms of diabetic nephropathy, but the exudative lesions are largely of diagnostic interest only.

**Diffuse glomerulosclerosis** is found in most patients who have had their disease for more than 10 years. It takes the form of thickening of the basement membranes of the glomerular capillaries throughout their entire length and is part and parcel of diabetic microangiopathy. Under the electron microscope, thickening of the glomerular basement membrane can be detected within a few years of the onset of diabetes, sometimes without any associated change in renal function. Associated with the alterations in the basement membrane is a diffuse increase in the mesangial matrix and mesangial cell proliferation. The membrane thickening and matrix deposits are PAS-positive. The basement membrane lesions almost always begin in the vascular stalk and sometimes appear to be continuous with the hyaline arteriolosclerosis in the afferent and efferent arterioles (Fig. 4–7). When the diffuse glomerulosclerosis becomes marked, these patients manifest severe proteinuria and the glomerular cells exhibit loss of their foot processes. The nephrotic syndrome (p. 464), characterized by proteinuria, hypoalbuminemia, and edema, may ensue.

**Nodular glomerulosclerosis describes a glomerular lesion made distinctive by ball-like deposits of a laminated matrix within the mesangial core of the lobule** (Fig. 4–8). These nodules tend to develop in the periphery of the glomerulus, and since they arise within the mesangium, they push the peripheral capillary loops ahead of them. Often these patent loops create halos about the nodule. This lesion has also been called intercapillary glomerulosclerosis and **Kimmelstiel-Wilson lesion,** after the pioneers who described it. Nodular glomerulosclerosis occurs irregularly throughout the kidney and affects random glomeruli, as well as random lobules within a glomerulus. In advanced disease, many nodules are present within a single glomerulus, and most glomeruli become involved. The deposits are PAS-positive and contain mucopolysaccharides, lipids, and fibrils, as well as collagen fibers, and have the same composition as

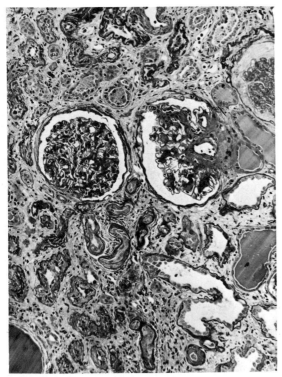

Figure 4–7. Diffuse glomerulosclerosis in a patient who had had diabetes for 16 years. The glomerulus at the right has marked axial thickening, fanning out from the vascular pole. The one on the left, caught in a less advantageous plane, has more delicate, diffuse glomerulosclerosis.

the matrix deposits of diffuse glomerulosclerosis. Often they contain trapped mesangial cells.

Nodular glomerulosclerosis is encountered in perhaps 10 to 35% of diabetics and is a major cause of morbidity and mortality. Like diffuse glomerulosclerosis, its appearance is related to the duration of the disease. Unlike the diffuse form, which may also be seen in association with old age and hypertension, **the nodular form of glomerulosclerosis is, for all practical purposes, highly suggestive of diabetes.**

In the great preponderance of cases, the nodular lesions are accompanied by diffuse glomerulosclerosis. Advanced arteriolosclerosis generally also is present. Whether the nodular lesion is simply an advanced stage of diffuse glomerulosclerosis or whether the processes are distinct is only of academic interest, since both are fundamentally lesions of the mesangium. Progression of these two lesions and their constant companion, arteriolosclerosis, usually leads to obliteration of the vascular channels in the glomerulus and to serious, sometimes fatal, impairment of renal function. As a consequence of glomerular sclerosis, the tubules suffer ischemia and are replaced by interstitial fibrous tissue. Both the diffuse and the nodular forms of glomerulosclerosis induce sufficient ischemia to cause overall fine scarring of the kidneys, marked by a finely granular cortical surface.

**Exudative lesions** take two forms. Glassy, homogeneous, strongly eosinophilic deposits in the parietal layer of Bowman's capsule, called "capsular drops," may hang

into the uriniferous space. Similar-appearing deposits, termed "fibrin caps," may develop over the outer surface of glomerular capillary loops, between the visceral epithelium of Bowman's capsule and the basement membrane. The nature of both of these lesions is obscure. The "fibrin caps" are somewhat misnamed since they contain all the plasma proteins but only a small amount of fibrin. Although no proof exists, both the capsular drop and the fibrin cap are attributed to excessive leakage of plasma proteins from glomeruli that were severely injured by either diffuse or nodular glomerulosclerosis.[32] The fibrin cap is nonspecific and may be encountered in other forms of glomerular disease. The capsular drop, although not pathognomonic, is virtually diagnostic of diabetes. Neither of these two lesions causes any impairment in renal function.

**Renal atherosclerosis and arteriolosclerosis** constitute only one part of the systemic involvement of vessels in diabetics. The kidney is one of the most frequently and severely affected organs. However, the changes in the arteries and arterioles are similar to those found throughout the body. **Hyaline arteriolosclerosis affects not only the afferent but also the efferent arteriole.** Such efferent arteriolosclerosis is rarely if ever encountered in nondiabetic persons and is virtually diagnostic of diabetes.

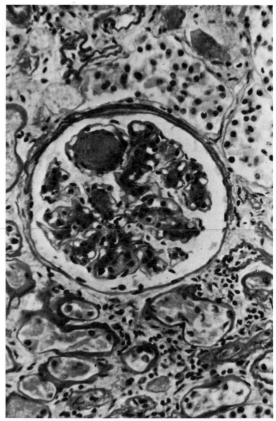

Figure 4–8. Nodular glomerulosclerosis in a patient who had had diabetes mellitus for 17 years. The nodule at the upper left of the glomerulus is surrounded by a patent capillary channel. Note the thickening of the basement membranes of the tubules.

**Pyelonephritis** is an acute or chronic inflammation of the kidneys that usually begins in the interstitial tissue and then spreads to affect the tubules and—possibly—ultimately the glomeruli. Both the acute and chronic forms of this disease occur in nondiabetics as well as in diabetics, and so they are described more fully on page 472. Suffice it to say here that acute pyelonephritis is essentially a bacterial suppurative inflammation that may cause abscesses. Chronic pyelonephritis often results from persistent or recurrent bacterial infections, but other complex etiologic factors may be involved (p. 474). These inflammatory disorders are more common in diabetics than in the general population, and once affected, diabetics tend to have more severe involvements.

One special pattern of acute pyelonephritis, **necrotizing papillitis,** is much more prevalent in diabetics than in nondiabetics. It is, however, **not limited to diabetics,** but is also seen with obstructions of the urinary tract as well as with analgesic abuse. As the term implies, necrotizing papillitis is an acute necrosis of the renal papillae (Fig. 4–9). Diabetics are particularly prone to develop this lesion owing to the combination of ischemia resulting from microangiopathy and increased susceptibility to bacterial infection. One or more papillae may be involved, bilaterally or unilaterally. The infarcted papilla may slough off and be excreted in the urine, permitting a clinical diagnosis by examination of the urinary sediment. In the diabetic, bilateral necrosis of all papillae is not uncommon. When many papillae are involved, papillary necrosis causes acute irreversible renal failure. This lesion is described more fully on page 474.

**Tubular lesions** are also encountered in diabetes mellitus. Perhaps the most striking is the deposition of glycogen within the epithelial cells of the distal portions of the proximal convoluted tubules (and sometimes in the descending loop of Henle). This lesion is variously termed glycogen infiltration, glycogen nephrosis, or Armanni-

Ebstein cells. The glycogen creates clearing of the cytoplasm of the affected cells. This condition is believed to be a reflection of severe hyperglycemia and glycosuria for a period of days or weeks prior to death. No tubular malfunction has been connected with this tubular change.

*Eyes.* Visual impairment, sometimes even total blindness, is one of the more feared consequences of long-standing diabetes. This disease is presently responsible for about 25% of all cases of acquired blindness in the United States. **The ocular involvement may take the form of retinopathy, cataract formation, or glaucoma.** Retinopathy, the most common pattern, consists of a constellation of changes that together are considered by many ophthalmologists to be virtually diagnostic of the disease. The lesion in the retina takes two forms—**nonproliferative** or background retinopathy and **proliferative retinopathy.** The former includes intraretinal or preretinal hemorrhages, retinal exudates, edema, venous dilatations, and, most importantly, thickening of the retinal capillaries (microangiopathy) and the development of microaneurysms. The retinal exudates can be either "soft" (microinfarcts) or "hard" (deposits of plasma proteins and lipids). The **microaneurysms** are discrete saccular dilatations of retinal-choroidal capillaries that appear through the ophthalmoscope as small red dots. The pathogenesis of retinal microaneurysms is not entirely clear. One view is that they represent dilatations at focal points of weakening resulting from degradation and loss of pericytes. In addition, retinal edema resulting from excessive capillary permeability might cause focal collapse, making the vessels vulnerable to aneurysmal dilatation. Although initially described in retinal capillaries, microaneurysms have also been found in glomerular and cardiac capillaries.[33] Thus, microaneurysms may be a generalized feature of the diabetic microcirculation.

The so-called **proliferative retinopathy** is associated with neovascularization and fibrosis. This lesion can lead

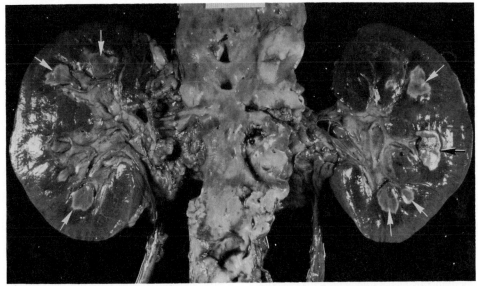

**Figure 4–9.** Bilateral necrotizing papillitis evidenced by the sharply demarcated areas of pale suppurative necrosis (*arrows*) in many pyramids of both kidneys.

to serious consequences, including blindness, especially when it involves the macula. Vitreous hemorrhages can result from rupture of the newly formed capillaries. It is of interest that about half of the patients with retinal microaneurysms also have nodular glomerulosclerosis. Conversely, **patients who have nodular glomerulosclerosis are almost certain to have retinal microaneurysms.**

**Nervous System.** The central and peripheral nervous systems are not spared by diabetes.[34] The most frequent pattern of involvement is a **peripheral, symmetric neuropathy** of the lower extremities that affects both motor and sensory function but particularly the latter. Such peripheral neuropathy may be accompanied by visceral neuropathy, producing disturbances in bowel and bladder function and sometimes sexual impotence. It has been suggested that the axon is the initial site of damage in the peripheral nerves, followed by Schwann cell injury and segmental demyelination. However, there is also evidence to support selective Schwann cell injury that is independent of axonal loss. These changes may be due to microangiopathy and increased permeability of the capillaries that supply the nerves as well as to direct axonal damage caused by alterations in metabolism (discussed later). Neuropathy generally is associated with poorly controlled diabetes, and there is some evidence that those who are under careful control have a lower incidence of this complication.

The **brain,** along with the rest of the body, develops widespread microangiopathy. Such microcirculatory lesions may lead to generalized neuronal degeneration. There is in addition some predisposition to cerebral vascular infarcts and brain hemorrhages, perhaps related to the hypertension often seen in diabetics. In addition, it must be remembered that both hypoglycemia and ketoacidosis may damage brain cells. Degenerative changes have also been observed in the spinal cord. None of the neurologic disorders, including the peripheral neuropathy, is specific for this disease.

**Other Organs.** **Hepatic fatty change** (discussed previously on p. 17) **is seen in many long-term diabetics.** In addition, glycogen vacuolation may be found in the nuclei of hepatic cells in about 10 to 20% of cases. **Degenerative changes are encountered in striated muscle,** perhaps related to the microangiopathy or to motor nerve degeneration. In addition to the changes already described in the dermal microcirculation, a variety of lesions may be encountered in the skin. **Skin infections,** manifestations of the vascular insufficiency and predisposition to infection of the diabetic, are perhaps the most common. **Xanthoma diabeticorum** refers to a localized collection in the dermis and subcutis of macrophages filled with lipid (foam cells or xanthoma cells), creating a firm, nontender, usually slightly yellow nodule. They are not specific for diabetes but are associated with all forms of hyperlipidemia. Another dermatologic change is known as **necrobiosis lipoidica diabeticorum.** This refers to a focal area of necrosis occurring within the dermis and subcutaneous tissues anywhere on the body. It is evident that diabetes is associated with widespread

anatomic changes, only a few of which are virtually pathognomonic. **"Insulitis," nodular glomerulosclerosis, retinopathy, and arteriolosclerosis in the efferent arterioles of the kidney are virtually diagnostic. Marked atrophy, hyperplasia or amyloid replacement of the islets is strongly suggestive.** Although individually some of these lesions may be found in nondiabetics, when present in combination, the anatomic diagnosis of diabetes can be made with a high level of certainty.

**RELATIONSHIP BETWEEN METABOLIC ABNORMALITIES AND COMPLICATIONS OF DIABETES MELLITUS.** The issue of whether the complications of long-standing diabetes (such as microangiopathy) are secondary to the metabolic derangements of the diabetic state or instead are a genetic concomitant unrelated to the metabolic abnormalities has been the subject of much discussion.[35, 36] This question is central not only to our understanding of the pathogenesis of the long-term complications but also to the rational management of diabetes. If metabolic abnormalities such as hyperglycemia are causally related to the complications of diabetes, it would be desirable to maintain "rigid" control of the carbohydrate intolerance. On the other hand, if the level of blood sugar does not affect the appearance or progression of renal vascular or neurologic changes, "heroic" efforts to maintain strict euglycemia (which entail considerable expense and patient inconvenience) may not be warranted. Although this issue is far from settled, *most of the available evidence suggests that the complications of diabetes mellitus are a consequence of associated metabolic derangements.*[37–39] Since hyperglycemia is the most obvious and consistent metabolic abnormality in diabetes mellitus, much interest has centered on elucidating the biochemical pathways by which elevated blood glucose may alter the structure and function of various tissues. Currently two mechanisms that link hyperglycemia to complications associated with long-standing diabetes are being investigated.

*1. Nonenzymatic Glycosylation.* This refers to the process by which glucose chemically attaches to the amino group of proteins without the aid of enzymes.[38] For example, nonenzymatic glycosylation of hemoglobin A (HbA) leads to the formation of $HbA_{1c}$, which normally constitutes about 4% of hemoglobin in red cells. The degree of nonenzymatic glycosylation is directly related to the level of blood glucose, and therefore the red cell $HbA_{1c}$ levels increase greatly in patients with diabetes mellitus. Since nonenzymatic glycosylation of HbA is irreversible and occurs continuously over the 120-day life span of the red cell, a single measurement of $HbA_{1c}$ level provides an index of the average blood glucose levels over the preceding two to four months. Thus it has been suggested that measurement of $HbA_{1c}$ levels may be a useful adjunct in the management of diabetes mellitus.[40] Although $HbA_{1c}$ is the most extensively investigated glycosylated protein, it is apparent that a variety of other structural and regulatory proteins undergo excessive glycosylation in patients with diabetes mellitus. Examples include serum albumin, collagen, basic myelin protein, and low-density lipoproteins. Glycosylation, it is postulated, alters the function of many proteins, thus contributing to various late complications of diabetes. In the case of small blood vessels, for example, abnormal glycosylation of collagen molecules in the basement membrane may favor trapping of plasma proteins such as albumin and immunoglobulins, leading eventually to thickening of the basement membranes (diabetic microangiopathy).

*2. Intracellular Hyperglycemia with Disturbances in Polyol Pathway.* In such tissues as lens and nerves, which do not require insulin for glucose transport, hyperglycemia leads to an increase in intracellular glucose. The excess glucose is metabolized to sorbitol, a polyhydroxyl alcohol (polyol), and eventually to fructose. The accumulated sorbitol and fructose lead to increased intracellular osmolarity, an influx of water, and eventually to osmotic cell injury. It is postulated that this mechanism is responsible for damage to Schwann cells and pericytes of retinal capillaries with resultant peripheral neuropathy and retinal microaneurysms, respectively. In the lens, osmotically imbibed water causes swelling and opacity. That this pathway of glucose-mediated cellular injury may contribute to ocular and neurologic complications of diabetes is supported by preliminary studies in which administration of a drug that inhibits the enzyme necessary for conversion of glucose to sorbitol (aldose reductase) resulted in clinical improvement.[41]

**CLINICAL CORRELATION.** The clinical manifestations of diabetes derive from the two major aspects of this disease: (1) the metabolic derangement and (2) the vascular and organ involvements. The insulin-dependent diabetic is likely to manifest prominent signs and symptoms referable to the metabolic problem early in the course of the disease. Ketoacidosis is an ever-present threat. Sometimes the disease is unsuspected until this medical emergency develops. The classic presentation involves the "three polys"—polyuria, polydipsia, and polyphagia. The hyperglycemia leads to glycosuria, which in turn induces an osmotic diuresis *(polyuria)*. This obligatory water loss, combined with the hyperosmolarity resulting from the increased levels of glucose in the blood and interstitial fluids, tends to deplete intracellular water, which is of particular significance in the osmoreceptors of the thirst centers of the brain. Thus arises the intense thirst *(polydipsia)* often seen in these patients. An increased appetite *(polyphagia)* may also be present, the cause of which is poorly understood. Weight loss and muscle weakness result from the widespread catabolic effects. The combination of polyphagia and weight loss is paradoxical and should always raise the suspicion of diabetes. In summary, then, *the deranged metabolism of diabetes—particularly marked*

*in IDDM—is manifested clinically as polyuria, polydipsia, polyphagia, weight loss, and weakness, and biochemically as hyperglycemia and glycosuria.* Ketoacidosis, with coma, may occur at any time.

Type II diabetes mellitus may also present with polyuria and polydypsia, but unlike Type I diabetes, the patients are often older (over 40 years) and frequently obese. In some cases medical attention is sought because of unexplained weakness or weight loss. Frequently, however, the diagnosis is made by routine blood or urine testing in asymptomatic individuals. Although patients with NIDDM also have metabolic derangements, these are usually relatively mild and controllable, and so this form of the disease is not often complicated by ketoacidosis unless intercurrent infection or stress imposes new burdens. In both forms of long-standing diabetes, atherosclerotic events such as myocardial infarction, cerebrovascular accidents, gangrene of the leg, and renal insufficiency are the most threatening and most frequent concomitants.

The changes in the glomerular basement membrane that are caused by diabetes mellitus induce proteinuria sometimes sufficient to cause the nephrotic syndrome (p. 464). In addition, elevated blood pressures are found in up to 80% of diabetics, especially in those who are obese. Increased vascular resistance secondary to the generalized large and small vessel disease may contribute to the hypertension. *The combination of diabetes mellitus, hypertension, and edema (resulting from proteinuria) is known as the Kimmelstiel-Wilson (K-W) syndrome.* Although the ocular and neurologic complications do not contribute to the mortality caused by this disease, they bedevil the sufferer with loss or impairment of vision and all manner of sensory and motor nerve deficits.

Diabetics are also plagued by an enhanced susceptibility to infections such as tuberculosis, pneumonia, pyelonephritis, and those affecting the skin. Collectively, such infections cause the deaths of about 5% of diabetic patients. The basis for this susceptibility is probably multifactorial; impaired leukocyte functions (p. 59) as well as poor blood supply secondary to vascular disease are involved. A trivial infection in a toe may be the first event in a long succession of complications (gangrene, bacteremia, and pneumonia) that ultimately lead to death.

Life expectancy for the diabetic is shortened by approximately seven to nine years.[42] Patients with IDDM have a greater chance of dying from their disease than do those with NIDDM. The causes of death in order of importance are myocardial infarction, renal failure, cerebrovascular disease, atherosclerotic heart disease, and infections, followed by a large number of other complications more common in the diabetic than in the nondiabetic (e.g., gangrene of an extremity or mesenteric thrombosis). Fortunately, hypoglycemia and ketoacidosis are rare causes of death today. It is sad to close with the note that the diabetic's life expectancy has not significantly improved over the past three decades and, as mentioned at the outset, this disease continues to be one of the top 10 "killers" in the United States. It is hoped that islet cell transplantation, which is still in the experimental stage, will lead to the cure of diabetes mellitus. Even then, the full benefit of islet cell replacement can be derived only early in the course of diabetes, before the myriad vascular complications have set in. Perhaps with good metabolic control it will be possible in future to postpone the complications of long-standing diabetes until islet cell transplantation becomes a practical treatment.

## GOUT

Gout is a genetic disorder of uric acid metabolism that leads to hyperuricemia and consequent acute and chronic arthritis.[43] The recurrent but transient attacks of acute arthritis are triggered by the precipitation into the joints of monosodium urate (MSU) crystals from supersaturated body fluids. Over the span of years, the progressive accumulation of urates and recurrent attacks of inflammation lead to chronic destructive arthritis. MSU crystals deposit in and around the joints as well as other tissues, creating inflammatory foci known as *tophi*—the morphologic hallmark of gout. Whatever its pathophysiology, *the primary biochemical requirement for the development of clinical gout is hyperuricemia.*

Elevation of serum uric acid can result from a variety of biochemical defects in diverse clinical settings. Gout is therefore a heterogeneous disorder that can be classified into several etiologic and biochemical groups. Our discussion will start with the pathogenetic classification of gout, followed by the morphologic changes that are common to most groups.

**PATHOPHYSIOLOGY AND CLASSIFICATION OF GOUT.** Gout is traditionally classified (Table 4–2) as primary when the basic metabolic defect is unknown or when the main manifestation of a known defect is hyperuricemia and gout. Approximately 90% of all cases of gout fall into this category, and this therefore will be the major focus of our discussion. Secondary gout refers to those cases in which the hyperuricemia is secondary to some other acquired or genetic disorder. In these patients gout is not the main clinical disorder.

Before we consider the pathogenetic mechanisms involved in the elevation of plasma uric acid, a clear distinction should be made between hyperuricemia and gout. A plasma urate value above 7 mg/100 ml is considered elevated, since this exceeds the saturation value for urate in plasma. By this definition 2 to 18% of the Western population has hyperuricemia, but the incidence of gout ranges from 0.13 to 0.37%. Obviously, other factors that remain poorly understood must be involved in the development of gout.

**Table 4–2. CLASSIFICATION OF GOUT**

| Clinical Category | Metabolic Defect |
|---|---|
| *Primary Gout (90% of cases)* Enzyme defects unknown (85 to 90% of primary gout) | 1. Overproduction of uric acid  a. Normal excretion (majority)  b. Increased excretion (minority) 2. Underexcretion of uric acid with normal production |
| Known enzyme defects—e.g., partial HGPRT deficiency (rare) | Overproduction of uric acid |
| *Secondary Gout (10% of cases)* 1. Associated with increased nucleic acid turnover—e.g., leukemias | Overproduction of uric acid with increased urinary excretion |
| 2. Chronic renal disease | Reduced excretion of uric acid with normal production |
| 3. Inborn errors of metabolism—e.g., complete HGPRT deficiency (Lesch-Nyhan syndrome) | Overproduction of uric acid with increased urinary excretion |

*In primary gout, elevation of the level of serum uric acid can be due to its overproduction, reduced excretion, or a combination of both.* In metabolic studies, increased synthesis of uric acid is found in over two thirds of patients.[44] In the remaining third, there is no evidence of excessive uric acid production, but there is a primary renal abnormality that selectively impairs excretion of even normal amounts of uric acid. From the clinical standpoint it is important to establish in a given patient whether there is associated excessive excretion of uric acid in the urine, since those with hyperuricaciduria have a much higher risk of developing renal stones. When 24-hour urinary excretion of uric acid is measured, excessive output (>600 mg/day on purine-free diet) is seen only in 10 to 20% of all patients.[45] In summary, on the basis of uric acid synthesis and excretion, there are the following three subsets of *primary gout* (Table 4–2): (1) a majority with overproduction and no increased urinary excretion (relative underexcretion), (2) a minority of patients with overproduction and increased urinary excretion, and (3) a significant minority (30%) with no overproduction but with underexcretion.

Although excessive purine biosynthesis occurs in over two thirds of those with gout, the precise metabolic defect leading to excessive production can be identified in only a minority of cases. Consideration of the mechanisms involved in excessive synthesis of purines and uric acid requires an understanding of their metabolism.[43] Purine nucleotides (e.g., guanylic acid and inosinic acid) can be synthesized de novo or by the so-called salvage pathways (Fig. 4–10). The starting substrate for the de novo pathway is ribose-5-phosphate, which is converted through a series of intermediates into inosinic acid and other

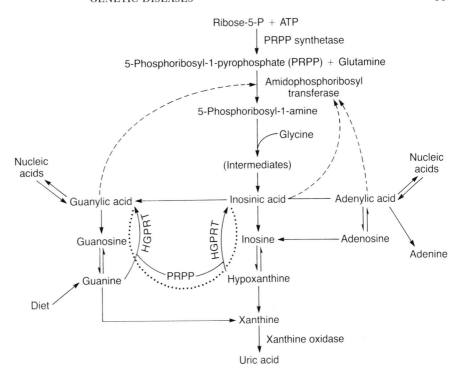

Figure 4–10. Uric acid production. Broken lines denote negative feedback, and the dotted circle indicates the salvage pathway. (Modified from German, D. C., and Holmes, E. W.: Hyperuricemia and gout. Med. Clin. North Am. 70:419, 1986.)

purine nucleotides. The rate-limiting step in this pathway is the conversion of 5-phosphoribosyl-1-pyrophosphate (PRPP) to 5-phosphoribosylamine. This reaction is catalyzed by the enzyme amidophosphoribosyltransferase. The purine nucleotides that are the products of this process exert allosteric inhibition of this key enzyme. The starting point of the salvage pathway consists of free purines, which are obtained from diet or breakdown of nucleic acids. Of particular interest in this pathway is the generation of guanylic acid and inosinic acid in the presence of the enzyme hypoxanthine-guanine phosphoribosyltransferase (HGPRT):

$$\text{Guanine} + \text{PRPP} \longrightarrow \text{Guanylic acid}$$
$$\text{Hypoxanthine} + \text{PRPP} \longrightarrow \text{Inosinic acid}$$

It should be noted that the PRPP utilized in these reactions is also a key substrate in the de novo pathway. Factors serving as control points in these metabolic reactions are the availability of required substrates, particularly PRPP, and the activity of involved enzymes, especially HGPRT and amidophosphoribosyltransferase. Deficiency of the enzyme HGPRT, although rare, will be described briefly since it is a well-characterized inborn error of metabolism associated with hyperuricemia and gout.

Complete lack of HGPRT gives rise to the *Lesch-Nyhan syndrome*. This X-linked genetic condition, seen only in males, is characterized by the excretion of excessive amounts of uric acid, severe neurologic disease with mental retardation, and self-mutilation. Typical gouty arthritis is neither common nor a prominent clinical feature, and hence the Lesch-Nyhan syndrome is considered an example of secondary gout. Because there is an almost complete lack of HGPRT, the synthesis of purine nucleotides by the salvage pathway is blocked. This has two effects: an accumulation of PRPP and reduced feedback inhibition of the amidophosphoribosyltransferase. Both of these conditions have the effect of augmenting purine biosynthesis (by the de novo pathway), resulting eventually in excess production of the end product, uric acid.

Less severe deficiencies of this enzyme ("partial" HGPRT deficiency, Table 4–2) may occur, and these patients present clinically with severe gouty arthritis, beginning in adolescence, that is associated in some cases with mild neurologic disease.

Informative as these genetic disorders may be in the understanding of the pathways of purine metabolism, collectively they account for less than 15% of cases with overproduction of uric acid. In the vast majority of patients with primary gout, the cause of excessive uric acid synthesis is unknown.

As in the case of primary gout, the hyperuricemia of *secondary gout* can result from overproduction or underexcretion of uric acid (Table 4–2). Most cases of secondary gout associated with excessive production result from the increased breakdown of cells and nucleic acid turnover such as occurs in myeloid metaplasia, chronic myeloid leukemia, polycythemia vera, and acute myelogenous and lymphocytic leukemias.

An understanding of the renal abnormality responsible for reduced excretion of uric acid requires that we briefly review normal uric acid excretion. Uric acid is freely filtered across the glomerulus, but 98 to 100% is reabsorbed in the early part of the proximal convoluted tubules. The major excretory mechanism, therefore, involves secretion of the urate back into the tubular lumen by a more distal region of the proximal tubule. In primary gout, "underexcretors" seem to have a defect in the tubular secretion of uric acid; the tubular cells in such cases require a plasma urate concentration 1 to 2 mg/100 ml higher than that required by the normal individual to achieve a comparable rate of excretion. Reduced excretion of uric acid such as occurs with chronic renal diseases or following administration of drugs may then produce secondary gout. Particularly implicated among the drugs are thiazide diuretics, presumably due to their effect on tubular transport of uric acid.[43] In all cases of secondary gout, the metabolic pool of uric acid is increased and may lead to disease indistinguishable from the primary idiopathic form.

**INHERITANCE.** It should be obvious from our discussion that primary gout is merely a common clinical term for a heterogeneous group of biochemical disorders. As such, more than one mode of genetic transmission may be expected. The most common form of primary gout, which predominantly affects males, is believed to have a polygenic or multifactorial mode of inheritance. Environmental factors such as drugs, dietary levels of purines, and alcohol often act in concert with genetic factors. The male preponderance has been attributed to the fact that before menopause women have lower serum concentrations of urate. An autosomal-dominant pattern of inheritance has also been reported in some families. In gout associated with HGPRT deficiency, transmission is X-linked, as already described.

**MORPHOLOGY.** The distinctive morphologic as well as clinical features of gout are (1) acute arthritis, (2) chronic tophaceous arthritis, and (3) tophi in soft tissues.

The **acute arthritis** takes the form of an acute inflammatory synovitis made distinctive by the microcrystals of urates in the joint effusion. In order of frequency, the joints in the following regions are involved, although ultimately any joint in the body may be affected: great toe (90% of patients), instep, ankle, heel, knee, and wrist.

The inflammatory response in the joints is initiated by the formation of MSU crystals within the synovial fluid and possibly within the synovial membrane.[46] Two mechanisms are believed to trigger the inflammatory response: (1) interaction of the crystals with neutrophils and (2) activation of Hageman factor (Fig. 4–11). MSU crystals are chemotactic, bringing forth a neutrophilic response. Phagocytosis of MSU crystals by the neutrophils leads to a series of reactions, one of the earliest being the release of a chemotactic glycoprotein from the neutrophils. This augments the local accumulation of polymorphonuclear leukocytes and phagocytosis of MSU crystals. The ingested crystals damage the lysosomal membrane, causing intracellular leakage of enzymes, which eventually destroys the leukocyte, thus pouring the lysosomal contents into the joint fluid. As discussed in the chapter on

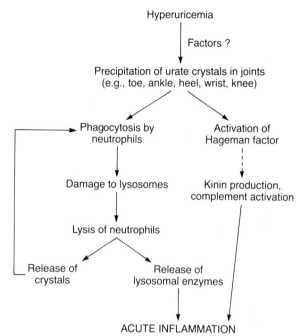

Figure 4–11. Pathogenesis of acute gouty arthritis.

inflammation (p. 41), lysosomes contain enzymes that are potent stimulators of the inflammatory response and that are capable of degrading tissue components such as collagen and elastin. Recent evidence suggests that urate crystals promote the generation and release of highly toxic free radicals from neutrophils, which add further to the tissue injury.[47] Once the crystals are released from the injured neutrophils they are recycled, creating a vicious circle.[48] Activation of the Hageman factor by the urate crystals can initiate production of a host of other mediators of the inflammatory response, including the kinins and complement fractions (p. 38). As a result of the inflammatory process, the synovial membranes are congested, swollen, and heavily infiltrated with neutrophils, macrophages, lymphocytes, and lesser numbers of plasma cells. When the episode of crystallization abates and the formed crystals are resolubilized, the acute attack remits.

Although the sequence of events as outlined is generally accepted, several questions remain unanswered. What initiates crystallization of urates in joint spaces? Why are certain peripheral joints preferentially involved? Why is there no correlation between the serum level of uric acid and occurrence of gouty arthritis? The marked predilection of acute gout for peripheral joints may relate to their lower temperature, since solubility of urates is significantly reduced as the temperature is lowered. The normal temperature of the ankle joint is 29°C, whereas in the knee joint it is 33°C. Solubility of the urate crystals in the joint fluid is also affected by its content of proteoglycans, hyaluronic acid, and chondroitin sulfate.[49] Alterations in the normal structure or concentration of various proteoglycans may therefore be an important factor in the pathogenesis of acute gouty arthritis. Such alterations

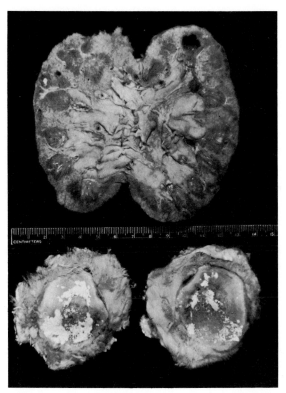

Figure 4–12. Urate depositions in gout. Several white urate deposits are seen within the pyramids of the opened kidney. Below, the white encrustations are seen on the articular surfaces of the patellae.

serve them in histologic sections. When preserved, they are demonstrable with routine or, more effectively, with silver staining techniques. The crystals are brilliantly anisotropic with polarized light microscopy.

Although the formation of tophi can be reasonably related to hyperuricemia, there exists a poorly understood association between cardiovascular disease, obesity, and gout. Without going into the perplexing plethora of details, we can state that (1) gouty and hyperuricemic patients tend to have an increased risk of hypertension, atherosclerosis, and their attendant complications;[50, 51] (2) hyperuricemic patients tend to be 10 to 14 kg heavier than controls;[52] and (3) the association between hypertension and gout cannot be explained on the basis of coexistent obesity[53] or impaired renal function.[50] Hypertension and obesity thus appear to be independently associated with gout. Undoubtedly hypertension contributes to the increased frequency of coronary artery disease seen in patients with gout.

Other than the joints, **the kidney** is the most commonly involved organ in gout.[54] Three types of lesions directly related to gout may be seen. (1) The most common is **"urate nephropathy"** resulting from the deposition of MSU crystals in the medullary interstitium, the pyramids, and papillae (Fig. 4–12). In time, distinctive microtophi with a typical foreign-body giant cell reaction are formed.

may be genetic or acquired—for example, by repeated joint trauma.

**Chronic arthritis** evolves from the continued precipitation of urates in the recurrent attacks of acute arthritis. The urates produce heavy encrustations on the articular surface, and some deposits penetrate deeply (Fig. 4–12). Large aggregations of urates are now formed within the subarticular bone or in the soft tissues about the joint. These deposits create the pathognomonic tissue lesion of gout—**the tophus. The tophus is a mass of crystalline or amorphous urates surrounded by an intense inflammatory reaction of macrophages, lymphocytes, and fibroblasts. Large foreign-body type giant cells, which are often wrapped around masses of precipitated salts, are very prominent** (Fig. 4–13). As tophi develop in joints, the articular cartilage and the underlying bone are eroded and progressive destruction of the joint ensues, simulating the changes of advanced osteoarthritis. Indeed, secondary osteoarthritis often supervenes in gouty arthritis.

Tophi are also likely to develop in the periarticular ligaments, tendons, connective tissues, olecranon and patellar bursae, and the ear lobes. Less frequently they appear in the kidneys; skin of the fingertips, palms, or soles; nasal cartilages; aorta; myocardium; and aortic or mitral valves. Very rarely, tophi develop in the central nervous system, eyes, tongue, larynx, penis, and testes.

Urate crystals are water soluble, and nonaqueous fixatives such as absolute alcohol are necessary to pre-

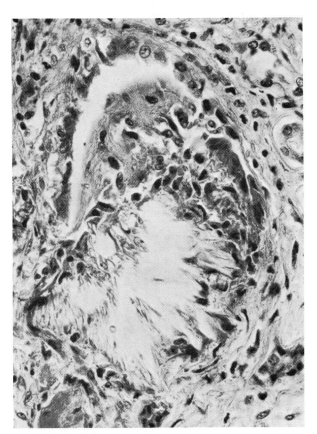

Figure 4–13. A tophus of gout. The deposit of urate crystals is surrounded by an inflammatory reaction of fibroblasts, occasional lymphocytes, and giant cells.

Tophus formation in the cortex is rare. (2) Acute obstructive renal failure resulting from **intratubular deposition of free uric acid crystals** is a well-known complication in patients with myeloproliferative disorders. These cases of secondary gout are associated with severe hyperuricaciduria, especially at initiation of chemotherapy, when massive nucleic acid breakdown occurs. (3) **Uric acid stones** are formed, particularly in subjects excreting more than 1100 mg of uric acid per day. In such cases the incidence of stones approaches 50% and secondary complications of obstructive uropathy such as pyelonephritis are also increased. In addition to these lesions, nephrosclerosis due to the increased prevalence of hypertension may also appear. It should be pointed out that urate nephropathy, which is the commonest renal lesion, does not result in renal functional impairment per se. Rather, when functional impairment appears it is most closely correlated with hypertension (and nephrosclerosis), urinary obstruction, and aging.[55] Indeed it has been suggested that increased ingestion of lead (by way of "moonshine" whiskey contaminated with lead) and the resulting renal injury may be involved in the pathogenesis of renal functional impairment seen in some patients with gout.[56] Contrary to earlier reports, there is no distinctive glomerular lesion associated with gout.

**CLINICAL CORRELATION.** From the clinical standpoint, gout has many faces. It may disclose its presence by a severe attack of arthritis early in its course, but equally often it smolders as a subclinical disease. Three stages have been delineated. *Stage 1 is designated as hyperuricemic asymptomatic gout.* Silent hyperuricemia is present in 25 to 33% of relatives of patients with the overt disease. *Stage 2 is acute gouty arthritis,* characterized by flare-ups that may last a few days to weeks but are followed by complete remissions (intercritical periods) ranging from months to years. *Stage 3—chronic tophaceous gout—*is the likely sequel to years of recurrent acute arthritis. Persistent disabling joint disease may develop within a few years or only after many decades of acute attacks. Involvement of the kidney by one or more of the mechanisms cited above gives rise to proteinuria, passage of gravel, and azotemia. Indeed, about 20% of those with chronic gout die of renal failure.

Gout can be a satisfying disease to the physician because the correct diagnosis and appropriate therapy have much to offer the patient.

# MENDELIAN DISORDERS (DISEASES CAUSED BY SINGLE GENE DEFECTS)

Single gene defects (mutations) follow the well-known mendelian patterns of inheritance. Thus, the conditions they produce are often called "mendelian disorders." The number of known mendelian disorders has grown rapidly to approximately 3000. Although individually rare, together they account for

approximately 1% of all adults admitted to hospitals and about 5% of all pediatric hospital admissions. Table 4–3 lists some of the more common mendelian disorders and their prevalence. Many of these will be discussed in this chapter; most of the remaining are described elsewhere in the text. First, however, we will briefly review some general concepts of medical genetics.

Mutations involving single genes follow one of three patterns of inheritance: (1) autosomal dominant, (2) autosomal recessive, and (3) X-linked. "Dominant" implies that effects of the mutant gene will be clinically manifest when the individual has a single dose of the mutant gene (or is heterozygous for it), whereas "recessive" implies that the trait is manifest only if a double dose of the mutant gene is present (homozygous state). Recessive X-linked mutant genes are expressed almost always in the male, even though only one copy is present, since there is no normal copy present on the Y chromosome. The male is said to be *hemizygous* for genes on the X chromosome.

Although gene expression is usually described as dominant or recessive, it should be remembered that in some cases both alleles of a gene pair may be fully expressed in the heterozygote—a condition called *codominance.* Histocompatibility and blood group antigens are good examples of codominant inheritance as well as *polymorphism.* The latter implies the existence of multiple allelic forms of a single gene.

Another topic of interest to the geneticist is the wide variation in the expression of genes. *Two common forms associated with autosomal dominant inheritance are recognized:* (1) When individuals who have a mutant gene fail to express it, the trait is said to demonstrate *reduced penetrance.* Penetrance is expressed in mathematical terms; thus 50% pene-

**Table 4–3. PREVALENCE OF SELECTED MONOGENIC DISORDERS AMONG LIVEBORN INFANTS***

| Disorder | Estimated Prevalence |
|---|---|
| *Autosomal Dominant* | |
| Familial hypercholesterolemia | 1 in 500 |
| Polycystic kidney disease | 1 in 1250 |
| Huntington's disease | 1 in 2500 |
| Hereditary spherocytosis | 1 in 5000 |
| Marfan's syndrome | 1 in 20,000 |
| *Autosomal Recessive* | |
| Sickle cell anemia | 1 in 625 (U.S. blacks) |
| Cystic fibrosis | 1 in 2000 (Caucasians) |
| Tay-Sachs disease | 1 in 3000 (U.S. Jews) |
| Phenylketonuria | 1 in 12,000 |
| Mucopolysaccharidoses (all types) | 1 in 25,000 |
| Glycogen storage diseases (all types) | 1 in 50,000 |
| Galactosemia | 1 in 57,000 |
| *X-linked* | |
| Duchenne muscular dystrophy | 1 in 7000 |
| Hemophilia | 1 in 10,000 |

*From Wyngaarden, J. B., and Smith, L. H., Jr.: Cecil Textbook of Medicine. 17th ed. Philadelphia, W. B. Saunders Co., 1985.

trance indicates that 50% of those who carry the gene express the trait. The factors that affect penetrance are not clearly understood, but this possibility is of obvious importance in genetic counseling. (2) In contrast to penetrance, if a trait is seen in all the individuals carrying the mutant gene but is expressed differently among individuals, the phenomenon is called *variable expressivity*. For example, polydactyly may be expressed in the toes or in the fingers as one or more extra digits.

A single gene mutation may lead to many phenotypic effects (*pleiotropy*) and, conversely, mutations at several genetic loci may produce the same trait (*genetic heterogeneity*). For example, Marfan's syndrome, which results from a basic defect in connective tissue, is associated with widespread effects involving the skeleton, eye, and cardiovascular system, all of which stem from a common abnormality in connective tissues. On the other hand, profound childhood deafness, an apparently homogeneous clinical entity, results from 16 different types of autosomal recessive mutations. Recognition of genetic heterogeneity is not only important in genetic counseling but also facilitates the understanding of the pathogenesis of common disorders, such as diabetes mellitus (p. 86).

## BIOCHEMICAL BASIS OF MENDELIAN DISORDERS

Mendelian disorders result from genetic errors involving single genes, implying that these diseases result from a primary abnormality in a *single protein molecule*. However, single gene disorders may have complex pathogeneses, due either to pleiotropy or to secondary and tertiary effects, somewhat like the "domino effect." In sickle cell anemia, for example, the basic error is the production of an abnormal beta chain of hemoglobin resulting from a single substitution of valine for glutamic acid in the sixth amino acid position. The entire clinical syndrome, including seemingly unrelated phenomena such as anemia, microinfarcts, chronic skin ulcers, and nephropathy, can be explained on the basis of the primary hemoglobin abnormality. One must hasten to add that unlike sickle cell disease, in which the biochemical error has been precisely identified, in the vast majority of single gene disorders we are ignorant not only of the precise biochemical abnormality but also of the genesis of the resultant lesions. Relatively common disorders such as cystic fibrosis (p. 106) and adult polycystic kidney disease (p. 484) are two such examples.

With the recognition that *a single mutation = a single protein defect*, one can examine the categories of proteins that may be altered and the biochemical consequences of such alterations. Broadly speaking, three kinds of proteins may be affected by mutation—enzymes, structural proteins, and regulatory

proteins. To some extent the pattern of inheritance of the disease is related to the kind of protein affected by the mutation. In general, *diseases resulting from mutations involving enzyme proteins are inherited as autosomal recessives*. In such cases, equal amounts of the normal as well as the defective enzyme are synthesized in the heterozygotes, and usually the natural "margin of safety" ensures that cells with half their usual complement of the enzyme will function normally. On the other hand, *mutations involving key structural proteins, such as collagen, or those involving regulatory proteins, such as membrane receptors, are usually dominant*. The biochemical derangements underlying autosomal dominant diseases are generally much more complex and difficult to characterize.

To aid our understanding of the pathogenesis of mendelian disorders, we can classify the mechanisms of single gene disorders into four categories: *(1) enzyme defects and their consequences; (2) defects in membrane receptors and transport systems; (3) alterations in the structure, function, or quantity of nonenzyme proteins, and (4) mutations predisposing to unusual reactions to drugs*. It should be understood that this is a provisional classification, subject to modification as the currently unknown biochemical basis of a large number of diseases begins to unfold.

**ENZYME DEFECTS AND THEIR CONSEQUENCES.** Mutations may result in the synthesis of a defective enzyme or in a reduced amount of a normal enzyme. In either case, the consequence is a metabolic block. Figure 4–14 provides an example of an enzyme reaction in which the substrate S is converted by intracellular enzymes $E_1$, $E_2$, and $E_3$ into an end product (P) through intermediates $I_1$ and $I_2$. In this proposal the final product P exerts feedback control on enzyme $E_1$. A minor pathway producing small quantities of $M_1$ and $M_2$ also exists. The biochemical consequences of an enzyme defect in such a reaction may lead to two major consequences: (1) *Accumulation of the substrate*, which, depending upon the site of block, may be accompanied by accumulation of one or both intermediates. Moreover, an increased concentration of $I_2$ may stimulate the minor pathway and thus lead to an excess of $M_1$ and $M_2$. Under these conditions tissue injury may result if the precursor, the intermediates, or the products of alternate minor pathways are toxic in high concentrations. For example, in galactosemia, the deficiency of galactose-

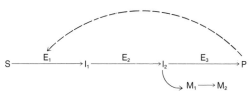

**Figure 4–14.** A schema illustrating the conversion of a substrate (S) to the end product (P), through several intermediates (I), brought about by enzymes (E). P exerts feedback inhibition of $E_1$. M denotes products of minor pathways.

1-phosphate uridyltransferase leads to the accumulation of galactose and consequent tissue damage. A deficiency of phenylalanine hydroxylase results in the accumulation of phenylalanine. Excessive accumulation of complex substrates within the lysosomes due to deficiency of degradative enzymes is responsible for a group of diseases generally referred to as *lysosomal* storage diseases (p. 111). (2) *An enzyme defect can lead to a metabolic block and a decreased amount of end product* that may be necessary for normal function. For example, a deficiency of melanin may result from lack of tyrosinase, which is necessary for the biosynthesis of melanin from its precursor tyrosine. This results in the clinical condition called albinism, to be discussed later. If the end product is a feedback inhibitor of the enzymes involved in the early reactions (in Fig. 4–14 it is shown that P inhibits $E_1$), the deficiency of the end product may permit overproduction of intermediates and their catabolic products, some of which may be injurious at high concentrations. A prime example of a disease with such an underlying mechanism is the Lesch-Nyhan syndrome, already discussed. (3) *There may be failure to inactivate a tissue-damaging substrate.* Alpha-1-antitrypsin is an enzyme that is synthesized and secreted by the liver. It is the main protease inhibitor in the serum, and its chief function is to inactivate neutrophil elastase. A point mutation in the coding region of the alpha-1-antitrypsin gene leads to the formation of a mutant protein that fails to be secreted from the liver. In patients with reduced serum levels of alpha-1-antitrypsin, the elastic tissue in the walls of pulmonary alveoli falls prey to the destructive activity of neutrophil elastase, leading eventually to emphysema (p. 419).

**DEFECTS IN RECEPTORS AND TRANSPORT SYSTEMS.** Many biologically active substances have to be actively transported across the cell membrane. This is generally achieved by one of two mechanisms—initial binding to a specific receptor site followed by internalization, or via a "carrier" protein. A genetic defect in a receptor-mediated transport system is exemplified by familial hypercholesterolemia, in which defective transport of low-density lipoproteins (LDL) into the cells leads secondarily to excessive cholesterol synthesis by complex intermediary mechanisms, discussed later. In Hartnup's disease, on the other hand, the transport system for tryptophan (and certain other amino acids) across the intestinal cells is defective. Since tryptophan is a precursor of the vitamin nicotinamide, symptoms of pellagra (p. 246) develop.

**ALTERATIONS IN THE STRUCTURE, FUNCTION, OR QUANTITY OF NONENZYME PROTEINS.** Genetic defects resulting in alterations of structural proteins often have widespread secondary effects, as exemplified by sickle cell disease (p. 354). Indeed, the hemoglobinopathies, of which sickle cell disease is one, best exemplify this category because all are characterized by defects in the globin molecule. Over 300 abnormal hemoglobins have been identified, most resulting from point mutations in the structural genes that code for the amino acid sequence in the globin chain. Other examples of genetically defective structural proteins that we shall discuss in this chapter involve collagen and are exemplified by Marfan's and Ehlers-Danlos syndromes.

**GENETICALLY DETERMINED ADVERSE REACTIONS TO DRUGS.** Certain genetically determined enzyme deficiencies are unmasked only after exposure of the affected individual to certain drugs. This special area of genetics, called pharmacogenetics, has been discussed in a recent review.[57] The classic example of drug-induced injury in the genetically susceptible individual is associated with a deficiency of the enzyme glucose-6-phosphate dehydrogenase (G6PD). Under normal conditions, G6PD deficiency does not result in disease, but on administration of the antimalarial drug primaquine, a severe hemolytic anemia results in the individual with G6PD deficiency (p. 354).

Despite the usefulness of a pathogenetic classification based on the nature of the underlying biochemical defect, mendelian disorders are generally classified according to their mode of inheritance, a tradition that is followed in the succeeding sections.

## AUTOSOMAL DOMINANT CONDITIONS

Autosomal dominant disorders are transmitted from one generation to the next; both males and females are affected and both can transmit the condition. When an affected person marries an unaffected individual, half of their children (on the average) will have the disease. It is important to remember that in every autosomal dominant disorder some patients do not have affected parents. Such patients owe their disorder to new mutations involving either the egg or the sperm from which they were derived. Their siblings would neither be affected nor incur an increased risk of developing the disease. The proportion of patients who develop the disease due to a new mutation is related to the effect of the disease on reproductive capability. If a disease markedly reduces reproductive fitness, most cases would be expected to result from new mutations, as is the case for example with achondroplasia, a form of dwarfness. Some other features that characterize autosomal dominant disorders are as follows:

○ Clinical features can be modified by reduced penetrance and variable expressivity.

○ In many conditions there is delayed age of onset: symptoms and signs do not appear until adulthood (as in Huntington's disease).

○ Mutations usually involve complex structural proteins, such as collagen, or those that function as regulatory proteins, such as LDL. Some examples are discussed next.

## Marfan's Syndrome

This autosomal dominant disorder is characterized by defective formation of collagen and elastic fibers. The precise nature of the fiber defect still is not clear but in all likelihood involves inadequate or inappropriate cross-linking, which reduces elasticity and fiber strength. Although inhibition of the cross-linking enzyme lysyl oxidase (p. 56) leads to a Marfan-like syndrome in experimental animals, there is no deficiency of this enzyme in the human disorder. Attention is therefore focused on possible abnormalities in the structure of collagen. Detailed study of collagen and cloned collagen genes isolated from an affected individual have revealed a mutation in the pro-α2(I) gene, resulting in the synthesis of abnormal collagen molecules that fail to form normal cross-links.[58, 59] In other cases a primary defect in the organization of elastin fibers has been noted.[60] It seems likely, therefore, that Marfan's syndrome is genetically heterogeneous, i.e., it may result from several distinct mutations involving collagen or elastin genes.

*Individuals with Marfan's syndrome have manifestations relating to three systems—skeletal, visual, and cardiovascular.* These patients have a slender, elongated habitus with abnormally long legs and arms; spider-like fingers (arachnodactyly); a high, arched palate; and hyperextensibility of joints. President Lincoln had a marfanoid appearance. The lens in the eye may suffer dislocation because of weakness of its suspensory ligaments. Most serious, however, are the involvements of the cardiovascular system. Defective cross-linking of collagen or elastica, or both, in the tunica media of the aorta predisposes to aneurysmal dilatation and dissecting aneurysms (p. 302). The cardiac valves, especially the mitral and tricuspid, may be excessively distensible and regurgitant (floppy valve syndrome), giving rise to congestive cardiac failure. Death may occur at any age from aortic rupture. Although some patients with this disorder survive into the seventh and eighth decades, the average age at death is 30 to 40 years.

## Familial Hypercholesterolemia

This disease is perhaps the most common of all mendelian disorders; the frequency of heterozygotes is 1 in 500 in the general population. *It is caused by a mutation in the gene specifying the receptor for low-density lipoprotein (LDL)*, the major transport form of cholesterol in the plasma. An understanding of this disorder has resulted largely from the elegant work of Michael Brown and Joseph Goldstein, who received the 1985 Nobel Prize for their work on the LDL receptors. We shall begin our discussion with a brief review of the normal process of LDL transport and metabolism (Fig. 4–15). Approximately 85 to 90% of circulating LDL is removed from the plasma by a receptor-mediated transport process. Although they are widely distributed on many cell types, approximately 75% of the LDL receptors are located on hepatocytes. The first step in the transport of LDL involves binding to the cell surface receptor, followed by its endocytotic internalization. Within the cell the endocytic vesicles fuse with the lysosomes and the LDL molecule is enzymically degraded, resulting ultimately in the release of free cholesterol into the cytoplasm. The cholesterol is not only utilized by the cell for membrane synthesis but also takes part in intracellular cholesterol homeostasis by a sophisticated system of feedback control. First, it suppresses cholesterol synthesis by inhibiting the activity of the enzyme 3-hydroxy-3-methylglutaryl (3HMG) CoA reductase, which is the rate-limiting enzyme in the synthetic pathway. Second, the cholesterol activates the enzyme cholesterol acyltransferase, which favors esterification and storage of excess cholesterol. Third, the cholesterol suppresses the synthesis of cell surface LDL receptors, thus protecting cells from excessive accumulation of cholesterol.[61] Mutations in the LDL-receptor gene impair intracellular transport and catabolism of the LDL, resulting in the accumulation of LDL-cholesterol in the plasma. In addition, the absence of LDL receptors on the liver cells leads to increased synthesis of

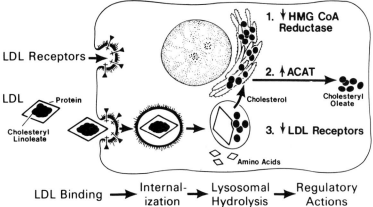

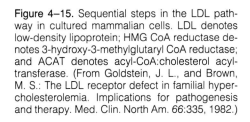

Figure 4–15. Sequential steps in the LDL pathway in cultured mammalian cells. LDL denotes low-density lipoprotein; HMG CoA reductase denotes 3-hydroxy-3-methylglutaryl CoA reductase; and ACAT denotes acyl-CoA:cholesterol acyltransferase. (From Goldstein, J. L., and Brown, M. S.: The LDL receptor defect in familial hypercholesterolemia. Implications for pathogenesis and therapy. Med. Clin. North Am. 66:335, 1982.)

LDL by complex alterations in lipoprotein metabolism.[62] Thus patients with familial hypercholesterolemia develop excessive levels of serum cholesterol owing to the combined effect of reduced catabolism and excessive biosynthesis.

Familial hypercholesterolemia is an autosomal dominant disease. Heterozygotes have a two- to threefold elevation of plasma cholesterol levels, whereas homozygotes may have in excess of a fivefold elevation in concentration of plasma cholesterol. Although their cholesterol levels are elevated from birth, the heterozygotes remain asymptomatic until adult life, when they develop cholesterol deposits (xanthomas) along tendon sheaths and premature atherosclerosis, resulting in coronary artery disease. Homozygous individuals are much more severely affected, developing cutaneous xanthomas in childhood and often dying of myocardial infarction by the age of 15 years.

At least three types of mutations affecting the LDL receptor have been recognized: (1) receptor-negative disease, characterized by a lack of receptors (heterozygotes have a 50% reduction in receptors); (2) receptor-defective disease, characterized by defective cellular binding of LDL, which is reduced to about 10% of the normal level in homozygous individuals; and (3) internalization defect, characterized by failure to internalize normally bound LDL.

It should be emphasized that familial hypercholesterolemia is only one of several forms of hyperlipoproteinemias, most of which are not genetically determined (p. 289).

### Neurofibromatosis (Recklinghausen's Multiple Neurofibromatosis)

Recklinghausen's disease is an autosomal dominant condition that can be diagnosed entirely by clinical criteria.[63] Most distinctive is the appearance of *multiple neurofibromas*, usually in the form of pedunculated nodules protruding from the skin. The neurofibromas are discrete, generally unencapsulated, soft nodules. Although derived from Schwann cells, they contain a tangled array of all the elements found in peripheral nerves, i.e., Schwann cells, neurites, and fibroblasts. Similar tumors ranging from microscopic to monstrous masses may occur in every conceivable site (along nerve trunks, the cauda equina, cranial nerves, in the retroperitoneum, orbit, tongue, and gastrointestinal tract, for example). In addition, most patients have pigmented skin lesions known as *café au lait* spots. Sometimes these overlie a neurofibroma. Infrequently, patients with Recklinghausen's disease have only the café au lait spots, an example of variable expressivity of a genetic defect. Another characteristic feature is the presence of pigmented iris hamartomas called *Lisch nodules*. They do not present any clinical problems but are helpful in establishing the diagnosis.

Besides being a disfiguring condition (the storied "elephant man" was a victim), neurofibromatosis may be extremely serious, either by virtue of the location of a lesion (e.g., within the cranial vault) or because one or more of the benign neurofibromas becomes transformed into a malignant neoplasm (in approximately 10 to 15% of patients). Usually the neurogenic sarcomas arise in the large nerve trunks of the neck or extremities. Infrequently, patients with this condition have other associated, presumably genetic disorders, including congenital malformations, pheochromocytomas, medullary carcinomas of the thyroid gland, and intracranial neoplasms. It is of interest that nearly half of these patients have no affected relatives and are therefore thought to have new mutations.

## AUTOSOMAL RECESSIVE DISORDERS

Since autosomal recessive disorders result only when both alleles at a given genetic locus are mutants, such disorders are characterized by the following features: (1) the trait does not usually affect the parents, but siblings may show the disease; (2) siblings have a one-in-four chance of being affected, i.e., the recurrence risk is 25% for each birth; (3) if the mutant gene occurs with a low frequency in the population, there is a strong likelihood that the proband is the product of a consanguineous marriage. In contrast to those of autosomal dominant diseases, the following features generally apply to most autosomal recessive disorders.

○ The expression of the defect tends to be more uniform.
○ Complete penetrance is common.
○ Age of onset is frequently early in life.
○ In many cases enzyme proteins are affected by the mutation.

Although by definition recessive genes are not expressed in heterozygotes, often the heterozygous state can be identified by appropriate tests. In the case of enzyme defects, heterozygotes may possess reduced amounts of the normal enzyme. Identification of heterozygotes is helpful for genetic counseling. Since most of the enzymes affected in the inherited inborn errors of metabolism are present in fibroblasts or red cells, these cell types are often used in carrier detection. Cells obtained by amniocentesis are also used to detect many inborn errors of metabolism before birth (p. 125).

Here we will discuss some of the more frequent autosomal recessive diseases. Many others in this category, including sickle cell disease and other hemoglobinopathies, thalassemias, and alpha-1-antitrypsin deficiency, are discussed elsewhere in this book.

### Cystic Fibrosis (CF)

Cystic fibrosis is a systemic disease of infancy or childhood in which there is a fundamental defect in the secretory processes of all forms of exocrine glands.[64] *Most consistently involved are the exocrine sweat glands and mucus glands. The sweat contains abnormally high levels of sodium and chloride, and the mucus glands produce abnormally viscid secretions.*[65] In earlier studies, attention was focused on the striking morphologic abnormalities in the pancreas evoked by the inspissated mucus within the ducts, and so sometimes this condition is still called "fibrocystic disease of the pancreas," or "mucoviscidosis." Largely a disease of whites, it is rarely encountered in blacks (and then principally among those in the United States). It is equally rare among those of Oriental and Mongolian descent. Approximately 1 in 2000 live births in the United States are affected with this condition, and cystic fibrosis is the most common lethal genetic disease in this country.

**PATHOGENESIS.** Theories abound and are surrounded by controversy. Any credible hypothesis must explain (1) the generalized involvement of exocrine glands while other tissues are spared, (2) the morphologic normality of these glands before they are damaged by the disease itself, and (3) the elevation in sweat sodium and chloride levels, which is the only consistent biochemical abnormality in cystic fibrosis. The genetics of this condition suggests that all characteristics of the disease must result from a single abnormal enzyme or protein. However, despite intensive research no unifying biochemical defect has been found. Increased concentration of proteins and the resulting hyperviscosity has been variously ascribed to primary defects in the transport of calcium or sodium ions or, alternatively, to impaired regulation of glandular secretions due to abnormalities in the autonomic nervous system. Progress in unraveling the biomolecular defect in cystic fibrosis has been hampered because the defective gene or its product have yet to be identified. However, recent rapid progress in its mapping offers hope that the elusive CF gene may be well within our reach. By utilizing recombinant DNA techniques and somatic cell genetics it has been possible to locate the CF gene on the long arm of chromosome 7.[66] There is every reason to believe the gene itself will soon be identified, which will offer not only insights into the pathogenesis of CF but a reliable method for prenatal diagnosis and carrier detection.

**MORPHOLOGY.** The anatomic changes in cystic fibrosis are highly variable and depend on the age of onset and severity of expression of this genetic disorder. Pancreatic abnormalities are present in approximately 80% of patients. These may consist only of accumulations of mucus, leading to dilatation of ducts; in more advanced cases the ducts may become totally plugged, causing atrophy of the exocrine glands (Fig. 4–16). The ducts may be converted into cysts separated only by islets of Langerhans and an abundant fibrous stroma, a picture giving rise to the designation "fibrocystic disease of the pancreas." Loss of pancreatic secretion may lead to severe malabsorption, particularly of fats. A resultant lack

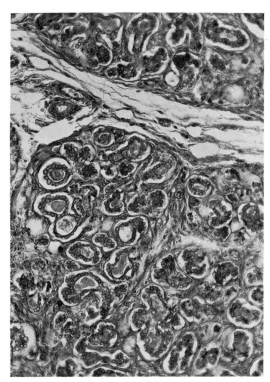

**Figure 4–16.** Cystic fibrosis of pancreas. The ducts are dilated and plugged with mucin, and the parenchymal glands are totally atrophic and replaced by fibrous tissue. (From Robbins, S. L., Cotran, R. S., and Kumar, V.: Pathologic Basis of Disease. 3rd ed. Philadelphia, W. B. Saunders Co., 1984, p. 494.)

of vitamin A, a fat-soluble vitamin, may then contribute to squamous metaplasia of the linings of the ducts. Changes similar to those in the pancreas may develop in the salivary glands. Pulmonary lesions are the most serious aspect of this disease. Retention of abnormally viscid mucin within the small airways leads to dilatation of bronchioles and bronchi with secondary infection, so that severe chronic bronchitis (p. 416), bronchiectasis (p. 423), and lung abscesses (p. 434) are frequent sequelae. *Pseudomonas aeruginosa* is the most commonly isolated pathogen in CF patients; *Haemophilus influenzae, Escherichia coli,* and *Klebsiella* sp. occur less frequently. For reasons not clear, the mucoid form of *P. aeruginosa,* rarely found in non-CF patients, is found in more than 50% of those who have the disease. The subtended pulmonary parenchyma may undergo emphysema (p. 417) or atelectasis (p. 414). Obstruction of the small bowel secondary to impacted viscid mucin (meconium ileus) is not an uncommon complication in newborns. In approximately 25% of patients, inspissation of mucin within the bile ducts impairs the excretion of bile, adding to the malabsorption problems. In time, biliary cirrhosis (p. 592) may develop, but in only about 2% of patients. The exocrine glands of the male reproductive tract are affected and in adults this often leads to sterility.

The clinical manifestations of this condition are extremely varied and range from mild to severe, from onset at birth to onset years later, and from syndromes that are predominantly gastrointestinal to those that appear to be cardiopulmonary. As many as 15% of the cases come to clinical attention at birth or soon after because of an attack of meconium ileus. More commonly, manifestations of malabsorption (e.g., large, foul stools, abdominal distention, and poor weight gain) appear during the first year of life. The faulty fat absorption may induce deficiency states of the fat-soluble vitamins, resulting in manifestations of avitaminosis A, D, or K. If the child survives these hazards, pulmonary problems such as chronic cough, persistent lung infections, obstructive pulmonary disease, and cor pulmonale may make their appearance. Persistent pulmonary infections are responsible for 80 to 90% of the deaths. With improved control of infections, more patients are now surviving to adulthood; the median life expectancy for females and males is approximately 23 and 28 years, respectively.[64] Most males (90%), however, are infertile due to blockage of vas deferens, epididymis, and seminal vesicles.

The diagnosis of CF is based on clinical findings and the biochemical abnormalities in sweat. A properly administered and interpreted sweat test is crucial to the diagnosis. An increase in sweat electrolytes (often the mother makes the diagnosis because baby tastes salty) along with one or more major clinical features is necessary for diagnosis. Until recently there has been no reliable test for detection of heterozygotes or for antenatal diagnosis, but as mentioned above, localization of the CF gene is likely to change this dismal state of affairs in the near future.

### Phenylketonuria (PKU)

*Homozygotes with this autosomal recessive disorder classically have a total lack of phenylalanine hydroxylase, leading to phenylketonuria.* Affected babies are normal at birth but within a few weeks develop a rising plasma phenylalanine level, which in some way impairs brain development. Usually by six months of life severe mental retardation becomes all too evident; fewer than 4% of untreated phenylketonuric children have IQ values greater than 50 to 60. About one third of these unfortunate children are never able to walk, and two thirds cannot talk. Seizures, other neurologic abnormalities, decreased pigmentation of hair and skin, and eczema often accompany the mental retardation in untreated children. Once established, the mental deficit is irreversible, but if PKU is recognized promptly and the

patient is placed on a low phenylalanine diet, the hyperphenylalaninemia can be prevented and the retardation of brain development avoided. A number of screening procedures are routinely used to detect phenylketonuria.[67]

*The biochemical abnormality in PKU is an inability to convert phenylalanine into tyrosine.* In the normal child, less than 50% of the dietary intake of phenylalanine is necessary for protein synthesis. The rest is converted to tyrosine by the phenylalanine hydroxylase system, which has several components in addition to the enzyme phenylalanine hydroxylase (Fig. 4–17). With a block in phenylalanine metabolism, due to lack of phenylalanine hydroxylase, minor shunt pathways come into play, yielding phenylpyruvic acid, phenyllactic acid, phenylacetic acid, and *o*-hydroxyphenylacetic acid, which are excreted in large amounts in the urine in PKU. Some of these abnormal metabolites are excreted in the sweat, and phenylacetic acid in particular imparts a strong musty or "mousy" odor to affected infants. It is believed that these metabolites contribute to the brain damage in PKU.

This inborn error of metabolism is quite common in those of Scandinavian descent and is distinctly uncommon in blacks and in Jews. As with all inborn errors of metabolism, a number of variants have been identified. In addition to the classic homozygous disease described previously, there is a condition in which some patients have only modest elevations of phenylalanine levels, without any associated neurologic abnormalities. This pattern of so-called benign hyperphenylalaninemia occurs with a less complete deficiency of phenylalanine hydroxylase. Presumably multiple mutant alleles may exist at the phenylalanine hydroxylase locus; only those mutations that result in severe deficiency of the enzyme result in classic PKU. This distinction is important clinically, since those with benign hyperphenylalaninemia do not develop the stigmata of classic PKU but may be picked up as "positive" in the widely used Guthrie screening test. Measurement of serum phenylalanine levels is necessary for differentiating benign hyperphenylalaninemia and PKU.[67] In other variant forms, accounting for 3 to 10% of all cases with PKU, enzymes other than phenylalanine hydroxylase are affected. These include patients who lack dihydropteridine reductase (DHPR, Fig. 4–17). Like those with classic PKU, they are also unable to metabolize phenylalanine, but in addition they have associated abnormalities of tyrosine and tryptophan metabolism, since DHPR is

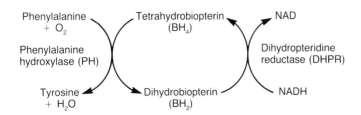

Figure 4–17. The phenylalanine hydroxylase system. (From Robbins, S. L., Cotran, R. S., and Kumar, V.: Pathologic Basis of Disease. 3rd. ed. Philadelphia, W. B. Saunders Co., 1984, p. 490.)

required for hydroxylation of these two amino acids. It is clinically important to recognize these variant forms of PKU because they cannot be treated by the dietary control of phenylalanine levels. The concomitant impairment of tyrosine and tryptophan hydroxylation leads to disturbance in the synthesis of neurotransmitters, and hence neurologic damage is not arrested despite normalization of phenylalanine levels.[68]

### Galactosemia

Galactosemia is an autosomal recessive disorder of galactose metabolism. Normally, lactose, the major carbohydrate of mammalian milk, is split into glucose and galactose in the intestinal microvilli by lactase. Galactose is then converted to glucose in three steps, as is detailed in Figure 4–18. *Two variants of galactosemia have been identified. The more common variant is a total lack of galactose-1-phosphate uridyl transferase involved in Reaction 2. The rare variant arises from a deficiency of galactokinase involved in Reaction 1.* Galactokinase deficiency leads to a milder form of the disease not associated with mental retardation, which will not be considered in our discussion. As a result of the transferase lack, galactose-1-phosphate accumulates in many locations, including the liver, spleen, lens of the eye, kidney, heart muscle, cerebral cortex, and erythrocytes. Alternative metabolic pathways are activated, leading to the production of galactitol, which also accumulates in the tissues.[69] Heterozygotes may have a mild deficiency but are spared the clinicomorphologic consequences of the homozygous state.

The liver, eyes, and brain bear the brunt of the damage. The early-appearing **hepatomegaly** is largely due to fatty change, but in time widespread scarring that closely resembles the cirrhosis of alcohol abuse may supervene (p. 584). **Opacification of the lens (cataracts)** develops, probably because the lens imbibes water and swells as galactitol, produced by alternate metabolic pathways, accumulates and increases its tonicity. **Nonspecific alterations appear in the central nervous system,** including loss of nerve cells, gliosis, and edema, particularly in the dentate nuclei of the cerebellum and the olivary nuclei of the medulla. Similar changes may occur in the cerebral cortex and white matter.

There is still no clear understanding of the mechanism of injury to the liver and brain. Toxicity has been imputed to galactose-1-phosphate. Alternatively, galactitol has been indicted as the toxic product. It is also possible that the abnormal galactose metabolism interferes with the formation of galactose-containing cerebral lipids.

Almost from birth these infants fail to thrive. Vomiting and diarrhea appear within a few days of milk ingestion. Jaundice and hepatomegaly usually become evident during the first week of life and may seem to be a continuation of the physiologic jaundice of the newborn. The cataracts develop within a few weeks, and within the first 6 to 12 months of life, mental retardation may be detected. Even in untreated infants the mental deficit is usually not as severe as that of phenylketonuria. Accumulation of galactose and galactose-1-phosphate in the kidney impairs amino acid transport, resulting in aminoaciduria. There is increased frequency of fulminant *E. coli* septicemia.

*Most of the clinical and morphologic changes can be prevented by early removal of galactose from the diet for at least the first two years of life.* Control instituted soon after birth prevents the cataracts and liver damage and permits almost normal mental development. When galactosemia is recognized later, the changes in the lens and liver (if cirrhosis has not occurred) may be reversible, but the mental retardation is irreversible. The diagnosis can be suspected by the demonstration of a reducing sugar other than glucose in the urine, but tests that directly identify the deficiency of the transferase in leukocytes and erythrocytes are more certain. Antenatal diagnosis is possible in cultured fibroblasts derived from amniotic fluid.

### Albinism

Albinism need be mentioned only briefly since, happily, it is not a serious clinical disorder. It represents the hereditary inability to synthesize melanin. There are a great many genetic variants of albinism, most of which are transmitted as autosomal recessives, but certain pedigrees suggest dominant transfer and others, X-linked transmission.[70] In some genetic variants the absence of pigmentation results from a deficiency of tyrosinase. In others the precise defect is not known. Tyrosinase, you may recall, is involved in the conversion of tyrosine to 3,4-dopa necessary for the synthesis of melanin. The lack of pigmentation of skin, hair, sclera, and iris is only of consequence

(Reaction 1) Galactose + ATP $\xleftarrow{\text{Galactokinase}}$ Galactose-1-phosphate + ADP

(Reaction 2) Galactose-1-phosphate + UDP glucose $\xleftarrow{\text{Galactose-1-phosphate uridyl transferase}}$ UDP galactose + glucose-1-phosphate

(Reaction 3) UDP-galactose $\xleftarrow{\text{UDP-galactose-4-epimerase}}$ UDP-glucose

Figure 4–18. Conversion of galactose to glucose.

insofar as it permits light to pour through the unpigmented iris and sclera, thus causing retinal injury, and the absence of melanin pigmentation of the skin makes these patients vulnerable to skin cancer (including malignant melanomas).

### Wilson's Disease

This autosomal recessive disorder of copper metabolism is characterized by three principal features: (1) excessive deposits of copper in liver cells, leading in time to a form of cirrhosis; (2) degenerative changes in the brain, hence the synonym "hepatolenticular disease"; and (3) a pathognomonic greenish-brown ring (Kayser-Fleischer ring) at the limbus of the cornea.[71] The nature of the metabolic error is as yet unestablished. Two possibilities have been suggested: (1) There may be a deficiency in the hepatic synthesis of the copper-binding protein ceruloplasmin. With a deficiency of ceruloplasmin, large amounts of copper are loosely bound to albumin. Ready dissociation of this albumin complex permits copper to be deposited in the tissues of the body, particularly in the liver, brain, and cornea. However, the recent observation that the genes for Wilson's disease and ceruloplasmin are located on two different chromosomes renders this possibility very unlikely.[72] (2) There may be a deficiency in the biliary excretion of copper, due to a still-undefined abnormality in hepatic copper metabolism. This is now believed to be the primary defect, accompanied by a secondary suppression of ceruloplasmin synthesis by free unexcreted copper within the liver cells. In any event, *a normal or slightly lowered serum copper level, a well-defined decrease in serum ceruloplasmin, and an increase in albumin-bound copper are characteristic of Wilson's disease*. The critical diagnostic feature is the biochemical burden of copper ions in a liver sample.

Wilson's disease may present predominantly hepatic, neurologic, or psychiatric symptoms. The liver disease rarely manifests prior to five to six years age, and in many cases the first symptoms are noted in adulthood. Hepatic involvement may present as an acute self-limited disease resembling viral hepatitis or may evolve rapidly into fulminant hepatitis. In many patients the onset is more insidious, mimicking chronic active hepatitis (p. 579) or, alternatively, as cirrhosis with associated portal hypertension and gradually developing hepatocellular failure. The histologic changes in the liver are as varied as the clinical picture.[73] Early in the course there is cytoplasmic fatty change accompanied by glycogen accumulation in the nuclei. At a later stage, hepatocellular necrosis is observed, accompanied by the formation of hyaline deposits very similar to those seen in the liver of an alcohol abuser. Electron microscopy discloses an accumulation of copper in the hepatic cell lysosomes as well as mitochondrial abnormalities. Scarring is a consequence of the hepatocellular necrosis, and in time cirrhosis develops; it may take the

form of either a fine delicate network of fibrous tissue or massive scars resembling postnecrotic cirrhosis (p. 590).

If the liver disease does not prove fatal, involvement of the brain usually appears during the second decade (p. 752). The most dramatic findings are cavitations in the lenticular nucleus, in the tip of the frontal lobe, and, rarely, in the dentate nucleus of the cerebellum. This is accompanied by brownish discoloration and often atrophy of the basal ganglia. Histologically, there is an increase in the number of Alzheimer type II and multinucleated Alzheimer type I astrocytes. Degeneration of nerve cells and astrocytes in these areas leads to cavitations. The Kayser-Fleischer ring results from deposits of copper in the cornea; they can usually be seen with the naked eye but may require slit-lamp examination. Aminoaciduria and glycosuria as well as other renal tubular abnormalities are virtually always present in patients who have developed neurologic disease.

Happily, despite the fact that the basic metabolic defect is unknown, it is possible to prevent the development of hepatic and brain disease, or in any event significantly improve the condition of patients with established disease by treatments (penicillamine, chelating agents) that reduce the stores of copper in the tissues. The disease can be recognized at an asymptomatic stage by the low serum ceruloplasmin level, which should be sought in children with a family history of this disorder.

### Glycogen Storage Disorders (Glycogenoses)

An inherited deficiency of any one of the enzymes involved in glycogen synthesis or degradation can result in the excessive accumulation of glycogen or some abnormal form of glycogen in various tissues. The type of glycogen stored, its intracellular location, and the tissue distribution of the affected cells vary, depending upon the specific enzyme deficiency. Whatever the tissue or cells affected, the glycogen is most often stored within the cytoplasm or sometimes within nuclei. One variant, type II (Pompe's disease), is a form of *lysosomal storage disease* because the missing enzyme is localized to lysosomes. Most glycogenoses are inherited as autosomal recessive diseases, as is common with "missing enzyme" syndromes. One variant, type VIII, is X-linked recessive.

The biochemical consequences of individual enzyme deficiencies can best be appreciated in the context of normal glycogen metabolism, which is illustrated schematically in Figure 4–19 but is dealt with in detail in specialized texts.[74] Only a few comments on glycogen metabolism that are of particular relevance to the understanding of glycogen storage diseases are in order. Glycogen is a very large polysaccharide of glucose (molecular weight, 250,000 to 100,000,000 daltons). A specific enzyme (amylo-1,4:1,6-transglucosidase) is necessary to initiate

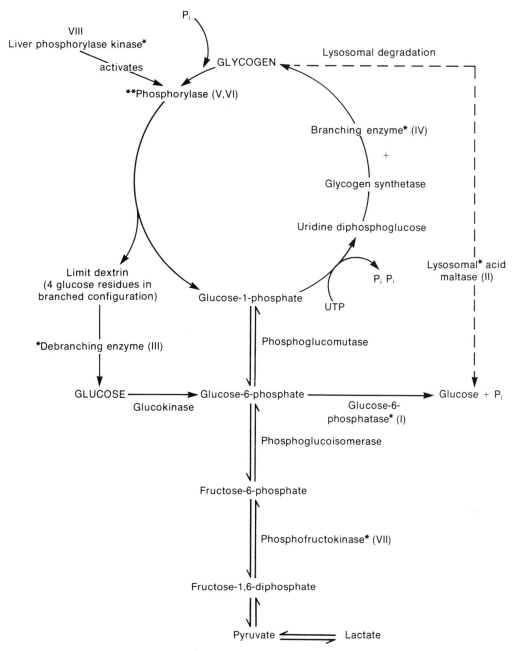

**Figure 4–19.** Pathways of glycogen metabolism. Asterisks mark the enzyme deficiencies associated with glycogen storage diseases. Roman numerals indicate the type of glycogen storage disease associated with the given enzyme deficiency. Types V and VI result from deficiencies of muscle and liver phosphorylases, respectively. (After Howell, R. R.: The glycogen storage diseases. *In* Stanbury, J. B., et al. [eds.]: Metabolic Basis of Inherited Disease. 5th ed. New York, McGraw-Hill, 1983, p. 144.)

branching during synthesis. Conversely, during degradation the phosphorylases split glucose-1-phosphate from the branches until about four glucose residues remain on each branch, leaving a branched oligosaccharide called limit dextrin. This can be further degraded only by the debranching enzyme (amylo-1,6-glucosidase). In addition to traveling these major metabolic pathways, glycogen is also broken down in the lysosomes by acid maltase; if the lysosomes are deficient in this enzyme, the membrane-enclosed glycogen is not accessible to degradation by

the cytoplasmic enzymes such as phosphorylases. All the glycogenoses are rare, and the eight recognized forms are summarized in Table 4–4. Diagnosis is usually established by estimation of enzyme activity in the appropriate tissues.

### Lysosomal Storage Diseases

Lysosomes, as is well known, contain a variety of hydrolytic enzymes that are involved in the breakdown of complex substrates, such as sphingolipids

**Table 4–4. PRINCIPAL FEATURES OF THE GLYCOGENOSES**

| | Type | Enzyme Deficiency | Morphologic Changes | Clinical Manifestations |
|---|---|---|---|---|
| I | Hepato-renal—von Gierke's disease | Glucose-6-phosphatase | *Hepatomegaly*—intracytoplasmic accumulations of glycogen and small amounts of lipid; intranuclear glycogen. *Renomegaly*—intracytoplasmic accumulations of glycogen in cortical tubular epithelial cells. | Failure to thrive, stunted growth, hepatomegaly, and renomegaly. Hypoglycemia due to failure in glucose mobilization, often leading to convulsions. Hyperlipidemia and hyperuricemia resulting from deranged glucose metabolism; many patients develop gout. Mortality approximately 50%. |
| II | Generalized glycogenosis—Pompe's disease | Lysosomal glucosidase (acid maltase) | *Mild hepatomegaly*—ballooning of lysosomes with glycogen creating lacy cytoplasmic pattern. *Cardiomegaly*—glycogen within sarcoplasm and sometimes membrane-bound. *Skeletal muscle*—similar to heart. | Massive cardiomegaly, muscle hypotonia, and cardiorespiratory failure within 2 years. |
| III | Cori's disease | Debrancher system | Mild to marked *hepatomegaly*—cells similar to those of type I. Mild to moderate *cardiomegaly*—cells similar to those of type II. *Skeletal muscle*—similar to that of type II. | Similar to type I but usually milder. Compatible with normal longevity. |
| IV | Brancher glycogenosis | Amylo-1,4:1,6 transglucosidase (brancher enzyme) | *Accumulation of abnormal glycogen (amylopectin) in liver cells, cardiac and skeletal muscle, and brain.* Intracytoplasmic accumulations of a hyaline, fibrillar, PAS-positive material that is diastase resistant. In time, development of *cirrhosis* of liver. | Hepatomegaly, splenomegaly, ascites, and liver failure. Very rare and lethal. |
| V | McArdle's syndrome | Muscle phosphorylase | *Skeletal muscle only*—sarcoplasmic accumulations of glycogen similar to those of type II. | Painful cramps associated with strenuous exercise. Myoglobinuria occurs in 50% of cases. Onset in adulthood (>20 years). Muscular exercise fails to raise lactate level in venous blood. Compatible with normal longevity. |
| VI | Hers' disease | Liver phosphorylase | *Only hepatomegaly*—scattered cytoplasmic vacuoles, occasionally lipid vacuoles; no intranuclear glycogen. | Hepatomegaly. Mild clinical course. |
| VII | Tarui's disease | Phosphofructokinase | *Only skeletal muscle* and erythrocytes studied—sarcoplasmic glycogen similar to that in type II. | Similar to type V. Very rare. |
| VIII | | Deficient activity of phosphorylase kinase | *Hepatomegaly*—similar to that in type VI. | X-linked recessive. Hepatomegaly and mild clinical course. |

and mucopolysaccharides, into soluble end products. These large molecules may be derived from the turnover of intracellular organelles that enter the lysosomes by autophagocytosis (p. 22), or they may be acquired from outside the cells by phagocytosis. With an inherited lack of a lysosomal enzyme, catabolism of its substrate remains incomplete, leading to the accumulation of the partially degraded insoluble metabolite within the lysosomes (Fig. 4–20). As might be expected, these missing-enzyme syndromes are inherited as autosomal recessive disorders, and the storage of insoluble intermediates occurs mainly in cells of the mononuclear phagocyte system, since they ingest and degrade senescent red cells, leukocytes, and other tissue breakdown products.

The numerous lysosomal storage diseases can be divided into broad categories based on the biochem-ical nature of the substrates and the accumulated metabolites (Table 4–5). Within each group there are several entities, each resulting from the deficiency of a specific enzyme. Fortunately, for both medical students and the diseases' potential victims, most of these conditions are very rare, and their detailed description is better relegated to specialized texts and reviews.[75, 76] Only a few of the more common sphingolipidoses and mucopolysaccharidoses (Table 4–5) will be considered here. Type 2 glycogen storage disease, also a lysosomal disorder, was discussed earlier.

**GAUCHER'S DISEASE.** There are three autosomal recessive variants of this condition. Common to all three is variably deficient activity of a glucocerebrosidase that normally cleaves the glucose residue from ceramide. This leads to an accumulation of glucocer-

Figure 4–20. A schematic diagram illustrating the pathogenesis of lysosomal storage diseases. In the example illustrated, a complex substrate is normally degraded by a series of lysosomal enzymes (1, 2, and 3) into soluble end products. If there is a deficiency of one of the enzymes (e.g., 3), catabolism is incomplete and insoluble intermediate metabolites accumulate in the lysosomes.

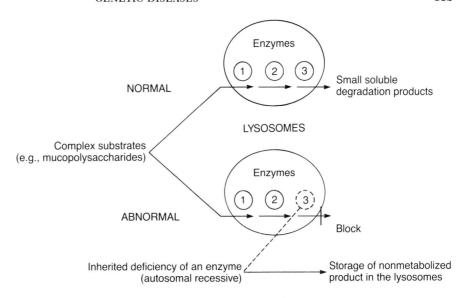

ebrosides in the reticuloendothelial cells and the formation of so-called Gaucher cells. Normally the glycolipids derived from the breakdown of blood cells, particularly erythrocytes, are sequentially degraded. In Gaucher's disease the degradation stops at the level of glucocerebrosides, which in transport through the blood as macromolecules are engulfed by the phagocytic cells of the body, especially those in the liver, spleen, and bone marrow. *These phagocytes (Gaucher cells) become enlarged, sometimes*

*up to 100 μm in size, and develop a pathognomonic cytoplasmic appearance, characterized as "wrinkled tissue paper"* (Fig. 4–21). No distinct vacuolation is present. Electron microscopy indicates that the distinctive cytoplasmic morphology represents secondary lysosomes or residual bodies filled with tubular structures and fibrils. Gaucher cells also stain positively with PAS stain because of the presence of carbohydrates.

One variant, *type I, also called the adult form, accounts for 80% of cases of Gaucher's disease.* It is characterized by hepatosplenomegaly and the absence of central nervous system involvement. The spleen often enlarges massively, filling the entire abdomen. Gaucher cells are found in the liver, spleen, lymph nodes, and bone marrow. Marrow replacement and cortical erosion may produce radiographically visible skeletal lesions as well as a reduction in the formed elements of blood. Hypersplenism (p. 404) also contributes to the anemia and leukopenia. Type I has a predilection for Ashkenazi Jews, and, unlike other variants, is compatible with long life. The type II variant is highly lethal, affects children by six months of age, and is characterized by severe central nervous system involvement. Although liver and spleen are also involved, the clinical features are dominated by neurologic disturbances. The major brain changes comprise lipid-laden periadventitial cells and loss of neurons, which themselves do not show lipid storage.

The type III (juvenile) variant involves the brain as well as viscera, but the course is intermediate between those of types I and II. The three variants are believed to result from distinct mutations affecting the activity of glucocerebrosidase. Type I is associated with reduction but not complete lack of enzyme activity, whereas in type II there is virtually no detectable glucocerebrosidase in tissues.

The level of glucocerebrosidase in leukocytes or cultured fibroblasts is helpful in diagnosis and the

## Table 4–5. LYSOSOMAL STORAGE DISORDERS

| Disease | Enzyme Deficiency | Major Accumulating Metabolite |
|---|---|---|
| **Glycogenoses** | | |
| Type 2—Pompe's disease | Lysosomal glucosidase | Glycogen |
| **Sphingolipidoses** | | |
| $G_{M1}$—gangliosidoses | $G_{M1}$ ganglioside β-galactosidase | $G_{M1}$ ganglioside, galactose-containing oligosaccharides |
| $G_{M2}$—gangliosidoses: Tay-Sachs disease | Hexosaminidase A | $G_{M2}$ ganglioside |
| Gaucher's disease | Glucocerebrosidase | Glucocerebroside |
| Neimann-Pick disease | Sphingomyelinase | Sphingomyelin |
| **Mucopolysaccharidoses** | | |
| MPS 1 H (Hurler) | α-L-iduronidase | Heparan sulfate Dermatan sulfate |
| MPS II (Hunter) (X-linked recessive) | L-iduronosulfate sulfatase | Heparan sulfate Dermatan sulfate |
| **Glycoproteinoses** | Enzymes involved in degradation of oligosaccharide side chains of glycoproteins (several) | Several, depending on specific enzyme |

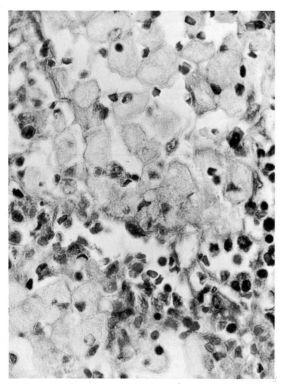

**Figure 4–21.** The spleen in Gaucher's disease. The large vacuolated cells have a ground-glass appearance and contain some faint wavy lines, creating some resemblance to wrinkled tissue paper.

detection of heterozygotes. Prenatal diagnosis is possible by amniocentesis.

**NIEMANN-PICK DISEASE.** This designation includes a constellation of hereditary syndromes characterized by the accumulation of sphingomyelin in phagocytic cells and often in the central nervous system as well. *Sphingomyelin, a constituent of all membranes (including those of organelles) accumulates because of a deficiency of the lysosomal enzyme sphingomyelinase,* which is required for the cleavage of sphingomyelin into ceramide and phosphorylcholine. The excess sphingomyelin is incorporated into all phagocytic cells, usually within secondary lysosomes. The phagocytic cells become stuffed with droplets or particles of the complex lipid, imparting a fine vacuolation or foaminess to the cytoplasm (Fig. 4–22). For reasons not yet clear, there is also usually a concomitant intracellular accumulation of cholesterol. Because of their high content of phagocytic cells, the organs most severely affected are the spleen, liver, bone marrow, lymph nodes, and lungs. As with Gaucher's disease, splenic enlargement may be striking. The spleen and lymph nodes in particular are virtually replaced by masses of foam cells, which cause considerable enlargement of these structures. The central nervous system is also involved in the most frequent variant of this disorder. In such cases the neurons are enlarged and vacuolated due to storage of lipids. The entire central nervous system,

including spinal cord and ganglia, are involved in this tragic, inexorable process. Involvement of the retinal neurons is responsible for the appearance of a cherry-red spot in the macula. This region, which is devoid of neurons, appears bright red, in contrast with the surrounding lipid-infiltrated retinal cells. Based on the distribution of lesions and associated clinical features, Niemann-Pick disease has been classified into five variants, designated types A through E. Type A, the most common, has just been described. It relentlessly destroys CNS function, and infants usually die within the first three to four years of life. Estimation of sphingomyelinase activity in the leukocytes or cultured fibroblasts can be used for diagnosis of suspected cases as well as for detection of carriers. Antenatal diagnosis is possible by the use of cultured fibroblasts obtained by amniocentesis.

**TAY-SACHS DISEASE ($G_{M2}$ GANGLIOSIDOSIS TYPE 1).** Gangliosidoses are characterized by accumulation of gangliosides, principally in the brain, due to a deficiency of a catabolic lysosomal enzyme. Depending upon the ganglioside involved, these disorders are subclassified into $G_{M1}$ and $G_{M2}$ categories. Tay-Sachs disease is by far the commonest of all gangliosidoses and is characterized by deficiency of the enzyme hexosaminidase A, which is necessary for the degradation of $G_{M2}$. The brain is principally affected since it is most involved in ganglioside metabolism. *The storage of $G_{M2}$ occurs within neurons, axon*

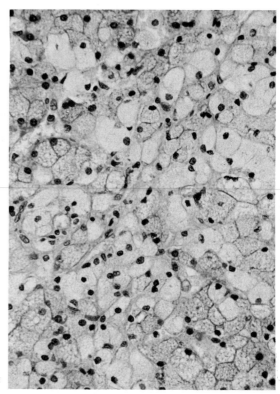

**Figure 4–22.** Niemann-Pick disease. The foamy vacuolation of the cells in the spleen results from accumulations of sphingomyelin.

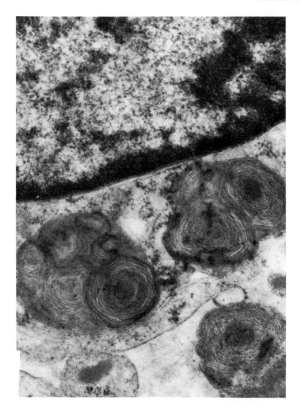

Figure 4–23. Portion of a neuron under the electron microscope shows prominent lysosomes with whorled configurations. Part of the nucleus is shown above. (Courtesy of Dr. Joe Rutledge, Southwestern Medical School, Dallas, Texas. From Robbins, S. L., Cotran, R. S., and Kumar, V.: Pathologic Basis of Disease. 3rd ed. Philadelphia, W. B. Saunders Co., 1984, p. 145.)

*cylinders of nerves, and glial cells throughout the central nervous system.* Affected cells appear swollen, possibly foamy and not dissimilar from those in Niemann-Pick disease. Electron microscopy reveals a whorled configuration within lysosomes (Fig. 4–23). These anatomic changes are found throughout the central nervous system (including the spinal cord), peripheral nerves, and autonomic nervous system. The retina is usually involved and discloses the characteristic cherry-red spot in the fovea of the macula. Occasionally minimal visceral involvement is encountered in Tay-Sachs disease, usually in the form of lipid inclusions in the parenchymal cells of the liver and lipid-laden foam cells in the spleen and lung.

Like the other lipidoses, Tay-Sachs disease is most common among Ashkenazi Jews, in whom the frequency of heterozygous carriers is estimated to be 1 in 30. Heterozygotes can be reliably detected by estimating the level of hexosaminidase A in the serum. Antenatal diagnosis is possible, and the detection of Tay-Sachs disease in the fetus is widely viewed as an indication for therapeutic abortion. Those unfortunate infants who are born suffer from mental retardation, blindness, and severe neurologic

dysfunctions, which lead to certain death within two to three years.

### *Mucopolysaccharidoses (MPS)*

*This group of diseases is characterized by defective degradation and therefore storage of mucopolysaccharides in various tissues.* You may recall that mucopolysaccharides form a part of ground substance and are synthesized in the connective tissues by fibroblasts (p. 56). Most of the mucopolysaccharide is secreted into the ground substance, but a certain fraction is degraded within lysosomes. Several enzymes are involved in this catabolic pathway; it is the lack of these enzymes that leads to accumulation of mucopolysaccharides within the lysosomes. Several clinical variants of MPS, classified numerically from MPS I to MPS VII, have been described, each resulting from the deficiency of one specific enzyme. Within a given group (e.g., MPS I, characterized by a deficiency of α-L-iduronidase) subgroups exist that result from *different* mutant alleles at the same genetic locus. Thus, the severity of enzyme deficiency and the clinical picture even within subgroups is often different. *The mucopolysaccharides that accumulate within the tissues include dermatan sulfate, heparan sulfate, keratan sulfate, and, in some cases, chondroitin sulfate.*

*In general the MPS are progressive disorders, characterized by involvement of multiple organs, including liver, spleen, heart, and blood vessels.* Most of them are associated with coarse facial features, clouding of the cornea, joint stiffness, and mental retardation. Urinary excretion of the accumulated mucopolysaccharides is often increased. All of the MPS except one are inherited as autosomal recessives; one variant, called Hunter syndrome, is an X-linked recessive. Of the seven recognized variants, only two well-characterized syndromes will be discussed briefly. Details of others may be found in specialized texts.[75]

*Hurler syndrome, also called MPS I H, results from a deficiency of α-L-iduronidase.* Affected children have a life expectancy of six to ten years. Like patients with most other forms of MPS, they develop coarse facial features associated with skeletal deformities, creating an appearance referred to as "gargoylism." Death is often due to cardiac complications resulting from the deposition of mucopolysaccharides in the coronary arteries and heart valves. Accumulation of dermatan sulfate and heparan sulfate is seen in cells of the mononuclear phagocyte system, in fibroblasts, and within endothelium and smooth muscles cells of the vascular wall. The affected cells are swollen and have clear cytoplasm, resulting from the accumulation of PAS-positive material within engorged, vacuolated lysosomes. Lysosomal inclusions are also found in neurons, accounting for mental retardation. Although most of the clinical features can be explained on the basis of excessive storage of mucopolysaccharides, joint stiffness, for example, probably results from disturbances in collagen synthesis, which occur secondary to derangement in the ground substance.

The other variant of MPS, called *Hunter's syndrome*, differs from Hurler syndrome in its mode of inheritance (X-linked), the absence of corneal clouding, and often its milder clinical course. Like the Hurler syndrome, *the accumulated mucopolysaccharides in the Hunter syndrome are heparan and dermatan sulfates, but this results from a deficiency of L-iduronate sulfatase.* Despite the difference in enzyme deficiency, an accumulation of identical substrates occurs, since breakdown of heparan and dermatan sulfates requires both L-iduronidase and the sulfatase; if either one is missing, further degradation is blocked.

## X-LINKED DISORDERS

Sex-linked, better known as X-linked, disorders are transmitted by heterozygous carrier females virtually only to sons, who of course are hemizygous for the X chromosome. Heterozygous females rarely express the full phenotypic change owing to the presence of the paired normal allele. However, because of the inactivation of one of the X chromosomes in females (discussed later) it is remotely possible for the normal allele to be inactivated in the vast majority of cells, permitting full expression of the disease in heterozygous females. An affected male does not transmit the disorder to sons, but all daughters are carriers. Sons of heterozygous women have, of course a one-in-two chance of receiving the mutant gene. To date, no Y-linked diseases are known. Save for determinants dictating male differentiation, the only characteristic that may be located on the Y chromosome is the not altogether unpleasant attribute of "hairy ears."

There are a very few X-linked dominant diseases. Their inheritance pattern is characterized by transmission of the disease to 50% of the sons and daughters of an affected heterozygous female. An affected male cannot transmit the disease to his sons, but all daughters are affected. One example of such a disease is vitamin D–resistant rickets.

X-linked recessive disorders are much less common than those arising in autosomal mutations. Some of the more important conditions having this mode of transmission are presented elsewhere—glucose-6-phosphate dehydrogenase deficiency (p. 360), hemophilia A, hemophilia B (p. 400), and agammaglobulinemia (p. 173). Some variants of inborn errors of metabolism have already been cited as being X-linked—for example, the Lesch-Nyhan syndrome and one form of mucopolysaccharidosis (Hunter's syndrome). Other X-linked disorders, such as Fabry's disease, Duchenne's and Becker's muscular dystrophies, and nephrogenic diabetes insipidus, are too rare for inclusion here. Without regrets we can proceed, then, to the next category of genetic disease.

# DISORDERS WITH VARIABLE MODES OF TRANSMISSION

## *Hereditary Malformation*

Congenital malformations may be familial and genetic or may be acquired by exposure to teratogenic agents *in utero*. Hereditary malformations are associated with several modes of transmission. Certain common congenital malformations are multifactorial disorders, whereas others are transmitted by single mutant genes; still others are caused by chromosomal aberrations. Some of the multifactorial defects that have a frequency of one or more per 1000 births are listed in Table 4–6. These disorders run in families and present significant risks to blood relatives. As already discussed, the more genes an individual shares with the affected family member (proband), the higher is the probability that the individual will develop the malformation. Thus, first-degree relatives of an individual with a hereditary harelip have a 35 to 40 times greater chance of being similarly affected than do control populations; the risk for second-degree relatives is sevenfold, and for third-degree relatives threefold. In some malformations of multifactorial origin, environmental influences that contribute to the expression of the disease can be identified. For example, in the infant with a genetic vulnerability to congenital hip dislocation, premature weight-bearing or trauma may unmask the problem. The importance of recognizing these multifactorial traits lies, then, in the possibility of controlling environmental factors contributing to the expression of the disorder. Other hereditary malformations are transmitted by single mutant genes. For the most part, these monogenic errors of morphogenesis take the form of localized lesions affecting a single organ or system (e.g., the fingers, eyes, or small intestine). Alterations associated with several abnormal karyotypes almost invariably comprise widespread malformations; the best examples are the autosomal

Table 4–6. MALFORMATIONS OCCURRING IN AT LEAST 1 IN 1000 BIRTHS*

| Diagnosis | Incidence/1000 Births |
|---|---|
| Cleft lip (with or without cleft palate) | 1.0 |
| Congenital heart defects | 6.0 |
| Pyloric stenosis | 3.0 |
| Anencephaly | 2.0 |
| Spina bifida cystica | 2.5 |
| Congenital dislocation of the hip | 1.0 |

*Modified from Carter, C. O.: Genetics of common single malformations. Br. Med. Bull. *32*:21, 1976.

trisomies (e.g., Down's syndrome) presented later in this chapter.

The importance of detecting the underlying cause of congenital malformations in genetic counseling is obvious, especially since some syndromes that closely resemble each other have different modes of transmission. It is also important to exclude nongenetic causes of congenital malformation, such as fetal exposure to teratogenic drugs and viruses.

### Ehlers-Danlos Syndromes (EDS)

Ehlers-Danlos syndromes are characterized by defects in collagen synthesis and structure. As such they belong to the same general category as Marfan's syndrome but are discussed here because of variable modes of transmission of the different types. All of them are single gene disorders, but the mode of inheritance, as we shall see, encompasses all three of the mendelian patterns. This should not be surprising, since biosynthesis of collagen is a complex process that may be disturbed by genetic errors affecting the structural genes or the genes coding for the enzymes necessary for posttranscriptional events, such as cross-linking of collagen fibers. Since abnormalities of collagen biosynthesis underlie all the variants of EDS, it is advisable to review collagen synthesis, discussed in Chapter 2. We should recall here that on the basis of chemical analyses, at least five distinct types of collagen have been found in humans. They have characteristic tissue distribution and are the products of different genes. To some extent the clinical heterogeneity of EDS can be explained on the basis of mutation in different collagen genes.

Eight clinical variants of EDS are recognized. Since defective collagen is present in all of the variants, certain clinical features are common to all, including hyperelasticity of skin and often extreme susceptibility to bruising and trauma of the skin. In many variants, the joints are hypermobile, allowing an extreme degree of contortion (the proverbial India-rubber man). The distinctive features of the individual variants, including patterns of inheritance, are summarized in Table 4–7. For details, the reader should refer to two recent reviews.[58, 77]

### Neoplasia

Neoplasia is another disorder that may involve inconstant genetic influence. Here the mutation may be germinal and hereditary or it may be somatic, as will be discussed on page 208. In this discussion it will be pointed out that ultimately the induction of cancer may well involve one or more mutations in somatic cells. Susceptibility to environmental oncogenic agents (chemicals, radiation, or viruses) is known to be conditioned by the genetic constitution. The development of a cancer, then, may well be a mutational event imposed by some environmental carcinogenic influence on a fertile genetic soil.

## CYTOGENETICS—THE NORMAL KARYOTYPE

Before we can embark upon the discussion of chromosomal aberrations, a brief outline of the methods utilized in the study of human chromosomes may

Table 4–7. THE EHLERS-DANLOS SYNDROMES

| Name | Clinical Features | Biochemical Defect |
|---|---|---|
| **Autosomal Dominant Syndromes** | | |
| EDS 1 | Classic skin and joint features: all severe; pregnancy often terminates prematurely due to rupture of membranes. | Unknown |
| EDS II | Skin and joint features: all mild. | Unknown |
| EDS III | Joints: severe, generalized hyperextensibility; skin abnormalities, minimal. | Unknown |
| EDS VIII | Skin and joint features: mild to moderate. Severe generalized periodontitis; premature loss of teeth | Unknown |
| **Autosomal Recessive Syndromes** | | |
| EDS IV (ecchymotic type) | Severe bruisability, very thin skin; rupture of bowel and muscular arteries. Joints normal. | Deficient synthesis of type III collagen, due to several distinct mutations in pro-α1(III) gene, especially in tissues containing smooth muscles. |
| EDS VI (ocular type) | Skin and joint features: moderate to severe. Sclera: thin, blue, and rupture easily. | Deficiency of enzyme lysyl hydroxylase. Hydroxylation of lysine necessary for lysyl-derived cross linkages. |
| EDS VII | Skin and joint features: moderate to severe. Short stature, dislocation of joints common. | Deficiency of procollagen-N-peptidase, necessary for conversion of procollagen to collagen fibrils. In some cases mutant pro-α2(I) gene. |
| **X-linked Recessive Syndrome** | | |
| EDS V | Skin features: moderately severe; joints affected mildly. Floppy mitral valve. | Possible deficiency of cross-linking enzyme lysyl oxidase. |

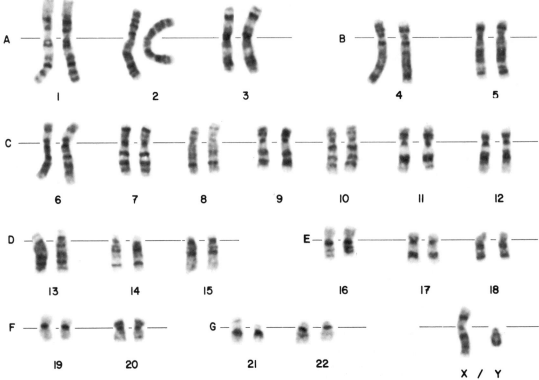

Figure 4–24. A normal male karyotype with G-banding. (Courtesy of Dr. Patricia Howard-Peebles, Department of Pathology, Southwestern Medical School, Dallas, Texas.)

be helpful. The usual procedure is to arrest mitosis in cultured cells in metaphase by the use of colchicine and to stain the chromosomes in the metaphase spread. The stained chromosomes are photographed and arranged in pairs; the composite picture so produced is called a *karyotype*. Karyotyping is the basic tool of the cytogeneticist. The normal human karyotype reveals 23 pairs of chromosomes, of which 22 pairs are autosomes and one pair is the sex chromosomes—XX in females and XY in males. Since the position of the centromere is a constant feature of each chromosome, this characteristic has been used to classify human chromosomes into three types: *metacentric* if the centromere is central, *submetacentric* if the centromere is somewhat off center, *acrocentric* if the centromere is near the end. The chromosome pairs are numbered 1 through 23 on the basis of decreasing size and arranged into seven groups (A to G). Group A includes the largest chromosomes (1, 2, and 3), and group G, the smallest autosomes (21 and 22 and the Y chromosome, which is also small). Within a group, the centromeres of all the chromosomes have more or less similar locations.

Prior to 1970 the techniques utilized in karyotyping resulted in solid dark staining of the chromosomes, which did not allow easy distinction between chromosomes of similar size and morphology (e.g., autosomes 4 and 5). In the 1970s, major advances in the study of chromosomes occurred with the introduction of special staining techniques called banding. Al-

though several banding techniques have been described, staining with Giemsa stain (G banding) is the one most commonly employed. With banding techniques, each chromosome can be seen to possess a distinctive pattern of 200 to 500 alternating light and dark bands of variable widths (Fig. 4–24). With recent improvements (high-resolution banding), up to 2000 bands can be recognized on some chromosomes. The use of banding techniques allows certain identification of each chromosome, as well as precise localization of structural changes in the chromosomes, to be described later.

Another technique that has been extremely useful in the study of chromosomes, particularly in gene mapping, is cell hybridization or cell fusion. The cell hybrids sequentially lose chromosomes until stability is achieved. Thus, correlation of a chromosomal loss with loss of specific phenotypic markers (such as enzymes) allows assignment of genes dictating the phenotypic characteristics to the specific chromosome. Regional assignment is achieved by using human cells having translocated chromosomes induced by quantitated doses of x-irradiation. An elegant map of the human genome has been published recently.[78]

## CYTOGENETIC DISORDERS

Chromosomal abnormalities are much more frequent than is generally appreciated. It is estimated that approximately 1 of 160 newborn infants has some form of chromosomal abnormality.[79] The figure is much higher in fetuses who do not survive to term. It is estimated that in 50% of first-trimester abortions the fetus has a chromosomal abnormality. Cytogenetic disorders may result from alterations in the number or structure of chromosomes and may affect autosomes or sex chromosomes.

**NUMERICAL ABNORMALITIES.** In humans the normal chromosome count is 46 (i.e., 2n = 46). Any exact multiple of the haploid number (n) is called a euploid. Chromosome numbers such as 3n and 4n are called *polyploid.* Polyploidy generally results in a spontaneous abortion. Any number that is not an exact multiple of n is called *aneuploid.* The chief cause of aneuploidy is nondisjunction of a homologous pair of chromosomes at the first meiotic division or a failure of sister chromatids to separate during the second meiotic division. The latter may also occur during somatic cell division, leading to the production of two aneuploid cells. Failure of pairing of homologous chromosomes followed by random assortment (anaphase lag) can also lead to aneuploidy. When nondisjunction occurs at the time of meiosis, the gametes formed have either an extra chromosome (n + 1) or one less chromosome (n − 1). Fertilization of such gametes by normal gametes would result in two types of zygotes—trisomic, with an extra chromosome (2n + 1), or monosomic (2n − 1). Monosomy involving an autosome is incompatible with life, whereas trisomies of certain autosomes and monosomy involving sex chromosomes are compatible with life. These, as we shall see, are usually associated with variable degrees of phenotypic abnormalities. *Mosaicism* is a term used to describe the presence of two or more populations of cells in the same individual. In the context of chromosome numbers, postzygotic mitotic nondisjunction would result in the production of a trisomic and a monosomic daughter cell; the descendants of these cells would then produce a mosaic. As we shall discuss later, mosaicism affecting sex chromosomes is common, whereas autosomal mosaics are not.

**STRUCTURAL ABNORMALITIES.** Structural changes in the chromosomes usually result from chromosome breakage followed by loss or rearrangement of material. Structural changes are usually designated using a cytogenetic "shorthand" in which "p" (petit) denotes the short arm of a chromosome and "q" the long arm. Each arm is then divided into numbered regions (1, 2, 3, and so on) from centromere outwards, and within each region the bands are numerically ordered (Fig. 4–25). Thus 2q34 indicates chromosome 2, long arm, region 3, band 4. Loss and gain of material is denoted by − and +, respectively. The causes of breakage so far as we know are the same as those giving rise to other genetic mutations. Three autosomal recessive syndromes in which chromosomal breakage occurs frequently have been identified: Fanconi's anemia, Bloom's syndrome, and ataxia telangiectasia. The patterns of chromosomal rearrangement following breakage (diagrammed in Fig. 4–26) are as follows:

*Translocation* implies transfer of a part of one chromosome to another nonhomologous chromosome. The process is usually reciprocal (i.e., fragments are exchanged between two chromosomes). In genetic shorthand, translocations are indicated by *t* followed by the involved chromosomes in numerical order—for example, t(14q; 21q). When the entire broken fragments are exchanged, the resulting balanced reciprocal translocation (Fig. 4–26) is not harm-

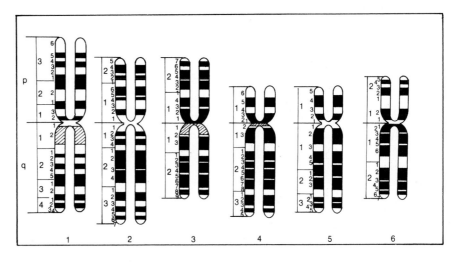

Figure 4–25. Diagrammatic representation of mid-metaphase chromosome bands to indicate nomenclature of arms, regions, and bands. (After Yunis, J. J., and Chandler, M. S.: The chromosomes of man—Clinical and biologic significance. A review. Am. J. Pathol. 8:466, 1977.)

☐ Negative or pale-staining G bands

■ Positive G bands

▨ Variable bands

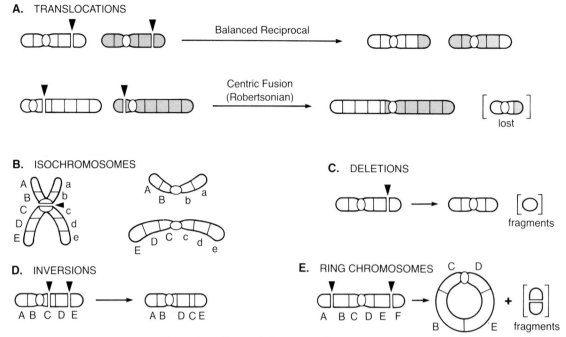

**Figure 4–26.** Types of chromosomal rearrangements.

ful to the carrier, who has the normal number of chromosomes and the full complement of genetic material. However, during gametogenesis, abnormal (unbalanced) gametes will be formed, resulting in abnormal zygotes. A special pattern of reciprocal translocation involving two acrocentric chromosomes is called *centric fusion type* or *Robertsonian translocation*. Typically the breaks occur close to the centromere, affecting the short arm in one and the long arm in the other. Transfer of the segments leads to one very large chromosome and one extremely small one (Fig. 4–26). Often the short fragments are lost. In this case the carrier has 45 chromosomes, but the amount of genetic information lost is so small that it is compatible with survival. However, difficulties arise during gametogenesis (Fig. 4–27), resulting in the formation of unbalanced gametes, which could lead to Down's syndrome in the offspring.

*Isochromosomes* result when the centromere divides horizontally rather than vertically, yielding two new chromosomes.

*Deletion* involves loss of a portion of a chromosome. A single break may delete a terminal segment. Two interstitial breaks, with reunion of the proximal and distal segments, may result in loss of an intermediate segment. The isolated fragment, which lacks a centromere, almost never survives and thus many genes are lost.

*Inversions* occur when there are two interstitial breaks in a chromosome and the segment reunites after a complete turnaround.

A *ring chromosome* is a variant of a deletion. Following the loss of segments from each end of the chromosome, the arms unite to form a ring.

It is apparent that some of these abnormal morphologies can be readily recognized in a metaphase spread, but an inversion or a subtle deletion might be missed without the aid of banding techniques.

Against this background, we can turn first to some general features of chromosomal disorders, followed by some specific examples of diseases involving changes in the karyotype.

○ Chromosomal disorders may be associated with lack (deletion, monosomy), excess (trisomy), or abnormal rearrangements (translocations) of chromosomes.

○ In general, loss of chromosomal material produces more severe defects than gains.

○ Excess chromosomal material may result from a complete extra chromosome (trisomy) or part of an extra chromosome (Robertsonian translocation).

○ Imbalances of sex chromosomes (excess or loss) are much better tolerated than similar imbalances of autosomes.

○ Sex chromosomal disorders often produce subtle abnormalities, sometimes not detected at birth. Infertility, a common manifestation, cannot be diagnosed until adolescence.

○ In most cases chromosomal disorders result from de novo changes—i.e., parents are normal and risk of recurrence in sibs is low. However, an important but uncommon exception to this principle is exhibited by the translocation form of Down's syndrome.

## AUTOSOMAL DISORDERS

Three autosomal trisomies (21, 18, and 13) and one deletion syndrome (cri du chat) resulting from partial deletion of the short arm of chromosome 5 were first identified over a decade ago. Within the past few years, several additional trisomies[80] and deletion syndromes have been described. Most of these disorders are quite uncommon, and all are characterized by clinical features that should permit ready recognition. Some of the features of the four most common entities are presented in Table 4–8. Only trisomy 21 occurs with sufficient frequency to merit further consideration.

### Down's Syndrome (Trisomy 21)

Down's syndrome is the most common of the chromosomal disorders. About 92 to 95% of the affected individuals have trisomy 21, so their chromosome count is 47. As mentioned earlier, the most common cause of trisomy and therefore of Down's syndrome is meiotic nondisjunction. The parents of such children have a normal karyotype and are normal in all respects. *Maternal age has a strong influence on the incidence of Down's syndrome. It occurs* once in 1550 live births in women under the age of 20 years, in contrast to 1 in 25 live births for mothers over 45 years of age.[81] The correlation with maternal age suggests that in most cases the meiotic nondisjunction of chromosome 21 occurs in the ovum. The reason for the increased susceptibility of the ovum to nondisjunction may lie in the fact that all ova are present from birth and as such are vulnerable to potentially harmful environmental influences. The increasing incidence of nondisjunction with age may be related to cumulative exposure to such environmental influences. However, recent evidence suggests that in 20 to 25% of patients with trisomy 21 the extra chromosome is paternal in origin.[80] No effect of paternal age has been found in these cases.

In about 4% of all patients with Down's syndrome, the extra chromosomal material is not present as an extra chromosome but as a translocation of the long arm of chromosome 21 to chromosome 22 or 14. Such cases are usually familial, and the translocated chromosome is inherited from one of the parents who is most frequently a carrier of a Robertsonian translocation. The consequences of the mating of a 14–21 translocation carrier (who may be phenotypically normal, with a chromosome count of 45) and a normal individual are depicted in Figure 4–27. Although

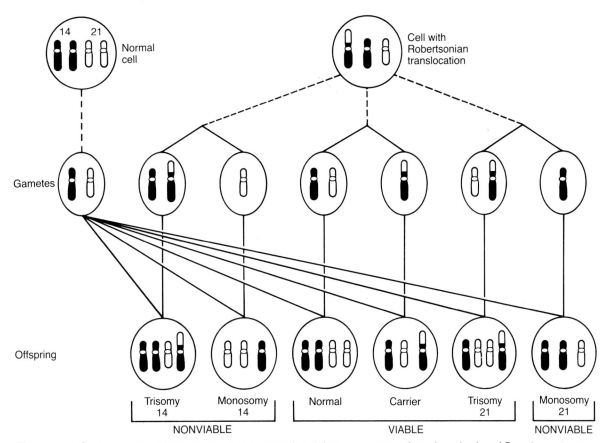

Figure 4–27. Consequences of Robertsonian translocation (14–21) on gametogenesis and production of Down's syndrome.

**Table 4–8.** DISORDERS ASSOCIATED WITH THE AUTOSOMES*

| Disorder | Examples of Karyotypes | Approximate Incidence | Maternal Age | Clinical Signs in Newborns |
|---|---|---|---|---|
| ***Down's Syndrome*** | | 1 in 700 births | | 1. Mental retardation |
| | | | | 2. Flat facial profile; epicanthic folds |
| | | | | 3. Congenital heart defects |
| Trisomy 21 type | 47,XX, +21 | About 95% of cases | Increased | 4. Muscle hypotonia |
| | 47,XY, +21 | | | 5. Hyperflexibility |
| | | | | 6. Lack of Moro reflex |
| | | | | 7. Abundant neck skin |
| Translocation type | 46,XX, − 14, + t(14q;21q) | 3 to 4% of cases | Normal | 8. Dysplastic ears |
| | | | | 9. Horizontal palmar crease |
| | 46,XX, − 22, + t(21q;22q) | | | 10. Dysplastic pelvis (by x-ray) |
| | | | | 11. Dysplastic middle phalanx (by x-ray) |
| Mosaic type | 46,XX/47,XX, +21 | 2 to 3% of cases | Normal | 12. Predisposition to acute leukemia |
| ***Edward's Syndrome*** | | 1 in 5000 births | | 1. Mental retardation and failure to thrive |
| Trisomy 18 type | 47,XX, +18 | 90% of cases | Increased | 2. Prominent occiput |
| | 47,XY, +18 | | | 3. Micrognathia and low-set ears |
| | | | | 4. Hypertonicity |
| Translocation type | 46,XX, − D, + t(Dq;18q) | Rare | Normal | 5. Flexion of fingers (index over third) |
| | | | | 6. Cardiac, renal, and intestinal defects |
| Mosaic type | 46,XX/47,XX, +18 | 10% of cases | Normal | 7. Short sternum and small pelvis |
| | | | | 8. Abduction deformity of hip |
| ***Patau's Syndrome*** | | 1 in 6000 births | | 1. Microcephaly and mental retardation |
| | | | | 2. Scalp defect |
| Trisomy 13 type (arhinencephaly) | 47,XX, +13 | Over 80% of cases | Increased | 3. Microphthalmia |
| | 47,XY, +13 | | | 4. Harelip and cleft palate |
| | | | | 5. Polydactyly |
| Translocation type | 46,XX, − 13, + t(Dq;13q) | 10% of cases | Normal | 6. Rocker-bottom feet |
| | | | | 7. Abnormal ears |
| | | | | 8. Apneic spells and myoclonic seizures |
| Mosaic type | 46,XX/47,XX, +13 | 5% of cases | Normal | 9. Cardiac dextroposition and interventricular septal defects |
| | | | | 10. Extensive visceral defects |
| ***Cri du Chat (Cat-cry) Syndrome*** | 46,XX,5p − | 1 in 50,000 births | Normal | 1. Mental retardation |
| | 46,XY,5p − | | | 2. Microcephaly and round facies |
| | | | | 3. Mewing cry |
| | | | | 4. Epicanthic folds |

*After Robbins, S. L., Cotran, R. S., and Kumar, V.: Pathologic Basis of Disease. 3rd ed. Philadelphia, W. B. Saunders Co., 1984, p. 127.

theoretically the carrier has a 1 in 3 chance of bearing a *live* child with Down's syndrome, the observed frequency of affected children in such cases is much lower. The reasons for this discrepancy are not well understood. Approximately 2% of Down's patients are mosaics, usually having a mixture of 46 and 47 chromosome cells. These result from mitotic nondisjunction of chromosome 21 during an early stage of embryogenesis. Symptoms in such cases are variable and milder, depending upon the proportion of abnormal cells.

The clinical features of Down's syndrome are listed in Table 4–8. The combination of epicanthic folds and flat facial profile accounted for the older, unfortunate designation "mongolian idiocy." Although Down's syndrome is a leading cause of mental retardation, the degree of mental retardation is variable, with IQs varying from 25 to 80. Congenital malformations are common and quite disabling. Approximately 40 to 60% of patients with trisomy 21 are afflicted by cardiac malformations, which are responsible for most of the deaths in early childhood. The

chromosomal unbalance in some undefined manner also increases the risk of developing acute leukemias.

Although the overall prognosis for individuals with Down's syndrome has improved remarkably in the recent past as the result of control of infections, even now 40% die by the age of 10 years. The majority survive into adulthood. A few of those who survive into middle age have a predisposition to develop premature Alzheimer's disease (p. 746).

## SEX CHROMOSOMAL DISORDERS

A number of abnormal karyotypes involving the sex chromosomes, ranging from 45,XO to 49,XXXXY, are compatible with life. Indeed, males who are phenotypically normal have been identified with two and even three Y chromosomes. Such extreme karyotypic deviations are not encountered with the autosomes. In large part this latitude relates to two facts: (1) lyonization of X chromosomes and (2) the scant amount of genetic information carried by the Y

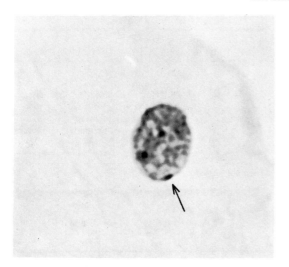

**Figure 4–28.** The Barr body (sex chromatin) is seen within the nucleus attached to the nuclear membrane at the five o'clock position *(arrow)*.

chromosome. The consideration of lyonization must begin with the *Barr body*, or *sex chromatin*. This refers to a distinctive clump of chromatin in the interphase nuclei of all somatic cells in females. It can be readily identified in smears of buccal squamous epithelial cells as a darkly staining mass lying adjacent to the nuclear membrane (Fig. 4–28).

Although sex chromatin is present in all somatic cells of a normal female, it can be demonstrated only in about 50% of the cells in a buccal smear. In 1962 Lyon proposed that *the X, or Barr, body represents one genetically inactivated X chromosome.* This inactivation occurs early in fetal life, about 16 days after conception, and randomly inactivates either the paternal or the maternal X chromosome in the cluster of primitive cells representing the developing zygote. Once inactivated, the same X chromosome remains genetically neutralized in all of the progeny of these cells. Moreover, it is now established that *all but one X chromosome is inactivated and so a 48,XXXX female has three X, or Barr, bodies and only one active X chromosome.* This phenomenon explains why normal females do not have a double dosage (as compared with the male) of phenotypic attributes coded by the X chromosome. Lyon's hypothesis also explains why normal females are mosaics, containing two cell populations—one with an active maternal X, the other with an active paternal X. This can be easily demonstrated if a female is heterozygous for an X-linked gene. For example, there are many variant genes (all X-linked) for glucose-6-phosphate dehydrogenase, which govern a comparable number of distinctive G6PD enzymes. If a number of fibroblasts from such a woman are cloned, two different populations containing two distinctive forms of G6PD can be demonstrated.

Extra Y chromosomes are readily tolerated because the only information known to be carried on the Y chromosome appears to relate to male differentia-

tion.[82] It might be noted that whatever the number of X chromosomes, the presence of a Y invariably dictates the male phenotype. Male somatic cells carry a Y (sometimes called F) body in interphase nuclei analogous to the X body in the female. The Y body appears as a small, brightly fluorescent spot in interphase nuclei stained with fluorescent dyes and examined with the ultraviolet microscope. The genes for male differentiation are located on the short arm of the Y.

The disorders arising in aberrations of sex chromosomes are detailed in Table 4–9. Three of the most common conditions are described briefly.

### Klinefelter's Syndrome

This syndrome is best defined as male hypogonadism that occurs when there are at least two X chromosomes and one or more Y chromosomes.[83] Although the following description applies to most of the patients, it should be noted that Klinefelter's syndrome is associated with a wide range of clinical manifestations. In some it may be expressed only as hypogonadism, but most patients have a distinctive body habitus with an increase in length between the soles and the pubic bone, which creates the appearance of an elongated body. Reduced facial and body hair and gynecomastia are also frequently noted. The testes are markedly reduced in size, sometimes to only 2 cm in greatest length. Along with the testicular atrophy, the serum testosterone levels are lower than normal, and urinary gonadotropin levels are normal or elevated. Most patients are 47,XXY and are therefore sex chromatin–positive. This karyotype results from nondisjunction of sex chromosomes during meiosis. The extra X chromosome may be of maternal or paternal origin. Advanced maternal age and history of irradiation of either parent may contribute to the meiotic error resulting in this condition. Approximately 15% of patients show mosaic patterns, including 46,XY/47,XXY, 47,XXY/48,XXXY, and variations on this theme. The presence of a 46,XY line in mosaics is usually associated with a milder clinical condition.

The principal clinical effect of this syndrome is sterility. Only rare patients, presumably mosaics with a large proportion of 46,XY cells, are fertile. The sterility is due to impaired spermatogenesis, sometimes to the extent of total azoospermia. A variety of testicular tubular alterations may be present. Some patients have hyalinization of tubules, so that they appear as ghost-like structures in tissue section. Others have rare, apparently normal testicular tubules mixed with atrophic tubules having virtually no spermatogenic germ cells, the so-called *tubule dysgenesis* pattern. Still others have very embryonic-appearing tubules, as though development had been arrested in early fetal life. In all forms, Leydig cells are prominent, owing to either hyperplasia or apparent increase related to loss of tubules. Klinefelter's syn-

**Table 4–9. DISORDERS ASSOCIATED WITH THE SEX CHROMOSOMES**

| Disorder | Examples of Karyotype | Chromatin Pattern | Approximate Incidence | Maternal Age | Clinical Signs |
|---|---|---|---|---|---|
| *Klinefelter's syndrome* | 47,XXY<br>46,XY/47,XXY | +<br>+ | 1 in 1000 male births | Slightly increased | 1. Testicular atrophy and azoospermia<br>2. Increase in sole–os pubis length<br>3. Gynecomastia<br>4. Female distribution of hair<br>5. Mild mental retardation |
| *Turner's syndrome (classic)*<br>Defective second X chromosome<br><br><br><br><br>Mosaicism | 45,X<br>46,XXp –<br>46,XXq –<br>46,XXr<br>46,X,i(Xq) (isochromosome)<br>46,XX/45,X | Negative<br>+ (small)<br>+ (small)<br>+<br>+ (large)<br><br>Usually + | 1 in 3000 female births | Normal<br><br>Normal<br>Normal<br>Normal<br>Normal<br><br>Normal | 1. Short stature<br>2. Primary amenorrhea<br>3. Webbing of the neck<br>4. Cubitus valgus<br>5. Peripheral lymphedema<br>6. Broad chest and widely spaced nipples<br>7. Low posterior hairline<br>8. Pigmented nevi<br>9. Coarctation of the aorta |
| *Triple X females*<br>Variants | 47,XXX<br>48,XXXX | + +<br>+ + + | 1 in 1000 female births<br>Rare | Increased | 1. Mental retardation<br>2. Menstrual irregularities<br>3. Many normal and fertile |
| *Double Y males* | 47,XYY | Negative | Rare | Normal | 1. Phenotypically normal<br>2. Most over 6 feet tall<br>3. "Increased aggressive behavior"(?) |

drome is sometimes associated with mental retardation. However, the degree of intellectual impairment is typically mild and in some cases undetectable. The reduction in intelligence is correlated with the number of extra X chromosomes. Thus, in patients with the most common variant (XXY), intelligence is nearly normal, but in those with rare variant forms involving additional X chromosomes, significantly subnormal levels of intelligence as well as more severe physical abnormalities are found.

### XYY Males

This type of chromosomal abnormality results from nondisjunction at the second meiotic division during spermatogenesis. Most of these individuals are phenotypically normal, although they may be somewhat taller than usual, but they have been reported to display antisocial behavior. However, this remains a controversial issue and requires long-term prospective studies for definite resolution.

### Turner's Syndrome

This syndrome, characterized by primary hypogonadism in phenotypic females, results from partial or complete monosomy of the short arm of the X chromosome. In approximately 55% of the patients, the entire X chromosome is missing, resulting in a 45,X karyotype. These patients are the most severely affected, and the diagnosis can often be made at birth or in early childhood. Typical clinical features asso-

ciated with 45,X Turner's syndrome include significant growth retardation leading to abnormally short stature (below third percentile); webbing of the neck; low posterior hairline; cubitus valgus (an increase in the carrying angle of the arms); shield-like chest with widely spaced nipples; high, arched palate; lymphedema of hands and feet; and a variety of congenital malformations (such as horseshoe kidney and coarctation of the aorta). Affected girls fail to develop normal secondary sex characteristics, the genitalia remain infantile, breast development is inadequate, and little pubic hair appears. Most have primary amenorrhea, and morphologic examination of the ovaries discloses white "streaks" of fibrous stroma devoid of follicles. Ovarian estrogen levels are low, and the loss of feedback inhibition leads to elevated levels of pituitary gonadotropin. Intelligence is usually normal but may be slightly reduced.

Approximately 45% of patients with Turner's syndrome are either mosaics (with one of the cell lines being 45,X) or have deletions of the small arm of one X chromosome. Combinations of deletions and mosaicism are reported (Table 4–9). Such patients may have many chromatin-positive cells. It is important to appreciate the karyotypic heterogeneity associated with Turner's syndrome since it is responsible for significant variations in the phenotype. In contrast to the patients with monosomy X described above, those that are mosaics or deletion variants may have an almost normal appearance and may present only with primary amenorrhea.

From our earlier discussion it might be expected

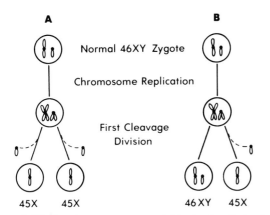

**Figure 4–29.** Sex chromosome aneuploidy due to mitotic chromosome loss. *A*, Both copies of the paternally derived Y chromosome are lost owing to anaphase lagging at the first cleavage division, resulting in Turner's syndrome, 45X. *B*, Only one copy of the Y chromosome is lost at the first cleavage division, resulting in sex chromosome mosaicism 45X/46XY. (From Smith, L. H., and Thier, S. O.: Pathophysiology: The Biologic Principles of Disease. 2nd ed. Philadelphia, W. B. Saunders Co., 1985, p. 71.)

that the 45,X karyotype may result from meiotic nondisjunction or a mitotic error (anaphase lag) during the first cell division of the zygote. The available evidence suggests that the X chromosome retained in patients with the 45,X karyotype is of maternal origin. Furthermore, it seems that the loss of the paternal sex chromosome occurs following fertilization, during the first cleavage divisions, as depicted in Figure 4–29.

## PRENATAL DIAGNOSIS

The last 10 years have witnessed the extension of medical genetics to the unborn child. Amniocentesis, used in prenatal diagnosis, involves aspiration of amniotic fluid early in pregnancy. The aspirated fluid contains cells (fibroblasts) of fetal origin that can be utilized for diagnostic procedures. Three types of analyses can be performed with fetal cells obtained by amniocentesis: (1) analysis of karyotype, (2) biochemical analysis for the presence of enzyme activity, and (3) analysis of abnormal gene structure. Each of these and their applications will be discussed briefly.

Cytogenetic studies on amniotic cells are relatively straightforward and involve principles and methods discussed earlier in this chapter. All of the numerical and most of the structural abnormalities of chromosomes can be detected by culture of fibroblastic cells obtained by amniocentesis. The commonest indication for chromosomal analysis is the risk of Down's syndrome associated with advanced maternal age. Previous trisomy in a sibling or a translocation in a parent are other indications. Fetal sexing is helpful when there is a high risk of serious X-linked recessive disease in the male fetus (e.g., Duchenne's muscular dystrophy). It should be remembered, of course, that identification of the male sex does not establish the

diagnosis, since 50% of male children of a carrier mother are likely to be normal.

Biochemical analysis of cells obtained from amniotic fluid can be used to detect several inborn errors of metabolism. For example, disorders such as Tay-Sachs disease, in which the product of the gene of interest is normally expressed in fibroblasts, can be diagnosed by assaying the level of the relevant enzyme in cultured fetal fibroblasts. However, in many relatively common genetic diseases (exemplified by hemoglobinopathies and PKU), the products of the corresponding normal genes are expressed only in specialized cells that are not readily obtained by amniocentesis. Thus PKU cannot be diagnosed antenatally by assay of fetal fibroblasts since even normal fibroblasts lack phenylalanine hydroxylase. Until recently this proved to be a major limitation in prenatal diagnosis. With the advent of recombinant DNA techniques, however, it is now possible to detect alterations in gene structure directly at the level of DNA, and hence the technical barriers to widespread application of prenatal diagnosis are rapidly crumbling. Indeed, the strides made in this area of medical genetics have brought into focus a major ethical dilemma: should one attempt prenatal diagnosis of a disorder that has a delayed onset after birth but for which there is currently no treatment? We can leave these complex issues to medical ethicians. Here we will present an outline of the procedure employed in the diagnosis of sickle cell anemia, to illustrate the principles of molecular biology that are utilized in the detection of genetic diseases.

As will be detailed in a later chapter, sickle cell anemia results from a mutation in the gene coding for the β-globin chain of hemoglobin. Before we "walk" through the steps involved in the detection of the mutant β-globin gene, it would be helpful to recapitulate some of the techniques commonly employed in the analysis of gene structure (Fig. 4–30).[84]

○ Large molecules of DNA can be cleaved by a series of bacterial enzymes called *restriction endonucleases.* Each restriction enzyme recognizes a short, specific sequence of base pairs (usually four to six in length) and cuts the DNA wherever that sequence occurs.

○ Digestion of the genomic DNA with a given restriction enzyme results in the production of a mixture of DNA fragments of different lengths and molecular weights. Subjecting the mixture to gel electrophoresis results in separation of the fragments based on their size.

○ The fragments are transferred from the gels to sheets of nitrocellulose filter paper by a technique commonly called "Southern blotting."

○ The DNA fragment containing a given gene can be detected by molecular hybridization to a synthetic DNA fragment (cDNA) that is complementary in structure to the gene of interest. cDNA is prepared by reverse transcription of the appropriate messenger RNA. For example, cDNA for glo-

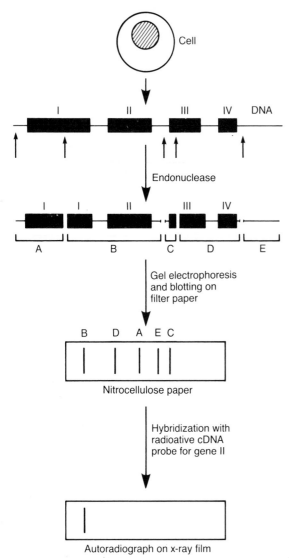

Figure 4–30. Detection of genes by Southern blot analysis. Four genes (I–IV), located on a long stretch of DNA, are represented by black boxes. Arrows indicate the sites of cleavage by a given restriction endonuclease. The restriction fragments produced are labeled A through E. On electrophoresis the restriction fragments migrate according to size, and hence the largest fragment (B) and the smallest fragment (C) are maximally separated. It should be noted that on nitrocellulose paper the fragments would not be visible, and the lines are only indications of their relative positions. Visualization of the fragment containing a given gene is accomplished by its hybridization with a radioactive cDNA probe. (Modified from Smith, L. H., and Thier, S. O.: Pathophysiology: The Biologic Principles of Disease. 2nd ed. Philadelphia, W. B. Saunders Co., 1985, p. 87.)

bin gene is made from globin m-RNA extracted from reticulocytes. The radiolabeled cDNA probe, when applied to the nitrocellulose filter, hybridizes only to the DNA fragment that contains the gene of interest. The position of the radioactive cDNA (and therefore the gene of interest) is revealed by autoradiography.

With this background, we can describe the application of these techniques in the diagnosis of sickle cell anemia. Figure 4–31 illustrates the partial orga-

nization of the β-globin gene. Repeated reference should be made to this figure to facilitate the understanding of the following discussion. It may be noted that there are three sites recognized by the restriction enzyme Mst II in the normal β-globin gene (HbA). Distances between these three sites are indicated in kilobases (1 Kb = 1000 bases). The mutation in sickle cell anemia involves a change in a single base pair near the 5′ end of the β-globin gene. This mutation has two effects: it replaces valine for glutamic acid at position 6 of the β-globin protein and at the same time abolishes the Mst II recognition site located at the 5′ end of the β-globin gene exon. When DNA from a normal individual is digested with Mst II and hybridized with the radioactive 1.15 Kb cDNA probe, a single 1.15 Kb fragment that reacts with the probe is detected on Southern blot analysis. (Although another 0.2 Kb fragment is also formed, it does not hybridize with the 1.15 Kb cDNA probe used, owing to lack of complementary sequences.) On the other hand, Mst II digestion of DNA obtained from amniotic cells of a patient with homozygous sickle cell

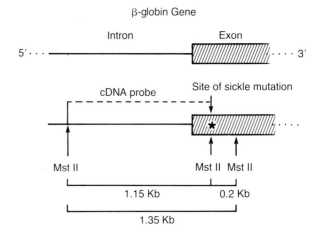

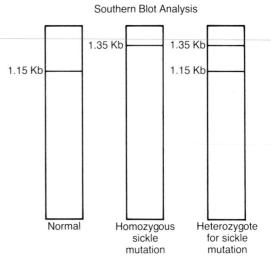

Figure 4–31. Application of Southern blot analysis in the diagnosis of sickle cell anemia.

anemia would not lead to the formation of the normal 1.15 Kb and 0.2 Kb DNA fragment, owing to the loss of one Mst II site. Instead, a single 1.35 Kb fragment that hybridizes with the 1.15 Kb cDNA probe would be formed. In individuals heterozygous for the sickle mutation, the normal chromosome would yield a 1.15 Kb fragment whereas the chromosome carrying the mutation would give rise only to the 1.35 Kb band. Thus the Southern blot analysis would reveal two fragments, 1.15 Kb and 1.35 Kb, that migrate separately owing to different size (and molecular weight) but each able to hybridize with the 1.15 Kb cDNA probe.

Although this method is extremely useful in the antenatal diagnosis of sickle cell anemia and several other disorders, it can be readily appreciated that this technique requires a knowledge of the mutant gene product and the primary genetic defect at the nucleotide level. In many common genetic diseases such as cystic fibrosis, such information is still not available. Since we do not know the product of the normal "CF gene" or the cells in which the product is expressed, it is not possible to produce cDNA probes. Despite these handicaps, remarkable progress is being made in the prenatal diagnosis of CF and other diseases in which the identity of mutant genes is unknown. This has been possible because polymorphisms in the structure of DNA linked to the "mutant" genes have been found, and these have led to alterations in the lengths of restriction fragments when the DNA is digested with appropriate enzymes. Details of these techniques, often referred to as restriction fragment length polymorphisms (RFLP), are beyond our scope and can be found in specialized texts and reviews.[84, 85]

Finally we come to the end of this chapter. Although the number of genetic disorders presented may have seemed endless, with the present rate of identification of new syndromes, consider the plight of future generations of medical students.

## References

1. Berg, K. (ed.): Medical Genetics—Past, Present, Future. New York, Alan R. Liss, Inc., 1985, p. 1.
2. Anderson, W. F.: Expectations from recombinant DNA research. In Wyngaarden, J. B., and Smith, L. H., Jr.: Cecil Textbook of Medicine. 17th ed. Philadelphia, W. B. Saunders Co., 1985, p. 132.
3. Bennett, P. H.: The diagnosis of diabetes: New international classification and diagnostic criteria. Ann. Rev. Med. 34:295, 1983.
4. Barnett, A. H., et al.: Diabetes in identical twins: A study of 200 pairs. Diabetologia 20:57, 1981.
5. Cudworth, A. G., and Wolf, E.: Genetic basis of type I (insulin-dependent) diabetes. In Gupta, S. (ed.): Immunobiology of Clinical and Experimental Diabetes. New York, Plenum Medical, 1984, p. 271.
6. Thompson, M. P., et al.: Purification and partial characterization of a putative mediator of insulin action of cyclic-AMP–dependent protein kinase. Mol. Cell. Biochem. 62:67, 1984.
7. Truglia, J. A., et al.: Insulin resistance: Receptor and post-binding defects in human obesity and non-insulin-dependent diabetes mellitus. Am. J. Med. 79 (Suppl. 2B):13, 1985.

8. Craighead, J. E.: Immunopathology of type I diabetes mellitus. Lab. Invest. 53:119, 1985.
9. Huber, A. A., and MacPherson, B. R.: Viruses and insulin dependent diabetes mellitus. In Gupta, S. (ed.): Immunobiology of Clinical and Experimental Diabetes. New York, Plenum Medical, 1984, p. 295.
10. Craighead, J. E.: Current views on the etiology of insulin-dependent diabetes mellitus. N. Engl. J. Med. 299:1439, 1978.
11. Oldstone, M. B. A., et al.: Virus persists in β-cells of islets of Langerhans and is associated with chemical manifestations of diabetes. Science 224:1440, 1984.
12. Yoon, J., et al.: Virus induced diabetes mellitus. Isolation of a virus from the pancreas of a child with diabetic ketoacidosis. N. Engl. J. Med. 300:1173, 1979.
13. Srikanta, S., et al.: First-degree relatives of patients with type I diabetes mellitus. Islet cell antibodies and abnormal insulin secretion. N. Engl. J. Med. 313:461, 1985.
14. Gepts, W., and Le Compte, P. M.: Pathology of type I (juvenile) diabetes. In Volk, B. W., and Arquilla, E. R. (eds.): The Diabetic Pancreas. 2nd ed. New York, Plenum Medical, 1985, p. 337.
15. Nerup, J., et al.: Autoimmunity. In Gupta, S. (ed.): Immunobiology of Clinical and Experimental Diabetes. New York, Plenum Medical, 1984, p. 351.
16. Bottazzo, G. F., et al.: In situ characterization of autoimmune phenomena and expression of HLA molecules in the pancreas in diabetic insulitis. N. Engl. J. Med. 313:353, 1985.
16A. Eisenbarth, G. S.: Type I diabetes mellitus. A chronic autoimmune disease. N. Engl. J. Med. 314:1360, 1986.
17. Stiller, C. R., et al.: Effects of cyclosporine immunosuppression in insulin-dependent diabetes mellitus of recent onset. Science 223:1362, 1984.
18. Unger, R. H., and Orci, L.: Glucagon and the A Cell physiology and pathophysiology. N. Engl. J. Med. 304:1518, 1575, 1981.
19. Raskin, P., and Unger, R. H.: Hyperglucagonemia and its suppression. Importance in metabolic control of diabetes. N. Engl. J. Med. 299:1366, 1978.
20. Sherwin, R. S., and Felig, P.: Hyperglucagonemia in diabetes. N. Engl. J. Med. 299:433, 1978.
21. Barnes, A. J., et al.: Persistent metabolic abnormalities in diabetes in the absence of glucagon. Diabetologia 13:71, 1977.
22. Volk, B. W., and Wellmann, K. F.: Pathogenetic considerations of type II diabetes. In Volk, B. W., and Arquilla, E. R. (eds.): The Diabetic Pancreas. 2nd ed. New York, Plenum Medical, 1985, p. 265.
23. DeFronzo, R. A., et al.: New concepts in the pathogenesis and treatment of non-insulin-dependent diabetes mellitus. Am. J. Med. 74(Suppl. 1A):52, 1983.
24. Vracko, R., and Benditt, E. P.: Manifestations of diabetes mellitus—Their possible relationships to an underlying cell defect. Am. J. Pathol. 75:204, 1974.
25. Olefsky, J. M., et al.: Mechanisms of insulin resistance in non-insulin-dependent (type II) diabetes. Am. J. Med. 79(Suppl. 3B):12, 1985.
26. Editorial: Vascular complications in diabetes mellitus. N. Engl. J. Med. 302:399, 1980.
27. Wellmann, K. F., and Volk, B. W.: Islets of Langerhans: Structure and function in diabetes. Pathobiol. Annu. 10:105, 1980.
28. Colwell, J. A., et al.: New concepts about the pathogenesis of atherosclerosis in diabetes mellitus. Am. J. Med. (Suppl.) Nov. 30, 1983, p. 67.
29. Sandek, C. D., and Eder, E. H.: Lipid metabolism in diabetes mellitus. Am. J. Med. 66:843, 1979.
30. Mustard, J. F., and Packham, M. A.: Platelets and diabetes mellitus. N. Engl. J. Med. 311:665, 1984.
31. Salinas-Madrigal, L., et al.: Glomerular and vascular "insudative" lesions of diabetic nephropathy: Electron microscopic observations. Am. J. Pathol. 59:369, 1970.
32. Bloodworth, J. M. B., Jr.: Diabetes mellitus, extrapancreatic pathology. In Bloodworth, J. M. B., Jr. (ed.): Endocrine Pathology. Baltimore, Williams & Wilkins Co., 1968, p. 330.

33. Factor, S. M., et al.: Capillary microaneurysms in the human diabetic heart. N. Engl. J. Med. 302:384, 1980.

34. Brown, M. G., et al.: Diabetic neuropathy. Ann. Neurol. 15:2, 1984.

35. Kilo, C.: Value of glucose control on preventing complications of diabetes. Am. J. Med. 79(Suppl. 3B):33, 1985.

36. Feldt-Rasmussen, B., et al.: Kidney function during 12 months of strict metabolic control in insulin-dependent diabetic patients with incipient nephropathy. N. Engl. J. Med. 314:665, 1986.

37. Steffes, M. W.: Study of kidney and muscle biopsy specimens from identical twins discordant for type I diabetes mellitus. N. Engl. J. Med. 312:1283, 1985.

38. Brownlee, M., et al.: Non-enzymatic glycosylation and pathogenesis of diabetic complications. Ann. Intern. Med. 101:527, 1984.

39. Clements, R. S., and Bell, D. S. H.: Complications of diabetes. Prevalence, detection, current treatment, and prognosis. Am. J. Med. 79(Suppl 5A):2, 1985.

40. Goldstein, D. E.: Is glycosylated hemoglobin clinically useful. N. Engl. J. Med. 310:384, 1984.

41. Proceedings of a Symposium: Diabetic complications and role of aldose reductase inhibition. Am. J. Med. 79(Suppl 5A):1, 1985.

42. Bale, G. S., and Entmacher, P. S.: Estimated life expectancy of diabetics. Diabetes 26:434, 1977.

43. German, D. C., and Holmes, E. W.: Hyperuricemia and gout. Med. Clin. North Am. 70:419, 1986.

44. Wyngaarden, J. B., and Kelley, W. N.: Gout. In Stanbury, J. B., et al. (eds.): The Metabolic Basis of Inherited Disease. 5th ed. New York, McGraw-Hill, 1983, p. 1043.

45. Boss, G. R., and Seegmiller, J. E.: Hyperuricemia and gout. Classification, complication and management. N. Engl. J. Med. 300:1459, 1979.

46. Dieppe, P. A.: Crystal deposition and inflammation. Q. J. Med. (new ser. L) 3:309, 1984.

47. Salerno, C., et al.: Urate crystal-induced superoxide radical production by human neutrophils. Adv. Exp. Med. Biol. 165(Part A):189, 1984.

48. Ginsberg, M. H., et al.: Urate crystal-dependent cleavage of Hageman factor in human plasma and synovial fluid. J. Lab. Clin. Med. 95:497, 1980.

49. Katz, W. A.: Deposition of urate crystals in gout: Altered connective tissue metabolism. Arthritis Rheum. 18:751, 1975.

50. Gibson, T., et al.: Hypertension, renal function and gout. Postgrad. Med. J. 55(Suppl.):21, 1979.

51. Fessel, W. J.: Hyperuricemia in health and disease. Semin. Arthritis Rheum. 1:275, 1972.

52. Fessel, W. J., et al.: Correlates and consequences of asymptomatic hyperuricemia. Arch. Intern. Med. 132:144, 1973.

53. Fessel, W. J.: High uric acid as an indicator of cardiovascular disease: Independence from obesity. Am. J. Med. 68:401, 1980.

54. Weeden, R.R., and Batumen, V.: Tubulointerstitial nephritis induced by heavy metals and metabolic disturbances. In Cotran, R. S., et al. (eds.): Tubulointerstitial Nephropathies. Contemporary Issues in Nephrology. Vol. 10. New York, Churchill Livingstone, 1983, p. 212.

55. Reif, M. C., et al.: Chronic gouty nephropathy: A vanishing syndrome. N. Engl. J. Med. 304:535, 1981.

56. Weeden, R. R.: Lead and gouty kidney. Am. J. Kid. Dis. 2:559, 1983.

57. Vessel, E. S.: Genetic host factors: Determinants of drug response. N. Engl. J. Med. 313:261, 1985.

58. Prockop, D. J., and Kivirikko, K. I.: Heritable disease of collagen. N. Engl. J. Med. 311:376, 1984.

59. Henke, E., et al.: A 38 base pair insertion in the pro alpha 2(I) gene of a patient with Marfan's syndrome. J. Cell. Biochem. 27:169, 1985.

60. Perejda, A., et al.: Marfan's syndrome: Structural, biochemical, and mechanical studies of aortic media. J. Lab. Clin. Med. 106:376, 1985.

61. Goldstein, J. L., and Brown, M. S.: The LDL-receptor defect in familial hypercholesterolemia. Implications for pathogenesis and therapy. Med. Clin. North Am. 66:335, 1982.

62. Grundy, S. M.: Pathogenesis of hyperlipoproteinemia. J. Lipid Res. 25:1611, 1984.

63. Riccardi, V. M.: Von Recklinghausen neurofibromatosis. N. Engl. J. Med. 305:1617, 1981.

64. McLusky, I., et al.: Cystic fibrosis. Curr. Probl. Pediatr. 15(6):1, and 15(7):1, 1985.

65. Kopelman, H., et al.: Pancreatic fluid secretion and protein hyperconcentration in cystic fibrosis. N. Engl. J. Med. 312:329, 1985.

66. Newmark, P.: Testing for cystic fibrosis. Nature 318:309, 1985.

67. Nyhan, W. L.: Neonatal screening for inherited disease. N. Engl. J. Med. 313:43, 1985.

68. Bickel, H.: Differential diagnosis and treatment of hyperphenylalaninemia. Prog. Clin. Biol. Res. 177:93, 1984.

69. Segal, S.: Disorders of galactose metabolism. In Stanbury, J. B., et al. (eds.): The Metabolic Basis of Inherited Disease. 5th Ed. New York, McGraw-Hill, 1983, p. 167.

70. Witkop, C. J.: Depigmentations of the general and oral tissues and their genetic foundations. Ala. J. Med. Sci. 16:327, 1979.

71. Sternlieb, I.: Wilson's disease: Indications for liver transplants. Hepatology 4:155, 1984.

72. Frydman, M., et al.: Assignment of the gene for Wilson's disease to chromosome 13: Linkage to the esterase D locus. Proc. Natl. Acad. Sci. USA 82:1819, 1985.

73. Stromeyer, F. W., and Ishak, K. G.: Histology of the liver in Wilson's disease. Am. J. Pathol. 73:12, 1980.

74. Howell, R. R., and Williams, J. C.: The glycogen storage disease. In Stanbury, J. B., et al. (eds.): Metabolic Basis of Inherited Disease. 5th ed. New York, McGraw-Hill, 1983, p. 144.

75. Stanbury, J. B., et al. (eds.): Metabolic Basis of Inherited Disease. 5th ed. New York, McGraw-Hill, 1983, p. 751.

76. Glew, R. H., et al.: Lysosomal storage diseases. Lab. Invest. 53:250, 1985.

77. Pinnell, S. R., and Murad, S.: Disorders of collagen. In Stanbury, J. B., et al. (eds.): Metabolic Basis of Inherited Disease. 5th ed. New York, McGraw-Hill, 1983, p. 1425.

78. ISCN 1981: An international system for human cytogenetic neomenclature 1981. Birth Defects. Original Article Series Vol. 17, 1982.

79. Hamerton, J.: Cytogenetic disorders. N. Engl. J. Med. 310:314, 1984.

80. Hassold, T. J., and Jacobs, P. A.: Trisomy in man. Ann. Rev. Genet. 18:69, 1984.

81. Thompson, J. S., and Thompson, M. W.: Genetics in Medicine. 3rd ed. Philadelphia, W. B. Saunders Co., 1980, p. 152.

82. Kidd, K. K.: The search for ultimate cause of maleness. N. Engl. J. Med. 313:260, 1985.

83. Emery, A. E., and Rimoin, D. L. (eds.): Principles and Practice of Medical Genetics. New York, Churchill Livingstone, 1983, p. 201.

84. Sklar, J.: DNA hybridization in diagnostic pathology. Hum. Pathol. 16:654, 1985.

85. Francomano, C. A., and Kazazian, H. H. Jr.: DNA analysis in genetic disorders. Ann. Rev. Med. 37:377, 1986.

# 5

# Disorders of Immunity

Immunity and immunologic disorders are to contemporary medicine what bacteriology and bacterial diseases were to the medical world at the turn of the century. New diseases, new immunologic insights into the causation of "old diseases," and new vistas of immunotherapy permeate the contemporary medical literature. More than ever it has become apparent that dependent as humans are on the immune system for survival, so vulnerable are they to the wide-ranging disorders in its function. On the one extreme, immunodeficiency states render them easy prey to infectious diseases. At the other extreme, a hyper-reactive immune apparatus may seemingly run amok, reacting against "self" to induce life-threatening disease. Put more succinctly, the disorders range from those caused by "too little" to those caused by "too much" immunologic reactivity. To encompass this spectrum, the various immunologic conditions will be considered under the following four headings:

1. Immunologic mechanisms of tissue injury.
2. Autoimmune diseases.
3. Possible immune disorders.
4. Immunodeficiency diseases.

The important prototypes in each category will be considered in the following sections, but first a recapitulation of the organization of the immune system and the recent major advances in our understanding of lymphocytes and their functions will be presented. We will also review the highlights of histocompatibility genes, since they are intimately related to immune responses against self- and non-self-antigens, which in turn result in autoimmune diseases and rejection of transplants, respectively.

As is well known, immunologic responsiveness involves two major effector mechanisms: humoral antibodies derived from the B (bursa-dependent) lymphocytes, and cell-mediated mechanisms that involve T (thymus-dependent) lymphocytes. Approximately 60 to 70% of the small lymphocytes in the circulating blood are T cells, and 10 to 20% are B cells. Most of the remaining 10 to 15% of the lymphocytes are not identifiable as T cells or B cells and were previously called "null cells" for want of a better name. However, recent studies indicate that most of the so-called null cell population is composed of a novel class of effector cells called natural killer (NK) cells, which will be described later in this section. In addition to lymphocytes, cells of the mononuclear phagocyte system, represented by monocytes in the peripheral blood and macrophages in the tissues, play an important role in the induction of both cellular and humoral immunity and in the expression of certain T cell–mediated reactions.

In the last decade major advances have occurred in our understanding of lymphocyte biology. In large part these breakthroughs have resulted from the merging of several new technologies. Foremost among these has been the development of monoclonal antibodies, which are secreted by clonal progeny of a single B cell that has been immortalized by fusion with a cancerous myeloma cell. With the use of monoclonal antibodies it has been possible to define functionally distinct subsets of lymphocytes, particularly T cells. The analysis of T cell subpopulations has provided insights into the pathogenesis of lethal disorders such as the acquired immune deficiency syndrome (AIDS). By the combined application of monoclonal antibodies and fluorescence-activated cell sorting, it has been possible to isolate lymphocyte subsets to virtual homogeneity. Several subpopulations of purified lymphocytes can be expanded to large numbers in vitro by using the newly discovered growth factor interleukin 2 (IL-2). As with several other biologically active molecules, the gene for IL-2 has been cloned and inserted into *Escherichia coli* for large-scale production of this lymphokine. Cloned lymphocyte populations propagated in recombinant IL-2 have not only proved invaluable in dissecting the complexities of the immune system but also hold the promise of being useful in the immunotherapy of cancer. Lastly, recent advances in molecular biology have led to rapid progress in unraveling the genetic basis of antigen recognition—a process fundamental to all immune responses. Details of these rapidly advancing areas of research are beyond our scope and may be found in recent reviews.[1-3] In the following section we will briefly allude to the information derived from recent studies as it relates to various cells of the immune system.

## T LYMPHOCYTES

T lymphocytes arise from precursors in the bone marrow that migrate to the thymus, where they undergo differentiation into mature T cells and then leave the thymus. Mature T cells circulate in the blood and thoracic duct lymph and also seed peripheral lymphoid tissues such as the *paracortical areas of lymph nodes and periarteriolar sheaths of the spleen.* T cells are long-lived and form a large recirculating pool of cells. With the use of monoclonal antibodies it has been possible to define several cell surface markers on T cells (Table 5–1). Some, such as T3 and T11, are present on all peripheral T cells, whereas others define functionally distinct subsets. For example, T4 and T8 antigens are expressed on two nonoverlapping subsets of peripheral T cells. Those cells positive for the T4 antigen (T4+ cells) constitute approximately 60% of mature T cells, whereas T8 is expressed on about 30% of T lymphocytes. Thus in normal healthy individuals, the T4/T8 ratio is approximately 2. This may be altered in various disease states, as will be discussed later in this chapter. Although initially discovered as markers for T cells, many of these molecules have now been shown to be intimately associated with T-cell functions, of which there are two broad categories:

**Table 5–1. T-CELL SURFACE ANTIGENS DEFINED BY MONOCLONAL ANTIBODIES**

| Antibody Designation | Antigen Designation* | Comments |
|---|---|---|
| T1 Leu-1 | CD5 | Present on all T cells, peripheral and intrathymic |
| T3 Leu-4 | CD3 | Present on all peripheral T cells; associated with T cell antigen receptor |
| T4 Leu-3 | CD4 | Present on 60% of peripheral T cells; marker for T-helper cells |
| T6 Leu-6 | CD1 | Absent from mature T cells; present on 70% of thymus cells |
| T8 Leu-2 | CD8 | Present on 30% of peripheral T cells; marker for cytotoxic T cells |
| T10 | — | Present on 5% of peripheral T cells and 95% of thymus cells |
| T11 Leu-5 | CD2 | Present on all T cells, peripheral and intrathymic; reacts with sheep red blood cell (E) receptor on T cells |

*Based on International Workshop on Human Leukocyte Differentiation Antigens.

1. *Cellular immune reactions.* These include several phenomena in which T cells serve as pivotal effector cells. Examples are cytolytic (killer) T cells (Tc), which are generated against foreign histocompatibility antigens, virus-infected cells, and some tumor cells. Tc, like all T cells, are T3+, but in addition they are also T8+. Another expression of cell-mediated immunity is the delayed hypersensitivity reaction (to be described later), that is mediated by T4+ cells.

2. *Regulatory functions.* In addition to their role as effector cells, T cells also serve to modulate the responses mediated by other T and B cells. This regulatory function can be expressed as facilitation or suppression of an immune response. Accordingly, *T-helper cells,* which are largely T4+, provide "help" to precursors of Tc and B cells by secreting "helper factors" such as IL-2. *T-suppressor cells,* on the other hand, serve to dampen both cellular and humoral immunity. Suppression is mediated by a subset of T8+ cells that differs from the T8+ cytotoxic T cells.

As alluded to earlier, there is accumulating evidence that cell surface molecules defined by the commonly employed monoclonal anti–T cell antibodies such as anti-T3, anti-T4, and anti-T8 are involved in the activation or function, or both, of T cells. This is best exemplified by the T3 molecular complex. Present on all T cells, T3 is closely associated with the T-cell receptor (TCR) for antigen.[1] TCR remained elusive for several years and has only recently been identified as a disulfide-linked heterodimer made up of an α and β polypeptide chain. Although the TCR is distinct from immunoglobulins that are known to function as the antigen receptors utilized by B cells, recent studies indicate that the genetic organization of the TCR is remarkably similar to that of immunoglobulins. Figure 5–1 depicts a portion of human chromosome 7 on which the genes for the β-chain of the T-cell receptor are located. It may be noted that the β-chain of the TCR is assembled from four separate genes, each belonging to a group of genes segregated into four regions. These are designated V, D, J, and C (to indicate Variable, Diversity, Joining, and Constant segments). As might be expected, every somatic cell contains the T-cell receptor genes (in the so-called germ-line configuration shown in Fig. 5–1), but they are expressed only in T lymphocytes. Transcription of the TCR genes is preceded by a remarkable phenomenon called *gene rearrangement*, whereby one gene each from the V, D, and J regions comes to lie next to each other by elimination of the intervening DNA. The rearranged DNA is then transcribed to form m-RNA. During processing of the m-RNA, the intervening sequences between the VDJ and the C regions are spliced off, so that the products of the VDJ and C regions come together. The α-chain is synthesized in an analogous manner. The phenomenon of the TCR gene rearrangement, which occurs only in T cells, has enormous theoretical and practical significance.

○ It provides a mechanism by which it is possible to have numerous antigen-specific clones of T cells. Since a complete α- and β-chain of the T-cell receptor is produced by a combination of one of the several genes in each of the V, D, J, and C regions, it is possible to generate enormous diversity in the TCR. Each TCR, resulting from a specific combinational rearrangement of the α- and β-chain genes, has a unique genetically determined structure that is specific only for one of a myriad of antigens.

○ At a practical level, the knowledge that each T cell has a unique DNA rearrangement makes it possible to distinguish polyclonal (non-neoplastic) proliferations of T lymphocytes from monoclonal (neoplastic) proliferations.[3] The technique of Southern blot analysis (described on p. 125) is utilized for such studies.

## B LYMPHOCYTES

The B lymphocytes constitute a distinct set of cells specialized for antibody production. Their progenitors are also marrow stem cells. In fowl, B-cell precursors migrate to the bursa of Fabricius, where they undergo maturation. The mature B cells synthesize surface immunoglobulin (sIg) and migrate from the bursa to the peripheral lymphoid tissues, where

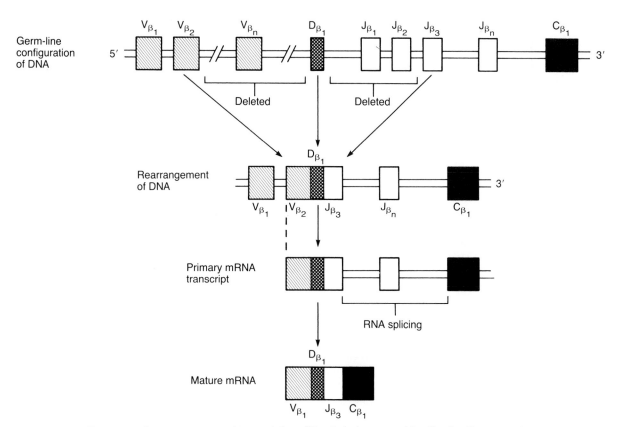

**Figure 5–1.** Rearrangement and transcription of the β-chain genes of the T-cell antigen receptor.

they aggregate in the form of follicles. Mammals do not possess a bursa of Fabricius, and the identity of the central lymphoid organ for B-cell maturation in humans remains unresolved. As with T cells, a variety of monoclonal antibodies directed against the surface molecules of B cells have been described.[4] These include anti-B1, -B2, and -B4 antibodies that define different stages of B-cell differentiation.

Upon appropriate antigenic stimulation, B cells differentiate into plasma cells that secrete immunoglobulins, of which there are five distinct classes: IgM, IgG, IgA, IgE, and IgD. The first three account for more than 95% of the circulating immunoglobulins. IgE occurs in traces, except in certain immunologic disorders, and IgD is found predominantly on the surface of B cells, where it may play a role in antigen-induced B-cell differentiation.

It has been known for quite some time that monomeric IgM, present on the surface of all B cells, constitutes the antigen receptor of B cells. The specificity of the surface immunoglobulin is identical to that of the immunoglobulin that is secreted when the B cell becomes a plasma cell. The genetic basis of the diversity of the B cell repertoire (i.e., the existence of numerous B cells programmed to recognize only one antigen) has been clarified by recent analyses of immunoglobulin genes.[2] There are remarkable similarities in the organization of immunoglobulin genes and genes of the T-cell receptor. Thus in mice the immunoglobulin heavy chain is assembled from genes in the V, D, J, and C regions. There are approximately 200 $V_H$ (heavy), 12 $D_H$, and four $J_H$ segments. In addition, there are eight constant region genes ($C_\mu$, $C_\gamma$, $C_\delta$, and so on) corresponding to the immunoglobulin isotypes and their subclasses. Genes in the immunoglobulin light chain have a similar organization, except that they lack the D-region genes. During B-cell maturation there is rearrangement of the DNA, which leads initially to V-D-J joining (for heavy chain synthesis) and then transcription of the complete VDJ gene and one of the C genes (e.g., $C_\mu$ for IgM antibodies). Eventually a heavy chain that is the product of genes in the VDJ and C regions is synthesized. Given the numbers of genes in the V, D, and J regions for heavy chains and light chains, it is not difficult to estimate that antibodies with greater than $10^7$ specificities can arise by unique combinational rearrangements of the immunoglobulin genes! As mentioned earlier with respect to T cells, it is important to note the practical application of this knowledge. *Since in a given B cell and its progeny only one of the several million possible DNA rearrangements occurs, it is feasible to distinguish between clonal (neoplastic, p. 375) and polyclonal (reactive) proliferations of B cells by extracting the DNA and subjecting it to Southern blot analysis.*

In addition to the antigen receptor (sIg), receptors for the Fc portion of IgG (Fc receptor) and for fixed complement (C3b and C3d) are expressed on B cells.

The role of these receptors is not entirely clear, but it is suspected that they regulate antibody synthesis.

## MACROPHAGES

Macrophages are a part of the mononuclear phagocyte system and as such their origin, differentiation, and role in inflammation was discussed in Chapter 2. Here we need only to emphasize that macrophages play several roles in the immune response.

○ First, they are required to process and present antigen to immunocompetent T cells. The presence of class II HLA antigens (p. 133) on the macrophages is considered critical for their antigen-presenting function. Since T cells (unlike B cells) cannot be triggered by free antigen, presentation of antigens by macrophages or other antigen-presenting cells (e.g., Langerhans' cells, discussed below) is obligatory for induction of cell-mediated immunity.

○ They produce interleukin 1 (IL-1), which promotes the differentiation of both T and B lymphocytes.[6] It should be noted that IL-1 has multiple targets and numerous other effects, some of which are described elsewhere in this text (Chapter 2, p. 50; Chapter 3, p. 80; Chapter 5, p. 145).

○ Macrophages lyse tumor cells by secreting toxic metabolites and proteolytic enzymes and as such may play a role in immunosurveillance.

○ Macrophages are important effector cells in certain forms of cell-mediated immunity, such as the delayed hypersensitivity reaction.

## NATURAL KILLER CELLS

In recent years, much interest has focused on a novel cell type called the natural killer (NK) cell. These cells are capable of lysing a variety of tumor cells, virus-infected cells, fungi, and some normal cells. In contrast to T and B lymphocytes, *NK cells do not require prior sensitization for expression of their function.*[6, 7] NK activity is markedly augmented both in vitro and in vivo by interferons and IL-2. In human peripheral blood, NK cells constitute approximately 15% of the total lymphocyte population and have a characteristic morphologic appearance that has earned the name *large granular lymphocytes.* They are somewhat larger than small lymphocytes and contain multiple azurophilic granules in the cytoplasm. The granules, believed to contain the lytic moiety, are devoid of myeloperoxidase and nonspecific esterases that characterize neutrophil and macrophage granules, respectively. Although NK cells share some cell surface antigens with macrophages and T cells and possess Fc receptors, they are believed to be distinct from mature T cells, B cells, and myeloid cells. As with other lymphoid cells, several monoclonal antibodies that react with NK cells have been developed. The ones most useful for practical identification of NK cells are Leu-11 and NKH-1. Because of their ability to lyse a wide range of tumor cells and virus-infected cells in vitro without prior sensitization, NK cells are considered to provide the first line of defense against tumors and virus infections. Furthermore, IL-2 and interferons, which are currently under evaluation as antitumor agents, may act at least in part by their ability to stimulate NK cells in vivo.

## DENDRITIC AND LANGERHANS' CELLS

These include a population of cells that have dendritic cytoplasmic processes and large amounts of class II HLA antigens on their cell surfaces. Dendritic cells are found in lymphoid tissues and Langerhans' cells occur in the epidermis. Both these cell types are extremely efficient in antigen presentation, and according to some they are the most important antigen-presenting (accessory) cells in the body. Unlike macrophages, they are poorly phagocytic, and hence they do not possess antimicrobial or scavenger cell activities.[8]

## HISTOCOMPATIBILITY ANTIGENS—HLA COMPLEX

The ability to distinguish between "self" and "non-self" is one of the fascinating properties of the immune system. Nowhere is this more evident than in organ transplantation, where human dexterity and skill have overcome the major technical hurdles in transplantation surgery; however, it has not been possible to thwart the rejection of non-self. *The term "rejection" in this context encompasses all those immunologic reactions that lead to the destruction of a transplant by a recipient who is genetically nonidentical to the donor.* It is obvious that for the rejection to occur the lymphoid system of the recipient must recognize foreign (non-self) antigens in the donor tissue. These cell surface antigens, which evoke rejection of transplants, are called *histocompatibility (or transplantation) antigens;* the genes that code for these antigens are called *histocompatibility genes.* Among histocompatibility genes, one set that codes for the strong transplantation antigens is closely linked and clustered together on a small region of the genome, called the *major histocompatibility complex* (MHC). The MHC of humans is located on chromosome 6 and is called the HLA (human lymphocyte antigen) complex.[9] The corresponding region in the mouse is called the H-2 complex.

Based on their chemical structure, tissue distribution, and function, the MHC gene products are classified into three categories. *Class I antigens* are coded by three closely linked loci designated HLA-

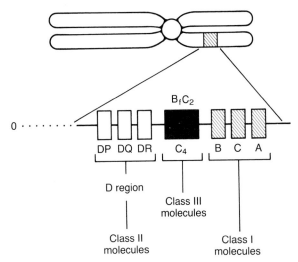

Figure 5–2. Schematic representation of the HLA complex and its subregions on human chromosome 6.

A, -B, and -C (Fig. 5–2). These molecules are glycoproteins of 45,000 molecular weight and are present on virtually all nucleated cells and platelets. *Class II antigens* are coded for in a region known as HLA-D.[10] These antigens were initially defined by a phenomenon called the *mixed lymphocyte reaction,* which occurs when lymphocytes from two individuals who differ at the HLA-D region are cultured together in vitro. T lymphocytes from one individual recognize ("see") foreign class II antigens on the cells of the other individual and respond by proliferation. If there is genetic identity at the HLA-D region, proliferation does not occur. Recent studies have identified three subregions, DP, DQ, and DR, within the originally defined HLA-D region.

*Class II antigens* differ from class I antigens in several respects. Chemically, they exist as bimolecular complexes made up of an α- and a β-chain. Unlike class I antigens, their tissue distribution is quite restricted; they are found mainly on antigen-presenting cells (monocytes/macrophages, dendritic cells), B cells, and some activated T cells. However, recent studies suggest that several other cell types, such as fibroblasts and renal tubular epithelial cells, can be induced to express class II antigens by γ-interferon, a lymphokine produced by activated T cells.

*Class III proteins* are those components of the complement system (C2, C4, and Bf) that are coded for within the MHC. Although genetically linked to class I and II antigens, class III molecules do not act as histocompatibility (transplantation) antigens and will not be discussed further.

A feature shared by class I and class II genes is the high degree of polymorphism (i.e., each gene exists in multiple allelic forms). Each of the several alleles at these loci is designated by a number, such as HLA-A1, HLA-B5, and so forth. (Those alleles that have not been fully characterized are identified by a W—e.g., HLA-BW4.) *All class I determinants and most (but not all) of the class II determinants evoke the formation of humoral antibodies in genetically nonidentical individuals.* This makes it possible to type these antigens by conventional serologic techniques such as antibody- and complement-mediated lysis. Sera of multiparous women (who are immunized by the paternal antigens of the fetus) have traditionally served as a useful source of such anti-HLA antibodies. However, it is now possible to raise monoclonal anti-HLA antibodies by immunizing rodents with human cells.

As mentioned above, certain class II antigens cannot be defined serologically at present. They are detected by the mixed lymphocyte reaction described earlier and are designated HLA-D antigens, to distinguish them from the serologically defined D-region antigens. Since HLA antigens form an allelic series, an individual inherits only one determinant from each parent and can have no more than two different antigens for every locus. Thus, cells of a heterozygous individual will express six different class I HLA antigens, three of maternal origin and three of paternal origin. Due to the polymorphism at the major HLA loci, innumerable combinations of antigens can exist, and therefore each individual in a noninbred population is likely to have a more or less unique antigenic profile, like a fingerprint on the cell surface. This complexity constitutes a formidable barrier to organ transplantation.

**SIGNIFICANCE OF THE MHC.** 1. The *importance of MHC-coded antigens in organ transplantation* has already been mentioned. Rejection mechanisms will be discussed in a later section. It should be obvious, however, that matching the donor and recipient for the HLA antigens, thereby reducing antigenic disparity, is likely to improve the chances of graft survival. HLA typing is therefore an important step in selecting appropriate donor-recipient combinations for transplantation.

2. *Regulation of cell-to-cell interaction in the immune response.* Although histocompatibility antigens were discovered by investigating transplant rejections, it is highly unlikely that MHC genes and antigens evolved to frustrate the transplant surgeon! A physiologic role for the HLA complex, especially class II antigens, is to facilitate interaction among lymphocytes and between lymphocytes and macrophages in the process of an immune response. For example, as alluded to earlier, T-helper cells (T4+) can recognize antigen only in association with class II antigens on the surface of macrophages and other antigen-presenting cells.

3. *Role in host defense against viral infections.* Cytotoxic (killer) T cells (T8+) can lyse virus-infected cells by a process that is extremely important in the control of a variety of infections, including influenza, vaccinia, herpes, and measles. Killer T cells can recognize viral antigens only in association with self class I molecules, a phenomenon called HLA-restricted killing (Fig. 5–3 and p. 144). Thus class I HLA antigens provide specific sites that are modified by virus infection and constitute the target antigen for T cell–mediated lysis of the infected cells. The presence of class I HLA antigens on somatic cells can therefore be viewed as evolutionary, helping to eliminate virus-infected cells; since virtually any cell type in the body can be infected by a virus, it makes "good sense" to have widespread expression of class I HLA antigens.

4. *Regulation of immune response.* It is well known that the magnitude of the immune response is under genetic control. The genes that regulate the immune response (Ir genes) are mapped within the HLA-D region, and indeed many of the cell surface class II antigens are believed to be the products of Ir genes. How class II antigens influence the immune reactivity of an individual is not fully understood. It is conceivable that class II genes regulate immune responses by affecting the manner in which antigen is presented to T cells. Thus a given class II antigen (X) and a nominal antigen (A) may associate in a nonimmunogenic form on the surface of an antigen-presenting cell in an individual who inherits the class II antigen X. On the other hand, a genetically distinct class II antigen (Y) may form a highly immunogenic A-Y complex and trigger a vigorous immune response (Fig. 5–4).

**ASSOCIATION OF HLA WITH DISEASE.** Data are rapidly accumulating that suggest a linkage between HLA antigens and many human diseases (Table 5–2). As an example, individuals who possess HLA-B27 antigen have an 87-fold greater risk of developing ankylosing spondylitis than do individuals lacking this antigen. It appears, therefore, that HLA genes are somehow related to disease susceptibility. The mechanism of such susceptibility is poorly understood, but certain possibilities have been suggested:

1. *Involvement of immune-response genes.* Since the magnitude of the immune response is regulated by Ir genes, it is possible that certain HLA-linked Ir genes may be associated with hyperresponsiveness to common allergens. Thus individuals with certain HLA profiles may be predisposed to develop immunologically mediated diseases. Since several autoimmune diseases show linkage with alleles in the HLA-D region, Ir genes within the HLA-D region may regulate the generation of autoantibodies.

2. *Direct participation of HLA macro-molecules in disease.*[11] There are two possible mechanisms by which HLA molecules may participate directly in disease. First, pathogens may share a cross-reacting antigen with HLA and be protected from an immune response by the host's tolerance for self-HLA antigens ("molecular mimicry"). Second, certain HLA molecules may provide receptors for viruses, and this may either facilitate virus-cell interaction or, alternatively, provide a target for host immune cells to destroy virus-infected cells. In the former case, the presence of a given HLA type would favor virus-induced

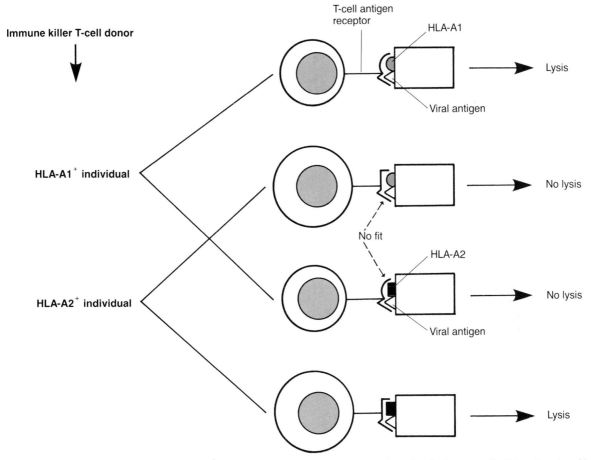

**Figure 5–3.** Schematic illustration of the role of HLA antigens in the lysis of virus-infected cells by cytotoxic T lymphocytes. Note that the cytotoxic T cells from HLA-A1- or HLA-A2-positive donors can recognize and lyse only those virus-infected parenchymal cells that carry self-HLA antigens (HLA-restricted killing).

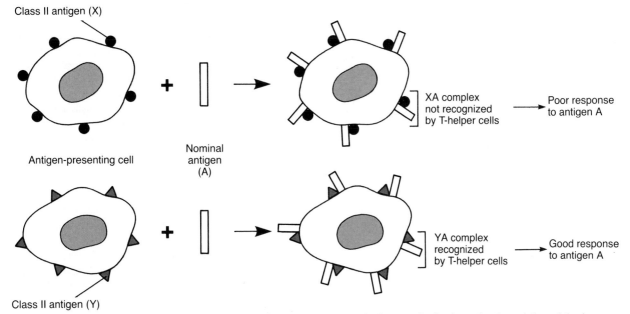

**Figure 5–4.** Schematic illustration of the proposed role of class II antigens in the genetically determined regulation of the immune response. As explained in the text, the magnitude of the immune response against a given antigen (A) may be determined by the nature of class II gene products expressed on the antigen-presenting cell.

**Table 5–2.** ASSOCIATION OF HLA
WITH DISEASE

| Disease | HLA Allele | Relative Risk |
|---|---|---|
| Ankylosing spondylitis | B27 | 87.4 |
| Postgonococcal arthritis | B27 | 14.0 |
| Acute anterior uveitis | B27 | 14.6 |
| Rheumatoid arthritis | DR4 | 5.8 |
| Chronic active hepatitis | DR3 | 13.9 |
| Primary Sjögren's syndrome | DR3 | 9.7 |
| Insulin-dependent diabetes | DR3 | 5.0 |
|  | DR4 | 6.8 |
|  | DR3/DR4 | 14.3 |
| Hemochromatosis | A3 | 8.2 |
| 21-Hydroxylase deficiency | BW47 | 15.0 |

disease, whereas in the latter case it would favor removal of virus-infected cells. It is important to note that diseases such as hemochromatosis, which are not associated with any obvious immunologic derangement, also have association with specific HLA profiles (p. 594). Thus, the HLA system may also be involved in nonimmunologic functions related to the cell surface, such as receptors and transport proteins.

# IMMUNOLOGIC MECHANISMS OF TISSUE INJURY

Immunologic responses (humoral or cell-mediated) to antigens of either endogenous or exogenous sources can cause tissue-damaging reactions. Classically these are called *hypersensitivity reactions* and the resultant tissue lesions *hypersensitivity disease.* The term hypersensitivity, however, is somewhat misleading; it implies abnormal or excessive sensitivity to an antigen. However, hypersensitivity disease may result from perfectly usual or normal immune responses to an antigen (e.g., the rejection of tissue grafts from antigenically dissimilar donors). A better designation for hypersensitivity diseases might be "diseases resulting from immunologically mediated tissue-damaging reactions," but alas, this is too cumbersome a designation.

The antigens that give rise to tissue-damaging immune reactions may be exogenous, homologous, or autologous. This distinction is of value because it indicates that some disorders—those due to exogenous antigens—are essentially environmental and as such are theoretically preventable. Poison ivy contact dermatitis could be eradicated as a disease by avoidance of contact with the plant, as could hay fever by avoiding inhalation of plant pollens. On the other hand, many of the most important immune diseases are caused by homologous and autologous antigens intrinsic to humans. The disorders triggered by homologous antigens result from the genetic and antigenic dissimilarities between individuals. Transfusion reactions are examples of immunologic disorders evoked by homologous antigens. Appropriate crossmatching of donor and recipient does preclude such reactions. The third category of disorders, those incited by autologous antigens, comprises the important group of autoimmune diseases to be discussed later. These diseases appear to arise because of the emergence of immune reactions against self-antigens.

Hypersensitivity diseases (Table 5–3) are best classified on the basis of the immunologic mechanism mediating the disease.[12] This approach is of great value, since it clarifies the manner in which the immune response ultimately causes tissue injury and disease. In Type I disease the immune response releases vasoactive amines and lipid mediators that affect vascular permeability and smooth muscles in various organs. In the Type II disorder humoral antibodies participate directly in injuring cells by predisposing them to phagocytosis or to lysis. Type III disorders are best remembered as "immune complex disease"; here humoral antibodies bind antigens and activate complement. The fractions of complement then attract neutrophils. Ultimately it is the activated complement and the release of neutrophilic enzymes and other toxic moieties (e.g., oxygen metabolites) that produce the tissue damage. Type IV disorders are examples of tissue injury in which cell-mediated immune responses with sensitized lymphocytes are the ultimate cause of the cellular and tissue injury. Each of these immunologic mechanisms is presented in the succeeding sections.

**Table 5–3.** MECHANISMS OF IMMUNOLOGICALLY MEDIATED DISORDERS

| Type | | Prototype Disorder | Immune Mechanism |
|---|---|---|---|
| I | Anaphylactic type | Anaphylaxis, some forms of bronchial asthma | Formation of IgE (cytotropic) antibody → release of vasoactive amines and other mediators from basophils and mast cells |
| II | Cytotoxic type | Autoimmune hemolytic anemia, erythroblastosis fetalis, Goodpasture's disease | Formation of IgG, IgM → binds to antigen on target cell surface → phagocytosis of target cell or lysis of target cell by C8,9 fraction of activated complement or antibody-dependent cellular cytotoxicity (ADCC) |
| III | Immune complex disease | Arthus reaction, serum sickness, systemic lupus erythematosus, certain forms of acute glomerulonephritis | Antigen-antibody complexes → activated complement → attracted neutrophils → release of lysosomal enzymes and other toxic moieties |
| IV | Cell-mediated (delayed) hypersensitivity | Tuberculosis, contact dermatitis, transplant rejection | Sensitized thymus-derived T lymphocytes → release of lymphokines and T cell–mediated cytotoxicity |

## Type I Hypersensitivity (Anaphylactic Type)

*Type I hypersensitivity is a rapidly occurring reaction that follows the combination of an antigen with antibody previously bound to the surface of mast cells and basophils.* In humans, Type I reactions are mediated by IgE antibodies (also called reaginic antibodies); in other species, IgG antibodies can mediate anaphylactic reactions. The basic sequence of events in the pathogenesis of this form of hypersensitivity begins with the initial exposure to certain antigens (often called allergens). The allergen stimulates IgE production by B cells, a process that requires the assistance of T-helper cells and is under the regulatory influence of T-suppressor cells. The IgE is strongly cytophilic for mast cells and basophils, which possess high affinity receptors for the Fc portion of IgE. Once IgE is bound to the surface of mast cells, the individual is primed to develop Type I hypersensitivity. Reexposure to the same antigen results in fixing of the antigen to cell-bound IgE, initiating a series of reactions that lead to release of several powerful mediators that are responsible for the clinical features of Type I hypersensitivity (Fig. 5–5). The mediator release requires that adjacent IgE molecules on the surface of mast cells and basophils be cross-linked by binding to a multivalent antigen. The cross-linking of cell-bound IgE induces a membrane signal that initiates two parallel and independent processes (Fig. 5–6)—one leading to mast cell degranulation with discharge of preformed or *primary mediators* and the other involving de novo synthesis and release of *secondary mediators* such as arachidonic acid metabolites.[13]

**PRIMARY MEDIATORS.** These are contained within the mast cell granules and include: (1) *histamine,* which causes increased vascular permeability, vasodilatation, bronchial smooth muscle contraction, and increased secretion of mucus; (2) *chemotactic factors* for eosinophils (ECF-A) and neutrophils (NCF); and (3) *neutral proteases* that can cleave complement and kininogens to generate other inflammatory mediators (p. 41).

**SECONDARY MEDIATORS.** These are generated by sequential reactions in the mast cell membranes that lead to activation of phospholipase $A_2$, an enzyme that acts on membrane phospholipids to yield *arachidonic acid* (p. 39).[14] This, you may recall, is the parent compound from which leukotrienes and prostaglandins are derived by the 5-lipoxygenase and cyclooxygenase pathways, respectively. Each of these will be considered separately. Leukotrienes are extremely important in the pathogenesis of Type I hypersensitivity. *Leukotrienes $C_4$ and $D_4$* are the most potent vasoactive and spasmogenic agents known. On a molar basis they are several thousand times more active than histamine in increasing vascular permeability and causing bronchial smooth muscle contraction. Because their release is slower than that of histamine, in the past they were designated as slow-reactive substance of anaphylaxis (SRS-A). *Leukotriene $B_4$* is highly chemotactic for neutrophils, eosinophils, and monocytes. Among the arachidonic acid metabolites generated by the cyclooxygenase pathway, prostaglandin $D_2$ is the most abundant mediator produced by the human lung mast cells.[15] It causes intense bronchospasm as well as increased mucus secretion. Platelet activating factor (PAF-acether, p. 41) is another secondary mediator that causes platelet aggregation and release of histamine. Although its production is also initiated by the activation of phospholipase $A_2$, it is not a product of arachidonic acid metabolism. In summary, a variety of chemotactic, vasoactive, and spasmogenic compounds listed in Table 5–4 mediate Type I hypersensitivity reactions. These compounds are released rapidly from sensi-

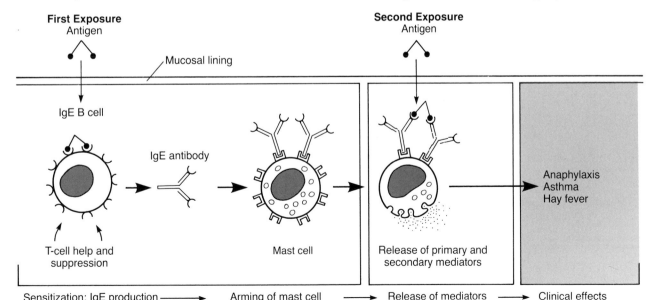

**First Exposure**
Antigen

Mucosal lining

**Second Exposure**
Antigen

IgE B cell

IgE antibody

T-cell help and suppression

Mast cell

Release of primary and secondary mediators

Anaphylaxis
Asthma
Hay fever

Sensitization: IgE production ⟶ Arming of mast cell ⟶ Release of mediators ⟶ Clinical effects

**Figure 5–5.** Sequence of events leading to Type I hypersensitivity. (Modified from Roitt, I., et al.: Immunology. New York, Gower Medical Publishing, 1985, p. 19.2.)

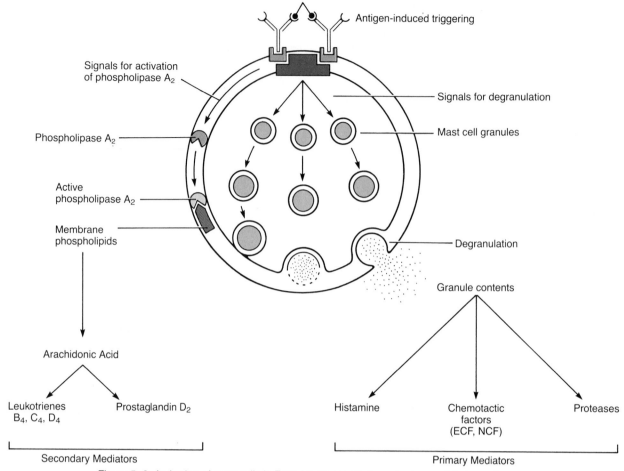

**Figure 5–6.** Activation of mast cells in Type I hypersensitivity and release of their mediators.

tized mast cells and are believed to be responsible for the intense immediate reactions associated with conditions such as bronchial asthma. However, in many individuals, the "allergic" reaction recurs within hours, without additional exposure to antigen. These so-called late-phase reactions are believed to involve activated leukocytes (neutrophils, eosinophils, and macrophages) that are attracted to the reaction site during the early response.[16] It may be recalled (p. 41) that, like mast cells, these other leukocytes can synthesize many of the secondary mediators listed above.

A Type I reaction may occur as a systemic disorder or as a local reaction. Often this is determined by the route of antigen exposure. Systemic (parenteral) administration of protein antigens (such as antisera) and drugs (such as penicillin) results in *systemic anaphylaxis*. It should be remembered that once the individual is primed, the challenge dose of antigen may be extremely small (as for example, the tiny amounts used in skin testing for various forms of allergies). Within minutes after exposure, itching, hives, and skin erythema appear, followed shortly thereafter by striking respiratory difficulty resulting presumably from constriction of respiratory bronchioles. Thus the principal organ affected is the lung, more specifically the smooth musculature of the pulmonary blood vessels and the respiratory passages. Pulmonary obstruction is accentuated by hypersecretion of mucus. Laryngeal edema may cause obstruction of the upper airway. In addition, the musculature of the entire gastrointestinal tract may

**Table 5–4.** SUMMARY OF THE ACTIONS OF MAST CELL MEDIATORS

| Action | Mediator | Source |
|---|---|---|
| *Chemotaxis* | Leukotriene B$_4$ | Arachidonic acid |
| | Eosinophil chemotactic factor of anaphylaxis | Mast cell granules |
| | Neutrophil chemotactic factor | Mast cell granules |
| *Vasoactive* (vasodilatation, increased permeability) | Histamine | Mast cell granules |
| | PAF-acether | Membrane lipids |
| | Proteases that activate complement and kinins | Mast cell granules |
| *Smooth muscle spasm* | Leukotriene C$_4$ | Arachidonic acid |
| | Leukotriene B$_4$ | Arachidonic acid |
| | Histamine | Mast cell granules |
| | Prostaglandin D$_2$ | Arachidonic acid |

be affected, with resultant vomiting, abdominal cramps, and diarrhea. The patient may go into shock and even die within the hour. At autopsy the findings may be surprisingly few, consisting principally of pulmonary edema and hemorrhages, sometimes accompanied by hyperdistention of the lungs and right-sided cardiac dilatation.

*Systemic anaphylaxis is an important condition to bear in mind, since it is capable of causing death within minutes.* It has been estimated, for example, that as many as 20% of individuals treated with penicillin develop varying degrees of sensitivity to the drug, each of whom is a potential candidate for an anaphylactic attack.

Local reactions generally occur on the skin or mucosal surfaces when they are the sites of antigenic exposure. The common forms of skin and food allergies, hay fever, and certain forms of asthma are examples of localized anaphylactic reactions. Presumably the synthesis of IgE occurs in the regional lymphoid tissues and local fixation to mast cells occurs. Susceptibility to localized Type I reactions appears to be genetically controlled, and the term *atopy* is used to imply familial predisposition to such localized reactions. Family history is often present in patients who suffer from nasobronchial allergy (including hay fever and some forms of asthma). However, neither the number of genes involved nor the mode of inheritance is clear.

Before we close the discussion of Type I hypersensitivity, it should be noted that the IgE antibodies are not merely "villains" that cause much human discomfort and diseases. They also play an important protective role in several parasitic infections.[17] IgE antibodies are regularly produced in response to many helminthic infections. Figure 5–7 provides a schematic illustration of the process by which IgE antibodies serve to inflict damage on the schistosome larvae. Some points worthy of note in this schema are:

○ IgE-sensitized mast cells do not cause direct damage to the parasites. Instead, they attract other leukocytes such as eosinophils by release of chemotactic factors.
○ In addition to mast cells, eosinophils, platelets, and some macrophages possess Fc receptors for IgE.
○ IgE-armed leukocytes attach to the surface of parasites and inflict damage by a variety of mechanisms. For example, eosinophils are capable of mediating antibody-dependent cellular cytotoxicity (described later); macrophages, on the other hand, release toxic oxygen metabolites and lysosomal enzymes.

### Type II Antibody-Dependent (Cytotoxic) Hypersensitivity

Unlike all other hypersensitivity reactions, in Type II the source of the antigen is *always* homologous or

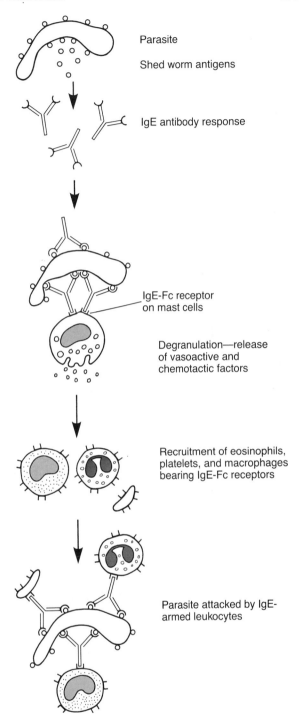

Parasite

Shed worm antigens

IgE antibody response

IgE-Fc receptor on mast cells

Degranulation—release of vasoactive and chemotactic factors

Recruitment of eosinophils, platelets, and macrophages bearing IgE-Fc receptors

Parasite attacked by IgE-armed leukocytes

Figure 5–7. IgE-mediated destruction of parasites.

autologous. The target antigens are either normal or altered cell surface components. Two different antibody-dependent mechanisms are involved in this type of hypersensitivity.

COMPLEMENT-MEDIATED CYTOTOXICITY. In this pattern, antibody reacts with a cell surface antigen, leading to fixation of complement and cell lysis. In addition, cells coated with antibodies become susceptible to phagocytosis, a process also favored by fixation of complement (p. 34). Blood cells are most commonly damaged by this mechanism, but antibodies can be directed against other tissue elements—e.g., glomerular basement membrane in Goodpasture's syndrome (p. 463). Clinically, antibody-mediated reactions occur in the following situations: (1) *Transfusion reactions*, in which red cells from an incompatible donor are destroyed after being coated with antibodies normally present in the recipient directed against blood group antigens. (2) *Rhesus incompatibility*, in which an Rh-negative mother is sensitized by red cells from an Rh-positive baby. The maternal Rh antibodies can cross the placenta and cause destruction of the Rh-positive fetal red cells. The resulting syndrome is called *erythroblastosis fetalis* (p. 362). (3) Some individuals develop antibodies against their own blood elements, resulting in autoimmune hemolytic anemia, agranulocytosis, or thrombocytopenia. The possible reasons for such autoantibody formation are discussed in a later section (p. 150).

**ANTIBODY-DEPENDENT CELL-MEDIATED CYTOTOXICITY (ADCC).** This is the other possible mechanism involved in Type II reactions. Many cell types that bear receptors for the Fc portion of IgG cause the lysis of target cells coated with IgG antibody. Presumably this interaction involves the Fc receptors of the killer cells, which engage the Fc portion of the antibody coating the target cell (Fig. 5–8). *Lysis of the target cell requires contact and is energy dependent but does not involve phagocytosis or fixation of complement.* ADCC can be mediated by a variety of cell types that bear Fc-IgG receptors. These include neutrophils, eosinophils, macrophages, and K cells.

**ADCC**

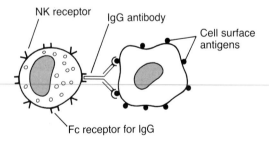

**NATURAL KILLING**

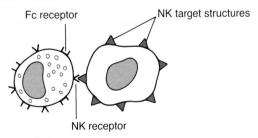

**Figure 5–8.** Antibody-dependent and antibody-independent lysis mediated by natural killer cells.

The last designation has been used for cells that bear Fc receptors but lack surface markers of T cells, B cells, or macrophages ("null cells"). It is now believed that most of the so-called K cells are actually NK cells that can kill their targets by two different mechanisms (Fig. 5–8): (1) spontaneous cytotoxicity that does not involve antibodies or Fc receptors, discussed in an earlier section (p. 132), and (2) lysis of antibody-coated target cells via Fc receptors. Both direct cytotoxicity and ADCC may be relevant to the antitumor activity of NK cells. Although in most cases IgG antibodies are involved in ADCC, in certain instances (for example, eosinophil-mediated ADCC against parasites, discussed above) IgE antibodies are utilized.

## Type III (Immune Complex–Mediated) Hypersensitivity

This type of hypersensitivity is mediated by antigen-antibody (immune) complexes that initiate an acute inflammatory reaction in the tissues. Activation of complement and accumulation of polymorphonuclear leukocytes are important components of immune complex–mediated tissue injury. The formation of immune complexes can be initiated by exogenous antigens, such as bacteria and viruses, or by endogenous antigens, such as DNA. Pathogenic immune complexes are either formed in the circulation and then deposited in the tissues or formed at extravascular sites where antigen may have been planted (in situ immune complexes). Some forms of glomerular diseases in which immune complexes are formed in situ on the glomerular basement membrane are discussed in Chapter 14. There are two patterns of immune complex–mediated injury. In one the complexes are deposited in various tissues of the body, thus causing a systemic pattern of injury. In the other the injury is localized to the site of formation, within a tissue or organ, of the complexes. Although the mechanism of tissue injury is the same, the sequence of events and the conditions leading to the formation of the immune complexes are different. We will, therefore, consider these two patterns separately.

**SYSTEMIC IMMUNE COMPLEX DISEASE (SERUM SICKNESS TYPE).** For the sake of simplicity, the pathogenesis of systemic immune complex disease can be resolved into three phases:[18] (1) formation of antigen-antibody complexes in the circulation and (2) deposition of the immune complexes in various tissues, thus initiating (3) an inflammatory reaction in dispersed sites throughout the body (Fig. 5–9). Acute serum sickness is the prototype of a systemic immune complex disease; it was at one time a frequent sequel to the administration of large amounts of foreign serum (e.g., horse antitetanus serum) used for passive immunization. It is now seen infrequently and in different clinical settings. For example, in a recent report 11 out of 12 patients who were injected with horse-antithymocyte globulin for treatment of aplastic

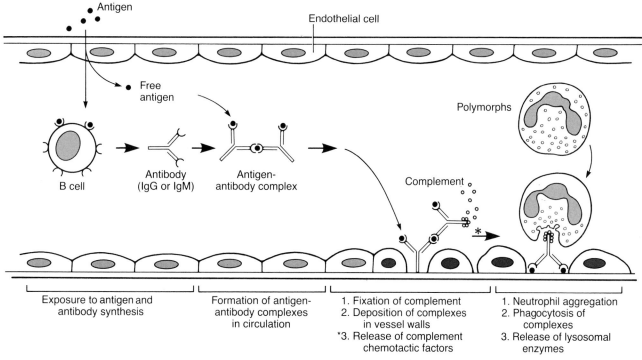

**Figure 5–9.** Schematic illustration of the sequence of events in systemic Type III (immune complex) hypersensitivity.

anemia developed serum sickness.[19] Approximately five days after the serum injection, antibodies directed against the serum components are produced; these react with the antigen still present in the circulation to form antigen-antibody complexes (the first phase). The mere formation of immune complexes in the circulation does not necessarily give rise to immune complex disease; indeed, immune complexes are often formed during many immune responses, and they are removed from the circulation by the mononuclear phagocyte system. The factors that determine whether immune complex formation will lead to tissue deposition and disease are not fully understood, but two possible influences are listed below:

○ Size of the complexes seems to be important. Very large complexes formed in great antibody excess are rapidly removed from the circulation by the MPS cells and are therefore relatively harmless. The most pathogenic complexes are of small or intermediate size, circulate longer, and bind less avidly to phagocytic cells.

○ Since the mononuclear phagocyte system normally serves to filter out the circulating immune complexes, its overload or intrinsic dysfunction increases the probability of persistence of immune complexes in circulation and tissue deposition.

Tissue injury does not occur unless the circulating immune complexes are extravasated into various tissues (second phase). For reasons not entirely clear, the favored sites of immune complex deposition are kidneys, joints, skin, heart, serosal surfaces, and small blood vessels. For complexes to leave the microcirculation there must be an increase in vascular permeability, mediated by small amounts of IgE induced shortly after administration of the antigen. Thus, a miniature Type I (anaphylactic) reaction ensues, which results in the release of histamine and platelet-activating factor. The latter induces platelet aggregation and release of their amines—histamine and serotonin—which increase vascular permeability (p. 37) and allow the complexes to enter the vessel wall. This transient Type I reaction has been appropriately called the "anaphylactic trigger." Although this mechanism explains the vascular localization of the complexes, it fails to account for their tissue distribution. Localization in the kidney could be explained in part by the filtration function of the glomerulus, with trapping of the circulating complexes in the glomeruli. Localization of immune complexes in the kidney is also affected by the charge on the antigen or antibody. Positively charged complexes tend to be attracted to the inner surface of the glomerular basement membrane, which carries a negative charge. In diseases such as systemic lupus erythematosus the predilection for renal deposition may be dictated by the affinity of the antigen (DNA) for the collagen in the basement membrane of the glomerulus. However, there is at present no satisfactory explanation for the peculiar localization of immune complexes in the other sites of predilection. Once complexes are deposited in the tissues they initiate an acute inflammatory reaction (phase three). It is during this phase (approximately 10 days after antigen administration) that clinical features such as fever, urticaria, arthralgias, lymph node enlargement, and proteinuria appear. Central to the pathogenesis of tissue injury is the fixation of complement by the complexes, resulting in the activation of the complement cascade and release of biologically active fragments (p. 38). It should be recalled that complement activation releases anaphylatoxins (C3a and C5a), which increase vascular permeability and yield chemotactic factors for polymorphonuclear leukocytes. Phagocytosis of immune complexes by the accumulated neutrophils results in the release of lysosomal enzymes, such as neutral proteases, which can digest basement membranes, collagen, elastin, and cartilage. Tissue damage may also be mediated by free oxygen radicals produced by activated neutrophils. The released lysosomal enzymes serve to perpetuate the inflammatory process (p. 41). Immune complexes have other effects as well: they lead to aggregation of platelets and activation of Hageman factor, both of which augment the inflammatory process (Fig. 5–10). Microthrombi formed by platelet aggregation and initiation of clotting also contribute to the tissue injury by producing local ischemia.

It should be clear from the above that only complement-fixing antibodies (i.e., IgG and IgM) are involved in Type III hypersensitivity. The important role of complement in the pathogenesis of the tissue injury is supported by the observation that experimental manipulations that deplete serum complement levels greatly reduce the severity of the lesions, as does depletion of neutrophils. During the active phase of the disease, consumption of complement induces low serum levels.

The morphologic consequences of immune complex injury are dominated by acute necrotizing vasculitis, microthrombi, and superimposed ischemic necrosis accompanied by acute inflammation of the affected organs. The necrotic vessel wall takes on a smudgy eosinophilic appearance called "fibrinoid necrosis" (Fig. 5–11). Immune complexes can be visualized in the tissues, usually in the vascular wall, by both electron microscopy and immunofluorescence. In due course the lesions tend to resolve, especially when brought about by a single large exposure to antigen (e.g., acute serum sickness and acute poststreptococcal glomerulonephritis, p. 468). However, chronic immune complex disease develops when there is persistent antigenemia or repeated exposure to the antigen. This occurs in several human diseases, such as systemic lupus erythematosus, which is associated with persistent exposure to autoantigens. Often, however, despite the fact that the morphologic changes and other findings suggest immune complex disease, the inciting antigens are unknown. Included in this category are rheumatoid arthritis, polyarteritis nodosa, membranous glomerulonephritis, and several vasculitides.

**LOCAL IMMUNE COMPLEX DISEASE (ARTHUS REACTION).** *The Arthus reaction may be defined as a localized area of tissue necrosis resulting from acute immune complex vasculitis.* The reaction can be produced experimentally by injecting an antigen into the skin of a previously immunized animal. Antibodies against the antigen are therefore already present in the circulation. *Because of the large excess of antibodies, immune complexes are formed; these are precipitated at the site of injection, especially within vessel walls, where the injected antigen is immediately bound to the circulating antibodies.* Once the complexes are formed, the subsequent events are very similar to those described in the systemic pattern.

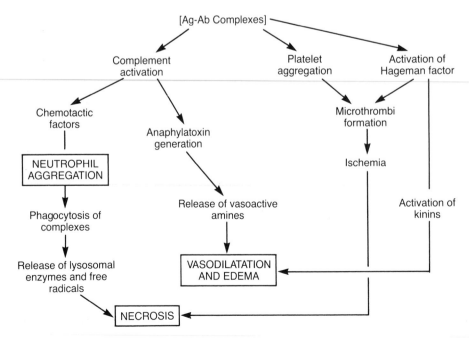

Figure 5–10. Schematic representation of the pathogenesis of immune complex–mediated tissue injury. The morphologic consequences are depicted as boxed areas.

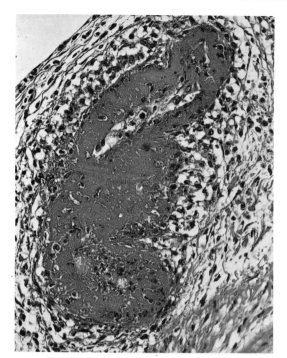

Figure 5–11. Immune complex vasculitis—acute fibrinoid necrosis of walls of small vessels. (From Robbins, S. L., Cotran, R. S., and Kumar, V.: Pathologic Basis of Disease. 3rd ed. Philadelphia, W. B. Saunders Co., 1984, p. 169.)

Histologically, there is a severe necrotizing vasculitis and intense accumulation of neutrophils. Intrapulmonary Arthus-type reactions seem to be responsible for a number of diseases in humans, including farmer's lung, a hypersensitivity reaction to molds that grow on hay.

## Type IV (Cell-Mediated) Hypersensitivity

This type of hypersensitivity is mediated by cells rather than antibodies. *Two types of reactions are involved in Type IV hypersensitivity, delayed hypersensitivity and cell-mediated cytotoxicity.* In both cases, the reaction is initiated by the exposure of sensitized T cells to the specific antigen, but the subsequent events are different. In delayed hypersensitivity there is recruitment of other cells, especially macrophages, which are the major effector cells. In cell-mediated cytotoxicity, on the other hand, sensitized T cells themselves assume the effector function. Although the final mode of expression of the two reactions is different, it is important to note that antigen-sensitized T cells are crucial to both the forms, as will be evident in the following discussions.

**DELAYED-TYPE HYPERSENSITIVITY.** *The classic example of a delayed hypersensitivity reaction is a positive Mantoux reaction (tuberculin test) elicited in an individual already sensitized to the tubercle bacillus by a prior infection* (p. 437). Following the intracutaneous injection of tuberculin, a local area of

erythema and induration begins to appear at eight to 12 hours, reaches a peak (approximately 1 to 2 cm in diameter) in two to seven days, and thereafter slowly subsides. The extremely sensitive individual may develop a larger area of induration and even central necrosis. Histologically, cutaneous delayed hypersensitivity in humans is characterized by emigration of lymphocytes and monocytes from dermal venules, producing a perivascular "cuffing" (Fig. 5–12). There is an associated increased microvascular permeability resulting from the formation of interendothelial gaps. Not unexpectedly, there is an escape of plasma proteins, which gives rise to dermal edema and deposition of fibrin.[20] In fully developed lesions, the lymphocyte-cuffed venules show marked endothelial hypertrophy and, in some cases, hyperplasia. In extremely sensitive individuals there is endothelial cell necrosis and a significant accumulation of neutrophils as well. As previously mentioned in Chapter 2, granulomatous inflammation is also an expression of delayed hypersensitivity. With certain persistent or nondegradable antigens, the initial perivascular mononuclear cell infiltrate is replaced by granulomas over a period of two to three weeks. This change is associated with the transformation of the emigrated monocytes into epithelioid cells that form cohesive aggregates recognized as granulomas (p. 47).

The sequence of events in delayed hypersensitivity, as exemplified by the tuberculin reaction, begins

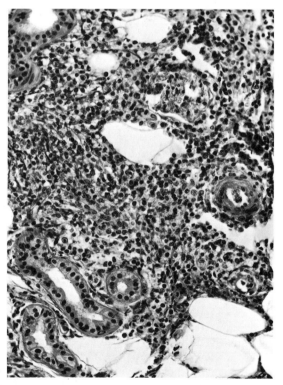

Figure 5–12. A tuberculin reaction in the dermis. There is infiltration of lymphocytes and macrophages about the small vessels and skin adnexa.

with the first exposure of the individual to tubercle bacilli. T4[+] lymphocytes recognize antigens of tubercle bacilli in association with class II antigens on the surface of macrophages that have ingested the mycobacteria. This sensitization process leads to the formation of "memory" T cells that remain in the circulation for long periods, sometimes years. Upon intracutaneous injection of tuberculin in such an individual, the specific-memory T cells interact with the antigens and are activated (i.e., they undergo blast transformation and proliferation). These changes are accompanied by the secretion of a number of biologically active factors referred to as lymphokines, each with its own activity.[21] Two of the well-known lymphokines are macrophage migration inhibition factor (MIF) and macrophage-activating factor. As their names indicate, they serve to immobilize macrophages at the reaction site and activate them, enhancing their ability and their capacity for intracellular destruction of pathogens. Many other lymphokines, detected primarily by diverse functional assays, have been described. It is not yet clear how many chemically distinct molecules are involved. Some of the important lymphokines and their properties are listed below:

○ Macrophage migration inhibition factor (MIF), a glycoprotein of 30,000 molecular weight.
○ Chemotactic factors for neutrophils, monocytes, and eosinophils.
○ Gamma-interferon, which like other interferons has antiviral activity, but in addition is also a macrophage-activating factor. γ-IFN also increases the expression of class II antigens on a variety of cell types, including macrophages, endothelial cells, and fibroblasts.
○ Interleukin-2. This substance, previously called T cell growth factor because of its ability to enhance growth and clonal expansion of T lymphocytes is now known to stimulate a variety of cell types, including B cells and NK cells.[22] IL-2 acts on its target cells via IL-2 receptors.
○ Lymphotoxins, which kill tumor cells and may be involved in antitumor immunity.
○ Vasoactive factors that increase vascular permeability. These have not been well characterized but are probably important in the emigration of cells during delayed hypersensitivity reactions.

It is important to point out that although the generation of lymphokines is the result of a very specific interaction between the antigen and the sensitized T cells, the effects of lymphokines are not antigen-specific. For example, macrophages activated by tuberculoprotein develop increased activity not only against tubercle bacilli but also against several unrelated bacteria. This type of hypersensitivity is a major mechanism of defense against a variety of intracellular pathogens, including mycobacteria, fungi, and certain parasites, and may also be involved in transplant rejection and tumor immunity.

**T CELL–MEDIATED CYTOTOXICITY.** In this variant of

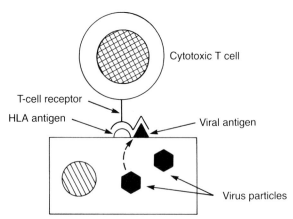

**Figure 5–13.** Schematic illustration of the role of HLA antigens in the lysis of virus-infected cells by cytotoxic T lymphocytes.

Type IV hypersensitivity, sensitized T cells (T8[+]) can themselves kill antigen-bearing target cells. Such effector cells are called cytotoxic T lymphocytes (CTLs). CTLs, directed against cell surface histocompatibility antigens, play an important role in graft rejection, to be discussed later in this chapter. They also play a role in resistance to virus infections, as alluded to earlier. Infection of cells with a virus leads to alterations in the cell surface HLA antigens, possibly by a physical association between the viral proteins and HLA molecules. *The modified HLA antigens differ from normal self-HLA antigens ("altered self") and so evoke cytotoxic T cells capable of killing virus-infected target cells* (Fig. 5–13). The lysis of infected cells before viral replication is completed leads in due course to the elimination of the infection. It is believed that many tumor-associated antigens (p. 200) may also be modified self-antigens, with the alteration induced by oncogenic agents. CTLs therefore may also be involved in tumor immunity. For lysis to occur, the CTL must first recognize its target via the T-cell antigen receptor; this step brings the CTL and the target cell in close contact. The lytic signal is delivered quite rapidly and does not involve complement; after target cell lysis, the CTL is free to move on and kill other target cells. It must be emphasized that cell lysis by CTL is antigen specific, and innocent bystander cells are not killed.[23]

### Transplant Rejection

Rejection of organ transplants is a complex immunologic phenomenon that involves both cell-mediated and antibody-mediated responses, both of which are targeted on the HLA antigens in the graft.[23a]

**T CELL–MEDIATED REJECTION.** The classic acute rejection, which occurs within 10 to 14 days in nonimmunosuppressed recipients, is largely the result of cell-mediated immunity. As already mentioned, this involves delayed hypersensitivity and T cell–mediated cytotoxicity. The generation of CTL in response to HLA-incompatible organ grafts is depicted schematically in Figure 5–14. This reaction starts when the recipient's lymphocytes encounter foreign HLA antigens on the surface of cells in the graft. It is believed that the donor lymphoid cells ("passenger lymphocytes"), especially dendritic cells contained within the grafts, are the most important immunogens, since they are rich in both class I and class II antigens. The T4+-helper T-cell subset is triggered into proliferation by recognition of the class II specificities; this is similar to the mixed lymphocyte reaction that occurs in vitro (p. 133). At the same time, precursors of T8+ CTL ("pre-killer T cells"), which bear receptors for class I HLA antigens, differentiate into mature CTLs. This process of differentiation is complex and incompletely understood. Involved are interactions of antigen-presenting cells, T-cell subsets, and soluble factors such as IL-1 and IL-2 (Fig. 5–14). Once mature CTLs are generated, they lyse the grafted tissue. In addition to the specific cytotoxic T cells, lymphokine-secreting T cells are also generated by sensitization, as in the delayed hypersensitivity reaction. This leads to increased vascular permeability and local accumulation of

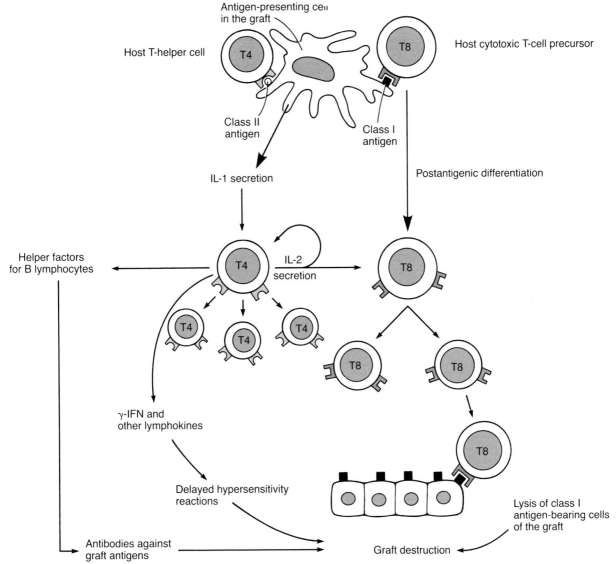

**Figure 5–14.** Schematic representation of events that lead to the destruction of histoincompatible grafts. Class I and class II antigens of the graft donor are recognized by T8+ cytotoxic T cells and T4+ helper cells, respectively, of the host. The interaction of the T4+ cells with class II antigens leads to the release of interleukin 1 (IL-1) from the antigen-presenting cells. IL-1 promotes the proliferation of T4+ cells and the release of interleukin 2 (IL-2) from the cells. IL-2 further augments the proliferation of T4+ cells and also provides helper signals for the differentiation of class I–specific T8+ cytotoxic cells. In addition to IL-2, a variety of other soluble mediators (lymphokines) that promote B-cell differentiation and participate in the induction of a local delayed hypersensitivity reaction are produced by T4+ helper cells. Eventually, several mechanisms converge to destroy the graft: (1) lysis of cells that bear class I antigens by T8+ cytotoxic T cells, (2) antigraft antibodies produced by sensitized B cells, and (3) nonspecific damage inflicted by macrophages and other cells that accumulate as a result of the delayed hypersensitivity reaction.

mononuclear cells (lymphocytes and macrophages) as previously described. According to some investigators, the delayed hypersensitivity with its attendant microvascular injury, tissue ischemia, and destruction mediated by accumulated macrophages is an important mechanism of graft destruction.[20]

**ANTIBODY-MEDIATED REJECTION.** There is little doubt that T cells are of paramount importance in the rejection of organ transplants. This is supported by the inability of T cell–deprived animals to reject allografts. However, antibodies can also mediate rejection, and this process can take two forms. (1) *Hyperacute rejection* occurs when *preformed antidonor antibodies are present in the circulation of the recipient.* Such antibodies may be present in a recipient who has already rejected a kidney transplant. Multiparous women who develop anti-HLA antibodies against paternal antigens shed from the fetus may also have preformed antibodies to grafts taken from their husbands or children. Prior blood transfusions from HLA nonidentical donors can also lead to presensitization, since platelets and white cells are particularly rich in HLA antigens. In such circumstances rejection occurs immediately after transplantation, since the circulating antibodies react with and deposit rapidly on the vascular endothelium of the grafted organ. Complement fixation occurs and an Arthus-type reaction follows. (2) Even in nonsensitized individuals, anti-HLA humoral antibodies develop concurrently with T cell–mediated rejection. These antibodies are particularly important in mediating *late acute rejection* in recipients who have been treated with immunosuppressive drugs following transplantation. The immunosuppressive drugs suppress T cell responses, but some formation of antibodies continues, causing damage by ADCC and complement fixation with the formation of immune complexes. In most cases, the major target of antibody-mediated damage is the vascular endothelium. Superimposed on the immunologically mediated vascular damage are platelet aggregation and coagulation, adding ischemic insult to the injury.

**MORPHOLOGY OF REJECTION REACTIONS.** Based on morphology and the mechanisms involved, rejection reactions have been classified as hyperacute, acute, and chronic.

The morphologic changes in these patterns will be described as they relate to renal transplants. Similar changes would be encountered in any other vascularized visceral organ transplant.

*Hyperacute Rejection.* This may occur within minutes or a few hours in presensitized individuals. **Basically, it is characterized by widespread acute arteritis and arteriolitis, thrombosis of vessels, and ischemic necrosis. As indicated earlier, this pattern of rejection is mediated largely by humoral antibodies, which evoke an Arthus-like reaction.** As a consequence of the arterial lesions, the graft never becomes vascularized and it undergoes ischemic necrosis. The renal allograft becomes mottled, dusky, and flaccid and loses its arterial

pulsation within minutes of establishing the vascular connections. Virtually all arterioles and arteries exhibit characteristic acute fibrinoid necrosis of their walls, with narrowing or complete occlusion of the lumens by precipitated fibrin and cellular debris. Deposits of IgG, IgM, complement, and fibrin can be demonstrated within the vessel walls. The glomeruli are large and swollen and contain deposits of fibrinoid as well as granular debris and fragments of cells within the vascular lumens. Immunoglobulins, C3, and fibrin can be demonstrated within these glomerular deposits. Acutely involved glomeruli may also be infiltrated with neutrophils if the kidney is left in situ for more than a few minutes. Tubular cells undergo ischemic necrosis, and usually the interstitial tissue is edematous and infiltrated with neutrophils and occasional lymphocytes and macrophages. Sometimes, in the less florid hyperacute reactions, vacuolation of endothelial cells and of intimal muscle cells appears in small to medium-sized arteries. This may produce intimal thickening resembling atherosclerosis (Fig. 5–15). Obviously, the hyperacute rejection results in prompt, irreversible destruction of the graft.

*Acute Rejection.* This may occur within days of transplantation in the untreated recipient or may appear suddenly months or even years later, when immunosuppression has been employed and terminated. As suggested

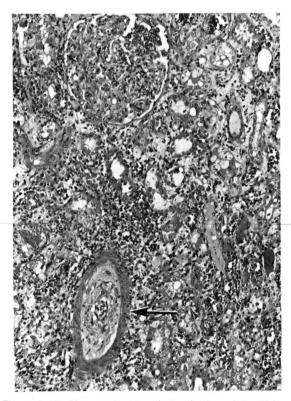

Figure 5–15. Hyperacute transplant rejection of the kidney. There is extensive interstitial edema and leukocytic infiltration. The glomerulus at the top is partially necrotic. The blood vessel (*arrow*) is virtually occluded by marked subintimal edema and fibrosis, and the small cleared spaces in the intima contain lipid. There is extensive damage to the tubular epithelial cells.

earlier, acute graft rejection is a combined process in which both cellular and humoral tissue injury play parts. In any one patient, one or the other mechanism may predominate. Histologically, humoral rejection is associated with vasculitis, whereas cellular rejection is marked by an interstitial mononuclear cell infiltrate.

**Acute cellular rejection** is most commonly seen within the initial months after transplantation and is often accompanied by the abrupt onset of clinical signs of failure of renal function. Histologically, there may be extensive interstitial mononuclear cell infiltration and edema, as well as mild interstitial hemorrhage. In humans, the mononuclear cell infiltrate consists primarily of medium-sized and small lymphocytes along with some large blast-like lymphocytes. Immunoperoxidase staining reveals both T4+ and T8+ cells, as might be expected from the earlier discussion of graft rejection. Plasma cells are also seen in long-standing cases. Glomerular and peritubular capillaries contain large numbers of mononuclear cells, which may also invade the tubules and cause focal tubular necrosis. In the absence of an accompanying arteritis, these cellular rejections respond promptly to immunosuppressive therapy.

*Acute rejection vasculitis (humoral rejection)* may also be present in the acute reaction after transplantation or when immunosuppressive therapy is discontinued. The histologic lesions consist of necrotizing arteritis with endothelial necrosis; neutrophilic infiltration; deposition of immunoglobulins, complement, and fibrin; and thrombosis. The process may evolve to extensive glomerular necrosis and cortical arteriolar thrombosis, with resulting cortical infarction. Almost all of the patients so affected will also have evidence of acute cellular rejection. More common than this acute type of vasculitis is so-called subacute vasculitis, which is characterized by marked thickening of the intima by a cushion of proliferating fibroblasts, myocytes, and foamy macrophages, often leading to luminal narrowing or obliteration. The thickened intima may be infiltrated by scattered neutrophils and mononuclear cells, and the walls of most of these arteries have deposits of immunoglobulin and complement.

*Chronic Rejection.* Since most instances of acute graft rejection are more or less controlled by immunosuppressive therapy, chronic changes are commonly seen in the renal allograft (Fig. 5–16). Patients with chronic rejection present clinically with a progressive rise in serum creatinine level (an index of renal dysfunction) over a period of four to six months. The vascular changes consist of dense intimal fibrosis, principally in the cortical arteries; the lesion probably is the end stage of the patterns of arteritis described in acute and subacute stages. These vascular lesions result in renal ischemia manifested by glomerular obsolescence, interstitial fibrosis, and tubular atrophy and shrinkage of the renal parenchyma. Together with the vascular lesions, the kidneys usually have interstitial mononuclear cell infiltrates containing large numbers of plasma cells and numerous eosinophils. This is taken as an indication of chronic cell-mediated rejection, but in truth it must be said that identification of the pathogenetic mechanisms in chronic graft rejection is

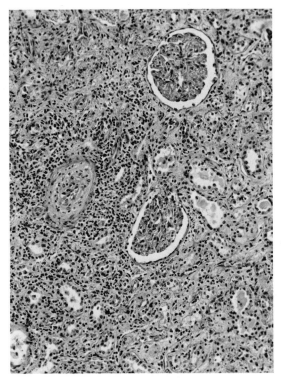

Figure 5–16. Chronic transplant rejection of the kidney. There is marked tubular atrophy, increased interstitial fibrosis, and mononuclear cell infiltration. The vessel at left center has a markedly thickened wall and virtual obliteration of the lumen. The glomeruli show some ischemic axial thickening.

much more difficult than it is in the acute forms; it is further complicated by the contribution of ischemic damage to progressive renal dysfunction.

**METHODS OF INCREASING GRAFT SURVIVAL.** We are still far from the utopia in which diseased organs can be replaced as easily as worn-out automobile parts. Intensive efforts have been made to devise strategies that will prevent graft rejection, and some attempts are closer to practical application than are others. The approaches to improving graft survival can be classified into three categories: (1) *HLA typing and matching*, (2) *immunosuppression of the recipient*, and (3) *previous blood transfusions*.

Since HLA antigens are the major targets in transplant rejection, better matching of the donor and the recipient would, of course, improve graft survival. Obviously, monozygotic twins are the most perfectly matched and are ideal donors for each other. Since the HLA genes of maternal or paternal origin are closely linked, they tend to be inherited en bloc (together called a haplotype). It can be readily appreciated that within a family, there is a 25% chance that two siblings will be HLA-identical (share both haplotypes), an additional 50% will share one haplotype, and 25% will share no haplotype. Parents share one haplotype with all children and differ at the other. The benefits of HLA-matching are most dramatic in intrafamilial (living related donor) kidney transplants. For example, transplants from HLA-identical siblings have a survival rate of 90% at one year, compared with 56% if donor and recipient do not share either haplotype. However, the effects of HLA-matching on graft survival in renal transplants from cadavers are much less dramatic and depend on several variables, including the class of HLA antigens matched, ethnic composition of the population under study (relatively homogeneous versus heterogeneous), and concurrent immunosuppressive therapy. The details of these complexities are beyond our scope and may be found in recent reviews.[24, 25] Only the salient points will be summarized here:

○ Class I matching (HLA-A and B) contributes modestly (~20% better survival) to cadaver graft success in some centers. In other centers, the beneficial effect is minimal.

○ Class II matching results in a definite improvement of graft survival, but the degree of improvement is variable in different populations. It should be recalled that class II antigens trigger T-helper cells, an event that is believed to be important in the induction of alloresponses.

○ Effective immunosuppression, discussed below, often masks any beneficial effects of HLA-matching.

Immunosuppression of the recipient is a practical necessity in all organ transplantation except in the case of identical twins. Even in transplants from HLA-identical siblings, there are minor non-HLA antigenic differences that can evoke a rejection reaction, albeit mild. Drugs and antilymphocyte serum are the two common modes of immunosuppression employed. Among drugs, cyclosporin has emerged as a powerful and effective tool in preventing organ transplant rejection.[26] It suppresses T cell–mediated immunity, and, as alluded to above, HLA-mismatched renal grafts often fare as well as HLA-matched grafts when cyclosporin is employed for immunosuppression. However, the use of cyclosporin is limited by its significant renal toxicity. Another avenue for immunosuppression currently under trial is the administration of monoclonal antibodies to T-cell subsets. Immunosuppression definitely improves graft survival, but it renders the individual vulnerable to opportunistic infections. Often an immunosuppressed patient dies of disseminated and refractory infections rather than organ failure.

Paradoxical as it may seem, *previous blood transfusions* have been definitely proved to be of benefit in enhancing survival of renal transplants from cadavers. Although blood transfusions carry a definite risk of presensitization, thereby rendering some recipients unsuitable for transplantation, such a risk is small, contrary to earlier expectations.[27] At present there is no satisfactory explanation for the transfusion effect, but in view of the distinct improvement that it confers on graft survival, pretransplant blood transfusion is a routine procedure in most kidney transplant programs.

It would, of course, be ideal if a state of specific unresponsiveness to the donor antigens could be achieved. Transplantation tolerance would have the merit of preventing graft rejection without impairing the immune response to infectious agents. Highly successful methods have been devised to induce transplantation tolerance in laboratory animals; however, none have reached the clinic as yet.

**TRANSPLANTATION OF HEMATOPOIETIC CELLS.** Transplantation of bone marrow is a form of therapy increasingly employed for hematologic malignancies, aplastic anemias, and certain immune deficiency states. The recipient is given large doses of irradiation either to destroy the malignant cells (e.g., leukemias) or to create a graft bed (aplastic anemias), and the destroyed bone marrow is restored by marrow transplantation. Two major problems complicate this form of transplantation: graft-versus-host disease (GVH) and rejection of the transplant. *Graft-versus-host disease* occurs when immunologically competent cells or their precursors are transplanted into recipients who are immunologically crippled because of the primary disease or from prior treatment with drugs or irradiation. When such recipients receive normal bone marrow cells from allogeneic donors, the immunocompetent T cells derived from the donor marrow recognize the recipient's tissue as "foreign" and react against them. This results in the generation of cytotoxic lymphocytes and lymphokine-secreting T cells, which are detrimental to the recipient's tissues. The resulting syndrome, graft-versus-host disease, is potentially lethal. HLA-matching reduces the severity of GVH but does not eliminate the syndrome, since the donor T cells react against minor histocompatibility antigens that lie outside the HLA locus. As a possible solution to this problem, T cells are depleted from the donor marrow by pretreatment with anti-T3 antibodies and complement. This protocol has proved to be the proverbial two-edged sword: GVH is reduced but there is increased incidence of graft failures. It seems that the schizophrenic T cells not only mediate GVH but are also in some manner required for the engraftment of the transplanted bone marrow stem cells.

# AUTOIMMUNE DISEASES

An immune reaction against "self-antigens"—autoimmunity—is now a well-established cause of disease. In recent years a growing list of diseases has been attributed to autoimmunity. However, caution must be exercised in assigning an autoimmune etiology to every disease in which autoantibodies can be demonstrated. It should be remembered that autoantibodies can be formed in response to injured, antigenically altered tissues. Moreover, autoantibodies can be demonstrated in a surprisingly large number of persons, particularly older individuals, who are apparently entirely free of autoimmune disease.

The designation of a condition as an autoimmune disease should therefore be based on (1) evidence of an autoimmune reaction, (2) the judgment that the immunologic findings are not merely secondary, and (3) the lack of any other identified cause for the disorder.

Despite uncertainties, a number of conditions have been designated as autoimmune diseases (Table 5–5). They range from *single organ–* or *single cell–type disorders*, which involve specific immune reactions directed against one particular organ or cell type, to *multisystem diseases*, characterized by lesions in many organs, associated usually with a multiplicity of autoantibodies or cell-mediated reactions, or both. In most of the latter diseases the pathologic changes are found principally within the connective tissue and blood vessels of the various organs involved. Thus, these diseases were once called "collagen-vascular diseases" or "connective tissue diseases." As will be seen, the autoimmune reactions in these systemic diseases are not specifically directed against the constituents of connective tissue or blood vessels, but these older designations remain useful, since they connote widespread lesions affecting many organs and systems.

The immunologic evidence that the diseases listed in Table 5–5 are indeed the result of autoimmune reactions is more compelling for some than for others. With systemic lupus erythematosus, the presence of a multiplicity of autoantibodies logically explains many of the observed changes. Moreover, the auto-antibodies can be identified within the lesions by immunofluorescent and electron microscopic techniques. Few would dispute the assumption that systemic lupus erythematosus is an autoimmune disease.

Table 5–5. AUTOIMMUNE DISEASES

| Single Organ or Cell Type | Systemic |
|---|---|
| *Probable* | *Probable* |
| Hashimoto's thyroiditis | Systemic lupus erythematosus |
| Autoimmune hemolytic anemia | Rheumatoid arthritis |
| | Sjögren's syndrome |
| Autoimmune atrophic gastritis of pernicious anemia | Reiter's syndrome |
| | *Possible* |
| Autoimmune encephalomyelitis | Polymyositis-dermatomyositis |
| Autoimmune orchitis | Systemic sclerosis (scleroderma) |
| Goodpasture's syndrome* | Polyarteritis nodosa |
| Autoimmune thrombocytopenia | |
| Insulin-dependent diabetes mellitus | |
| Myasthenia gravis | |
| Graves' diseases | |
| *Possible* | |
| Primary biliary cirrhosis | |
| Chronic active hepatitis | |
| Ulcerative colitis | |
| Membranous glomerulonephritis | |

*Target is basement membrane of glomeruli and alveolar walls.

In many others, such as polyarteritis nodosa, an immunologic basis of tissue injury can be established with reasonable certainty, but the nature of the autoantigen is not established. Indeed, in some cases the antigen may be exogenous, as we shall discuss later in this chapter.

Only the systemic autoimmune diseases are considered in this chapter. The single-target involvements are more appropriately discussed in the chapters dealing with specific organs. Before describing individual disorders we will consider the general nature of self-tolerance and theories about its loss.

## SELF-TOLERANCE

Immunologic tolerance is defined as a state in which the individual is incapable of developing an immune response against a specific antigen. Tolerance obeys the same laws of antigen specificity that apply to other immune responses; thus it is restricted to the antigens used to induce tolerance. *Self-tolerance refers to lack of immune responsiveness to the individual's own tissue antigens*. Obviously, self-tolerance is necessary for our tissues to live harmoniously with an army of lymphocytes. What mechanisms prevent anti-self reactivity in healthy individuals? Two major mechanisms are believed to exist (Fig. 5–17). According to one, termed *clonal deletion*, normal adults lack either or both T and B lymphocytes that can recognize self-antigens. It is proposed that any potential self-reactive lymphocytes are "deleted" from the lymphoid system during embryogenesis. Indeed, mice exposed to a foreign antigen in utero or in the early neonatal period become tolerant to that particular foreign antigen (as if it were a self-antigen). When such animals reach adulthood, lymphocytes reactive with the tolerated antigen cannot be detected.

If clonal deletion were the only mechanism responsible for self-tolerance, one would predict that lymphocytes that can recognize self-antigens would never be found in normal healthy adults. However, this is clearly not the case. B lymphocytes that can specifically recognize and bind to normal body constituents such as thyroglobulin, collagen, myelin basic protein, and DNA can be detected in normal humans. Therefore it is suggested that *active suppression of autoreactive lymphocytes* is an important factor in maintaining self-tolerance. A variety of mechanisms, both humoral and cellular, have been suggested as inhibitors of autoimmunity.[28] Much interest, however, is focused on T-suppressor cells as mediators of self-tolerance. In experimental models, it is possible to demonstrate that the activity of both T-helper cells and antibody-producing B cells can be suppressed by T-suppressor cells. Thus the physiologic function of T-suppressor cells may relate to regulation of immune responses to heterologous as well as self-antigens. The association between dysfunction or loss of T-

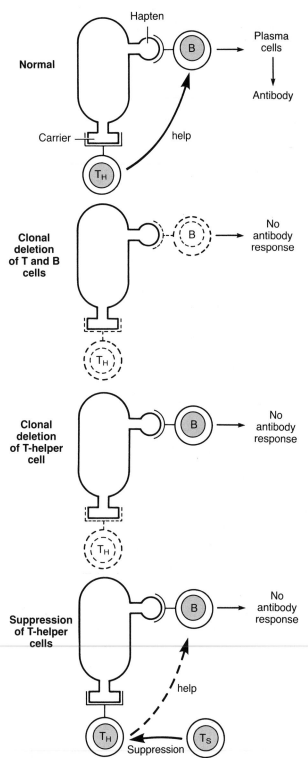

**Figure 5–17.** Schematic illustration of the T- and B-cell interactions involved in normal antibody response and the proposed mechanisms of self-tolerance.

suppressor cells and the emergence of autoimmunity, seen in animal models and in some human autoimmune diseases, supports such a concept of self-tolerance.

In summary, prevention of autoimmunity is so vital to survival that at least two major mechanisms have evolved to protect ourselves from our "protectors." Deletion of autoreactive clones appears to be the major mechanism of self-tolerance during the development of the lymphoid system. However, since approximately $10^{11}$ new lymphocytes of diverse specificities (some of them autoreactive) are generated every day in a normal adult, the odds heavily favor the possibility that some autoreactive lymphocytes will "leak" through the barrier of clonal deletion. Such autoreactive cells would then have to be restrained by suppressor mechanisms.

### Cellular Basis of Tolerance

Before we can discuss the mechanisms underlying autoimmune disease, it is necessary to review the cellular basis of tolerance. You may recall that antibody responses against several protein antigens require the cooperation of T-helper cells and B cells. Most self-antigens can be visualized as hapten-carrier complexes (Fig. 5–17). The antibody-forming B cells recognize the haptenic determinants and form anti-hapten antibody, but this process can occur only if the T-helper cells recognize the carrier determinants and send appropriate activating signals to the hapten-specific B cells. It follows that lack of an immune response can result from a deletion or suppression of either B cells or T-helper cells, or both. With respect to self-antigens, it is believed that the tolerance is maintained largely at the level of the T cells. Thus fully competent autoreactive B cells are kept in check due to the presence of T-suppressor cells reactive against T-helper cells or, alternatively, clonal deletion of T-helper cells.

## MECHANISMS OF AUTOIMMUNE DISEASE

Breakdown of one or more of the mechanisms of self-tolerance can unleash an immunologic attack on tissues that leads to the development of autoimmune diseases. Although immunocompetent cells are undoubtedly involved in mediating the tissue injury, we do not know the precise influences that initiate their reactions against "self," but genetic factors and infectious agents, particularly viruses, are thought to be important. First the mechanisms involved in the breakdown of self-tolerance will be discussed, followed by the genetic and viral factors.

### Loss of Self-Tolerance

This can be best understood in the context of the mechanisms invoked in the maintenance of self-tolerance.

**BYPASS OF T-HELPER CELL TOLERANCE.** Tolerance to self-antigens, as discussed earlier, is often associated with unresponsive carrier-specific T-helper cells

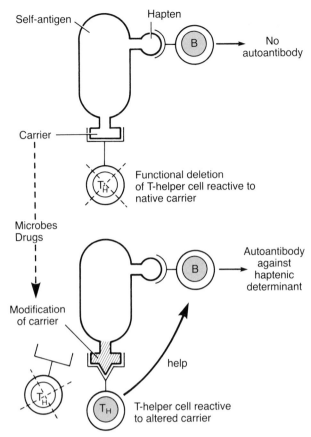

**Figure 5–18.** Tolerance to self-antigens due to lack of T-cell help, and the loss of self-tolerance by T-helper–cell bypass.

and with fully competent hapten-specific B cells. Therefore, this form of tolerance may be overcome, if the need for tolerant T-helper cells is bypassed or substituted. This can be accomplished in one of several ways:

1. *Modification of the molecule.* If the carrier determinant of a self-antigen is modified, it may acquire new antigenic specificities, which will be recognized as foreign by nontolerant clones of T-helper cells (Fig. 5–18). These could then cooperate with the hapten-specific B cells, leading to formation of autoantibodies. Modification of the carrier may result from complexing of self-antigens with drugs or microorganisms. For example, autoimmune hemolytic anemia, which occurs after the administration of certain drugs, may result from drug-induced alterations in the red cell surface (p. 361). Partial degradation of an autoantigen such as collagen could expose new carrier determinants; such degradation may be brought about by lysosomal enzymes (e.g., in rheumatoid arthritis).

2. *Cross reactions.* These may occur between some human antigens and certain microbes if they share haptenic specificities. Normally, no autoantibody against the self-hapten is formed, owing to T-helper cell tolerance. However, infecting microorganisms may trigger an antibody response by pre-

senting the cross-reacting hapten in association with their own carrier, which would be recognized by nontolerant T-helper cells. Antibody capable of reacting with the infecting organisms and normal tissues would thus be formed. Such may be the case in rheumatic heart disease, which follows infection with certain streptococci.[29] Streptococcal M protein appears to be a hapten that cross-reacts with sarcolemmal antigens of heart muscle.

3. *Polyclonal B-cell activation.* Several microorganisms and their products (especially endotoxins) can act as powerful stimulants of B cells. In experimental models, the need for T-helper cells can be bypassed by lipopolysaccharide (endotoxin)–induced stimulation of hapten-specific B cells. Such an event could follow infection with gram-negative bacteria. Infection of B cells with Epstein-Barr virus (EBV) could also achieve the same effects since human B cells bear receptors for EBV.

**ABNORMALITIES IN THE REGULATION OF THE IMMUNE RESPONSE.** Since T-suppressor cells are considered important in keeping autoreactive B cells in check, loss of such a regulatory influence may allow formation of autoantibodies. There is some evidence that premature decline in the function of T-suppressor cells is associated with the appearance of autoantibodies in (NZB × NZW) $F_1$ hybrid mice. These mice develop a disease resembling human lupus erythematosus. Defects in several other immunoregulatory pathways, such as abnormalities in lymphokine secretion, and the presence of anti-idiotypic antibodies have also been invoked. For a discussion of these and other proposed examples of immunodysregulation that may initiate autoimmunity, the reader is referred to specialized texts and reviews.[28, 30]

**RELEASE OF SEQUESTERED ANTIGENS.** Certain self-antigens may remain completely sequestered from the immune system so that tolerance does not develop against them. If trauma or disease were to release such antigens, an autoimmune response could occur. This may explain the genesis of autoimmune orchitis, which follows release of spermatozoa from injured testes. However, most antigens formerly believed to be sequestered can be found in the circulation in small quantities, and a state of T-cell tolerance may exist. The effect of trauma could be related to the release of modified antigens capable of bypassing T-cell tolerance.

### Genetic Factors in Autoimmunity

There is little doubt that genetic factors play a significant role in the predisposition to autoimmune diseases.[30] This conclusion is derived from two lines of evidence:

○ Familial clustering of several human autoimmune diseases such as systemic lupus erythematosus, autoimmune hemolytic anemia, and autoimmune thyroiditis.

○ Linkage of several autoimmune diseases with HLA, especially HLA-DR antigens.

We discussed previously (p. 134) the presence of immune-response (*Ir*) genes in the D-region of the HLA complex. Conceivably, certain *Ir* genes may facilitate immune responses against autoantigens. Individuals who possess such genes would therefore be at greater risk of developing autoimmune disease when appropriately stimulated with self-antigens. Certain genotypes may also constitute fertile soils for the initiation of abnormal immune responses by environmental agents. Included among such agents are microorganisms, particularly viruses, which have the unenviable position of being the prime suspects in most diseases of obscure etiology.

### Viruses in Autoimmunity

The suspicion that viruses play an etiologic role in autoimmunity derives largely from studies of the spontaneous autoimmune disease affecting NZB and NZW mice and their F₁ hybrids. Type C viruses and their antigens are present in various tissues of NZB mice throughout a substantial portion of their life spans and, moreover, viral antigens are found in the immune complexes in glomerular lesions. Theoretically, viruses could trigger autoimmune disease by several of the mechanisms outlined earlier. Viruses may modify self-carriers and help bypass T-cell tolerance, may act as B-cell adjuvants (e.g., EBV), or may infect and inactivate T-suppressor cells. Indeed, some virus genomes may become incorporated in the DNA of the host's cells to thus cause somatic mutations and production of cells not recognized as "self." Although there is no dearth of possible (and some plausible) mechanisms by which viruses can initiate autoimmunity, there is as yet no clear evidence to support such events in humans.

Against this general background we turn to the individual systemic autoimmune diseases. Although each disease is discussed separately, it will be apparent that there is considerable overlap in their clinical, serologic, and morphologic features. Indeed, in some instances the term "overlap syndrome" best describes the patient's condition.

## SYSTEMIC LUPUS ERYTHEMATOSUS (SLE)

This is a febrile, inflammatory, multisystem disease of protean manifestations and variable behavior.[31] It is best characterized by the following features: (1) *Clinically*, it is an unpredictable, remitting, relapsing disease of acute or insidious onset that may involve virtually any organ in the body; however, it principally affects the skin, kidneys, serosal membranes, joints, and heart. (2) *Anatomically*, all sites of involvement have in common vascular lesions with fibrinoid deposits. (3) *Immunologically*, the disease involves a bewildering array of antibodies of presumed autoimmune origin, especially antinuclear antibodies. The

clinical presentation of SLE is so variable and bears so many similarities to other autoimmune connective tissue diseases (rheumatoid arthritis, polymyositis-dermatomyositis, and others) that it has been necessary to develop diagnostic criteria (Table 5–6). If a patient demonstrates four or more of the criteria during any interval of observation, the diagnosis of SLE is established.[32]

At one time SLE was considered to be a fairly rare disease. Better methods of diagnosis and an increased awareness that it may be mild and insidious, however, have made it evident that its prevalence may be as high as one case per 2500 in certain populations.[33] There is a strong female preponderance—about 10 to 1. It usually arises in the second and third decades of life but may become manifest at any age, even in early childhood.

**ETIOLOGY AND PATHOGENESIS.** A mountain of evi-

---

**Table 5–6.** THE 1982 REVISED CRITERIA FOR THE CLASSIFICATION OF SLE*

1. Butterfly rash
2. Discoid lupus
3. Photosensitivity
4. Oral ulcers
5. Arthritis
6. Serositis
   a. Pleuritis: rub heard by a physician or pleural effusion, or
   b. Pericarditis: documented by ECG or rub, or evidence of pericardial effusion
7. Renal disorder
   a. Persistent proteinuria > 0.5 gm/dl per day
   b. Cellular casts: may be red cell, hemoglobin, granular, tubular, or mixed
8. Neurologic disorder
   a. Seizures: in the absence of offending drugs or known metabolic derangements
   b. Psychosis in the absence of offending drugs
9. Hematologic disorder
   a. Hemolytic anemia: with reticulocytosis or
   b. Leukopenia: 4,000 cells/μL on two or more occasions or
   c. Lymphopenia: 1,500 cells/μL on two or more occasions or
   d. Thrombocytopenia: 100,000/μL in the absence of offending drugs
10. Immunologic disorder
    a. Positive LE cell preparation or
    b. Anti-DNA: presence of antibody to untreated DNA in abnormal titer or
    c. Anti-Sm: presence of antibody to Sm nuclear antigen or
    d. False-positive STS known to be positive for at least six months and confirmed by TPI or FTA tests
11. Antinuclear antibody. An abnormal titer of antinuclear antibody by immunofluorescence or an equivalent assay at any point in time and in the absence of drugs known to be associated with "drug-induced lupus" syndrome

NOTE: STS = Serologic test for syphilis, TPI = treponemal inhibition, FTA = fluorescent treponemal antibody.

*The proposed classification is based on 11 criteria. For the purpose of identifying patients in clinical studies, a person shall be said to have SLE if any four or more of the 11 criteria are present serially or simultaneously, during any interval of observation. From Tan, E. M., et al.: The 1982 revised criteria for the classification of systemic lupus erythematosus. Arthritis Rheum. 25:1271, 1982. Reprinted from Arthritis and Rheumatism Journal, copyright 1982. Used by permission of the American Rheumatism Association.

Table 5–7. THE ANA-DISEASE CORRELATES, SHOWING PER CENT FREQUENCY
OF SPECIFIC ANAs IN VARIOUS DISEASES (BOXED ENTRIES
INDICATE HIGH CORRELATION)*

| Nature of Antigen | Antibody System | Disease, % Positive | | | |
|---|---|---|---|---|---|
| | | SLE | Systemic Sclerosis | Sjögren's Syndrome | Polymyositis |
| Many nuclear antigens (DNA, RNA, proteins) | "Generic" ANA (Indirect immunofluorescence) | >95 | 70–90 | 50–80 | 40–60 |
| Native DNA | Anti-double-stranded DNA | 60 | <5 | <5 | <5 |
| Small nuclear RNAs (Smith antigen) | Anti-Sm | 30 | <5 | <5 | <5 |
| Nuclear RNA | SS-A | 25 | <5 | 70 | 10 |
| Nuclear RNA | SS-B | 15 | <5 | 60 | <5 |
| Nuclear protein | Scl-70 | <5 | 30–40 | <5 | <5 |
| t-RNA synthetase | Jo-1 | <5 | <5 | <5 | 30–50 |

*Modified from Tan, E. M., et al.: ANA in systemic rheumatic disease. Postgrad. Med. 78:141, 1985, and McCarty, G. A.: Autoantibodies and their relation to rheumatic diseases. Med. Clin. North Am. 70:237, 1986.

dence points toward an autoimmune pathogenesis for SLE, but the cause or causes of the bewildering array of autoimmune reactions in these patients still allude us. First we shall present some of the immunologic findings, followed by the theories that attempt to explain their origins.

A host of autoantibodies, some of which may react with several targets, have been identified against both nuclear and cytoplasmic components of cells. *Antinuclear antibodies (ANA)* are directed against several nuclear antigens and can be grouped into four categories[34] (1) *antibodies to DNA,* (2) *antibodies to histones,* (3) *antibodies to nonhistone proteins bound to RNA,* (4) *antibodies to nucleolar antigens.* Several techniques are employed to detect ANAs. Clinically, the most commonly utilized method is indirect immunofluorescence, which detects a variety of nuclear antigens including DNA, RNA, and proteins (*generic ANA*). The pattern of nuclear fluorescence suggests the type of antibody present in the patient's serum. Four basic patterns are recognized:

○ *Homogeneous or diffuse staining* usually reflects antibodies to deoxyribonucleoprotein, histone, and, occasionally, double-stranded DNA.

○ *Rim or peripheral staining* patterns are most commonly indicative of antibodies to double-stranded DNA.

○ *Speckled pattern* refers to the presence of uniform or variable-sized speckles. It is one of the most commonly observed patterns of fluorescence and therefore the least specific. It reflects presence of antibodies to non-DNA nuclear constituents such as antibodies to histones and ribonucleoproteins.

○ *Nucleolar pattern* refers to the presence of a few discrete spots of fluorescence within the nucleus and represents antibodies to nucleolar RNA. This pattern is reported most often in patients with systemic sclerosis.

It must be emphasized, however, that the patterns are not absolutely specific for the type of antibody. The immunofluorescence test for ANA is quite sensitive for the detection of SLE, but it is not specific.

Table 5–7 shows that the ANAs detected by this technique are present not only in SLE but also in several other related autoimmune diseases. Furthermore, approximately 10% of normal individuals have low titers of these antibodies.

Detection of antibodies to specific nuclear antigens requires specialized techniques. Of the approximately 30 nuclear antigen-antibody systems,[35] some that are clinically useful are listed in Table 5–7. It will be noted that *antibodies to double-stranded DNA and the so-called Smith (Sm) antigen are virtually diagnostic of SLE.*

Although antibodies to double-stranded DNA are highly specific for SLE, recent studies have challenged the conventional wisdom that native DNA is the immunogen that triggers the formation of anti-DNA antibodies.[36] Doubts arose when it was found that monoclonal anti-DNA autoantibodies derived from lupus patients could react not only with DNA but also with RNA, certain polynucleotides, and even with phospholipids. The "polyspecificity" of the monoclonal anti-DNA antibodies is best explained by reactivity to an antigenic determinant that recurs in different molecules. One such epitope is believed to reside in the sugar-phosphate backbone that is common to several polynucleotides and certain phospholipids. Indeed, it has been possible to produce monoclonal antibodies that bind to DNA by immunizing mice with certain phospholipids. By contrast, it has been difficult to induce anti-DNA antibodies when native DNA was used as an immunogen.[30] With respect to the pathogenesis of autoimmunity in SLE, these results imply that:

○ Anti-DNA antibodies in SLE arise not in response to DNA (which is poorly immunogenic) but by autoimmunization against other immunogens (phospholipids?) that share determinants with DNA.

○ The array of autoantibodies produced in SLE may not be as broad as is suggested by their different biologic activities. Thus a single autoantibody may register as an ANA, as an anticoagulant (due to reactivity with phospholipids essential for clotting, p. 69), or as a false-positive result in the VDRL test for syphilis (p. 626).

Given the presence of all these autoantibodies, we still know little about the mechanism of their emergence. Three converging lines of investigation hold center stage today: genetic predisposition, a fundamental abnormality in the immune system, and some nongenetic (environmental) factors.

**GENETIC FACTORS.** The evidence that supports a genetic predisposition takes many forms.

○ There is a high rate of concordance (69%) in monozygotic twins.[37]

○ Family members have an increased risk of developing SLE.

○ In North American Caucasian populations there is a positive association between SLE and the DR-2, DR-3 genes of the HLA-complex.

The role of HLA genes in the pathogenesis of SLE can only be a matter of speculation at present. As discussed earlier (p. 134) *Ir* genes within the HLA-D region regulate the magnitude of the immune response against several antigens. Conceivably, such regulation may extend to immune responses against self-antigens. It should be noted, however, that many immune disorders other than SLE are associated with HLA-DR3, and many individuals with this genotype are clinically unaffected. It follows therefore that the genes in the *D region confer only a general predisposition to autoimmunity, and, more importantly, other (nongenetic) factors must act to convert the genetic susceptibility to clinical disease.*

**NONGENETIC FACTORS.** The impact of nongenetic factors in initiating autoimmunity is best exemplified by the occurrence of an SLE-like syndrome in patients receiving several *drugs* such as procainamide and hydralazine. Most patients treated with procainamide for over six months develop antinuclear antibodies, and clinical features of SLE appear in 15 to 20%. *Sex hormones* seem to exert an important influence on the occurrence of SLE. Androgens appear to protect, whereas estrogens seem to favor the development of SLE. Witness the overwhelming female preponderance (10:1) of the disease. As with many other diseases of unknown etiology, *viruses* have been suspected as the cause of SLE. The major impetus for the viral hypothesis has come from the studies of the lupus-like disease in NZB mice (p. 152). However, evidence for a role of viruses in human SLE is very tenuous. Despite claims to the contrary, virus particles cannot be reproducibly demonstrated in tissues of lupus patients, and viral antigens have not been shown in immune complexes.

**IMMUNOLOGIC FACTORS.** With the host of autoantibodies that have been described, it will come as no surprise that *B-cell hyperactivity is fundamental to the pathogenesis of SLE.* There is overwhelming evidence that B cells are "turned on" in patients with SLE.[31] The activation of B cells is polyclonal, and as such there is *increased production of antibodies to*

*both self- and non-self-antigens.* What is the basis of B-cell hyperactivity? In theory, excessive B-cell activation could result from an intrinsic defect in B cells, excessive stimulation by T-helper cells, or a defect in T-suppressor cells that fail to dampen the B-cell response. Recent studies with several murine models of SLE and analyses of immune cell populations in patients with SLE reveal that B-cell hyperactivity arises by diverse mechanisms, and evidence implicating each of the three mechanisms listed above has been uncovered.[28, 37] Thus it appears that SLE is a syndrome that can result from several different forms of immunologic derangements. As with different animal models, a genetically determined defect in T-helper cells may be paramount in some patients, whereas in others, a combination of intrinsic B-cell hyperactivity and decreased activity of T-suppressor cells may be critical to the formation of autoantibodies.

Regardless of the exact sequence by which autoantibodies are formed, they are clearly the mediators of tissue injury. Most of the visceral lesions are mediated by immune complexes (Type III hypersensitivity). DNA–anti-DNA complexes can be detected in the glomeruli. It is believed that free DNA binds first to the basement membrane, followed by the formation of DNA–anti-DNA complexes *in situ.* Low levels of serum complement and granular deposits of complement and immunoglobulins in the glomeruli further support the immune complex nature of the disease. On the other hand, autoantibodies against red cells, white cells, and platelets mediate their effects via Type II hypersensitivity. There is no evidence that antinuclear antibodies, which are involved in immune complex formation, can permeate intact cells. However, if cell nuclei are exposed, the ANAs can bind to them. In tissues, nuclei of damaged cells react with antinuclear antibodies, lose their chromatin pattern, and become homogeneous, to produce so-called *LE bodies* or *hematoxylin bodies.* Related to this phenomenon is the *LE cell, which is seen only in vitro. Basically, the LE cell is any phagocytic leukocyte (neutrophil or macrophage) that has engulfed the denatured nucleus of an injured cell* (Fig. 5–19). The demonstration of LE cells involves the microscopic examination of white cells in vitro. If the withdrawn blood is agitated, a sufficient number of leukocytes can be damaged to thus expose their nuclei to ANAs. The binding of ANAs to nuclei denatures them, and subsequent fixation of complement renders antibody-coated nuclei strongly chemotactic for phagocytic cells. The LE cell test is positive in up to 70% of the patients with SLE. However, with newer techniques for detection of ANA, this test is now largely of historical interest.

*To summarize, SLE appears to be a multifactorial disease involving complex interactions among genetic, hormonal, and environmental factors, all of which presumably act in concert to produce pronounced B-cell activation, resulting in the production of several*

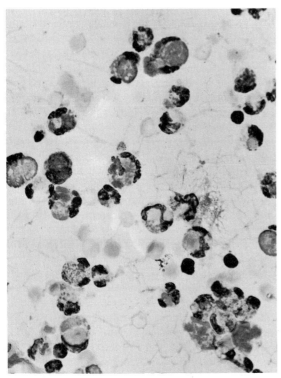

Figure 5–19. Lupus erythematosus (LE) cells. Homogeneous inclusions representing denatured nuclei are seen in many of the polymorphonuclear leukocytes.

*polyspecific autoantibodies.* Each factor may be necessary but not enough per se for the expression of disease, and the relative importance of various factors may vary in different individuals.

**MORPHOLOGY.** The morphologic changes in SLE result largely from the formation of immune complexes in a variety of tissues. SLE is therefore a systemic disease with protean manifestations. Although many organs may be involved, some are affected more than others (Table 5–8). We will discuss changes in small blood vessels that are common to all the affected tissues and the

**Table 5–8.** DISTRIBUTION OF LESIONS IN SLE

| Site of Lesion | Approximate Percentage of Cases |
|---|---|
| Joints* | 95 |
| Kidneys* | 60 |
| Heart* | 50 |
| Serous membranes* | 40 |
| Skin | 80 |
| Lymph node enlargement | 60 |
| Gastrointestinal tract | 30 |
| Central nervous system | 30 |
| Liver | 25 |
| Spleen | 20 |
| Eyes | 20 |
| Lungs | 15 |
| Peripheral nervous system | 10 |

*Lesions cause major clinical findings.

specific anatomic lesions in the organs most frequently involved.

An **acute necrotizing vasculitis** affecting small arteries and arterioles classically is present in most affected tissues and organs. The arteritis is characterized by necrosis and fibrinoid deposits within the vessel walls. Immunoglobulins, DNA, the third component of complement (C3), and fibrinogen have been found in the fibrinoid deposits within the arterial and arteriolar lesions. At a later stage, the involved vessels undergo fibrous thickening with luminal narrowing. Frequently, a perivascular lymphocytic infiltrate is present, sometimes accompanied by significant edema and an apparent increase in ground substance. Foci of fibrinoid deposits in microscopic areas of necrosis are typically found within the interstitial tissue of affected organs. These foci of necrosis are presumably caused by vascular lesions.

**Skin lesions** are prominent clinical findings in these patients. Classically, the lesion is an erythematous or maculopapular eruption over the malar eminences and bridge of the nose, creating a "butterfly" shape. Microscopically the areas of involvement show liquefactive degeneration of the basal layer of the epidermis, edema at the dermoepidermal junction, swelling and apparent fusion of collagen fibers, and an acute necrotizing vasculitis with fibrinoid deposits in dermal vessels. In an occasional patient the rash may occur on the neck, chest, back, or abdomen and may even be purpuric, bullous, or vesicular.

Deposits of immunoglobulin and complement can be seen along the dermoepidermal junction, in both the involved and the uninvolved parts of the skin. The presence of granular immunoglobulin deposits in the uninvolved skin is considered highly specific for SLE and helps in differentiating it from other immunologic diseases with skin involvement.[38] Twenty to 30% of patients develop so-called **discoid lupus.** This takes the form of erythematous raised patches with adherent keratotic scaling, which may progress to atrophic scarring. These lesions may be present anywhere on the body. Discoid lesions may be present without the characteristic systemic involvement of SLE, but about 50% of cases eventually progress to SLE.[39]

**Serosal membranes,** particularly the pericardium and pleura, may exhibit a variety of changes ranging from serous effusions or fibrinous exudation in acute cases to fibrous opacification in chronic cases. During the acute stages of serositis there is microscopic evidence of edema, focal vasculitis with perivascular lymphocytic infiltration, and foci of fibrinoid necrosis, sometimes containing LE bodies. These microscopic changes may be present without grossly visible alterations in the serosal membranes.

The **heart,** when involved, may display quite characteristic small vegetations on the valves, known as **Libman-Sacks endocarditis.** This **nonbacterial verrucous endocarditis** takes the form of single or multiple irregular warty deposits on any valve in the heart. The individual vegetations range from 1 to 3 mm in size (Fig. 5–20). **Perhaps the most distinctive feature of this endocar-**

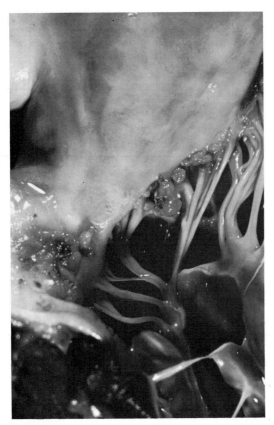

Figure 5–20. Libman-Sacks endocarditis of the mitral valve in lupus erythematosus. The small vegetations attached to the margin of the valve leaflet are easily seen.

ditis is the location of the vegetations on either surface of the leaflets (i.e., on the surface exposed to the forward flow of the blood or on the underside of the leaflet). Histologic examination of these lesions reveals deposits of fibrinoid associated with a surrounding mononuclear inflammatory reaction. At a later phase, there may be collagenization of the areas of inflammation. Not surprisingly, such fibrinoid contains a variety of plasma proteins, including immunoglobulins. Elsewhere in the heart, the interstitial connective tissue may contain foci of vasculitis, deposits of fibrinoid, mononuclear infiltrates, and focal poolings of ground substance in the interstitial tissue of the myocardium.

**Kidney** involvement is one of the most important anatomic features of SLE, since renal failure is the major cause of death in these patients. Although the kidney appears normal by light microscopy in 30 to 40% of cases, almost all cases of SLE show some renal abnormality if examined by immunofluorescence and electron microscopy.[40] According to the WHO morphologic classification of lupus nephritis, five patterns are recognized: (1) normal by light, electron, and immunofluorescent microscopy (class I), which is quite rare; (2) mesangial lupus glomerulonephritis (class II); (3) focal glomerulonephritis (class III); (4) diffuse proliferative glomerulonephritis (class IV); and (5) membranous glomerulonephritis (class V).

**Mesangial lupus nephritis** is associated with mild clinical symptoms. It occurs in approximately 10% of the patients. There is a slight increase in the mesangial matrix and cellularity. However, granular mesangial deposits of IgG and C3 are almost invariably present, even in minimally affected glomeruli. Such deposits presumably represent the earliest change, since filtered immune complexes aggregate primarily in the mesangium, where they may be catabolized. Not infrequently, therefore, other alterations (to be described) are superimposed on the mesangial changes.

**Focal glomerulonephritis** implies involvement of only portions of fewer than 50% of glomeruli. Typically one or several glomerular lobules within an otherwise normal glomerulus exhibit swelling and proliferation of endothelial and mesangial cells, foci of acute capillary necrosis infiltrated with neutrophils, and sometimes fibrinoid deposits and intracapillary thrombi. This form of change is seen in about 30% of the initial biopsies. Focal lesions are usually associated with mild clinical manifestations such as microscopic hematuria and some proteinuria.

**Diffuse proliferative glomerulonephritis** is the most common form of renal lesion, affecting 45 to 50% of patients. The anatomic changes are dominated by proliferation of endothelial, mesangial, and, sometimes, epithelial cells. Thus there is hypercellularity of the glomeruli. Sometimes macrophages and the proliferation of epithelial cells fill Bowman's space to create crescent-shaped masses of cells, not surprisingly referred to as "crescents." In time these changes lead to sclerosis of the glomeruli. Most or all glomeruli are involved in both kidneys, and almost always entire glomeruli are affected. Thickening of the basement membrane may be present, but it is generally not as prominent nor as uniform as in membranous glomerulonephritis.

**Membranous glomerulonephritis** is the designation given to glomerular disease in which the principal histologic change consists of widespread thickening of the capillary wall ("wire loop lesions") (Fig. 5–21). Membranous glomerulonephritis associated with SLE is very similar if not identical to that encountered in idiopathic membranous glomerulopathy and is described more fully on page 466. Thickening of glomerular capillary walls is the consequence of both the increased deposition of basement membrane-like material and the presence of irregular clumps of immune complexes deposited on the basement membrane. Usually necrosis, thrombi, and neutrophils are not prominent in membranous disease, and such increased cellularity as is present is mesangial in origin. In advanced cases glomerular sclerosis may supervene. This form of glomerular lesion is seen in 10% of the cases.

The pathogenesis of all forms of glomerulonephritis involves the deposition of DNA–anti-DNA complexes within the glomeruli. The immune deposits are seen within the mesangium as well as in subendothelial and subepithelial locations. **The subendothelial location of immune deposits in diffuse proliferative glomerulonephritis is particularly characteristic of SLE** during the acute stages of the disease. As a consequence of

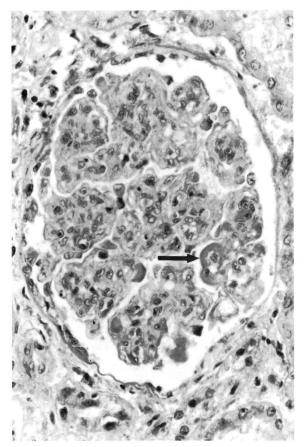

Figure 5–21. Lupus nephritis. A glomerulus with "wire loop" thickening of the basement membrane. (Courtesy of Dr. Fred Silva, Department of Pathology, Southwestern Medical School, Dallas, Texas.)

the increased cellularity and basement membrane alterations, the capillary lumens are narrowed or even obliterated, leading to ischemic injury to tubules and interstitial fibrosis. Kidneys so affected may be normal in size and color during the acute stages but sometimes are enlarged, pale, and dotted with punctate cortical hemorrhages. When glomerular sclerosis supervenes, contraction and a diffuse, fine cortical granularity appear.

Interstitial and tubular lesions are also seen in SLE. In approximately 50% of patients, granular deposits composed of immunoglobulin and complement are present around the tubules.[41] Immune complex–mediated tubular injury leads to diffuse interstitial fibrosis.

**Joint involvement,** although very common clinically, is usually not associated with striking anatomic changes nor with joint deformity. When present it consists of swelling and a nonspecific mononuclear cell infiltration in the synovial membranes, occasionally accompanied by some increase in ground substance and focal areas of fibrinoid necrosis in the subepithelial connective tissue. Grossly the synovial membranes may appear reddened, opaque, and somewhat thickened. Erosion of the membranes and destruction of articular cartilage such as occurs with rheumatoid arthritis is exceedingly rare. For

this reason, even in advanced cases, permanent disabling joint disease is very uncommon in SLE.

The **spleen** may be of normal size or moderately enlarged. Capsular fibrous thickening is common, as is follicular hyperplasia. Plasma cells are usually numerous in the pulp and can be shown to contain immunoglobulins of the IgG and IgM varieties. One of the most constant alterations in spleens of both normal and abnormal size is a marked perivascular fibrosis, producing so-called **onion-skin lesions** around the central penicilliary arteries (Fig. 5–22). Immunoglobulins have been localized in these lesions also.

**Lymph nodes** often are enlarged throughout the body because of nonspecific reactive changes principally within the follicular centers. Plasma cells may be seen in the perifollicular collars.

Many **other organs and tissues** may be involved. The changes consist essentially of acute vasculitis of the small vessels, foci of mononuclear infiltrations, and fibrinoid deposits. Acute necrotizing vasculitis in the brain and spinal cord may lead either to microinfarcts or microhemorrhages.

**CLINICAL MANIFESTATIONS.** The diagnosis of SLE may be obvious in a young female with a classic butterfly rash over the face, fever, pain but no deformity in one or more peripheral joints (feet, ankles, knees, hips, fingers, wrists, elbows, shoulders), pleuritic chest pain, and photosensitivity. However, in many patients the presentation of SLE

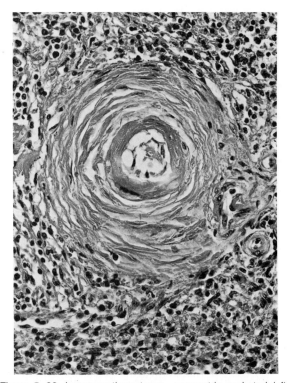

Figure 5–22. Lupus erythematosus—concentric periarterial fibrosis in the spleen. (From Robbins, S. L., Cotran, R. S., and Kumar, V.: Pathologic Basis of Disease. 3rd ed. Philadelphia, W. B. Saunders Co., 1984, p. 184.)

is subtle and puzzling, taking forms such as a febrile illness of unknown origin, abnormal urinary findings, or joint disease masquerading as rheumatoid arthritis or rheumatic fever. Antinuclear antibodies can be found in virtually 100% of patients. However, ANAs can also be found in 50 to 80% of those with Sjögren's syndrome, in 80% with systemic sclerosis, and in 15 to 25% with adult rheumatoid arthritis, as well as in patients with other autoimmune disorders. As mentioned earlier, anti-DNA antibodies are considered highly diagnostic of SLE, and their titer seems to be correlated with the severity of renal disease. A variety of clinical findings may point toward renal involvement, including hematuria, red cell casts, proteinuria, and, in some cases, the classic nephrotic syndrome (p. 464). Varying levels of azotemia and renal failure are encountered in those with diffuse proliferative or membranous glomerulonephritis, or both. In most patients focal glomerulonephritis produces recurrent hematuria and mild proteinuria, but approximately 30% of patients with focal lesions develop renal failure. The hematologic derangements mentioned (Table 5–6) may in some cases be the presenting manifestation as well as the dominant clinical problem. In still others, mental aberrations, including psychosis or convulsions, may constitute prominent clinical problems. In addition, patients with SLE often have small retinal exudates (cytoid bodies) and such nonspecific complaints as malaise, anorexia, vomiting, and weakness.

The course of SLE is extremely variable and virtually unpredictable. Some unfortunate individuals have an acute onset and follow a progressively downhill course to death within months. More often the disease is characterized by flare-ups and remissions spanning a period of years and even decades. Acute attacks are usually treated by adrenocortical steroids or immunosuppressive drugs, and these drugs often control the acute manifestations. With cessation of therapy the disease usually recurs and is exacerbated. The prognosis appears to have improved significantly in the recent past; approximately 70% of patients are alive 10 years after the onset of illness. In some part this apparent improvement derives from the earlier diagnosis and the recognition of milder forms of the disease. In addition to renal failure, other important causes of death are diffuse central nervous system involvement, intercurrent infections, and uncontrolled acute febrile illness.

## RHEUMATOID ARTHRITIS

Rheumatoid arthritis (RA) is a systemic, chronic inflammatory disease that affects principally the joints and sometimes many other organs and tissues throughout the body as well. More specifically, *the disease is characterized by a nonsuppurative proliferative synovitis, which in time leads to the destruction of articular cartilage and progressive disabling arthritis.* When extra-articular involvement develops—for example, of the skin, heart, blood vessels, muscles, and lungs—RA assumes more than a passing resemblance to SLE, scleroderma, and polymyositis-dermatomyositis, and, along with these entities, is sometimes referred to as a "connective tissue disease."

RA is a very common condition and is variously reported (depending on diagnostic criteria) to affect 0.5 to 3.8% of women and 0.1 to 1.3% of men in the United States. It usually has its onset in young adults but may begin at any age. It is three to five times more common in women than in men.

**ETIOLOGY AND PATHOGENESIS.** Rheumatoid arthritis is caused by persistent and self-perpetuating inflammation resulting from immunologic processes taking place in the joints. As is the case with most autoimmune diseases, the trigger that initiates the immune reaction remains unidentified. Various infectious agents such as EBV have been suspected, but the evidence is fragmentary. Since the immunologic mechanisms leading to the inflammation of the joints are the best understood aspect of the pathogenesis of this disease, these will be discussed first, to be followed by a consideration of the genetic factors and finally the possible role of infectious agents.

Both humoral and cell-mediated immune responses are involved in the pathogenesis of rheumatoid arthritis (Fig. 5–23).[42] Most patients have elevated levels of serum immunoglobulins, and virtually all patients have an antibody called rheumatoid factor (RF) directed against the Fc portion of autologous IgG. IgM is the major immunoglobulin class constituting RF; it can be identified in the serum of approximately 80% of patients (seropositive patients). In addition to IgM, RF activity is also found in association with IgG and IgA immunoglobulins. Although the precise role of circulating IgM rheumatoid factor in the pathogenesis of the arthritis is not defined, since it is not found in joints, there is a correlation between its titer in the serum and the clinical severity of the disease.[43] IgG rheumatoid factor, on the other hand, is found within the diseased joints and is believed to be involved in the pathogenesis of the arthritis. Since this form of RF is itself an IgG molecule, it can act both as an antigen and antibody. This results in the self-association of RF molecules (Fig. 5–24) and the formation of immune complexes that can fix complement. There follows the well-known train of events that characterize Type III hypersensitivity of the Arthus type (p. 142). Phagocytosis of the complexes by attracted polymorphs, synovial lining cells, and macrophages results in the release of lysosomal enzymes, including neutral proteases and collagenases. These enzymes damage the synovial lining and the articular cartilage as well. Several observations support this mechanism of joint injury. IgG–anti-IgG complexes are found regularly in the synovial spaces. IgG RF can be formed in situ by the plasma cells infiltrating the

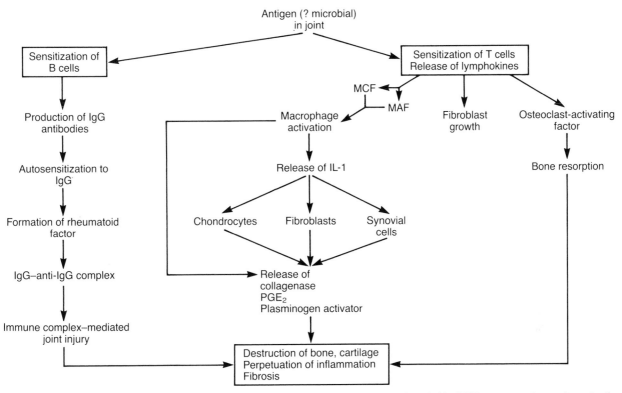

**Figure 5–23.** Role of humoral and cellular immunity in the pathogenesis of rheumatoid arthritis. MCF = macrophage-chemotactic factor; MAF = macrophage-activating factor.

synovium. Immune complexes can be detected in the synovial membrane, and the level of complement in the synovial fluid is low.

Although the schema outlined above is seductive, many questions remain unanswered. What triggers the formation of RF? Why is the major damage localized to joints? Indeed, it has been questioned whether the formation of RF and immune complexes is central to the pathogenesis of rheumatoid arthritis. RF is present in the serum (albeit less consistently) during the course of many chronic infections such as bacterial endocarditis. These observations have led to the suggestion that T cells and delayed hypersensitivity reactions also play a role in the immunopathogenesis of rheumatoid arthritis. Although B cells

and plasma cells are found in the synovial membrane, the infiltrating T cells outnumber them. Most of these are T4⁺, suggesting that they belong to the helper subset. The activated T cells produce lymphokines that activate macrophages, promote growth of fibroblasts, and cause bone resorption. Activated macrophages in turn produce a host of factors, including collagenases and IL-1, that contribute to joint destruction (Fig. 5–23). Interleukin-1 has wide-ranging effects on chondrocytes, synovial cells, and fibroblasts, causing these cells to liberate prostaglandins and collagenases. Thus sensitized T cells can unleash a series of reactions that ultimately destroy the integrity of the joint. What leads to the T-cell sensitization in the joint is not clear.[44] One thing is

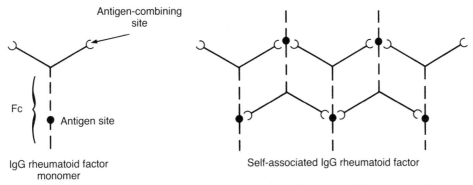

**Figure 5–24.** Schematic illustration of self-associating IgG rheumatoid factor molecules.

certain—persistent inflammation, regardless of its cause, leads to the proliferation of granulation tissue (pannus), which invades the articular cartilage and causes relentless destruction of joints.

*Genetic factors* affect the occurrence of rheumatoid arthritis. A significant association of rheumatoid arthritis with HLA-DR4 has been reported.[45] In all likelihood genetic factors are related to their modulating effects on the immune response.

Finally, we come to the elusive *infectious agent* that may be responsible for the persistent infection or the initiation of the autoimmune response. Although several infectious agents have been implicated in the etiology of RA, much interest has focused on EBV.[44] Antibodies directed against an EBV-associated nuclear antigen have been reported in the serum of 65 to 93% of cases of rheumatoid arthritis and in only 10 to 29% of cases of other forms of arthritis. EBV-transformed B cells from patients with rheumatoid arthritis produce RF in culture.[46, 47] Despite these findings, the question remains—is EBV infection an epiphenomenon or a causal factor in rheumatoid arthritis? So we must leave it that although the *joint damage in RA is of immunologic origin and appears to occur in genetically predisposed individuals, the precise trigger that initiates the apparent autoimmune reaction is still unknown.*

**MORPHOLOGY.** RA is a systemic disease that can cause significant damage to many organs. Its most destructive effects are seen in the joints. Classically, it produces symmetric arthritis, which affects principally the small joints of the hands and feet, ankles, knees, wrists, elbows, shoulders, temporomandibular joints, and sometimes the joints of the vertebral column. Strikingly, the hip joints are seldom involved, except in severe, advanced disease. The process begins as a nonspecific inflammatory synovitis characterized by swelling and hypertrophy of the synoviocytes and the underlying connective tissues. More advanced chronic synovitis shows (1) proliferation of synovial lining cells as well as subjacent cells, often with palisading of the synoviocytes; (2) marked hypertrophy of the synovium, with the formation of villi (finger-like projections); (3) lymphocytic and plasma cell infiltration (with perivascular predilection), sometimes with formation of lymphocytic nodules; (4) focal deposits of fibrinoid; and (5) foci of cellular necrosis (Fig. 5–25). The highly vascularized, inflammatory, reduplicated synovium that covers the articular cartilaginous surfaces is known as a **pannus** (mantle). With full-blown inflammatory joint involvement, periarticular soft tissue edema usually develops, which is classically manifested first by fusiform swelling of the proximal interphalangeal joints. Later, swelling of other affected joints may appear. With progression of the disease, the articular cartilage subjacent to the pannus is eroded and in time virtually destroyed. The subarticular bone may also be attacked and eroded. Eventually the pannus fills the joint space, and subsequent fibrosis and calcification may cause permanent ankylosis. A number of additional changes occur simultaneously.

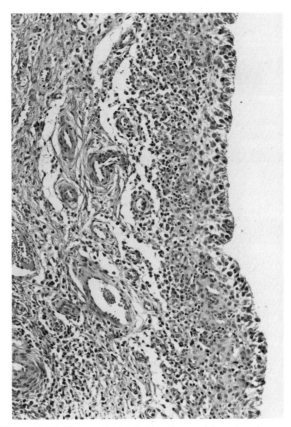

Figure 5–25. Rheumatoid arthritis—the evolving chronic synovitis. Palisaded synoviocytes constitute the surface seen on the right. The subjacent chronic inflammatory mononuclear infiltrate and increased vascularization are evident.

Early in the disease the synovial fluid is increased in volume, becomes turbid because of the inflammatory infiltrate of neutrophils, and loses some of its mucin content (thus forming a poor mucin clot when mixed with dilute acetic acid). The contained leukocytes exhibit granular inclusions of phagocytized immune complexes. Joint motion may cause erosion of the exuberant pannus, leading to bleeding and fibrin clots. The eroded, devascularized cartilage may undergo calcification and fragmentation, adding foreign bodies to the inflammatory process. Osteoarthritis may supervene and compound the articular disability. The periarticular inflammatory response may lead to local myositis, followed by muscle atrophy, and is sometimes accompanied by more remote focal myositis in the form of collections of lymphocytes, plasma cells, and occasional epithelioid cells. Collectively, then, the musculoskeletal lesions in progressive disease cause marked motor disability and even permanent crippling disease.

**Rheumatoid subcutaneous nodules** eventually appear in about one quarter of patients; the nodules usually occur along the extensor surface of the forearm or within the olecranon bursa. They are firm, nontender, oval or rounded masses varying in size to up to 2 cm in diameter. Less commonly these nodules appear in the Achilles tendons, on the back of the skull, overlying the ischial tuberosities, or along the tibia. They are characterized by a focus of central necrosis surrounded by a palisade of connective tissue cells and macrophages. Sometimes the central focus of necrosis contains deposits of fibrinoid. About the connective tissue palisade there is usually an infiltrate of lymphocytes and occasional plasma cells. Rheumatoid nodules may also involve the viscera, including lung, spleen, pericardium, and the heart valves.

As it is a systemic disease, a number of other structures may be affected in RA.[44] Acute necrotizing vasculitis may involve small or large arteries. Serosal involvement may manifest itself as fibrinous pleuritis, pericarditis, or both conditions. Lung parenchyma may be damaged by progressive interstitial fibrosis. Ocular changes such as uveitis and keratoconjunctivitis (similar to those seen in Sjögren's syndrome) may be prominent in some cases.

CLINICAL COURSE. Although rheumatoid arthritis is basically a symmetric polyarticular arthritis, the joint involvement may be associated with constitutional symptoms, such as weakness, malaise, and low-grade fever. Many of these systemic manifestations result from the release of IL-1. Occasionally, in children there is an "unexplained" high fever. The arthritis first appears insidiously, with aching and stiffness of the joints, particularly in the morning. Although the small joints of the hand (particularly the proximal interphalangeal and metacarpophalangeal joints) usually are affected first, other joints become involved in most cases and sometimes virtually all of the joints of the body, even the hips, are affected. As the disease advances the joints become enlarged, motion is limited, and even complete ankylosis may appear. The fingers may become virtually immobilized in a claw-like position with ulnar deviation. At this stage of the disease, anemia is common. The vasculitis may give rise to Raynaud's phenomenon, chronic leg ulcers, and gastrointestinal mucosal erosions, and indeed may cause infarctions in the brain, heart, or intestines. It is obvious that with such multisystemic involvement rheumatoid arthritis must be differentiated from systemic lupus erythematosus, scleroderma, polymyositis-dermatomyositis, and rheumatic fever, as well as other forms of arthritis. Critical to this differential diagnosis are the following: (1) characteristic radiographic findings; (2) sterile, turbid synovial fluid with decreased viscosity, poor mucin clot formation, and inclusion-bearing leukocytes; and (3) rheumatoid factor (85 to 90% of patients). It must be appreciated, however, that rheumatoid factor may also be present with SLE, sarcoidosis, leprosy, syphilis, tuberculosis, bacterial endocarditis, and other diseases associated with persistent antigenemia.

The clinical course of RA is highly variable. After approximately 10 years, the disease in about half of the patients becomes stabilized or may even regress. Most of the remainder pursue a chronic, remitting, relapsing course. After 15 to 20 years, approximately 10% of patients become permanently and severely crippled. RA is an important cause of reactive amyloidosis. This complication develops in 5 to 10% of these patients, particularly those with protracted severe disease.

### Variants of Rheumatoid Arthritis

Two variants of rheumatoid arthritis merit brief characterization. *Juvenile RA*, previously called *Still's disease*, affects children and shows a peak incidence between the ages of one and three years. The disease often has an acute febrile onset and systemic manifestations. Leukocytosis (15,000 to 25,000 cells/mm$^3$), hepatosplenomegaly, lymphadenopathy, and skin rash are common. Rheumatoid factor, however, is present only infrequently. In about one third of patients the disease is monoarticular. Unlike the classic form of rheumatoid arthritis, 50% of patients with juvenile RA experience complete remission. *Felty's syndrome* comprises the triad of polyarthritis, splenomegaly, and leukopenia. In these patients the hematologic problems often dominate the clinical picture.

## SPONDYLOARTHROPATHIES

For years, several entities in this group of disorders were considered variants of rheumatoid arthritis. However, careful clinical, morphologic, and genetic studies have revealed fundamental differences that distinguish these disorders from rheumatoid arthritis and hence they are segregated from it.[48] The spondyloarthropathies are characterized by the following features:

○ Pathologic changes affect primarily the site of ligamentous attachments to bone rather than synovium.
○ Involvement of the sacroiliac joints along with peripheral inflammatory arthropathy.
○ Absence of rheumatoid factor.
○ Association with HLA-B27.

This group of disorders includes several clinical subsets of which ankylosing spondylitis is the prototype. Others included in this category are psoriatic arthropathy, spondylitis associated with inflammatory bowel diseases, and reactive arthropathies (that follow infections by *Yersinia* and *Salmonella*). There is a considerable overlap in these conditions, and they are distinguished from each other according to the particular peripheral joint involved and associated extraskeletal manifestations (urethritis, conjunctivitis, uveitis). As mentioned earlier, sacroiliitis is common to all. Although the seronegative spondyloarthropathies are believed to be caused by immunologic mechanisms, their pathogenesis remains obscure.

## SYSTEMIC SCLEROSIS (SS)

Although the designation "*scleroderma*" is time-honored, this disorder is better called "systemic sclerosis" (SS) since it is characterized by inflammatory and fibrotic changes throughout the interstitium of many organs in the body. *Although skin involvement is the usual presenting symptom and eventually appears in approximately 95% of cases, it is the visceral involvement—of the gastrointestinal tract, lungs, kidneys, heart, and striated muscles—that produces the major disabilities and threatens life.* The disease may begin at any age, from infancy to the advanced years of life, but most often commences in the third to fifth decades. Women are affected about three times more often than men.

In recent years, systemic sclerosis has been subclassified into two groups on the basis of its clinical course.[49]

○ *Diffuse scleroderma*, characterized by widespread skin involvement at onset, with rapid progression and early visceral involvement.

○ *CREST syndrome* (p. 163), with relatively limited skin involvement often confined to fingers and face. Involvement of the viscera occurs late, and hence in general the disease in these patients has a relatively benign course.

**ETIOLOGY AND PATHOGENESIS.** SS is a disease of unknown etiology. Although traditionally grouped with the autoimmune diseases, the evidence supporting an immunologic basis of this condition is indirect. Two other possible pathogeneses have also received consideration: an alteration in collagen synthesis and a primary microvascular abnormality.

Although widespread collagenous sclerosis is a hallmark of this disease, the collagen itself is not abnormal. Fibroblasts from patients with SS synthesize twice as much collagen as normal fibroblasts, but they also produce normal amounts of collagenase, indicating normal collagen degradation.[50] Thus, increased biosynthesis of normal collagen is established, but what triggers the fibroblasts to choke the tissues with collagen remains unknown. The ability of lymphokines to attract fibroblasts and promote collagen synthesis has generated interest in the possible role of immunologic factors in the pathogenesis of systemic sclerosis.[51] Early skin lesions of SS show infiltration of the dermis with T lymphocytes before fibrosis occurs,[52] and some patients manifest T-cell sensitization to collagen. Conceivably, a delayed hypersensitivity to collagen might initiate a vicious circle of lymphokine release and more collagen production. The presence of nonspecific serologic abnormalities such as hypergammaglobulinemia (50% of cases), antinuclear antibodies (70 to 90% of cases), and rheumatoid factor (25% of cases) points to a possible role for disordered humoral immunity as well. Recently two antinuclear antibodies more or less unique to systemic sclerosis have been described.[35] One of these, called Scl-70 (Table 5–7), is present in 30 to 40% of patients with the diffuse variant of SS, whereas the other, an anticentromere antibody, is found in 50 to 70% of the patients with the CREST syndrome.

Finally, it has been suggested that SS is a primary disease of the microvasculature[53] that results from recurrent injury to the endothelium. A serum factor cytotoxic to endothelial cells has been described in some but not all cases. Telltale signs of increased platelet activation (e.g., increased level of circulating platelet aggregates) have also been noted. According to this view, repeated cycles of endothelial injury followed by platelet aggregation leads to release of platelet factors that trigger periadventitial fibrosis and eventual ischemic injury caused by widespread narrowing of the microvasculature. This simple and otherwise attractive hypothesis fails to explain the host of immunologic abnormalities noted in SS, and hence the mystery surrounding the pathogenesis of SS persists.

**MORPHOLOGY.** Virtually any organ may be affected in SS, but the most prominent changes are found in the skin, musculoskeletal system, gastrointestinal tract, lungs, kidneys, and heart.[54]

The changes in the **skin** almost always begin in the fingers and distal regions of the upper extremities and extend proximally to involve the upper arm, shoulders, neck, and face. In advanced cases the entire back and abdomen as well as the lower extremities may be affected. The earliest changes consist only of some dermal edema and possibly some increased ground substance, but as the disease advances, there is considerable increase in dermal collagen, with epidermal atrophy and loss of skin adnexa (Fig. 5–26). The walls of dermal capillaries and arterioles are markedly thickened and hyalinized. The fingers may take on a tapered, claw-like appearance, and the dermal fibrosis may result in limitation of motion in the joints. The sclerotic atrophy of the tips of the fingers often causes resorption of the terminal phalanges of the fingers. Focal and sometimes diffuse subcutaneous calcifications may develop, especially in patients with the CREST syndrome. Recurrent traumatic ulcerations associated with chronic ischemia due to vascular occlusion may progress to autoamputation of the fingers. The face may take on the appearance of a drawn mask. A variety of superimposed changes may appear, including vitiligo and hyperpigmentation.

The **gastrointestinal tract** is affected in over half the patients. The most common manifestation consists of progressive atrophy and fibrosis of the esophageal wall, involving principally the submucosa and muscularis. This may be accompanied by atrophy and ulceration of the overlying mucosa. Almost invariably the small vessels in these areas show progressive thickening of their walls, accompanied by a perivascular infiltrate of lymphocytes. Similar atrophy and fibrosis may occur in the stomach and small bowel. Only rarely is the colon affected.

In the **musculoskeletal system** both joints and muscles are affected. Early in the disease a nonspecific inflammatory synovitis may appear, resembling the early stages of rheumatoid arthritis. With progression, the synovium undergoes collagenous sclerosis, followed in some cases by some bony resorption of the subjacent bone. At the same time there is sclerosis in the periarticular

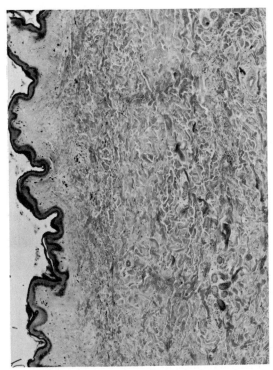

Figure 5–26. Systemic sclerosis. Atrophy of the skin, with dense sclerosis of dermal tissue and atrophy of skin adnexa. (From Robbins, S. L., Cotran, R. S., and Kumar, V.: Pathologic Basis of Disease. 3rd ed. Philadelphia, W. B. Saunders Co., 1984, p. 191.)

connective tissues that limits joint motion. Destruction of joints, such as occurs with rheumatoid arthritis, is quite rare. Focal inflammatory infiltrates followed by fibrosis may appear in the skeletal muscles, and many of these patients develop muscle atrophy.

The **lungs** often develop diffuse interstitial fibrosis of the alveolar septa, accompanied by progressive thickening of the walls of the smaller pulmonary vessels. The fibrosis may lead to the production of microcysts. Thus patients with SS may develop lesions indistinguishable from those of idiopathic pulmonary fibrosis (honeycomb lung, p. 428).

The **kidneys** frequently (66% of cases) are damaged by a variety of lesions, but it is difficult to interpret the nature of the renal lesions, since many patients with SS and renal involvement have severe hypertension, known to induce renal injury. The principal changes are found in small arteries, which show concentric intimal proliferation, deposition of acid mucopolysaccharides, reduplication of the internal elastic lamina, and hyalinization. Although these vascular changes resemble those found in malignant hypertension, it should be noted that in SS they are restricted to vessels that are 150 to 500 μm in diameter, and, moreover, they are not always associated with hypertension. Indeed, hypertension is seen in only 30% of the cases; in 7 to 10% it takes the form of malignant hypertension. In those with hypertension the lesions in the kidney are more severe and often include fibrinoid necrosis of arterioles, focal necrosis of glomeruli, and microinfarcts. Other glomerular changes are nonspecific,

such as localized basement membrane thickening and an increase in the mesangium. About half of the patients die of renal failure.

The **heart** may have focal interstitial fibrosis, principally in the perivascular areas, and occasionally there are perivascular infiltrates of lymphocytes and macrophages. Small intramyocardial arteries and arterioles may show vascular thickening. Because of the changes in the lungs, right-sided cardiac hypertrophy (cor pulmonale, p. 338) is often present.

**Other sites** may be affected, particularly nerve trunks, possibly related to microvascular lesions with ischemic and fibrotic alterations in the perineurium.

**CLINICAL COURSE.** It must be apparent from the described anatomic changes that systemic sclerosis has many of the features of rheumatoid arthritis, SLE, and, as will be described, dermatomyositis. It is, however, *distinctive in its striking cutaneous changes*. Most patients first develop Raynaud's phenomenon, which may be present prior to the appearance of the more definitive changes in the skin. The progressive collagenization of the skin leads to atrophy of the hands, with increasing stiffness and eventually complete immobilization of the joints. The disability becomes more generalized as the trunk and extremities are affected. Muscular weakness and atrophy soon make their appearance, perhaps as a result of limitation of motion imposed by the cutaneous changes or possibly as a result of intrinsic involvement of the joints and muscles as they suffer progressive interstitial fibrosis. Difficulty in swallowing and gastrointestinal symptoms are inevitable consequences of the changes in the esophagus and lower gut. Malabsorption may appear if the submucosal and muscular atrophy and fibrosis involve the small intestine. Dyspnea and chronic cough reflect the pulmonary changes, and often these patients develop the so-called *stiff lung syndrome*. With advanced pulmonary involvement, secondary pulmonary hypertension may develop, leading in turn to right-sided cardiac dysfunction. Renal functional impairment secondary to both the advance of SS and the concomitant malignant hypertension frequently is marked.

Patients with the so-called CREST syndrome are characterized by Calcinosis, Raynaud's phenomenon, Esophageal dysmotility, Sclerodactyly, and Telangiectasia. Raynaud's phenomena is frequently the presenting feature and is associated with limited skin involvement confined to the fingers and face. These two features may be present alone for decades before the appearance of distinctive visceral lesions.

The course of systemic sclerosis is difficult to predict. In most patients, the disease pursues a steady, slow, downhill course over the span of many years, with gradual evolution of the cutaneous lesions and progressive deformity. Many develop crippling limitation of motion of various joints. In the absence of renal involvement, the life span may be normal.

The overall five-year survival ranges from 35 to 70%. The survival of patients with the CREST syndrome is significantly better than that of patients with the usual diffuse progressive disease.

## POLYMYOSITIS (DERMATOMYOSITIS)

Polymyositis is a chronic inflammatory myopathy of uncertain cause.[55] When a skin rash is also present it is called dermatomyositis. Clinically, the disease is characterized by symmetric muscle weakness and variable degrees of pain, swelling, or atrophy of affected muscles, often accompanied by a rash about the eyes, face, and extensor surfaces of the limbs. The disease may occur at any age from infancy to late life; there are bimodal peaks in the age groups of five to 15 and 50 to 60 years.

The clinical expression of inflammatory myopathies is extremely varied and hence they have been subclassified as follows:
○ Adult polymyositis (without skin involvement).
○ Adult dermatomyositis (muscle and skin involvement).
○ Polymyositis or dermatomyositis with malignancy.
○ Childhood dermatomyositis.
○ Polymyositis or dermatomyositis with other connective tissue disorders, such as SLE, systemic sclerosis, or Sjögren's syndrome.

The detailed clinicopathologic features of these subgroups may be found in specialized texts and reviews.[55, 56] Only the more distinctive features that distinguish these subgroups will be presented here.

Among the various subsets, one that is most sharply distinguished from the others is *childhood dermatomyositis*. In this group of patients there is widespread vasculitis involving the skin and the gastrointestinal tract. As a result, bowel infarction with perforation and skin ulceration are prominent clinical features, in addition to the myositis. The other group that deserves special mention is the one with associated malignancy. Visceral cancers are present in 10 to 20% of the patients. Those with dermatomyositis are at greater risk than those without skin involvement. The most common associations are with carcinomas of breast and ovary in females, and of the lung and gastrointestinal tract in males.

**ETIOLOGY AND PATHOGENESIS.** The conviction that polymyositis-dermatomyositis is of immunologic origin is growing stronger. This is based in part on "guilt by association," because the clinical and anatomic features in some cases overlap with those of other connective tissue diseases with better established immunopathogeneses (i.e., Sjögren's syndrome, rheumatoid arthritis, and SLE). Autoantibodies such as rheumatoid factor and antinuclear antibodies have been found in some cases. Recent studies suggest that antibodies to the Jo-1 antigen, which is a subunit of transfer RNA, are found primarily in patients with polymyositis.[35] Whether an-

tibodies play any role in pathogenesis is unknown except possibly in childhood dermatomyositis. The widespread vasculitis seen in this condition seems to be mediated by immune complexes that can be identified in the affected blood vessels. Cell-mediated immunity has also been implicated in the pathogenesis of polymyositis-dermatomyositis. Supporting this view is the presence of helper and cytotoxic T lymphocytes in the inflammatory infiltrate. These lymphocytes may damage the muscle fibers by cell-mediated cytotoxicity or by soluble lymphotoxins, which are released upon contact with the muscle antigens. What initiates the autosensitization is as obscure as it is in other autoimmune diseases. As usual, microbial agents are prime suspects because of sporadic reports of elevated antibody titers to viruses (Coxsackie B), and *Toxoplasma gondii*.[55] However, firm evidence linking any infectious agent to the causation of polymyositis is lacking.

**MORPHOLOGY.** The major anatomic features of polymyositis-dermatomyositis are muscle involvement and skin rash. Initially, the involved muscles are only slightly swollen and edematous. In advanced cases, affected muscles become pale gray, atrophic, and fibrous. Sometimes focal calcifications appear. Histologically, any or all of the following features may be present: necrosis of muscle cells, phagocytosis of muscle cell fragments, regenerative activity resulting in basophilia of muscle cells with the appearance of large prominent sarcolemmal nuclei and nucleoli, variation in individual fiber size, and, usually, a prominent mononuclear inflammatory infiltrate in the sites of involvement (Fig. 5–27). Immunocytochemical studies reveal that most of the infiltrating cells are T lymphocytes that also bear class II antigens, suggesting that they are activated.[57]

The skin rash seen in approximately 40% of patients may be quite variable or it may be virtually diagnostic. The classic rash takes the form of a lilac or heliotrope discoloration of the upper eyelids, with periorbital edema, accompanied by a scaling erythematous eruption or dusky red patches over the knuckles, elbows, knees, medial malleoli, forehead, face, neck and upper chest, and back. Histologically, dermal edema is seen in the early stages, with mononuclear infiltrates surrounding the dermal vessels. The changes are followed in the later stages by fibrosis and sometimes calcification.

In children, and in some acute involvements in adults, widespread necrotizing vasculitis may be present, involving the lungs, kidneys, heart, and other organs. This vasculitis is reminiscent of that encountered in polyarteritis. These acute lesions may lead to vascular fibrosis. Transitory arthritis may appear during the acute phases of the disease, but chronic synovitis is rare.

**CLINICAL COURSE.** Polymyositis-dermatomyositis has, as its principal clinical finding, symmetric muscular weakness that is sometimes insidious but sometimes acute in onset. Acute cases are often febrile. *The diagnosis cannot be entertained in the absence of muscular involvement.* It usually begins proximally

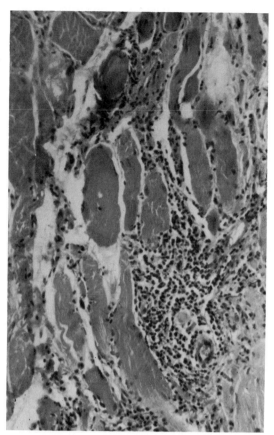

Figure 5–27. A focus in skeletal muscle in polymyositis-dermatomyositis, showing loss of some fibers and irregular adjacent atrophy and hypertrophy of others. The inflammatory infiltrate is entirely mononuclear.

in the shoulders and pelvic girdles and may then extend to the neck and eventually to the distal extremities. This pattern is not invariable. Frequently, weakness of the striated muscles of the pharynx leads to difficulty in swallowing. In advanced cases, the muscular atrophy and fibrosis may be totally disabling. The skin rash may or may not be diagnostic. Occasionally, patients exhibit Raynaud's phenomenon or rheumatoid manifestations. As mentioned, there is considerable overlap of symptoms with SLE, systemic sclerosis, and rheumatoid arthritis, and, indeed, sometimes these diseases coexist. Moreover, it is hardly necessary to point out that many other muscle disorders (e.g., myasthenia gravis and the muscular dystrophies) may also require differential diagnosis. Bohan and Peter[58] cite five major criteria that help to define polymyositis-dermatomyositis. These include (1) proximal muscle weakness; (2) characteristic changes on muscle biopsy; (3) elevated muscle enzymes in the serum (creatine phosphokinase, aldolase, transaminases, and lactic dehydrogenase); (4) electromyographic abnormalities; and (5) a characteristic skin rash.

The course is characterized by remissions and exacerbations. Approximately 60% of the patients recover completely with immunosuppressive therapy.[56] In the rest the disease slowly progresses over many years to death.

## SJÖGREN'S SYNDROME

*Sjögren's syndrome is a clinicopathologic entity characterized by dry eyes (keratoconjunctivitis sicca) and dry mouth (xerostomia) resulting from immunologically mediated destruction of the lacrimal and salivary glands.* It occurs as an isolated disorder (primary form), also known as the sicca syndrome, or more often in association with another autoimmune disease (secondary form). Among the associated disorders, rheumatoid arthritis is the most common, but some patients have SLE, polymyositis, systemic sclerosis, vasculitis, or thyroiditis.[59]

**ETIOLOGY AND PATHOGENESIS.** Several lines of evidence support a role of B-cell dysfunction in the pathogenesis of Sjögren's syndrome, which is second only to SLE in its multiplicity of serum autoantibodies. Hypergammaglobulinemia is virtually always present, and most patients have rheumatoid factor in their sera, even in the absence of demonstrable rheumatoid arthritis. Approximately 50 to 80% of patients have antinuclear antibodies, and about 25% show positive results in the LE cell test. A majority of patients (~70%) with primary Sjögren's syndrome possess autoantibodies to two nuclear antigens, designated SS-A and SS-B. Anti–SS-B antibodies are considered specific for Sjögren's syndrome, since they are not commonly found in association with other autoimmune diseases (Table 5–7). A host of additional antibodies have been identified in these patients, including autoantibodies to thyroglobulin, thyroid microsomes, gastric parietal cells, mitochondria, salivary duct cells, and other autologous antigens. The basis for all of these humoral immune reactions is still unclear; as with SLE, primary B-cell hyperactivity has been implicated. A role for T cells in the pathogenesis of Sjögren's syndrome is indicated by immunohistochemical studies of the inflammatory cells within the salivary and lacrimal glands. The infiltrate contains predominantly T cells of the helper phenotype,[60] but some cytotoxic T cells are also found. It is tempting to speculate that the helper T cells aid both local formation of antibodies and activation of cytotoxic T cells, but firm evidence is lacking.

Genetic factors also play a role in the pathogenesis of Sjögren's syndrome. Patients with the primary form of the disease show increased frequency of HLA-DR3, whereas those with associated rheumatoid arthritis show a positive correlation with HLA-DR4. These genetic studies suggest that despite several clinical similarities, patients with primary and secondary forms of Sjögren's syndrome constitute distinct subsets.

**MORPHOLOGY.** The keratoconjunctivitis and xerostomia are the consequence of extensive damage to the lacrimal and salivary glands. Other secretory glands, including those in the nose, pharynx, larynx, trachea, bronchi, and vagina, may also be involved. When involved, all exhibit an intense lymphocytic and plasma cell infiltration and destruction of the native architecture, similar to the changes encountered in Hashimoto's thyroiditis (p. 679) (Fig. 5–28). Sometimes the lymphoid infiltrates create germinal follicles. These changes may be confused with lymphomatous invasion and, in some instances, true neoplastic transformation occurs.

The lack of tears in the eyes resulting from the secretory lesions leads to drying of the corneal epithelium, which becomes inflamed, eroded, and ulcerated. The oral mucosa may atrophy, with inflammatory fissuring and ulceration. Dryness and crusting of the nose may lead to ulcerations and even perforation of the nasal septum. When the respiratory passages are involved, secondary laryngitis, bronchitis, and pneumonitis may appear. Atrophic gastritis (p. 514) also may appear. One third of the patients exhibit a tubulointerstitial nephritis associated with a mononuclear cell infiltrate in the interstitium, leading to defects in tubular function. Glomerular lesions are uncommon.

**CLINICAL COURSE.** Sjögren's syndrome predominantly affects females over 40 years of age. As was noted at the outset, in approximately 60% of patients it is associated with other "connective tissue dis-

eases." The diagnosis of primary Sjögren's syndrome can be made readily by the lack of moisture and by the secondary changes in the eyes and oral cavity. Some patients have mild arthritis, neuropathy, and Raynaud's phenomenon. Functional renal tubular defects, when present, include renal tubular acidosis, uricosuria, phosphaturia, and generalized aminoaciduria, characteristic of Fanconi's syndrome. With the possible exception of anti–SS-B antibodies, serologic findings do not allow differentiation among the related "connective tissue diseases." Of particular interest is the development of B-cell lymphomas, reported in seven of 134 patients with the disease; this represents a relative risk (observed/expected cases) of 44.[61]

In addition, some patients have had lesions designated as "pseudolymphomas." These comprise marked inflammatory hyperplastic changes within the salivary glands, bordering on the appearance of lymphoid cancer. It would therefore appear that, in this disorder of probable immunologic origin, lymphoid hyperactivity may in time give rise to abnormal pseudolymphomatous proliferations and in some cases to true malignant lymphoid tumors.

## POLYARTERITIS NODOSA

Polyarteritis nodosa, sometimes called *periarteritis nodosa*, is a disease of medium to small-sized arteries characterized by necrotizing inflammation of these vessels. The arteritis is peculiarly focal, random, and episodic, often producing vascular obstruction and sometimes infarctions in the organ or tissue supplied. This unpredictability results in extremely variable clinical manifestations, reflecting the sites of involvement.

Polyarteritis nodosa belongs to a group of vasculitis syndromes that is characterized by necrotizing inflammatory changes in the blood vessels. A classification of vasculitis is presented in Chapter 10. Since morphologic changes within the affected vessels are very similar in many of the vasculitides, the diagnosis of polyarteritis requires not only appropriate morphologic changes but also exclusion of other forms of arteritis by consideration of the clinical setting. It will be noted that the so-called classic polyarteritis, to be described here, differs from other related vasculitides by the absence of pulmonary involvement.

**ETIOLOGY AND PATHOGENESIS.** Determining the origin of a poorly defined condition is bound to be an unsatisfactory exercise. The possibility must be borne in mind that the disorder now referred to as polyarteritis may represent a number of etiologically separate entities.

A variety of observations suggests that polyarteritis and the related group of necrotizing vasculitides (p. 295) are induced by immunologic mechanisms. *The histologic lesions are strongly reminiscent of those in*

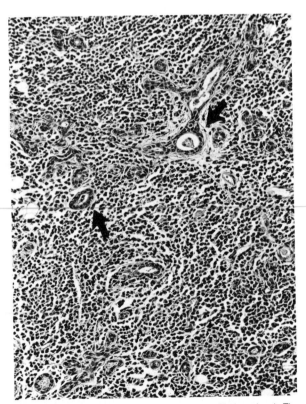

Figure 5–28. Sjögren's syndrome—submandibular gland. The intense lymphocytic and plasma cell infiltration virtually obscures the native architecture. Only a few residual ducts (*arrows*) can be identified.

*the Arthus reaction, which, you may recall, is caused by immune complexes.* Furthermore, necrotizing vasculitis is found in SLE and rheumatoid arthritis, diseases in which immune complexes clearly play a pathogenetic role. Immunoglobulins and complement can be localized in the vascular wall, but one must be cautious in the interpretation of such data, since it is difficult to rule out nonspecific seepage of plasma proteins following vascular injury. The best evidence supporting a role for immune complexes is the high incidence of hepatitis B surface antigen (HBsAg) in the blood and circulating HBsAg-antiHBs immune complexes in the sera of patients with polyarteritis. HBs antigen, immunoglobulin, and complement have also been demonstrated in the vascular lesions.[62] Hepatitis B virus is believed to be the initiating agent in approximately one third of cases. Presumably, the remaining two thirds are caused by similar immune complex mechanisms initiated by as yet undefined antigens. Hypersensitivity vasculitis (p. 296), which resembles polyarteritis nodosa, is often associated with ingestion of drugs such as sulfonamides and penicillin. Conceivably, drugs act as haptens and, after combining with serum proteins, induce antibody and immune complex formation.

**MORPHOLOGY.** The focal necrotizing lesions of polyarteritis nodosa may be found in any artery of medium to small size. In a series of autopsies, the sites of predilection were as follows: kidneys (80%), heart (70%), liver (65%), and gastrointestinal tract (50%); for obscure reasons the lungs are rarely involved. The inflammatory necroses are randomly distributed in curiously localized, sharply demarcated segments of the artery. Sometimes they involve only a portion of the circumference. In the acute phase of the lesion, the vessel may show subtle thickening and periarterial edema. Later, progressive fibrosis may create discrete **nodulations** at the sites of involvement. Microscopically, the pattern is that of an acute necrotizing inflammation beginning in the intima and inner portion of the media and extending in both directions to involve ultimately the entire thickness of the arterial wall, including the adventitia (Fig. 5–29). During the acute phase of the disease, fibrinoid deposits are prominent in the necrotic vessel walls. At this time, there is an acute inflammatory reaction in which eosinophils may be quite numerous. There is in addition destruction of the elastica, particularly the internal elastic lamina. Thrombosis and rupture are potential sequelae. This acute lesion is later converted into an area of fibroblastic thickening of the involved segment, sometimes with organized obliteration of the lumen and striking periarterial fibrosis. At this stage elastic tissue stains are valuable in diagnosis, since they can disclose loss or fragmentation of the internal elastic lamina. Aneurysmal dilatation of the injured wall may occur but is not common. It should be stressed that individual lesions of varying stages of development—from the earliest inflammatory changes to dense collagenization—may coexist in the same patient at the same time, suggesting that whatever the underlying mechanism may be, it acts asynchronously throughout

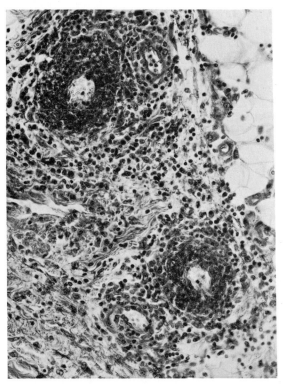

Figure 5–29. Two small arteries disclose an acute necrotizing angiitis that has virtually destroyed the vessel walls. There is an extensive perivascular inflammatory infiltrate.

the body. The principal importance of these arterial lesions is their production of ischemic injury and infarction of tissues and organs. The kidneys bear the brunt of such injury, and in addition to the infarctions, they may also develop foci of glomerular necrosis.

**CLINICAL COURSE.** Polyarteritis is one of the few diseases in the so-called autoimmune group that affects males more frequently than females (2:1). It is apparent that the clinical signs and symptoms of this disease are likely to be as varied as the sites of involvement. Indeed, the diagnosis is often reached by exclusion or because of the erratic multisystem involvement. In all suspected cases, the diagnosis must be confirmed by histologic examination of affected blood vessels. Tender muscles, skin lesions, and subcutaneous nodules are advantageous sites for biopsy.

Polyarteritis nodosa may be of acute onset or may arise insidiously. Most cases pursue a protracted course, with recurrent flare-ups of activity. During the acute phase, the patient often shows systemic manifestations such as malaise, fever, weakness, and weight loss. Renal involvement is one of the prominent manifestations and a major cause of death. Hematuria, albuminuria, and sudden costovertebral angle pain may herald focal necroses in the kidneys. Hypertension is a common accompaniment and may sometimes precede clinically apparent renal disease. Vascular lesions in the gastrointestinal tract produce a wide variety of symptoms, including abdominal pain, diarrhea, and melena. Peripheral neuritis or spinal cord involvement is quite frequent.

The course and outcome of this disease are completely unpredictable. Sometimes it is an acute process that subsides within a few weeks or months, never to recur. More often, the disease persists, with recurrent exacerbations over a course of years, until some vital organ is destroyed. With immunosuppressive therapy, 55% of patients survive five years.

## WEGENER'S GRANULOMATOSIS

This is a rare disorder characterized by (1) *focal acute necrotizing vasculitis*, affecting virtually any vessel in any organ of the body but showing a predilection for the respiratory tract, kidneys, and spleen; (2) *acute granulomatous necrotizing lesions of the respiratory tract*, including the nasal and oral cavities, paranasal sinuses, larynx, tracheobronchial tree, and lung parenchyma; and (3) *necrotizing focal or diffuse proliferative glomerulonephritis*, which if untreated develops into rapidly progressive glomerulonephritis (p. 469).[63] The vascular lesions are nearly identical to those of polyarteritis nodosa, with fibrinoid necrosis of the vessel wall and diffuse polymorphonuclear and eosinophilic infiltrations. However, it can be distinguished from polyarteritis both by the involvement of smaller arteries and veins and by prominent pulmonary effects. The respiratory involvement takes the form of areas of central necrosis surrounded by a zone of inflammatory cells, giant cells, and fibroblasts. Thus the lesions resemble granulomas of tuberculosis. The etiology of Wegener's granulomatosis is unknown, but it is generally accepted that the lesions represent immunologically mediated tissue injury.

Most of these patients present with the insidious development of purulent rhinorrhea and epistaxis, often interpreted as chronic sinusitis. At one time the usual outcome was death from renal failure within a few months. In recent years, however, the use of cytotoxic drugs has dramatically altered the prognosis, and long-term remission can now be expected in over 90% of cases.

## POSSIBLE IMMUNE DISORDERS

Immunologic mechanisms are suspected of contributing to a large number of diseases in addition to those already described in this chapter. Some of these entities will be discussed in the chapters dealing with individual organs and systems. One disease—amyloidosis—requires description at this point. New observations provide strong evidence that some derangement in the immune apparatus underlies this disease, and as a systemic disease it cannot be assigned to any single organ or system.

## AMYLOIDOSIS

Amyloid is an abnormal proteinaceous substance that is deposited between cells in many tissues and organs of the body in a variety of clinical disorders. Since its first recognition, it has been delineated by its morphologic appearance on light microscopy. With usual tissue stains, amyloid appears as an intercellular pink translucent material. At one time it was thought to be starch-like, hence the designation "amyloid"; however, it is now known to be composed of protein.

Despite the striking morphologic uniformity of amyloid in all cases, *it is quite clear that amyloid is not a single chemical entity.* There are two major and several minor biochemical forms. These are deposited by several different pathogenetic mechanisms, and therefore amyloidosis should not be considered a single disease; rather, it is a group of diseases sharing in common the deposition of similar-appearing proteins. At the heart of the morphologic uniformity is the remarkably uniform physical organization of amyloid protein, which we will consider first. This will be followed by a discussion of the chemical nature of amyloid.

**PHYSICAL NATURE OF AMYLOID.** By electron microscopy, amyloid appears to be made up largely of nonbranching fibrils of indefinite length with a width of approximately 7.5 to 10 nm. The fibrils may appear singly, in laterally aggregated bundles, or in an interlocking meshwork. X-ray crystallography and infrared spectroscopy demonstrate a characteristic pattern described as a "β-pleated sheet conformation," which is unique among fibrillar mammalian proteins.[64] This conformation (Fig. 5–30), seen regardless of the clinical setting or the chemical composition, is responsible for the distinctive staining and optical properties of amyloid (to be discussed later). In other words, any fibrillar protein deposited in tissues that yields a β-pleated sheet will be rec-

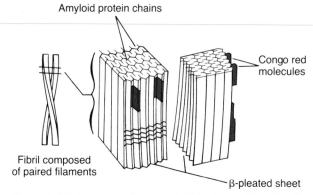

Figure 5–30. Structure of an amyloid fibril, depicting the β-pleated sheet structure and binding sites for the Congo red dye, which is used for diagnosis of amyloidosis. (After Glenner, G. G.: Amyloid deposit and amyloidosis. The β-fibrilloses. N. Engl. J. Med. 52:148, 1980, by permission of The New England Journal of Medicine.)

ognized as amyloid. In addition to the fibrils, a nonfibrillar pentagonal substance (P component) is a minor component of all amyloid deposits.

**CHEMICAL NATURE OF AMYLOID.** *Two major chemical classes of amyloid have been identified, one composed of immunoglobulin light chains called AL (amyloid light chain), the other made up of a nonimmunoglobulin protein designated AA (amyloid associated). These proteins are antigenically distinct and, as we shall discuss later, are deposited in different clinical disorders.* Immunoglobulin amyloid fibril protein (AL) is made up of complete immunoglobulin light chains, the N-terminal fragment of light chains, or both. You may recall that there are two types of immunoglobulin light chains, λ and κ; most frequently it is the λ light chain that gives rise to AL. Glenner and coworkers have demonstrated that proteolytic digestion of λ light chains in vitro can yield a fibrillar precipitate that has the typical ultrastructure and conformation of amyloid fibrils.[65] The AL protein amyloid is associated with B-cell dyscrasias and is produced by immunoglobulin-secreting cells. The other major form of amyloid fibril protein (AA) can be described as a unique nonimmunoglobulin protein with molecular weight of 8500. AA fibrils are believed to be derived from a larger precursor protein in the serum called SAA (serum amyloid–associated protein) which serves as the protein component (apoprotein) of a high-density lipoprotein. SAA behaves as an acute phase reactant, its serum concentration increasing a thousand times within 24 hours of an inflammatory stimulus. As will be pointed out, AA protein is the major component of the amyloid deposited secondary to chronic inflammatory diseases.[66]

Two other biochemically distinct proteins have been found in amyloid deposits.[64] Amyloid deposited within medullary carcinomas of the thyroid appears to share chemical structure with the hormone calcitonin. It is believed that this form of amyloid (designated $AE_t$) is derived by precipitation of a calcitonin precursor secreted by the tumor cells (see also p. 687). The normal plasma protein prealbumin seems to be the major protein constituent of amyloid in several disorders. These include certain forms of familial amyloidosis, senile cardiac amyloidosis, and senile cerebral amyloidosis. The nonfibrillar P component described earlier is a normal serum alpha$_1$-glycoprotein that bears a striking structural homology to C-reactive protein, a well-known acute phase reactant. Serum P component has an affinity for purified amyloid fibrils, and its presence in amyloid deposits is responsible for the positive staining with PAS that led early observers to believe that amyloid was a saccharide.

**CLASSIFICATION OF AMYLOIDOSIS.** Classifications of amyloidosis are notoriously unsatisfactory. This is not surprising, since amyloidosis as defined by morphologic features is not a single disease but a disease complex. Many classifications are based largely on tissue distribution (generalized versus localized) and the presence or absence of an identifiable predisposing condition (secondary versus primary amyloidosis). The classification presented here attempts to take into account the associated clinical settings, anatomic distribution, and chemical composition of amyloid (Table 5–9).[64, 67]

*Immunocyte Dyscrasias with Amyloidosis.* Amyloidosis in this category (sometimes called "primary") is systemic in distribution and results from deposition of immunoglobulin light chains (AL), produced by aberrant clones of B cells. In the United States this is the most common form of amyloidosis.[68] The best example in this category is amyloidosis associated with multiple myeloma, which is a malignant neoplasm of plasma cells (p. 391). This disorder is characterized by proliferation of neoplastic plasma cells in the bone marrow, often producing multiple osteolytic lesions in the skeleton. The malignant plasma cells are monoclonal and therefore secrete a

**Table 5–9. CLASSIFICATION OF AMYLOIDOSIS***

| Clinicopathologic Category | Commonly Used Equivalents | Major Fibril Protein | Chemically Related Protein |
|---|---|---|---|
| A. *Systemic amyloidosis* | Generalized amyloidosis | | |
|    1. Immunocyte dyscrasias with amyloidosis | Primary amyloidosis, amyloidosis associated with multiple myeloma | AL | Immunoglobulin light chains |
|    2. Reactive systemic amyloidosis | Secondary amyloidosis | AA | SAA |
|    3. Heredofamilial amyloidosis | — | | |
|      a. Neuropathic forms (several)—e.g., Portuguese type | | $AF_p$ | Prealbumin |
|      b. Non-neuropathic forms—e.g., familial Mediterranean fever (FMF) | | AA | SAA |
| B. *Localized amyloidosis* | | | |
|    1. Senile—e.g., cardiac | — | $AS_c$ | Prealbumin |
|    2. Endocrine—e.g., amyloid in medullary carcinoma of thyroid | — | $AE_t$ | Calcitonin |

*After Glenner, G. G.: Amyloid deposit and amyloidosis. The β-fibrilloses. N. Engl. J. Med. *302*:1283, 1980, and Husby, G.: A chemical classification of amyloid. Correlation with different types of amyloidosis. Scand. J. Rheumatol. 9:60, 1980.

single species of immunoglobulin (monoclonal gammopathy) producing an M (myeloma) protein spike on serum electrophoresis. In addition to complete immunoglobulin molecules, the plasma cells may also synthesize and secrete only the λ or κ light chains, also known as Bence Jones proteins. These are present in the blood of up to 70% of patients with multiple myeloma, but amyloidosis develops in only 6 to 15% of all cases. Most of those who develop amyloidosis do have Bence Jones proteins. However, it is clear that free light chain production, although necessary, by itself is not sufficient to produce amyloidosis. It is believed that the quality of the light chain produced ("amyloidogenic potential") and the subsequent handling (degradation?) are important factors that determine whether the Bence Jones proteins will be deposited as amyloid.

The great majority of patients in this category do not have classic multiple myeloma but do show evidence of monoclonal gammopathy. Bence Jones proteins with or without monoclonal immunoglobulins are found in the serum, and there is modest increase in the number of plasma cells in the bone marrow. Unlike myeloma, however, there are no skeletal lesions. Clearly, these patients have an underlying dyscrasia of plasma cells, which has been dubbed "covert" myeloma by some experts. However, the exact relationship to multiple myeloma is not clear. In addition to these two groups, a smaller number of patients with a variety of the other B-cell neoplasms, such as macroglobulinemia, nodular lymphoma, and immunoblastic lymphadenopathy, may also develop amyloidosis.

*Reactive Systemic Amyloidosis.* The amyloid deposits in this group are systemic in distribution and are composed of AA protein. This category is commonly referred to as *"secondary amyloidosis,"* since it is believed to be secondary to chronic inflammatory conditions. However, the term is best avoided, since chemically distinct amyloid described in the previously mentioned category is also "secondary" to underlying immunocyte dyscrasias. *The unifying feature of various conditions that predispose to reactive systemic amyloidosis is protracted breakdown of cells, resulting in most cases from a chronic inflammatory disorder.* Before the advent of antimicrobial chemotherapy, diseases such as tuberculosis, chronic osteomyelitis, and bronchiectasis were the common culprits, and in many parts of the world infectious disease is still the number one cause of amyloidosis. In the United States, however, diseases such as rheumatoid arthritis, other connective tissue disorders, ulcerative colitis, and neoplasms (e.g., Hodgkin's disease) are emerging as the leading predisposing conditions. As mentioned, AA protein, which is deposited as amyloid, is derived from SAA, a precursor protein in the serum.

*Heredofamilial Amyloidosis.* This group includes several mendelian disorders characterized by widespread deposits of amyloid in the tissues. *The best*

*characterized is familial Mediterranean fever, which is inherited as an autosomal recessive.* Affected individuals are of Armenian, Sephardic Jewish, and Arabic origins. The amyloid fibrils are composed of AA protein. This may be related to the recurrent bouts of inflammation of the joints and serosal surfaces that characterize this condition. Several other heredofamilial forms have been recognized. These are extremely rare and are designated by the principal organs involved; for example, the neuropathic forms are characterized by involvement of nerves (Table 5–9).

*Localized Amyloidosis.* This is a heterogeneous group, in terms of both chemical composition of amyloid and clinical presentation. One of the following sites may be involved in the form of nodular deposits: lungs, larynx, skin, urinary bladder, or tongue. Often infiltrates of plasma cells are found around the nodules, and at least in some cases the amyloid consists of AL protein. Local deposits of amyloid are also sometimes found within tumors of the endocrine system. Medullary carcinoma of the thyroid is one such example in which the amyloid is chemically related to calcitonin, a hormone secreted by the tumor cells. Aging, even in the absence of specific disease, is sometimes associated with deposits of amyloid in isolated organs. Senile cardiac amyloidosis can be sufficiently severe to give rise to clinical symptoms.

**PATHOGENESIS.** Although the precursors of the two major amyloid proteins have been identified, several aspects of their origins are still not clear. In reactive systemic amyloidosis, it appears that chronic tissue destruction and inflammation leads to elevated SAA levels (Fig. 5–31). SAA is synthesized by the liver cells under the influence of interleukin-1. However, increased production of SAA by itself is not sufficient for the deposition of amyloid. As mentioned earlier, elevation of serum SAA levels is common in inflammatory states but in most instances does not lead to amyloidosis. It is believed that SAA is normally degraded to soluble end products by the action of monocyte-derived enzymes. Conceivably, individuals who develop amyloidosis have an enzyme defect resulting in incomplete breakdown of SAA, thus generating insoluble AA molecules. In the case of immunocyte dyscrasias, the source of the precursor proteins is well defined, and amyloid material can be derived in vitro by proteolysis of immunoglobulin light chains.[65] But we still do not know why only a fraction of those with circulating Bence Jones proteins develop amyloidosis. Again, defective proteolytic degradation has been invoked, but firm evidence is lacking.

**MORPHOLOGY.** There are no consistent or distinctive patterns of organ or tissue distribution of amyloid deposits in any of the categories cited. Nonetheless, a few generalizations can be made. Amyloidosis secondary to chronic inflammatory disorders tends to yield the most

Figure 5–31. Proposed scheme of the pathogenesis of amyloid fibrils.

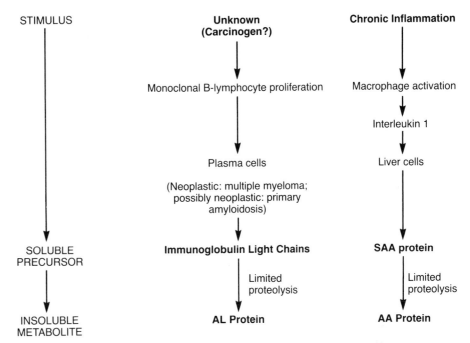

STIMULUS

Unknown (Carcinogen?)

Chronic Inflammation

Monoclonal B-lymphocyte proliferation

Macrophage activation

Interleukin 1

Plasma cells

Liver cells

(Neoplastic: multiple myeloma; possibly neoplastic: primary amyloidosis)

SOLUBLE PRECURSOR

Immunoglobulin Light Chains

SAA protein

Limited proteolysis

Limited proteolysis

INSOLUBLE METABOLITE

AL Protein

AA Protein

severe systemic involvements. Kidneys, liver, spleen, lymph nodes, adrenals, and thyroid, as well as many other tissues, are classically affected. Although immunocyte-associated amyloidosis cannot reliably be distinguished from the secondary form by its organ distribution, more often it involves the heart, gastrointestinal tract, respiratory tract, peripheral nerves, skin, and tongue. In addition, bizarre distributions, such as amyloidosis of the eye and musculoskeletal system, are encountered more often in patients with immunocyte-associated amyloidosis. However, the same organs affected by reactive systemic amyloidosis (secondary amyloidosis), including kidneys, liver, and spleen, may also contain deposits in the immunocyte-associated form of the disease.

The localization of amyloid deposits in the **heredofamilial syndromes** is quite varied. In familial Mediterranean fever the amyloidosis may be widespread, involving the kidneys, blood vessels, spleen, respiratory tract, and, rarely, liver. The localization of amyloid in the remaining hereditary syndromes can be inferred from the designation of these entities. **Localized organ amyloidosis** has already been characterized.

Whatever the clinical disorder, the amyloidosis may or may not be apparent on macroscopic examination. Often small amounts are not recognized until the surface of the cut organ is painted with iodine and sulfuric acid. This yields a mahogany-brown staining of the amyloid deposits. When amyloid accumulates in larger amounts, frequently the organ is enlarged, and the tissue appears gray with a waxy, firm consistency. **Histologically, the deposition always begins between cells,** often closely adjacent to basement membranes. As the amyloid progressively accumulates, it encroaches on the cells. In time the depositions surround and destroy the trapped native cells. In the immunocyte-associated form, perivascular and vascular localizations are common.

**The histologic diagnosis of amyloid is based almost entirely on its staining characteristics. The most commonly used staining technique utilizes the dye Congo red, which under ordinary light imparts a pink or red color to amyloid deposits. Under polarized light the Congo red–stained amyloid shows a green birefringence.** This reaction is shared by all forms of amyloid and is due to the crossed β-pleated configuration of amyloid fibrils. AA and AL amyloid can be distinguished in histologic sections. AA protein loses affinity for Congo red after incubation of tissue sections with potassium permanganate, whereas AL proteins and other chemical forms of amyloid do not.[69] Immunoperoxidase staining with specific antisera directed toward various chemical forms of amyloid is also useful in diagnosis. Other histochemical reactions less specific for amyloid include metachromasia following staining with crystal or methyl violet and fluorescence after staining with thioflavine T and S. **It should be emphasized that demonstration of a birefringence after Congo red staining is the most specific histochemical tool for the routine diagnosis of amyloidosis.**

Since the pattern of organ involvement in different clinical forms of amyloidosis is variable, each of the major organ involvements will be described separately.

**Amyloidosis of the kidney** is the most common and the most serious involvement in the disease. Grossly, the kidney may appear unchanged, it may be abnormally large, pale, gray, and firm, or it may be reduced in size. Microscopically, the amyloid deposits are found principally in the glomeruli, but they are also present in the interstitial peritubular tissue as well as in the walls of the blood vessels. The glomerulus first develops focal deposits within the mesangial matrix and diffuse or nodular thickenings of the basement membranes of the capillary loops. Subsequently, the fibrils appear to stream through and obscure the basement membrane, appearing on both the epithelial and the endothelial sides.[70] With progression, the deposition encroaches on the capillary lumens and eventually leads to total obliteration of the vascular tuft (Fig. 5–32). The interstitial peritubular deposits frequently are associated with the appearance of amorphous pink casts within the tubular lumens, presumably of proteinaceous nature. In cases of myeloma-associated amyloid, the casts may exhibit the typical staining reactions of amyloid, suggesting that they are composed of AL proteins. Blood vessels of all sizes may develop deposits of amyloid within their walls, often causing marked vascular narrowing. It is this vascular narrowing that presumably leads to the contracture of the kidneys, mentioned previously.

**Amyloidosis of the spleen** often causes moderate or even marked enlargement (200 to 800 gm). For obscure reasons, one of two patterns may develop. The deposits may be virtually limited to the splenic follicles, producing tapioca-like granules on gross examination **("sago spleen"),** or the involvement may affect principally the splenic sinuses and eventually extend to the splenic pulp, forming large, sheet-like deposits **("lardaceous spleen").** In both patterns, the spleen exhibits increased consistency and often reveals, on the cut surface, the pale gray, waxy deposits in the distribution described.

**Amyloidosis of the liver** may cause massive enlargement, up to such extraordinary weights as 9000 gm. In such advanced cases, the liver is extremely pale, grayish, and waxy on both the external surface and the cut section. Histologically, the deposits appear first in the space of Disse and then progressively enlarge to encroach on the adjacent hepatic parenchyma and sinusoids. The trapped liver cells are literally squeezed to death and are eventually replaced by sheets of amyloid.

**Amyloidosis of the heart** may occur either as an isolated organ involvement or as part of a systemic distribution. When accompanied by systemic involvement, it is usually associated with immunocyte dyscrasias. The isolated form **(senile amyloidosis)** is usually confined to individuals of advanced age. The deposits may not be evident on gross examination, or they may cause minimal to moderate cardiac enlargement. The most characteristic gross findings are gray-pink, dewdrop-like subendocardial elevations, particularly in the atrial chambers. However, on histologic examination, in addition to these focal subendocardial accumulations, deposits are frequently found throughout the myocardium, beginning between myocardial fibers and eventually causing their pressure atrophy. Vascular involvement and subpericardial accumulations may also be present. In advanced cases, the myocardial aggregates may cause considerable loss of muscle fibers, with attendant derangements of the cardiac conduction system and cardiac contractility. Cardiac failure is an important cause of death in amyloidosis.

**Amyloidosis of the endocrine organs,** particularly of the adrenals, thyroid, and pituitary, is common in advanced systemic distributions. In this case also, the amyloid deposition begins in relation to stromal and endothelial cells and progressively encroaches on the parenchymal cells. Surprisingly, large amounts of amyloid may be present in any of these endocrine glands without apparent disturbance of function. The adrenal must be almost totally replaced before hypofunction is manifested and, hence, amyloidosis is an uncommon cause of Addison's disease (hypoadrenalism) (p. 695).

**Other organs** may be involved. Indeed, no organ or tissue of the body is exempt. Deposits may be encountered in the upper and lower respiratory passages, sometimes in nodular masses. The gastrointestinal tract is a relatively favored site, in which amyloid may be found at all levels, sometimes producing tumorous masses that must be distinguished from neoplasms. Depositions in the tongue may produce macroglossia. On the basis of the frequent involvement of the gastrointestinal tract in systemic cases, gingival, intestinal, and rectal biopsies are commonly employed in the diagnosis of suspected cases. Congo red staining and polarization microscopy should be employed in all cases to detect trace amounts, which may be limited to the vascular walls within the tissue examined. The skin, eye, and nervous system are also affected. Indeed, amyloid deposits in the peripheral nerves are among the prominent manifestations of one of the hereditary forms of this disease. As was previously mentioned, involvement of the arterial and arteriolar walls may be found in any site in the body.

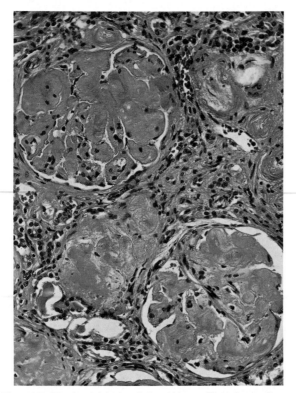

Figure 5–32. Amyloidosis of the kidney. The glomeruli are obliterated by the amorphous amyloid deposit. The vessels (*upper right*) are also virtually occluded by the deposition within their walls.

**CLINICAL CORRELATION.** Amyloidosis may be an unsuspected finding at autopsy in a patient having no apparent related clinical manifestations, or it may be responsible for serious clinical dysfunction and even death. All depends on the particular sites or organs affected and the severity of the involvement. Nonspecific complaints such as weakness, fatigue, and loss of weight are the most common initial symptoms. Later in the course, amyloidosis tends to manifest itself in one of several ways—by renal disease, hepatomegaly, splenomegaly, or cardiac abnormalities. Renal involvement is often the major cause of symptoms in reactive systemic amyloidosis (secondary amyloidosis). It is usually manifested by proteinuria that may be severe enough to induce the nephrotic syndrome (p. 464). Advancement of the renal disease may lead to renal failure, which is an important cause of death in these patients. The hepatosplenomegaly rarely causes significant clinical dysfunction, but it may be the presenting finding. Cardiac amyloidosis may represent an isolated organ involvement or be part of a systemic distribution seen most often in patients with underlying plasma cell dyscrasias. The most severe forms of cardiac amyloidosis are seen in aged individuals, usually in the eighth and ninth decades of life, as isolated organ involvement. The intramyocardial deposits may manifest themselves as conduction disturbances or an apparent cardiomyopathy. Cardiac arrhythmias are an important cause of death in cardiac amyloidosis. In one large series, 40% of the patients with AL amyloid died of cardiac disease.[68]

The diagnosis of amyloidosis may be suspected from the clinical signs and symptoms and from some of the findings mentioned. However, more specific tests must often be employed for definitive diagnosis. Biopsy followed by Congo red staining is the most important tool in the diagnosis of amyloidosis. In general, biopsy is taken from the organ suspected to be involved. For example, renal biopsy is useful in the presence of urinary abnormalities. Rectal and gingival biopsies are positive for amyloid in up to 75% of cases with generalized amyloidosis. In suspected cases of immunocyte-associated amyloidosis, serum and urinary protein electrophoresis and immunoelectrophoresis should be performed. Bone marrow in such cases usually shows plasmacytosis, even if skeletal lesions of multiple myeloma are not present.

The outlook for patients with generalized amyloidosis is poor, and the mean survival time after diagnosis ranges from one to three years. When the disease is associated with immunocytic dyscrasias, cytotoxic drugs have been used to treat the underlying disorder.

# IMMUNODEFICIENCY DISEASES

The more we learn about the immune system, the more complex it becomes. No less complex is the classification of immunodeficiency states. At one time, in blissful ignorance, these were simply categorized as a lack of B cells or T cells or sometimes of both forms of cells; but alas, many new subtleties have emerged. For example, it is now appreciated that ineffective immune responses may be caused not merely by lack of lymphocytes but also by disorders of immunoregulatory circuits. Despite many complexities, the immunodeficiencies can be broadly subdivided into primary diseases of genetic origin and those secondary to some underlying disorder. Our discussion will begin with a brief account of the primary immunodeficiencies, to be followed by more detailed description of the acquired immunodeficiency syndrome, the most devastating example of secondary immunodeficiency.

## PRIMARY IMMUNODEFICIENCY STATES

Primary immunodeficiency states are experiments of nature that have greatly helped our understanding of the ontogeny and regulation of the immune system. They usually come to attention early in life because of the vulnerability of the child to recurrent infections. Although these immune disorders are relatively uncommon, they are often devastating, and the infections are often fatal. A few of the more common ones will be characterized.

### X-Linked (Congenital) Agammaglobulinemia—Bruton's Disease

This disorder is the counterpart in humans of the immune defect produced in birds by neonatal bursectomy. The basic defect is a failure of pre-B cells to differentiate into mature B cells. At the molecular level, the defect seems to reside in an inability to effect orderly and productive rearrangement of immunoglobulin genes.[71] It is one of the more common forms of primary immunodeficiency. As an X-linked disease, it is seen almost entirely in males, but sporadic cases have been described in females. It usually does not become apparent until about six months of age, when maternal immunoglobulins are depleted. In most cases, recurrent bacterial infections such as acute and chronic pharyngitis, sinusitis, otitis media, bronchitis, and pneumonia call attention to the underlying immune defect. Almost always the causative organisms are *Haemophilus influenzae*, *Streptococcus pyogenes*, *Staphylococcus aureus*, or the pneumococci. Most viral and fungal infections are handled normally, but there are some important exceptions to this generalization. These patients seem to be very susceptible to hepatitis and enterovirus infections. They are also at increased risk for the development of *Pneumocystis carinii* pneumonia. These observations indicate a role for antibodies in resistance against certain agents that are traditionally considered to be eliminated only by cell-mediated immunity. The classic form of this disease has the following characteristics: (1) B cells are absent or remarkably decreased in the circulation, and the serum levels of all classes of immunoglobulins are depressed. Pre-B cells are found in normal numbers in bone marrow. (2) The germinal centers of lymph nodes, Peyer's patches, the appendix, and tonsils are underdeveloped or rudimentary. (3) There is a remarkable absence of plasma cells throughout the body. (4) The T-cell system and cell-mediated reactions are entirely normal.

Autoimmune diseases occur with increased frequency in patients with Bruton's disease. Nearly half of these children develop a condition similar to rheumatoid arthritis that clears remarkably with restitutive gamma-globulin therapy. Similarly, lupus erythematosus (p. 152), dermatomyositis (p. 164), and other autoimmune disorders are more common in these patients.

### Thymic Hypoplasia (DiGeorge's Syndrome)

This disorder results from a lack of thymic influence on the immune system. *The thymus is usually rudimentary and T cells are deficient or absent in the circulation. They are similarly depleted in the thymus-dependent areas of the lymph nodes and spleen* (p. 130). Thus infants with this defect are extremely vulnerable to viral and fungal infections as well as to those bacterial infections requiring T and B cell cooperation for the synthesis of protective antibodies. The parathyroid glands are also either hypoplastic or totally absent, often leading to tetany from hypocalcemia. The evidence suggests some embryonic defect in the development of the third and fourth pharyngeal pouches, from which both the thymus and parathyroids are derived. The mode of inheritance of this condition is uncertain, and, indeed, it may well represent a nonhereditary mutation arising during embryogenesis. Only rarely is more than one child in a family affected. The B cell system and serum immunoglobulins are entirely unaffected. Most of these infants have additional developmental defects affecting the face, ears, heart, and great vessels, adding further evidence of a developmental origin. Transplantation of thymic tissue has been successful in some of these infants. Isolated deficiency of thymus without hypoparathyroidism and other congenital anomalies has been called *Nezelof's syndrome*. The immunologic characteristics of this condition are similar to those of DiGeorge's syndrome.

### Severe Combined Immunodeficiency (Swiss-Type Agammaglobulinemia)

Severe combined immunodeficiency represents a constellation of syndromes all having in common variable defects in both humoral and cell-mediated immune responses.[72] Several variants have been identified, all quite rare. Most affected individuals have marked lymphopenia with a deficiency of both T and B cells. Others have normal numbers of B cells, which are nonfunctional due to lack of T-cell help. Still others have normal numbers of circulating lymphocytes that bear the cell surface markers of very immature intrathymic T cells. In all cases, however, the thymus is hypoplastic and fetal in type, or it may be absent. Lymph nodes are difficult to find, markedly reduced in size, and lack both germinal centers, which normally contain B cells, and the paracortical T cells. The lymphoid tissues of the tonsils, gut, and appendix are also markedly hypoplastic.[73] About 50% of patients with the autosomal recessive type of severe combined immunodeficiency have a lack of adenosine deaminase (ADA), an enzyme involved in purine metabolism. In these patients, T-cell deficiency is more profound than B-cell deficiency. ADA levels are low in all the tissues, including red blood cells. It is believed that deficiency of this enzyme leads to accumulation of adenosine and deoxy-ATP, which are toxic to lymphocytes, particularly of the T-cell lineage.[74]

A second, X-linked syndrome is essentially the same, except that the lymphopenia is less severe, ADA is not lacking, and the prognosis is slightly better.

Infants with these severe immunologic handicaps are vulnerable to all forms of viral, fungal, and bacterial infections, and most die within the first year of life. A number of patients with severe combined immunodeficiency with or without ADA deficiency have been successfully treated by transplantation of normal histocompatible bone marrow cells, suggesting that these patients have normal thymus and bursa-equivalent tissues and that the basis of their T- and B-cell deficiency is defective lymphoid stem cells. In ADA-deficient patients, enzyme replacement by infusion of normal erythrocytes results in immunologic improvement in some but not all patients.[74]

### Isolated Deficiency of IgA

This is the commonest of all the primary immunodeficiency diseases, occurring in about one in 700 individuals. Both serum and secretory IgA are deficient. Although most individuals with this condition are asymptomatic, some present with a variety of symptoms, including respiratory infections, chronic diarrhea, and atopic disorders such as asthma. There is also a significant association with autoimmune diseases, the basis of which is not entirely clear. Recent reports suggest that some individuals previously classified as selectively IgA deficient are also deficient in IgG2 and IgG4 subclasses of immunoglobulin G. This subgroup of patients is particularly prone to develop infections.[75] Most commonly this defect appears in sporadic form; when familial, no consistent pattern of inheritance can be discovered. The pathogenesis of IgA deficiency seems to involve a block in the terminal differentiation of IgA-secreting B cells. Serum antibodies to IgA are found in approximately 44% of the patients. Whether this observation is of any etiologic significance is unknown, but it has important clinical implications. When transfused with blood containing normal levels of IgA, some of these patients develop severe, sometimes fatal anaphylactic reactions.

### Common Variable Immunodeficiency

This relatively common but poorly defined derangement probably represents a heterogeneous group of disorders. It may be congenital or acquired, sporadic or familial (with an inconstant mode of inheritance). The feature common to all patients is hypogammaglobulinemia, generally affecting all the antibody classes but sometimes only IgG. About two thirds of the patients have *normal levels of circulating B cells*, which can recognize antigens and proliferate but fail to differentiate into plasma cells. Histologically the B-cell areas—i.e., the lymphoid follicles in the nodes, spleen, and the gut—are markedly hyperplastic. These histologic findings support the notion that B cells can proliferate in response to antigen recognition. Several types of immunologic abnormalities have been found in such patients—an intrinsic inability of B cells to differentiate, even when provided with T-helper cells; lack of T-helper cells; excessive T-suppressor cells; and an inability to secrete intracytoplasmic immunoglobulin.[76] The symptoms are those of antibody deficiency—i.e., recurrent bacterial infections. Infestation with the intestinal parasite *Giardia lamblia* is also quite common and may lead to a sprue-like syndrome. Another peculiar feature is the occurrence in multiple organs of noncaseating granulomas without any known microbial cause. These patients also display a high incidence of autoimmune diseases.

### Immunodeficiency with Thrombocytopenia and Eczema (Wiskott-Aldrich Syndrome)

This condition is selected for presentation because it demonstrates the complexity of the immunologic findings in some patients with primary immune deficiency syndromes. The Wiskott-Aldrich syndrome is an X-linked recessive disease characterized by eczema, thrombocytopenia, and recurrent infections. Classically, these patients show a poor antibody response to polysaccharide antigens (for example, those derived from pneumococcus types I and II). Serum concentrations of IgM are classically low, whereas IgG levels are normal. Serum IgE and IgA levels are greatly elevated in some patients. With time, a progressive loss of cell-mediated immunity develops. But despite all of these defects, the number of circulating lymphocytes may be normal or near normal. Only when there is well-developed loss of T-cell function is lymphopenia found. The pathogenesis of this form of immunodeficiency is obscure, but much of the evidence is compatible with a defect in antigen handling or recognition. Here, then, is an example of an immunodeficiency in the presence of adequate numbers of immunocompetent cells. Encouraging results have been achieved in the treatment of this syndrome by bone marrow transplantation.[77]

## SECONDARY IMMUNODEFICIENCIES

These disorders are sometimes encountered in patients with malnutrition, infection, cancer, renal diseases, Hodgkin's disease, and sarcoidosis. They may also occur secondary to the use of immunosuppressive drugs such as corticosteroids and cancer therapeutic agents. Many of these secondary states can be accounted for by loss of immunoglobulins (as in proteinuric renal diseases), inadequate synthesis of immunoglobulins (as in malnutrition), or loss of lymphocytes (as may occur with drugs and systemic infections), but other mechanisms may also be operative. As a group, the secondary immunodeficiencies are more common than the disorders of genetic origin. Here we will discuss only the acquired immunodeficiency syndrome that has assumed epidemic proportions in the last five years.

### Acquired Immunodeficiency Syndrome (AIDS)

In June 1981, the Centers for Disease Control (CDC) of the United States reported that five young male homosexuals had contracted *Pneumocystis carinii* pneumonia in the Los Angeles area. Two of the patients died. The report of these cases signaled the beginning of an epidemic of a disease characterized by profound immunosuppression associated with opportunistic infections, Kaposi's sarcoma, or both, which has come to be known as acquired immunodeficiency syndrome (AIDS). As of August 1986, more than 20,000 patients with AIDS had been reported in the United States, and, based on serologic data, it is estimated that approximately 1,500,000 individuals have been infected with HTLV-III, the virus believed to cause AIDS. With a problem of this magnitude, it might be expected that there is a rapidly growing body of literature devoted to AIDS. Here we will summarize only the salient epidemiologic, etiologic, immunologic, and clinical features of this new scourge, realizing fully that many of the statements will be out of date before the ink is dry on the printed page.[78]

**EPIDEMIOLOGY.** For epidemiologic and surveillance studies, the CDC defines a case of AIDS as a "disease at least moderately predictive of a defect in cell-mediated immunity, occurring in a person with no known cause for diminished resistance to that disease."[79] Such diseases are classified into five etiologic categories (Table 5–10). With the emerging evidence implicating human T-cell lymphotropic virus-III

**Table 5–10.** OPPORTUNISTIC INFECTIONS AND NEOPLASMS COVERED BY THE CDC SURVEILLANCE DEFINITION OF AIDS

**Protozoal and Helminthic Infections**
Cryptosporidiosis (intestinal)
*Pneumocystis carinii*, causing pneumonia
Strongyloidosis, causing pneumonia, central nervous system infection, or disseminated infection
Toxoplasmosis, causing pneumonia or central nervous system infection

**Fungal Infections**
Candidiasis, causing esophagitis
Cryptococcosis, causing central nervous system infection

**Bacterial Infections**
"Atypical" mycobacteriosis, causing disseminated infection

**Viral Infections**
Cytomegalovirus, causing pulmonary, intestinal, or central nervous system infection
Herpes-simplex virus, causing chronic mucocutaneous, pulmonary, gastrointestinal, or disseminated infection
Progressive multifocal leukoencephalopathy (presumed to be caused by papovavirus)

**Cancers**
Kaposi's sarcoma in persons under 60 years
Lymphoma limited to the brain

(HTLV-III) as the primary cause of AIDS, the CDC has suggested a revision of the case definition to include other opportunistic infections and neoplasms such as disseminated histoplasmosis and diffuse B-cell lymphomas, if they occur in a patient who has serologic or virologic evidence of HTLV-III infection.[80] Although the AIDS epidemic was initially described in the United States and this country has the largest patient population, AIDS has now been reported from over 40 countries around the world.

Epidemiologic studies in the United States have identified six groups at risk for developing AIDS:

○ *Homosexual or bisexual males* comprise by far the largest group, accounting for 73% of the reported cases.

○ *Intravenous drug abusers* with no previous history of homosexuality comprise the next largest group, with about 17% of the total number of patients.

○ *Hemophiliacs*, especially those who receive large amounts of factor VIII concentrates, make up 1% of the AIDS patients.

○ The remaining three risk groups, which include *recipients of multiple blood transfusions, infants born of parents belonging to the first three high-risk groups*, and *heterosexual contacts of members of high-risk groups*, together constitute approximately 4% of the AIDS population.

Approximately 5% of AIDS patients have not been shown to be members of any of the risk groups mentioned above. Half of these patients (2.5% of total) are recent immigrants from Haiti and central Africa, where most AIDS cases have not been associated with the known risk factors.

**ETIOLOGY AND PATHOGENESIS.** There is now over-whelming evidence that AIDS is caused by a transmissible agent, believed to be a virus that has been variously called HTLV-III, lymphadenopathy associated virus (LAV), or AIDS-related virus (ARV).[78] In an attempt to unify the nomenclature, a group of international experts has recently suggested the name human immunodeficiency virus (HIV).[81] Pending widespread usage of the new terminology, it is likely that for some time the AIDS virus will continue to be referred to as HTLV-III/LAV. Several characteristics of this virus have been defined[82]:

○ It belongs to the family of human retroviruses, which includes at least two other members, HTLV-I, and HTLV-II. All contain the enzyme reverse transcriptase.

○ Like HTLV-I, it has a selective affinity for T-helper/inducer lymphocytes that are identified by the T4 or Leu-3 phenotypic marker.[83] It is believed that the T4 molecule is a receptor for HTLV-III/LAV, thus accounting for its tropism.

○ Unlike HTLV-I, which immortalizes T4 cells and causes a T-cell leukemia (p. 389), HTLV-III/LAV is cytolytic for helper T cells and is therefore profoundly immunosuppressive.[84]

The evidence linking HTLV-III/LAV with the etiology of AIDS is strong.[82, 85] The virus has been isolated repeatedly from the lymphoid cells and bodily fluids (semen, saliva, and spinal fluid) of patients with AIDS and those at risk of developing AIDS. In no instance has HTLV-III/LAV been recovered from a normal donor. Antibodies to HTLV-III/LAV have been found in more than 90% of patients with AIDS; by contrast, antibodies are found in less than 1% of healthy populations outside the defined risk groups. Furthermore, a retrovirus STLV-III that cross-reacts serologically with HTLV-III/LAV causes an AIDS-like disease in macaques. Based on accumulating evidence summarized in several recent publications,[78, 86] the natural history of HTLV-III/LAV infection and the subsequent development of AIDS can be outlined as follows.

Transmission of the AIDS virus occurs through one or more of four routes: *sexual contact, intravenous drug administration by contaminated needles, administration of blood and blood products*, and *passage of the virus from infected mothers to their newborns.* Venereal transmission is clearly the predominant mode of spread in the United States. In homosexual men, increased number of sexual partners is associated with greatly increased risk of infection. It is believed that the virus is carried in lymphocytes present in the semen and enters the recipient's body through abrasions in the rectal mucosa. Heterosexual transmission, although less frequent, is also well documented and may become increasingly important in the spread of AIDS.[87] It has been noted in female sexual partners of hemophiliacs and intravenous drug abusers with AIDS, and, conversely, there is also evidence supporting transmission from female prostitutes to their male partners. *Transfusion-associated*

AIDS has been caused by as little as one unit of whole blood, but it is more often related to transfusion of pooled blood components from multiple donors, as is the case with hemophiliacs, who receive lyophilized factor VIII concentrates. Finally, *transplacental passage of HTLV-III/LAV* may account for the transmission of AIDS from infected mothers to their newborns. Conceivably, mother-to-infant transmission may also occur by breast-feeding or other close mother-infant contact. The mode of spread in Haitian immigrants in the United States is not clear. Most of them do not share the known risk factors common to other AIDS victims. It has been suggested that heterosexual transmission is more common in this group, but much remains to be known.

Because of the dismal outlook for patients with AIDS, there has been much concern in the lay public and among health care workers regarding the spread of HTLV-III/LAV outside the high-risk groups. However, to date there is no evidence that AIDS can be transmitted by casual contact, even within a family unit.[88] Furthermore, occupational exposure to patients infected with HTLV-III/LAV does not seem to pose a serious risk to health care workers.

The precise sequence of events after exposure to the virus is not entirely clear. As indicated earlier, the virus infects T4 lymphocytes, but other cells, especially monocytes, may also be infected. The initial response to the virus seems to be the formation of antibodies, which can be detected in the serum within four to seven weeks after parenteral infection. What happens after seroconversion is an area of much uncertainty. One possible sequence of events, leading eventually to full-blown AIDS, is illustrated in Figure 5–33. Until more information becomes available, several qualifying statements must be made.

○ There is a long and variable latent period between seroconversion and the clinical expression of AIDS. The current estimates of the incubation period vary from two to five years.

○ It is not proven that all individuals who have been infected (as indicated by positive results on antibody tests) will develop AIDS. In one study, 34%

of the seropositive homosexual men developed AIDS during a three-year follow-up.[89] Because of the long incubation period, additional follow-up will be required to ascertain the precise frequency of seropositive individuals who develop AIDS.

○ The intermediate outcomes of HTLV-III infection (e.g., seropositive healthy carrier, lymphadenopathy without opportunistic infections) may in some cases be stages in the progression of AIDS, whereas in others they may be stable end points of uncertain duration and clinical relevance.

**CLINICAL FEATURES.** Clinically, the typical patient is a young homosexual male presenting with fever, weight loss, and persistent generalized lymphadenopathy. Pneumonia caused by the opportunistic protozoon *Pneumocytis carinii*, which very rarely affects healthy individuals, is seen in approximately 50% of cases. A variety of other (often multiple) opportunistic pathogens, including *Aspergillus, Candida, Cryptococcus*, cytomegalovirus, *Toxoplasma*, atypical mycobacteria, and herpes viruses, have also been found in these patients (Table 5–10). About 26% of the patients present with Kaposi's sarcoma, a multicentric neoplasm that is extremely rare in the United States (p. 309). Unlike the sporadic cases, Kaposi's sarcoma in patients with AIDS follows an aggressive clinical course characterized by widespread involvement of the skin and early involvement of the lymph nodes and viscera.[90] In addition to Kaposi's sarcoma, several other tumors (mostly lymphoid) have also been reported in AIDS patients. These include diffuse high-grade undifferentiated non-Hodgkin's lymphoma, Hodgkin's disease, and Burkitt's lymphoma. Recent studies indicate that the central nervous system is frequently affected in patients with AIDS. In addition to opportunistic infections and neoplasms, several distinct neurologic syndromes, such as subacute encephalitis, have been reported.[91] These are believed to be caused by direct infection with HTLV-III/LAV, since viral sequences can be demonstrated in the brain by hybridization studies. Thus it appears that in addition to lymphocytes, the nervous system is also a target of HTLV-III infection (p. 731).[92]

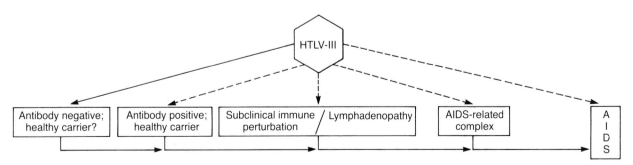

Figure 5–33. Natural history of human T-cell lymphotropic virus type III (HTLV-III) infection. Available data suggest a number of intermediate outcomes of HTLV-III infection, which are shown here. In some cases, these outcomes appear to represent stages of a progressive immunodestructive process. In others, these may be stable outcomes of uncertain duration and clinical relevance. (Modified from Blattner, W. A., et al.: Epidemiology of human T-lymphotropic virus type III and the risk of acquired immunodeficiency syndrome. Ann. Intern. Med. *103*:665, 1985.)

In addition to showing the full-blown syndrome characterized by opportunistic infections and neoplasms, many individuals belonging to the high-risk groups present with persistent generalized lymphadenopathy and nonspecific constitutional symptoms such as recurrent fever, weight loss, and diarrhea. This constellation of clinical features has been called *AIDS-related complex* (ARC) since HTLV-III/LAV and antibodies against it can be detected in over 80% of these patients. As mentioned earlier, in one study 34% of such patients developed AIDS in three years of follow-up. Whether everyone with the ARC will eventually develop AIDS is not known. It is conceivable that HTLV-III/LAV infection produces a wide spectrum of clinical disorders (Fig. 5–33), and in some patients, the AIDS-related complex represents an end point with no further progression.

**IMMUNOLOGIC FEATURES.** As might be surmised from the clinical picture, there is a profound suppression of cell-mediated immunity in AIDS.[93] Central to the disturbed immunity appears to be the infection and subsequent destruction of the T4 inducer/helper lymphocytes by HTLV-III/LAV (Table 5–11). Loss of T4 cells leads to an inversion of the ratio of T4 lymphocyte to T8 lymphocytes in the peripheral blood. It may be recalled that the normal T4/T8 ratio is approximately 2 (p. 130), whereas in patients with AIDS and AIDS-related complex a ratio of 0.5 is not uncommon. Although the inversion of T4/T8 ratio is a particularly consistent finding in AIDS, it should be noted that it is not diagnostic.

The loss of T4 cells has ripple effects on the function of other cells of the immune system (Fig. 5–34), since T4 cells are the source of lymphokines such as IL-2, γ-IFN, macrophage chemotactic factor, and B-cell growth factor. For reasons not entirely clear, the B cells of AIDS patients are polyclonally activated, resulting in hypergammaglobulinemia. However, they are unable to mount a normal antibody response when challenged with a new antigen. Thus humoral immunity is also impaired.

**MORPHOLOGY.** The anatomic changes in tissues are neither specific nor diagnostic.[94, 95]

Biopsies of the enlarged lymph nodes from patients with the AIDS-related complex reveal nonspecific lymphoid hyperplasia involving the follicles, paracortex, and sinusoidal histiocytes. Presumably, these are reactions to infectious agents that occur prior to the onset of severe immunologic failure. With the onset of full-blown AIDS, there is marked lymphoid cell depletion in the lymph nodes, spleen, and the thymus. Changes related to opportunistic infections are widespread and may involve virtually every organ. Because of profound immunosuppression, the inflammatory response to infections may be sparse or atypical. For example, in the lungs mycobacteria do not evoke granuloma formation due to failure of T-cell immunity. In the empty-looking lymph nodes, the presence of infectious agents or neoplasms, or both, may not be readily apparent. Changes in the central nervous system, caused possibly by direct cytopathic effects of HTLV-III/LAV, are common. These include subacute encephalitis, brain atrophy, and degenerative changes in the spinal cord. In this context it is interesting to note that the HTLV-III genome is related to visna, a nononcogenic retrovirus (lentivirus) responsible for a slow neurologic disease in sheep.

Since the discovery of AIDS in 1981, the concerted efforts of epidemiologists, immunologists, and molecular biologists have resulted in spectacular advances in our understanding of this disorder. Despite all this progress, however, the prognosis of patients with AIDS remains dismal. Approximately 50% of those who were afflicted during the initial epidemic in the early 1980s are dead. With time, true mortality figures are likely to approach 100%. Although the causative virus has been identified, many hurdles remain to be crossed before a vaccine can be developed. Recent molecular analyses have revealed an alarming degree of polymorphism in viral isolates from different patients, thus rendering the task of producing a vaccine remarkably difficult. Since no effective drug therapy is yet available, efforts to stem the tide of the AIDS epidemic are focused largely on preventive measures. These include avoidance of sexual contact with persons with clinical or laboratory evidence of infection. To prevent transfusion-associated AIDS, all blood collected for donation in the United States is tested for the presence of anti-HTLV-III/LAV antibodies. Since seropositive samples are discarded, the incidence of AIDS in recipients of blood transfusion should decline rapidly. Factor VIII concentrates that were prepared before serologic testing for HTLV-III/LAV became available are being heat-treated to inactivate any contaminating virus. Together these measures will prevent the occurrence of AIDS in less than one third of those at

---

**Table 5–11. ABNORMALITIES OF IMMUNE FUNCTION IN AIDS***

**Lymphopenia**
Predominately due to a selective defect in the helper/inducer subset (OKT 4, Leu-3) of T lymphocytes; inversion of T4/T8 ratio

**Decreased in vivo T-cell Function**
Susceptibility to neoplasms
Susceptibility to opportunistic infections
Decreased delayed-type hypersensitivity

**Altered in vitro T-cell Function**
Decreased blast transformation
Decreased alloreactivity
Decreased specific cytotoxicity
Decreased ability to provide help to B lymphocytes

**Polyclonal B-cell Activation**
Elevated levels of total serum immunoglobulins and circulating immune complexes
Inability to mount a de novo serologic response to a new antigen
Refractoriness to the normal in vitro signals for B-cell activation

*Modified from Fauci, A. S., et al.: Acquired immunodeficiency syndrome: Epidemiologic, clinical, immunologic, and therapeutic considerations. Ann. Intern. Med. *100*: 92, 1984.

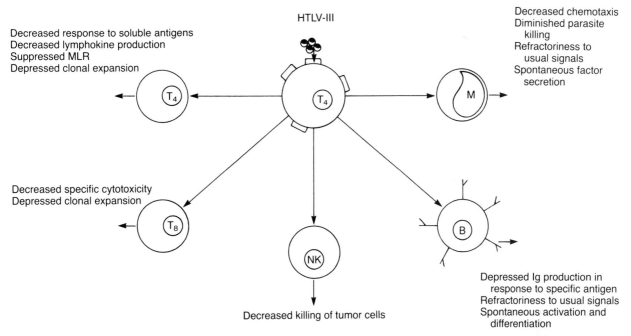

HTLV-III

Decreased response to soluble antigens
Decreased lymphokine production
Suppressed MLR
Depressed clonal expansion

Decreased chemotaxis
Diminished parasite
  killing
Refractoriness to
  usual signals
Spontaneous factor
  secretion

Decreased specific cytotoxicity
Depressed clonal expansion

Depressed Ig production in
  response to specific antigen
Refractoriness to usual signals
Spontaneous activation and
  differentiation

Decreased killing of tumor cells

**Figure 5–34.** Modulation of the human immune system by direct infection by human T-lymphotropic virus type III (*HTLV-III*) of the T4 helper/inducer lymphocyte subset. Infection with HTLV-III results in diverse functional defects due to the central role of the helper/inducer cell on other immune functions. These defects result in a lack of inductive function for other T cells, cytotoxic cells (natural killer [*NK*] and T8), and monocytes (*M*) and a lack of helper function for the B cell (*B*). MLR = mixed lymphocyte response. (From Bowen, D. L., et al.: Immunopathogenesis of the acquired immunodeficiency syndrome. Ann. Intern. Med. *103*:704, 1985.)

risk. Until an effective therapy or vaccine is developed, the major preventive measures must necessarily involve modification of sexual behavior.

## References

1. Fitch, F. W.: T-cell clones and T-cell receptors. Microbiol. Rev. *50*:50, 1986.
2. Tonegawa, S.: Molecules of the immune system. Sci. Am. *253*:122, 1985.
3. Editorial: T-cell receptors. N. Engl. J. Med. *313*:576, 1985.
4. Anderson, K. C., et al.: Expression of human B-cell associated antigens on leukemias and lymphomes: A model for B cell differentiation. Blood *63*:1424, 1984.
5. Oppenheim, J. J., et al.: There is more than one interleukin-1. Immunol. Today *7*:45, 1986.
6. Natural killer cells. Immunol. Rev. *44*:1, 1979.
7. Trinchieri, G., and Perussia, B.: Human natural killer cells: Biologic and pathologic aspects. Lab. Invest. *50*:489, 1984.
8. Grey, H. M., and Chestnut, R.: Antigen processing and presentation to T cells. Immunol. Today *6*:101, 1985.
9. Hood, L., et al.: Genes of the major histocompatibility complex. Ann. Rev. Immunol. *1*:529, 1983.
10. Bach, F.: The HLA class II genes and products: The HLA-D region. Immunol. Today *6*:89, 1985.
11. Turek, P. J., et al.: Molecular variants of the HLA-B27 antigen in healthy individuals and patients with spondyloarthropathies. Immunol. Rev. *86*:71, 1985.
12. Roitt, I.: Essential Immunology. 5th ed. Oxford, Blackwell Scientific Publications, 1984, p. 233.
13. Wasserman, S. I.: Mediators of immediate hypersensitivity. J. Allergy Clin. Immunol. *72*:101, 1983.
14. Barnes, N. C., and Costello, J. F.: Mast cell derived mediators in asthma: Arachidonic acid metabolites. Postgrad. Med. *76*:140, 1984.
15. Hardy, C. C., et al.: The bronchoconstrictor effect of inhaled prostaglandin $D_2$ in normal and asthmatic men. N. Engl. J. Med. *311*:209, 1984.
16. Naclerio, R. M., et al.: Inflammatory mediators in later antigen-induced rhinitis. N. Engl. J. Med. *313*:65, 1985.
17. Capon, A., et al.: From parasites to allergy: A second receptor for IgE. Immunol. Today *7*:15, 1986.
18. Gilliland, B. C.: Serum sickness and immune complexes. N. Engl. J. Med. *311*:1435, 1984.
19. Lawley, T. J., et al.: A prospective clinical and immunologic analysis of patients with serum sickness. N. Engl. J. Med. *311*:1407, 1984.
20. Dvorak, H. F., et al.: Cellular and vascular manifestations of cell-mediated immunity. Hum. Pathol. *17*:122, 1986.
21. Cohen, S.: Physiologic and pathologic manifestations of lymphokine action. Hum. Pathol. *17*:112, 1986.
22. Robb, R. J.: Interleukin-2: The molecule and its function. Immunol. Today *5*:203, 1984.
23. Goldfarb, R. H.: Cell-mediated cytotoxic reaction. Hum. Pathol. *17*:138, 1986.
23a. Mason, D. W., and Morris, P. J.: Effector mechanisms in allograft rejection. Ann. Rev. Imm. *4*:119, 1986.
24. Zmijewski, C. M.: Human leukocyte antigen matching in renal transplantation: Review and current status. J. Surg. Res. *38*:66, 1985.
25. Ting, A., and Morris, P. J.: The role of HLA-matching in renal transplantation. Tissue Antigens *25*:225, 1985.
26. The Canadian Multicenter Transplant Group: A randomized clinical trial of cyclosporine in cadaveric renal transplantation: Analysis at three years. N. Engl. J. Med. *314*:1219, 1986.
27. Fine, R. N. (Moderator): Renal transplantation update. Ann. Intern. Med. *100*:246, 1984.
28. Theofilopoulos, A. N.: Autoimmunity. *In* Stites, D. P., et al. (ed.): Basic and Clinical Immunology. 5th ed. Los Altos, Lange Medical Publications, 1984, p. 1952.
29. Williams, R. C., Jr.: Rheumatic fever and the streptococcus. Another look at molecular mimicry. Am. J. Med. *75*:127, 1983.

30. Shoenfeld, Y., and Schwartz, R. S.: Immunologic and genetic factors in autoimmune disease. N. Engl. J. Med. *311*:1019, 1984.

31. Pisetsky, D. S.: Systemic lupus erythematosus. Med. Clin. North Am. *70*:337, 1986.

32. Tan, E. M., et al.: The 1982 revised criteria for the classification of systemic lupus erythematosus. Arthritis Rheum. *25*:1271, 1982.

33. Michet, C. J., Jr., et al.: Epidemiology of systemic lupus erythematosus and other connective tissue diseases in Rochester, Minnesota, 1950 through 1979. Mayo Clin. Proc. *60*:105, 1985.

34. Tan, E. M., et al.: ANA's in systemic rheumatic disease. Diagnostic significance. Postgrad. Med. *78*:141, 1985.

35. McCarty, G. A.: Autoantibodies and their relation to rheumatic diseases. Med. Clin. North Am. *70*:237, 1986.

36. Schwartz, R. S.: Monoclonal lupus autoantibodies. Immunol. Today *4*:68, 1983.

37. Steinberg, A. D., et al.: Systemic lupus erythematosus: Insights from animal models. Ann. Intern. Med. *100*:714, 1984.

38. Harrist, T. J., and Mihm, M. C., Jr.: The specificity and clinical usefulness of the lupus band test. Arthritis Rheum. *23*:479, 1980.

39. Gilliam, J. N., and Sontheimer, R. D.: Skin manifestations of S.L.E. Clin. Rheum. Dis. *8*:207, 1982.

40. Silva, F. G.: The nephropathies of systemic lupus erythematosus. *In* Rosen S. (ed.): Contemporary Issues in Surgical Pathology. Vol. 1. Pathology of Glomerular Diseases. New York, Churchill Livingstone, 1983, p. 79.

41. McCluskey, R. T., and Colvin, R.: Immunologic aspects of renal tubular and interstitial disease. Ann. Rev. Med. *29*:530, 1978.

42. Decker, J. L., et al.: Rheumatoid arthritis: Evolving concepts of pathogenesis and treatment. Ann. Intern. Med. *101*:810, 1984.

43. Christian, C. L., and Paget, S. A.: Rheumatoid arthritis. *In* Samter, M. (ed.): Immunological Diseases. 3rd ed. Boston, Little, Brown and Co., 1978, p. 1061.

44. Krane, S. M., and Simon, L. S.: Rheumatoid arthritis. Clinical features and pathogenetic mechanisms. Med. Clin. North Am. *70*:263, 1986.

45. Griffin, A. J., et al.: HLA-DR antigens and disease expression in rheumatoid arthritis. Ann. Rheum. Dis. *43*:218, 1984.

46. Ng, K. C., et al.: Anti-RANA antibody: A marker for seronegative and seropositive rheumatoid arthritis. Lancet *1*:447, 1980.

47. Slaughter, L., et al.: In vitro effects of Epstein-Barr virus on peripheral blood mononuclear cells from patients with rheumatoid arthritis and normal subjects. J. Exp. Med. *148*:1429, 1978.

48. Calin, A.: Seronegative spondyloarthritides. Med. Clin. North Am. *70*:323, 1986.

49. Medsger, T. A., Jr.: Systemic sclerosis (scleroderma), eosinophilic fascitis, and calcinosis. *In* McCarty, D. J. (ed.): Arthritis and Allied Conditions. Philadelphia, Lea & Febiger, 1985, p. 994.

50. Uitto, J., et al.: Scleroderma. Increased biosynthesis of triple helical type I and type III procollagens associated with unaltered expression of collagenase by skin fibroblasts in culture. J. Clin. Invest. *64*:921, 1979.

51. Jiminez, S. A.: Cellular immune dysfunction and pathogenesis of scleroderma. Semin. Arthritis Rheum. *13*:104, 1983.

52. Padula, S. J., et al.: Cell-mediated immunity in rheumatic disease. Hum. Pathol. *17*:254, 1986.

53. LeRoy, E. C.: Pathogenesis of systemic sclerosis. J. Invest. Dermatol. *79*(Suppl. 1): 875, 1982.

54. D'Angelo, W. A., et al.: Pathologic observations in systemic sclerosis (scleroderma). Am. J. Med. *46*:428, 1969.

55. Mastaglia, F. L., and Ojeda, V. J.: Inflammatory myopathies. Ann. Neurol. *17*:215, 1985.

56. Ansell, B. M. (ed.): Inflammatory disorders of muscle. Clin. Rheum. Dis. *10*:1, 1984.

57. Arahata, K., and Engel, A. G.: Monoclonal antibody analysis of mononuclear cells in myopathies. Ann. Neurol. *16*:193, 1984.

58. Bohan, A., and Peter, J. B.: Polymyositis and dermatomyositis. N. Engl. J. Med. *292*:343, 405, 1975.

59. Moutsopoulos, H. M. (Moderator), NIH conference: Sjögren's syndrome (sicca syndrome): Current issues. Ann. Intern. Med. *92*(Part 1):212, 1980.

60. Fox, I., et al.: Primary Sjögren's syndrome: Clinical and immunopathologic features. Semin. Arthritis Rheum. *14*:77, 1984.

61. Kassan, S. S., and Gardy, M.: Sjögren's syndrome: An update and overview. Am. J. Med. *64*:1037, 1978.

62. Cupps, T. R., and Fauci, A. S.: The Vasculitides. Philadelphia, W. B. Saunders Co., 1981, pp. 1–211.

63. Fauci, A. S., et al.: Wegener's granulomatosis: Prospective clinical and therapeutic experience with 85 patients over 21 years. Ann. Intern. Med. *98*:76, 1983.

64. Glenner, G. G.: Amyloid deposit and amyloidosis. The β-fibilloses. N. Engl. J. Med. *52*:148, 1980.

65. Glenner, G. G., et al.: Creation of amyloid fibrils from Bence Jones proteins in vitro. Science *174*:712, 1971.

66. Kisilevsky, R.: Amyloidosis: A familiar problem in the light of current pathogenetic developments. Lab. Invest. *49*:381, 1983.

67. Husby, G.: A chemical classification of amyloid. Correlation with different types of amyloidosis. Scand. J. Rheumatol. *9*:60, 1980.

68. Kyle, R. A., and Greipp, P. R.: Amyloidosis (AL): Clinical and laboratory features of 229 cases. Mayo Clin. Proc. *58*:665, 1983.

69. van Rijswijk, M. H., and van Heusden, C. W. G. J.: The potassium permanganate method. A reliable method for differentiating amyloid AA from other forms of amyloid in routine laboratory practice. Am. J. Pathol. *97*:43, 1979.

70. Suzuki, Y., et al.: The mesangium of renal glomerulus. Electron microscopic studies of pathologic alterations. Am. J. Pathol. *43*:555, 1963.

71. Rosen, R., et al.: The primary immunodeficiencies. N. Engl. J. Med. *311*:235, 1984.

72. Gelfand, E. W., and Dosch, H. M.: Diagnosis and classification of severe combined immunodeficiency disease. Birth Defects *19*:65, 1983.

73. Berry, C. L.: Histopathological findings in the combined immunity-deficiency syndrome. J. Clin. Pathol. *23*:193, 1970.

74. Mitchell, B. S., et al.: Purinogenic immunodeficiency disease: Clinical features and molecular mechanisms. Ann. Intern. Med. *92*:826, 1980.

75. Ugazio, A. G., et al.: Recurrent infections in children with selective IgA deficiency. Birth Defects *19*:169, 1983.

76. White, W. B., and Balow, M.: Modulation of suppressor-cell activity by cimetidine in patients with common variable hypogammaglobulinemia. N. Engl. J. Med. *312*:198, 1985.

77. Parkman, R., et al.: Correction of Wiskott-Aldrich syndrome by allogeneic bone-marrow transplantation. N. Engl. J. Med. *298*:921, 1978.

78. Melby, M.: The natural history of human T lymphotropic virus-III infection: The cause of AIDS. Br. Med. J. *292*:5, 1986.

79. Castro, K. G., et al.: The acquired immunodeficiency syndrome: Epidemiology and risk factors for transmission. Med. Clin. North Am. *70*:635, 1986.

80. Centers for Disease Control: Revision of the case definition of acquired immunodeficiency syndrome for national reporting—United States. Ann. Intern. Med. *103*:402, 1985.

81. Coffin, J., et al.: Human immunodeficiency virus. Science *232*:692, 1986.

82. Gallo, R. C., and Wong-Staal, F.: A human T lymphotropic retrovirus (HTLV-III) as the cause of acquired immunodeficiency syndrome. Ann. Intern. Med. *103*:679, 1985.

83. Kalish, R. S., and Schlossman, S. F.: The T4 lymphocyte and AIDS. N. Engl. J. Med. *313*:112, 1985.

84. Zagury, D., et al.: Long-term culture of HTLV-III infected T cells: A model of cytopathology of T-cell depletion in AIDS. Science 231:850, 1986.

85. Montagnier, L.: Lymphadenopathy-associated virus: From molecular biology to pathogenicity. Ann. Intern. Med. 103:689, 1985.

86. Blattner, W. A., et al.: Epidemiology of human T-lymphotropic virus type III and the risk of the acquired immunodeficiency syndrome. Ann. Intern. Med. 103:665, 1985.

87. Lederman, M. M.: Transmission of the acquired immunodeficiency syndrome through heterosexual activity. Ann. Intern. Med. 104:115, 1986.

88. Sande, M. A.: Transmission of AIDS. The case against casual contagion. N. Engl. J. Med. 314:380, 1986.

89. Goeddert, J. J., et al.: Three-year incidence of AIDS in five cohorts of HTLV-III–infected risk group members. Science 231:992, 1986.

90. Volberding, P. A.: Kaposi's sarcoma and the acquired immunodeficiency syndrome. Med. Clin. North Am. 70:665, 1986.

91. Anders, K. H., et al.: The neuropathology of AIDS. UCLA experience and review. Am. J. Pathol. 124:537, 1986.

92. Sharer, L. R., et al.: Pathologic features of AIDS encephalopathy in children. Evidence for LAV-HTLV-III infection of brain. Hum. Pathol. 17:271, 1986.

93. Bowen, D. L., et al.: Immunopathogenesis of the acquired immunodeficiency syndrome. Ann. Intern. Med. 103:704, 1985.

94. Urmacher, C., and Nielsen, S.: The histopathology of the acquired immune deficiency syndrome. Pathol. Annu. (Pt. 1) 20:197, 1985.

95. Liu, P. I., et al.: Morphologic alterations in the lymphoreticular system in acquired immunodeficiency syndrome. Ann. Clin. Lab. Sci. 15:212, 1985.

# 6

# Neoplasia

The study of neoplasia is the study of benign and malignant tumors, more properly known as neoplasms. The importance of this area of study needs no documentation. In the United States, currently over 400,000 deaths are caused each year by malignant neoplasms (cancers); only cardiovascular disease exacts a higher toll. Even more anguishing than the mortality is the emotional and physical suffering inflicted by these neoplasms. The only hope for controlling this dreadful scourge lies in learning more about its origins and vulnerabilities. And, indeed, great progress has been made, leading one eminent investigator to say recently, "Perhaps the puzzle of cancer is not as complex as we had all feared."[1] This chapter deals with the basic biology of neoplasia, namely, the nature of benign and malignant neoplasms, as well as the agents known to cause cancers in animals and humans and their cellular interactions. In the succeeding chapter, the clinical aspects of neoplasms will be considered.

*Neoplasia literally means new growth.* A neoplasm, as defined by Willis, is "an abnormal mass of tissue the growth of which exceeds and is uncoordinated with that of the normal tissues and persists in the same excessive manner after the cessation of the stimuli which evoked the change.[2] *Fundamental to the origin of all neoplasms is loss of responsiveness to normal growth controls.* Neoplastic cells continue to replicate apparently oblivious to the regulatory influences that control normal cell growth. In addition, neoplasms have two other characteristics. They seem to behave as parasites and compete with normal cells and tissues for their metabolic needs. Thus, neoplasms may flourish in patients who are otherwise wasting. Neoplasms also enjoy a certain degree of autonomy, and more or less steadily increase in size regardless of their local environment and the nutritional status of the host. To an extent, then, they are uncontrolled growths. Their autonomy, however, is by no means complete. Some neoplasms require endocrine support, and, indeed, such dependencies can sometimes be exploited to the disadvantage of the neoplasm. Moreover, all are critically dependent on the host for their nutrition and blood supply. To place neoplastic growth in perspective, non-neoplastic controlled proliferations must be considered first.

# Non-neoplastic Proliferation

In an earlier chapter, alterations in cell size and volume—*hypertrophy* and *atrophy*—were discussed (p. 23 and p. 24). These cellular changes, the former an increase in cell size and volume, the latter a decrease in cell size and volume, are basically adaptive responses permitting cells to survive in an altered milieu. Neither cellular change constitutes a proliferative reaction. Here we are concerned with *non-neoplastic cellular proliferations—regeneration, hyperplasia, metaplasia, and dysplasia* (Fig. 6–1). All differ from neoplastic growth because all are *controlled* and abate when the inciting stimulus ceases. Nonetheless, as proliferative processes they constitute soils in which neoplasia may arise. Although each of the patterns may exist in relatively "pure" form, there is much overlap. Thus, hyperplastic cells may simultaneously undergo metaplasia, and, similarly, dysplasia may coexist with metaplasia. Regeneration has already been considered on page 50, so only the remaining three require further description.

## HYPERPLASIA

*Hyperplasia is characterized by an increase in the number of cells in a tissue or organ.* Hyperplasia can

**Hyperplasia**

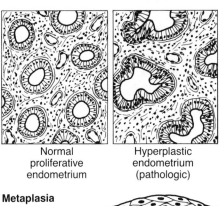

Normal proliferative endometrium

Hyperplastic endometrium (pathologic)

**Metaplasia**

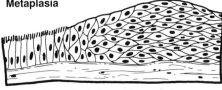

Metaplastic bronchial epithelium

**Dysplasia**

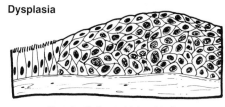

Dysplastic bronchial epithelium

**Figure 6–1.** Schematic comparison of hyperplasia, metaplasia, and dysplasia—all non-neoplastic processes.

only occur in tissues or organs composed of cells capable of mitotic division in postembryonic life. Neurons and striated muscle cells, for example, are incapable of hyperplastic division. The genetic programs in striated muscle cells (including myocardial cells) do not permit them to enter the M phase in the cell cycle. They may synthesize organelles and DNA and undergo hypertrophy but block in the $G_2$ phase and so cannot divide. In contrast, neoplasia may arise in any of the cell types (or their precursor cells) in the body. Hyperplastic tissues and organs have more cells that are normal in size, so they have an increased volume that cannot be differentiated macroscopically from the increased volume induced by hypertrophy. Indeed, hypertrophy and hyperplasia may occur concurrently in response to the same stimuli in tissues composed of cells capable of dividing (e.g., the thyroid).

Hyperplasia may occur under physiologic or pathologic conditions. *Physiologic hyperplasia* can be divided into *hormonal* and *compensatory* types. *Hormonal hyperplasia* is best exemplified by the glandular proliferation of the female breast at puberty and during pregnancy and lactation. Analogously, the smooth muscle cells in the gravid uterus undergo hyperplasia and simultaneously hypertrophy in response to the increased circulating levels of ovarian steroids during pregnancy. The hormonal mechanisms inducing cell division are only partially understood. This much is known: the normal cell types in the body responsive to steroid hormones possess receptors to both estrogen and progesterone. Steroids probably bind to receptors in the cytoplasm. The ligands are translocated to the nucleus, where they initiate synthetic programs involving, very likely, both DNA and messenger RNA, leading to cellular and nuclear enlargement culminating in cell division.

*Compensatory hyperplasia* is seen in the remaining kidney when the other is removed or destroyed by disease. The renal enlargement is the consequence of an increase in the size of the individual nephrons, which in turn is produced largely by hyperplasia of tubular epithelial cells and glomerular enlargement. New nephrons or glomeruli are not formed. The trigger initiating this reaction is not known but presumably involves increased work demand on the remaining kidney.

The best examples of *pathologic hyperplasia* are (1) endometrial hyperplasia, (2) thyroid hyperplasia, and (3) epidermal hyperplasia. Endometrial hyperplasia is usually the consequence of excessive estrogen stimulation, whether it is due to an ovarian dysfunction with an imbalance between estrogen and progesterone synthesis, an ovarian neoplasm, which elaborates estrogens, or chronic use of estrogenic drugs. Thyroid hyperplasia is encountered in primary hyperthyroidism, also known as Graves' disease. In this condition, thyroid-stimulating immunoglobulins appear for mysterious reasons and bind to thyrotropic hormone receptors on the thyroid acinar cells to thus mimic the trophic stimulatory action of the pituitary hormone. The proliferative process causes, as would be expected, enlargement of the thyroid gland and with it, excessive elaboration of thyroid hormone. Epidermal hyperplasia is seen with chronic irritation or abrasion of the skin and underlies the formation of a callus. Presumably the abrasion causes the loss of surface epithelial cells followed by regeneration, which overshoots to produce the excessive thickening. *All of these forms of pathologic hyperplasia are controlled proliferations that cease when the inciting stimulus abates to thus respond to normal growth controls.* However, depending on the severity of the hyperplastic process, they constitute fertile soils in which neoplasia may arise. As will be pointed out later, carcinogenic (cancer-producing) influences have their greatest effect on proliferating cells. It is estimated that 3 to 25% of patients with severe endometrial hyperplasia (atypical adenomatous hyperplasia) later develop endometrial cancer.[3] Thus hyperplasias have two clinical significances: *(1) by and of themselves they may produce clinical disease (e.g., endometrial bleeding, thyroid hyperfunction), and (2) they incur an increased risk of neoplasia, which, however, is much less than that associated with metaplasia and dysplasia.*

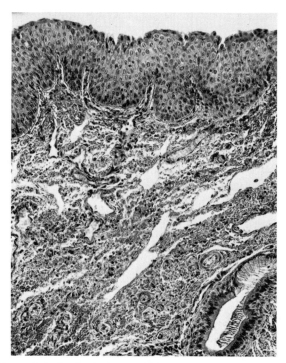

**Figure 6–2.** Tracheal mucosa. The normal columnar, mucus-secreting lining epithelium (similar to that seen in the gland at lower right) has been totally replaced by stratified squamous cells.

## METAPLASIA

Metaplasia is another form of controlled, abnormal cell growth. It is essentially characterized by an *adaptive substitution of one type of adult or fully differentiated cell for another type of adult cell.* For example, under conditions of chronic irritation or inflammation, the more delicate and vulnerable ciliated, pseudostratified columnar epithelium of the bronchi and bronchioles may be replaced by more rugged stratified squamous epithelium. The pseudostratified columnar cells probably do not themselves undergo conversion to squamous cells, but rather the reserve cells within the respiratory epithelium develop along new pathways of differentiation.

Metaplasia may occur in both epithelial and connective tissue cells. In the epithelia it usually takes the form of substitution of a stratified squamous epithelial surface for a columnar mucus-secreting surface. This pattern of metaplasia is seen in the gallbladder, trachea, bronchi or bronchioles, endocervical glands, and excretory ducts of any gland of the body, whenever these sites are chronically inflamed or irritated (Fig. 6–2). A deficiency of Vitamin A (a retinol) is an important cause of epithelial metaplasia leading to keratinizing stratified squamous epithelium in the respiratory passages and in the renal calyces and pelves. How the deficiency exerts these effects is not known, but there are speculations

that retinoids control gene expression and thus cellular differentiation.[4]

Connective tissue metaplasia may be encountered after injury to soft tissue. Scarring is sometimes followed by metaplasia of fibroblasts to osteoblasts, and bone may thus be formed in the area of injury. Similar osseous metaplasia may be seen in traumatic injury to muscle, producing a lesion known as "myositis ossificans." Epithelial metaplasia is almost always reversible, but the connective tissue metaplasias that form bone are usually irreversible and leave permanent markers at the site of old injury.

Teleologically, metaplasia most often represents an adaptive or protective response insofar as the squamous metaplastic epithelium is better able to survive in its adverse environment than was the preceding columnar or pseudostratified epithelium. However, the change is not without drawbacks, because, for example, it implies loss of ciliary and mucus protective functions of the normal columnar epithelium in the respiratory tract.

Often the metaplastic transformation is quite orderly and, in fact, may faithfully reproduce an epithelial architecture that exactly resembles normal squamous epithelium. At times, however, particularly when there is persistent chronic irritation or inflammation, the metaplastic epithelium is somewhat disorderly—i.e., the cells vary slightly in size and shape, do not have the usual orientation to each other, and may have slight variations in nuclear size and chromaticity. Such changes are called "*atypical metaplasia*"; they represent a transition between the orderly pattern of metaplasia and the disorderly pattern of dysplasia. Atypical squamous metaplasia of the bronchial epithelium in cigarette smokers is a frequent forerunner of squamous cell bronchogenic carcinoma.

## DYSPLASIA

In the spectrum of non-neoplastic (i.e., controlled) proliferations, dysplasia is the most disorderly. Frequently it is the forerunner of a cancer, although the causes for this important transition are by no means clear. Dysplasia is encountered principally in the epithelia. *It comprises a loss in the uniformity of the individual cells, as well as a loss in their architectural orientation.* Dysplastic cells exhibit considerable pleomorphism (variation in size and shape) and often possess deeply stained (hyperchromatic) nuclei, which are abnormally large for the size of the cell. Mitotic figures are more abundant than usual, although almost invariably they conform to normal patterns. Frequently the mitoses appear in abnormal locations within the epithelium. Thus, in dysplastic stratified squamous epithelium, mitoses are not confined to the basal layers and may appear at all levels and even in surface cells. There is considerable architectural anarchy. For example, the usual progressive maturation of tall cells in the basal layer to flattened squames on the surface may be lost and replaced by a disordered scrambling of dark basal-appearing cells throughout the entire thickness of the epithelium (Fig. 6–3).

*Dysplasia is characteristically associated with protracted chronic irritation or inflammation.* Classically it is encountered in the cervix, respiratory passages, oral cavity, and gallbladder. Chronic infection is an antecedent of cervical dysplasia. Dysplasia in the respiratory passages is encountered in chronic bronchitis or bronchiectasis and is notably present in the airways of habitual cigarette smokers. In the gallbladder, gallstones and chronic inflammation of the gallbladder wall frequently precede dysplastic change.

*Dysplasia is potentially reversible, and therefore presumably remains under control. When the inciting stimulus is removed, the dysplastic alterations revert*

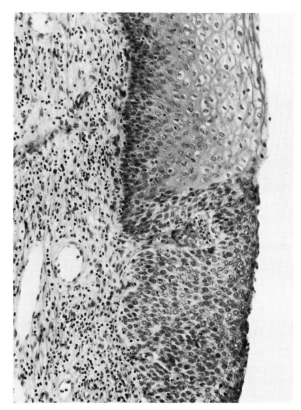

**Figure 6–3.** Dysplasia of the cervical mucosa. The normal epithelium above relatively suddenly changes into the dysplastic epithelium below. The dysplastic cells are smaller, more crowded, and there is loss of the orderly maturation of the surface layers.

*to normal.* However, this is an extremely important type of cell change, particularly in the bronchial and cervical epithelium, because malignant transformation sometimes supervenes. Why this occurs is still unknown. It is possible that within the dysplastic epithelium the more frequent mitoses provide a higher chance of mutation, with the production of aberrant cells freed from regulation. Alternatively, the influences inducing the dysplastic atypicalities when sufficiently prolonged or severe ultimately serve as promotors in the carcinogenic process. Whatever the mechanism, dysplasia is an ominous alteration having grave potential.

# Neoplasia

In common medical usage a neoplasm is often referred to as a "tumor" and the study of tumors is called "oncology" (from *oncos*, tumor, and *logos*, study of). Strictly speaking, a tumor is merely a swelling that could be produced by, among other things, edema or hemorrhage into a tissue. However, the term "tumor" has now come to be applied almost

solely to neoplastic masses that may cause swellings on the body surface; use of the term for non-neoplastic lesions has almost disappeared. In oncology the division of neoplasms into benign and malignant categories is most important. This categorization is based on a judgment of a neoplasm's potential clinical behavior. A tumor is said to be benign when its cytologic and gross characteristics are considered relatively innocent, implying that it will remain localized, cannot spread to other sites, and is, therefore, generally amenable to local surgical removal and survival of the patient. It should be noted, however, that benign tumors can produce more than localized lumps, and sometimes they are responsible for serious disease, as will be pointed out (p. 213).

*Malignant tumors are collectively referred to as cancers*, derived from the Latin word for crab—it adheres to any part that it seizes upon in an obstinate manner, like the crab. "Malignant," as applied to a neoplasm, implies that it can invade and destroy adjacent structures and spread to distant sites (metastasize) to cause death. Obviously, not all cancers pursue so malignant a course. Some are discovered early and are successfully treated. But the designation "malignant" constitutes a red flag.

## NOMENCLATURE

All tumors, benign and malignant, have two basic components: (1) the parenchyma, made up of proliferating neoplastic cells, and (2) the supporting stroma, made up of connective tissue, blood vessels, and possibly lymphatics. As will be seen, *it is the parenchyma of the neoplasm that largely determines its biologic behavior and is the component from which the tumor derives its name*. The stroma, however, carries the blood supply and provides support for the growth of parenchymal cells and is therefore crucial to the growth of the neoplasm.

The nomenclature of tumors is based on the parenchyma. Most benign tumors are composed of parenchymal cells that closely resemble the tissue of origin. Mesenchymal tumors are classified by their histogenesis. They are designated by attaching the suffix "-oma" to the cell type from which the tumor arises. A benign tumor arising in fibrous tissue is termed a fibroma; a benign cartilaginous tumor is a chondroma. Benign tumors of epithelial origin are classified sometimes on the basis of their microscopic and sometimes on the basis of their macroscopic patterns. Others are classified by their cells of origin. *Adenoma is the term applied to benign epithelial neoplasms producing gland patterns and to those derived from glands but not necessarily reproducing gland patterns*. A benign epithelial neoplasm growing in gland-like patterns arising from renal tubular cells would be termed an adenoma, as would a mass of benign epithelial cells producing no glandular patterns but having its origin in the adrenal cortex. Benign epithelial neoplasms growing on any surface that produce microscopic or macroscopic finger-like fronds are designated *papillomas*. Benign tumors protruding from a mucosal surface as in the gut are termed *polyps*. Some benign tumors form large cystic masses, as in the ovary, and are referred to as *cystadenomas*. If papillary projections are formed on the epithelial linings of these cystic tumors, they may be further qualified as *papillary cystadenomas*.

The nomenclature of malignant tumors essentially follows that of benign tumors, with certain additions. *Malignant neoplasms arising in mesenchymal tissue or its derivatives are called sarcomas*. A cancer of fibrous tissue origin is a fibrosarcoma, and a malignant neoplasm composed of chondrocytes is a chondrosarcoma. Thus sarcomas are designated by their histogenesis—i.e., the cell type of which they are composed. *Malignant neoplasms of epithelial cell origin are called carcinomas*. It must be remembered that the epithelia of the body are derived from all three germ layers; thus, a malignant neoplasm arising in the renal tubular epithelium (mesoderm) is a carcinoma, as are the cancers arising in the skin (ectoderm) and lining epithelium of the gut (endoderm). It is evident, then, that mesoderm may give rise to epithelial carcinomas and mesenchymal sarcomas. Carcinomas may be further qualified. *Squamous cell carcinoma* would denote a cancer in which the tumor cells resemble stratified squamous epithelium, and *adenocarcinoma*, a lesion in which the neoplastic epithelial cells grow in gland patterns. Sometimes the tissue or organ of origin can be identified, as for instance in the designation of renal cell adenocarcinoma, or in cholangiocarcinoma, which implies an origin from bile ducts. Sometimes the tumor grows in a very embryonic or undifferentiated pattern and must be called poorly differentiated carcinoma.

The parenchymal cells in a neoplasm, benign or malignant, more or less resemble each other as though all had been derived from a single progenitor. Indeed it appears that most (but not all) neoplasms are of monoclonal origin, as will be documented later. However, in some instances, the stem cell may undergo *divergent differentiation creating so-called mixed tumors*. The best example is the mixed tumor of salivary gland origin. These tumors have obvious epithelial components dispersed throughout an apparent fibromyxoid stroma sometimes harboring islands of cartilage or bone. All of these diverse elements are thought to derive from epithelial or myoepithelial cells, or both, in the salivary glands, and hence the preferred designation of these neoplasms is *pleomorphic adenoma*. The schizophrenic mixed tumor should not be confused with a *teratoma* containing recognizable mature or immature cells or tissues representative of more than one germ layer and sometimes all three. Teratomas take origin from totipotential cells such as are normally present in the ovary and testis and sometimes abnormally present in sequestered midline embryonic rests. Such cells obviously have the capacity to differentiate into all of the cell types to be found in the adult body and so not surprisingly may give rise to neoplasms mimicking in a helter-skelter fashion bits of bone, epithelium, muscle, fat, neural tissue, and others. When all the component parts are well differentiated it is a *benign (mature) teratoma*; when less well differen-

Table 6–1. NOMENCLATURE OF TUMORS*

| Tissue of Origin | Benign | Malignant |
|---|---|---|
| **I. Composed of one parenchymal cell type** | | |
| A. Tumors of mesenchymal origin | | *Sarcomas* |
| (1) Connective tissue and derivatives | Fibroma | Fibrosarcoma |
| | Myxoma | Myxosarcoma |
| | Lipoma | Liposarcoma |
| | Chondroma | Chondrosarcoma |
| | Osteoma | Osteogenic sarcoma |
| (2) Endothelial and related tissues | | |
| Blood vessels | Hemangioma | Angiosarcoma |
| | Capillary | |
| | Cavernous | |
| Lymph vessels | Lymphangioma | Lymphangiosarcoma |
| Synovia | | Synovioma (synoviosarcoma) |
| Mesothelium (lining cells of body cavities) | | Mesothelioma |
| Brain coverings | Meningioma | Invasive meningioma |
| Glomus | Glomus tumor | |
| (3) Blood cells and related cells | | |
| Hematopoietic cells | | Myelogenous leukemia |
| | | Monocytic leukemia |
| Lymphoid tissue | | Malignant lymphomas |
| | | Lymphocytic leukemia |
| | | Plasmacytoma (multiple myeloma) |
| Langerhans' cells | | Histiocytosis X |
| Monocyte-macrophage | | ? Histiocytic lymphoma |
| | | ? Hodgkin's disease |
| (4) Muscle | | |
| Smooth muscle | Leiomyoma | Leiomyosarcoma |
| Striated | Rhabdomyoma | Rhabdomyosarcoma |
| B. Tumors of epithelial origin | | *Carcinomas* |
| (1) Stratified squamous | Squamous cell papilloma | Squamous cell or epidermoid carcinoma |
| (2) Basal cells of skin or adnexa | | Basal cell carcinoma |
| (3) Skin adnexal glands: | | |
| Sweat glands | Sweat gland adenoma | Sweat gland carcinoma |
| Sebaceous glands | Sebaceous gland adenoma | Sebaceous gland carcinoma |
| (4) Epithelial lining | | |
| Glands or ducts—well-differentiated group | Adenoma | Adenocarcinoma |
| | Papilloma | Papillary carcinoma |
| | Papillary adenoma | Papillary adenocarcinoma |
| | Cystadenoma | Cystadenocarcinoma |
| Poorly differentiated group | | Medullary carcinoma |
| | | Undifferentiated carcinoma (simplex) |
| (5) Respiratory passages | | Bronchogenic carcinoma |
| | | Bronchial "adenoma" |
| (6) Neuroectoderm | Nevus | Melanoma (melanocarcinoma) |
| (7) Renal epithelium | Renal tubular adenoma | Renal cell carcinoma (hypernephroma) |
| (8) Liver cells | Liver cell adenoma | Hepatoma (hepatocellular carcinoma) |
| (9) Bile duct | Bile duct adenoma | Bile duct carcinoma (cholangiocarcinoma) |
| (10) Urinary tract epithelium (transitional) | Transitional cell papilloma | Papillary carcinoma |
| | | Transitional cell carcinoma |
| | | Squamous cell carcinoma |
| (11) Placental epithelium | Hydatidiform mole | Choriocarcinoma |
| (12) Testicular epithelium (germ cells) | | Seminoma |
| | | Embryonal carcinoma |
| **II. More than one neoplastic cell type—mixed tumors—usually derived from one germ layer** | | |
| (1) Salivary glands | Pleomorphic adenoma (mixed tumor of salivary gland origin) | Malignant mixed tumor of salivary gland origin |
| (2) Renal anlage | | Wilms' tumor |
| **III. More than one neoplastic cell type derived from more than one germ layer—teratogenous** | | |
| (1) Totipotential cells in gonads or in embryonic rests | Mature teratoma, dermoid cyst | Immature teratoma |

*From Robbins, S. L., Cotran, R. S., and Kumar, V.: Pathologic Basis of Disease. 3rd ed. Philadelphia, W. B. Saunders Co., 1984, p. 217.

tiated, an *immature potentially or overtly malignant teratoma.*

The specific names of the more common forms of neoplasms are presented in Table 6–1. Some glaring inconsistencies may be noted. Witness the use of the terms synovioma, mesothelioma, hepatoma, melanoma, and seminoma for malignant neoplasms. These inappropriate usages are firmly entrenched in medical terminology; but perhaps it is irrational to expect humans to be rational.

There are additional instances of inappropriate terminology. The *hamartoma* is a localized overgrowth of mature cells normally found in an organ. The cells in the hamartoma, although mature and normal, do not re-create the normal organization of the tissue in which they are found. Thus one may see a mass of disorganized hepatic cells, blood vessels, and possibly bile ducts within the liver, or there may be a disorganized accumulation of cells indigenous to the spleen, creating an apparent tumor within the spleen. The designation hamartoma is appropriate inasmuch as the aggregation of cells may create a small tumor, but the lesion is not a true neoplasm; rather, it is a form of congenital anomaly. Another misnomer is the term *choristoma*. This congenital anomaly is better described as a *heterotopic rest* of cells. For example, a small nodule of very well developed and normally organized pancreatic substance may be found in the submucosa of the stomach, duodenum, or even small intestine. This heterotopic rest may be replete with islets of Langerhans as well as exocrine glands. The term choristoma, connoting a neoplasm, imparts to the heterotopic rest a gravity far beyond its usual trivial significance. In all probability the rest merely reflects an embryogenic defect. Regrettably, neither life nor the terminology of neoplasms is simple, but the terminology has importance because it is the language by which the nature and significance of tumors are categorized.

# CHARACTERISTICS OF BENIGN AND MALIGNANT NEOPLASMS

Nothing is more important to the patient with a tumor than being told "It is benign." In most instances such a prediction can be made with remarkable accuracy based upon long-established clinical and anatomic criteria, but some neoplasms defy easy characterization. Certain features may point to innocence and others to malignancy. Moreover, in a few instances there is not perfect concordance between the appearance of a neoplasm and its biologic behavior. However, these problems are not the rule and there are generally reliable criteria by which benign and malignant tumors can be differentiated. These differences will be discussed under the following headings:

1. Differentiation and anaplasia
2. Rate of growth—tumor progression
3. Encapsulation versus invasion
4. Metastasis

## DIFFERENTIATION AND ANAPLASIA

Differentiation and anaplasia refer only to the parenchymal cells that constitute the proliferating pool and bulk of most neoplasms. The stroma, as noted earlier, is critical to the growth of tumors but does not aid in the separation of benign from malignant ones. The amount of stromal connective tissue does, however, determine the consistence of a neoplasm. Certain cancers induce a dense, abundant fibrous stroma (*desmoplasia*) making them hard, so-called scirrhous, tumors. It is the parenchyma that is the "cutting edge" of a neoplasm. *The differentiation of parenchymal cells refers to the extent to which they resemble their normal forebears, both morphologically and functionally.* Differentiation in multicellular organisms involves the expression in particular types of cells of certain genetic programs and the repression of others. In general, in highly differentiated specialized cells, the genetic programs for replication are repressed; *in neoplasia, these programs are reactivated and differentiation may occur without loss of replicative ability.*

*Benign neoplasms are composed of well-differentiated cells that resemble very closely their normal counterparts.* Thus, the lipoma is made up of mature fat cells laden with cytoplasmic lipid vacuoles and the chondroma of mature cartilage cells that synthesize their usual cartilaginous matrix, evidence of both morphologic and functional differentiation. Thus, some alteration, genetic or epigenetic, must have occurred to account for loss of growth control, but the remaining programs of differentiation are essentially unaltered. In well-differentiated benign tumors, mitoses are extremely scant in number and are of normal configuration. One can only speculate that the tumor achieved its size by prolongation of the lifespan of the neoplastic cells, which fail to differentiate further and die, or perhaps by a marked expansion of the replicating cell pool, cycling at a slow rate.

*Cancers are characterized by a wide range of parenchymal cell differentiation, from those surprisingly well differentiated to those completely undifferentiated* (Fig. 6–4). The term anaplasia literally means "to form backward." It implies dedifferentiation or loss of the structural and functional differentiation of normal cells. However, we now appreciate that most, if not all, cancers arise from reserve cells in tissues, and so failure of differentiation accounts for undifferentiated tumors rather than dedifferentiation of specialized cells. *Malignant neoplasms composed of undifferentiated cells are said to be anaplastic.* It is a matter of semantics whether one also applies such terms as "minimal to moderate anaplasia" to well-differentiated cancers. Clearly, even in these lesions

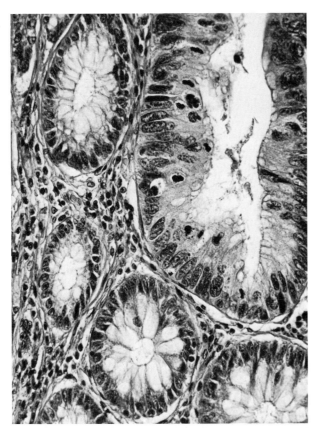

**Figure 6–4.** Histologic detail of well-differentiated adenocarcinoma of the colon. The normal colonic glands are at left and below and the cancerous gland is at upper right. Compare the normal cells having basal small nuclei and apical vacuoles with the cancerous cells having pleomorphic nuclei and virtually lacking secretory vacuoles.

there has been loss of some feature of differentiation to account for the escape from growth controls. To this extent, there is some lack of differentiation in all cancers, but it may not be evident at the usual morphologic and functional levels save for the evidence of uncontrolled proliferation. In any event, when lack of differentiation or anaplasia is evident in a tumor, it is almost certainly a malignant neoplasm and therefore *anaplasia is a marker of cancer.* But, as pointed out, not all cancers are obviously anaplastic.

*Anaplastic cells display marked pleomorphism, i.e., marked variation in size and shape. This pleomorphism exceeds that found in dysplastic cells* (Fig. 6–5). Characteristically the nuclei are extremely hyperchromatic and large. The nuclear-cytoplasmic ratio may approach 1:1 instead of the normal 1:4 or 1:6. Giant cells may be formed that are considerably larger than their neighbors and possess either one enormous nucleus or several nuclei. Anaplastic nuclei are variable and bizarre in size and shape. The chromatin is coarse and clumped, and nucleoli may be of astounding size. More important, the mitoses are often numerous and distinctly atypical; anarchic multiple spindles may be seen that sometimes can

be resolved as tripolar or quadripolar forms, often with one spindle enormously large and the others puny and abortive (Fig. 6–6). Also, anaplastic cells may fail to develop recognizable patterns of orientation to each other. They may grow in sheets, with total loss of communal structures, such as gland formations or stratified squamous architecture. Thus, anaplasia is the most extreme disturbance in cell growth encountered in the spectrum of cellular proliferations. It is placed in some perspective in Table 6–3, p. 197. The changes of anaplasia provide the basis for the Papanicolaou (cytologic) test for cancer, described on page 224.

Electron microscopic studies of neoplastic cells have yielded no great surprises.[5] Well-differentiated cells, whether from benign or malignant neoplasms, deviate little from their normal forebears. With loss of differentiation in cancer cells, there is progressively more marked accentuation of the nuclear chromatin in clumps along the membrane, simplification of the rough endoplasmic reticulum, an increase of free ribosomes and greater pleomorphism of the mitochondria. Various organelles may be reduced in size or number or distributed throughout the cell in

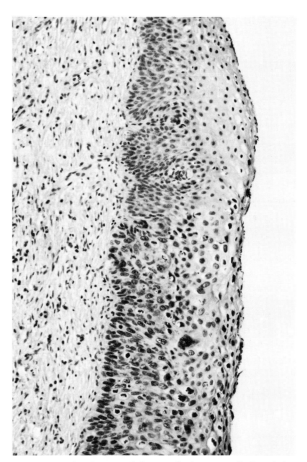

**Figure 6–5.** Carcinoma of the cervical mucosa before it has penetrated the underlying cervical tissue. The normal cervical mucosa above is replaced below by anaplastic cells having marked pleomorphism.

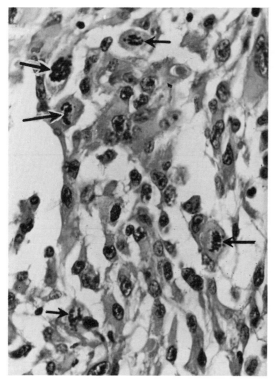

**Figure 6–6.** Atypical mitoses in a rapidly growing carcinoma of the pancreas. The disorganized mitotic figures (*arrows*) reflect the anarchic reproduction of anaplastic tumor cells.

abnormal patterns. Malignant cells on the whole have greater mobility than normal cells, possibly contributing to their invasiveness.[6] Not surprisingly then, it is often possible to visualize microfilaments of actin and myosin, as well as microtubules containing tubulin. *Intermediate filaments*, which are thought to integrate the organelles within cells, also can often be visualized. The various types of filaments and the types of tumors in which they are found are presented in Table 6–2. The demonstration of these intermediate filaments by immunohistochemical methods (immunofluorescence and immunoperoxidase techniques) has greatly improved the identification of many cancers, particularly when cytologic features are otherwise not entirely clear-cut, as will be pointed out on page 225.[7]

Turning to the functional differentiation of neoplastic cells, as you might presume, the better the differentiation of the cell, the more completely they retain the functional capabilities found in their normal counterparts. Thus, benign neoplasms and indeed well-differentiated cancers of endocrine glands frequently elaborate the hormones characteristic of their origin. Well-differentiated squamous cell carcinomas of the epidermis elaborate keratin just as well-differentiated hepatocellular carcinomas elaborate bile. Indeed, there are few differences in the enzyme profiles of well-differentiated tumor cells from their normal counterparts. As one descends the scale of differentiation, enzymes and specialized pathways of metabolism are lost and the cells as it were undergo functional simplification. Highly anaplastic undifferentiated cells then, whatever their tissue of origin, come to resemble each other more than the normal cells from which they have arisen, a phenomenon referred to as *biochemical convergence*. However, in some instances unanticipated functions emerge. Some cancers may elaborate fetal proteins (antigens) not produced by the comparable cells in the adult (p. 226). Analogously, cancers of nonendocrine origin may assume hormone synthesis to produce so-called "ectopic hormones." For example, bronchogenic carcinomas may produce adrenocorticotropic hormone, parathyroid-like hormone, insulin, and glucagon, as well as others.[8] More will be said about these phenomena later (p. 215), but for here it suffices to state that in the process of cancerous transformation, either repressed genes are derepressed or new DNA sequences are formed. *Despite exceptions, the more rapidly growing and the more anaplastic a tumor, the less likely there will be specialized functional activity.*

In summary, the *cells in benign tumors are almost always well differentiated and resemble their normal cells of origin; the cells in cancers are more or less differentiated but some loss of differentiation is always present.*

## RATE OF GROWTH—TUMOR PROGRESSION

It is common knowledge that most benign tumors grow slowly and that most cancers grow much faster to eventually spread locally and to distant sites (metastasize) and cause death. However, there are many exceptions to this generalization, and some benign tumors grow more rapidly than some cancers.[9] For example, the rate of growth of leiomyomas (benign smooth muscle tumors) of the uterus is influenced by the circulating levels of estrogens. Thus, they may rapidly increase in size during pregnancy and conversely cease growing or even atrophy and become largely fibrocalcific following menopause. Other influences such as adequacy of blood supply and possibly pressure constraints also may affect the growth rate of benign tumors. Adenomas of the pituitary gland locked into the sella turcica have been observed to suddenly shrink in size. Presumably they undergo a wave of necrosis as their progressive enlargement compresses their blood supply. Noting these varia-

**Table 6–2.** INTERMEDIATE FILAMENTS AND THEIR DISTRIBUTION

| | |
|---|---|
| *Keratins* | Carcinomas |
| | Mesothelioma |
| *Desmin* | Muscle tumors, smooth, striated |
| *Vimentin* | Mesenchymal tumors, some carcinomas |
| *Glial Filaments* | Gliomatous tumors |
| *Neurofilaments* | Neuronal tumors |

bles, it is nonetheless true that most benign tumors under clinical observation for long periods of time increase in size slowly over the span of months to years and there is some variation in rate of growth from one neoplasm to another.

*The rate of growth of cancers correlates in general with their level of differentiation.* Thus there is wide variation. Some grow relatively slowly, and indeed there are exceptional instances when they come almost to a standstill when they undergo increased differentiation to revert to benign neoplasms.[10] Even more exceptionally, cancers (particularly choriocarcinomas) have spontaneously disappeared as they become totally necrotic, leaving only secondary metastatic implants. However, with the exception of these rarities, most cancers progressively enlarge over time—some slowly, others rapidly—but the notion that they "emerge out of the blue" is not true. Many lines of experimental and clinical evidence document that most, perhaps all cancers, take years and possibly decades to evolve into clinically overt lesions.

We know from many types of observations that most cancers are monoclonal in origin (i.e., arise from the clonal expansion of a single cell) but some are polyclonal. One proof of monoclonality is as follows. Glucose-6-phosphate-dehydrogenase (G6PD), of which there are many isoenzymes, is encoded by a gene on the X chromosome. Recall that in women there is random inactivation of one X chromosome in all cells of the female embryo at the blastocyst stage (p. 123). Thus, all organs in the female are composed of two populations of cells, one population having an active X chromosome of maternal origin and the other of paternal origin. In some women, more often black women, the two X chromosomes each encode a different G6PD isoenzyme. Most neoplasms in these women express only a single isoenzyme, strongly suggesting that they are monoclonal in origin. If the tumors were polyclonal, chance alone would dictate expression of both variants[11] (Fig. 6–7).

In the case of a monoclonal neoplasm, how long does it take for the single cell to give rise to a clinically overt mass? This depends on (a) the doubling time of the cell and its progeny, (b) the fraction of accumulating cells that remain viable and in the replicating pool, and (c) the rate at which cells are shed and lost to the growing lesion. Without going into elaborate details, it suffices that the doubling time of cancer cells is extremely variable and sometimes longer than their normal forebears. Moreover, *there is continuous shedding of cells as well as maturation and death, which may account for an 80 to 90% loss from the replicating pool.*[12] Thus the growth of a single cell into a 1-cm mass requires many years. An important point from these considerations should be underscored—*the number of mitoses in a cancer is not a reliable index of growth rate because increase in size involves more than loss*

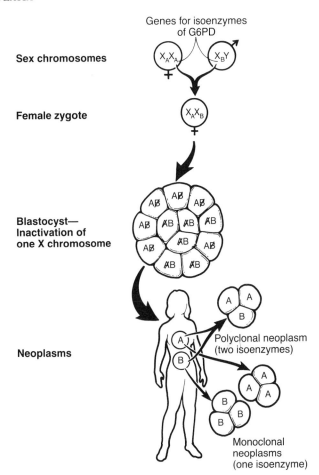

**Figure 6–7.** Diagram depicting the use of isoenzyme cell markers as supportive evidence of the monoclonality of some neoplasms.

*of growth controls; also involved are shedding and failure in maturation and death of cells.*

Clinical observations of patients with carcinoma of the cervix confirm the slow rate of evolution of this form of cancer. Cytologic studies permit the identification of "early" cervical carcinomas while still confined to minute foci within the epithelium—*carcinoma in situ.* At this stage, the lesion might well be clinically inapparent. The peak incidence of these in situ lesions occurs in women approximately 25 to 30 years of age, but the peak incidence of a clinically visible mass is about 10 to 15 years later (as discussed more fully on p. 637). We may conclude that the overt cancer is only the tip of the iceberg preceded by years of subsurface evolution.

Factors other than cell kinetics modify the rate of growth. Most important among these are blood supply. The importance of blood supply has been emphasized by the studies of Folkman.[13] He showed in experimental animal models that tumor cells in culture can grow in the absence of vascularization only up to nodules in the range of 1 to 2 mm in diameter.

However, when these nodules are implanted in tissue and develop a blood supply from the surrounding tissues, further growth ensues. It was then possible to isolate a soluble *tumor angiogenesis factor (TAF)* produced by the tumor cells accounting for the neovascularization. Macrophages that infiltrate a tumor apparently also elaborate angiogenic substances. Blood supply then is critical to tumor growth. Lack of adequate blood supply may indeed cause tumors to undergo necrosis, particularly in the centers of evolving masses (and their metastases) most remote from the vascular supply of the surrounding native tissue. Quite recently a "tumor necrosis factor" has been described, elaborated by activated monocytes-macrophages.[14] Whether it plays a role in vivo is uncertain. But, in any event, necrosis may in some instances cause the tumor and its metastases to decrease in size. Usually, however, the margins remain viable. Hormones influence the growth rate, particularly in cancers arising in hormonally responsive tissues (e.g., breast, uterus, endometrium, ovary, and prostate). As pointed out earlier, the normal cells in such locations have steroid receptors, as do many of the cancers, and so carcinomas of the breast may sometimes become explosive in their growth during pregnancy; conversely, the use of antiestrogenic agents or surgical removal of the ovaries and sometimes adrenals and pituitary gland may markedly slow the growth of breast carcinomas. Unfortunately, however, such hormonal manipulations rarely are more than palliative measures. Suffice it that *host factors influence growth rate.*

We come now to the phenomenon of *tumor progression* and its impact on rate of growth. The cells of all fully evolved cancers, even those of monoclonal origin, are heterogeneous. *Subsets can be identified having differences in their karyotypes, invasiveness, hormonal responsiveness, metastatic capabilities, growth rate, and susceptibility to antineoplastic drugs.* These differences appear to arise from new mutations in the genetically unstable replicating cells of the evolving neoplasm or from the variable expression of genes in different subsets.[15] The progressive acquisition of these attributes is referred to as *progression.* Moreover, each of these cancerous attributes appears to arise independently, so one particular clone of cells may acquire an increased growth rate while another may gain the capacity to invade or to metastasize.[16] Although a fully evolved cancer is therefore composed of a heterogeny of clones, certain ones having greater replicative capacity may dominate. On the basis of this independent assortment of tumorous attributes, some cancers have the capacity to invade but may not be able to metastasize (for example, the basal cell carcinoma). Conversely, some ovarian carcinomas may seed (metastasize) throughout the peritoneal cavity but not be able to invade the organs on which they have become implanted. Thus, the rate of growth of a neoplasm may increase with time as the more vigorous clones of

cells having shorter cell cycles or longer life spans gain a selective advantage. Tumor progression adds yet another variable to the growth rate of cancers.

## ENCAPSULATION—INVASION

*A benign neoplasm stays localized at its site of origin. It does not have the capacity to infiltrate, invade, or metastasize to distant sites, as do cancers.* As fibromas and adenomas, for example, slowly expand, *most develop an enclosing fibrous capsule that separates them from the host tissue.* This capsule is probably derived from the stroma of the native tissue as the parenchymal cells atrophy under the pressure of the expanding tumor. The stroma of the tumor itself may also contribute to the capsule (Figs. 6–8 and 6–9). However, it should be emphasized that *not all benign neoplasms are encapsulated.* The leiomyoma of the uterus, for example, is quite discretely demarcated from the surrounding smooth muscle by a zone of compressed and attenuated normal myometrium, but there is no well-developed capsule. Nonetheless, a well-defined cleavage plane exists around these lesions. A few benign tumors are neither encapsulated nor discretely defined. This is particularly true of some of the vascular benign neoplasms of the dermis. These exceptions are

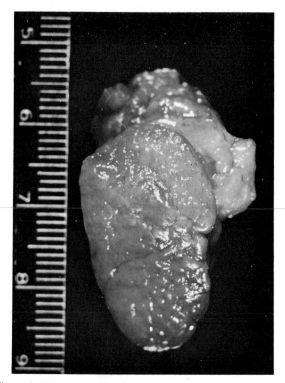

Figure 6–8. A gross view of a fibroadenoma of the breast. The discrete tumor bulges above the level of the surrounding breast substance as it extrudes from its tight encapsulation. (From Robbins, S. L., Cotran, R. S., and Kumar, V.: Pathologic Basis of Disease. 3rd ed. Philadelphia, W. B. Saunders Co., 1984, p. 223.)

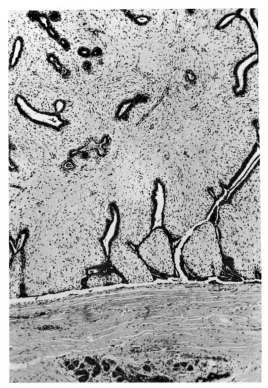

Figure 6–9. A microscopic view of the fibroadenoma of the breast seen in Figure 6–8. The fibrous capsule (*below*) separates the sharply delimited tumor mass from the surrounding breast substance. (From Robbins, S. L., Cotran, R. S., and Kumar, V.: Pathologic Basis of Disease. 3rd ed. Philadelphia, W. B. Saunders Co., 1984, p. 223.)

sure generated by an enlarging tumor mass could facilitate permeation of contiguous normal structures, much more is involved—witness the tendency for certain malignant neoplasms of the gut to widely permeate the bowel wall without bulging into the lumen and follow the path of least resistance. Some studies of the phenomenon suggest that *three steps are involved in invasion: (a) attachment of cancerous cells, (b) local proteolysis, and (c) locomotion.*[17] Normal tissues are separated into compartments by basement membranes and interstitial stroma. The basement membrane is largely composed of type IV collagen, proteoglycans, and glycoproteins such as laminin. According to Liotta, invasiveness involves the generation of laminin receptors by cancer cells, which permits their attachment to surrounding structures and is followed by their synthesis of proteases, mainly collagenases, thus opening pathways into the interstitial stroma for tumor cell locomotion and migration into surrounding normal tissues, as depicted in Figure 6–11.[18] In this connection, certain structures in the body are notably resistant to tumor invasion (e.g., cartilage and arterial walls). Both tissues are compact and resistant to degradative enzymes because they elaborate antiproteases. *This*

pointed out only to emphasize that *although encapsulation is the rule in benign tumors, the lack of a capsule does not imply that a tumor is malignant.* Occasionally, benign tumors, the lipoma for example, may rupture through delicate capsules to extend pseudopods into the surrounding tissue. The pseudopods are usually clearly attached to the main mass, grow along a broad front, and are not easily confused with the infiltrative growth of malignant neoplasms.

*Cancers grow by progressive infiltration, invasion, destruction, and penetration of the surrounding tissue* (Fig. 6–10). They do not develop capsules. There are, however, occasional instances in which a slowly growing malignant tumor deceptively appears to be encased by the stroma of the surrounding native tissue, but usually microscopic examination will reveal tiny, crab-like feet penetrating the margin and infiltrating adjacent structures. This invasion tends to occur along anatomic planes of cleavage. The infiltrative mode of growth makes it necessary to remove a wide margin of surrounding normal tissue when surgical excision of a malignant tumor is attempted. The surgeon must have knowledge of the invasive potential of the various forms of cancer, since there are striking differences among them.

The invasiveness of cancer cells is a complex phenomenon still under study. Although expansile pres-

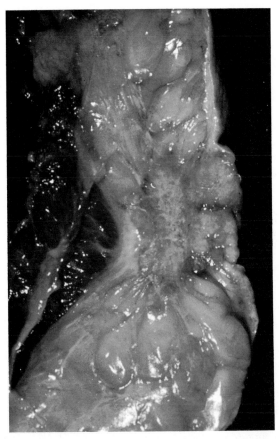

Figure 6–10. A close-up view of the cut surface of a cancer of the female breast. The infiltrative tumor has eroded through the skin (*right*) and its crab-like extensions pull on the adjacent fat and dark pectoral muscles (*left*).

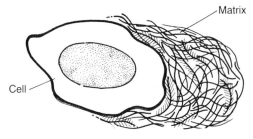

Attachment of tumor cell

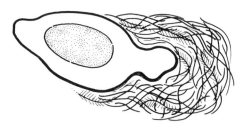

Release of proteases by cell

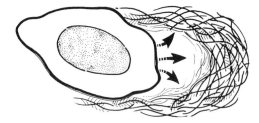

Tumor cell migration

**Figure 6–11.** A representation of one possible mechanism of cancer invasiveness.

*concept of invasiveness is buttressed by the observations that (a) basement membranes in proximity to tumor cells are frequently disrupted,[19] (b) cancer cells have increased locomotory capacities, and (c) they are less cohesive and therefore able to detach themselves from their origins. In passing we might* note that loss of cohesiveness implies some alteration in tumor cell surfaces, which is a characteristic feature of the cancerous phenotype (discussed later).

## METASTASIS

The term *metastasis* connotes the development of secondary implants (*metastases*) discontinuous with the primary tumor, possibly in remote tissues (Fig. 6–12). *The properties of invasiveness and, even more so, metastasis more unequivocally identify a neoplasm as malignant than any of the other neoplastic attributes. Not all cancers have the ability to metastasize.* The notable exceptions are basal cell carcinoma of the skin and most primary tumors of the central nervous system. Although these neoplasms are highly invasive in their primary sites of origin, they rarely metastasize. It is evident then that the properties of invasion and metastasis are separable.

Metastases are already present in about one half of all patients with cancers by the time of diagnosis.[20] In general, the more anaplastic and the larger the primary neoplasm, the more likely metastatic spread. However, exceptions abound. For example, extremely small in situ cancers infrequently have been known to metastasize, and conversely, some large, ugly lesions may not have spread. Dissemination strongly prejudices, if it doesn't preclude, the possibility of cure of the disease, so it is obvious that, short of prevention of cancer, no achievement would confer greater benefit on patients than methods to prevent metastasis. Accordingly, the process has been intensively studied, and much has been learned.[21, 22] Because so much is still controversial, only an overview of the immensely complex sequence will be presented here.

*Malignant neoplasms disseminate by one of three pathways: (1) seeding within body cavities, (2) lymphatic spread, and (3) hematogenous spread.* Although direct transplantation of tumor cells, as, for

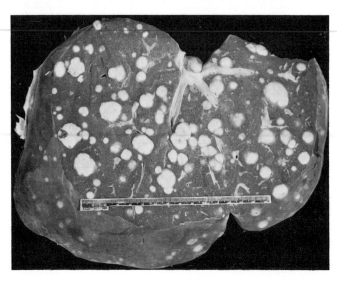

**Figure 6–12.** A liver studded with metastatic cancer.

example, on surgical instruments or on the surgeon's gloves, may theoretically occur, happily in clinical practice, it is exceedingly rare and, in any event, it is an artificial mode of dissemination.

*Seeding of cancers occurs when neoplasms invade a natural body cavity.* Carcinoma of the colon may penetrate the wall of the gut and reimplant at distant sites in the peritoneal cavity. A similar sequence may occur with lung cancers in the pleural cavities. This mode of dissemination is particularly characteristic of cancers of the ovary, which often cover the peritoneal surfaces widely. Strangely, the implants may literally glaze all peritoneal surfaces and yet not invade the underlying parenchyma of the abdominal organs. Here again is an instance of the ability to reimplant elsewhere that appears to be separable from the capacity to invade. Neoplasms of the central nervous system such as the medulloblastoma and ependymoma may penetrate the cerebral ventricles and be carried by the cerebrospinal fluid to reimplant on the meningeal surfaces, either within the brain or in the spinal cord. Strangely, however, a cancer arising in the mucosa of an organ system almost never reimplants at a lower level, as, for example, from the renal pelvis into the urinary bladder or from the stomach into the colon.

*Lymphatic spread is more typical of carcinomas, whereas the hematogenous route is favored by sarcomas.* However, there are numerous interconnections between the lymphatic and vascular systems, and so all forms of cancer may disseminate through either or both systems.[23] The pattern of lymph node involvement depends principally on the site of the primary neoplasm and the natural lymphatic pathways of drainage of the site. Thus, bronchogenic carcinomas arising in the respiratory passages metastasize first to the regional bronchial lymph nodes and then to the tracheobronchial and hilar nodes. Carcinoma of the breast usually arises in the upper outer quadrant and first spreads to the axillary nodes. Medial lesions may drain through the chest wall to the nodes along the internal mammary artery. Thereafter, in both instances the supra- and infraclavicular nodes may be seeded. In some cases, the cancer cells appear to traverse the lymphatic channels within the immediately proximate nodes to be trapped in subsequent lymph nodes, producing so-called *skip metastases*. Indeed, the cells may traverse all of the lymph nodes to ultimately reach the vascular compartment via the thoracic duct. Involved in lymphatic dissemination are the same features that characterize invasiveness—i.e., attachment to lymphatic basement membranes, release of degradative enzymes, and ameboid penetration into the channel. In this manner, the cancer cells travel as emboli and not as continuous intralymphatic extensions from the primary lesion.

At one time it was standard surgical practice, when resecting a cancer, to attempt to excise all of the regional lymph nodes, particularly when they were enlarged. More recently, the nodes in the primary area of drainage are sampled to ascertain possible involvement. For most cancers the prognosis is much the same with one to three involved nodes and only worsened with four or more positive nodes. Moreover, prophylactic excision, as it is called, of all primary nodes is fruitless for reasons already cited; cancer cells may traverse or bypass primary nodes to involve more distant ones. Furthermore, enlargement of nodes in proximity to a primary neoplasm may not imply cancerous involvement. The necrotic products of the neoplasm and possibly tumorous antigens (p. 200) often evoke reactive changes in the nodes, such as enlargement and hyperplasia of the follicle (lymphadenitis) and proliferation of reticulum cells and sinus reticuloendothelial cells (sinus histiocytosis). Thus, nodal enlargement does not necessarily imply cancerous spread.

*Hematogenous spread* is the most feared consequence of a cancer. It is the favored pathway for sarcomas, but carcinomas are by no means shy about using it. The development of hematogenous metastases is a surprisingly complex process that has been likened to a stairway, in which each step must be successfully mounted before the next step can be taken (depicted in Fig. 6–13). Indeed in the experimental animal, only about 0.1% of cancer cells injected into a vein successfully complete the climb to produce implants. Analogously, in humans, cancer cells have been observed in the circulating blood in patients without metastatic disease. It is not necessary to delve into all the details of this complex process, and so only a few significant features will be emphasized.[24] It begins with invasion of veins by the primary neoplasm (arteries are much more resistant) and the formation of tumor emboli. Certain types of cancers have a high propensity for growing in continuity within veins. The renal cell carcinoma may grow within the renal vein in a solid column of cells that occasionally extends up the inferior vena cava to enter the right side of the heart in a long, unbroken, snake-like cord. Hepatocellular carcinomas also frequently invade the portal and hepatic veins. Surprisingly, despite such behavior, there is sometimes no hematogenous dissemination. Even with these exceptions, most hematogenous spread occurs via emboli. Critical to the formation of emboli is cancer cell detachment, a function of alteration in cell surfaces with reduction of their cohesiveness.[25] Several or many tumor cells may clump together to form slightly larger masses, or they may attach to platelets and sometimes be enclosed within a fibrin mesh. The emboli then drain through the venous pathways to arrest in capillary beds, where they may or may not successfully penetrate the walls of the vessels to grow into implants. Thus cancers arising in the abdominal cavity characteristically spread to the liver, and neoplasms draining through the caval systems reach the lungs. However, many features complicate this simplistic view. As already noted, most cells are de-

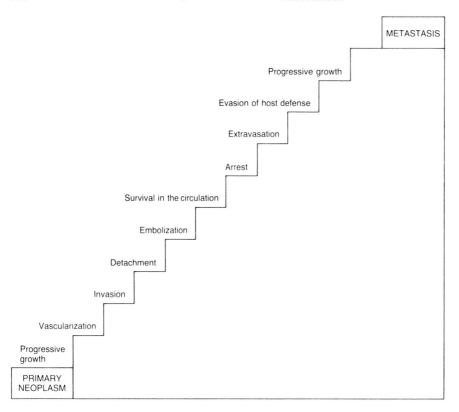

Figure 6–13. Essential steps in the formation of a metastatic lesion. Failure to complete any of the steps will lead to no secondary growth. (Drawn from Hart, I. R., and Fidler, I. J.: The implications of tumor heterogeneity for studies on the biology and therapy of cancer metastasis. Biochim. Biophys. Acta 651:37, 1981. Reproduced with permission.)

stroyed within the circulation. Whether they simply perish by themselves because they cannot survive in isolation or are destroyed by immune mechanisms such as natural killer cells or activated macrophages (as described on p. 216) is not clear. Indeed, from the earlier discussion of tumor progression, it is evident that invasiveness and the ability to metastasize are independent attributes that may or may not have emerged in the clonal evolution of a cancer.

Many observations suggest that *mere anatomic localization of the neoplasm and natural pathways of venous drainage do not wholly explain the systemic distributions of metastases.* For example, prostatic carcinoma preferentially spreads to bone, bronchogenic carcinomas tend to involve the adrenals and the brain, and neuroblastomas spread to the liver and bones. Cell surface properties, most likely receptors, on the cancer cells or on the endothelial cells appear to underlie such distributions.[15] Ingeniously, it has been possible to select sublines from a variety of cancers—notably the B-16 mouse melanoma—that will selectively "home" to specific organs such as the lung, liver, brain, or ovary. In the case of a "lung subline" it can be shown that irrespective of where the cancer cells are introduced into the vascular system, they selectively "home" to the lung. When normal lung tissue is implanted into the thigh of the animal, the cancer cells unerringly colonize it and the native lungs. The fact that this "homing" attribute relates to the cell surface is documented by the ability to transfer "lung preference" to other cancer cell lines by fusing onto them vesicles of plasma membrane shed by pulmonary homing sublines (Fig. 6–14). Conversely, it has long been observed that malignant neoplasms rarely metastasize to skeletal muscles and seldom to the spleen. Although this could be attributable to what has been called "unfavorable soil," conceivably it may relate to the lack of receptor interactions between tumor cells and endothelial cells in these tissues. However, despite all of the foregoing considerations, the localization of metastases cannot be predicted with any form of cancer. Evidently many tumors have not read all of the experimental literature. Moreover, the precise point in the natural course of the disease when metastases are likely to appear is highly variable and unpredictable. But it can be said—*the larger and the more undifferentiated and anaplastic the primary tumor, the greater likelihood of hematogenous dissemination.*

In conclusion, the various features discussed in the preceding sections, as summarized in Table 6–3, permit the differentiation of benign and malignant neoplasms.

## GRADING AND STAGING OF CANCER

Methods to quantify the probable clinical aggressiveness of a given neoplasm and, further, to express its apparent extent and spread in the individual patient are necessary for comparisons of end results of various therapeutic modalities. The results of treating extremely small, highly differentiated thyroid

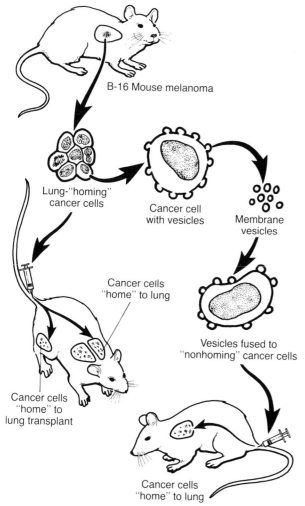

**Figure 6–14.** Experimental model documenting the preferential localization in lung tissue of the B-16 mouse melanoma.

B-16 Mouse melanoma

Lung-"homing" cancer cells

Cancer cell with vesicles

Membrane vesicles

Cancer cells "home" to lung

Vesicles fused to "nonhoming" cancer cells

Cancer cells "home" to lung transplant

Cancer cells "home" to lung

cancer may be classified as Grade I, II, III, or IV with increasing anaplasia. Criteria for the individual grades vary with each form of neoplasia and so will not be detailed here. Moreover, difficulties in establishing clear-cut criteria have led increasingly to descriptive characterizations—e.g., well-differentiated adenocarcinoma with no evidence of vascular or lymphatic invasion, or highly anaplastic sarcoma with extensive vascular invasion, and so forth. Thus grading of cancers has proved of less clinical value than their staging.

*The staging of cancers is based on the size of the primary lesion, its extent of spread to regional lymph nodes, and the presence or absence of metastases.* Widely used is a so-called *TNM system* for each type of cancer—T for primary tumor, N for regional lymph node involvement, and M for metastases. This method of staging is applicable to all forms of neoplasia.[26] A specific neoplasm would be characterized using this system as T1, T2, T3, or T4, with increasing size of the primary lesion; N0, N1, N2, or N3, to indicate progressively advancing nodal disease; and M0 or M1 according to whether there are distant metastases. As will be seen, the Stage T1 is often further subdivided to indicate those lesions that are in situ and those with minimal local invasion. Unfortunately, other systems are also sometimes used that employ a different nomenclature. The cancers are divided into Stages 0 to IV, incorporating the size of primary lesions as well as the presence of nodal spread and of distant metastases.[27] Examples of the application of these two staging systems will be cited in later chapters. It is worth noting here, however, that the staging of neoplastic disease in the patient has assumed great importance in the selection of the best form of therapy for the patient.

Against this background of the structure and behavior of neoplasms, we can turn to some considerations of its nature and origins.

adenocarcinomas that are localized to the thyroid gland will be different from those obtained from treatment of highly anaplastic thyroid cancers that have invaded the neck organs.

*The grading of a cancer attempts to establish some estimate of its aggressiveness or level of malignancy based on the cytologic differentiation of tumor cells and the number of mitoses within the tumor.* The

## ATTRIBUTES OF TRANSFORMED (CANCEROUS) CELLS

*When normal cells are exposed in vitro to carcinogenic agents, be they chemicals, viruses or radiant*

**Table 6–3.** COMPARISONS BETWEEN BENIGN AND MALIGNANT TUMORS*

| Characteristics | Benign | Malignant |
|---|---|---|
| Differentiation—anaplasia | Well-differentiated; structure may be typical of tissue of origin | Some lack of differentiation with anaplasia; structure is often atypical |
| Rate of growth | Usually progressive and slow; may come to a standstill or regress; mitotic figures are rare and normal | Erratic and may be slow to rapid; mitotic figures usually numerous and abnormal |
| Encapsulation—invasion | Usually encapsulated, but rarely capsule is lacking; generally cohesive and expansile | Invasive without encapsulation; usually infiltrative, but may be seemingly cohesive and expansile |
| Metastasis | Absent | Frequently present; the larger and more undifferentiated the primary, the more likely metastases |

*From Robbins, S. L., Cotran, R. S., and Kumar, V.: Pathologic Basis of Disease. 3rd ed. Philadelphia, W. B. Saunders Co., 1984, p. 229.

*energy, they acquire a variety of phenotypic altera-
tions conferring on them cancerous attributes and
are said to have undergone transformation.* The
specific features characterizing transformation will be
presented later, but ultimately it confers on cells the
ability to produce a cancerous lethal neoplasm when
introduced into an appropriate host. *Transformation
does not occur all at once, but rather appears to be
the selective acquisition of increased growth vigor
and escape from controls by sequential clones (referred to as "immortalization") until finally the fully
transformed cancerous state is achieved.* During the
process some attributes may be acquired before others and so some of the clones, while phenotypically
altered, may not yet be tumorigenic; therefore, *transformation of normal cells into the malignant phenotype constitutes the beginning of tumor progression.*
Still unresolved is the central question—are the
changes the consequence of a succession of mutational events or could they be epigenetic in origin,
perhaps related to activation or suppression of successive genes? Although we shall return later to this
fundamental question, it suffices for now that the
weight of evidence suggests that this multistage process involves multiple genes and multiple mechanisms.[28] Whatever the underlying mechanism, cell
proliferation is required to "fix" the transformed state
permanently. Selection may be involved in this process (i.e., the preferential survival of clones having
the greatest proliferative potential). In the absence
of cell proliferation, transformation in vitro is reversible. What then are the phenotypic attributes involved in transformation? In the following discussions
they will be divided arbitrarily into (1) altered growth
properties, (2) morphologic changes, (3) karyotypic
changes, (4) antigenic changes, (5) metabolic deviations, and (6) altered surface features. *It is important
to note that none of these deviations from the norm
is invariably present in all transformed cells and so
none can be construed as a reliable marker of the
cancerous phenotype. The ultimate criterion of complete transformation is the capacity to form tumors
when implanted into appropriate hosts.*

## CHANGES IN GROWTH PROPERTIES

The alterations in cell growth incurred in transformation can be summarized as follows:

○ *Apparent escape from regulatory controls.* Normal
cells grown in culture containing serum continue
to divide until they form a confluent monolayer,
at which time further replication ceases because of
"contact inhibition" or "density-dependent inhibition." Transformed cells are not "contact inhibited"
and are less subject to "density-dependent inhibition of growth" (possibly reflecting lowered requirements for supportive growth factors such as
are present in serum). Thus, when transformed
cells are grown in culture, they pile up in multilayered, disorderly masses (Fig. 6–15).

○ *Failure to maturate.* By not undergoing terminal

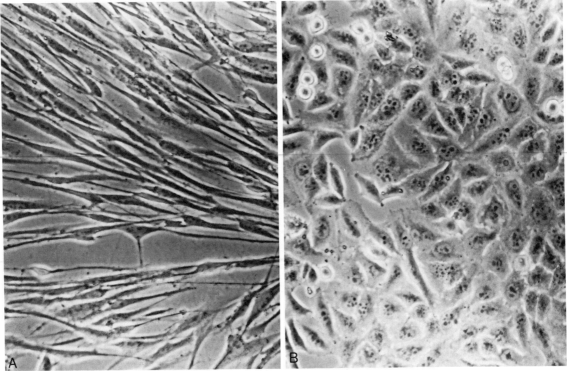

Figure 6–15. *A,* Orderly, oriented growth in culture of normal fibroblasts. Compare with disoriented, random growth of transformed fibroblasts in *B.* (Courtesy of Dr. Tom Wright, Brigham and Women's Hospital and Harvard Medical School, Boston, MA.)

differentiation and cell death, transformed cells retain for longer periods of time their viability and capacity to replicate and accumulate.

○ *Transformed cells are "immortal."* Normal cells capable of being maintained in subculture undergo only a finite number of cell divisions before they perish; transformed cells can be subcultured indefinitely (some have been maintained for decades).

○ *Transplantability.* Fully transformed cells can be grown in vitro in artificial culture media; they have lowered requirements for serum. They can also be introduced into syngeneic hosts without difficulty, in contrast to normal differentiated cells.

All of these characteristics confer a growth advantage on transformed cells vis-à-vis normal cells.

## MORPHOLOGIC CHANGES

In the discussion of differentiation and anaplasia, the cancerous phenotype was noted to be marked by alterations in cell morphology. For example, transformed fibroblasts no longer assume orderly bipolar spindle shapes but have more variegated shapes, sometimes with multipolar profiles. Although morphologic alterations, when present, strongly suggest that transformation is in process or has been achieved, their absence does not deny it, nor is their presence a reliable marker.

## KARYOTYPIC CHANGES

As you know, alterations in the karyotype only become evident when some major mutational event has occurred. Although current banding techniques (p. 117) permit high resolution analysis of the substructure of individual chromosomes, the absence of an apparent chromosomal change does not preclude the possibility of an abnormality involving one or more genes that is beyond present means of resolution. Nonetheless, alterations in the karyotype have now been identified in a great many transformed and cancerous cells and there is a strong possibility that gene changes are present in all. The demonstrated alterations take the forms of abnormal numbers of chromosomes and abnormalities in specific chromosomes, mainly involving translocations and deletions. *In certain types of neoplasms in humans the karyotypic abnormality is nonrandom and common, which strongly suggests that it is a primary event in the development of the malignant state. Such observations and others underlie the current widely held proposition that the origins of cancers lie within particular genes—"oncogenes"* (discussed later, p. 208). However, it should be cautioned that cytogenetic abnormalities may merely reflect fragile sites within chromosomes vulnerable to breaks and rearrangements in a rapidly replicating population. More-

over, even when a nonrandom, potentially "primary alteration" has appeared, tumor progression is often accompanied by ever greater karyotypic deviation.[29] Thus the karyotype may vary somewhat among the many clones making up a fully evolved cancer. Nonetheless, it is usually possible to identify a modal pattern and nonrandom abnormalities and to differentiate them from secondary changes.

It would only be confusing to attempt to detail all of the observed karyotypic abnormalities now recorded for the many types of human cancers and transformed cells. Many will be described with the later consideration of specific forms of neoplasia. Some generalizations and examples will suffice for now.

Specific karyotypic aberrations have been associated with most leukemias and lymphomas, but progress has been much slower with solid tumors.[30] *Most notable and first described is the Philadelphia (Ph¹) chromosome in chronic myelogenous leukemia (CML), comprising a reciprocal and balanced translocation (no genetic material is lost) between chromosome 22 and, usually, 9 (and in a small percentage, a translocation to other chromosomes).* As a consequence, chromosome 22 appears somewhat abbreviated. *This change is present in over 90% of cases of CML and indeed constitutes a reliable marker of the disease.* The Ph¹ chromosome can be identified in the myeloblastic, erythroblastic, and megakaryocytic lines of cells. Indeed, the few cases of CML lacking the Ph¹ tend to be more resistant to therapy and have a worse prognosis. As we see later (p. 209), a putative oncogene is present at or close to the breakpoint in chromosome 9, suggesting that a shift in the location of the oncogene is fundamental to the development of CML.[31] Another example, in *over 90% of the instances of Burkitt's lymphoma (BL), the cells have a translocation usually between chromosomes 8 and 14, and less often between 8 and 2 or 22.* Once again an apparent oncogene has been assigned to the breakpoint on chromosome 8 (Fig. 6–16).[32] Analogous karyotypic abnormalities have been associated with many other varieties of leukemia and lymphoma.

Although some apparently nonrandom abnormalities have been associated with certain solid tumors (e.g., small cell lung carcinoma, neuroblastoma, carcinoma of the ovary, and meningioma), most solid cancers have not yet yielded apparent primary cytogenetic alterations. Nonetheless, aneuploidy, hyperdiploidy, and abnormal chromosome morphology is commonly present. It is possible that some of these aberrations are secondary abnormalities that may have played some role in the progressive acquisition of cancerous behavior, but analysis of many clones derived from a single solid tumor may reveal a modal pattern. However, it is important to stress that a significant number of solid tumors appear to be diploid; whether subtle gene changes are present has not yet been established. It is, however, relevant that in some forms of familial tumors identical specific

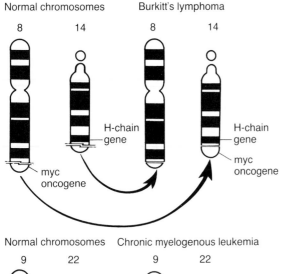

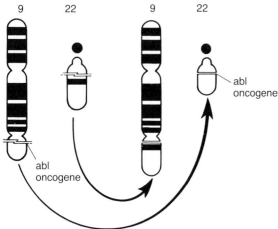

Figure 6–16. The chromosomal translocations with associated oncogenes in chronic myelogenous leukemia and Burkitt's lymphoma.

nonrandom changes have been identified in the neoplasms borne by all members of the family.[33, 33a]

## ANTIGENIC CHANGES

The issue of whether cancerous cells in humans bear antigens that are different from those of normal cells and can be recognized by the immune system of the host has long been and remains highly controversial.[34] The controversy has its roots in the extrapolation of results obtained in animal model systems to humans. Nonetheless, a few generalizations can be made.

○ Cancers in animals induced by oncogenic viruses and chemical carcinogens possess tumor antigens that evoke "immune" responses.

○ Spontaneous tumors in animals are weakly, if at all, immunogenic, but more sensitive methods using highly specific monoclonal antibodies may modify this conclusion.

○ There are hints that some cancers in humans evoke

defensive reactions, but it is not clear that these are specific immune responses.

○ Such defensive reactions as can be demonstrated in humans are likely to be triggered by tumor-associated antigens shared by histogenetically similar neoplasms.

○ There is no unequivocal evidence that human cancers possess unique tumor-specific antigens.

In experimental model systems, tumor antigenicity is generally assessed by (a) the ability of an animal to resist a tumor implant following previous exposure to live or killed tumor cells, (b) the ability of a non-tumor-bearing animal to resist a challenge when infused with immunocompetent cells from a tumor-bearing syngeneic host, and (c) the in vitro demonstration of tumor cell growth inhibition or destruction by cell-mediated or humoral effectors derived from tumor-bearing animals. Using these approaches it has been possible to document that viral and chemically induced cancers in experimental animals often have two types of antigens: tumor-specific antigens (TSA), present only on tumor cells and different from those expressed by normal cells, and tumor-associated antigens (TAA), present in tumor cells but also in normal tissues. Because these tumor antigens, when administered to a normal animal, can induce resistance to a tumor implant, they are sometimes referred to as TSTA or TATA (tumor-specific or tumor-associated transplantation antigens).

*Tumors induced by both RNA and DNA viruses generally express strong antigens, which are membrane associated and are shared by all tumors induced by the same virus.* Some viral tumors develop individually unique "private" antigens. In addition, DNA viruses often induce nuclear antigens that do not participate in resistance to tumors but are involved in the transformation of normal cells into tumor cells (discussed later).[35] *Chemically induced tumors express "private" antigens, not shared by other tumors induced by the same chemical even in the same animal.* These antigens are not as effective in evoking immunity as those induced by viruses. In a few instances, it has been shown that the antigens in chemically induced neoplasms are the consequence of an endogenous retrovirus common in mice and as such are not "private" antigens.[36] Spontaneous neoplasms in animals as mentioned are, in general, not immunogenic or weakly immunogenic, but this could reflect a lack of sensitivity of the assay methods.

The evidence that human cancers express tumor antigens is at best equivocal. It derives largely from the observations that certain cancers evoke significant lymphocytic infiltrates. These infiltrates are thought to be composed of immunocompetent cells, since in general these tumors carry a somewhat better prognosis than those neoplasms unassociated with lymphocytic responses. In addition the evidence comes from in vitro assays, demonstrating the capacity of lymphocytes and sera from tumor patients to inhibit the growth or cause lysis of tumor cells in culture.[37]

The cancers yielding the strongest evidence for the existence of tumor antigens are melanocarcinomas, neuroblastomas, Burkitt's lymphoma, leukemia, osteogenic sarcomas, and cancers of the colon. But these antigens are shared by similar tumors in other hosts, i.e., they are associated with the histogenetic type of tumor rather than with the individual neoplasm. Furthermore, they appear to represent differentiation antigens particular to the differentiation stage at which the cancer cells are arrested. Normal embryonic cells bear similar antigens. Supporting this view is the recent suggestion that certain antigens in the major histocompatibility complex, not normally expressed in adult cells, may emerge in the course of malignant transformation.[38] Apparently, genetic programs repressed in differentiated cells are derepressed in the course of transformation. In this context certain cancers express embryonic antigens—e.g., yolk sac and hepatocellular carcinomas often elaborate alpha-fetoprotein (p. 226), and carcinomas of the colon as well as many other forms of cancer frequently produce carcinoembryonic antigen (p. 226). These oncofetal antigens are of little functional importance in the induction of a tumor rejection reaction. In conclusion, such antigens as may be elaborated by certain spontaneous cancers in humans are common antigens shared by other similar tumors and by differentiating normal cells. Perhaps neoplasms express these antigens in greater quantity than normal differentiating cells. Whether the antigens in spontaneous neoplasms, whatever their nature, evoke specific immune responses is still controversial because, as will be pointed out later, much of the host defense against tumors may be effected by nonspecific macrophage and natural killer cell activity (discussed on p. 216).

## METABOLIC CHANGES

Several generalizations can be made. (1) None of the observed biochemical aberrations in cancer cells can be construed as hallmarks of cancer. (2) The better the differentiation of the cancer cell, the more nearly its enzyme profile resembles that of its normal forebears. (3) The more anaplastic and undifferentiated the tumor cell, the greater the deviation from the enzyme system of the normal cell. (4) *Ultimately all primitive anaplastic cells converge on a common simplified metabolic and enzyme pattern* sometimes referred to as "the biochemical convergence of tumors." As always the question arises—is the observed aberration fundamental to the carcinogenic process or is it a secondary attribute? A few of the observations follow.

Warburg observed that cancer cells exhibit an unusually high rate of anaerobic metabolism even in the presence of oxygen—so-called aerobic glycolysis—which is now recognized as a characteristic of all rapidly growing cells, neoplastic and non-neoplastic.[39]

Similarly, "the biochemical convergence of tumors" reveals no profound insights into the nature of cancer. Weinhouse[40] has aptly stated, "The highly neoplastic cell which has been transplanted many generations is like a stripped down racing car in which other metabolic activities have been subordinated to the overwhelming compulsion to divide." Although the enzyme profiles of differentiated cancers generally resemble those of normal cells, the levels of some enzymes may be depleted, whereas others are increased. In experimental chemical liver carcinogenesis it has been shown that enzyme changes appear early in the process of hepatocellular carcinogenesis.[41] Particularly common is increased synthesis and release of various degradative enzymes as well as activators of plasminogen. Many other metabolic and biochemical deviations might be mentioned, such as production of fetal antigens (mentioned earlier), membrane changes (to be discussed), and the ectopic production of hormones, but it suffices that none appears to be fundamental to the cancerous phenotype.

## CELL SURFACE AND MEMBRANE CHANGES

A host of surface and membrane alterations have been described involving aspects of surface specializations (microvilli, pseudopodia), the biochemical makeup of the plasma membrane, and many other features. Only a few of the more significant will be mentioned.[15]

○ *Alterations in membrane glycoproteins.* Changes include loss or shedding of the glycoprotein fibronectin and increased lectin agglutinability—lectins are agents that agglutinate cells by cross-linking sugars on adjacent cells. Lectin agglutinability has been correlated with metastatic potential.

○ *Loss of cohesiveness and adhesiveness.*[25] This phenomenon might be mediated by several mechanisms, including a decrease in fibronectin, lectin, or matrix receptors. In passing, it might be noted that shedding of cells underlies the Papanicolaou cytologic test.

○ *Synthesis and release of growth factors.* By feedback, cell growth is promoted—so-called autocrine stimulation.

○ *Synthesis of particular types of surface receptors.* Such changes may act in the response of cancerous cells to growth factors and may also play a role in preferential localization of metastases.

○ *Impaired cell-to-cell communication.* This could result from abnormalities in membrane gap junctions or from intracellular unresponsiveness to membrane-derived signals.[42]

○ *Elaboration and release of degradative enzymes.* These enzymes include proteases such as fibrinolysins involved in invasiveness and metastasis (p. 193).

○ *Elaboration and release of plasminogen activator.*
○ *Elaboration and release of procoagulant factors.* This phenomenon is associated with particular types of cancers, producing the hypercoagulable state, e.g., venous thrombosis, DIC (p. 395).
○ *Enhanced transmembrane transport of nutrients and metabolites.* By this method, cell replication is facilitated.

The asocial behavior of transformed cancer cells, escape from controls, invasiveness, and ability to metastasize (i.e., the malignant phenotype) may well be attributable to surface changes that constitute the interface between the cancer cells and their immediate environment. Indeed it has been said that in the last analysis, "Cancer is a membrane disease."

## CARCINOGENIC AGENTS AND THEIR CELLULAR INTERACTIONS

Neoplastic transformation of cells can be achieved in vitro and cancers induced in experimental animals by a variety of agents, principally chemical carcinogens, oncogenic viruses, and radiant energy. Moreover, certain chemicals and radiation have been shown to be responsible for some cancers in humans, and the evidence implicating viruses grows stronger daily. No attempt will be made to present the entire catalogue of known carcinogens; only some of the more important prototypes follow, particularly as they shed light on the possible mechanisms of cancer induction.

### CHEMICAL CARCINOGENS

It is now about 200 years since the London surgeon Sir Percival Pott correctly attributed scrotal skin cancer in chimney sweeps to chronic exposure to soot. A few years later, based on this observation, the Danish Chimney Sweeps Guild ruled that its members must bathe daily. No public health measure since that time has achieved so much in the control of a form of cancer! Nonetheless, these dramatic results lay unnoted for over a century, until Yamagiwa and Ichikawa in 1915 reawakened interest in Pott's observation by inducing cancer in a rabbit's ear with the repeated application of coal tar. Subsequently, Kennaway and Cook, in a monumental feat, extracted 50 grams of a chemically pure carcinogen, 3,4-benzpyrene, from *two tons* of crude coal tars. These pioneering observations documented the carcinogenicity of polycyclic aromatic hydrocarbons. Since then, hundreds of chemicals have been shown to be carcinogenic in animals.[43, 44]

The following pertinent observations have emerged from the study of chemical carcinogens:

1. They are of extremely diverse structure and include both natural and synthetic products.
2. Some are **direct-reacting** and require no chemical transformation to induce carcinogenicity, but others are **indirect-reacting** and become active only after metabolic conversion. Such agents are referred to as **procarcinogens** and their active end products are called **ultimate carcinogens**.

3. All chemical carcinogens, both the direct-reacting and the ultimate carcinogens, are highly reactive electrophiles (have electron-deficient atoms) that react with the electron-rich atoms in RNA, cellular proteins, and, mainly, DNA.

4. The carcinogenicity of many chemicals, particularly weak carcinogens, is augmented by agents that by themselves have little if any cancerous activity. Such augmenting agents are referred to as **promoters**. However, strong carcinogens have no requirement for promoting agents.

5. The transforming effects of carcinogens on DNA are permanent and irreversible. However, the effects of promoters are transient, reversible, and appear to involve epigenetic mechanisms.

6. Several chemical carcinogens may act in concert or with other types of carcinogenic influences (e.g., viruses or radiation) to induce neoplasia—cocarcinogenesis.

Some of the major agents are presented in Table 6–4. Only a few comments are offered on some.

### Table 6–4. MAJOR CHEMICAL CARCINOGENS*

**Direct-Acting Carcinogens**
*Alkylating agents*
Beta-propiolactone
Dimethyl sulfate
Diepoxybutane
Anticancer drugs (cyclophosphamide, chlorambucil, nitrosoureas, and others)
*Acylating agents*
1-Acetyl-imidazole
Dimethylcarbamyl chloride

**Procarcinogens that Require Metabolic Activation**
*Polycyclic and heterocyclic aromatic hydrocarbons*
Benz(a)anthracene
Benzo(a)pyrene
Dibenz(a,h)anthracene
3-Methylcholanthrene
7,12-Dimethylbenz(a)anthracene
*Aromatic amines, amides, azo dyes*
2-Naphthylamine (beta-naphthylamine)
Benzidine
2-Acetylaminofluorene
Dimethylaminoazobenzene (butter yellow)
*Natural plant and microbial products*
Aflatoxin $B_1$
Griseofulvin
Cycasin
Safrole
Betel nuts
*Others*
Nitrosamine and amides
Vinyl chloride, nickel, chromium
Insecticides, fungicides
Polychlorinated biphenyls (PCBs)

*Modified from Robbins, S. L., Cotran, R. S., and Kumar, V.: Pathologic Basis of Disease. 3rd ed. Philadelphia, W. B. Saunders Co., 1984, p. 237.

## Direct-Acting Agents

These substances as noted require no metabolic conversion to become carcinogenic. They are in general weak carcinogens and, depending on time-dosage considerations, may not produce tumors. However, they have importance because some of them are cancer chemotherapeutic drugs (e.g., alkylating agents) that have successfully cured, controlled, or delayed recurrence of certain types of cancer (e.g., leukemia, lymphoma, Hodgkin's disease, ovarian carcinoma) only to later evoke a second form of cancer, usually leukemia. This tragic consequence has been called a "Pyrrhic victory" which becomes less of a victory when their initial use has been for non-neoplastic disorders such as rheumatoid arthritis and Wegener's granulomatosis.[45] The risk of induced cancer is low but dictates the need for the judicious use of such agents.

## Indirect-Acting Agents

This designation indicates that the chemicals require metabolic conversion before they become active. Some of the most potent indirect chemical carcinogens—the *polycyclic hydrocarbons*—are present in fossil fuels. Benz(a)anthracene will produce cancer wherever it is applied—painted on the skin it will induce skin cancers, injected subcutaneously it induces fibrosarcomas. Polycyclics are also produced in the combustion of organic substances. For example, benzo(a)pyrene and other carcinogens are formed in the high-temperature combustion of tobacco in cigarette smoking. These products are implicated in the role of cigarette smoking in lung cancer. Polycyclic hydrocarbons may also be produced from animal fats in the process of broiling meats and are present in smoked meats and fish. The principal active products in many hydrocarbons are epoxides, which form covalent bonds with molecules in the cell, principally DNA, but also with RNA and proteins.[46]

Another class of indirect agents are the *aromatic amines and azo dyes*. Beta-naphthylamine has been responsible, before its carcinogenicity was recognized, for a 50-fold increased incidence of bladder cancers in workers heavily exposed in the aniline dye and rubber industries.[47] Many other occupational carcinogens are discussed on page 273. Benzidine, another aromatic amine, was once used in medicine for testing for occult blood in the stools. Some of the azo dyes were developed to color food—e.g., butter yellow to make margarine more enticing, and scarlet red for maraschino cherries. What price esthetics? Most of the aromatic amines and azo dyes are converted into ultimate carcinogens in the liver by the cytochrome P-450 oxygenase systems and therefore in experimental animals induce hepatocellular carcinomas.

A few *other agents* merit brief mention. *Nitros-amines* and amides have aroused great concern because of the evidence that they can be formed endogenously in the acidic conditions of the stomach. Various amines derived from food may undergo nitrosation with nitrites that have been added to food as preservatives or derived from nitrates by bacterial action.[48] Repeatedly the question has been raised whether nitroso compounds could account for the increased incidence of gastric carcinoma in some populations. Nitroso compounds are also present in tobacco smoke and following absorption could lead to cancers in a variety of organs. *Aflatoxin $B_1$* is of interest because it is a naturally occurring agent produced by some strains of aspergillus, a mold that grows on improperly stored grains and nuts. There is a strong correlation between the dietary level of this food contaminant and the incidence of hepatocellular carcinoma in some parts of Africa and the Far East. However, there is an even stronger correlation between the prevalence of infection with hepatitis B virus and hepatocellular carcinoma. Thus it is not certain whether the aflatoxin acts as a cocarcinogen or instead as an immunosuppressant or promoter. The controversy over the role of saccharin and cyclamates in the induction of cancer is pointed out on page 251. Finally attention should be called to vinyl chloride, arsenic, nickel, chromium, insecticides, fungicides, and PCBs as potential carcinogens in the workplace and about the house.

## Mechanisms of Action of Chemical Carcinogens

The study of chemical carcinogens has provided many insights into the fundamental nature of carcinogenesis. These insights can be summarized as follows:

○ *The great majority of chemical carcinogens are mutagens as can be documented in bacterial assay systems.[49] Thus, they bind directly to DNA and to specific sites within the molecule, inducing miscoding errors during transcription and replication.[50]* However, this does not exclude the possibility that in some instances binding to RNA or cytoplasmic proteins may also take place and be carcinogenic. As corroboration for DNA as the primary target, normal cells can be converted to cancer cells by transfection (transfer of genes by recombinant DNA techniques) of DNA from chemically transformed cells.

○ *The carcinogenicity of chemical agents is dose-dependent, and multiple fractional doses over time have the same oncogenicity as a single comparable dose.* The time interval between fractional doses can be considerably extended (within limits) and thus the critical carcinogenic effect, which has been termed *initiation*, is virtually irreversible.

○ *The carcinogenicity of chemical agents can be significantly enhanced by the subsequent adminis-*

tration of so-called promoters such as phorbol esters, which themselves are nontumorigenic, or virtually nontumorigenic. Strong carcinogens or sufficiently large doses of weak initiators may not require the action of promoters. But in all cases subeffective doses of initiators can be made to yield cancers by the action of promoters, which appear to interact with membrane receptors to stimulate cell replication.

○ *To be effective the promoter must follow the initiator.* When the order is reversed, there may be no tumor yield or a much reduced yield depending on the total dose of initiator. Fractional doses of promoters when widely spaced are without effect, indicating that their action is reversible. On the other hand, when the intervals are not too prolonged, the promoting effect is additive.[51]

○ *The initiation-promotion two-stage sequence has given rise to the recognition that carcinogenesis involves more than a single event.*

○ *Two or more initiators, be they chemical agents, oncogenic viruses, or radiant energy, may act in concert to induce malignant transformation, referred to as cocarcinogenesis.* Thus subeffective doses of one may be synergized by the actions of one or more additional influences.

From these observations, a seductive picture is beginning to emerge. It seems most likely that initiators interact with DNA to induce a mutation that is more or less irreversible. Subsequent exposure to initiators may introduce new mutations leading ever closer to the brink. Promoters, by inducing cell replication, may permit selection of the most aberrant clone or clones and thereby permanently "fix" the transformed state. In the process of cell replication, successive clones of cells develop ever greater genetic errors. Presumably the first mutation may involve "immortalization" and release from growth controls, creating more opportunity for subsequent mutational and oncogenic events. Indeed, it is known that cells already having abnormalities in the genome (as in many genetic syndromes) are particularly susceptible to the effects of initiators or promoters. Thus it appears that *carcinogenesis involves multiple stages, multiple genes, and probably multiple mechanisms.*[28]

There are additional lessons to be learned from chemical carcinogenesis. Because the sequential effects of chemical carcinogens can be additive and because multiple subeffective dosages of cocarcinogens may be tumorigenic, *there is no "safe" threshold level.* Moreover, in humans, promoters may be as important in the induction of cancer as initiators because the effects of initiators are prolonged and lurk in the background, awaiting any promoting influence. However, in experimental systems it can be proved that when a subeffective dose of carcinogen is not followed for some long time by either an additional exposure to a carcinogen or to a promoter, the cells may revert to normal. Thus the mutational error can be repaired as discussed on page 276.

## ONCOGENIC VIRUSES

A large number of viruses have been proved to be oncogenic in a wide variety of animals, ranging from amphibia to our first "cousins" the primates, and the evidence grows ever stronger that certain forms of human cancer are of viral origin. They fall into two classes—single-stranded RNA viruses and double-stranded DNA viruses.[52, 53] In the following discussion, the better characterized agents most intensively studied will be presented first, followed by a consideration of the important insights they have provided into the mechanism(s) of carcinogenesis (and, necessarily, some of the studies in experimental animals). The major agents documented to cause cancer in animals and suspected of being involved in human neoplasia are presented in Table 6–5.

**RNA VIRUSES.** These agents were formerly called oncornaviruses (ONCOgenic-RNA VIRUSES). The seminal studies of Baltimore and of Temin and Mizutani showed that all these viruses possess an RNA-dependent DNA polymerase, more commonly known as *reverse transcriptase,* which allows reverse transcription of viral RNA into virus-specific DNA.[54, 55] Hence these agents are now known as *retroviruses.* The DNA transcript may then be incorporated within the genome of the cell in the form of a virogene or provirus. Some RNA viruses (e.g., leukemia viruses) are so-called defective—their virogenes are replication-defective and require a helper virus. Others such as the avian sarcoma virus are nondefective; their virogenes are capable of synthesizing more virus, and the cell infection is called "productive." The outcome of cell infection by all oncogenic viruses, including DNA agents, depends on the high degree of viral specificity for cell type and species and on host resistance and other factors. Thus DNA agents may cause cytolysis, latent infection, or transformation. In general, cells that are permissive and support viral replication undergo cytolysis; cells that are nonpermissive may or may not undergo transformation. Unlike the case with DNA agents, cells transformed by retroviruses may bear demonstrable viral particles and the virus may be passaged, but sometimes only if there is concomitant helper virus. As will be shown later, the entire viral RNA is not necessary for transformation; only a fragment when incorporated into the genome of the host cell may suffice. Indeed, it has been possible to dissect the viral RNA and its DNA transcript and show that only a single gene—*an oncogene*—is necessary for transformation. Furthermore, long, terminal repeat (LTR) sequences at each end of the viral RNA (containing regulatory sequences for expression of genetic material) may do the same.[56] This surprising finding led to the recognition that retroviruses not possessing oncogenes may nonetheless be capable of transforming cells, albeit slowly (p. 206). Viruses having oncogenes effect transformation relatively quickly and are known as "acutely transforming" agents.

**Table 6–5.** SELECTED ONCOGENIC VIRUSES

| Agent | Type of Neoplasia | Strength of Evidence |
|---|---|---|
| **RNA** | | |
| *In animals* | | |
| Avian sarcoma (Rous) virus (ASV) | Fibrosarcoma in avian and various mammalian species | Proven |
| Abelson leukemia virus | Lymphosarcoma/leukemia in mice | Proven |
| Leukemia viruses | Leukemia in mice, cats, gibbon ape | Proven |
| Murine mammary tumor virus (MMTV) | Breast cancers in young mice | Proven |
| *In humans* | | |
| Human T-cell leukemia virus (HTLV-1) | T-cell leukemia/lymphoma | Almost certain |
| Mammary tumor virus | Breast carcinoma | Weak |
| Uncharacterized agents | Leukemias, lymphomas | Weak |
| **DNA** | | |
| *In animals* | | |
| Papovaviruses, polyomavirus | Variety of epithelial and mesenchymal tumors in hamsters, rats, mice | Proven |
| Simian vacuolating virus (SV-40) | Sarcomas in leukemia, lymphoma in hamsters, mice, and rats; transforms monkey cells in culture | Proven |
| Adenoviruses of human and animal origin | Sarcomas in hamsters, rats, mice; transforms cells of various origin | Proven |
| Herpesviruses (HSV, many strains) | Tumors in frogs; leukemia/lymphoma in fowl, guinea pigs, monkeys | Proven |
| *In humans* | | |
| Human papillomavirus (HPV—many strains) | Common warts and closely related condylomata | Proven |
| | Squamous cell carcinoma in hereditary epidermodysplasia verruciformis | Almost certain |
| | Vulvar and cervical carcinoma | Uncertain |
| Herpesviruses | | |
|   HSV-2 | Vulvar and cervical carcinoma | Uncertain |
|   Epstein-Barr virus (EBV) | African Burkitt's lymphoma, nasopharyngeal carcinoma | Probable |
|   Cytomegalovirus (CMV) | Kaposi's sarcoma | Weak |
| Hepatitis B virus (HBV) | Hepatocellular carcinoma | Probable |

**DNA VIRUSES.** There are major differences between the oncogenic DNA viruses and retroviruses. The former do not have reverse transcriptases, and so the viral DNA or a portion of it is directly incorporated within the genome of susceptible cells. In contrast to the case with the retroviruses, cells undergoing transformation by the DNA viruses cannot replicate more virus; multiplication of virus causes cytolysis. Thus it is apparent that infectious virus cannot be isolated from cells transformed by DNA viruses and, moreover, the oncogenicity of DNA viruses appears to depend on the protracted interaction of viral genome and host-cell genome and the suppression of viral replicative function. Identification of oncogenic DNA viruses within transformed cells must depend then either on the detection of footprints such as genetic sequences within the transformed cells homologous to the genome of the virus or on the presence of viral related antigens. Indeed, many of the DNA oncogenic agents produce T (tumor) antigens or analogous proteins that appear to be important in the transforming function of the agents.[57] As with the retroviruses, cell transformation or cancer induction in vivo occurs in association with integration of a part or all of the viral DNA into the genome of the host's cells.

### Mechanisms of Viral Carcinogenesis

Deeper penetrations have been made into the biomolecular events involved in retroviral cell transformation and cancer induction than is the case with the DNA viruses. In particular, the very small agents, such as the avian sarcoma retrovirus and certain murine leukemia retroviruses, have permitted correlation between individual viral genes and their functions. Several lines of evidence have documented that some of the retroviruses contain a single gene responsible for cell transformation. Such genes are referred to as v-oncogenes (v-oncs). Unexpected was the finding that *the normal genome of nearly all species in the biologic kingdom (including humans) harbors genes called proto-oncogenes or cellular oncogenes (c-oncs), referred to by Bishop as the "enemies within."*[58] They are closely homologous to v-oncs. The conservation of c-oncs throughout evolution in species as diverse as yeast and humans suggests that they have essential roles, probably in cell differentiation or in regulation of cell division.[59] Many lines of evidence strongly suggest that acutely transforming retroviruses emerged by capture, incorporation, and modification of cellular oncogenes during evolutionary development.[60] Indeed, the genome of normal cells is believed to contain more than one and possibly many proto-oncogenes. Thus the following conclusions about retroviral carcinogenesis are possible.

○ "Acutely transforming retroviruses" that have v-oncogenes acquired them during evolution by capture and perhaps modification of c-oncogenes (c-oncs).

○ Retroviruses lacking a v-oncogene may cause cancer by inducing mutation of c-oncs.

○ Retroviral promoter sequences (e.g., *LTR*), when inserted adjacent to a c-oncogene, may cause cancer by overexpression of the c-onc.

○ Retroviruses may also cause cancer by mutation and inactivation of cellular regulatory genes, thereby causing overexpression of c-oncs.

We shall return later to the function of these viral oncogenes and their cellular counterparts, but suffice for now that some synthesize a single polypeptide with tyrosine kinase activity that appears to be a receptor for growth factors (see later). Other transforming proteins are not kinases; some have homology with well-defined normal growth factors, and others have also been identified. An attempt to depict the various pathways leading to the activation of cellular oncogenes is offered in Figure 6–17.

With regard to the DNA agents, their modes of action are still uncertain. In most instances, the viral DNA is inserted into the host cell genome. However, fragments of the viral DNA suffice to induce transformation, suggesting that the transforming function is restricted to certain viral genes. These genes are not "captured" cellular oncogenes, as is the case with retroviruses.[61] With the polyoma and SV-40 viruses, the products of these DNA segments are responsible for the production of nuclear T antigens, which are requisite for cell transformation. Mutants faulty in production and activity of T antigens are incapable of transformation. Papilloma and adenoviruses do not encode T antigens but instead other virus-specified unique proteins necessary for transformation. Thus, as in the case with retroviruses, neoplastic cells transformed by DNA viruses often produce transforming proteins. Critical to the emergence of tumors in vivo is the level of host resistance, possibly immunologic. Thus it has been proposed that the function of transforming proteins, particularly the T antigens, is to govern the level of susceptibility of transformed cells to host defenses.[62]

### Relationship of Oncogenic Viruses to Human Cancer

More is said on this topic with the later consideration of specific forms of neoplasia, and so only a few comments are indicated. To begin at the end, *no form of human cancer has unequivocally been proved to be of viral origin*, although that goal seems tantalizingly close. Only the trivial benign common wart and closely related condylomata enjoy or suffer this distinction, since they are caused by human papillomaviruses. Nonetheless, in the hereditary condition epidermodysplasia verruciformis, characterized by numerous flat warts, there is a high tendency for one or more of the warts to become cancerous. As indicated in Table 6–5 (p. 205), there are varying

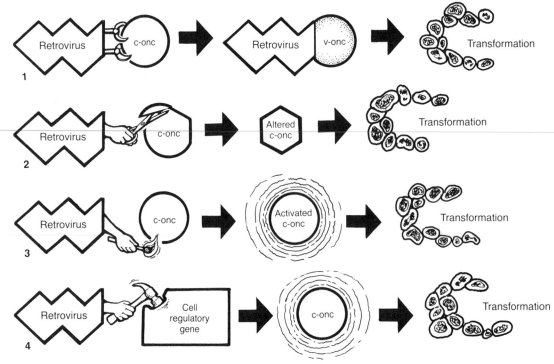

Figure 6–17. Potential pathways (discussed in text) by which retrovirus induces cancerous transformation.

levels of evidence linking a relatively few other forms of human cancer to the oncogenic viruses, but as mentioned, the evidence grows stronger with each passing month.[63] The strongest relationship is the linking of an uncommon form of T-cell leukemia/lymphoma to a unique retrovirus, HTLV-I.[64] The details of the evidence are presented on page 388. Interestingly, HTLV-III is strongly linked to the production of AIDS, characterized by viral invasion of T-lymphocytes (p. 175). Other retroviruses have been associated with, for example, breast carcinoma and certain forms of leukemia and lymphoma, but the documentation is very tenuous.

An incriminating finger has been pointed at several of the DNA agents. There is a substantial body of evidence linking the Epstein-Barr virus (EBV, one of the herpes groups) to the endemic African form of Burkitt's lymphoma (p. 372). Interestingly, this virus is known to cause infectious mononucleosis. There are suggestions that immunologic incompetence, perhaps caused by concomitant malaria, accounts for its oncogenicity in Africa. A similar lymphoma occurs infrequently throughout the world (including the United States) but it is uncertain whether the EBV is implicated in its causation. Significantly, the cells in all Burkitt's lymphomas are characterized by a translocation between chromosomes 8 and, usually, 14. What then are the roles of the virus and the translocation? It is hypothesized that the EBV stimulates proliferation of lymphoid cells by conferring "immortality" on them, setting the stage for the activation of a cellular oncogene located near the breakpoint on chromosome 8.[65] The EBV has also been linked to nasopharyngeal cancer by serologic and hybridization studies revealing viral sequences in the tumor cells. One additional example is the association of herpes simplex virus type II with cervical carcinoma. Here the evidence is largely inferential, as is detailed on page 638. It comprises largely elevated titers to viral antigens and the putative finding of viral DNA sequences in the cancer cells of some patients. However, it is unclear as to whether the viral findings point to an etiologic relationship or merely concomitant infection in patients with tumors. A few other instances in which viruses have been associated with human malignancies were mentioned in Table 6–5 (p. 205) but without convincing documentation. Nonetheless, the recent studies about the role of cellular genes in the origins of cancer (to be detailed later) raise the possibility that viruses may play roles, possibly by their actions on proto-oncogenes, in many forms of human malignant disease.

## RADIATION CARCINOGENESIS

*Radiation, whatever its source—sunlight, x-rays, nuclear fission, radionuclides—is an established carcinogen.*[66] The evidence is so voluminous that only a few examples will suffice. Many of the pioneers in the development of roentgen rays developed skin cancers. Among persons with fair skin, there is a linear correlation between intensity of exposure to sunlight and skin cancer—squamous cell carcinoma, basal cell carcinoma, and malignant melanoma.[67] Miners of radioactive elements have suffered a tenfold increased incidence of lung cancers. The follow-up of survivors of the atomic bombs dropped on Hiroshima and Nagasaki has disclosed a markedly increased incidence of leukemia—principally acute and chronic myelocytic leukemia—after an average latent period of about seven years. Decades later, the leukemia risk in those heavily exposed is still above the level for control populations, as is the mortality rate from thyroid, breast, colon, pulmonary carcinoma and others.[68] Even therapeutic irradiation has been documented to be carcinogenic. Thyroid cancers have developed in approximately 9% of those exposed during infancy and childhood to head and neck irradiation.[69] The previous practice of treating a form of arthritis of the spine known as ankylosing spondylitis with therapeutic irradiation has yielded a ten- to twelvefold increase in the incidence of leukemia years later. Thus, it is abundantly clear that radiation is a potent oncogen.

It is known that radiant energy has the potential of producing mutations and even killing cells, but how does it exert its carcinogenicity? This question remains largely unanswered, but two facts are well established. First, the tumors appear only after a long latent period during which successive generations of clones have developed. This cell replication may be requisite for permanent fixation of the radiation-induced injury and possibly for its amplification. Second, the radiation initiation is generally irreversible but at low dosage levels is amenable to repair (p. 276). Thus tumors may or may not appear when fractional doses are received by cells, depending on dosage, length of the intervals, and capacity of the cells to repair in the intervals. The lack of clear understanding of these modifying factors and the wide variable individual susceptibility makes it impossible to establish "safe" tolerable levels of radiation exposure. This is a principal concern of regulatory agencies and of those who live in proximity to sources of radiant energy (e.g., nuclear energy installations and waste dumps) adding to the inevitable background exposure to sunlight and cosmic radiation.

As mentioned, the ultimate mechanism of radiation carcinogenicity is not understood. Only a few speculations will be offered: (1) radiation-induced mutations may activate proto-oncogenes or, by damaging control regions, permit overexpression of proto-oncogenes; (2) radiation mutations may render cells vulnerable to other carcinogenic influences (e.g., viruses); (3) radiation might cause cell killing, permitting survivors to proliferate and thereby become vulnerable to oncogenic influences; and (4) amplification over time of radiation-induced mutations might ultimately lead to the neoformation of cellular oncogenes. Whatever the mechanism, it is clear that radiation has induced cancers in humans and that its effects are additive, making it clear that its therapeutic and diagnostic medical uses, important as they undoubtedly are, are not without hazard—"Be sure the treatment is not worse than the disease."

## OTHER CARCINOGENS

Cancers have been induced in experimental animals by plastic films, methylcellulose, metal foils, and chronic irritation. However, in all of these instances, the question arises as to whether these interventions provoke cell replication and therefore serve as promoters rather than true initiators. Repeatedly cases are brought to the courts in which the victim of an auto accident or an industrial mishap, who later developed a neoplasm at a site of trauma, contends that the injury evoked the cancer. There is no experimental evidence to support the contention that a single trauma is carcinogenic. More important and relevant is the issue of hormone-associated cancers.[70] Estrogens are of particular concern because of the well-documented increased incidence of endometrial cancer in women taking various forms of exogenous estrogens. Similarly, the development of vaginal adenocarcinoma in young women born of mothers who had taken stilbestrol (an estrogenic agent) during pregnancy is another well-established association. This subject is discussed more fully on page 636, but the weight of evidence favors the view that steroids serve as promoters. In whatever manner, they are potent agents having the potential to lead to an increased frequency of cancer in target organs. Asbestos is a well-established carcinogen inducing an increased incidence of lung carcinomas, mesotheliomas, and other forms of cancer (p. 452). The litany could be extended, but it is clear that we "swim in a sea of carcinogens."

## UNIFYING THEORY OF CARCINOGENESIS

It is almost impossible not to be lured by the rapidly accumulating evidence into attempting a unifying theory of the origins of cancer. *It strongly suggests that the secrets of cancer lie within normal cells themselves in the form of proto-oncogenes (c-oncs).* But how these genes are transformed into activated oncogenes and how they ultimately bring about the phenotypic alterations characteristic of cancer remain mysteries, although there are hints. Not so long ago it was said that "cancer is not a single disease, but rather the wide variety of cancers in humans constitute a family of diseases having diverse

origins." However, identical genetic changes have now been identified in many widely differing types of cancer, although some forms are associated with particular specific gene changes.[1] Before presenting some of this evidence, it must be admitted that the age-old controversy about epigenetic versus genetic mechanisms has not yet been laid to rest, and so first a few brief details about the epigenetic theory will be presented.

## EPIGENETIC ABERRANT DIFFERENTIATION HYPOTHESIS

The thesis that the cancer phenotype represents aberrant differentiation of normal cells involving epigenetic mechanisms is not totally lacking in support. Recall the widely differing phenotypes of normal cells in the adult body, all possessing the identical genome derived from the fertilized ovum. Moreover, this phenotype is heritable—liver cells make liver cells, and adrenal cortical cells make adrenal cortical cells. The "turning on and off" of genes presumably accounts for this variable differentiation. Conceivably, aberrant differentiation yields cancer cells retaining embryonic characteristics capable of active replication and tumorigenesis. Mention was made earlier of the expression of alpha-fetoproteins by germ cell tumors and carcinoembryonic antigen by a variety of cancers, principally colonic carcinoma. Aberrant differentiation involving derepression of genes must account for this production of embryonic proteins and the synthesis of hormones and other bioactive products by tumors of nonendocrine origin. But the strongest documentation that cancer cells do not necessarily bear mutations are the remarkable studies of Illmensee and Mintz.[71] These workers introduced mouse teratocarcinoma cells into normal embryos at the blastocyst stage. Completely normal mosaic mice were achieved whose tissues were derived from the genomes of both the normal embryonic cells and the tumor cells. The genome of the teratocarcinoma cells was intact![72] The epigenetic hypothesis then struggles on, but whether it is solely capable of inducing cancer or instead acts in concert with genetic mechanisms remains a question.

## GENETIC HYPOTHESIS

The belief that the origins of cancer lie within cellular genes grows ever stronger. The proposed model in simplified terms is as follows.[73] *All eukaryotic cells contain cellular oncogenes. Inappropriate overexpression of these genes, or point mutations activating them causes the cell to produce stimulatory growth factors or in some way deranges normal regulatory controls. The quantitative or qualitative changes in the expression of the genome may be brought about by carcinogenic influences—*

*chemicals, viruses, radiation—or by spontaneous random mutations.*

The background for the cellular oncogene model begins with the retroviruses. Intensive studies utilizing hybridization techniques and genetic engineering (splitting viral genome into small segments and cloning genes in bacterial plasmids) have shown that many retroviral genomes have a single gene that, when introduced into appropriate cell types, induces malignant transformation. Currently about 30 viral oncogenes (v-oncs) have been identified, each given a specific designation; for example, *src* for the Rous sarcoma viral agent, *sis* for the simian sarcoma virus, *myc* for the myelocytomatosis agent, and *ras* (there being three subtypes) for rat sarcoma viruses.[74, 75] The field exploded with the discovery that the *sequences in the cellular oncogenes are closely homologous to the v-oncs and that normal cells contain more than a single c-onc, sometimes homologous to more than one v-onc.* The homology and other evidence strongly points (as cited) to "capture" of cellular genes during evolution by acutely transforming retroviruses. The search for transforming DNA sequences in experimentally induced cancers (by all oncogenic agents) and in human "spontaneous" cancers has yielded rich dividends. Discrete, transforming sequences have been identified in a variety of tumor cell lines, including human carcinomas of the prostate, bladder, lung, colon, and pancreas; sarcomas; leukemias; lymphomas; and neuroblastomas.[76] Significantly, the nontumorous cells in these hosts did not have the transforming sequences. Many of these transforming sequences derived from human cancers proved to be closely homologous to v-oncs, in particular one of the *ras* oncogenes. Others are unrelated to identified v-oncs. Even more surprising, the same *ras* oncogene was present in cancers as diverse as lymphomas, leukemias, colon and prostate carcinoma, sarcomas, and neuroblastomas. *Thus it appears that cellular oncogenes, under appropriate circumstances (or perhaps we should say unfortunate circumstances), can be induced to evoke cancers.* Indeed, retroviruses lacking an oncogene when inserted into the genome of the host cell presumably are oncogenic by a mutational or promotor effect on indigenous cellular genes. Further proving the oncogenicity of the c-oncs, small DNA sequences from *normal* cells (presumably harboring one or more of these genes), when introduced by transfection into a "normal" cell line in culture, have induced transformation.[77]

*The question arises—does oncogenesis involve overexpression, or amplification of cellular oncogenes, or instead alteration (mutation) of them?* Studies suggest that all of these potential mechanisms may be operative.[61] Some human cancer cells contain many copies of certain oncogenes associated with increased expression, and the transforming proteins produced by the cellular oncogenes are present in increased amount.[78] Moreover, as pointed out earlier,

mere insertion of a long terminal repeat (LTR) segment found adjacent to the viral genes acting as a promoter or enhancer when in proximity to a cellular oncogene induces neoplastic transformation.[79] Conceivably, the viral insertion may impair cell regulatory sequences, permitting overexpression of one or more proto-oncogenes.[80] But direct impingement on the cellular gene producing a mutation cannot be ruled out. *Indeed, in transforming sequences derived from human cancers, more often structural differences have been identified between the transforming c-oncs and the normal c-oncs.* To date, the alterations identified have been point mutations as simple as substitution of a single nucleotide, resulting in a gene product differing from the normal product in only a few amino acids. So it is thought that *all of the known environmental carcinogens exert their effects by altering the genetic code either affecting regulatory sequences or inducing mutations in cellular oncogenes to thus activate them.* Several mutagens may collaborate or act sequentially, explaining the synergism of various carcinogens—cocarcinogenesis. The proliferative effects of promoters may act by amplifying mutations in a replicating clone. But in addition the mutational event might be a random unfortunate accident.

Transpositions of genetic sequences are thought to be common in the human genome.[81] Most are without consequence, but some may have tragic consequences. In the case of Burkitt's lymphoma, there is an exchange of segments between chromosomes 8 and 14, as cited earlier (p. 199). The breakpoint on chromosome 8 is located at the region of a cellular oncogene (c-myc) that is transposed to a new location on chromosome 14, close to the region coding for the immunoglobulin heavy chain.[82] It was first postulated that c-myc came under the influence of actively transcribing genes, but present evidence indicates a subtle break (mutation) in the gene. Similarly, the Philadelphia chromosome involves a reciprocal translocation between chromosomes 9 and 22. The breakpoint on 9 is close to the *abl* oncogene, and so the transposition locates it in contact with a particular DNA sequence in 22, called *bcr* (breakpoint cluster region). The newly created "hybrid gene" codes for a tyrosine kinase that phosphorylates tyrosine at the plasma membrane (described below).[31] *In any event, activation of oncogenes may be the consequence of quantitative or qualitative perturbations.*

The fact that neoplastic transformation is very likely a multistage process involving tumor progression makes it unlikely that oncogenesis is related to a single mutational event. Not surprisingly then, two (and possibly more) activated oncogenes have been identified in some tumors.[83] American Burkitt's lymphoma, for example, carries both a *ras* and a *myc* oncogene, the latter activated by translocation. Thus it is theorized that activation of one is necessary for "immortalization" of the cell (providing replicative activity and escape from growth controls) and the second oncogene then confers cancerous phenotypic characteristics. Perhaps then the multistage evolution of human cancers and tumor progression involves two or more genetic changes such as the "turning on" of multiple genes or DNA rearrangements creating oncogenes.[82a] Such studies help to explain why cells already bearing a hereditary mutation as in Down's syndrome (p. 121) are particularly susceptible to oncogenesis.

Granting the existence of *cellular* oncogenes and their activation or conversion, how do they ultimately bring about the many phenotypic changes characteristic of cancer cells? Although some penetrations have been made, large black holes remain. It is, however, clear that all oncogenes do not produce the same product.[84] Some code for a kinase that selectively phosphorylates tyrosine at the plasma membrane. The cellular receptor for many well-defined growth factors (e.g., epidermal growth factor) has tyrosine kinase activity, and it is possible that the oncogene-produced receptor is either permanently "turned on" to growth or fails to respond to normal controls. Another product is homologous to one of the chains of the well-defined platelet-derived growth factor (PDGF), and there are still others, but all appear to play some role in cell division or its control. A proposed schema is presented in Figure 6–18. Thus it is possible that cells bearing activated oncogenes may synthesize factors or receptors potentiating or stimulating their own growth—"autocrine stimulation."[85]

*In sum, a wealth of evidence strongly suggests that cancer in animals and humans is at least in large part a genetic-mutational disease.* The strongest documentation comes from the transfection assays producing neoplastic transformation. Indeed, as will be seen in the next chapter, some cancers are hereditary, and hereditary factors contribute to the development of many others, again pointing to the genetic basis of malignant neoplasia. Thus *it is now possible to formulate a unifying hypothesis for the mode of action of all known carcinogenic influences by relating them to their ability to induce mutations in cells. Even in the absence of environmental influences, reshuffling of the DNA code, as by spontaneous translocations or other genetic errors, may impinge on cellular oncogenes and activate them or create new oncogenes.* But lest the "state-of-the-art" be oversimplified, to date only about 30% of human cancers studied have revealed oncogenes. Perhaps with time more will emerge, or as mentioned earlier, epigenetic mechanisms may also in some instances play roles.

Before closing this discussion, it must be pointed out that as with all diseases, host factors play roles. Age is important. The young are especially vulnerable to radiation carcinogenesis, and decades later thyroid carcinoma may emerge following radiation to and about the thyroid during infancy and childhood. The tendency for most cancers to arise in middle and late

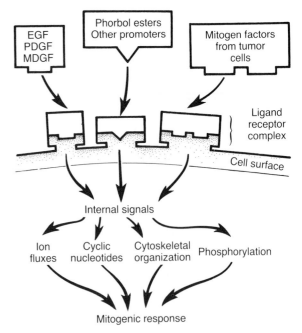

EGF = Epidermal growth factor

PDGF = Platelet-derived growth factor

MDGF = Macrophage-derived growth factor

**Figure 6–18.** Potential pathways by which external influences, membrane receptors, and internal signals induce cell growth.

life may well be attributable to the increased frequency of mitotic errors with aging. Alternatively, with the passing years, mechanisms capable of repair of DNA mutations may be slowed. We know the importance of repair mechanisms from the increased incidence of cancer in various hereditary DNA repair–deficiency syndromes (p. 276).[86] Thus the normal individual may sustain potentially oncogenic mutations that are repaired. Finally, the possible protective role of the immune system should be mentioned as a modifying host factor. Although this controversial subject is discussed in the subsequent chapter in more detail, it suffices that in conditions characterized by immunoincompetence there is an increased predisposition to cancer.

In conclusion, great strides have been made in unravelling the complexities of the origin(s) of cancer and the final goal seems almost within reach, but perhaps our reach is longer than our grasp.

### References

1. Weinberg, R. A.: *ras* Oncogenes and the molecular mechanisms of carcinogenesis. Blood 64:1143, 1984.
2. Willis, R. A.: The Spread of Tumours in the Human Body. 3rd ed. London, Butterworth, 1973.
3. Hertig, A. T., and Sommers, S. C.: Genesis of endometrial carcinoma. A study of prior biopsies. Cancer 2:946, 1949.

4. Sporn, M. B., and Roberts, A. B.: Role of retinoids in differentiation and carcinogenesis. J. Natl. Cancer Inst. 73:1381, 1984.

5. Allred, L. E., and Porter, K. R.: Morphology of normal and transformed cells. In Hynes, R. O. (ed.): Surfaces of Normal and Malignant Cells. New York, John Wiley & Sons, 1979, p. 21.

6. Gabbiani, G.: The cytoskeleton in cancer cells in animals and humans. Methods Achiev. Exp. Pathol., 9:231, 1979.

7. Walts, A. E., et al.: Keratins of different molecular weight in exfoliated mesothelial and adenocarcinoma cells—An aid to cell identification. Am. J. Clin. Pathol. 81:442, 1984.

8. Broder, L. E.: Hormone production by bronchogenic carcinoma. A review. Pathobiol. Annu. 9:205, 1979.

9. Hill, B. T.: The management of human "solid" tumours: Some observations on the irrelevance of traditional cell cycle kinetics and the value of certain recent concepts. Cell Biol. Int. Rep. 2:215, 1978.

10. Editorial: Reversal of cancer. Lancet 1:799, 1983.

11. Fialkow, P. J.: Clonal origin of human tumors. Biochim. Biophys. Acta 458:283, 1976.

12. Baserga, R.: The cell cycle. N. Engl. J. Med. 304:453, 1981.

13. Folkman, J.: Tumor angiogenesis. Adv. Cancer Res. 43:175, 1984.

14. Pennica, D., et al.: Human tumour necrosis factor: Precursor structure, expression and homology to lymphotoxin. Nature 312:724, 1984.

15. Nicolson, G. L.: Cell surface molecules and tumor metastasis. Regulation of metastatic phenotypic diversity. Exp. Cell Res. 150:3, 1984.

16. Foulds, L.: Neoplastic development. Vol. 1. New York, Academic Press, 1969.

17. Liotta, L. A., et al.: Role of collagenases in tumor cell invasion. Cancer Metastasis Rev. 1:277, 1982.

18. Liotta, L. A.: Tumor invasion and metastases: Role of the basement membrane. Am J. Pathol. 117:339, 1984.

19. Barsky, S. H., et al.: Loss of basement membrane components by invasive tumors but not their benign counterparts. Lab. Invest. 49:140, 1983.

20. Sugarbaker, E. V., and Ketcham, A. S.: Mechanisms and prevention of cancer dissemination: An overview. Semin. Oncol. 4:19, 1977.

21. Hart, I. R., and Fidler, I. J.: Cancer invasion and metastasis. Q. Rev. Biol. 55:121, 1980.

22. Knox, P.: Metastasis. Mol. Aspects Med. 7:269, 1984.

23. Fisher, E. R., and Fisher, B.: Circulating cancer cells and metastases. Int. J. Radiat. Oncol. Biol. Phys. 1:87, 1976.

24. Hagmar, B., et al.: Why do tumors metastasize? An overview of current research. Tumour Biol. 5:141, 1984.

25. Weiss, L., and Ward, P. M.: Cell detachment and metastasis. Cancer Metastasis Rev. 2:111, 1983.

26. Commission on Clinical Oncology of the Union Internationale Contre le Cancer (International Union Against Cancer): TNM Classification of Malignant Tumors. Geneva, International Union Against Cancer, 1968.

27. Copeland, M. M.: American Joint Committee on Cancer Staging and End Results reporting. Objectives and progress. Cancer 18:1637, 1965.

28. Weinstein, I. B., et al.: Multistage carcinogenesis involves multiple genes and multiple mechanisms. J. Cell Physiol. 3(Suppl.):127, 1984.

29. Wolman, S. R.: Karyotypic progression in human tumors. Cancer Metastasis Rev. 2:257, 1983.

30. Sandberg, A. A.: Chromosomes in human neoplasia. Curr. Probl. Cancer 8:1, 1983.

31. Stam, K.: Evidence of a new chimeric bcr/c-abl mRNA in patients with chronic myelocytic leukemia and the Philadelphia chromosome. N. Engl. J. Med. 313:1429, 1985.

32. Editorial: Molecular biology and lymphoma. Lancet 1:26, 1984.

33. Bolger, G. B., et al.: Chromosome translocation t(14;22) and oncogene (c—sis) variant in a pedigree with familial meningioma. N. Engl. J. Med. 312:564, 1985.

33a. Brodeur, G. M.: Molecular correlates of cytogenetic abnormalities in human cancer cells: Implications for oncogene activation. Prog. Hematol., 14:229, 1986.

34. Lachmann, P. J.: Tumor immunology: A review. J. R. Soc. Med. 77:1023, 1984.

35. Brodt, P.:Tumor immunology—Three decades in review. Annu. Rev. Microbiol. 37:447, 1983.

36. Lennox, E. S., et al.: Specific antigens on methylcholanthrene-induced tumors of mice. Transplant. Proc. 13:1759, 1981.

37. Hellström, I., and Hellström, K. E.: Cell-mediated reactivity to human tumor–type associated antigens: Does it exist? J. Biol. Response Mod. 2:310, 1983.

38. Brickell, P. M., et al.: Activation of a Qa/Tla class I major histocompatibility antigen gene is a general feature of oncogenesis in the mouse. Nature (London) 306:756, 1983.

39. Friedkin, M.: The biochemist's outlook on cancer research. Fed. Proc. 32:2148, 1973.

40. Weinhouse, S.: Enzyme activities in tumor progression. In Edsall, J. T. (ed.): Amino Acids, Proteins, and Cancer Biochemistry. New York, Academic Press, 1960, p. 109.

41. Farber, E.: Cellular biochemistry of the stepwise development of cancer with chemicals: G.H.A. Clowes Memorial Lecture. Cancer Res. 44:5463, 1984.

42. Trosko, J. E., et al.: Mechanisms of tumor promotion: Potential role of intercellular communication. Cancer Invest. 1:511, 1983.

43. Miller, J. A.: Carcinogenesis by chemicals: An overview—G.H.A. Clowes Memorial Lecture. Cancer Res. 30:559, 1970.

44. Weisburger, J. H., and Williams, G. M.: Metabolism of chemical carcinogens. In Becker, F. F. (ed.): Cancer: A Comprehensive Treatise. Vol. I. New York, Plenum Press, 1975, p. 185.

45. Calabresi, P.: Leukemia after cytotoxic chemotherapy—A Pyrrhic victory? N. Engl. J. Med. 309:1118, 1983.

46. Miller, E. C., and Miller, J. A.: Mechanisms of chemical carcinogenesis. Cancer 47:1055, 1981.

47. Goldwater, L. J., et al.: Bladder tumors in a coal tar dye plant. Arch. Environ. Health (Chicago) 11:814, 1965.

48. Bartsch, H., and Montesano, R.: Relevance of nitrosamines to human cancer. Carcinogenesis 5:1381, 1984.

49. Ames, B. N.: Identifying environmental chemicals causing mutations and cancer. Science 204:587, 1979.

50. Weinstein, I. B.: Current concepts and controversies in chemical carcinogenesis. J. Supramol. Struct. Cell Biochem. 17:99, 1981.

51. Pitot, H. C.: Triggering the cellular change to neoplasia. Urology 23 (Suppl.):9, 1984.

52. Wyke, J. A.: Oncogenic viruses. J. Pathol. 135:39, 1981.

53. Fenoglio, C. M., and Lefkowitch, J. H.: Viruses and cancer. Med. Clin. North Am. 67:1105, 1983.

54. Baltimore, D.: RNA-dependent DNA polymerase in virions of RNA tumour viruses. Nature 226:1209, 1970.

55. Temin, H. M., and Mizutani, S.: RNA-dependent DNA polymerase in virions of Rous sarcoma virus. Nature 226:1211, 1970.

56. Rhim, J. S.: Viruses as etiological factors in cancer. Cancer Detect. Prev. 7:9, 1984.

57. Rapp, F.: Current knowledge of mechanisms of viral carcinogenesis. CRC Crit. Rev. Toxicol. 13:197, 1984.

58. Bishop, J. M.: Enemies within: The genesis of retrovirus oncogenes. Cell 23:5, 1981.

59. Marx, J. L.: What do oncogenes do? Science 223:673, 1984.

60. Evan, G. I., and Lennox, E. S.: Retroviral antigens and tumours. Br. Med. Bull. 41:59, 1985.

61. Rapp, F.: Viral carcinogenesis. Int. Rev. Cytol. 15(Suppl.):203, 1983.

62. Lewis, A. M., Jr., and Cook, J. L.: A new role for DNA virus early proteins in viral carcinogenesis. Science 277:15, 1985.

63. Pagano, J. S.: DNA tumor viruses. Transplant. Proc. 16:419, 1984.

64. Editorial: HTLV-related disease. Lancet 2:319, 1983.

65. Klein, G.: Specific chromosomal translocations and the genesis of B-cell–derived tumors in mice and men. Cell 32:311, 1983.

66. Lyon, J. L.: Radiation exposure and cancer. Hosp. Pract. 19:159, 1984.

67. Houghton, A., et al.: Increased incidence of malignant melanoma after peaks of sunspot activity. Lancet 1:759, 1978.

68. Kohn, H. I., and Fry, R. J. M.: Radiation carcinogenesis. N. Engl. J. Med. 310:504, 1984.

69. Favus, M. J., et al.: Thyroid cancer occurring as a late consequence of head and neck irradiation. Evaluation of 1056 patients. N. Engl. J. Med. 294:1019, 1976.

70. Miller, A. B.: An overview of hormone associated cancers. Cancer Res. 38:3985, 1978.

71. Illmensee, K., and Mintz, B.: Totipotency and normal differentiation of single teratocarcinoma cells cloned by injection into blastocysts. Proc. Natl. Acad. Sci. U.S.A. 73:549, 1976.

72. Mintz, B.: Gene expression in neoplasia and differentiation. Harvey Lect. 71:193, 1978.

73. Bishop, J. M.: Cellular oncogenes and retroviruses. Annu. Rev. Biochem. 52:301, 1983.

74. Cooper, G. M., and Lane, M. A.: Cellular transforming genes and oncogenes. Biochim. Biophys. Acta 738:9, 1984.

75. Gordon, H.: Oncogenes. Mayo Clin. Proc. 60:697, 1985.

76. Land, H., et al.: Cellular oncogenes and multistep carcinogenesis. Science 222:771, 1983.

77. Schafer, R., et al.: Unstable transformation of mouse 3T3 cells by transfection with DNA from normal human lymphocytes. EMBO J 3:659, 1984.

78. Viola, M. V., et al.: Expression of *ras* oncogene p21 in prostate cancer. N. Engl. J. Med. 314:133, 1986.

79. Paul, J.: Oncogenes. J. Pathol. 143:1, 1984.

80. Green, A. R., and Wyke, J. A.: Anti-oncogenes. A subset of regulatory genes involved in carcinogenesis. Lancet 2:475, 1985.

81. Krontiris, T. G.: The emerging genetics of human cancer. N. Engl. J. Med. 309:404, 1983.

82. Croce, C. M., and Klein, G.: Chromosome translocations and human cancer. Sci. Am. 252:54, 1985.

82a. Editorial: Molecular mechanisms of tumour evolution. Lancet 1:780, 1986.

83. Cooper, G. M.: Activation of transforming genes in neoplasms. Br. J. Cancer 50:137, 1984.

84. Deuel, T. F., and Huang, J. S.: Roles of growth factor activities in oncogenesis. Blood 64:951, 1984.

85. Hunter, T.: The proteins of oncogenes. Sci. Am. 251:70, 1984.

86. Maher, V. C., and McCormick, J. J.: Role of DNA lesions and repair in the transformation of human cells. Pharmacol. Ther. 25:395, 1984.

# 7

# Clinical Aspects of Neoplasia

turbing, small lesions are often merely observed for significant increase in size. Analogously, leiomyomas of the uterus are extremely common. They can usually be palpated readily as discrete, round, firm tumors on pelvic examination. Follow-up of patients with these lesions over the span of years usually discloses little, if any, increase in size and indeed at the menopause they may begin to shrink. By contrast, leiomyosarcomas, which usually begin de novo and not in previous leiomyomas, increase in size over the span of months. If uterine neoplasms do not enlarge significantly under observation and are asymptomatic, the gynecologist, with the patient's understanding and approval, may elect not to remove them. A few other examples might be cited, but it suffices that *with a few exceptions all masses require anatomic evaluation.* But besides the concern neoplasms arouse, even benign ones may have many adverse effects. The sections that follow in this chapter consider (1) the effects of a tumor on the host, (2) the host's defense against tumors, (3) factors involved in the predisposition to neoplasia, (4) the laboratory diagnosis of neoplasms, and (5) brief descriptions of certain neoplasms common to all tissues (mesenchymal tumors) and skin tumors not presented elsewhere in this text.

## EFFECTS OF TUMOR ON HOST

Obviously, cancers are far more threatening to the host than are benign tumors. Nonetheless, both types of neoplasia may cause problems because of (a) location and impingement on adjacent structures, (b) functional activity such as hormone synthesis, (c) the production of bleeding and secondary infections when they ulcerate through adjacent natural surfaces, and (d) the initiation of acute symptoms by either rupturing or becoming infarcted. Any metastasis has the same potential. Cancers may also be responsible for cachexia (wasting) or paraneoplastic syndromes.

*Location* is of critical importance with both benign and malignant tumors. A small (1 cm) pituitary adenoma can compress and destroy the surrounding normal gland and give rise to hypopituitarism, and a 0.5-cm leiomyoma in the wall of the renal artery may lead to renal ischemia and serious hypertension. A

Ultimately the importance of neoplasms lies in their effects on people. All tumors, even the benign, may cause morbidity and mortality. Moreover, every new growth requires careful appraisal lest it be cancerous. This differential comes into sharpest focus with "lumps" in the female breast. Both cancerous and many benign disorders of the female breast present as palpable masses. In fact, benign lesions are more common than cancers. Although clinical evaluation may suggest one or the other, "the only unequivocally benign breast mass is the excised and anatomically diagnosed one." This is equally true of all neoplasms. There are, however, instances when adherence to this dictum must be tempered by clinical judgment. Subcutaneous lipomas, for example, are quite common and readily recognized by their soft, yielding consistence. Unless they are uncomfortable, subject to trauma, or aesthetically dis-

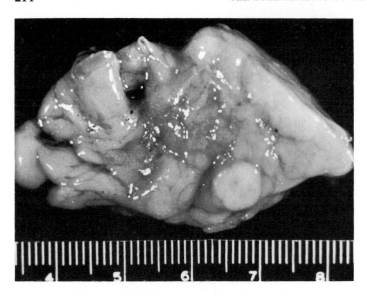

Figure 7–1. A graphic example of the potential significance of a benign tumor. An islet cell adenoma less than 1 cm in diameter was responsible for fatal hypoglycemia in a young adult.

comparably small carcinoma within the common bile duct may induce fatal biliary tract obstruction.

*The production of hormones* is seen with both benign and malignant neoplasms arising in endocrine glands. The adenoma or carcinoma arising in the beta cells of the islets of the pancreas often produces hyperinsulinism, sometimes fatal (Fig. 7–1). Analogously, some adenomas or carcinomas of the adrenal cortex elaborate corticosteroids (for example, aldosterone, which induces sodium retention, hypertension, and hypokalemia). Surprisingly, the functioning adenoma, wherever it arises, may induce a life-threatening endocrinopathy even though it may be less than 1 cm in diameter, and indeed such hormonal activity is more likely with a well-differentiated benign tumor than with a corresponding carcinoma.

Ulceration through a surface with consequent *bleeding or secondary infection* needs no further comment, but a few less obvious ramifications might be mentioned. The neoplasm, benign or malignant, that protrudes into the gut lumen may get caught in the peristaltic pull to telescope the neoplasm and its site of origin into the downstream segment of gut—intussusception (p. 536)—leading to ulceration of the mucosa or, even worse, intestinal obstruction or infarction.

Neoplasms may give rise to *acute medical emergencies* when they suddenly become infarcted or rupture. The cystic teratoma (dermoid cyst) of the mobile ovary may mysteriously twist, become infarcted, and produce severe abdominal pain. The rapidly expanding tumor, usually in some subcapsular location as for example in the liver, may spontaneously, or following slight trauma, rupture to cause massive, possibly fatal, intraperitoneal bleeding.

It is evident that tumors create many problems, not only due to their need for removal or eradication but also in many other ways.

## CANCER CACHEXIA

In the terminal stages of advanced cancer, patients commonly suffer progressive loss of body fat and lean body mass accompanied by profound weakness, anorexia, and anemia. This wasting syndrome is referred to as cachexia. Usually, an intercurrent infection brings a blessed end to the slow deterioration. There is in general some correlation between the size and extent of spread of the cancer and the severity of the cachexia. Small localized cancers therefore are generally silent and produce no cachexia, but there are rare exceptions.

The origins of cancer cachexia are obscure. Wasted patients with any form of chronic illness have impaired immune defenses and so are prone to infections, which could explain some of the debilitation and fever-induced hypermetabolism. Ulcerative lesions may bleed, accounting in some part for the anemia and weakness. Understandably, grief and depression affect the appetite. So there are many potential bases for manifestations. But these simplistic explanations are not sufficient for all cases, and more subtle metabolic abnormalities have been proposed. Patients with cancer cachexia appear to have higher rates of whole body protein turnover than either noncancer patients or starved, normal subjects.[1] Concomitantly, there is a disproportionately increased rate of metabolism of all nutrients, often accompanied by a reduced food intake, that has been related to abnormalities in the sensation of taste and in the central control of appetite.[2] These metabolic abnormalities are not firmly established, but one fact is clear—the wasting is not attributable solely to the nutritional demands of the cancer. Rarely does the body burden of tumor represent more than a very small fraction of the total body mass, and no tumor grows more rapidly than the fetus.[3] Perhaps cachectin, a recently characterized molecule, is involved. This macrophage product acts to mobilize adipose tissues and may thus contribute to cachexia.[4] Thus much remains unknown about the origins of cancer cachexia, but the syndrome is all too real.

## PARANEOPLASTIC SYNDROMES

*Symptom complexes other than cachexia that appear in patients with cancer and that cannot be* readily explained either by the local or distant spread of the tumor or by the elaboration of hormones indigenous to the tissue of origin of the tumor are referred to as paraneoplastic syndromes. *They appear in 10 to 15% of patients with cancer, sometimes even before the tumor is discovered. The syndromes are diverse and are associated with many different tumors, as can be seen in Table 7–1. The most common syndromes are hypercalcemia, Cushing's syndrome, and nonbacterial thrombotic endocarditis; the neoplasms most often associated with these and*

**Table 7–1. PARANEOPLASTIC SYNDROMES***

| Clinical Syndromes | Major Forms of Underlying Cancer | Causal Mechanism |
|---|---|---|
| *Endocrinopathies* | | |
| Cushing's syndrome | Bronchogenic ("oat cell") carcinoma<br>Pancreatic carcinoma<br>Neural tumors | Adrenocorticotropin or ACTH-like substance |
| Hyponatremia | Bronchogenic carcinoma<br>Intracranial neoplasms | Antidiuretic hormone or ADH-like substance |
| Hypercalcemia | Bronchogenic squamous cell carcinoma<br>Breast carcinoma<br>Renal carcinoma | ?Parathyroid hormone or PTH-like substance<br>?Osteoclast activating factor<br>?Growth factors<br>?Prostaglandins, uncertain origin |
| Hyperthyroidism | Blood dyscrasias<br>Bronchogenic carcinoma<br>Prostatic carcinoma | Thyroid-stimulating hormone or TSH-like substance |
| Hypoglycemia | Fibrosarcoma<br>Other mesenchymal sarcomas<br>Hepatocellular carcinoma | Insulin or insulin-like substance |
| Carcinoid syndrome | Bronchial adenoma (carcinoid)<br>Pancreatic carcinoma<br>Gastric carcinoma | Serotonin, bradykinin, ?histamine |
| Polycythemia | Renal carcinoma<br>Cerebellar hemangioma<br>Hepatocellular carcinoma | Erythropoietin |
| *Nerve and Muscle Syndromes* | | |
| Myasthenia<br>Disorders of the central and peripheral nervous systems | Bronchogenic carcinoma<br>Breast carcinoma | ?Immunologic, ?toxic |
| *Dermatologic Disorders* | | |
| Acanthosis nigricans | Gastric carcinoma<br>Lung carcinoma<br>Uterine carcinoma | ?Immunologic, ?toxic |
| Dermatomyositis | Bronchogenic, breast carcinoma | ?Immunologic, ?toxic |
| *Osseous, Articular, and Soft Tissue Changes* | | |
| Hypertrophic osteoarthropathy and clubbing of the fingers | Bronchogenic carcinoma | Unknown |
| *Vascular and Hematologic Changes* | | |
| Venous thrombosis (Trousseau's phenomenon) | Pancreatic carcinoma<br>Bronchogenic carcinoma<br>Other cancers | ?Hypercoagulability |
| Nonbacterial thrombotic endocarditis | Advanced cancers | Hypercoagulability |
| Anemia | Thymic neoplasms | Unknown |
| Leukemoid reaction | Thymic neoplasms | Unknown |
| *Others* | | |
| Nephrotic syndrome | Various cancers | Tumor antigens, immune complexes |

*From Robbins, S. L., Cotran, R.S., and Kumar, V.: Pathologic Basis of Disease. 3rd ed. Philadelphia, W. B. Saunders Co., 1984, p. 256.

other syndromes are bronchogenic and breast cancers and hematologic malignancies. Cushing's syndrome as a paraneoplastic phenomenon is usually related to the ectopic production by the cancer of ACTH or ACTH-like polypeptides but rarely ectopic secretion of corticotropin-releasing factor.[5] However, the mediation of hypercalcemia, another common paraneoplastic syndrome, is poorly understood. There is substantial evidence that parathyroid hormone (PTH) is not involved, but the possibility of closely related peptides has not been completely excluded. Although other candidate products have been proposed (e.g., prostaglandins), favored today are transforming growth factors involved in the genesis of the neoplasm. They presumably bind to the parathyroid hormone receptors in bone to mimic the calcium-mobilizing action of parathormone.[6] Another possible mechanism for hypercalcemia is widespread osteolytic metastatic disease of bone mediated by osteoclast-activating factor, but it should be noted that hypercalcemia as a paraneoplastic syndrome may occur in the absence of skeletal metastases. Sometimes one tumor induces several syndromes concomitantly. Radioimmunoassays document, for example, that bronchogenic carcinomas may elaborate products identical to or having the effects of ACTH, ADH, parathyroid hormone, serotonin, and human chorionic gonadotropin as well as other bioactive substances.[7]

The molecular basis for the ectopic production of hormones or other bioactive substances by cancer cells is not well understood. At one time it was thought that most of this activity was associated with a particular histogenetic type of cancer composed of neurosecretory "small cells" belonging to the family of APUD cells (having the capacity for *Amine Precursor Uptake and Decarboxylation*). The APUD concept is discussed in detail on page 537, but for here it will suffice that APUD cells, widely distributed throughout the body in the gastrointestinal tract, biliary tract, airways, and many other sites, have the capacity to synthesize a variety of amine and polypeptide bioactive products, among them hormones or hormone-like substances.[8, 9] It was further proposed that the widely distributed APUD cells were all of neural crest origin. However, it is now appreciated that all neurosecretory cells are not of neural crest origin. Furthermore, all functionally active cancers are not "small cell" neoplasms. For example, although most bronchogenic carcinomas associated with Cushing's syndrome are of the oat cell type, hypercalcemia is most commonly caused by squamous cell bronchogenic carcinomas and is rare with oat cell tumors. So it appears that some hormonally active tumors are indeed APUDomas but in many instances ectopic hormone production constitutes the expression of new genetic programs, emanating from the alteration of the genotype characteristic of neoplastic transformation. It is unclear whether the new genetic programs emerge because of derepression of formerly repressed genes or because of the formation of new DNA sequences resulting from DNA rearrangements (e.g., chromosomal translocations), seen in many tumors (Fig. 7–2).[10]

Paraneoplastic syndromes may take many other forms, such as hypercoagulability leading to venous thrombosis and nonbacterial thrombotic endocarditis (discussed on p. 71) or the development of clubbing of the fingers and hypertrophic osteoarthropathy in patients with bronchogenic carcinomas (p. 708). Still others will be encountered in the consideration of the cancers of the various organs of the body.

# HOST DEFENSE AGAINST TUMORS

## TUMOR IMMUNITY

As was pointed out on page 200, animals with viral or chemically induced neoplasms bearing tumor-specific or tumor-associated antigens mount an immune response against it. It was natural to assume then that humans might do the same, particularly because there is substantial evidence that exogenous carcinogens probably contribute to the emergence of many cancers in humans (e.g., cigarette smoking and bronchogenic carcinoma, HTLV-I and T-cell lymphoma/leukemia). Indeed it was at the turn of the century that Ehrlich first referred to "positive mechanisms" capable of eliminating abnormal cells, which he proposed must arise throughout life. Formalization of this concept came later when Thomas[11] and subsequently Burnet[12] specifically used the term "immunosurveillance" to refer to recognition and destruction of "non-self" tumor cells on their appearance. It is obvious that immunosurveillance is imperfect, but the fact that some cancers escape detection as the mortality data clearly document does not preclude the possibility that others may have been aborted. Even if nascent cancers escape destruction, the greater antigenic challenge of developed neoplasms might evoke an immune response. It is necessary therefore to explore the following issues: (1) What is the nature of the immune response in animals and possibly in humans to tumors? (2) Does immunosurveillance exist in humans? (3) Do human cancers evoke an immune reaction and can it be exploited in the immunotherapy of them?

### Nature of Tumor Immunity

It is clear from animal experiments that *tumor immunity can be passively transferred by sensitized lymphoid cells but not by cell-free serum (i.e., it is mediated by cells)*. However, antibodies may participate, as is pointed out later. The specific types of cells that mediate the immunity have already been discussed in an earlier chapter (p. 132), and so it is

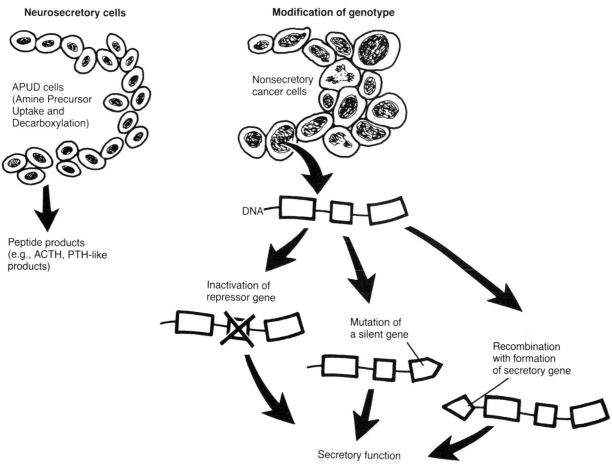

**Figure 7–2.** Possible origins of bioactive secretory products of cancers—on left, the APUD concept; on right, the carcinogenic alterations of the genome that might lead to "secretory genes."

necessary here only to characterize them briefly. Four basic categories are arguably involved:

1. *Specifically sensitized cytotoxic T cells*, capable of recognition of membrane-associated tumor antigens.

2. *Killer (K) cells*, a heterogeneous population possessing Fc receptors, capable of recognition and lysis of antibody-coated tumor cells by a process referred to as antibody-dependent cellular cytotoxicity (ADCC). Most ADCC activity against tumor cells is mediated by NK cells via their Fc receptors and specific antibodies.

3. *Macrophages*, both nonspecifically activated (e.g., endotoxin), and activated by immune T cell–derived gamma interferon, may kill tumor cells by two mechanisms: (a) ADCC and (b) the generation of cytotoxic products.

4. *Natural killer (NK) cells* capable of destroying tumor cells without specific sensitization (see also Fig. 5–8, p. 140).

Uncertainty persists about which of these cell types, if any, contributes to tumor immunity in humans, as is discussed later.[13]

*Humoral mechanisms* may also participate in tumor cell destruction, at least in animals. In experimental model systems tumor antigens evoke specific antibodies. These immunoglobulins can exert antitumor effects by two mechanisms: (1) activation of complement following binding to target cells to form the lytic C′8–9 complex or (2) they can coat tumor cells and render them vulnerable to ADCC by NK cells or macrophages. An attempt to depict various mechanisms of tumor immunity is offered in Figure 7–3.

Paradoxically, both cell-mediated and humoral mechanisms may inhibit the defensive immune response to a tumor. T-suppressor cells have a central role in the regulation of both cellular and humoral immunity to all antigens, and tumors are no exception. Suppressor T cells inhibit tumor immunity in some experimental systems and may play a similar role in humans.[14] Some years ago, before these suppressor cells had been well characterized, Prehn noted that co-cultivation of tumor cells in vitro with a small number of specifically-sensitized T cells *increased* the rate of growth of the tumor cells, whereas a higher ratio of T cells to tumor cells was inhibitory.[15] In retrospect, these observations underscore the delicate balance between tumor inhibition and tumor

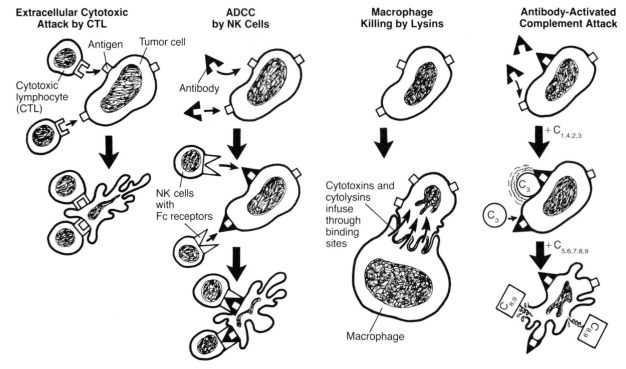

**Figure 7–3.** Potential mechanisms by which humoral and cellular immunity may destroy tumor cells.

promotion exerted by subsets of T cells. Humoral "blocking factors" may abrogate cell-mediated cytotoxicity. The nature of these factors is uncertain, but most of the evidence favors antigen-antibody complexes; circulating, shed tumor antigens may also play roles. Presumably, these factors operate by binding to and blocking either antigen sites on tumor cells or receptors on immunocompetent cells. In conclusion it appears the response of a host to its tumors may, on the one hand, be beneficial or, on the other hand, be detrimental by inhibiting any immune reactions.

### Immunosurveillance

To begin at the end, *there is no unequivocal evidence that humans enjoy a self-policing immune system.*[16] The strongest argument for its existence is the increased frequency of cancers in immunodeficient hosts. About 5% of individuals with a congenital immunodeficiency develop cancers, about 200 times the expected rate. Analogously, immunosuppressed transplant recipients have an increased frequency of malignancies. It should be noted that most (but not all) of these neoplasms are lymphomas, often immunoblastic lymphomas. Particularly illustrative is the X-linked recessive, combined-variable immunodeficiency disorder now termed XLP.[17] When affected boys develop an Epstein-Barr virus infection, it does not take the usual self-limited form of infectious mononucleosis but instead evolves into a chronic or sometimes fatal form of infectious mononucleosis or,

even worse, a malignant lymphoma. Studies indicate that excessive T-suppressor cell activity not only inhibits the normal immune response to the viral infection but presumably also favors the ultimate transformation of the reactive lymphoid hyperplasia into lymphoma.

It has also been argued that the frequency of cancers cannot be construed to invalidate the concept of immunosurveillance, because mechanisms for tumor escape may exist.

○ *Sneaking through.* Emerging cancers may present too small an antigenic challenge to evoke an effective immune response. Later the mass becomes too large for immunologic destruction.

○ *Shedding or modulation of tumor antigens.* Sufficient antigen shedding may inhibit recognition of tumor cells or, with tumor progression, new clones and new antigens may appear.

○ *Immunosuppression.* As noted earlier, several mechanisms may block the immune response.

○ *Genetic vulnerability.* Specific genetic immune deficiencies may induce a predisposition to cancer in particular individuals.

An equally impressive roster of observations challenges the concept of immunosurveillance. The commonest forms of cancers in immunosuppressed and immunodeficient patients are lymphomas, notably immunoblastic lymphomas, which could be the consequence of abnormal immunoproliferative responses to microbial infections or to the various therapeutic agents so commonly administered to these patients. An increased incidence of the most common forms of cancer—lung, breast, gastrointestinal tract—and multiple neoplasms might be anticipated in immunologic cripples but does not occur.[18] Moreover, "nude" mice lacking a thymus gland and cell-mediated immunity have no increased incidence of spontaneous tumors, nor are they more susceptible to chemically induced tumors, but it should be noted they have marked NK-cell activity. So the uncertainty about immunosurveillance continues.

### Tumor Immunity and Immunotherapy in Humans

The issue of an immune response to cancers in humans is a case of "the cup being half empty and half full." As you know, spontaneous human cancers do not express strong tumor-specific antigens. Nonetheless, as mentioned (p. 200), certain cancers evoke strong mononuclear cell reactions construed as defensive immunologic responses. In addition, in vitro assays yield evidence of cell-mediated and humoral responses to target tumor cells; these occur principally with a few specific forms of neoplasia, i.e., melanocarcinomas, neuroblastomas, Burkitt's lymphoma, leukemia, and osteogenic sarcoma.[19] Correlations have been drawn between the level of these responses, the presence or absence of "blocking factors," and the clinical course of these neoplasms.[20] Several features of these immune reactions should be noted. The immunity is cross-reactive among all patients bearing similar neoplasms, implying that the antigens are not tumor specific but rather tumor associated and shared by all histogenetically similar tumors. Could they be differentiation antigens?

In view of the uncertainty surrounding the expression of tumor-specific antigens on human tumors and consequently the relevance of "specific" immunity in immunosurveillance, much attention is focused on NK cells. The concept that the NK system may be an extremely important one as an antitumor mechanism is supported by several observations:[21]

○ NK cells do not require prior sensitization for efficient tumor cell lysis. Thus they can readily act as a "first line of defense" when the tumor burden is low.

○ Following activation with interferons and the lymphokine interleukin 2 (IL-2) NK cells can lyse cells from spontaneously arising human tumors. Such tumors are usually "nonimmunogenic" for the T and B cell systems.

○ In animal models, NK cells have been convincingly demonstrated to have antitumor activity in vivo, especially in controlling hematogenous metastases.

Interleukin 2 is also capable in vitro of activating cytotoxic T cells. Thus incubation of peripheral blood lymphocytes with IL-2 generates lymphokine-activated killer cells reactive against fresh human tumor cells. Clinical trials employing lymphokine-activated killer cells for immunotherapy are currently in progress.[22] To date, all clinical trials using other approaches, such as nonspecific activation of macrophages or immune sera drawn from tumor-bearing hosts, have not proved to be effective. Whether monoclonal antibodies can be developed for specific neoplasms, and whether they will open new avenues for the immunotherapy of human cancers, only time will tell.

## PREDISPOSITION TO NEOPLASIA

It is impossible, unfortunately or fortunately, to predict whether an individual will develop cancer. However, many influences relating both to the individual and to the individual's environment bear on this possibility. The most important ones follow.

### GEOGRAPHIC AND RACIAL FACTORS

Some perspective on the likelihood of developing a specific form of cancer can be gained from national incidence and mortality data. Overall, it is estimated that about 460,000 deaths were caused by cancer in the United States in 1985.[23] However, cancer is still overshadowed by heart disease, which causes nearly twice as many deaths annually. The cancer deaths represent approximately 23% of the total mortality; only six years ago it was about 21%. In some part this increase is the consequence of the better control of infectious diseases and the slow decline in the number of deaths caused by heart disease. But national data aside, calculations indicate that about one in four males and one in five females born in 1985 will eventually die of cancer.[24] The major killers are presented in Table 7–2.

Mortality data for a particular year do not tell the whole story because currently almost 50% of patients developing a cancer are alive five years later. Thus, many more patients are alive with cancer than die of it annually. Some are cured, others have long survival and die of intercurrent causes, and certain forms of malignant neoplasia represent incidental findings

**Table 7–2.** ESTIMATED CANCER DEATHS FOR MAJOR SITES—U.S. 1985*

| Males | | Females | |
|---|---|---|---|
| Organs | No. of Deaths | Organs | No. of Deaths |
| Lung | 87,000 | Lung | 38,600 |
| Colorectal | 29,000 | Breast | 38,400 |
| Prostate | 25,500 | Colorectal | 30,900 |
| Pancreas | 12,500 | Ovary | 11,600 |
| Lymphoma (including Hodgkins) | 11,500 | Lymphoma (including Hodgkins) | 10,800 |
| Leukemia | 9,500 | Leukemia | 7,700 |
| Stomach | 8,400 | Cervix Uteri | 6,800 |
| Urinary Bladder | 7,300 | | |

*Drawn from Silverberg, E: Cancer Statistics 1985. CA 35:19, 1985.

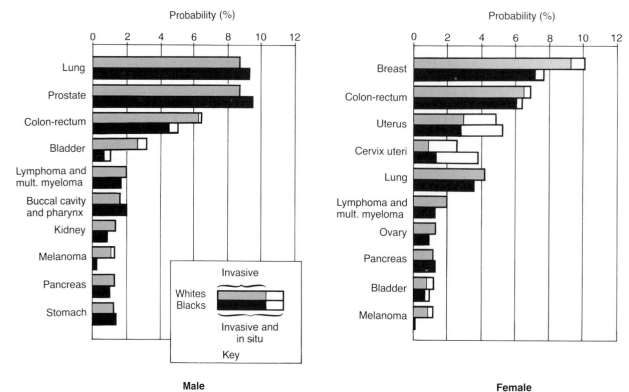

**Figure 7–4.** Probability at birth of eventually developing cancer of selected sites (whites and blacks). (Modified from Seidman, H., et al.: Probabilities of eventually developing or dying of cancer. CA *35*:36, 1985.)

rather than biologically malignant disease (e.g., microscopic foci of prostatic cancer). Therefore, to determine the likelihood of developing a cancer, we must look at probability estimates (Fig. 7–4). It can be seen that the probability of developing prostatic cancer is roughly equal to that of developing carcinoma of the lung, but the mortality data make clear that the latter is far more lethal than many minute prostatic lesions found incidentally. Also evident is the influence of race on the probability of developing specific forms of cancer. Whether the differences truly reflect racial predisposition or instead other factors such as environmental influences is not known.

The death rates of many forms of malignant neoplasia have changed in the past few decades (Table 7–3). To be particularly noted is the significant increase in the overall cancer death rate among males that is attributable largely to lung cancer. In contrast, the overall death rate among females has fallen slightly, owing mostly to the decline in death rates from cancers of the uterus, stomach, and liver. These welcome trends have more than counterbalanced the striking climb in the rate of lung cancer among females, not so long ago a relatively uncommon form of neoplasia in this sex. The declining death rate from uterine cancer can reasonably be attributed to the gratifying control of cervical carcinoma, made possible by the widespread use of cytologic smears for its

early detection while still curable. The decline in death rate of cancers of the liver and stomach in both sexes is, however, obscure, but speculations have been raised about decreasing exposure to dietary carcinogens.

Data on the death rates of specific forms of cancer among the nations of the world are also of interest; sometimes there are striking differences. For example, the age-adjusted death rate in 1975 for cancer of the breast per 100,000 women was 22 in the United States, 28 in England and Wales, 26 in the Netherlands and in Scotland, but, in striking contrast, only 5 in Japan. Conversely, the death rate for stomach carcinoma in both males and females is about seven times higher in Japan than in the United States. Liver cell carcinoma is relatively infrequent in the United States but is the number one cancer-killer among many African native populations. Nearly all of the evidence indicates that these geographic differences are environmental rather than genetic in origin. For example, Nisei (second-generation Japanese living in the United States) have mortality rates for certain forms of cancer that are intermediate between those of natives of Japan and of Americans of native lineage, and the two rates come ever closer with each passing generation. Yet enigmas remain—the death rate from breast carcinoma in females is significantly higher in Denmark than in Sweden, yet environmental differences between these two countries are not immediately apparent. Geographic differences are of great interest because they may contain clues to the causes of cancer.

## AGE

As everyone knows, the frequency of cancer increases with age. Most of the mortality occurs between the ages of 55 and 75 and then declines along with the population base over the age of 75. The strongest effect of age is seen with prostatic cancer. Relatively uncommon in the first half of life, the cancer rises in prevalence to about 40 to 50% at age 70 and progressively faster thereafter (fortunately many are incidental lesions—p. 620). However, it should be noted that cancer is no stranger among the young; it causes slightly more than 10% of all deaths among children under the age of 15. The major cancer-killers in children in approximate decreasing

order of importance are leukemia, tumors of the central nervous system, lymphomas, soft tissue sarcomas, and bone sarcomas. Although cancer at any age is lamentable, it is particularly tragic when it strikes those with "so much life to live." But dramatic therapeutic results are now being achieved with some of the childhood malignancies; an example is acute lymphocytic leukemia—over 50% survive more than five years, and many apparently are cured of their disease. Unfortunately, many other forms of childhood neoplasia have not yielded as much to methods of treatment, and so cancer remains a principal cause of death in the young and in the elderly.

## ENVIRONMENTAL INFLUENCES

No one escapes some exposure to carcinogenic influences. They lurk in the ambient environment, in the workplace, in food, and in personal practices.

**Table 7–3. 25-YEAR TRENDS IN AGE-ADJUSTED CANCER DEATH RATES PER 100,000 POPULATION, 1951–53 TO 1976–78\***

| Sex | Sites | 1951–53 | 1976–78 | Percent Changes | Comments |
|---|---|---|---|---|---|
| Male | All Sites | 171.9 | 215.7 | + 25 | Steady increase mainly due to lung cancer. |
| Female | All Sites | 146.4 | 136.1 | − 7 | Slight decrease. |
| Male | Bladder | 7.2 | 7.2 | † | Slight fluctuations; overall no change. |
| Female | Bladder | 3.1 | 2.1 | − 32 | Some fluctuations; noticeable decrease. |
| Male | Breast | 0.3 | 0.3 | † | Constant rate. |
| Female | Breast | 26.0 | 27.1 | + 4 | Slight fluctuations; overall no change. |
| Male | Colon & Rectum | 25.8 | 26.4 | † | Slight fluctuations; overall no change. |
| Female | Colon & Rectum | 24.8 | 20.0 | − 19 | Slight fluctuations; noticeable decrease. |
| Male | Esophagus | 4.7 | 5.4 | + 15 | Some fluctuations; slight increase. |
| Female | Esophagus | 1.2 | 1.5 | † | Slight fluctuations; overall no change in females. |
| Male | Kidney | 3.4 | 4.7 | + 38 | Steady slight increase. |
| Female | Kidney | 2.1 | 2.2 | † | Slight fluctuations; overall no change. |
| Male | Leukemia | 7.9 | 8.8 | + 11 | Early increase, later leveling off. |
| Female | Leukemia | 5.4 | 5.2 | † | Slight early increase, later leveling off. |
| Male | Liver | 6.7 | 4.8 | − 28 | Some fluctuations. Steady decrease in both sexes. |
| Female | Liver | 7.6 | 3.6 | − 53 | |
| Male | Lung | 25.5 | 69.3 | + 172 | Steady increase in both sexes due to cigarette smoking. |
| Female | Lung | 5.0 | 17.8 | + 256 | |
| Male | Oral | 5.9 | 5.8 | † | Slight fluctuations; overall no change in both sexes. |
| Female | Oral | 1.5 | 2.0 | † | |
| Female | Ovary | 8.1 | 8.6 | + 8 | Steady increase, later leveling off. |
| Male | Pancreas | 8.6 | 11.2 | + 30 | Steady increase in both sexes, then leveling off. Reasons unknown. |
| Female | Pancreas | 5.5 | 7.1 | + 29 | |
| Male | Prostate | 21.0 | 22.6 | + 8 | Fluctuations all through period; overall no change. |
| Male | Skin | 3.1 | 3.4 | † | Slight fluctuations; overall no change in both sexes. |
| Female | Skin | 1.9 | 1.9 | † | |
| Male | Stomach | 22.8 | 9.3 | − 59 | Steady decrease in both sexes; reasons unknown. |
| Female | Stomach | 12.3 | 4.3 | − 65 | |
| Female | Uterus | 20.0 | 8.7 | − 57 | Steady decrease. |

\*From American Cancer Society: Cancer Facts and Figures, 1983, p. 11.
†Percent changes not listed because they are not meaningful.

Environmental carcinogens abound. They can be as universal as sunlight (p. 275), be found particularly in urban settings (as, for example, asbestos), or be limited to a type of occupation (as is detailed on p. 273). Certain features of the diet have also been implicated as possible predisposing influences (p. 250), but the documentation consists largely of epidemiologic association rather than cause and effect. Among the possible environmental influences, the most distressing are those incurred in personal practices, notably cigarette smoking (described on p. 253 and p. 446) and chronic alcohol consumption, discussed on page 267. The risk of cervical cancer is also linked to age at first intercourse and the number of sex partners (pointing to a possible causal role for venereal transmission of an oncogenic virus). Suffice it that there is no escape; it seems that everything one does to earn a livelihood, to subsist, or for pleasure, turns out to be fattening, immoral, illegal, or—more disturbing—possibly carcinogenic.

## HEREDITY

Because cancer is destined to occur in one out of four or five individuals, nearly all families have at least one afflicted first- or second-degree relative. Understandably, the question is often asked—"Is cancer an inherited disease?" Regrettably there is no simple answer. A predisposition to a few uncommon forms of cancer can be hereditary, transmitted by an autosomal dominant germinal mutation (Table 7–4). Individuals inheriting the germinal mutation are at significantly increased risk but are not inevitably destined to develop the neoplasm. The retinoblastoma provides the best example. About 40% of all cases are attributable to a germinal mutation; the remainder are nonhereditary. The retinal tumors are bilateral in about one third of all cases. Bilaterally affected individuals are highly likely to be carriers of a germinal mutation, but whether it is a new one or hereditary cannot be determined except by pedigree analysis. But in either event about 50% of the offspring of bilaterally affected survivors are likely to develop the tumor(s). The unaffected 50% either did not inherit the germinal mutation or it was not expressed in neoplasia because, as pointed out in the previous chapter, more than a single mutation, perhaps several, may be requisite for the emergence of a cancer. Nonetheless, a child of a bilaterally affected parent has a 100,000-fold greater chance of developing a retinoblastoma than does a child in the general population.[25] The retinoblastoma can be taken as an example of the other autosomal dominant disorders.

Besides the dominantly inheritable cancerous and precancerous disorders, there is a small group of autosomal recessive conditions (Table 7–4) collectively referred to as "chromosome instability syndromes" and characterized by some deficiency in DNA-repair mechanisms, which increase the predisposition to cancer (p. 276).[26] Homozygotes with xeroderma pigmentosum, for example, have the fully expressed condition, which includes a strong predisposition to sunlight-induced melanocarcinomas and basal cell and squamous cell carcinomas of the skin in addition to other non-neoplastic cutaneous and ocular abnormalities. Heterozygotes, who of course are much more common, do not express the complete clinical condition but nonetheless have a predisposition (albeit less marked) to sunlight-induced malignancies of the skin. Indeed, they probably account for a significant portion of the genetic predisposition

### Table 7–4. HEREDITARY CANCEROUS AND PRECANCEROUS DISORDERS*

| Disorder | Predominant Tumors |
|---|---|
| **Autosomal Dominant Inheritance** | |
| Retinoblastoma | Retinoblastoma, sarcomas—orbital (following radiation) and at remote sites |
| Neurofibromatosis | Neurogenic sarcoma, acoustic neuroma, pheochromocytoma |
| Familial polyposis coli | Colonic cancer, adenomatous polyps |
| Gardner's syndrome | Colonic cancer, adenomatous polyps |
| Peutz-Jeghers syndrome | Controversial whether predisposes to colonic cancer |
| Hereditary multiple endocrine neoplasia syndrome—type I (MEN I) | Tumors of the pituitary gland, parathyroid gland, and pancreatic islet cells |
| Multiple endocrine neoplasia syndrome—type II (MEN II) | Medullary carcinoma of the thyroid, pheochromocytoma, and parathyroid disease |
| Multiple endocrine neoplasia syndrome—type III (MEN III) | Variant MEN II (see p. 701) |
| Cutaneous malignant melanoma | Cutaneous malignant melanoma, other cancers |
| Von Hippel-Lindau disease | Hemangioblastoma of cerebellum, hypernephroma, and pheochromocytoma |
| Wilms' tumor | Wilms' tumor |
| Cancer-family syndrome | Adenocarcinomas (primarily of the colon and endometrium) |
| Breast cancer in association with other malignant neoplasms | Breast cancer, ovarian carcinoma, sarcoma, leukemia, and brain tumor |
| **Autosomal Recessive Inheritance** | |
| Chromosome instability syndromes | |
| Xeroderma pigmentosum | Basal and squamous cell carcinoma of skin, malignant melanoma |
| Fanconi's anemia | Leukemia and lymphoma |
| Bloom's syndrome | Acute leukemia |
| Ataxia telangiectasia | Acute leukemia, lymphoma, and possibly gastric cancer |
| Turcot's syndrome | Colonic polyps, cancer, and brain tumors |

*From Robbins, S. L., Cotran, R. S., and Kumar, V.: Pathologic Basis of Disease. 3rd ed. Philadelphia, W. B. Saunders Co., 1984, p. 264.

to various forms of skin cancer in the general population.

All the well-defined conditions already discussed account for only a small fraction of the total burden of malignant neoplasia. What can be said about the influence of heredity on the large preponderance of malignant neoplasms? To begin with, as pointed out in the preceding chapter, the evidence is strong that carcinogenesis involves one or, more likely, several mutations in the genome. It follows therefore that the altered phenotype, represented by the appearance of a neoplasm, involves some alteration in the genotype of the tumorous cells. To this extent most, and possibly all, malignancies are genetic in origin.[27] However, whether all individuals who develop a cancer have genotypes that are particularly vulnerable to critical mutations is unknown. There can be no doubt that certain individuals have greater predisposition to cancer than others. Not all heavy cigarette smokers develop bronchogenic carcinoma. Furthermore, epidemiologic studies indicate that lung cancer is more common among both nonsmoking and smoking relatives of lung cancer patients than it is in comparable controls. Familial predisposition has also been noted with carcinoma of the breast, colon, ovary, prostate, and uterus and with melanocarcinomas. Indeed, with each of these types of neoplasia, specific families have been identified in which there appear to be Mendelian patterns of inheritance.[28] Rare families have an increased predisposition to diverse forms of cancer ranging from sarcomas of soft tissues and bone to breast carcinoma.[29] However, *with most forms of malignancy, well-defined familial influences can be identified in only a few instances.* We may conclude therefore with the following generalizations:

○ Most individuals with cancer have no well-defined familial predisposition, and the development of the tumor must be viewed as the result of chance, possibly influenced by environmental factors.

○ An autosomal dominant or recessive mutation predisposing to certain forms of cancer is relatively uncommon.

○ Even in the absence of specific germinal mutations, some genotypes appear to be particularly vulnerable to the development of oncogenic mutations.

○ The extent of the familial input can be suspected by the number of close relatives affected and the number of family members having multiple cancers.

○ Early age at appearance of the tumor and multiple cancers in an individual suggest hereditary influence; e.g., the appearance of breast carcinomas, premenopausally, particularly when bilateral.

*Heredity and environment can be viewed then as the two ends of a spectrum of predisposing influences.* At the extremes are those neoplasms developing because of a strong hereditary component and those related to heavy exposure to environmental carcinogens, but in between are the great majority resulting from varying proportions of heredity and environment.

## CLINICAL DISORDERS

Besides the genetic influences described above, certain clinical conditions are well-recognized predispositions to the development of malignant neoplasia. Sometimes they are referred to as "*precancerous disorders.*" This designation is unfortunate because it implies a certain inevitability, but in fact although they may increase the likelihood, in most instances, cancer does not always develop during the lifetime of the individual. Brief citation of the chief conditions follows:

○ *Persistent regenerative cell replication*—i.e., squamous cell carcinoma in the margins of a chronic skin fistula, or a long-standing unhealing skin wound; hepatocellular carcinoma in cirrhosis of the liver (particularly certain forms).

○ *Hyperplastic and dysplastic proliferations*—i.e., endometrial carcinoma in atypical endometrial hyperplasia; bronchogenic carcinoma in the dysplastic bronchial mucosa of habitual cigarette smokers.

○ *Chronic atrophic gastritis*—i.e., gastric carcinoma in pernicious anemia.

○ *Chronic ulcerative colitis*—i.e., an increased incidence of colorectal carcinoma in long-standing disease.

○ *Leukoplakia of the oral cavity, vulva, and penis*—i.e., increased risk of squamous cell carcinoma.

○ *Tubular and villous adenomas of the colon*—i.e., high risk of becoming colorectal carcinoma.

In this context, *in general, benign neoplasms do not become transformed into malignancies.* Tumorous masses known to be present for years and decades are found ultimately to be benign. There are exceptions. On occasion a pleomorphic adenoma (mixed salivary gland tumor) that has been present for years is found to have a cancerous focus. The question always arises: was the malignant neoplasm of low growth potential taken to be a benign lesion, or was there a focus of malignancy from the outset masked by the accompanying benign tumor? Colorectal carcinomas arise in preexisting adenomatous polyps. Other examples might be offered, but it suffices that they are the exceptions and not the rule.

# LABORATORY DIAGNOSIS OF CANCER

## HISTOLOGIC AND CYTOLOGIC METHODS

The laboratory diagnosis of cancer is, in most instances, not difficult. The two ends of the benign-malignant spectrum pose no problems; however, in the middle lies a "no man's land" where wise men tread cautiously. This issue has been sufficiently emphasized in the preceding chapter; here the focus is on the roles of the clinician (often a surgeon) and the pathologist in facilitating the correct diagnosis.

Clinicians tend to underestimate the important contributions they make to the diagnosis of a neoplasm. Clinical data are invaluable for optimal pathologic diagnosis. Radiation changes in the skin or mucosa can be similar to cancer. Sections taken from a healing fracture can mimic remarkably an osteosarcoma. Moreover, the laboratory evaluation of a lesion can be only as good as the specimen made available for examination. It must be adequate, representative, and properly preserved. Several sampling approaches are available: (1) excision or biopsy, (2) needle aspiration, and (3) cytologic smears. When excision of a small lesion is not possible, selection of an appropriate site for biopsy of a large mass requires awareness that the margins may not be representative and the center largely necrotic. Analogously with disseminated lymphoma (involving many nodes), those in the inguinal region draining large areas of the body often have reactive changes that may mask neoplastic involvement. Appropriate preservation of the specimen is obvious, yet it involves such issues as prompt immersion in a usual fixative (for example, formalin solution) or instead preservation of a portion in a special fixative (e.g., glutaraldehyde) for electron microscopy or prompt refrigeration to permit optimal hormone or receptor analysis. In the case of breast carcinoma, assays for estrogen and progesterone receptors provide guidelines for possible hormonal therapeutic interventions. Requesting "quick-frozen section" diagnosis is sometimes desirable, for example in determining the nature of a breast lesion or in evaluating the margins of an excised cancer to ascertain that the entire neoplasm has been removed. This method allows sectioning of a "quick-frozen" sample and permits histologic evaluation within minutes. It is then possible with, for example, a breast biopsy to determine whether the lesion is malignant and may require wider excision or sampling of axillary nodes for possible spread. The patient is thereby saved the expense and trauma of a subsequent operation. In experienced, competent hands, frozen-section diagnosis is highly accurate, but there are particular instances when the better histologic detail provided by the more time-consuming routine methods is needed—for example, when extremely radical surgery, such as the amputation of an extremity, may be indicated. Better to wait a few days despite the drawbacks than to perform inadequate or unnecessary surgery. Fortunately, except for the rare instances of rapidly growing sarcomas (usually in children), there is no evidence that cutting into a neoplasm followed by a few days' delay between biopsy and definitive surgery imposes any additional danger of dissemination of the tumor.

*Fine-needle aspiration* of tumors provides another approach that is growing in popularity. This procedure is most commonly employed with breast, prostate, and thyroid tumors but sometimes with others. It obviates the need for surgery and its attendant ramifications, but the process is essentially blind and the validity of the diagnosis rests heavily on the accuracy of the sampling. Radiographic methods are often used therefore to guide the insertion of the biopsy needle. Moreover, interpretation of the minute tissue fragment or the aspirated cells (using essentially cytologic methods) is more difficult than evaluation of excised lesions having architectural and cytologic details.

*Cytologic (Papanicolaou) smears* provide yet another method for the detection of cancer. This approach is widely used for the discovery of carcinoma of the cervix, often at an in situ stage, but it is also used with many other forms of suspected malignancy, such as endometrial carcinoma, bronchogenic carcinoma, bladder and prostatic tumors, and gastric carcinomas; for the identification of tumor cells in abdominal, pleural, joint, and cerebrospinal fluids; and, less commonly, with other forms of neoplasia. It was pointed out earlier that cancerous cells have a range of levels of differentiation and have lowered cohesiveness and adhesiveness, leading to their being shed into fluids or secretions (Fig. 7–5). Based on their cellular (particularly, nuclear) details, exfoliated cells can be categorized as:

| | |
|---|---|
| Class I: | Normal |
| Class II: | Few atypical cells—repeat |
| Class III: | Dysplasia—sometimes subdivided into mild, moderate, and severe |
| Class IV: | Carcinoma in situ |
| Class V: | Overt cancer |

Cytologic interpretation requires a great deal of expertise but can yield with cervical smears nearly 100% correct positive diagnosis; i.e., false-positives are rare. However, there is a significant fraction of false-negative diagnosis, owing largely to sampling errors. Smears for other types of tumors (e.g., lung, stomach, prostate) are more difficult to evaluate. Nonetheless, with all a positive finding almost always provides strong evidence of the existence of a cancer. It should be emphasized, however, that *all positive findings are best confirmed by biopsy and histologic examination before therapy is instituted.* A negative report does not exclude the presence of a malignancy. The gratifying control of cervical cancer is the best testament to the value of the cytologic method.

It is well beyond our scope to delve into the technical details of the *anatomic diagnosis of cancer.* Only a brief "statement-of-the-art" will be made. Up to the relatively recent past, it was in some part science and in large part art, depending heavily on subjective judgments of histologic visual images. Involved was, and to some extent still is, the Solomonic judgment of when the level of cytologic atypia is sufficient to demand the diagnosis of cancer. Great advances have been made recently. Electron microscopy, immunoelectron microscopy, histochemistry, immunocytologic methods, and most recently, analyses of the DNA code of the presumptive tumor cells have added considerable objectivity to the laboratory diagnosis of cancer. A few examples will be illustrative. Electron microscopy revealing slender, elongated surface pseudopodia combined with immunofluorescence or immunoperoxidase methods using specific antibodies to identify the intermediate filaments of cytokeratin point almost certainly to a mesothelioma, differentiating it from other histologically similar types of neoplasia such as adenocarcinomas and sarcomas.[30] Immunofluorescence or immunoperoxidase methods and antibodies, preferably monoclonal, for specific immunoglobulin chains permit the segregation of B cells from T cells in the differential diagnosis of lymphomas and lymphocytic leukemias. Furthermore, the monoclonality of B-cell lesions can be established by the fact that all cells bear similar light chains documenting that the nodal enlargement is neoplastic rather than polyclonal and reactive. Further specificity can be achieved with anti-idiotype antibodies, which indeed are now being exploited as a therapeutic tool in the hope of destroying the malignant cells.[31] Most recently, diagnostic specificity has been extended to the use of DNA molecular probes. It is now possible with recombinant techniques to identify the rearranged genes of specific forms of lymphoid cancer, such as those coding for T-cell receptors, proving the monoclonality of T-cell lymphomas or leukemias.[32] Thus molecular

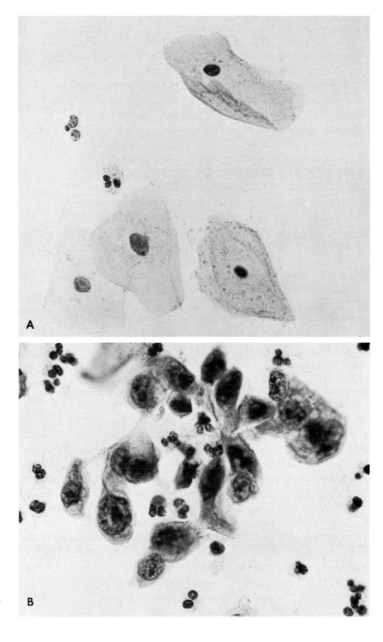

**Figure 7–5.** Papanicolaou smears of cervical cytology. *A*, Normal squames. *B*, Cancer cells (Class V).

biology has moved from the laboratory to the bedside, and with it the diagnosis of malignant neoplasia has progressed from the level of "eyeballing" to the precision offered by molecular genetics.[33]

## BIOCHEMICAL ASSAYS

Biochemical assays for tumor-associated enzymes, hormones, and other tumor "markers" in the blood cannot be construed as modalities for the diagnosis of cancer; however, they contribute to finding cases and in some instances are useful in determining the effectiveness of therapy. The application of these assays will be considered with many of the specific forms of neoplasia discussed in other chapters, so only a few examples will suffice here. Prostatic carcinoma can be suspected when elevated levels of acid phosphatase are found in the blood. Regrettably, the levels become significantly raised only when the tumor is advanced (as is detailed on p. 623) and so the false-negative rate is high. Radioimmunoassays for circulating hormones may point to the presence of tumors in the endocrine system and in some instances to the ectopic production of hormones by nonendocrine tumors (p. 215).

A host of circulating "tumor markers" have been described, and new ones appear every year.[34] Only a few have stood the test of time and proved to have clinical usefulness. *The two best established are carcinoembryonic antigen (CEA) and alpha-fetoprotein (AFP).*[35] CEA, normally produced in embryonic tissue of the gut, pancreas, and liver, is a complex glycoprotein that is elaborated by many different neoplasms. Depending on the serum level adopted as a significant elevation, it is variously reported to be positive in 60 to 90% of colorectal, 50 to 80% of pancreatic, and 25 to 50% of gastric and breast carcinomas. Much less consistently, elevated CEA has been described in other forms of cancer. Regrettably, in almost all types of neoplasia the level of elevation is correlated with the body burden of tumor and so highest levels are found in those with advanced metastatic disease. Moreover, CEA elevations have also been reported in many benign disorders, such as alcoholic cirrhosis, hepatitis, ulcerative colitis, Crohn's disease, and others. Occasionally levels of this antigen are elevated in apparently healthy smokers. Thus, CEA assays lack both specificity and the sensitivity required for the detection of early cancers. But they are still useful in providing presumptive evidence of the possibility of colorectal carcinoma because this tumor yields the highest CEA levels, and the assay is particularly useful in the detection of recurrences following excision.[36] With successful resection of the tumor, CEA disappears from the serum; its reappearance almost always spells the beginning of the end (p. 558).

The other well-established tumor marker is alpha-fetoprotein (AFP).[35] Elevated circulating levels are encountered in adults with cancers arising principally in the liver and from yolk sac remnants. Less regularly it is elevated in teratocarcinomas and embryonal cell carcinomas of the testis, ovary, and extragonadal sites and, occasionally, in cancers of the stomach and pancreas. As with CEA, benign conditions including cirrhosis, hepatitis, and pregnancy (especially with fetal distress or death) may cause modest elevations of AFP. There is then a problem with both specificity and sensitivity, but the marker may still provide presumptive evidence of a hepatocellular carcinoma, for example, and is of value in the follow-up of therapeutic interventions. More details are found on page 599. This cursory overview suffices to indicate the many laboratory approaches in use for the detection and diagnosis of tumors.

# MESENCHYMAL AND SKIN TUMORS

Most of the clinically significant forms of benign and malignant neoplasia will be presented in the chapters dealing with specific organs and systems. A few, such as mesenchymal tumors of connective tissue and smooth muscle origin, are so ubiquitous they do not fit into any specific organ presentation and so are considered here. Neoplasms of the skin are also presented here because they are not considered elsewhere in this text.

## CONNECTIVE TISSUE TUMORS

Tumors arising in connective tissue occur throughout the body. They may take origin from fibrocytes, fibroblasts, or the specialized derivatives of mesenchymal tissue, such as fat and muscle.

### *Lipoma and Liposarcoma*

The lipoma is an extremely common, usually innocuous tumor. It generally appears in subcutaneous locations (neck, trunk, face, hands, and feet) and less often in the retroperitoneum, mediastinum, skeletal muscles and gastrointestinal tract.

Usually the **lipoma** is a 3.0- to 5.0-cm, soft, round to lobulated mass of fatty tissue enclosed within a very delicate capsule. The capsule is often so thin that it is easily ruptured during removal. Histologically, these lesions are indistinguishable from normal adipose tissue and the designation "tumor" is only merited by the tumorous accumulation of fat cells enclosed within a delicate capsule. Localized collections of fat not discretely encapsulated may appear in such sites as the spermatic cord, mediastinum, and omentum. These lesions probably represent bizarre, aberrant accumulations of fat that are not truly neoplastic. The distinction between these localized overgrowths and true neoplasia is at best arbitrary and academic.

**Liposarcomas** are extremely pleomorphic histologically.[37, 38] They have been subdivided into (1) well-differentiated lesions (readily mistaken for lipomas); (2) myxoid liposarcoma having an abundant mucopolysaccharide ground substance in which are scattered primitive stellate mesenchymal cells and occasional vacuolated lipomatous cells; (3) round cell liposarcomas composed of highly undifferentiated small cells having hyperchromatic nuclei, among which are scattered vacuolated cells referred to as lipoblasts; and (4) a pleomorphic pattern having marked anaplasia with numerous tumor giant cells and only sometimes cells bearing fatty vacuoles. A helpful diagnostic feature, when present, is the large cytoplasmic diastase-resistant PAS-positive granules seen in scattered neoplastic cells. The origin of these granules is unclear, but they are more typical of pleomorphic liposarcoma than of other soft tissue sarcomas. The pleomorphic pattern is basically a neoplasm of primitive mesenchymal cells. The well-differentiated and myxoid liposarcomas are usually locally invasive but rarely metastasize. The other two forms are highly aggressive lesions that metastasize widely and yield less than a 20% five-year survival rate following resection.

### Fibroma and Fibrosarcoma

Fibroblasts are ubiquitous and can arise not only from other fibroblasts but also from fibroblastic differentiation of primitive mesenchymal cells that are widely scattered in the body. It is surprising therefore that fibromas and fibrosarcomas are uncommon neoplasms. An intermediate category of fibromatoses is more frequent, but these growths are most often located in proximity to the musculoskeletal system (p. 721).

True **fibromas** are seldom located outside of the ovaries and gastrointestinal tract. A closely related lesion, the neurofibroma, is derived from Schwann cells and is found along nerve trunks. The true **fibroma** appears as a rubbery, gray, discrete, encapsulated mass. On transection, the surface is glistening and gray-white and usually devoid of hemorrhage or necrosis. Histologically, the lesion is composed of mature fibrocytes or fibroblasts having no distinctive orientation. Intercellular collagen may be abundant or scant. As benign lesions, fibromas display no anaplasia and few, if any, mitoses. Special stains, such as silver impregnation techniques, will demonstrate reticulin laid down by the fibroblasts, or the phosphotungstic acid–hematoxylin stain may reveal delicate, wavy fibroglial fibrils elaborated by the fibroblast, which is a means of differentiating these spindle cell tumors from those of muscle origin.

**Fibrosarcomas** are the malignant counterparts of fibromas. These tumors may occur anywhere in the body but are perhaps most frequent in the soft tissues of the extremities and in the retroperitoneum. They occur as bulky, soft, pearly gray-white infiltrative masses. On transection, the tumor has a characteristic raw fish-flesh appearance. Often there are areas of necrosis or hemorrhage, reflecting the rapidity of growth that outstrips the blood supply. Histologically, these lesions have variable degrees of anaplasia. Some of the better differentiated fibrosarcomas are made up of mature looking fibroblasts and show occasional mitoses and some slight cellular pleomorphism. At the other end of the spectrum, the anaplastic fibrosarcomas rate among the wildest appearing neoplasms in the body. Massive tumor giant cells, with huge single or multiple nuclei, may be present. Mitoses may be frequent and are often atypical and totally chaotic. Such anarchic tumors are extremely treacherous, and local recurrence often frequently follows inadequate primary resection. As lesions made up of multipotential mesenchymal cells, areas of myxomatous, lipomatous, and chondroosteomatous differentiation are sometimes present.

## SMOOTH MUSCLE TUMORS

### Leiomyoma and Leiomyosarcoma

The *leiomyoma* is a benign tumor of smooth muscle origin. It may arise anywhere in the body, such as the wall of the intestinal tract or the walls of arteries, but it is particularly common in the uterus and is described in greater detail on page 644. The uterine variety is undoubtedly the most common visceral neoplasm in women.

The **leiomyomas** that arise outside the uterus tend, on the whole, to be small lesions that rarely exceed 2.0 to 3.0 cm in diameter. They are composed of bands of mature smooth muscle cells closely resembling their normal counterparts.

The **leiomyosarcoma** rarely arises in a leiomyoma but more often begins de novo. In common with all cancers the cells display variability in size and shape and the other characteristics already cited in the discussion of anaplasia (Fig. 7–6). These tumors too are described in more detail on page 644. Differentiation from a fibrosarcoma can be difficult; a strong positive immunostain for the intermediate filaments—desmin—would denote a leiomyosarcoma.

## SKIN TUMORS

Three types of lesions will be considered here: (1) squamous cell carcinoma, (2) basal cell carcinoma, and (3) pigmented lesions—nevi, lentigo maligna, and melanomas.

Skin cancer in general is the most common form of malignant neoplasia. It has been estimated that almost half of all people who reach 65 years of age have had or will have at least one skin cancer. Fortunately, 90% of these lesions are curable by adequate local excision. Among the skin cancers, 30%

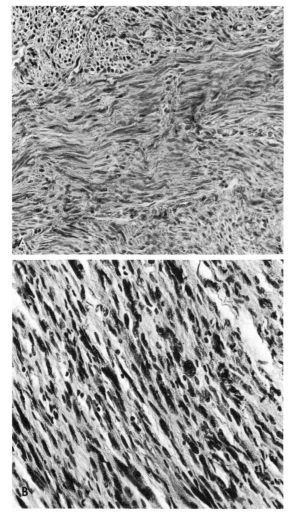

Figure 7–6. A comparison of the well-differentiated histology of a leiomyoma (*above*) and a leiomyosarcoma (*below*).

## Squamous Cell (Epidermoid) Carcinoma

Squamous cell carcinomas may arise in any stratified squamous epithelium or mucosa that has undergone squamous metaplasia. Thus this form of cancer may occur, for example, in the tongue, lips, esophagus, cervix, vulva, vagina, bronchus, or urinary bladder. On oral or vulval mucosal surfaces, leukoplakia is an important antecedent. Most squamous cell carcinomas, however, arise in the skin (90 to 95%). Fair-skinned, blond individuals who have outdoor occupations are particularly likely to develop this form of cancer. Often the tumors are preceded by so-called actinic (solar) keratosis, a form of dysplasia or anaplasia of the epidermal cells. Arsenic and coal tars have also been implicated in their causation. Protracted chronic inflammation constitutes yet another predisposing influence and so this form of cancer is sometimes encountered in the margins of long-standing draining sinuses and in old x-ray or burn scars. Sometimes the neoplasm does not appear until decades after the x-ray or thermal injury.

The earliest recognizable lesion, the in situ carcinoma, appears as a well-defined small (1 to 2 cm) red-brown plaque with slightly elevated firm margins. Often the surface is scaly owing to hyperkeratinization. On moist mucosal surfaces where keratinization is unusual, the patch may be red and oozing. The in situ stage is followed by progressive invasion and expansion of the tumor, creating a firm, elevated plaque. This is often followed by central ulceration yielding a necrotic crater, rimmed by firm margins. Histologically, the in situ tumor reveals complete replacement of the normal epidermal thickness by atypical cells, showing the classic features of variation in cell and nuclear size and in morphology accompanied by hyperchromatic nuclei, which sometimes bear numerous and possibly abnormal mitotic figures well above the basal zone. Progressive penetration of the basement membrane and invasion of the dermis or underlying connective tissue follows in the form of tongue-like penetrations (Fig. 7–7).

are squamous cell carcinomas, about 60% are basal cell carcinomas, and approximately 2% are melanocarcinomas. The residual 8% includes various uncommon forms of cancer too rare to merit description here. Over 90% of the common skin tumors (squamous and basal cell carcinomas) occur on the head and neck regions most heavily exposed to the sun, whereas melanomas tend to occur on the back, which also receives bouts of heavy sun exposure during vacation periods. The frequency of all these forms of skin cancer is higher in those living in southern latitudes than in inhabitants of the northern hemisphere. There is therefore epidemiologic evidence implicating the ultraviolet radiation of sunlight in their causation.[39] Recall that certain hereditary conditions, the chromosome instability syndromes such as xeroderma pigmentosum characterized by defective DNA-repair systems, make these individuals particularly predisposed to sunlight-induced skin cancers.

Approximately 80% of these cancers are extremely well differentiated and are composed of readily recognized keratinocytes forming keratin pearls (concentric laminated keratinous layers). The burrowing, invasive strands and nests of cells in the well-differentiated lesions tend to replicate the organization of the normal epidermis; basal cells occupy the perimeter of these nests, and there is progressive maturation of the cells in the centers of the islands. Thus the central regions of these tumor nests are often keratinized and sometimes form "horn cysts." The residual 20% of squamous cell carcinomas show varying levels of loss of differentiation; some are totally undifferentiated with marked anaplasia, giant cell formation, numerous mitoses, and no keratinization.

The prognosis is more dependent on the location, size, and depth of penetration of the tumor than on the level of anaplasia. Skin lesions tend to be discov-

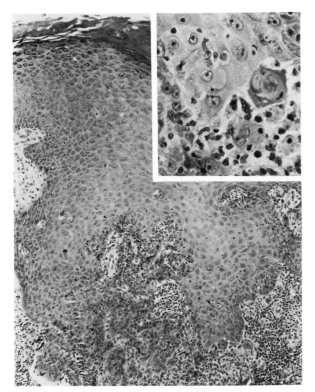

Figure 7–7. Squamous cell carcinoma of the skin. The penetrating tongues of tumor are seen below. Inset shows a keratinous pearl. (Courtesy of Dr. George F. Murphy, Brigham and Women's Hospital and Harvard Medical School, Boston, MA.)

Grossly these lesions begin as tiny, firm, elevated nodules with an intact overlying surface, and they progressively become small plaques. Even small lesions (less than 1 cm) soon develop central ulcerations, which are characteristically rimmed by a pearly raised border (rodent ulcers). Some show varying degrees of pigmentation, which makes them superficially resemble nevi. Neglected lesions may be locally penetrating, ulcerative, and destructive, but in general their progression is slow and indolent, spanning many months to years.

Histologically, basal cell carcinomas usually appear as invasive clusters or strands of compact, darkly chromatic, spindled cells that in the plane of section may have no connection with the overlying epidermis or adnexa. On cross section the strands create numerous nests or islands having a peripheral array of palisaded basal cells that strongly resemble their normal forebears and which enclose a uniform collection of spindled forms (Fig. 7–8). Giant cells, striking anaplasia, and mitotic figures are conspicuously absent. There are a large number of variations on this basic theme. Some lesions grow as solid masses, invading the dermis or deeper structures. Others are cystic or produce pseudoglandular lacy patterns, and still others show maturation of the basal cells to produce keratin-lined microcysts, termed basosquamous carcinoma. Some of these tumors are pigmented, containing melanin granules within many of the epidermal cells.

ered when relatively small, and less than 2 to 5% of patients have metastases to regional nodes. Resection then can be curative. Squamous cell carcinomas arising in the lung have usually metastasized to regional nodes and perhaps more widely at the time of diagnosis, and up to 50% of those arising on most mucosal surfaces and in chronic skin injuries have already metastasized at least to regional nodes by the time a diagnosis is made. For these the prognosis depends on extent of spread and completeness of excision of the primary tumor and its extensions.

## Basal Cell Carcinoma

*Basal cell carcinomas* almost never metastasize. These cancers arise in the basal cells of the pilosebaceous adnexa and occur only on the skin. Mucosal surfaces lacking these adnexa, such as the lips, tongue, and cervix, are never primary sites. As with the squamous cell carcinoma, these cancers tend to occur in those over 40 with fair skin. Blacks and Orientals are seldom affected. Although sunlight is considered to be a predisposing influence, for unexplained reasons these tumors are more frequent on the eyelids and bridge of the nose (rich in adnexal glands) than on the sun-exposed backs of hands and forearms. Use of arsenicals also increases the risk of basal cell carcinoma.

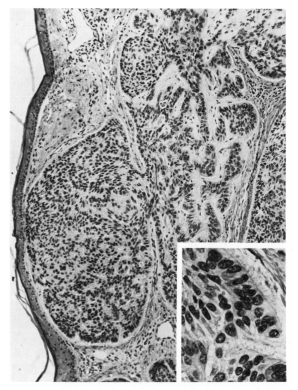

Figure 7–8. Basal cell carcinoma of the skin. Normal epidermis is at left. The nests and strands of invasive tumor cells are penetrating into the subcutaneous tissue. Inset lower right reveals the peripheral palisade. (Courtesy of Dr. George F. Murphy, Brigham and Women's Hospital and Harvard Medical School, Boston, MA.)

Although most basal cell carcinomas are unicentric, on occasion multiple foci of tumor are separated by small zones of normal intervening epidermis. Usually, however, such multicentricity is confined to a localized area (1 to 3 cm) of the skin.

Surgical excision, irradiation, or adequate cauterization will cure most basal cell carcinomas. Even when the neoplasm extends to the margins of surgical excision, only one third of these recur. These continue to extend and produce more difficult clinical problems. Ultimately, however, all are amenable to total cure. The presence of keratinization in a basal cell carcinoma does not alter its biologic behavior, and so basosquamous patterns do not assume the significance of the more ominous squamous cell carcinomas, which may metastasize.

### Pigmented Nevi

Some clinicians refer to any colored lesion of the skin as a nevus, including those of vascular origin. Here the term "nevus" is restricted to lesions composed of modified melanocytes (nevus cells) of neural crest origin. All types of nevi at some point in their course have excess melanin pigmentation, which makes them tan-brown distinctive skin lesions. *They can be divided into three categories: (1) common acquired nevi; (2) less frequent subtypes, including congenital giant nevus, blue nevus, and compound nevus of Spitz (spindle and epithelioid cell nevus, halo nevus); and (3) dysplastic nevi.* Although all may give rise to melanocarcinomas (more commonly referred to as melanomas), the risk is significantly greater with congenital giant nevi and dysplastic nevi. Only the common acquired and dysplastic nevi will be described.

*Common acquired nevi* are often referred to as "moles." They are extremely frequent lesions found in greater or lesser numbers (average 10 to 40) on most white individuals. The evolution of acquired nevi strongly suggests that they are focal developmental aberrations of melanocytes rather than true neoplasms.[40] Absent at birth, they first appear in early childhood and become more frequent in middle adult life (most on the trunk); then progressively disappear. Those on the extremities, particularly on the palms and soles, are apt to persist. The basis for this regional variation is unclear.

All common nevi begin as small (1 to 2 mm) uniformly tan to brown, almost black, macules. They gradually enlarge but rarely exceed 1 cm in diameter, and some become slightly elevated. **Characteristically they have distinct rounded borders.** Those on the trunk generally over the course of time become depigmented and transformed into pink or flesh-colored papules, whereas those on the extremities, as mentioned, often persist. Thus, to quote Greene and coworkers, "most people enter life free of nevi and leave with relatively few."[41]

There is an orderly histologic progression accompa-

nying the macroscopic evolution, particularly with trunk nevi. At the outset the tiny lesions are composed of nests of nevus cells, which are basically rounded melanocytes having ovoid nuclei without prominent nucleoli, located within the epidermis at the dermoepidermal junction (**junctional nevus**). They usually contain cytoplasmic granules of melanin. As moles enlarge and become slightly raised, nests of neval cells appear in the dermis along with the intraepidermal nests (**compound nevus**) (Fig. 7–9). Over the course of time, particularly in trunk nevi, the intraepidermal nests disappear (**intradermal nevus**). Concomitantly, the nevus cells in the dermis become more spindled and possibly dendritic; they differentiate along neural lines and simultaneously lose the ability to synthesize melanin. In this manner, the nevus becomes depigmented and transformed into a flesh-colored papule. This evolution is depicted in Figure 7–10. Nevi on the extremities tend not to undergo this orderly "maturation" and persist as junctional or compound lesions.

*Dysplastic nevi* may arise de novo or in common acquired nevi when they fail to undergo orderly "maturation." They have important differences from common acquired nevi: (1) although most do not progress to melanoma, the risk is significantly greater than with common nevi; (2) other members of the

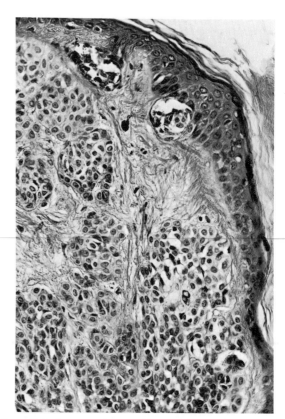

Figure 7–9. Compound nevus. Nests of nevus cells are present both at dermoepidermal junction and within dermis. (From Robbins, S. L., Cotran, R. S., and Kumar, V.: Pathologic Basis of Disease. 3rd ed. Philadelphia, W. B. Saunders Co., 1984, p. 1276.)

Figure 7–10. The usual transition of the common, acquired junctional nevus into the compound nevus and then finally into the intradermal nevus. Note the differences in the locations of the neval cells.

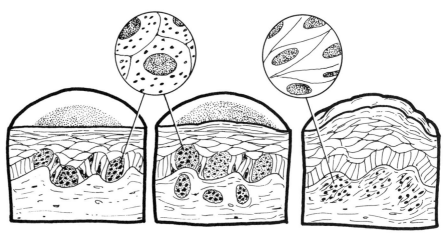

Junctional　　　　Compound　　　　Intradermal

family may have similar lesions, indicating that some individuals with these lesions have the *"familial dysplastic nevus syndrome"*; and (3) they differ both macroscopically and microscopically from common nevi and may be difficult to differentiate from melanomas.

Dysplastic nevi occur not only in the same locations as common nevi but also on the scalp, buttocks, and female breasts. **They tend to be larger macules (greater than 1 cm in diameter) and, unlike ordinary moles, have indistinct irregular borders and a variegated tan to dark brown to pink color.** This macroscopic appearance, as will become evident, is similar to that of some melanomas. In familial settings, the individual may have 25 to 75% dysplastic lesions. Histologically, they appear to represent arrest of the evolution of the ordinary mole at the junctional or compound stage. But the melanocytes also have varying degrees of atypia and dysplasia, which in some instances borders on a superficial spreading melanoma (discussed later).[40]

*Relationship of nevi to melanomas.* Ask three dermatologists about the risk of transformation of a particular type of nevus into a melanoma and you will get four answers. Without going into the confusing controversy, the weight of evidence supports the following generalizations:

○ Most melanomas arise de novo, but fully one third arise in preexisting nevi.

○ Individuals having many common acquired nevi have a significantly greater risk of melanoma (roughly proportional to the number of nevi) than individuals having no nevi.[42] Nonetheless, only a small fraction of 1% of common moles become cancerous.

○ Congenital giant nevi are at greater risk than ordinary moles; about 10% eventually become cancerous, indeed often before the patient reaches age 10.

○ Dysplastic nevi are the most ominous and are thought to be 100-fold more likely than ordinary

moles to become melanomas. In the individual, the risk is proportional to the number of dysplastic nevi (hence the great risk with the familial nevus syndrome).[43] However, this view is stoutly denied by some investigators who contend that the dysplastic nevus is simply a variant of common nevus and is not more likely to become a melanoma.[44]

### Lentigo Maligna

The lentigo maligna (melanotic freckle of Hutchinson) lies at the interface between a dysplastic nevus and a superficial spreading melanoma. It tends to appear on the face but sometimes occurs on other sun-exposed areas of the skin as a large (up to 6 cm) brown-black "ink stain." For years the atypical melanocytes may appear only dysplastic in their intraepidermal location. These cells tend to spread radially along the basal layer of the epidermis and are variable in size and shape (rounded to fusiform) and have enlarged, hyperchromatic nuclei. Cytoplasmic melanin granules are usually evident, and in some cases dermal macrophages become filled with phagocytosed pigment. Eventually, however, the cells become overtly anaplastic and penetrate the dermis. At this stage the lesion is referred to as *lentigo maligna melanoma*, a close relative to the superficial spreading melanoma, to be described. Typically at this stage there is an intense dermal infiltrate of lymphocytes and macrophages.

### MELANOMA (MALIGNANT MELANOMA, MELANOCARCINOMA)

These uncommon forms of cancer arise most often in the skin but infrequently are seen in the oral cavity, esophagus, anus, vagina, meninges, conjunctiva, or retina. Although any age may be affected, the peak incidence is 40 to 60 years. An alarming increase in the incidence of lesions has been noted (second only to the rate of climb of bronchogenic carcinoma), particularly in the lower limbs of females, above the waist in males, and in the upper limbs of both sexes. This increase in frequency is attributed to the growing worship of a suntan with intense exposures to sunlight during the warm weather months.[39]

The "melanomaniacs" who have intensively studied these lesions have evolved a complex classification and even more complex terminology relating to various subtypes. Only the two most frequent subtypes will be described. It is proposed that the development of melanomas involves two patterns of growth—radial and vertical. Radial growth implies lateral spread, largely confined to the epidermis and perhaps with minimal dermal penetration. Vertical growth implies tumor progression and the emergence of a new clone having greater aggressiveness, resulting in downward spread into the dermis and subjacent layers.[40] These two patterns of growth have significantly different clinical consequences. In the radial phase the melanomas have little if any capacity for metastases, but unfortunately vertical growth brings with it the ugly potential of all anaplastic cancers. From the clinical standpoint, it is usually possible to distinguish macroscopically these two growth phases.

In some melanocarcinomas radial growth predominates for months to years before becoming invasive, and so these lesions have been called **superficial spreading melanomas.** The superficial spread rarely exceeds 4 cm in greatest diameter. **They appear as flat to raised, brown to black lesions having several distinctive characteristics: (1) focal areas of red, white, or blue coloration and (2) irregular, ill-defined serpiginous margins, sometimes with tongue-like extensions or satellite lesions.** This gross appearance should make them distinctive from the sharply circumscribed, uniformly tan-brown common nevi with their regular rounded contours, but the shape and color closely approximates those of some dysplastic nevi. Histologically this pattern is marked by anaplastic, usually pigment-laden melanocytes confined to the epidermis. Distinctive are the occasional isolated cells enclosed by a clear halo (Paget's cells) resembling those seen in Paget's disease of the breast (p. 666). In time, individual and nested tumor cells penetrate all layers of the epidermis up to the surface, sometimes with ulceration of the surface. At the same time the cells invade the dermis and ultimately move more deeply, and with this vertical growth they acquire the potential to metastasize. A variable dermal infiltrate of lymphocytes may be present along with pigment-laden macrophages.

**Some melanomas have a minimal radial phase and vertical growth is dominant (nodular melanomas).** They appear as small (1 to 3 cm), firm, raised variegated lesions marked by total involvement of the full thickness of the epidermis, sometimes with ulceration through the surface accompanied by penetration into the dermis and

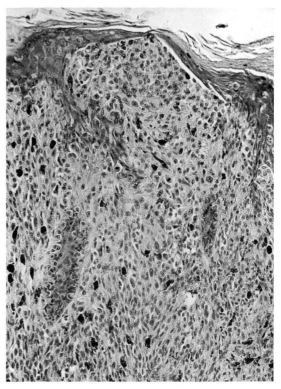

Figure 7–11. Nodular melanocarcinoma. The anaplastic cells have invaded the epidermis and have almost eroded through the surface. The dark cells are filled with melanin pigment.

more deeply (Fig. 7–11). Rarely the anaplastic melanocytes do not form pigment (amelanotic melanomas). Pigmented or not, these are **nodular melanomas** having the capacity to metastasize widely to almost any organ or tissue in the body. The metastases are usually brown to black but sometimes are nonpigmented with amelanotic primaries, on occasion even when the primary itself is deeply pigmented (attributed to the emergence of new clones lacking the ability to synthesize melanin).

Of major clinical importance are (1) the early recognition of malignant melanomas before they have penetrated deeply and acquired the potential to metastasize and (2) the prognosis of the lesions, based on the depth of penetration. Early recognition requires their differentiation from common nevi, based on the distinctive margins and pigmentary changes already described (Fig. 7–12). Warning signs are changes in size, conformation, and pigmentation and ulceration with bleeding. Much more difficult is their segregation from dysplastic nevi, and usually biopsy is required.[45] The prognosis following excision is largely determined by the depth of invasion. On this basis malignant melanomas have been classified into Levels I to V. It is sufficient here to indicate merely that Level I implies "confined to the epidermis," indicating that there is little likelihood of metastatic spread and an excellent prognosis, whereas Levels

Figure 7–12. Diagrammatic representation of gross appearances and cellular distributions of common nevus (*left*) and two patterns of melanoma.

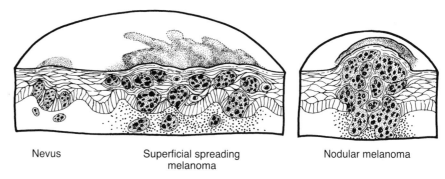

Nevus        Superficial spreading melanoma        Nodular melanoma

IV and V represent penetrations at least below the papillary dermis, yielding progressively poorer outlooks down to about 20 to 25% five-year survivals.[46] An alternative approach expresses the depth of invasion in millimeters. Although the level or thickness of a lesion is the most important prognostic index, other variables such as anatomic site of the lesion, mitotic rate, and lymphocytic response condition the outlook.[47] Early recognition is of critical importance because when these lesions are invasive they must be categorized as among the "ugliest" of cancers and may literally spray the body with implants.

## References

1. Jeevanandem, M., et al.: Cancer cachexia and protein metabolism. Lancet 1:1423, 1984.
2. Editorial: Cancer cachexia. Lancet 1:833, 1984.
3. Costa, G., and Donaldson, S. S.: Effects of cancer and cancer treatment on the nutrition of the host. N. Engl. J. Med. 300:1471, 1979.
4. Beutler, B., et al.: Identity of tumor necrosis factor and macrophage secreted factor cachectin. Nature 316:552, 1985.
5. Carey, R. M., et al.: Ectopic secretion of corticotropin-releasing factor as a cause of Cushing's syndrome. A clinical, morphologic, and biochemical study. N. Engl. J. Med. 311:13, 1984.
6. Mundy, G. R., et al.: The hypercalcemia of cancer. Clinical implications and pathogenic mechanisms. N. Engl. J. Med. 310:1718, 1984.
7. Gropp, C., et al.: Ectopic hormones in lung cancer. Ergebnisse der Inneren Medizin und Kinderheilkunde, Bd 53:133, 1984.
8. Pearse, A. G.: The diffuse neuroendocrine system and the APUD concept: related "endocrine" peptides in brain, intestine, pituitary, placenta and anuran cutaneous glands. Med. Biol. 55:115, 1977.
9. Gould, V. E., et al.: The APUD cell system and its neoplasms: Observations on the significance and limitations of the concept. Surg. Clin. North Am. 59:93, 1979.
10. Mendelsohn, G., and Baylin, S. B.: Ectopic hormone production—Biological and clinical implications. Prog. Clin. Biol. Res. 142:291, 1984.
11. Thomas, L.: Discussion. *In* Lawrence, H. S. (ed.): Cellular and Humoral Aspects of the Hypersensitive States. New York, Hoeber-Harper, 1959, p. 529.
12. Burnet, F. M.: The concept of immunological surveillance. Prog. Exp. Tumor Res 13:1, 1970.
13. Brodt, P.: Tumor immunology—three decades in review. Annu. Rev. Microbiol. 37:447, 1983.
14. Schatten, S., et al.: Suppressor T cells and the immune response to tumors. CRC Crit. Rev. Immunol. 4:335, 1984.
15. Prehn, R. T.: The immune reaction as a stimulator of tumor growth. Science 176:170, 1972.
16. Drew, S. I.: Immunological surveillance against neoplasia: An immunological quandary. Hum. Pathol. 10:5, 1979.
17. Purtilo, D. T.: Biology of disease. Defective immune surveillance in viral carcinogenesis. Lab. Invest. 51:373, 1984.
18. Schwartz, R. S.: Current concepts: Another look at immunological surveillance. N. Engl. J. Med. 293:181, 1975.
19. Hellstrom, I., and Hellstrom, K. E.: Cell-mediated reactivity to human tumor-type associated antigens: Does it exist? J. Biol. Response Mod. 2:310, 1983.
20. Carpentier, N. A., et al.: Circulating immune complexes and the prognosis of acute myeloid leukemia. N. Engl. J. Med. 307:1174, 1982.
21. Herberman, R. B.: Possible role of natural killer cells and other effector cells in immune surveillance against cancer. J. Invest. Dermatol. 83:137s, 1984.
22. Rayner, A. A., et al.: Lymphokine-activated killer (LAK) cells. Analysis of factors relevant to the immunotherapy of human cancer. Cancer 55:1327, 1985.
23. Silverberg, E.: Cancer statistics, 1985. CA 35:19, 1985.
24. Seidman, H., et al.: Probabilities of eventually developing or dying of cancer—United States, 1985. CA 35:36, 1985.
25. Gilbert, F.: Retinoblastoma and cancer genetics. N. Engl. J. Med. 314:1248, 1986.
26. Paterson, M. C.: Heritable cancer-prone disorders featuring carcinogen hypersensitivity and DNA repair deficiency. *In* Bartsch, H., and Armstrong, B. (eds.): Host Factors in Human Carcinogenesis. IARC Sci. Pub. 39:57, 1982.
27. Harnden, D. G.: The nature of inherited susceptibility to cancer. Carcinogenesis 5:1535, 1984.
28. Burt, R. W., et al.: Dominant inheritance of adenomatous colonic polyps and colorectal cancer. N. Engl. J. Med. 312:1540, 1985.
29. Mulvihill, J. J.: Clinical ecogenetics. Cancer in families. N. Engl. J. Med. 312:1569, 1985.
30. Erlandson, R. A.: Diagnostic immunohistochemistry of human tumors. Am. J. Surg. Pathol. 8:615, 1984.
31. Rankin, E. M., et al.: Treatment of two patients with B cell lymphoma with monoclonal anti-idiotype bodies. Blood 65:1373, 1985.
32. Knowles, D. M., II.: The human T-cell leukemias: Chemical, cytomorphologic, immunophenotypic and genotypic characteristics. Hum. Pathol. 17:14, 1986.
33. Sklar, J.: DNA hybridization in diagnostic pathology. Hum. Pathol. 16:654, 1985.
34. Metcalfe, S. M., and Jamieson, N. V.: A new tumour marker tested in 98 patients with bladder carcinoma. Ann. R. Coll. Surg. Engl. 66:399, 1984.
35. McIntire, K. R.: Tumor markers: How useful are they? Hosp. Pract. 19:55, 1984.
36. Minton, J. P., et al.: Results of a 400-patient carcinoembryonic antigen second-look colorectal cancer study. Cancer 55:1284, 1985.
37. Enzinger, F. M., and Winslow, D. J.: Liposarcoma—A study of 103 cases. Virchows Arch. (Pathol. Anat.) 335:367, 1962.

38. Enterline, H. T., et al.: Liposarcoma—A clinical and pathologic study of 53 cases. Cancer 13:932, 1960.

39. Fitzpatrick, T. B., and Sober, A. J.: Sunlight and skin cancer. N. Engl. J. Med. 313:818, 1985.

40. Clark, W. H., Jr., et al.: A study of tumor progression: The precursor lesions of superficial spreading and nodular melanoma. Hum. Pathol. 15:1147, 1984.

41. Greene, M. H., et al.: Acquired precursors of cutaneous malignant melanoma. The familial dysplastic nevus syndrome. N. Engl. J. Med. 312:91, 1985.

42. Green, A., et al.: Common acquired naevi and the risk of malignant melanoma. Int. J. Cancer 35:297, 1985.

43. Kraemer, K. H., et al.: Dysplastic naevi and cutaneous melanoma risk. (Letter) Lancet 2:1076, 1983.

44. Ackerman, A. B., and Mihara, I.: Dysplasia, dysplastic melanocytes, dysplastic nevi, the dysplastic nevus syndrome, and the relation between dysplastic nevi and malignant melanomas. Hum. Pathol. 16:87, 1985.

45. Friedman, R. J., et al.: Early detection of malignant melanoma: The role of physician examination and self-examination of the skin. CA 35:130, 1985.

46. Sondergaard, K.: Depth of invasion and tumor thickness in primary cutaneous malignant melanoma. A study of 2012 cases. Acta Pathol. Microbiol. Immunol. Scand. (A.) 93:49, 1985.

47. Day, C. L., et al.: Cutaneous malignant melanoma: Prognostic guidelines for physicians and patients. CA 32:113, 1982.

# 8

# Nutritional Disorders

It is a tragic irony that almost a fourth of the world's population hungers for food while an equal number eats too much or worries about the carcinogenicity, atherogenicity, or some other "-icity" of the diet. This maldistribution is all the more unconscionable because in fact the worldwide production of food is adequate for all. Nonetheless, it is estimated that as many as one billion individuals suffer from severe malnutrition and thousands die daily of starvation and allied disorders in Third World countries. Infants and young children bear the brunt of this grim mortality. In the great preponderance of instances the final event is an infection, often with diarrhea and severe fluid losses, because malnutrition severely reduces resistance—particularly immunologic—to microbial invaders. Often these hapless victims die, loaded with worms and other parasites. Contrast the infant mortality rates in developed countries, ranging around 10 deaths per 1000 live births, with those in excess of 200 per 1000 in developing countries.

Malnutrition is not restricted to the underdeveloped world nor is it always caused by a primary lack of food. It is encountered even in highly industrialized countries in pockets of poverty, among the infants and children of socioeconomically deprived families, and in the very elderly living alone; it is surprisingly common among alcoholics, drug addicts, and those with eating disorders (e.g., fear of obesity and anorexia nervosa). Patients hospitalized for long periods of time, especially when receiving parenteral feeding, are prime candidates for malnutrition. Several studies have found that over half of general medical and surgical patients hospitalized for more than two weeks develop stigmata of nutritional deficiency.[1] As noted, inadequate nutrition is not always caused by lack of food—so-called *primary malnutrition*. It may also arise from impairment in absorption, utilization, or storage; excessive losses (e.g., chronic catabolic febrile illnesses); or increased demands (e.g., pregnancy, rapid growth, and so on). In these circumstances it is referred to as *secondary malnutrition*.

The major topics to be covered here are protein-calorie malnutrition, avitaminoses, trace metal deficiencies, obesity, and the possible role of the diet in the causation of cancer. Iron deficiency and the relationship of the diet to atherosclerosis and other forms of disease are covered elsewhere.

## PROTEIN-CALORIE MALNUTRITION (PCM)

PCM, also called protein-energy malnutrition, is unquestionably the commonest, most disastrous form of malnutrition in the world. It is widespread in Third World countries; recall the mass starvation in Ethiopia brought to the world's attention in 1984. It is estimated that at least 25% of the children in these less favored areas, where 50% of all deaths occur before the age of five, suffer from PCM. In these locales, the basis for the PCM is all too apparent—inadequate food. Much milder forms of PCM may also be encountered in more affluent societies where its origins may be a primary deficiency of protein-calorie intake, owing to poverty or one of the other previously mentioned causes, or to a secondary deficiency state for one of the reasons cited earlier.

Two often overlapping PCM syndromes have been distinguished: (1) kwashiorkor and (2) marasmus. *Kwashiorkor* in the Ghanian language means "the sickness which the old one gets when the next baby is born" (i.e., when a child is deprived of breast-feeding and is fed a starchy fluid). In its advanced form, rarely encountered in developed countries, it is characterized by apathy; marked edema; "flaky-paint" hyperkeratotic or excoriated skin lesions, most often involving the extremities and face; dry, reddish or yellowish hair (sometimes in bands reflecting periods of deprivation—"flag-sign"); distended abdomen; and hepatomegaly (Fig. 8–1). Classically, there

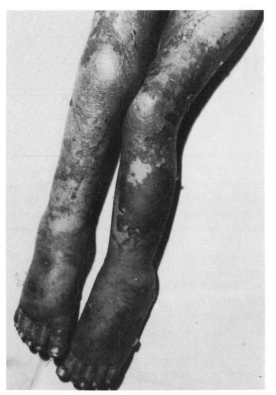

Figure 8–1. Kwashiorkor. Lower extremities of child showing the distinctive skin lesions and edema. (Courtesy of Dr. N. Scrimshaw, Massachusetts Institute of Technology; the Institute of Nutrition of Central America and Panama; and Science 133:2039, 1961. Copyright 1961 by the American Association for the Advancement of Science.)

is also marked hypoalbuminemia; a normochromic, normocytic anemia, unless other vitamin or iron deficiencies are also present; and a lymphopenia of variable severity, accompanied by depressed immune responsiveness, particularly in cell-mediated immunity. When not compounded by a lack of total calorie-energy intake (i.e., marasmus), kwashiorkor causes no significant retardation of growth. The milder forms of kwashiorkor, as seen in more affluent populations, are much more subtle and may comprise only hepatomegaly, mild hypoalbuminemia, anemia, and sometimes mild edema.

*Marasmus*, to put it bluntly, is the condition caused by starvation. In its flagrant form the child suffers from retardation or arrest of growth, loss of fat and muscle, and is transformed to a pathetic "bag of bones," with skin hanging loosely from emaciated extremities, a head too large for the scrawny torso, and an abdomen often infested with worms. Anemia and manifestations of multivitamin deficiencies are also present, but rarely is there edema.

The organ changes in these two syndromes principally involve the liver, gastrointestinal mucosa, and hematopoietic system. Kwashiorkor, but not marasmus, is characterized by fatty change in the liver, probably due to decreased synthesis of lipoproteins. There is no evidence

that these children ever develop cirrhosis, and with an adequate diet the fat in the liver completely disappears. The mucosa of the small bowel in kwashiorkor (rarely in marasmus) is usually atrophic and shows loss of microvilli and villi. There is an accompanying loss of small intestinal enzymes, most often manifested as disaccharidase deficiency. Thus these infants respond poorly to a diet of milk because of the enzyme deficiency. Despite the mucosal atrophy, no other absorptive defects are consistently present. An adequate diet and control of intercurrent infections permit recovery of the normal gastrointestinal mucosa. Anemia of the normochromic, normocytic type is almost always present in both marasmus and kwashiorkor. The anemia is often made worse by concomitant intestinal parasites, such as hookworms, that deprive the host of iron and folic acid; thus, the mixed changes of iron and folate deficiency anemia may develop. Alternatively, in kwashiorkor when protein therapy is administered, a folic acid or iron deficiency, or both, is unmasked. The bone marrow usually shows erythroid hypoplasia and a disturbed erythroid-myeloid ratio. Complete remission of all these changes in marasmus and kwashiorkor can be achieved with an adequate diet and control of infections.

Bacterial and parasitic infections plague malnourished infants and children who have marasmus or kwashiorkor. Infections are most often located in the gastrointestinal tract, but even the usual childhood infections may often prove fatal. This vulnerability is in large part related to impaired immune responses. In severe cases of marasmus and kwashiorkor there is marked atrophy of the thymus, usually with reduced numbers of T cells in the peripheral blood. The T-cell deficit is particularly marked in kwashiorkor and may be accompanied by deficient B-cell function.

It has long been held and probably remains valid that *marasmus is caused by a deficiency of total calories, whereas kwashiorkor appears when there is a deficiency of quality protein relative to the total calorie intake* (as may occur in developed countries with an unbalanced vegetarian diet). This classic view of kwashiorkor as a protein deficiency has been challenged on the grounds that there is a poor correlation between the severity of the edema and the serum albumin level[2] and by the contention that injury to the liver by dietary hepatotoxins (e.g., aflatoxins) or other nutritional insults must be present to explain the hypoalbuminemia and edema.[3] Despite these challenges, it has been observed repeatedly that marasmus in the child may be transformed into kwashiorkor by excessive losses of proteins, as occur during childhood infections, parasitism, or infectious diarrhea, or by feeding a marasmic child an adequate number of calories containing insufficient amounts of protein. Thus there appears to be a close relationship between the two syndromes, and often they overlap, suggesting closely related origins.[4]

In the usual case of protein-energy malnutrition, if the omnipresent infections can be controlled and an adequate diet restored, the course of both children and adults is toward complete recovery; "catch-up growth" will in time usually restore normal height for age. There is, however, concern that a severe deficiency state during pregnancy and in the newborn may impose irreversible deficits of physical and intellectual development on the child.

# VITAMIN DEFICIENCIES

About 45 to 50 dietary nutrients are required for health, including nine amino acids, one or possibly two fatty acids, a large number of inorganic elements, and 13 vitamins—four fat-soluble agents and the remainder water soluble. Small amounts of four can be synthesized endogenously—vitamin D from precursor steroids, vitamin K and biotin by the intestinal microflora, and niacin from tryptophan, an essential amino acid. A deficiency of vitamins may be primary (i.e., dietary in origin) or secondary because of disturbances in intestinal absorption, transport in the blood, tissue storage, or metabolic conversion. For example, the B vitamins must first be converted into their active derivatives before they can function as coenzymes. Interference with such conversion would be manifest as a deficiency state despite an adequate dietary intake. On the other side of the coin, excesses of certain vitamins have well-defined adverse effects. Once again, the old adage is confirmed: "Too much of a good thing can be bad."

In the following sections, each of the major vitamins with well-defined deficiency or toxic syndromes is discussed individually, beginning with the fat-soluble vitamins. However, it should be emphasized that individual vitamin deficiencies are uncommon and indeed may be submerged in concomitant protein-calorie malnutrition. Nonetheless, to put the puzzle together, one must first deal with the individual pieces.

## VITAMIN A

Vitamin A is fat soluble and essential for the maintenance of vision and specialized (particularly mucus-secreting) epithelia. The term "vitamin A" is applied to a number of compounds collectively known as "retinoids" having at least partial vitamin A activity. The naturally occurring preformed vitamin is retinol, which can be oxidized in the body to the aldehyde retinal (also known as retinaldehyde) and retinoic acid. Preformed vitamin A is found in the diet almost exclusively in animal products (e.g., liver, milk, fish liver oils). Vegetables such as carrots and lettuce and other green, leafy edibles contain larger precursor carotenoids that undergo cleavage to yield vitamin A activity; the most important of these is beta-carotene, constituting in essence two linked retinols. There are also well over 1000 synthetic retinoids currently used in the treatment of certain dermatologic conditions and under study for the possible treatment and prevention of certain forms of cancer (discussed later). These also have at least partial vitamin A activity and are largely (but not entirely) devoid of the toxicity of naturally occurring retinol.

The details of the absorption and metabolism of vitamin A or carotenoids are available in a recent excellent review.[5] It suffices here that a large quantity is stored in the liver and can be mobilized to yield retinol, which is transported through the blood complexed to retinol-binding protein (RBP). Thus the body's needs can be satisfied despite a long period of deprivation by the hepatic stores. Nonetheless, a primary deficiency of vitamin A remains a major problem among children in developing countries, particularly throughout Southeast Asia, making it the prime cause of blindness in the world.[6] Secondary deficiencies, usually much milder than the primary deficiencies, may be encountered in any population because of malabsorption (biliary tract, pancreatic, and extensive intestinal disease), inadequate storage in the liver (diffuse liver disease), disturbed transport (diffuse hepatic disease with impaired synthesis of RBP), or excessive excretion (proteinuria with loss of vitamin-protein complex).

**DEFICIENCY CONSEQUENCES.** Best established is the role of vitamin A in the visual process. We owe to the Nobel laureate Dr. George Wald the understanding that retinal is the prosthetic group of the photosensitive pigments in rods and cones.[7] In light, photons produce a stereochemical conversion of retinal from a *cis* to a *trans* isomer with transduction of the light energy into a neural signal. Restoration of the pigment to the active form occurs automatically in the dark and is mediated by an isomerase with reversal of the conformational changes in retinal. But a small amount is degraded or lost, and so maintenance of vision requires a constant supply of vitamin A.

Thus **one of the earliest manifestations of vitamin A deficiency is impaired vision, particularly in reduced light (night blindness)**. With a protracted deficiency this condition is followed by a sequence of physical changes collectively referred to as **xerophthalmia** (dry eye). First there is dryness of the conjunctivae **(xerosis)** as the normal lachrymal and mucus-secreting epithelium is replaced by keratinized epithelium. This is followed by the build-up of keratin debris in small opaque plaques **(Bitot's spots)** and, eventually, erosion of the roughened corneal surface with softening and destruction of the cornea **(keratomalacia)** and total blindness.

Vitamin A (and retinoids) is also involved in the differentiation of a variety of non-neoplastic and neoplastic cells. With a protracted deficiency, normal, specialized epithelial cells, particularly in the eyes (as noted earlier), upper respiratory passages, and urinary tract, are replaced by keratinizing squamous cells. Loss of the mucociliary epithelium of the airways predisposes to secondary pulmonary infections. Desquamation of keratin debris in the urinary tract predisposes to renal and urinary bladder stones. Hyperplasia and hyperkeratinization of the epidermis with plugging of the ducts of the adnexal glands may produce follicular or papular dermatosis.

How the retinoids or vitamin A exert their effects on cell differentiation is unclear. A favored hypothesis invokes some action on genomic expression similar to that of steroid hormones, which modulate cell replication by binding to intracellular protein receptors that are then translocated to the nuclei.[8] *There is therefore great current interest in the possibility that vitamin A or its synthetic analogs might be used in the prevention or treatment of cancers.* Despite the numerous studies and varying approaches, no unassailable conclusions have been reached. There are reports that low serum retinol levels are associated with an increased incidence of lung cancer and, conversely, that elevated levels exert some protection against lung and other cancers, but other studies have failed to confirm these findings.[9] From a different vantage point, the topical application of various retinoids has been reported to produce regression of basal cell carcinomas, melanomas, and various premalignant hyperplasias of the skin and mucous membranes. Here again the benefits have been challenged by other studies. One benefit is well established. The retinoids are very effective in the treatment of acne, but not without certain risks mentioned subsequently.[10] An overview of the major consequences of vitamin A deficiency is offered in Figure 8–2.

**TOXICITY.** An excess of preformed vitamin A, or some of the synthetic analogs, has well-defined adverse effects. The rabbits of the world can take comfort that an excess of carotenes produces only carotenemia (harmless yellowing of the skin but not the sclerae). The clinical consequences of hypervitaminosis A include increased intracranial pressure with headache, nausea, vomiting, skeletal pain, hepatomegaly, impaired liver functions, and a variety of hematologic abnormalities. Even more distressing, some of the synthetic analogs such as those used for the treatment of acne, when given for prolonged periods during pregnancy, have caused a significant incidence of congenital malformations in the embryo.[11] This untoward consequence is highly important; acne rarely develops in females before the age of fertility.

## VITAMIN D

Fat-soluble vitamin D is necessary for normal skeletal development and mineralization in infants and children and for maintenance of normal bone remodeling in the adult. *A significant deficiency before closure of the epiphyses induces rickets, but in adults the deficiency leads to poorly mineralized osteopenic bone, a condition known as osteomalacia.* Vitamin D performs its role by maintaining calcium homeostasis.[12] More accurately, an active metabolite referred to as a "hormone" affects the mineralization of bone. Like many other hormones, it acts on specific receptors principally in the small intestine and bone to raise normal serum calcium levels, and in turn its formation is suppressed by increased levels of serum calcium in a classic feedback loop. Vitamin D is closely interrelated not only with calcium metabolism but also with that of parathyroid hormone (PTH) and

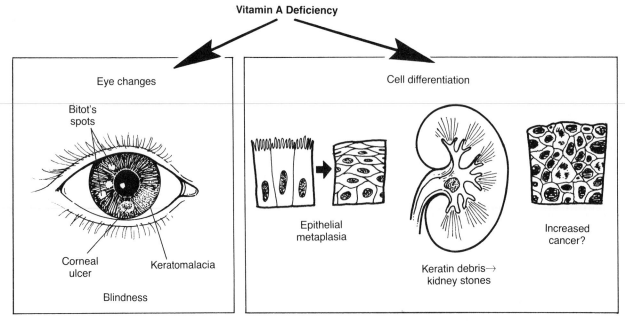

Vitamin A Deficiency

Eye changes

Bitot's spots

Corneal ulcer

Keratomalacia

Blindness

Cell differentiation

Epithelial metaplasia

Keratin debris→ kidney stones

Increased cancer?

**Figure 8–2.** Vitamin A deficiency. Its major consequences in the eye, in the production of keratinizing metaplasia of specialized epithelial surfaces, and its possible role in potentiating neoplasia.

phosphorus, all of which are involved in bone mineralization.

Endogenous synthesis of vitamin $D_3$ by ultraviolet irradiation of 7-dehydrocholesterol in the skin can provide adequate supplies in sunny climes. In the Northern Hemisphere, dietary augmentation is almost always needed. The diet also contains vitamin $D_3$, which occurs naturally in fish liver oils or as a supplement in milk and other foods, and vitamin $D_2$, derived from plant ergosterol. Both forms of the vitamin are identical in their metabolism and function and will henceforth be referred to as "vitamin D."

Metabolic conversion of vitamin D into its active hormone is depicted in Figure 8–3. Critical steps in this process are:

○ Transport of vitamin D to the liver from the skin or after intestinal absorption bound to an alpha-globulin binding protein (vitamin DBP).

○ Conversion by a hepatic vitamin D-25-hydroxylase in the microsomes or mitochondria to 25-(OH)D.

○ Transport to the kidney of the 25-(OH)D in the blood bound to vitamin DBP.

○ Conversion in the kidney of 25-(OH)D into $1,25(OH)_2D$, the active hormone (known as calcitriol), by a mitochondrial 1-alpha-hydroxylase.

○ Delivery of the $1,25(OH)_2D$ (calcitriol) to its target organs, the intestines and bones.

○ In the intestine, $1,25(OH)_2D$ enhances calcium absorption by a complex process—in part by increasing the synthesis of a mucosal cell calcium-binding protein.[13] It independently increases absorption of phosphates.

○ The actions of $1,25(OH)_2D$ on bone depend on the serum levels of calcium. On the one hand, by facilitating intestinal absorption, it maintains normal serum levels of calcium and phosphorus and thus provides for mineralization of bone. On the other hand, when the serum levels of calcium fall, the active hormone in concert with parathormone (PTH) mobilizes calcium from bone to restore normocalcemia. The action is mediated primarily by PTH; the vitamin D–hormone's role is permissive.

A complex of regulatory mechanisms involving parathormone and phosphorus also participates in fine-tuning calcium homeostasis. When hypocalcemia occurs, the parathyroid glands release increased amounts of hormone, which (1) accelerates the activity of the renal 1-alpha-hydroxylase to thus increase the amount of $1,25(OH)_2D$ synthesized, (2) mobilizes calcium from bone, (3) decreases renal excretion of calcium, and (4) increases renal excretion of phosphate. The serum level of calcium is restored but the hypophosphatemia may persist (Fig. 8–3). When hypercalcemia occurs, parathormone secretion is suppressed and along with it the synthesis of $1,25(OH)_2D$, and an alternative renal enzyme is activated with the synthesis of an inactive metabolite $24,25(OH)_2D$. A depressed level of phosphate also increases the amount of $1,25(OH)_2D$ synthesized, which also enhances phosphate absorption in the small intestine to thus maintain the normal serum ratio of calcium to phosphorus.

It is evident that the intestines, kidneys, and parathyroid glands all participate in vitamin D metabolism and in the maintenance of normal calcium and phosphate levels in the serum requisite for normal mineralization of bone.[14] Not surprisingly, then, *many dysfunctions may lead to rickets or osteomalacia* (Table 8–1). Only a few comments are necessary. The classic dietary vitamin D deficiency—rickets—is now uncommon in the western world owing to the widespread practice of food supplementation, but it is still encountered in impoverished, malnourished rural populations. By contrast, osteomalacia is common in both developing and developed countries when individuals survive into their later years. A marginal dietary intake of vitamin D in older individuals may contribute to this skeletal disorder. More likely, it is multifactorial in origin and also involves avoidance of sun exposure (and reduced endogenous synthesis), marginal dietary calcium intake, and possibly hormonal influence because the condition is particularly common in postmenopausal women. Malabsorption of the fat-soluble vitamin may occur at any age from infancy to advanced life, depending on the onset of the disorder impairing fat absorption. The many other potential causes of rickets or osteomalacia such as diffuse liver disease, renal failure, and the inherited systemic syndromes are too uncommon to merit further comment.

*Whatever the basis, a deficiency of vitamin D tends to cause hypocalcemia followed by the train of events*

## Table 8–1. CAUSES OF RICKETS OR OSTEOMALACIA

**Decreased Endogenous Synthesis of Vitamin**
 Inadequate exposure to sunlight
 Heavy melanin pigmentation of skin (blacks)

**Decreased Absorption of Fat-soluble Vitamin in the Intestine**
 Dietary lack
 Biliary tract, pancreatic, or intestinal dysfunction

**Enhanced Degradation of Vitamin D and 25(OH)D**
 Phenytoin, phenobarbital, rifampin

**Impaired Synthesis of 25(OH)D**
 Diffuse liver diseases

**Decreased Synthesis of $1,25(OH)_2D$**
 Advanced renal disease with failure
 Vitamin D–dependent rickets type I
  (inherited deficiency, renal 1-alpha-hydroxylase)
 ? Aging (postmenopausal)

**Target Organ Resistance to $1,25(OH)_2D$**
 Vitamin D–dependent rickets type 2
  (congenital lack of or defective receptors for active
  metabolite)

**Phosphate Depletion**
 Poor absorption—chronic use of antacids, which bind
  phosphates and render them insoluble
 Renal tubular disorders—acquired or genetic, causing
  increased excretion

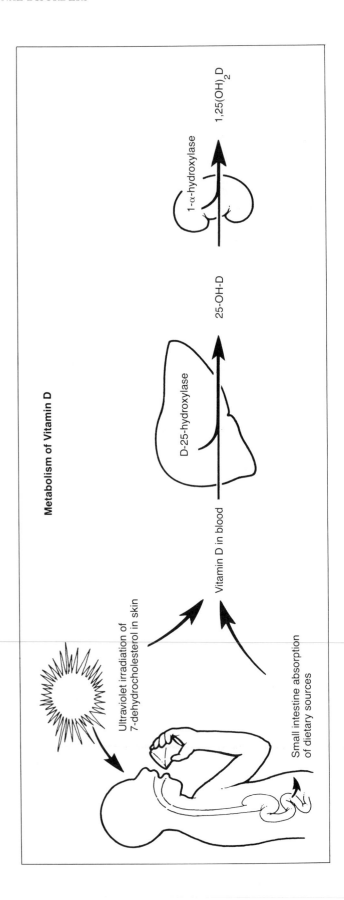

**Metabolism of Vitamin D**

Ultraviolet irradiation of 7-dehydrocholesterol in skin

Small intestine absorption of dietary sources

Vitamin D in blood

D-25-hydroxylase

25-OH-D

1-α-hydroxylase

1,25(OH)$_2$D

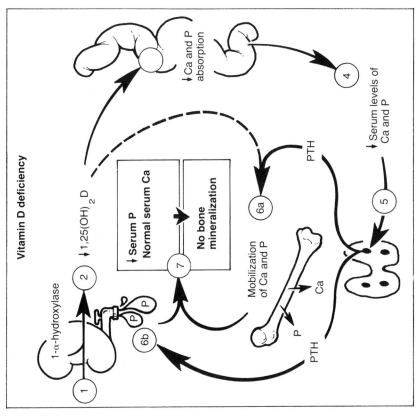

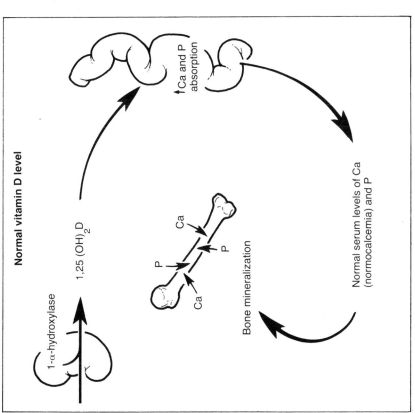

**Figure 8–3.** A schema of normal vitamin D metabolism (*above*) and function (*lower left*). With vitamin D deficiency (*lower right*), there is inadequate substrate for the renal hydroxylase (1) yielding a deficiency of 1,25(OH)₂D (2) and deficient absorption of calcium and phosphorus from the gut (3) with consequent depressed serum levels of both (4). The hypocalcemia activates the parathyroid glands (5), causing along with the D deficiency mobilization of calcium and phosphorus from bone (6a). Simultaneously, the PTH induces wasting of phosphate in the urine (6b). Consequently, the serum levels of calcium are normal or near normal but the phosphate is low, hence bone mineralization is impaired (7).

*discussed earlier, involving increased levels of 1,25(OH)₂D and PTH with its phosphate-wasting action on the kidney. Thus while the serum level of calcium may be restored to normal, the increased urinary phosphate excretion leads to hypophosphatemia and consequent impaired mineralization of bone. In passing it might be noted that calcium has many other critical functions in addition to bone mineralization—in blood clotting, regulating the level of neuromuscular irritability, maintenance of normal membrane permeability, and many other intracellular functions.*

**The basic change with both rickets and osteomalacia is an excess of poorly mineralized osteoid tissue leading in the former to deranged epiphyseal bone growth and in the latter to defective bone remodeling.**
The changes in rickets are as follows:

1. Failure of deposition of calcium and phosphate into the cartilage—i.e., failure of provisional calcification.

2. Failure of the cartilage cells to mature and disintegrate, with resultant overgrowth of cartilage.

3. Persistence of distorted, irregular masses of cartilage, many of which project into the marrow cavity.

4. Deposition of osteoid matrix on cartilaginous remnants, with formation of a disorderly, totally disrupted osteochondral junction (Fig. 8–4).

5. Abnormal overgrowth of capillaries and fibroblasts into the disorganized zone.

6. Bending, compression, and microfractures of soft, weakly supported osteoid and cartilaginous tissue, with resultant skeletal deformities.

The gross skeletal deformities depend to a large extent on the stress to which individual bones are subjected, which, in turn, is related to the age of the child. During infancy, the nonambulatory child places greatest stress upon the head and chest. Often, the abnormally soft cranium can be buckled under pressure, recoiling back into position with release of pressure. This clinical sign is known as **craniotabes**. An excess of osteoid tissue produces **frontal bossing** and a squared appearance to the head. Chest deformities include the **rachitic rosary**, caused by overgrowth of osteoid tissue at the costochondral junctions; the **pigeon-breast deformity**, resulting from collapse of the ribs with relative protrusion of the sternum; and **Harrison's groove**, produced by the inward pull on the ribs at the margin of the diaphragm. When the child with full-blown rickets begins to ambulate, additional deformities occur in the spine, pelvis, and long bones. Lumbar lordosis and bowing of the legs are common.

In adults the lack of vitamin D deranges normal bone remodeling that occurs throughout life. As you know, trabecular bone is constantly being resorbed, but new bone formation exactly balances the trabecular resorption to thus maintain the skeleton. The newly formed osteoid matrix laid down by osteoblasts is inadequately mineralized, thus producing the excess of persistent osteoid characteristic of **osteomalacia**. Although the contours of the bone are not affected, it is abnormally weak and

vulnerable to gross or microfractures, which are most likely to affect the vertebral bodies and femoral necks.

Histologically, the unmineralized osteoid can be visualized as a thickened layer of pink-staining matrix (in H and E preparations) about the more basophilic normally mineralized trabeculae.

Rickets, when well advanced, presents no clinical diagnostic challenge, but when less developed can be extremely subtle. The skeletal deformities when present are readily apparent. There may also be bone pain and muscle weakness. X-ray examination merely confirms the skeletal changes and may disclose abnormal radiolucence of the bones. Characteristically, the serum alkaline phosphatase level is elevated because of the osteoblastic activity; serum calcium and phosphorus levels may be either normal or low. The diagnosis of osteomalacia in adults is not simple. Predisposition to compression fractures of the vertebral bodies and fractures of other bones may raise the suspicion of this condition, but it is exceedingly difficult to estimate the adequacy of bony mineralization from routine diagnostic radiographs. Special techniques exist to quantitate the amount of calcium in the skeleton, but they are not widely available. Moreover, decreased bony mineralization is also encountered in osteoporosis and a few other disorders and so it is difficult to differentiate these various

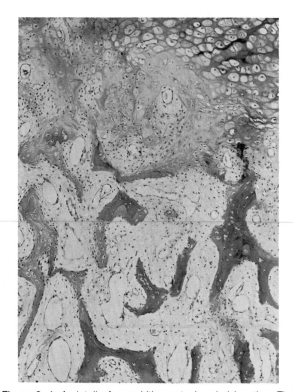

Figure 8–4. A detail of a rachitic costochondral junction. The palisade of cartilage is lost. Some of the trabeculae are old, well-formed bone, but the paler ones consist of unmineralized osteoid tissue. (From Robbins, S. L., Cotran, R. S., and Kumar, V.: Pathologic Basis of Disease. 3rd ed. Philadelphia, W. B. Saunders Co., 1984.)

*osteopenias* radiologically. Helpful in adults and in children with less advanced rickets are abnormally low serum levels of the vitamin D metabolites—25(OH)D and 1,25(OH)$_2$D.

*Hypervitaminosis D* induces hypercalcemia manifested by weakness, lethargy, headaches, and nausea. The elevated calcium levels in turn lead to hypercalciuria and metastatic calcifications in various sites throughout the body, particularly the kidneys, blood vessels, and lungs, as described on page 26.

## VITAMIN E

It was only in 1977 that it was said of this fat-soluble vitamin, "we are still faced with a vitamin looking for a disease with which it can have an honorable marriage."[15] Since then a lack of vitamin E has been associated with a more or less well-characterized disorder, but much remains to be clarified and so this presentation will be brief.

Vitamin E is one of the most widely available vitamins and is found in the form of tocopherols and related compounds in cooking oils, whole grains, and a wide variety of leafy green vegetables. Primary nutritional deficiencies therefore are only encountered in the severely malnourished suffering from multiple dietary problems. Secondary deficiencies are, however, encountered, particularly in neonates having any disorder that impairs fat absorption and causes steatorrhea (e.g., disease of the biliary tract, pancreas, or intestinal mucosa) or affects fat transport (e.g., abetalipoproteinemia). Controversy continues about whether premature infants have only marginal stores and require immediate supplementation.

*Most clearly documented is the role of vitamin E as an antioxidant*, stabilizing unsaturated lipids against auto-oxidation as by free radicals. The more polyunsaturates in the diet, the more E required. You already know the wide-ranging potential of free radicals in producing cell injury, notably membrane damage and denaturation of DNA. Although vitamin E does not function alone in protection against free radicals, it nonetheless plays a critical and important role. In passing we might note that selenium is a component of glutathione perioxidase, which complements the antioxidant function of vitamin E. A deficiency of vitamin E has at last been fairly clearly associated with a clinical syndrome encountered most often in children who also have biliary tract obstruction, abetalipoproteinemia, or some other steatorrheal disorder. The syndrome constitutes a spinocerebellar degeneration with loss of nerve fibers in the posterior spinal columns and "dying back" regressive changes in the related sensory neurons.[16] As a consequence, these children develop ataxia of gait, areflexia, and loss of position and vibratory sense. Whether or not the retinal degeneration and visual disturbances sometimes seen in these children is secondary to a lack of vitamin E or a concomitant lack of vitamin A remains uncertain. A deficiency of vitamin E has also been suspected to cause a hemolytic anemia, particularly in premature and newborn infants, but this view has been strongly challenged.[17]

Because of its well-defined antioxidant activity, vitamin E has been used in the treatment of a variety of conditions thought to be at least in part caused by oxidative or free radical injury (e.g., retrolental fibroplasia in premature infants exposed to high oxygen tensions in incubators), and it has been used in conjunction with oxygen in infants having severe respiratory problems and in those of low birth weight who have hemolytic anemia.[18] In all these situations, there is still uncertainty about the usefulness of the vitamin, but at least the dosages administered are small and not likely to be harmful. In contrast, an enormous volume of distorted hyperbole in the media "hustles" the use of megadoses of vitamin E as a cure-all for maintaining muscular and sexual vigor and the youthfulness of the skin as well as everything under it. To paraphrase an eminent physician: if it also facilitated getting rich, it would satisfy the major wants of American culture.[19] There is no evidence that megadoses of vitamin E provide any benefit except to its purveyors. This vain pursuit of youth and beauty would be amusing were it not for the many potential adverse effects, including decreased platelet aggregation, impaired wound healing, hepatomegaly, impaired fibrinolysis, and impairment of absorption of vitamin K. The consequences of vitamin E toxicity in the preterm child are even more threatening—renal failure, liver disease, thrombocytopenia, and even death.[20] Such risks clearly indicate that this vitamin is not to be trifled with.

## VITAMIN K

This fat-soluble vitamin is essential for the synthesis in the liver of the plasma coagulation factors II (prothrombin), VII, IX, and X. Thus a deficiency of vitamin K induces a bleeding tendency (hemorrhagic diathesis) that continues to be a major global cause of infant morbidity and mortality.[21] Specifically, *vitamin K is required for the post-translational carboxylation of glutamic acid residues on the coagulation factor precursor proteins*. Carboxylation provides calcium binding sites without which the precursors are functionally defective.[22] In the course of this carboxylation, vitamin K–epoxide is formed, which is then reconverted to vitamin K by a reductase. The existence of a vitamin K deficiency clinically can be determined by assays of the noncarboxylated prothrombin in the blood. This functionally inactive prothrombin is often referred to as PIVKA (*protein induced in vitamin K absence*). A less specific assay but one that is widely used clinically is the prothrombin time, which becomes longer than normal when a deficiency of vitamin K blocks the synthesis of prothrombin. However, the prothrombin time is also lengthened by diffuse liver disease. In passing we should note that protein C, an important inhibitor of coagulation (discussed on p. 67) is also vitamin K dependent, as are a few other less well understood proteins.

The normal intestinal flora synthesizes some vitamin K, but the amount that can be absorbed is small and does not obviate the need for dietary sources. Vitamin K is found in liver, cheese, butter, plants, vegetable oils, and, of particular revelance to the newborn, in human milk (but in smaller amounts than in most commercial formulas). Deficiency states may occur in adults but are much more common in the newborn and young infants. *In adults*, it is almost always a conditioned deficiency related to some form of diffuse liver disease that impairs both absorption of vitamin K and the synthesis of vitamin K–dependent proteins.[23] The long-term use of the anticoagulant warfarin (Coumadin) also may lead to a deficiency state. This drug derives its effectiveness as an anticoagulant by interfering with the reductase that reconverts vitamin K–epoxide to vitamin K and thus depletes the body's stores of the vitamin.

*The infant* is particularly vulnerable to vitamin K deficiency because its reserves are marginal and appear to depend on gestational maturity and the circulating levels of vitamin K in the mother. These reserves are gnerally believed to be sufficiently low to require prophylactic administration of vitamin K to all neonates to prevent the possible development of serious (e.g., intracranial) hemorrhages, but this practice is not universally accepted.[21] The neonatal levels of vitamin K are particularly low when the mother has been taking warfarin or anticonvulsant drugs such as barbiturates or phenytoin during pregnancy. In the first few months following birth, the vitamin K level in the infant reaches the normal adult value; however, this occurs more slowly in breast-fed infants than in those receiving formulas or cow's milk. A vitamin K deficiency may also be encountered after the first few months of life when there is (1) chronic warfarin exposure, (2) persistent diarrhea that superimposes decreased absorption and decreased synthesis by intestinal flora on top of marginal dietary intake, (3) any disorder that interferes with fat absorption (e.g., cystic fibrosis, diffuse liver disease, celiac disease), or (4) any disorder with extensive intestinal mucosal damage.

Whatever the cause of the deficiency state, it is marked by a predisposition to bleeding, which may range from the trivial (increased tendency to bruise or have nosebleeds) to the catastrophic (intracranial hemorrhage, which can be epidural, subarachnoid, subdural, intracerebral, or intracerebellar). Other patterns of bleeding include petechial hemorrhages, hematuria, melena, and excessive oozing from puncture sites. Within 12 hours after intravenous administration of some form of vitamin K, the prothrombin levels return to normal with disappearance of the bleeding tendency.

## B VITAMINS

The water-soluble B vitamins (or B complex) are often found together in such foods as yeast, grains, rice, vegetables, fish, and meats. The various members of this group function as essential coenzymes in intermediary metabolism, particularly in energy-releasing mechanisms and in hematopoiesis. The energy-releasing reactions provide the sources of the high-energy bonds of ATP, and so deficiencies of B vitamins tend to induce changes in tissues having high levels of metabolism and rapid turnover. Thus dermatitis, stomatitis, gastritis, and blood and bone marrow disorders are features common to many of the vitamin B deficiencies. Degenerative disorders of the brain and nerves are also characteristic of these deficiency states, because nervous tissue is totally dependent on glucose for its energy requirements. In hematopoiesis, vitamin $B_{12}$ and folates are essential for maturation of red cell precursors (and other rapidly proliferating cells). The B vitamins are water soluble and so their absorption is unaffected by malabsorption states except those that result from severe diarrhea or diffuse involvement of the intestinal mucosa.

With these brief remarks on a large subject, we turn to a consideration of the major members of the B complex.

### Thiamine (Vitamin B₁)

Thiamine, after conversion to thiamine pyrophosphate, serves as a crucial coenzyme in intracellular carbohydrate metabolism. It is critical to the pentosephosphate pathway and the tricarboxylic acid cycle. It also participates in a poorly defined manner in neural conduction. As a water-soluble vitamin, it is readily absorbed from dietary sources but only in a limited amount. Thus a continued supply is necessary. A deficiency worldwide on a dietary basis is seen only with severe malnourishment because this vitamin is readily available in whole grains, peas, beans, beef, pork, and nuts. In developed nations deficiencies are most commonly encountered in chronic alcoholics because of their poor nutrition in general and because alcohol interferes with intestinal absorption of thiamine. Surveys indicate that as many as one-quarter of chronic alcoholics admitted to general hospitals in the United States are deficient in thiamine. Much less frequently the deficiency is seen as a result of pernicious vomiting of pregnancy, long-term parenteral nutrition, or debilitating chronic illnesses that impair the appetite and predispose to vomiting. Because thiamine is required for carbohydrate metabolism, a marginal reserve may be converted to an acute deficiency syndrome with intensive intravenous glucose therapy unless thiamine is simultaneously administered.

*A deficiency of vitamin $B_1$ is known clinically as beriberi*. The principal targets affected are the heart, central nervous system, and peripheral nerves. For unknown reasons, in most instances only one of these targets is predominantly involved. Thus cardiac disease with failure may dominate (*wet beriberi*) or there may be involvement only of the nervous system (*dry beriberi*). Whatever the clinical pattern, there is usually concomitant anorexia, anemia (responsive to thiamine), and sometimes lactic acidosis because of interference with pyruvate metabolism in the pentose-phosphate pathway.

*Beriberi heart disease is marked by cardiac dilatation with four-chamber enlargement and pallor and flabbiness of the myocardium.* The histologic changes are unimpressive and inconstant and include interstitial myocardial edema, swelling of myofibers, and, rarely, individual myofibrillar necrosis. Often there is concomitant alcoholism, as noted, which also has cardiotoxicity, confusing the interpretation of the histologic findings. The valves and other features of the heart are unaffected, but occasionally mural thrombi are found in the markedly enlarged atrial appendages. This involvement of the heart often leads to cardiac failure, predominantly of the right side, and the consequent peripheral edema accounting for the designation "wet beriberi." Simultaneously, there is marked peripheral vasodilatation, which leads to a ruddy, warm, dry skin, a decrease in circulation time, and so-called high-output failure.[24]

*Involvement of the central nervous system produces the Wernicke-Korsakoff syndrome.*[25] Generally, Wernicke's encephalopathy precedes the development of Korsakoff's psychosis. *Wernicke's syndrome is marked by focal symmetrical subependymal areas of grayish discoloration and sometimes softening with congestion and possibly punctate hemorrhages about the third and fourth ventricles and aqueduct.* A favored location is the mammillary bodies. Histologically, the changes are variable and include hypertrophy and hyperplasia of small blood vessels, sometimes enclosed within fresh hemorrhage; degenerative changes up to necrosis of neurons; and degenerative changes in nerve fibers involving not only the myelin sheath but also the axon process. As a consequence, these patients classically have the triad of ocular abnormalities (most often nystagmus), ataxia, and confusion, to which is often added loss of equilibrium. Because only about 10% of chronic alcoholics develop the Wernicke-Korsakoff syndrome, individual predisposition is suspected, and indeed an abnormality of a thiamine-requiring enzyme has been observed in some patients with CNS involvement.[26]

With *Korsakoff's psychosis*, the cortical gray matter may be diffusely affected with brain swelling and edema and retrogressive changes in neurons. With such widespread CNS involvement, loss of memory, spontaneity, and initiative appear, often accompanied by confabulation (fabrication of stories).

*When involvement of the peripheral nerves occurs, it is usually symmetrical and takes the form of a* *nonspecific neuropathy with myelin degeneration and disruption of axons, involving motor, sensory, and reflex arcs* (p. 752). It usually first appears in the legs but may extend to the arms, and so classically these patients present with toe, foot, and wrist drop. The response to thiamine administration is variable and depends on the severity of the clinical dysfunction. In most instances, beriberi heart disease responds favorably to thiamine and other supportive measures. When diagnosed early, Wernicke's encephalopathy is curable, generally without residual effects, but a 10 to 20% fatality rate still prevails.[25] Fortunately, thiamine is without significant toxicity, and so massive doses can be given and may be necessary to starve off death. However, with Korsakoff's psychosis improvement is not common despite all therapeutic measures.

### Riboflavin (Vitamin B₂)

Riboflavin is an essential component of the coenzymes flavin mononucleotide (FMN) and flavin adenine dinucleotide (FAD), involved mainly in a wide variety of oxidation-reduction reactions in intermediary metabolism. Riboflavin sometimes incorporated within FAD is widely available in beef, poultry, fish, eggs, milk, and dairy derivatives. Thus a deficiency on the basis of inadequate diet is only encountered when there is, almost inevitably, a concurrent inadequacy of other essential nutrients, including vitamins, proteins, and calories. Secondary deficiencies, however, may occur with diffuse intestinal disease or the protracted use of psychotropic drugs that interfere with the production of FMN and FAD; chronic alcoholism; extensive injuries (burns, trauma); and severe, chronic debilitating disease.

The clinical signs of riboflavin deficiency are poorly defined and frequently are accompanied by manifestations of deficiencies of the other members of the B complex. When full-blown, *it presents as lesions involving the lips, tongue, skin, eyes, and bone marrow.* The lip lesions can be characterized as *angular stomatitis.* Pallor or redness appears at the angles of the lips and is followed by desquamation and painful fissuring. Essentially similar changes occur along the vermilion borders of the lips as well, a condition referred to as *cheilosis.* These changes are not specific and may be found also in aged individuals who show drooling and maceration of the lips and angles of the mouth. *The tongue lesion (glossitis) results from atrophy of the mucosa, with loss of filiform papillae* (Fig. 8–5). Often the fungiform papillae are enlarged, producing a pebbled appearance. Such atrophy of the tongue mucosa, along with a superficial submucosal inflammation, induces a bright red or magenta color. A *greasy, scaling dermatitis* may appear over the nasolabial fold and may extend in a butterfly distribution over the cheeks and face, particularly about the ears. Skin lesions also develop on the scrotum and vulva, and sometimes over the

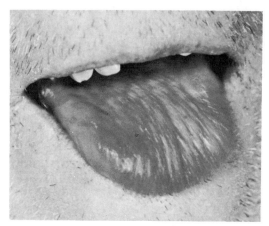

Figure 8–5. The glazed, shiny, atrophic tongue seen in riboflavin deficiency. (From Robbins, S. L., Cotran, R. S., and Kumar, V.: Pathologic Basis of Disease. 3rd ed. Philadelphia, W. B. Saunders Co., 1984.)

trunk and extremities. In this context, it should be noted that niacin deficiency (pellagra) also induces skin lesions, and frequently deficiencies of both nutrients exist. The changes in the eyes take the form of *interstitial keratitis* with vascularization and inflammation of the cornea, sometimes leading to ulceration or opacification. With severe deficiency states, the bone marrow becomes hypoplastic and induces a marked normocytic, normochromic anemia.

No toxicity has been associated with the use of large doses of riboflavin.

### Niacin

Niacin is the term employed for nicotinic acid and its derivatives (e.g., nicotinamide). It is required for the formation of the coenzymes nicotinamide adenine dinucleotide (NAD) and nicotinamide adenine dinucleotide phosphate (NADP), which participate in a wide variety of redox reactions involving carbohydrate, protein, and lipid metabolism, particularly cell respiration.

Unlike the other B vitamins, niacin can be endogenously synthesized from tryptophan. Thus a deficiency state can only develop when there is insufficient tryptrophan available for synthesis of niacin, coupled with a dietary deficiency of niacin (which is widely available in all varieties of meat, most vegetables, and grains). Other complexities may also lead to a deficiency state. High dietary levels of the amino acid leucine antagonize the synthesis of NAD and NADP. Chronic alcoholism impairs absorption of niacin, and diarrheal states may cause excessive losses. Finally, the carcinoid syndrome (p. 538) may be complicated by a deficiency of niacin because tryptophan is usurped for the synthesis of serotonin.

Whatever its basis, a deficiency of niacin leads to the clinical condition known as *pellagra* (*pelle*, "skin," and *agra*, "rough"), from time immemorial remembered by the three D's—*dermatitis, diarrhea, and dementia. The dermatitis is usually bilaterally symmetric and is found mainly on exposed areas of the body.* It may also occur in protected areas, such as the elbows and knees, and in the body folds. The changes comprise at first redness, thickening, and roughening of the skin, which may be followed by extensive scaling and desquamation, producing fissures and chronic inflammation. Depigmentation or increased pigmentation may develop, resulting in a mottled rash. Similar lesions may occur in the mucous membranes of the mouth and vagina. The *tongue often becomes red, swollen, and beefy,* reminiscent of the black tongue found in pellagrous animals. *The diarrhea is caused by atrophy of the columnar epithelium of the gastrointestinal tract mucosa, followed by submucosal inflammation. The atrophy may be followed by ulceration. The dementia is based upon regressive changes in the neurons of the brain, accompanied by degeneration of the tracts of the spinal cord.* In advanced cases, the spinal cord lesions come to resemble the alterations in the posterior spinal column in patients who have pernicious anemia caused by a deficiency of vitamin $B_{12}$. It is suspected, therefore, that the cord lesions in pellagrous patients reflect multiple B-vitamin deficiencies.

No serious overdosage effect has been identified, but when niacin is administered parenterally (not orally) it produces peripheral vasodilatation and the sensations of heat, flushing, and itching, which pass within an hour.

### Pyridoxine (Vitamin B₆)

The discussion of this vitamin can be brief because despite its important role as a coenzyme in the intermediary metabolism of amino acids and complex glycolipids, the clinical and anatomic consequences of a deficiency are not clearly delineated. A limited amount of pyridoxine can be synthesized by the bacterial flora of the gut. Moreover, pyridoxine and its analogs are widely available in vegetables, fruits, grains, meats, and other foodstuffs and so dietary deficiency is unusual. However, secondary deficiency states may be produced by long-term use of a variety of drugs, notably isoniazid (used in the treatment of tuberculosis). Alcoholism also may lead to deficiencies. In addition, there is a group of uncommon inborn errors of metabolism known as pyridoxine-dependency syndromes, which require massive doses of this vitamin. Whatever the setting, a lack of vitamin $B_6$ has been associated with dermatitis, glossitis, cheilosis, and, in infants and children, diarrhea, anemia, peripheral neuropathy, and sometimes convulsions—all reminiscent of those encountered in the deficiency states of the B vitamins already described.

Of recent date, a severe sensory neuropathy has been described in patients taking megadoses of pyridoxine in the ill-founded belief that it is "bodybuilding" or a remedy for the premenstrual syndrome.[27]

## Vitamin B₁₂ and Folate

A deficiency of vitamin $B_{12}$ and folate induces megaloblastic anemias that are remarkably similar but can be distinguished from each other by certain clinical findings and by specific laboratory tests. A lack of either vitamin leads to defective maturation of all proliferating cells, notably the precursors of red cells in the bone marrow. As a consequence, gigantism of these cells develops, as evidenced in the blood by abnormally large red cells (macrocytes). These anemias are discussed in detail on page 365 and so remarks here can be confined to a few nutritional comments.

A *deficiency of vitamin $B_{12}$* on a dietary basis occurs only among strict vegetarians, because animal proteins are the sole source of this vitamin. The animals in turn acquire the vitamin from the microorganisms growing in soil, water, and their intestinal tracts. Secondary deficiencies, however, occur in a number of specific clinical settings discussed on page 366. Prominent among them is so-called pernicious anemia, marked by inadequate gastric synthesis of intrinsic factor required for the intestinal absorption of vitamin $B_{12}$.

*Folate deficiency* occurs most commonly among pregnant women because of their increased needs for this nutrient. Although folates are abundant in nearly all natural foods, exposure of the food to 100°C for 15 minutes destroys it. Thus a daily diet containing some fresh or fresh-frozen uncooked fruit or vegetable is necessary to prevent folate deficiency. In affluent societies only chronic alcoholics and drug addicts have a sufficiently restricted diet to produce a folate deficiency in the absence of pregnancy.

## VITAMIN C

As is well known, a deficiency of vitamin C (ascorbic acid) in humans produces *scurvy*. Because this vitamin is water soluble and readily absorbed from the intestines, conditioned deficiencies are uncommon. Analogously, primary dietary deficiencies are rarely encountered in developed countries because the vitamin is abundant in foods (vegetables, liver, fish, milk, and notably citrus fruits). Moreover, stores of ascorbic acid under normal conditions are sufficient for long periods of negative balance. Nonetheless, dietary deficiencies are sometimes encountered in chronic alcoholics, rigid devotees of macrobiotic diets, the very elderly who live on a "tea and toast" diet, and the neglected, underprivileged poor of the world.

Vitamin C is a powerful antioxidant and so participates in wide-ranging redox reactions and in hydrogen ion transfer. It serves many important functions:
○ Synthesis of normal collagen
○ Synthesis of chondroitin sulfate
○ Maintenance of the folate pool
○ Facilitation of the absorption of nonheme iron and the mobilization of iron stored in cells
○ Synthesis of neurotransmitters
○ ? Maintenance of the mobility and phagocytic activity of neutrophils and macrophages

The most clearly established function of vitamin C is the activation of prolyl and lysyl hydroxylases from inactive precursors, providing for hydroxylation of procollagen.[28] Inadequately hydroxylated precursors cannot acquire stable helical configuration and cannot be adequately cross-linked (as discussed on p. 56) and so are poorly secreted from the fibroblast. Such inadequately cross-linked collagen as is produced lacks tensile strength, has increased solubility, and is more vulnerable to enzymatic degradation.[29] Collagen, normally having the highest content of hydroxyproline, is most affected, such as in blood vessels, accounting for the predisposition to hemorrhages in scurvy.[30]

The major clinical consequences of a deficiency of vitamin C can be deduced from its functions, particularly in the formation of normal collagen. **Thus scurvy is characterized by (1) weakened blood vessels, particularly microvessels having the least muscular support, (2) defective synthesis of osteoid (a derivative of collagen), and (3) impaired wound healing.** Other less prominent changes may also be present.

Even the minor trauma of daily life causes rupture of capillaries and venules with consequent hemorrhage. Rupture is, of course, most likely when venous pressures are increased. An example of this is the sudden rash of skin petechiae that develops distal to the cuff as the blood pressure is taken. Histologically, scorbutic vessels appear normal, since the alterations are submicroscopic. When hemorrhages occur, favored sites are the joints of the lower extremities (hemarthroses), subperiosteum, and skin (perifollicular hemorrhages about hair shafts, petechiae, and ecchymoses) (Fig. 8–6). Nosebleeds and hemorrhages into the conjunctivae, eyeballs, brain, and kidneys are also encountered. Bleeding into the gastrointestinal tract may produce melena. In addition, the gingivae characteristically become edematous, spongy, and

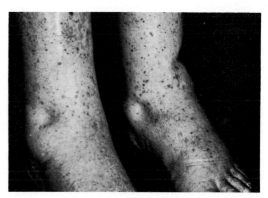

Figure 8–6. The lower extremities of a patient with marked malnutrition, nutritional edema, and petechial hemorrhages related to low levels of vitamin C. (From Robbins, S. L., Cotran, R. S., and Kumar, V.: Pathologic Basis of Disease. 3rd ed. Philadelphia, W. B. Saunders Co., 1984.)

hemorrhagic, presumably on the basis of vascular fragility. Secondary bacterial infections (gingivitis) often follow.

**Defective bone formation and maintenance result from the deficient elaboration of osteoid matrix, in turn related to the defect in collagen synthesis.** Mineralization remains normal. The palisade of cartilage cells is formed as usual and is provisionally calcified, but the osteoblasts are incapable of forming bone matrix. Resorption of the cartilage is then retarded and as a consequence, long, irregular spicules of overgrown cartilage project into the marrow shaft. The resultant disorganization of the epiphyseal line of growth is similar to that seen with rickets. The persistent cartilage ultimately becomes patchily or completely calcified, without the intermediate formation of osteoid matrix (Fig. 8–7). Since calcified cartilage is an inadequate structural substitute for normal bone, this poorly formed material is subject to compression and distortion by the stresses of weightbearing and muscle tension. Pathologic fractures may occur, complicated by the bleeding diathesis. Resorption of alveolar bone causes the teeth to loosen, fall out, or become malaligned.

**The failure of collagen formation is most directly evident in the poor wound repair of scorbutic patients.** Although fibroblastic proliferation occurs, the granulation tissue is relatively devoid of collagen. The reparative process results, then, in a loose cellular connective tissue of diminished tensile strength. Contributing to this poor wound healing is the bleeding tendency of the newly formed capillaries. Similarly, walling off of infections is inadequate with scurvy, so that abscesses are not surrounded by the normal collagenous barrier and the infection therefore is not sharply delimited.

Clinically, scurvy first becomes manifest by the insidious appearance of vague signs and symptoms, such as anorexia, weight loss, listlessness, and, in infants, retarded development. As the deficiency becomes worse a microcytic anemia appears, possibly related to the role of vitamin C in reducing dietary iron to the more absorbable ferrous state while maintaining the reduced state of stored iron so that it is more readily available. Occasionally, the anemia is megaloblastic and responds to folic acid. Ascorbic acid normally prevents the oxidation of tetrahydrofolate, so a lack of it leads to a decreased folate pool. Affected infants tend to lie quietly with their legs flexed onto the abdomen, presumably to relieve tension on the muscles, tendons, and fasciae. The first definitive findings usually result from the gingival changes and bleeding diathesis and include most strikingly perifollicular hemorrhages, petechiae, or ecchymoses in the skin. Intra-articular subperiosteal or intramuscular hemorrhages may cause painful swelling of a joint or extremity. Swollen, bleeding gums and loosening of the teeth often appear, and wounds heal poorly (Fig. 8–8). The diagnosis is made by x-rays (which reveal skeletal abnormalities and sometimes microfractures), low plasma levels of vitamin C, urinary excretion measurements following administration of vitamin C (saturation test), and increased capillary fragility (positive tourniquet test). Bleeding time and coagulation time are usually normal.

The *megadose controversy*—namely, the use of nonphysiologic quantities of vitamin C for the prevention and alleviation of the common cold and for the therapy of advanced cancer—has largely simmered down. Controlled studies do *not* reveal any consistent effect on the prevention or frequency of colds or in the relief of symptoms with the use of megadoses of vitamin C (grams/day).[31] Nonetheless, an occasional individual may experience some slight alleviation of symptoms, probably because large doses of vitamin C have a mild antihistamine effect. As to the prolongation of the life of patients with metastatic cancer, it has been established, with regret, that megadoses of vitamin C are without effect.[32] If vitamin C were without toxicity, its use in megadose quantities for the common cold and particularly for advanced cancer would be no cause for concern, but in large doses it predisposes to oxalate and urate urinary tract stones, potentiates aspirin-induced gastric erosions, interacts with the metabolism of some drugs, increases intestinal absorption of iron, and may lead to iron overload as well as sundry other forms of mischief.

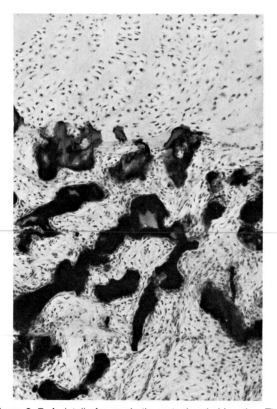

Figure 8–7. A detail of a scorbutic costochondral junction. The orderly palisade is totally destroyed. There is dense mineralization of the spicules present but no evidence of newly formed osteoid. (From Robbins, S. L., Cotran, R. S., and Kumar, V.: Pathologic Basis of Disease. 3rd ed. Philadelphia, W. B. Saunders Co., 1984.)

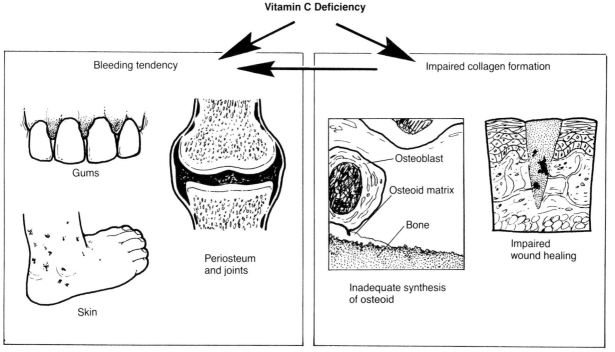

**Figure 8–8.** Vitamin C deficiency—its major consequences.

## TRACE ELEMENTS

Trace amounts of at least 14 inorganic elements are essential for life and health—iron, copper, cobalt, iodine, zinc, selenium, manganese, molybdenum, chromium, fluorine, silicon, nickel, tin, and vanadium. They serve a host of functions in redox reactions and as integral parts of many enzymes referred to as metalloenzymes. Consider only that both DNA and RNA polymerases are zinc metalloenzymes. With the exception of a dietary iodine deficiency, which is well known, a dietary lack of these elements is unusual on even a moderately adequate caloric intake. But secondary deficiency states have been characterized for iodine, zinc, copper, and selenium because of marginal dietary intake compounded by metabolic interferences, excessive losses, impaired intake, or competition between metal ions for receptor sites. Conversely, excessive exposures have been associated with toxicity. Zinc, copper, and selenium deficiencies will be described here briefly; iodine deficiency is discussed with disorders of the thyroid gland (p. 678).

*Zinc deficiency*, sometimes subclinical, is thought to be one of the most prevalent worldwide nutritional problems, exceeding the prevalence of vitamin deficiencies.[33] There are no body stores of this element, and there are well-recognized bases for conditioned deficiencies. In the Mideast, diets composed mostly of grains, cereals, and breads contain phytic acid, which chelates zinc and makes it nonabsorbable. Throughout the world various disease states may interfere with absorption or cause excessive losses

(e.g., alcoholism, cirrhosis of the liver, burns, renal disease, and gastrointestinal disorders). Zinc deficiency is also encountered in a rare genetic malabsorption syndrome and with protracted parenteral feeding.

The clinical manifestations range from various skin lesions (acrodermatitis enteropathica) to neurologic and psychiatric disturbances. They have been well described by Prasad, so only an overview is presented.[34] In children the essential clinical features are growth retardation to the point of dwarfism, hypogonadism in males, hepatosplenomegaly, mental lethargy, and dermatitis (bullous; pustular on extremities and oral and perineal regions). In adults, retardation of growth is obviously not apparent, but the remaining changes are present. Important at all ages is significant thymic atrophy and depression of T-cell function, thus rendering these individuals vulnerable to infections requiring cell-mediated immune responses (e.g., mycobacteria, viruses, helminths).

*Copper* is an essential element for hematopoiesis; connective tissue metabolism; the maintenance of vascular, neural, and skeletal integrity; and humoral immunity. The metal is a component of a wide variety of enzymes such as ferroxidase, which, among other functions, regulates the rate of iron uptake by transferrin and therefore the amount available for heme synthesis. Copper is also a component of cytochrome oxidase and certain of the superoxide dismutases important in quenching singlet oxygen free radicals. It participates in many other processes too numerous to detail. Ordinarily the diet contains ample quantities of copper, particularly in whole-grain cereals, legumes, meats, and shellfish. Overt deficiency therefore appears only in severely malnourished individuals, particularly premature infants; in adults and infants on prolonged parenteral feeding; with persistent intestinal malabsorption; with the long-term use of chelating agents; and in the rare autosomal recessive condition known by the intriguing name of Menkes' kinky hair disease (the hair indeed is like steel wool). In passing, we should note that an excess of copper produces Wilson's disease (p. 110). The major manifestation of copper deficiency in the absence of Menkes' disease is anemia, usually microcytic but sometimes megaloblastic, possibly accompanied by leukopenia and neutropenia. In a few well-developed cases, neurologic changes have been observed; they are related to the role of copper enzymes in myelin synthesis. Predisposition to aortic dissection (p. 302) and skeletal abnormalities have been observed in animals but have not been clearly documented in humans.

*Selenium deficiency* is well known in China as Keshan disease, presenting as a congestive cardiomyopathy mainly in children and young women.[35] Rare instances of selenium deficiency have been described in the Western world, marked principally by skeletal myopathy rather than cardiomyopathy. Selenium is a component of glutathione peroxidase which, like vitamin E, protects against peroxidative damage of membrane lipids. Whether this function relates to the myopathies is unclear.

## OBESITY

A casual walk down any city street in most Western countries confirms very quickly that obesity is a common problem. Its exact prevalence depends on the diagnostic criteria employed (and they are generally conceded to be imprecise). Satisfactory for clinical purposes and most widely used is weight relative to actuarial norm standards—with an arbitrary threshold of 20% overweight constituting obesity. Whatever the criteria, various surveys indicate that 25 to 30% of adults in the United States are overweight.[36] The prevalence increases with age, affects women more than men, and is becoming an increasingly more common problem among children and adolescents in the United States. The "fatties" of the world who have long suffered the derision of their leaner neighbors will be pleased to learn that a recent adoption study provides strong evidence that obesity is in some significant measure a hereditary trait.[37] This finding in no way mitigates the contribution of excess caloric intake to the problem but indicates that more is involved than merely "pigging out at the table."

Here our prime concern is the health implications of obesity. The major findings are as follows:[38]

○ Increases the overall prevalence of hypertension threefold, but in young adults (20 to 44 years of age), almost sixfold.

○ Increases the prevalence of diabetes threefold,

**Table 8–2.** VARIATION IN MORTALITY ACCORDING TO RELATIVE WEIGHT FOR MEN IN THE BUILD STUDY 1979

| Weight Relative to Average Weight | Mortality Ratio |
|---|---|
| *%* | |
| 65–75 | 105 |
| 75–95 | 93 |
| 95–105 (average) | 95 |
| 105–115 | 110 |
| 115–125 | 127 |
| 125–135 | 134 |
| 135–145 | 141 |
| 145–155 | 211 |
| 155–165 | 227 |

From NIH Consensus Development Panel on the Health Implications of Obesity: Health Implications of Obesity. Ann. Intern. Med. *103*:1073, 1985.

particularly Type II noninsulin-dependent diabetes.

○ Elevates the serum cholesterol level.

○ Increases the mortality from cancer of the colon, rectum, and prostate in males; and cancer of the gallbladder, biliary passages, breast (postmenopausal), uterus (including both cervix and endometrium), and ovaries in females.

○ Worsens the respiratory difficulties in those with chronic obstructive pulmonary disease.

○ Aggravates the severity of osteoarthritis of the weight-bearing joints.

○ Increases the incidence of gallbladder disease in females.

Notably absent from the above findings is coronary heart disease, because no consensus has yet developed. One would anticipate that with the increased prevalence of hypertension, hypercholesterolemia, and diabetes mellitus in obese patients, coronary heart disease would be significantly more prevalent. However, when these independent variables are rigorously excluded, studies have yielded inconsistent results. Nonetheless, the weight of evidence leans toward a positive relationship between obesity and coronary heart disease. But there is no doubt about its inducing cardiac enlargement, because of the expanded blood volume. The full impact of excessive storage of energy in the form of fat is most clearly documented in Table 8–2. It is evident that there is a linear correlation between the severity of the obesity and the risk of dying.

On the brighter side, there is substantial evidence that weight reduction lessens the prevalence and severity of hypertension and decreases heart size and consequent related cardiac disorders.[39] Analogously, it lessens the severity of the carbohydrate defect in diabetes and sometimes obviates the need for insulin.

## DIET AND CANCER

There is a widely prevalent belief, sometimes fear, that the Western diet—rich in meats, fats, cholesterol, and refined sugars and grains but low in fiber and heavily larded with additives—is responsible for many of the diseases in affluent societies. Witness the growing popularity of organically grown fruits and vegetables and of macrobiotic, vegetarian, and other special diets. Indeed, there is some basis for this concern. The striking differences in the prevalence rates of certain forms of cancer among countries was pointed out in an earlier chapter (p. 220). These variations have been attributed to environmental influences and, although many variables might be involved, there is substantial evidence from controlled animal studies that the diet materially modifies the incidence of spontaneous and induced cancers, raising the possibility that it might do the same in humans. What then can be said about diet and cancer in humans? Only this—the welter of evidence permits no firm conclusions but neither does it dispel all doubts. Attention has been focused on: (1) contaminants, derivatives, and additives; (2) the fat and protein content of the diet; and (3) the fiber content.

Additives and contaminants abound in the Western diet; a few examples follow. In earlier discussions the carcinogenicity of nitrosamines in experimental animals was pointed out (p. 203). Nitrites are added to some foods (e.g., processed meats) as a preservative. But in individuals with reduced levels of gastric acid, bacteria may also colonize the stomach and reduce nitrates in food and water to nitrites, which may then combine with amines and amides to form N-nitroso compounds.[40] Could nitroso compounds underlie the increased incidence of gastric carcinoma in some areas of the world? In Japan, for example, this form of neoplasia is five times more common than in the United States. Another dietary suspect, aflatoxins derived from moldy nuts and grains, has been implicated in the causation of liver cancer among rural African tribes (p. 203). However, an even stronger

correlation has been drawn with hepatitis B virus as the possible oncogen. This virus is widely prevalent in populations exposed to aflatoxins, and so it is uncertain whether the aflatoxins serve as cocarcinogens or instead in some way synergize the oncogenicity of the virus. Saccharin and cyclamates have also come under close scrutiny because they have in a few studies in animals produced bladder neoplasms when given at high dosages. Whether these artificial sweeteners, when administered to animals, are by themselves carcinogens or instead serve as "promoters" that enhance the action of other carcinogens remains uncertain.[41] But this issue is academic because there has been no convincing proof of the oncogenicity of artificial sweeteners in humans, even among diabetics who use them freely.

An incriminating finger has also been pointed at the meat, fat, and fiber content of the diet.[42] Epidemiologic surveys have shown a correlation between the level of consumption of meats—particularly animal fats—and the incidence of breast cancer.[43] On page 664 it is pointed out that high levels of estrogens are associated with an increased incidence of breast cancer in women. There is evidence that diets high in saturated fats increase the circulating levels of prolactin and enhance the conversion of steroids of adrenal origin into estrogenic compounds, particularly within fat depots—courtesy of diets laden with fats. A diet high in fat and low in fiber has also been implicated in the causation of colonic cancer. Since this subject is treated on page 556, it suffices here to indicate that the high level of dietary fat is postulated to undergo conversion to carcinogens in the gut and the lack of fiber is postulated to slow the transit time of the colonic contents and lower the level of protective adsorption of the putative carcinogens (Fig. 8–9). But nearly all of the evidence associating

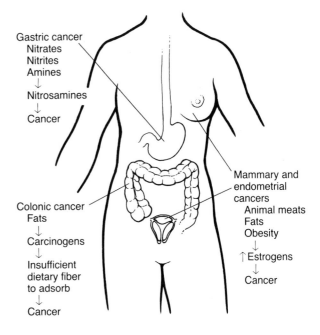

Figure 8–9. Some of the major concerns about the possible role of diet in the causation of certain forms of cancer.

the diet with the promotion (?causation) of cancer is epidemiologic and does not prove causality. Indeed, the diet may not be all bad.

As was pointed out (p. 238), there is some evidence that vitamin A and retinoids protect against cancer. The evidence is strongest for lung cancer, but an inverse relationship between vitamin A intake and cancers of the bladder, upper gastrointestinal tract, and breast has also been proposed. However, there is an equally impressive number of studies disagreeing with these findings. So much is still "iffy" that we should conclude this discussion by saying that, to date, there has been no proof that the diet can cause or protect against cancer. Nonetheless, the concern persists that anything as pleasurable as juicy steak and rich ice cream must in some way be evil.

## References

1. Butterworth, C. E., Jr., and Weinsier, R. L.: Malnutrition in hospital patients: assessment and treatment. *In* Goodhart, R. S., and Shils, M. E. (eds.): Modern Nutrition in Health and Disease. 6th ed. Philadelphia, Lea & Febiger, 1980, p. 667.
2. Golden, M. H. N.: Protein deficiency, energy deficiency, and the oedema of malnutrition. Lancet *1*:1261, 1982.
3. Editorial: Aflatoxins and kwashiorkor. Lancet 2:1133, 1984.
4. Waterlow, J. C.: Kwashiorkor revisited: The pathogenesis of oedema in kwashiorkor and its significance. Trans. R. Soc. Trop. Med. Hyg. 78:436, 1984.
5. Goodman, D. S.: Vitamin A and retinoids in health and disease. N. Engl. J. Med. *310*:1023, 1984.
6. Sommer, A.: Nutritional Blindness: Xerophthalmia and Keratomalacia. New York, Oxford University Press, 1982.
7. Wald, G.: The molecular basis of visual excitation. Nature *219*:800, 1968.
8. Chytil, F.: Liver and cellular vitamin A binding proteins. Hepatology 2:282, 1982.
9. Editorial: Vitamin A and cancer. Lancet 2:325, 1984.
10. Pochi, P. E.: Isoretinoin for acne: The experience broadens. N. Engl. J. Med. *313*:1013, 1985.
11. Lammer, E. J.: Retinoic acid embryopathy. N. Engl. J. Med. *313*:837, 1985.
12. Kumar, R.: Metabolism of 1,25-dihydroxyvitamin $D_3$. Physiol. Rev. *64*:478, 1984.
13. Audran, M., and Kumar, R.: The physiology and pathophysiology of vitamin D. Mayo Clin. Proc. *60*:851, 1985.
14. DeLuca, H. F.: Metabolism, physiology, and function of vitamin D. *In* Kumar, R. (ed.): Vitamin D: Basic and Clinical Aspects. Boston, Martinus Nijhoff Publishing, Kluwer Academic, 1984, p. 1.
15. Mason, K. E.: The first two decades of vitamin E. Fed. Proc. *36*:1906, 1977.
16. Harding, A. E., et al.: Spinocerebellar degeneration associated with a selective defect of vitamin E absorption. N. Engl. J. Med. *313*:32, 1985.
17. Zipursky, A.: Vitamin E deficiency anemia in newborn infants. Clin. Perinatol. *11*:393, 1984.
18. Bieri, J. G., et al.: Medical uses of vitamin E. N. Engl. J. Med. *308*:1063, 1983.
19. Kligman, A. M.: Vitamin E toxicity. Arch. Dermatol. *118*:289, 1982.
20. Lemons, J. A., and Maisels, M. J.: Vitamin E—How much is too much? Pediatrics 78:625, 1985.
21. Lane, P. A., and Hathaway, W. E.: Vitamin K in infancy. J. Pediatr. *106*:351, 1985.
22. Gallop, P. M., et al.: Carboxylated calcium-binding proteins and vitamin K. N. Engl. J. Med. *302*:1460, 1980.
23. Blanchard, R. A., et al.: Acquired vitamin K-dependent carboxylation deficiency in liver disease. N. Engl. J. Med. *305*:242, 1981.
24. Editorial: Cardiovascular beriberi. Lancet *1*:1287, 1982.
25. Reuler, J. B., et al.: Wernicke's encephalopathy. N. Engl. J. Med. *312*:1035, 1985.
26. Blass, J. P., and Gibson, G. E.: Abnormality of a thiamine-requiring enzyme in patients with Wernicke-Korsakoff syndrome. N. Engl. J. Med. *297*:1367, 1977.
27. Schaumburg, H., et al.: Sensory neuropathy from pyridoxine abuse. A new megavitamin syndrome. N. Engl. J. Med. *309*:445, 1983.
28. Levine, M.: New concepts in the biology and biochemistry of ascorbic acid. N. Engl. J. Med. *314*:892, 1986.
29. Levene, C. I., et al.: Scurvy. A comparison between ultrastructural and biochemical changes observed in cultured fibroblasts and the collagen they synthesize. Virchows Arch. [Cell Pathol.] 23:325, 1977.
30. Nimni, M. E.: Collagen: structure, function, and metabolism in normal and fibrotic tissues. Semin. Arthritis Rheum. *13*:1, 1983.
31. Coulehan, J. L.: Ascorbic acid and the common cold: reviewing the evidence. Postgrad. Med. *66*:153, 1979.
32. Moertel, C. G., et al.: High-dose vitamin C versus placebo in the treatment of patients with advanced cancer who have had no prior chemotherapy. N. Engl. J. Med. *312*:137, 1985.
33. Fraker, P. J.: Zinc deficiency: a common immunodeficiency state. Surv. Immunol. Res. 2:155, 1983.
34. Prasad, A. S.: Clinical manifestations of zinc deficiency. Annu. Rev. Nutr. 5:341, 1985.
35. Keshan Disease Research Group of the Chinese Academy of Medical Sciences: Epidemiologic studies on the etiologic relationship of selenium and Keshan disease. Chin. Med. J. (Engl.) 92:477, 1979.
36. Van Itallie, T. B.: Health implications of overweight and obesity in the United States. Ann. Intern. Med. *103*:983, 1985.
37. Stunkard, A. J., et al.: An adoption study of human obesity. N. Engl. J. Med. *314*:193, 1986.
38. NIH Consensus Development Panel on the Health Implications of Obesity: Health implications of obesity: NIH consensus development conference statement. Ann. Intern. Med. *103*:1073, 1985.
39. MacMahon, S. W., et al.: The effect of weight reduction on left ventricular mass: A randomized controlled trial in young, overweight hypertensive patients. N. Engl. J. Med. *314*:334, 1986.
40. Tannenbaum, S. R.: N-nitroso compounds: A prospective on human exposure. Lancet *1*:629, 1983.
41. Cohen, S. M., et al.: Promoting effect of saccharin and DL-tryptophan in urinary bladder carcinogenesis. Cancer Res. 39:1207, 1979.
42. Willett, W. C., and MacMahon, B.: Diet and cancer—An overview. N. Engl. J. Med. *310*:633 (Pt. 1); 697 (Pt. 2), 1984.
43. Wynder, E. L., and Rose, D. P.: Diet and breast cancer. Hosp. Pract. *19*(4):73, 1984.

# 9

# Environmental Disorders

All disease is either genetic or acquired in origin. Even those you are "born with" are modified by the environment—witness the hereditary deficiency of glucose-6-phosphate-dehydrogenase that remains asymptomatic until the ingestion of an oxidant drug induces a wave of hemolysis. In this context most diseases are at least in part environmental in origin. With our deteriorating environment they become more serious and affect more people every day. Indeed the worldwide problems of overpopulation, air and water pollution, loss of arable land, shortage of food, and dwindling sources of energy threaten the survival of humans on this planet.[1] The staggering death toll exacted by the drought and famine in Ethiopia in 1984 grimly underscores the magnitude of the crisis, one that has long been festering in many regions around the world. It is impossible within the limits of space to more than scratch the surface of all the "environmental disorders." Only a relatively few will be considered, largely those most prevalent in the Western world, documenting that most could be prevented or controlled by immediately available

measures. These disorders are considered under the headings of air pollution, disorders caused by chemicals and drugs, and physical agents.

## AIR POLLUTION

That we breathe an atmospheric "soup" laden with $CO_2$, $NO_2$, $SO_2$, ozone, various aerosolized metals, and sundry dusts is now an unpleasant reality of life in developed and developing nations. The air in urban areas, with their industries, is obviously the most heavily polluted, but air currents and the near universality of internal combustion engines on land, sea, and air disperse the pollution to all regions. Life would be difficult without such means of travel, but the price is high—as many as 300 different compounds are emitted from internal combustion engines. In this context, urban air in major United States cities has been judged to contain up to 1000-fold the rural levels of lead, zinc, carbon, and hydrocarbons.[2] Compounding the problem is the self-imposed air pollution of tobacco smoking.

The impact of the various air pollutants on human health is enormous and includes the causation of bronchitis, asthma, emphysema, specific occupational respiratory diseases, and cancer, notably of the lung. It has been difficult to segregate the effects of one pollutant from another because of variable individual sensitivity, varying levels of the many pollutants from time to time, the synergistic effects of one upon another, and the possibility of sequential effects of several agents. Best studied are the consequences of tobacco smoking and specific occupational dusts, the latter causing what are called *pneumoconioses*, as will be detailed in the subsequent sections.

### SMOKING

The data on the ill effects of cigarette smoking are awesome and grim. It is estimated that the annual excess mortality in the United States incurred by cigarette smoking is 350,000, more than the total loss of American lives in World War I, Korea, and Vietnam.[3] In 1979, the US Surgeon General's Report declared: "Cigarette smoking is the single most important environmental factor contributing to premature mortality in the United States."[4] The Royal

College of Physicians and many studies since that time have supported this conclusion. The morbidity and mortality related to cigarette smoking are almost linearly correlated with the number of cigarettes smoked daily and years of use. This is frequently expressed in terms of "pack-years" (i.e., one pack a day for 20 years equals 20 pack-years). One statistician calculated that among smokers for 5 to 8 years, each cigarette reduces life expectancy 5.5 minutes. There is some evidence that the current swing to filter-tip and "low-tar" cigarettes reduces the risk significantly, but how much awaits long-term analyses of their sole use.[3] Cigar and pipe smoking are not without risk, but it is significantly lower than that for cigarette smoking. Currently there is considerable concern about the deleterious effects of "passive smoking." Mild impairment of ventilatory function has been noted and even worse, a suggestion of an increased risk of cancer,[5] but further studies are necessary. Specific diseases related to tobacco smoking will not be dealt with here because they will be brought up in subsequent discussions. They are depicted in Figure 9–1; the major ones are shown on the left of the illustration. Some concept about the frequency of these disorders can be derived from the following data. The evidence linking cigarette smoking to lung cancer is nearly irrefutable, and lung cancer is the number one cause of cancer mortality among both males and females in the US in 1985.[6] Male smokers are about 10 times more likely to die of bronchogenic carcinoma than nonsmokers. Female smokers in the past have had about half the risk of male smokers, but changing practices may obliterate this difference. The risks involved in smoking two packs of cigarettes a day are three times higher than those of smoking one-half pack a day. The data are equally doleful in relation to cardiovascular deaths. Cigarette smoking is a major risk factor in the development of atherosclerosis and in the causation of coronary heart disease, particularly myocardial infarction, which is the number one cause of death in most industrialized countries. To add to this litany, the unborn child is not spared because smoking during pregnancy has been implicated in reduced birth weight and increased perinatal mortality. In the past few years, the attempt to escape these hazards has led to the growing use of smokeless tobacco such as snuff, chewing tobacco, or small bags of tobacco tucked into the cheek pouch. Regrettably, these practices have led to a striking increase in the incidence of squamous cell carcinoma in the gingiva and buccal mucosa (p. 228).

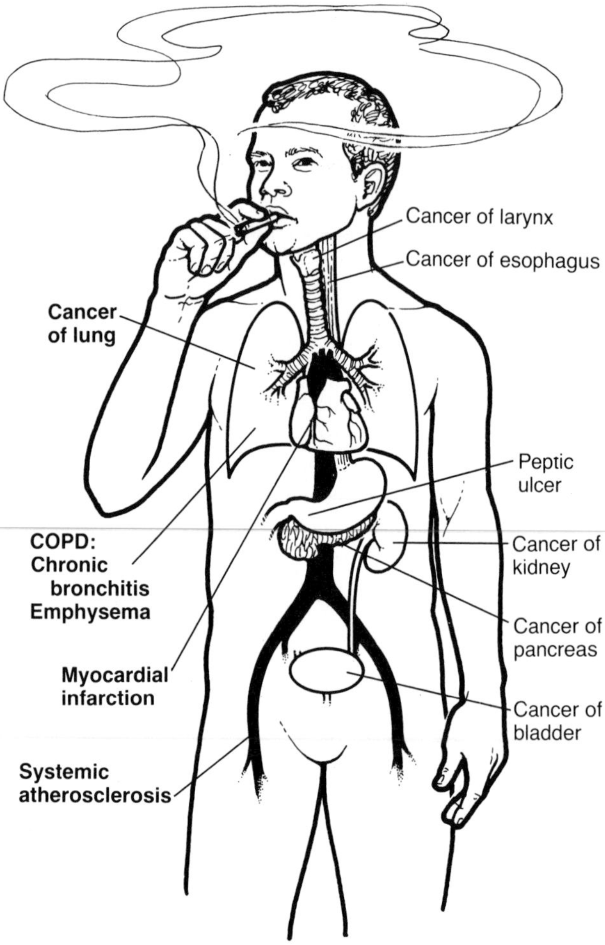

Smokers can "take heart" because "within a year of quitting the habit" the increased incidence of heart attacks in males under 55 years of age begins to fall and in two years reaches the basal level of nonsmokers.[7] In addition, a small drop in the number of deaths from bronchogenic carcinoma has just been noted among males but not among females. Is it too much to believe that all of the efforts to curb cigarette smoking have begun to pay off, that the decline in male deaths from lung cancer is the beginning of a trend, and that the same will soon happen with females? The conclusion is inescapable—cigarettes are veritable "coffin nails."

Figure 9–1. Depiction of the more common (*on the left*) and somewhat less common (*on the right*) adverse effects of smoking.

## PNEUMOCONIOSIS

In strict usage, the term "pneumoconiosis" means lung disease caused by inhaled dust. The definition has been broadened to encompass the lungs' reaction to any aerosol, including fumes, vapors, volatilized metals, and particulate matter. Although the pneumoconioses are generally referred to as occupational disorders, they are better considered environmental diseases, because air pollution is now a disturbing "fact of life" for all (as has been pointed out). Families of workers and urban dwellers particularly in the neighborhood of industries are also at increased risk. Safety regulations have largely controlled most of these industrial pollutants, but their diseases continue to be important causes of morbidity and mortality. Concurrent cigarette smoking not only aggravates the gravity of nearly all forms of pneumoconiosis, it compounds the risk.

*The development of pneumoconioses depends on four variables: (1) the concentration of the pollutant in the air, (2) the amount retained in the airways and lungs, (3) the size and shape of the contaminant,* and *(4) its solubility and physicochemical reactivity.* Fortunately, the normal ventilatory apparatus in humans possesses many remarkable clearance mechanisms.[8] The largest particles are filtered out by the vibrissae in the nares or settle or impact in the airways and are then removed by the "mucociliary escalator." The smallest particles, below 1 μm in diameter, are likely to reach the terminal alveolar ducts and air sacs (depicted in Fig. 9–2, later) but remain airborne to be exhaled. *It is the particles between 1 and 5 μm in diameter that present the greatest hazards* because they have a high resistance to airflow and are likely to impact or settle in the respiratory bronchioles or be trapped in the blind-end air sacs. Some are phagocytosed by type II pneumocytes or alveolar macrophages and carried off through lymphatics to nodes, but some remain to cause damage. So it is that size, shape, and concentration of the pollutant condition the amount retained in the respiratory system. Solubility and reactivity determine the nature of the pulmonary reaction. *The more soluble the agent, the more reactive it is and so the more likely an acute exudative pulmonary reaction. The relatively insoluble particles such as silica and asbestos tend to evoke fibrosing pneumoconioses.* Within this context, many different airborne pollutants induce disease; the most common are cited in Table 9–1. Only the more important will be discussed.

## COAL WORKERS' PNEUMOCONIOSIS (CWP)—PROGRESSIVE MASSIVE FIBROSIS (PMF)

After years of exposure, nearly every coal miner has focal pulmonary accumulations of coal dust. Under the microscope the focal blackenings can be resolved as aggregations of dust-laden macrophages about respiratory bronchioles, creating *coal macules,* the hallmark of CWP. The size and number of the macules depend on duration and intensity of exposure, the adequacy of the clearance mechanisms, and, particularly, the presence or absence of concurrent cigarette smoking. At first soft and minute, the macules develop a delicate fibrosis as they approach 1 cm in diameter and may then become visible in chest films as discrete radiodensities. Nonetheless

Table 9–1. DUST-INDUCED DISEASE

| Agent | Disease | Exposure |
|---|---|---|
| **Mineral Dusts** | | |
| Coal dust | Macules | Coal mining (particularly hard coal) |
| | Progressive massive fibrosis | |
| | Caplan's syndrome | |
| | ? Gastric carcinoma | |
| Silica | Silicosis | Foundry work, sandblasting, hard-rock |
| | Caplan's syndrome | mining, stone cutting, others |
| Asbestos | Asbestosis | Mining, milling, and fabrication; installation |
| | Pleural plaques | and removal of insulation |
| | Caplan's syndrome | |
| | Mesothelioma | |
| | Carcinoma of the lung, larynx, stomach, colon | |
| Beryllium | Acute berylliosis | Mining, fabrication |
| | Beryllium granulomatoses | |
| | ?Bronchogenic carcinoma | |
| Iron oxide | Siderosis | Welding |
| Barium sulfate | Baritosis | Mining |
| Tin oxide | Stannosis | Mining |
| **Organic Dusts that Induce Extrinsic Allergic Alveolitis** | | |
| Moldy hay | Farmer's lung | Farming |
| Bagasse | Bagassosis | Manufacturing wallboard, paper |
| Bird droppings | Bird-breeder's lung | Bird handling |
| **Organic Dusts that Induce Asthma** | | |
| Cotton, flax, hemp | Byssinosis | Textile manufacturing |
| Red cedar dust | Asthma | Lumbering, carpentry |
| **Chemical Fumes and Vapors** | | |
| Nitrous oxide, sulfur dioxide, ammonia, benzene, certain insecticides (e.g., cyanate gases) | Bronchitis | Occupational and accidental exposure |
| | Asthma | |
| | Pulmonary edema | |
| | Respiratory distress syndrome | |
| | Injury to exposed mucosal surfaces | |
| | Fulminating poisoning | |

they do not significantly derange the native pulmonary architecture and do not embarrass respiratory function or predispose to other pulmonary disease. However, they are precursors to progressive massive fibrosis (PMF), which supervenes in less than 5% of cases. It is well to understand that *the designation PMF is a generic term for any massive fibrosing pulmonary reaction that is initiated by any type of inhalational pollutant.* The line demarcating CWP from PMF is ill defined. PMF has been arbitrarily defined by clinicians as at least a single opacity on the chest x-ray that exceeds 1 cm in diameter. In anatomic terms, a lower limit of 2 cm has been set.[9]

At the other end of the spectrum of carbon dust accumulation is the nonoccupational *pulmonary anthracosis.* Innocuous, relatively trivial, focal blackenings are an almost inevitable stigma of urban life. They are particularly prominent in the habitual cigarette smoker. Like the coal macule, the focal accumulations of dust may drain through lymphatics to blacken the peribronchial and tracheobronchial lymph nodes. *Thus anthracosis, CWP, and PMF are ill-defined segments of a spectrum of progressively greater accumulation of carbon dust that ends in a clinically significant pneumoconiosis.*[10]

The **coal macule** is an aggregation of dust-laden macrophages, less than 2 cm but averaging 0.5 cm in diameter. They are fairly evenly distributed throughout the lung fields but have a predilection for the upper lobes, where they create dispersed focal blackenings. They develop by the deposition of coal dust in respiratory bronchioles or in air sacs, from where it is then carried by phagocytes toward the respiratory bronchioles. Thus the dust-laden macule is centered around the respiratory bronchiole (Fig. 9–2). Simultaneously, the macrophages drain through lymphatics to the regional lymph nodes and around the pulmonary arterioles and veins. A delicate collagenous fibrosis may develop in the peribronchiolar collections and with it the walls of the respiratory bronchioles may dilate, sometimes referred to as centrilobular emphysema (p. 417). Concurrent cigarette smoking exaggerates the coal macule and may add an element of bronchiolitis worsening the bronchiolar dilatation. However, in the absence of this compounding influence, the coal macule causes no significant damage to the pulmonary architecture.

**PMF develops on a background of CWP.** It is marked by rubbery to firm black nodules, some of which are at least 2 cm in diameter. The macules develop a delicate fibrosis that radiates out in strands to distort and destroy surrounding architecture, sometimes obliterating trapped airways and vessels. Unlike the case with CWP, the development of PMF results in significant ventilatory dysfunction and sometimes makes its victims respiratory cripples. The disease advances by enlargement, coalescence, and fibrosis of preexisting coal macules. In this manner, large areas of black scarring replace the native architecture, justifying the name "**black lung disease**" (Fig. 9–3). The lesions tend to be disposed in the lower regions of the upper lobes and upper zones of the lower lobes and, when located at the periphery of the lung, may induce a secondary fibrous pleuritis.[11] Sometimes the centers of the foci of scarring are cavitated and filled with an inky black fluid.

Histologically, the fibrous strands within a dust-laden nodule are arranged in a haphazard pattern and therefore are dissimilar from the concentric whorls seen in silicosis. However, polarized light may disclose some refractile crystals in the periphery of these lesions, suggesting some role for silica in the development of the more fibrotic nodules.

The basis for the transition of CWP into PMF is still not understood. Four mechanisms are entertained:

1. Enlarging burden of coal dust
2. Intercurrent tuberculosis
3. Exposure to silica
4. Immunologic mechanisms

Although the *magnitude of the burden of coal dust* cannot be ruled out as one basis for the development of PMF, there is no linear correlation between the severity of the dust accumulation and the appearance or severity of the fibrosing lesions of PMF.

In years past coal miners with PMF had a high incidence of *pulmonary tuberculosis.* However, neither organisms nor characteristic granulomas are found in the lesions, and improved health measures have dramatically reduced the frequency of tuberculosis in PMF.

*Concurrent exposure to silica,* which is often present in the coal deposits, cannot be ruled out and is an attractive theory to explain the fibrosing reaction because silicosis itself is marked by dense fibrosis.[12] However, PMF has been observed in carbon-electrode makers presumably exposed to pure volatilized carbon.

Currently favored are *immunologic mechanisms.* A higher incidence of non-organ-specific antibodies, rheumatoid factor, and antinuclear antibodies has been observed in miners with PMF than in those with simple CWP. Some workers develop rheumatoid arthritis and with it *Caplan's syndrome,* the appearance of distinctive giant pulmonary nodules 5

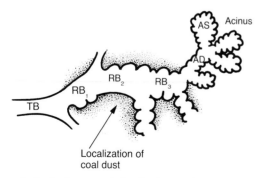

**Figure 9–2.** A diagram of the fundamental respiratory unit, indicating major locus of coal dust accumulation. TB = terminal bronchiole; RB = respiratory bronchiole; AD = alveolar duct; AS = alveolus.

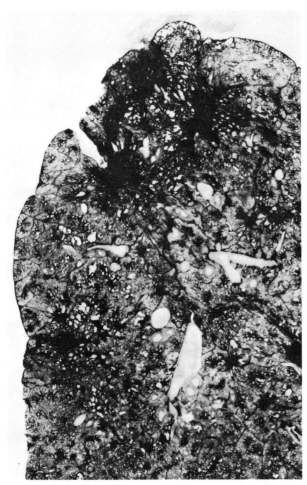

**Figure 9–3.** Progressive massive fibrosis superimposed on coal workers' pneumoconiosis. The large blackened scars are principally located in the upper lobe. Note extensions of scars into surrounding parenchyma and retraction of adjacent pleura. (Courtesy of Dr. Werner Laquer, Dr. Jerome Kleinerman, and the National Institute of Occupational Safety and Health. From Robbins, S. L., Cotran, R. S., and Kumar, V.: Pathologic Basis of Disease. 3rd ed. Philadelphia, W. B. Saunders Co., 1984, p. 434.)

is more a marker of a particular occupation than a disease. But PMF is a disabling disease manifested by worsening dyspnea and chronic cough raising dust-laden sputum; sometimes a jet-black viscid fluid is released as a cavity ruptures. With continued exposure the respiratory function deteriorates. However, unlike asbestosis and silicosis, PMF does not worsen in the absence of continued exposure to coal dust. The diagnosis depends upon (1) an occupational history, (2) demonstrable ventilatory impairment, and (3) the identification of nodular radiographic densities greater than 1 cm in diameter. *There is no increased incidence of bronchogenic carcinomas in coal workers in the absence of concurrent cigarette smoking.*[13] On the other hand, there may be a slightly increased incidence of carcinoma of the stomach—could it be related to swallowed hydrocarbons?

## SILICOSIS

Intense exposure to very finely divided silica is rare but evokes a massive pulmonary exudation within months that closely resembles pulmonary al-

cm or more in diameter that have concentric internal, fibrous laminations and are surrounded by a marked plasma-cell perivascular infiltrate. Immunoglobulins can often be identified in these lesions and so an immunologic origin is proposed. The concurrence of Caplan's syndrome lends some credence to an immunologic basis for PMF. Central to this thesis is immune-mediated aggregation of macrophages, their release of lysosomal enzymes, and their formation of free radicals as the basis for tissue injury and, at the same time, their release of fibroblast growth factors from macrophages as the basis for the fibrosis (Fig. 9–4). Other macrophage-derived factors could be responsible for expansion of the T helper-cell pool with polyclonal B-cell stimulation or suppression of regulatory T cells leading to the antibodies mentioned.

**CLINICAL COURSE.** Coal workers' pneumoconiosis

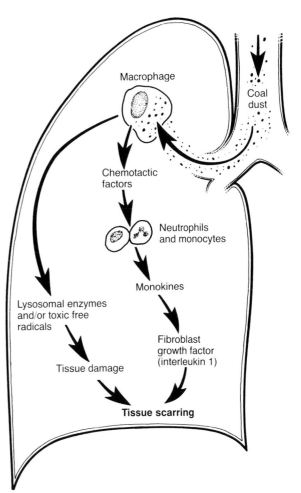

**Figure 9–4.** Favored theory of pathogenesis of the pulmonary fibrosis in PMF.

veolar proteinosis (p. 425). In many instances, the pulmonary changes resist therapy and prove fatal. *More often and implied by the term "silicosis" is a chronic fibrosing pneumoconiosis that is insidious in onset and relentlessly progresses long after exposure has ceased.* The most hazardous dust, varying from 1 to 5 μm in diameter and causing this chronic reaction, is encountered in sundry industrial operations including, among others, mining, quarrying, tunneling, sandblasting, foundry work, and pottery fabrication. In most instances, clinical evidence of disease only appears after 10 years of exposure, indicating that the changes evolve slowly. In high-risk occupations, 10 to 15% of 30-year workers are affected. *Caplan's syndrome (p. 256) may complicate chronic silicosis, and there is an increased risk of intercurrent tuberculosis.*

**PATHOGENESIS.** The precise mechanisms by which inhaled silica causes cellular and tissue injury and induces the formation of collagenizing fibrous pulmonary nodules are poorly understood. However, a few observations are well established.

○ The crystalline tetrahedral forms of silica are most fibrogenic (e.g., quartz, crystobalite, and tridymite); noncrystalline forms usually are not fibrogenic.

○ The dangerous particles between 1 and 5 μm in diameter are deposited in respiratory bronchioles and alveolar sacs. (Larger particles, such as beach sand, do not reach the lungs.)

○ Most retained particles are promptly ingested by pulmonary alveolar macrophages, followed by death of the phagocytes and release of the particles.

The mechanism of macrophage-killing is uncertain, but hypothesized are (1) membrane injury and calcium influx or (2) intracellular release of lysosomal enzymes. At the same time, the macrophages release chemotactic factors recruiting neutrophils and other macrophages to the focus of injury. The tissue injury is attributed to the release of lysosomal enzymes or formation of free radicals. Simultaneously, released fibroblast growth factors, like interleukin 1, may mediate the collagenous fibrosis typical of silicosis.[14]

A host of immunologic changes have also been observed, but it is not known whether they have central roles or instead are merely epiphenomena. Patients with silicosis have increased levels of serum immunoglobulins, autoantibodies, and immune complexes and show variable and inconstant cell-mediated changes.[15] Credence to a possible pathogenetic role for immunologic mechanisms is given by the increased frequency of autoimmune diseases, particularly rheumatoid arthritis and Caplan's syndrome (p. 256), in patients with chronic silicosis. An attempt to synthesize some of the pathogenetic influences is presented in Figure 9–5.[16]

**Classic silicosis** is characterized by dense fibrosing reactions, both in the pleura and in the lung substance. Typically there are either large collagenous pleural plaques or dense fibrous adhesions, which sometimes

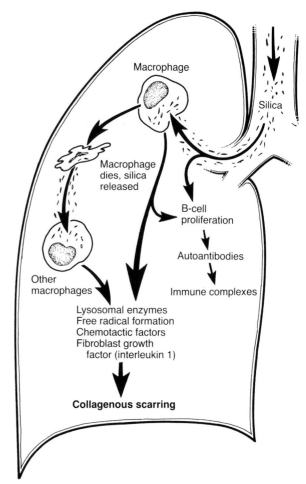

Figure 9–5. Silicosis. Postulated pathogenetic mechanisms leading to the collagenous pulmonary scarring.

extend throughout both pleural cavities. Gray-white, sometimes blackened (by coal dust) fibrotic nodules can be palpated in the lung substance and are seen on transection. They are most abundant in the apical and posterior parts of upper and lower lobes, but in advanced cases extend throughout the lungs (Fig. 9–6). These vary from a few millimeters in diameter to conglomerate masses that may replace an entire lobe. Often spicules of calcification are palpable within these areas of fibrosis. Similar nodules may appear in the draining lymph nodes. Subsequent calcification of them may yield, on chest film, peripheral "egg shell" densities in the involved nodes. A number of additional changes may be present, including irregular emphysema about the areas of scarring, honeycombing of segments of lung interposed between areas of scarring, subpleural bullae, and, when there is a concomitant tuberculous infection, foci of caseation, necrosis, and cavitation.

Histologically, **the fibrotic hyalinized nodules tend to show peripheral concentric collagenous laminations.** Continued layering of this fibrous tissue causes enlargement of the nodules and eventual coalescence of neighboring nodules to create massive collagenous scars. Foci of black coal dust pigment and calcification are

The degree of breathlessness is variable; it may become severe enough to incapacitate the patient or may remain relatively mild. Systemic symptoms are unusual with pure silicosis. However, the picture is often complicated by the development of concomitant rheumatoid arthritis with Caplan's syndrome, chronic bronchitis, emphysema, cor pulmonale (p. 338), or pulmonary tuberculosis. The incidence of intercurrent tuberculosis in patients with silicosis has dramatically fallen but it is still higher than that in the general population. *Unlike the case with asbestosis, there appears to be no increased risk of bronchogenic carcinoma or other forms of cancer in silicosis.*

## ASBESTOSIS AND ASBESTOS-RELATED DISEASES

Prolonged inhalation of asbestos dust may lead to a fibrosing interstitial pneumoconiosis—asbestosis—as well as to other forms of asbestos-related disease, notably fibrous pleural plaques, bronchogenic carcinoma, mesothelioma, and other forms of cancer (Table 9–2).[17] Asbestosis is slow to develop and therefore may not become clinically evident for decades after the last exposure. There is a clear correlation between the dose or duration of exposure and the development of clinical disease. Asbestosis is rarely encountered in industrial workers with less than 10 years of exposure, but it is encountered in about 10% of those with 10 to 20 years of exposure and in more than 50% of those with exposure times that exceed 40 years.[18] The correlation between the other asbestos-related lesions (e.g., bronchogenic carcinoma, pleural plaques, mesothelioma) and the pulmonary burden of dust or duration of exposure is less clear-cut. There is, then, concern about the effects of low dose exposure, particularly because there may be individual susceptibility and because of the near universality of asbestos air pollution in industrialized nations.

Asbestos is the generic term for a family of fibrous silicates that can be divided into curled serpentines and straight amphiboles. The serpentine chrysotile accounts for 90% of commercially used asbestos. Among the many amphiboles, crocidolite and amosite account for most of the remaining amounts of asbestos in industrial use. All types of fibers may induce asbestos-related diseases, but crocidolite is most strongly implicated in the induction of cancers. The greatest exposure to asbestos dust occurs in the mining, milling, and preparation of the raw minerals but it is widely incorporated into asbestos-cement pipes, flooring and roofing products, insulations, ceiling-board, brake linings, clutch facings, and innumerable other commercial fabrications. Some 300,000 workers in the US are engaged in the fabrication and use of asbestos products and in the demolition of buildings where these products were once used. Moreover, millions are exposed incidentally, particularly those who encounter asbestos workers at home

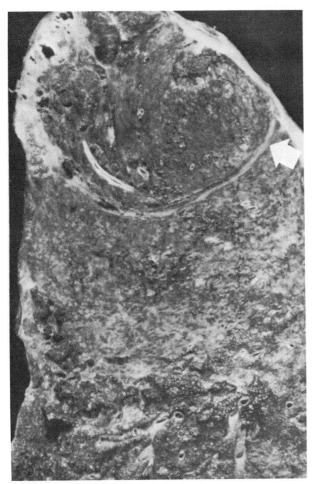

Figure 9–6. Advanced silicosis seen on transection of lung. Scarring is almost confluent, occupying most of upper lobe and contiguous region of lower lobe. Arrow indicates interlobar fissure. Several tuberculous cavities are present in apex. Note dense pleural thickening. (Courtesy of Dr. John Godleski, Brigham and Women's Hospital. From Robbins, S. L., Cotran, R. S., and Kumar, V.: Pathologic Basis of Disease. 3rd ed. Philadelphia, W. B. Saunders Co., 1984, p. 436.)

usually present in these scars; more importantly, **polariscopic study will disclose doubly refractile silica particles in the fine cleft-like spaces within the collagenous tissue.** Occasionally, doubly refractile crystals are seen within foreign body–type giant cells. Coexistent tuberculosis may be distinguished readily or with difficulty, depending upon whether well-formed tubercles with central caseation are present.

**CLINICAL COURSE.** In the early stages of classic chronic silicosis, the patient is asymptomatic. Frequently the disease is first discovered on a routine chest x-ray; the "snowstorm" appearance of the lungs, characteristic of the phase of fine nodularity, coupled with the occupational history, leads to the diagnosis. As the lungs become progressively fibrous, causing a marked decrease in their compliance and in gas diffusion, the first symptom—dyspnea on exertion—appears. This may not be noticeable until years after the disease has been discovered on chest x-ray.

**Table 9–2. ASBESTOS-RELATED DISEASE***

| Disease or Finding | Association with Asbestos Exposure | Comment |
|---|---|---|
| Asbestos body in lung tissue or sputum | Established | By itself, indicator of exposure only; does not indicate disease |
| Asbestosis (interstitial fibrosis) | Established | Combination of interstitial fibrosis and asbestos bodies required for diagnosis |
| Pleural effusion/fibrosis | Established | Frequently sanguineous/severe disease may produce functional abnormalities |
| Pleural plaques | Established | Sometimes incorrectly called "pleural asbestosis"; plaques over diaphragm and lower parietal pleura strongly suggestive of exposure |
| Lung carcinoma | Established | Histologic types similar to non-asbestos-related tumors; more frequent in lower lobes |
| Malignant mesothelioma | Established | |
| Cancer: Larynx, GI tract | Established | |
| Emphysema, chronic bronchitis | No established association | Presence of emphysema in persons with asbestos exposure is almost always attributable to smoking |

*From Churg, A., and Golden, J.: Current problems in the pathology of asbestos-related disease. Pathol. Ann. *17*(Pt. 2):33, 1982.

or in the workplace, but every urban dweller has some exposure to the mineral. No small wonder that there is anxiety about the welfare of children attending schools where asbestos was incorporated into insulation or ceilings.[19]

**PATHOGENESIS.** Although the initial events leading to the induction of asbestosis are well understood, the ultimate basis for the fibrogenicity of inhaled asbestos fibers is still a puzzle.[20, 21] This much is known:

○ Inhaled fibers less than 5 μm in length are the most pathogenic because they are carried in the airstream into the terminal airways and air sacs.

○ Some of the deposited particles are almost immediately engulfed by lining epithelial cells or pulmonary macrophages, but most remain free.

○ The macrophages containing the asbestos particles or the fibers themselves activate complement within the plasma layer lining alveolar surfaces to release C5a, a powerful chemoattractant for more pulmonary macrophages and neutrophils.[22]

○ The fibers engulfed by macrophages are coated with protein-iron complexes to create beaded, sometimes dumbbell-shaped, *"asbestos bodies"* (Fig. 9–7), but most fibers are not engulfed and so are not transformed. Nonasbestos particles of inorganic dust may be similarly coated, but these are called *"ferruginous bodies"* in order to differentiate them from those having a core of asbestos fiber.[23]

From this point the pathways leading to interstitial fibrosis are ill defined. One possibility is that the macrophages elaborate fibroblast growth factors. Alternatively, damage to the native pulmonary tissue from released lysosomal enzymes or macrophage-produced free radicals could incite an inflammatory-reparative fibrosing response. Also, chrysotile itself is cytotoxic in vitro. However, cell injury does not appear to be a prominent feature of the early lesion in asbestosis. Moreover, in vitro, chrysotile directly stimulates collagen synthesis by lung fibroblasts, raising yet another possibility. A host of immunologic

changes have also been observed, including hyper-gammaglobulinemia and circulating immune complexes, but their role remains uncertain.[15, 19] A synthesis of some of the possible events is provided in Figure 9–8. Moreover, often there is a history of heavy cigarette smoking, which further complicates the pathogenetic puzzle.

Epidemiologic studies leave no doubt that asbestos in some way is carcinogenic; studies in insulation workers have shown that asbestos-exposed smokers have a 50-fold greater incidence of bronchogenic

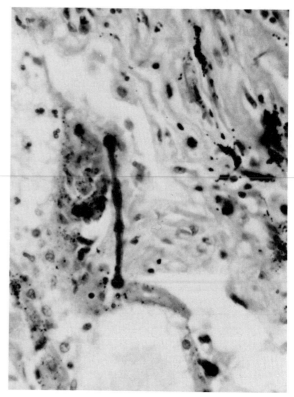

**Figure 9–7.** A high-power detail of an asbestos body, revealing the typical beading and knobbed ends.

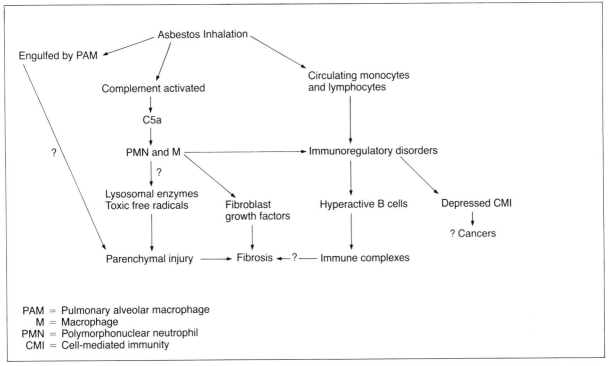

Figure 9–8. Possible pathogenesis of asbestosis. (Modified from deShazo, R. D.: Current concepts about the pathogenesis of silicosis and asbestosis. J. Allergy Clin. Immunol. 70:41, 1982.)

carcinoma, which is reduced to fivefold in asbestos-exposed nonsmokers.[24] However, it is not clear how it exerts this carcinogenic effect. One theory relative to bronchogenic carcinoma proposes that it acts as a promoter inducing cell proliferation and metaplastic epithelial changes with increasing susceptibility to environmental carcinogens.[25] Depressed cell-mediated immunity and loss of surveillance may predispose to the emergence of the cancers.

**MORPHOLOGY.** The various asbestos-associated lesions will be considered separately.[26, 27]

**Asbestosis** is a diffuse, chronic interstitial pneumonitis. **It is indistinguishable from other forms of chronic fibrosing interstitial pneumonia except for the presence of asbestos bodies**. The fibrosis begins about the respiratory bronchioles and alveolar ducts, changes reminiscent of those seen in cigarette smokers and called "small airways disease."[28] Then the fibrosis extends into the walls of adjacent alveolar sacs to create the characteristic chronic interstitial pneumonitis. Contraction of the fibrous tissue "distorts" the native architecture, creating enlarged air spaces enclosed within thick fibrous walls. In this way the affected regions become "honeycombed." Asbestos bodies can sometimes be found in the lungs of the general population; for the diagnosis of asbestosis, however, an accompanying interstitial fibrosis is necessary. Typically, the disease begins in the lower lobes and subpleurally, but the middle and upper lobes of the lungs are affected as the scarring becomes heavier. Simultaneously, the visceral pleura undergoes fibrous thickening and sometimes densely binds the lungs into the pleural cavities.

A number of complications may supervene. Large parenchymal nodules typical of Caplan's syndrome appear in a few patients having concomitant rheumatoid arthritis (p. 158). Pulmonary arteries and arterioles trapped within the scarring are narrowed and so may cause pulmonary hypertension and cor pulmonale. Concurrent cigarette smoking or exposure to coal dust leads to focal blackening of the lung.

**Parietal pleural plaques** that are sharply circumscribed and composed of hyalinized collagen lacking asbestos bodies are another asbestos-associated lesion. They may appear with or without overt asbestosis in the lungs. Typically **they are found on the dome of the diaphragm or on the anterior or posterolateral aspects of the thorax**. Sometimes they are encountered in the absence of apparent exposure, raising the possibilities that they may also have other origins or could be the consequence of very low levels of urban air pollution. In time the plaques may become calcified but rarely become adherent to the adjacent visceral pleura. They have no relationship to the subsequent development of malignant mesothelium.

**Various types of cancer** may develop in patients with significant exposure to asbestos dust. All are described in detail elsewhere. The most common form is bronchogenic carcinoma, having a fivefold increased risk (p. 446). There is a correlation between the severity of the pulmonary parenchymal fibrosis and the frequency of superimposed carcinomas; more importantly, concomitant cigarette smoking by asbestos workers multiplies the risk by 50! In contrast to the situation in nonexposed cigarette smokers in whom the most common pattern is squamous cell carcinoma, asbestos-related cancers tend to be (but not exclusively) adenocarcinomas. It is significant that the tumors usually appear long after exposure has ceased.

Until proved otherwise, a malignant mesothelioma (p. 452) means that there has been exposure to asbestos dust. This lesion is reported in about 2 to 3% of industrial workers who have had heavy exposure over extended periods, and it does not appear until 20 or even 50 years later. Cigarette smoking is not implicated in the genesis of malignant mesothelioma, nor has any other etiologic agent been clearly documented in humans.

Other forms of cancer (i.e., carcinoma of the larynx, gastrointestinal tract, kidney, ovary, and lymphomas) occur with increased frequency in asbestos workers. However, the associations are not strong.

CLINICAL CORRELATION. The clinical findings in asbestosis are nonspecific and are essentially those of any diffuse interstitial lung disease. Ventilatory insufficiency with shortness of breath is usually the first manifestation, at first provoked by minimal exertion; with the passage of time the dyspnea worsens and is present even at rest. These manifestations rarely appear before 10 years after the onset of exposure and, more commonly, 20 or more years later. The dyspnea is usually accompanied by a nonproductive cough. Hemoptysis is infrequent but when present should raise the suspicion of intercurrent bronchogenic carcinoma. It must be recalled that cigarette smoking also produces "small airways disease" and so, to an extent, can mimic these findings. Finger- and toe-clubbing (p. 708) develops in about 60 to 70% of patients. Chest films reveal irregular linear densities, particularly in the lower lobes bilaterally, and, with advancement of the pneumoconiosis, a honeycomb pattern develops. Other forms of chronic interstitial disease may produce identical changes, but when parietal fibrocalcific plaques are visualized on the chest film it points strongly to asbestos. Because of the nonspecificity of the clinical picture it is sometimes necessary to resort to lung biopsy to establish the diagnosis.

As noted previously, Caplan's syndrome may complicate the clinical course and should be suspected in those who have rheumatoid arthritis and circulating titers of rheumatoid factor or ANA. Other late-appearing complications of asbestos exposure are the many forms of cancer cited.

# BERYLLIOSIS

Beryllium dusts and vapors derived from the metal itself or its alloys, oxides, and hydroxides may cause pulmonary and systemic lesions. Depending on the concentration of the aerosol, particle size, and solubility, an acute or chronic disease may follow. *Acute berylliosis takes the form of a chemical pneumonitis; chronic berylliosis is marked by the formation of noncaseating granulomas indistinguishable from those of sarcoidosis and the hard tubercles of tuberculosis.*

Beryllium and its derivatives are currently used in the electrical, electronic, aerospace, and nuclear reactor industries and many others. The workers are not the only ones at risk; family members of workers and individuals living in proximity to these industries have also acquired berylliosis. Thus, low levels of exposure may induce disease. It has been shown that some workers exposed to levels of pollution apparently within the established regulatory standards have developed chronic disease.[29] There appears to be an apparent individual predisposition; fewer than 4% of those exposed in an industry develop lesions. Hypersensitization to the metal may be involved; patients with berylliosis often have a positive skin test for the metal, and frequently the disease is encountered in those who have returned to their hazardous occupation after a period of absence, suggesting that time is needed for the development of sensitivity. Additional evidence pointing to hypersensitization is the occasional development of an erythematous contact dermatitis in those working in beryllium industries. Some evidence suggests that the metal acts as a hapten, which becomes antigenic when complexed to native proteins.[30]

Although the lungs are the usual pathway of absorption of beryllium, infrequently skin wounds provide another point of entry, leading sometimes to beryllium lesions about the wound. Once absorbed in sufficient quantities, the metal in combination with protein is transported through the blood and is deposited throughout the body, particularly in the liver, spleen, and bones. Some, however, remains in the lungs. Thus, chronic berylliosis is not restricted to lesions of the lungs.

MORPHOLOGY. Chronic berylliosis, also known as beryllium granulomatosis, is characterized by focal granulomas within the alveolar septa and encroaching on the alveolar spaces. These granulomas bear a strong resemblance to those of sarcoidosis and tuberculosis and, indeed, may be indistinguishable.[31] The mimicry of sarcoidosis is heightened when the beryllium granuloma contains multinucleate giant cells harboring the distinctive inclusions also found in sarcoid lesions: (1) concentrically laminated Schaumann bodies (up to 50 $\mu$m in diameter) or (2) stellate acidophilic asteroids (p. 427). A third type of inclusion may also be present—a spiculated birefringent crystal 3 to 10 $\mu$m in length. Occasionally, however, the beryllium granulomas are distinctive from those of tuberculosis and sarcoidosis in that they contain necrotic centers with preserved and degenerating neutrophils. Sometimes these cells become so necrotic as to produce an acellular granular debris that strongly resembles caseous necrosis, making the differentiation from tuberculosis difficult. The degree of granuloma formation varies from case to case; sometimes granulomas are difficult to find. Similarly variable is the presence of an accompanying mononuclear interstitial infiltrate. In any case the regional nodes of drainage are commonly affected. Although the pleural surfaces may be thickened and fibrotic, they are usually not involved. In the lung the granulomas tend to become progressively fibrotic, thus inducing diffuse fibrous scarring.

Accompanying the chronic pulmonary lesions may be granulomatous involvement of the liver, kidney, spleen, lymph nodes, and skin. Chronic persistent ulcerations of the skin may develop at sites of scratches or injuries where beryllium has been introduced.

**Acute berylliosis** takes the form of a rapidly developing chemical pneumonitis with severe pulmonary edema.

**CLINICAL COURSE.** There is a latent period, usually from weeks to decades, between exposure and the development of clinical signs and symptoms. With heavy exposure the time lag is brief, leading to the acute pneumonitis described. This is manifested by the sudden onset of cough, dyspnea, fever, and constitutional symptoms such as malaise and weakness. Death sometimes occurs within a few weeks, although most patients recover.[31]

The chronic form of the disease may not appear before years of exposure. It produces manifestations similar to those of the other pneumoconioses, such as the insidious onset of dyspnea. Even with lung biopsy, the disease may be indistinguishable from sarcoidosis or tuberculosis, and in these cases, the diagnosis depends on epidemiologic and clinical factors, namely, a history of significant exposure, the presence of a diffusion defect, and consistent chest x-ray results.[32] The disease may progress inexorably to death, or it may subside, apparently spontaneously. Steroids have proved beneficial in arresting berylliosis. The prognosis is best when there are well-formed granulomas and a minimal interstitial infiltrate.[31] About 20% of the 836 cases (both acute and chronic types) in the Beryllium Case Registry in 1974 were fatal.

Opinions conflict about the carcinogenicity of beryllium, particularly with respect to bronchogenic carcinoma.[33] However, epidemiologic studies suggest a small increase in the frequency of lung cancer among industrially exposed workers.[34]

# DISORDERS CAUSED BY CHEMICALS AND DRUGS

Nearly all chemicals, including therapeutic drugs, have the potential of causing injury and sometimes death. Some are highly and promptly toxic and are referred to as poisons, but more commonly they reveal their potential only insidiously and after some time has elapsed. They range from individual hazards, such as adverse reactions to medications, to widespread pollutants, as is the case with lead. In the following sections some of these adverse reactions are presented under two headings—to therapeutic and to nontherapeutic agents.

## ADVERSE REACTIONS TO THERAPEUTIC AGENTS

Adverse reactions to therapeutic agents, more widely known as "adverse drug reactions" (ADRs), are often equated in the media with "bad medicine." Indeed they are all too frequent; they occur in about 3 to 4% of general hospital patients and are fatal in about one tenth of these instances.[35] Less frequently they are also encountered in ambulatory patients.[36] However, by no means are all ADRs "bad medicine." Often they represent well-recognized risks assumed by patients, family, and physician. For example, the patient with life-threatening leukemia may be administered a powerful cytotoxic drug to destroy the leukemic cells with full knowledge that the normal cells of the bone marrow may be simultaneously destroyed. If the marrow function does not recover promptly (with or without an autologous marrow transplant) following a course of one of these agents and the patient succumbs to an overwhelming bacterial infection potentiated by the profound neutropenia, the death could be considered an ADR because it is an unintended, undesired consequence of a form of drug therapy.[37] Thus "ADRs that count" are those that follow the unwarranted or incautious use of a medication, such as the allergic skin rash triggered by penicillin employed in some futile effort to abort a banal viral upper respiratory infection.[38]

Any drug may at one time or another be responsible for an ADR. Clearly it is not possible to comprehensively explore this "bottomless pit," but admirable surveys are available.[39] However, there is wide agreement that *four categories of therapeutics account for most serious ADRs—cardioactive, antibacterial, antineoplastic, and immunosuppressive agents.* It is apparent that all four categories would only come into use with serious disease. Indeed, often the ADR occurs because the more potent drugs in use today are capable of sustaining life in patients too sick to handle potent drugs. In an ironic sense, the increasing frequency of ADRs is a testament to "medical progress."

ADRS can be divided into the following categories.

### PREDICTABLE, DOSE-RELATED
*Overdosage*—e.g., digitalis toxicity in attempt to achieve maximal cardiotonic effect.

*Side-effect*—e.g., well-known toxicity of streptomycin for the inner ear; secondary infection incident to marrow depression in the treatment of leukemia.

### UNPREDICTABLE REACTION, NOT DOSE-RELATED
*Hypersensitivity*—e.g., antibody-mediated red cell hemolysis triggered by metabolites of penicillin; urticaria following injection of a foreign protein vaccine.

*Extension effect*—e.g., a profound drop in blood sugar following a small dose of insulin.

*Idiosyncratic reaction*—e.g., massive liver necrosis following exposure to halothane.

**Table 9–3.** SOME OF THE MORE COMMON
DRUG REACTIONS AND CAUSAL AGENTS

| Reaction | Major Offenders |
|---|---|
| **Blood Dyscrasias** (occur in almost half of all drug-related deaths) | |
| Granulocytopenia | Chloramphenicol |
| Thrombocytopenia | Quinidine |
| Hemolytic anemia | Methyldopa |
| Aplastic anemia | Isoniazid |
| Pancytopenia | Most cytotoxins |
| **Cutaneous Reactions** | |
| Ranging from urticaria, macules, papules, vesicles, and acne to exfoliative dermatitis | Antimitotics |
| | Antibiotics |
| | Hydantoin |
| | Phenindione |
| | Bromides |
| | Barbiturates |
| | Many others |
| **Renal Reactions** | |
| Acute tubular necrosis | Cyclosporine A |
| Tubulointerstitial nephritis | Analgesics |
| Glomerulonephritis | Penicillamine |
| Papillary necrosis | Phenacetin |
| Acute vasculitis | Sulfonamides |
| **Pulmonary Reactions** | |
| Diffuse alveolar damage | Bleomycin |
| Interstitial fibrosis | Nitrofurantoin |
| Edema | Busulfan |
| Acute vasculitis | Methotrexate |
| **Hepatic Reactions** | |
| Fatty change | Tetracycline |
| Hepatitis | Methyldopa |
| Cholestasis | Estrogens |
| Massive necrosis | Chlorpromazine; halothane |

These categories and the examples are merely intended to provide some concept of the diversity and scope of ARDs. Any organ or system may become the primary target, but a sampling of some of the more serious reactions and some of their common initiators is presented in Table 9–3.

## Analgesics

Tons of aspirin and other analgesics (e.g., phenacetin, acetaminophen) are freely consumed annually without awareness that they are not "unalloyed blessings." Aspirin overdose can produce serious, sometimes fatal poisoning; before safety packaging was instituted, as few as 6 to 12 adult-sized tablets of aspirin (approximately 2 to 4 gm) popped into the mouths of unsuspecting infants and children often proved fatal. A single dose of about 15 gm might be fatal in adults. *The acute toxicity takes the form of severe metabolic derangements.* At first respiratory centers are stimulated, producing a respiratory alkalosis as excessive amounts of $CO_2$ are blown off. Compensatory mechanisms then induce a metabolic acidosis with excessive excretion of bicarbonate, potassium, and water which leads potentially to fatal hypokalemia. Concomitantly, aspirin-induced gastritis induces severe vomiting and sometimes hemate-

mesis with additional losses of fluids, acid salts, and other electrolytes. The blood loss is compounded by the effect of aspirin on cyclooxygenase, which blocks the synthesis of prostacyclin ($PGI_2$) and thromboxane $A_2$, agents that play important roles in normal hemostasis (p. 66).

Less extreme overdosages with aspirin, although not necessarily fatal, may produce apparent hypersensitivity reactions that principally take the forms of erythematous, eczematous, or desquamative skin rashes; angioedema; urticaria; asthma; or even anaphylaxis. As is pointed out on page 570, the use of aspirin during viral illnesses has also been implicated in causing Reye's syndrome.[40]

Chronic consumption of therapeutic levels of aspirin is a potent factor in the development of gastritis (p. 513) and may contribute to gastric peptic ulceration (p. 516). When the total dosage of analgesics (usually taken as a proprietary mixture of aspirin, phenacetin, and acetaminophen) reaches the level of kilograms over the span of years, a potentially fatal renal lesion may appear known as analgesic-associated nephropathy (p. 476). Most of the evidence points to phenacetin or the combination of phenacetin and aspirin as the culprits, and so phenacetin has been withdrawn from the market in the United States but is still used elsewhere. Heavy use of phenacetin has also been suggested to cause bladder cancer.[41] It is clear that analgesics have their "other side."

## Barbiturates

The various barbiturates have long been favorites among those bent on escaping "the slings and arrows of outrageous fortune."[42] Indeed, in a 1977 report barbiturates were implicated in about 70% of all suicidal deaths involving therapeutic agents in the British Isles.[43] Not surprisingly, they are also major causes of ADRs, sometimes because of accidental overdosage and at other times during the administration of widely accepted therapeutic dosages. Extremely large amounts of the drug may be taken without suicidal intent because of what is called "drug automatism." An initial small dose of a barbiturate may induce sufficient mental depression or confusion to lead to repeated dosages that may build up to potentially fatal levels of the drug. Accidental and unintentional overdosages are responsible annually for over 15,000 deaths in the United States, making this highly useful therapeutic agent, along with the automobile and alcohol, one of the three prime causes of "unnatural" death.

Setting aside hypersensitivity reactions that may occur with any dosage, the levels of the various forms of barbiturates required to produce toxicity are extremely variable and are based on poorly understood individual susceptibility, the rate of accumulation of the particular formulation, its pharmacodynamics, and concurrent predisposing influences. Alcoholism is probably the most important predisposing influence, not only by adding to the confusion of the individual and thus favoring overdosage but also by impairing hepatic function, the principal site of metabolic detoxification of barbiturates. Analogously, any diffuse severe liver disease has a similar effect. All barbiturates have similar pharmacologic effects, but they vary in their rapidity of action. In general, *short-acting compounds declare their CNS-depressive effects relatively promptly, and as little as 3 gm at one time may be fatal within a few hours; after this time, the effects of nonlethal doses of short-acting barbiturates begin to wane. Long-acting barbiturates require two to three times the dosage of short-acting ones to have comparable effects, but the CNS depression is more prolonged, more difficult to reverse therapeutically, and therefore more often fatal.*

Based on the variables mentioned, the clinicoanatomic consequences of barbiturate toxicity range from profound CNS depression with fatal coma within a few hours to a variety of delayed nonfatal reactions that are perhaps related to drug sensitivity. When blood levels are high enough (beginning at about 2 mg/100 ml for short-acting agents) all neurons in the CNS are depressed, including, most importantly, the regulatory centers in the brain stem. Thus coma is accompanied by respiratory depression and sometimes depression of vasomotor control and cardiac rate. Death may result from worsening pulmonary edema with cyanosis or from shock, and in many instances, except for the pulmonary edema, there are no distinctive anatomic findings at necropsy. When the patient survives for a day or two, pulmonary edema becomes more evident and is often complicated by bacterial pneumonia; the vasomotor insufficiency may lead to acute renal tubular necrosis, oliguria, and azotemia. If death is to occur at this late stage, ischemic-hypoxic injury to the neurons throughout the CNS may be demonstrable. With near-fatal levels of intoxication or even with therapeutic levels, lesions of the skin and blood vessels may also appear. These are probably related to hypersensitivity reactions in which the drug or its metabolites act as haptens. The most common skin reaction is large, bullous vesicles—*barbiturate blisters*—that may become so generalized as to produce a widespread exfoliative dermatitis. Less severe cutaneous reactions may take the form of an eczematous dermatitis. *Systemic hypersensitivity angiitis* closely resembling polyarteritis nodosa can appear. The diagnosis of barbiturate intoxication, both clinically and anatomically, depends heavily on gas chromatographic identification of the agent in the blood or gastric contents because the clinical and anatomic changes are not distinctive.

## Exogenous Estrogens and Oral Contraceptives (OCs)

Because endogenous hyperestrinism is considered to be a factor in the development of endometrial and breast carcinomas, there has long been concern about the possible adverse effects of exogenous estrogens (usually used as replacement therapy in postmenopausal women) and estrogen-containing OCs. Although controversy persists about both agents, the accumulating data permit some reasonably reliable conclusions. First the findings relative to exogenous estrogens will be presented, followed by those relating to the OCs.

*Exogenous estrogens*, dependent on total dose and duration of use, increase the risk of carcinoma in some target organs more so than in others (Table 9–4). Besides their apparent oncogenicity, exogenous estrogens double the risk of the development of gallstones in women. Whether postmenopausal use increases or decreases the risk of cardiovascular disease, in particular myocardial infarction, remains uncertain. Within the recent past, two completely contradictory reports on this issue appeared as adjacent articles in the same journal.[49, 50]

*Oral contraceptives* are still evoking wide disagreement over their short- and long-term effects despite their use for well over two decades by millions of women (providing, one would think, an adequate population for study). Some of the difficulties stem from the differences in the absolute and relative estrogen and progestin content of the various OCs used. It has been claimed (and denied) that OCs having a high content of estrogen (more than 50 µm) induce hypercoagulability and a predisposition to thrombosis.[51] Attention also has been drawn to the possible tendency of the contained progestins to raise the blood pressure and at the same time decrease the blood level of high-density lipoproteins, both predisposing conditions for the development of atherosclerosis and coronary heart disease (p. 287). Arguable as all these hemodynamic effects may be, *it is well established that OCs as used in the past were and still are responsible for a death rate from circulatory disease that is five times greater than that among comparable nonusers.*

#### Table 9–4. ADVERSE EFFECTS OF EXOGENOUS ESTROGENS*

| Effect | Frequency |
|---|---|
| Endometrial carcinoma | Three- to eightfold increased risk in postmenopausal women (see ref. 45) |
| Vaginal adenosis | In adolescent offspring of women taking diethylstilbestrol during pregnancy |
| Vaginal clear-cell carcinoma | In approximately 0.1% of adolescent offspring of women taking diethylstilbestrol during pregnancy; usually superimposed on adenosis |
| Breast carcinoma | Findings vary from no increased risk (see ref. 46) to an approximate twofold increased risk with long-term high dosage (see ref. 47) |
| Ovarian carcinoma | More data needed, but suggest a two- to threefold increased risk (see ref. 48) |

*From Morrow, C. P.: The benefits of estrogen to the menopausal woman outweigh the risks of developing endometrial cancer. CA 34:220, 1984.

The major adverse cardiovascular effects of OCs are shown in Figure 9–9. Among the hazards, myocardial infarction and subarachnoid hemorrhage account for the largest part of the excess cardiovascular mortality. Some concept of the magnitude of the increased risk is provided in Table 9–5. To be noted, (1) *the risks do not apply equally to all women (those over 35 are at substantially higher risk); (2) cigarette smoking multiplies the hazard of thrombotic disease, particularly in those over 35; (3) the increased risk of cardiovascular death in nonsmoking women under the age of 35 is small; (4) most OCs in current use contain reduced levels of estrogens and progestins, expected to lower the risk of thrombotic complications; and (5) the morbidity and mortality entailed in the use of OCs must be balanced against the potential complications of unwanted pregnancies, the reliability and side effects of other forms of contraception, and the worldwide availability of other forms of contraception.*[52]

**Table 9–5.** CARDIOVASCULAR EFFECTS OF ORAL CONTRACEPTIVE USE—ANALYSIS OF 23,000 USERS*

| Disease | Standardized Mortality Rate (No. of Deaths) | | |
| --- | --- | --- | --- |
| | Current Users | Former Users | Controls |
| Ischemic heart disease | 13.0 | 4.1 | 2.0 |
| Subarachnoid hemorrhage | 7.3 | 10.2 | 2.3 |
| Cerebral thrombosis, hemorrhage, and embolism | 2.7 | 8.1 | 2.7 |
| Pulmonary embolism and venous thrombosis | 2.8 | 2.2 | 0.0 |
| Malignant hypertension | 0.0 | 2.5 | 0.0 |

*Modified from Royal College of General Practitioners Oral Contraception Study: Further analyses of mortality and oral contraceptive users. Lancet 1:541, 1981.

The *possible oncogenicity of OCs*, because of their estrogen content, is another area of concern. The literature is filled with claims and counterclaims but the following conclusions are generally accepted.

○ Endometrial cancer—no risk, may protect.[53]
○ Cervical cancer—no increased risk despite one contrary study.[54]
○ Ovarian cancer—protects against; the longer the use the greater the protection, which persists after OC use has been stopped.[55]
○ Breast cancer—controversial but little or no increased risk in the short term (5 to 10 years),[56] but long-term effects still under observation.
○ Benign proliferative breast disease and fibroadenoma of the breast—protects against.[58]

A few additional findings are of interest. Oral contraceptives appear to have a preventive effect against rheumatoid arthritis but may predispose to liver cell adenoma and (even more uncertainly) to hepatocellular carcinoma. The rarity of both forms of liver tumors and the fragility of the evidence call into question the significance of these risks.

One must conclude that OCs are like everything else; they have their good and their bad sides.

### Cancer Chemotherapeutic Drugs

It is already clear from the discussion of estrogens that therapeutic agents can be responsible for an increased incidence of cancer. Ironically, those most implicated are drugs used for cancer chemotherapy.[59] These tragic complications constitute Pyrrhic victories. Had the patient not survived the initial cancer, the second cancers could never have arisen, and it is possible that to some extent these complications reflect an underlying predisposition to neoplasia.

In most instances, drug-induced neoplasms are acute nonlymphocytic leukemias.[60] They have occurred principally in patients with neoplasms that are responsive to therapy, including Hodgkins' disease, non-Hodgkins' lymphoma, multiple myeloma, and carcinoma of the ovary, but sometimes they occur in

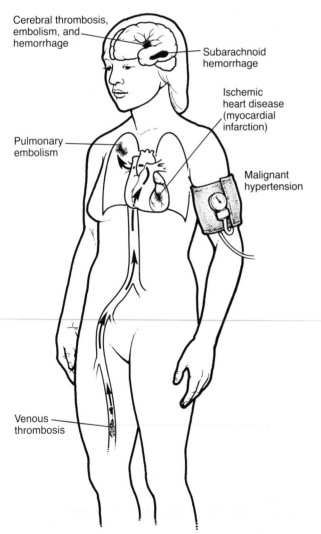

Cerebral thrombosis, embolism, and hemorrhage

Subarachnoid hemorrhage

Ischemic heart disease (myocardial infarction)

Pulmonary embolism

Malignant hypertension

Venous thrombosis

Figure 9–9. Oral contraceptives—their major cardiovascular adverse effects.

conditions less effectively controlled by the therapy (e.g., carcinoma of the breast, gastrointestinal cancer, and polycythemia vera).[61] On the basis of present evidence, the alkylating agents (e.g., melphalan and cyclophosphamide) pose the greatest risk because they have the potential of inducing mutations. In contrast, chemotherapeutic agents that function as antimetabolites to inhibit pyrimidine biosynthesis appear to be free of this untoward effect. The passage between Scylla and Charybdis is hazardous.

### Antibiotics and Immunosuppressants

*Antibiotics*, like all drugs, are two-edged swords—on the one hand they are frequently lifesaving in infectious diseases, but on the other hand they have many possible adverse effects. Indeed, it is not possible to give in detail all of their untoward potentials, and only some of the principal ones will be mentioned.

○ Antibiotic-related sensitivity reactions range from anaphylaxis to skin rashes.

○ New strains of drug-resistant organisms have emerged, particularly notable with the staphylococci, gonococci, and gram-negative enteropathogens.[62] These and other resistant strains pose grave problems and have given rise to serious epidemics, both in the community and within hospitals.

○ Destruction of the normal microflora of the body often provides the opportunity for proliferation of microbial opportunists that have the capacity to induce disease only in vulnerable hosts.

Such considerations make it evident that antibiotics can be "wolves in sheep's clothing."

*Immunosuppressants* make possible the present era of organ transplantation and are sometimes lifesaving in patients with immune-mediated diseases, but they too invoke risks. Some act mainly against immunocompetent cells (as is the case with glucocorticoids, azathioprine, and cyclosporine A) and thus predispose to infections by both pathogens and opportunists. Well recognized is the reactivation of quiescent tuberculosis by the long-term administration of high doses of steroids, which sometimes leads to fatal miliary dissemination of the infection. In the immunocompromised patient such microbes as cytomegalovirus, *Pneumocystis carinii*, and the fungi become serious risks. Another adverse effect of immunosuppressants is the development of lymphomas, particularly immunoblastic lymphoma. It is conjectured that destruction or inactivation of T-suppressor cells potentiates the emergence of these neoplasms. Many agents used for immunosuppression also have specific toxicity for particular organs. Azathioprine, for example, causes pulmonary toxic effects and may induce a diffuse interstitial pneumonitis.[63] Cyclosporine, a recently discovered "wonder" drug that acts selectively on cell-mediated immunity, has been shown to cause renal tubular necrosis and sometimes to induce kidney failure.[64]

## ADVERSE REACTIONS TO NONTHERAPEUTIC AGENTS

Among the many nontherapeutic substances that can cause disease, only a few of the more important can be considered.

### Ethyl Alcohol

The excessive consumption of ethanol is one of the principal medical and societal problems in the world. In most privileged populations it has assumed epidemic proportions, chiefly in adults but increasingly in teenagers and even children! It is estimated that alcohol abuse affects the quality and duration of life of 8 to 12% of the adult population of the United States. There is no satisfactory definition of what constitutes alcohol abuse. One wag defined an abuser of alcohol as "anyone that drinks as much as I do, whom I do not like." But more is involved than merely the level of consumption; poorly understood individual and genetic predispositions may account for the fact that among individuals having roughly comparable drinking habits, only a few suffer significant deleterious effects. Whatever the operative influences, alcohol consumption can be considered excessive when it adversely effects the intellectual, psychologic, or physical condition of the individual. The physical effects can be divided into those related to acute and to chronic alcoholism.

The clinical syndrome of *acute alcoholism* is too well known to require description. The level of intoxication is correlated directly with the blood alcohol level, which in turn is correlated with both the amount absorbed and its metabolism and excretion. Without going into great detail, it suffices that food, particularly milk and fatty substances in the stomach and small intestine, impedes absorption. After alcohol enters the bloodstream, only about 5 to 10% is excreted, unchanged, largely in the urine and breath (the basis of the breath test employed by law enforcement agents). The remainder is metabolized mainly in the liver and converted to acetaldehyde, but some may be metabolized by two other enzyme systems, as indicated in Figure 9–10. The rate-limiting enzyme in this process is hepatic alcohol dehydrogenase. In the normal nonhabituated individual the rate of metabolic breakdown is fairly constant and independent of its concentration in the blood. However, the rate can be increased by chronic alcoholism, which up to a point speeds the metabolic breakdown, presumably by enzyme induction. The rate can be decreased by diffuse liver disease. (Note—alcohol itself is a potent hepatotoxin.)

Among the many pathophysiologic effects of elevated blood levels of alcohol, those relating to the CNS are most important. Contrary to the notion that it "gives one a lift," *ethanol is a depressant of the CNS*. As the blood levels begin to rise there is first inhibition of subcortical regulatory pathways, leading

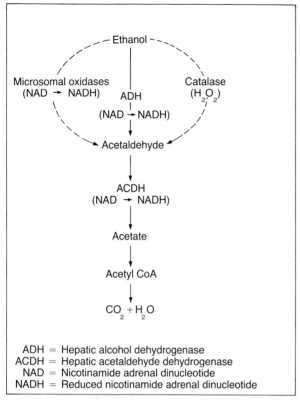

ADH = Hepatic alcohol dehydrogenase
ACDH = Hepatic acetaldehyde dehydrogenase
NAD = Nicotinamide adrenal dinucleotide
NADH = Reduced nicotinamide adrenal dinucleotide

**Figure 9–10.** Metabolism of alcohol: the major (rate-limiting) pathway is via ADH.

to hyperexcitability of cortical neurons and accounting for the characteristic behavior patterns so well known to every college student. At slightly higher levels (e.g., from four to five usual-sized drinks of whiskey), both mental and motor function are impaired, which converts the inebriate into an "unguided missile" when behind the wheel of a motor vehicle. With continued rise, cortical function is depressed and induces (with good luck) drowsiness, but at still higher levels the depressant effects extend to the brain stem and spinal cord, leading to coma and potentially to death.

Among the many other acute effects of alcohol is its toxicity for liver cells (p. 18).[65] After a simulated weekend "drinking spree," healthy young volunteers developed hepatic fatty changes. As is discussed later (p. 584), chronic ethanol consumption is the leading cause of cirrhosis of the liver in most industrialized nations. It is evident that the widely used "social lubricant" can "clog the gears."

*Chronic alcoholism* is even more insidious and damages nearly every organ and tissue in the body.[66] Some of these effects are related to nutrition, because alcohol in the gut impairs the intestinal absorption of many nutrients, notably folate and vitamin $B_{12}$. Moreover, it represents "empty calories" substituting for more beneficial foodstuffs. In addition, alcohol or one of its metabolites has direct toxicity. A high level of acetaldehyde, one metabolite of alcohol, has been implicated in injury to the liver, heart, and other organs. Attention has been directed recently to increased free radical activity in chronic alcoholics as another possible mechanism of tissue injury.[67] Whatever the mechanism, on average, *heavy drinkers have a shortened lifespan related principally to damage to the liver, brain, and heart.* As noted, alcohol is the leading cause of fatty change and cirrhosis in the liver in many cultures. Many different neurologic lesions may appear. Some are thought to be nutritional in origin; they include *Wernicke-Korsakoff syndrome (p. 752) and peripheral neuropathies.* Others are of uncertain pathogenesis, such as cerebral atrophy with intellectual impairment and cerebellar atrophy. The cardiovascular ramifications range widely. On the one hand, a few chronic alcoholics develop a cardiomyopathy (p. 341) attributed to direct injury to myocardial cells. On the other hand, it has been repeatedly shown that *moderate drinkers have less coronary heart disease than nondrinkers, but excessive consumption reverses this "protection."*[68] The beneficial effect has been attributed to increased levels of high-density lipoproteins (HDL) (p. 288).

A few additional implications of chronic alcoholism merit brief mention—increased vulnerability to infections, skeletal muscle myopathy analogous to the condition in cardiomyopathy, gastritis and peptic ulcers, acute and chronic pancreatitis, and an increased frequency of carcinoma of the oropharynx, larynx, esophagus, and possibly rectum and lung.[69] The litany could be extended, but it is evident that the cost of chronic alcohol abuse is more than its price.[70]

### Lead

Lead poisoning has been aptly termed "the silent epidemic." At one time considered to be largely an occupational hazard, it is now recognized as a widespread threat because of the growing awareness of the dangerously rising blood levels of lead in urban adults and children. This trend is particularly marked in children under five years of age, especially in black inner-city children from low-income families.[71] To place the problem in some perspective, the safe upper limit of blood levels of lead was once considered to be 70 µg/100 ml. However, substantial evidence indicates that much lower levels, down to 30 µg/100 ml, are associated with neuropsychologic and intelligence deficits in children.[72] Hematologic abnormalities may appear with levels below 30 µg/100 ml. In this context, blood lead levels exceeding 30 µg/100 ml were found in 4% of children that were aged 6 months to 5 years and in 18.6% of black inner-city children from low-income families.[71]

There are many potential environmental sources of lead. Automotive emissions once heavily contaminated the air; today the use of lead-free fuels is diminishing (but not totally removing) this source of pollution. Similarly, there are restrictions now on the use of lead paint in the United States, but many peeling and flaking dwellings built in past years remain. Lead is therefore in the dust of older deteriorating houses as well as in newsprint and ceramic decorations. Approximately 40% of inhaled lead is absorbed. Slightly acidic water passing through lead pipes becomes contaminated. Volatilized lead may contaminate the air in industries extracting, processing, and using lead or its products, and the risk is high for miners, smelter workers, welders, and ceramists. Burning storage batteries to recover the lead is particularly hazardous. Once absorbed, lead is stored in tissue, particularly in bones, and so small daily increments yield accumulations that by slow dissolution augment the level in the blood. Moreover, blood-borne lead crosses the placental barrier and exposes the unborn child to the potential of mental retardation.

Lead has many deleterious metabolic effects. It inhibits the incorporation of iron into heme, impairs the synthesis of globin, and inhibits delta-aminolevulinic acid dehydratase in red cells. Interference with the normal synthesis of hemoglobin leads to increased levels of protoporphyrin in the blood and excretion of delta-aminolevulinic acid in the urine. Lead has also been shown to inhibit adenylate cyclase in brains of experimental animals.[73]

The principal anatomic changes in lead poisoning are cited in Table 9–6. Clinically, the hematologic changes are the first and most constant. Other changes (e.g., those in the brain and skeleton) are found mainly in children. Brain changes are uncommon in adults. The CNS abnormalities are striking in children and range from subtle intellectual and psychologic deficits to severe brain swelling that can develop with alarming rapidity despite the slow ac-

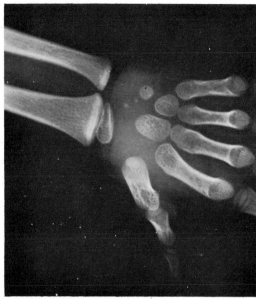

Figure 9–11. Lead deposits in the epiphyses of the wrist have caused a marked increase in their radiodensity so that they are as radiopaque as the cortical bone. (From Robbins, S. L., Cotran, R. S., and Kumar, V.: Pathologic Basis of Disease. 3rd ed. Philadelphia, W. B. Saunders Company, 1984, p. 455.)

cumulation of lead over years. Convulsions, coma, and death may follow a brief period of impaired brain function. In those who survive, residual neurologic effects are common. Peripheral neuropathy is more characteristic of lead poisoning in adults; it is exclusively motor and involves the most actively used muscles, so wrist-drop and foot-drop are typical signs. With chronic lead poisoning in children, the increased skeletal deposits may produce abnormal radiodensities of the epiphyseal regions (Fig. 9–11). Renal lesions may be associated with defective proximal tubular dysfunction (Fanconi's syndrome). For unexplained reasons severe abdominal colic is sometimes seen and can be mistaken for an acute surgical emergency. It has been alleged without substantial proof to be a direct result of lead on intestinal smooth muscle.

The major diagnostic features of lead poisoning at all ages are the basophilic red-cell stippling, elevated levels of blood protoporphyrin, and reduction in activity of delta-aminolevulinic acid dehydratase in red cells. There is also increased urinary excretion of delta-aminolevulinic acid. The levels of lead in the blood can be spuriously low because they are mainly an indicator of current absorption. When recognized early, lead poisoning can be reversed by appropriate measures, but left unrecognized it may permanently impair or even terminate the life of the victim.

### Drug Addiction

Addiction to "street" drugs, most obtained surreptitiously, has become a serious societal and medical

**Table 9–6. ANATOMIC FEATURES OF LEAD POISONING**

| | |
|---|---|
| Blood | *Anemia*, usually microcytic, hypochromic (related to impaired hemoglobin synthesis and increased red cell fragility)<br>*Basophilic stippling of red cells* (related to mitochondrial and ribosomal injury with ribosomal aggregation) |
| Nervous System | *Encephalopathy* (in children) with brain swelling, possibly demyelination of cerebral and cerebellar white matter, death of neurons, and astrocytic proliferation (poorly understood, may be related to impaired mitochondrial oxidative phosphorylation)<br>*Peripheral neuritis with demyelination* |
| Oral Cavity | *Gingival lead line* in adults with gingivitis (blue/black deposition of lead sulfide) |
| Kidneys | *Acid-fast intranuclear inclusions*, principally in proximal tubular cells (composed in part of lead-protein complexes) |
| Skeletal System | *Radiodense lead deposits* in epiphyses of children |

problem in the United States and many other affluent societies. It is estimated that there are at least 600,000 opioid addicts in the United States. In Great Britain, the number of new addicts has been rising by almost 40% per year since 1980.[74] The consequences of drug abuse are brought into stark relief by the finding in 1972 (probably valid today) that it was the leading cause of death in New York City in those between 15 and 35 years old.[75] The roster of agents used by addicts is known only to them, but of principal concern to the public and medical worlds are marijuana and heroin—the former because of its growing use among teenagers and because it often leads to more dangerous practices, and the latter because of its well-defined adverse physical effects. This is not to say that lysergic acid diethylamide (LSD), amphetamines, cocaine and "crack", phencyclidine hydrochloride (PCP or "angel dust"), and many other agents are not widely used or are without danger. Most addicts have used concurrently or sequentially so many drugs that it has been difficult to segregate the effects of each. This is less of a problem with marijuana because at first it is often the only agent used by the young individual, and heroin is now a major and widely available drug and so has been associated with striking and well-defined pathologic effects. Comments, therefore, will be restricted to these two.

*Marijuana* (cannabis), is currently a federally regulated agent in the United States, and therefore its possession or use is illegal, whether justified or not. A past survey points out that 72% of individuals between 15 and 25 years old have used cannabis[76] and so it has been said that "failure to experiment with cannabis by the age of 25 must be regarded as statistically deviant."[77] The psychoactive substance contained in the resin of the leaves and flowering tops of the plant is tetrahydrocannabinol (THC). Hashish also contains THC. As is well known, marijuana is usually smoked in home-made cigarettes ("joints"), during which THC is volatilized and absorbed through the respiratory tract. It is significant that a single "joint" contains 50 to 100 times more benzopyrene and other potentially carcinogenic hydrocarbons than is found in a tobacco cigarette. Habitual use not surprisingly has led to inflammatory changes in the upper and lower air passages and decreased vital capacity analogous to the effects of habitual cigarette smoking.[78] Will an increased incidence of lung cancer appear in time? Controlled studies also have found a significant correlation between heavy marijuana use during pregnancy and impaired fetal growth and development. Many other charges have been leveled at this agent, such as suppression of gonadal function, but none has been soundly established. Neither is there convincing evidence that prolonged use has permanent effects on the structure or function of the brain.[79] Despite the paucity of well-established physical effects, the use of cannabis during the early years of life is frequently

an initiation into other illicit drugs. It would seem prudent to heed the title of a recent book—*Keep Off the Grass.*[80]

*Heroin*, a derivative of morphine, is unquestionably the most common opioid in illicit use. In the drug traffic it is sold as a more or less white powder having a variable concentration of heroin (2 to 70%) that was "cut" (diluted) with quinine, lactose, talc, or other white powder. The drug may be "sniffed" or dissolved in fluid (in desperation, lavatory water has been used) and injected subcutaneously ("skin popping") or intravenously. Other than the trafficker's dubious word about how "good the stuff is," addicts cannot know the potency of the material they are about to "shoot," and so a favored method of "disposing" of a bothersome or nonpaying customer is to provide a particularly high concentration of heroin, which causes an acute overdosage. Moreover, tolerance builds up rapidly but also disappears within about two weeks, and the addict who returns to past practices after a period of abstinence (perhaps in jail) is at risk of overdosage.

Leaving aside the tragic behavioral and functional consequences of heroin addiction, it is associated with a wide range of physical effects.[81–83] *The consequences may be related to (1) the direct pharmacologic effect of the drug, (2) hypersensitivity reactions to the drug or the "cutting agent," (3) microbiologic contaminants, and (4) diseases contracted in the course of sharing hypodermic needles.* Up to the recent past the most feared communicable disease was viral hepatitis, but it has been displaced by the even more feared AIDS (p. 175). In a recent analysis at least 50% of intravenous-drug addicts were found to have serologic markers of HIV (human immunodeficiency virus), thought to be the causal agent of AIDS.[84] The range of effects of heroin will be considered by brief discussions of overdosage and changes in specific organs (Fig. 9–12).

*Overdosage* is the most common cause of death. About 20% of all cases are suicides or homicides; the remainder are presumably accidental. Death may occur with unbelievable suddenness—the victim may be found with the needle still in place. Deaths by overdosage are attributable to inhibition of medullary centers and profound depression of respiration, to arrhythmias or cardiac arrest (possibly related to the use of quinine as a diluting agent), or to hypoxia incident to the development of extreme pulmonary edema, perhaps as a manifestation of a hypersensitivity reaction.

*Skin abscesses, cellulitis, thrombosed veins or skin scarring, and hyperpigmentations over the course of veins—"tracks"*—are frequent telltales of heroin addiction. The skin infections have at times been the site of introduction of tetanus bacilli.

*Cardiovascular lesions* in the form of *septicemia* or *infective endocarditis* are secondary to microbial contamination of the injected "shot." The endocarditis may affect either side of the heart, usually conforms

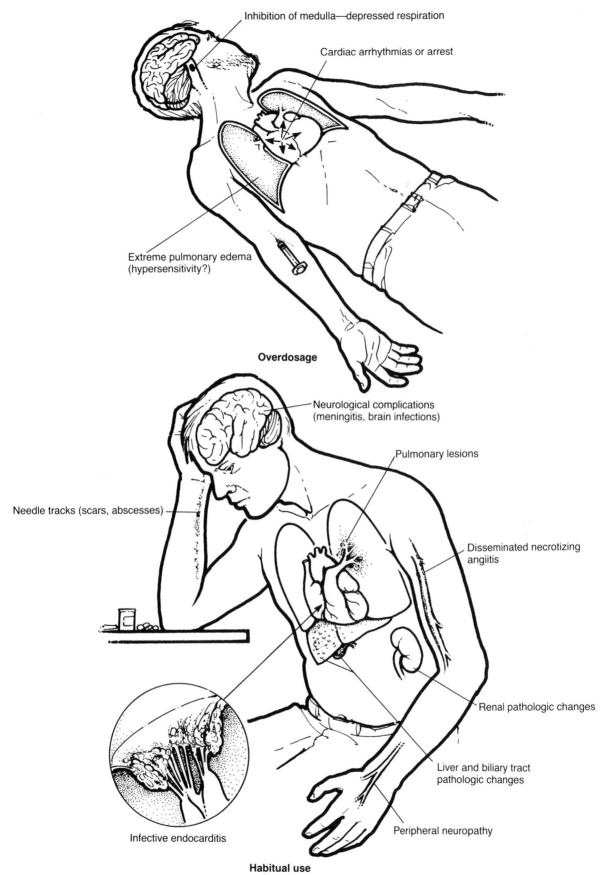

**Overdosage**

Inhibition of medulla—depressed respiration

Cardiac arrhythmias or arrest

Extreme pulmonary edema (hypersensitivity?)

**Habitual use**

Neurological complications (meningitis, brain infections)

Pulmonary lesions

Needle tracks (scars, abscesses)

Disseminated necrotizing angiitis

Renal pathologic changes

Liver and biliary tract pathologic changes

Peripheral neuropathy

Infective endocarditis

**Figure 9–12.** Depiction of the major consequences of drug addiction—overdosage (*above*) and less catastrophic consequences (*below*).

271

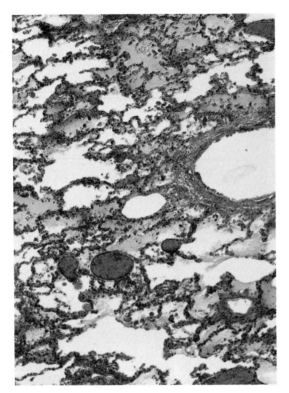

Figure 9–13. Patchy pulmonary edema and atelectasis of the alveoli of the lung in a heroin addict.

or chronic viral hepatitis.[86] Alcoholism is common in addicts and may contribute to the development of hepatic fatty change or cirrhosis. For obscure reasons, the gallbladder is frequently distended with thick bile and the portahepatic lymph nodes are often strikingly enlarged.

*Lymph nodes and spleen* may be somewhat enlarged owing to nonspecific inflammatory changes and, occasionally, granulomatous reactions induced by the cutting agents (Fig. 9–14).

*Renal changes* are frequently encountered in chronic addiction. Most characteristic is focal to diffuse sclerosing glomerulonephritis, progressing in some individuals to end-stage renal disease.[87] This form of glomerulopathy is a frequent complication of AIDS or may be attributable to immunologic reactions to the drug, its cutting agents, or microbial contaminants (notably hepatitis virus). Other forms of glomerulonephritis may also be encountered, including proliferative and membranoproliferative forms (p. 467).

*Neurologic complications* constitute another hazard. They include acute peripheral neuropathy, transverse myelitis, and various types of myopathy that are perhaps related to involvement of motor nerves. The microbial contamination of the injectate may also lead to meningitis or subdural and brain infections.

It is evident that the pursuit of addiction often leads to the hospital or, even worse, the grave.

to the "acute" pattern, and in its most distinctive form involves the previously normal tricuspid valve. *Staphylococcus aureus* and *Candida albicans* account for the infections in about two thirds of all cases.[85] *Disseminated necrotizing angiitis* resembling polyarteritis nodosa may develop apparently as a hypersensitivity reaction to the narcotic or its diluting agent. Alternatively, the angiitis may be related to hepatitis B viral infection and its circulating viral antigens and antibodies.

*Pulmonary lesions* are common. The most frequent form is pulmonary edema, sometimes hemorrhagic—"narcotic lung"—resembling the changes found in the adult respiratory distress syndrome (Fig. 9–13). A number of secondary complications may appear, including bronchopneumonia, focal atelectasis, aspiration of gastric contents, and more distinctively foreign body granulomas within the walls of pulmonary arteries or adjacent alveolar septa consequent to the injection of such "cutting agents" as talc (a silicate). The talc crystals are readily visualized by polarized light. Infrequently, thromboses and plexiform and angiomatoid lesions (residuals of organized thrombi) obstruct pulmonary blood flow and lead to cor pulmonale.

*Liver and biliary tract* lesions are present in 75 to 80% of addicts. Most often there are periportal infiltrations of mononuclear cells, reflecting bacteremias, sensitivity reactions to the drug or its cutting agents,

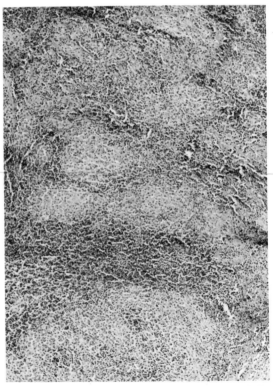

Figure 9–14. The pale foci are numerous granulomas within the spleen of a heroin addict.

## Industrial Carcinogens

According to the Environmental Protection Agency of the United States, of the approximately 50,000 substances in current commercial use, only about a fifth have been tested, and of these about 20% were labeled carcinogenic. However, in some instances, the evidence supporting this contention is open to challenge because in some part it is based on epidemiologic evidence of an increased incidence of certain forms of cancer in those who hold particular occupations or on experimental data using dosage schedules far beyond those that might be encountered in the workplace. Alternatively, it is based on evidence documenting the mutagenic activity of substances on the premise that most (not all) carcinogens are mutagens and that mutagenesis is often involved in experimental carcinogenesis. Although all of these approaches provide incriminatory evidence, they do not lead to certain proofs.[88] Nonetheless, there can be no challenge to the fact that occupational exposure has induced an estimated 1 to 5% of all human cancers.[89] However, it is impossible in a free-living population to rigorously rule out confounding influences such as cigarette smoking, diet, and genetic predisposition as causes for these cancers.

All of the substances that at one time or another have been indicted as occupational carcinogens cannot be covered here. Only a few of the best established associations are listed below with their principal occupational exposures.[90]

For further details, reference can be made to the review by Schottenfeld and Haas.[91]

## Other Nontherapeutic Agents

In addition to those substances already considered, many others have been known to cause disease and often death; they include arsenic, cyanide, insecticides, polychlorinated biphenyls (PCBs), and poisonous mushrooms (mainly *Amanita* species). Most constitute rare problems and so further brief comments will be restricted to only a few.

*Methyl alcohol* is widely used in solvents, paint removers, antifreezes, and Sterno. Absorption after ingestion or inhalation is followed by oxidation to formaldehyde and formic acid, the latter inhibiting hexokinase function and cellular respiration. The main targets of injury are the retinal and cortical neurons, leading to visual impairment and sometimes total blindness. With brain involvement, the occurrence of CNS depression may progress to coma or even death.

*Carbon monoxide* (CO) is an occasional cause of accidental death or suicide. It is no longer present in natural gas, but incomplete combustion of this gas may release CO. Carbon monoxide is also present in cigarette smoke and in coolants sometimes used in gas refrigerators; it is also emitted by internal combustion engines and industrial processes using fossil fuels. The affinity of CO for hemoglobin is 200 times greater than that of oxygen. This increased affinity yields carboxyhemoglobin, which impairs oxygen transport and leads to systemic hypoxia. *Acute poisoning* can develop within minutes when ambient air has a high CO content. Past sad experiences indicate that a car in a small, closed garage can create lethal levels within five minutes. Typically the blood turns cherry-red (owing to the carboxyhemoglobin) and induces striking hyperemia of the tissues. This is soon followed first by mental confusion that renders the victim incapable of self-help and then by progressively deepening coma and death. The main targets of the hypoxia are the neurons within the CNS. *Chronic low-dose poisoning* insidiously induces low-grade hypoxia, ultimately causing neuronal injury. The principal sites of damage are the basal ganglia, particularly the lenticular nuclei. In some instances, demyelinating lesions in the cerebral white matter develop, followed by cystic rarefactions. Hypoxic injury may also be encountered in the liver, kidney, and heart. Death may be due to depression of brain function or to renal, hepatic, or cardiac failure. Except in rare instances, the victim recovers but may be left with permanent neurologic damage.

*Mercury*, by combining with sulfhydryl groups, poisons enzymes and damages membranes. *Acute toxicity* from soluble mercuric salts, once a method of suicide, has almost disappeared. Mothers will be happy to know that when a child crunches a mercury thermometer in its mouth, the glass is more of a hazard than the metallic mercury, which is so insoluble as to be almost without toxicity. *Chronic toxicity* was once encountered in those who made felt hats and mirrors but now is seen in photoengravers and workers in the tool-hardening industry. Indeed, Lewis Carroll's enduring phrase "mad as a hatter" remains a testament to the use of mercury compounds

| Agent | Type of Cancer |
| --- | --- |
| Asbestos (p. 259) | Bronchogenic carcinoma, mesothelioma, others |
| Beta-naphthylamine (rubber, dye industries) | Bladder carcinoma |
| Benzene (rubber-cement workers, distillers, dye users) | Leukemia |
| Vinyl chloride (plastic industries) | Liver angiosarcoma |
| Arsenic (miners, insecticide makers and sprayers, chemical workers) | Skin, lung, liver carcinomas |
| Chromium (producers and processors exposed to volatilized gases) | Nasal cavity, sinuses, lung, and larynx cancers |
| Nickel (miners and processors exposed to volatilized gases) | Nasal, sinuses, lung cancers |
| Radioactive ores (miners exposed to dusts) | Lung and bone cancers, leukemia |

in the production of felt hats—workers often suffered from the neurologic effects of chronic mercury poisoning manifested by loss of memory, emotional instability, motor dysfunction, and deafness. In some instances coma and death followed. These neurologic changes in chronic poisoning reflect scattered foci of atrophy in the cerebral cortex, principally in the occipital lobes, and cerebellar atrophy resulting from loss of neurons and subsequent gliosis. Chronic intoxication may also cause gingival discoloration resembling a "lead line" and renal damage in the form of nephrotoxic nephritis (p. 476) and glomerulonephritis. Distinctive of the damaged kidneys is heavy proteinuria with tubular reabsorption of protein, leading to the formation of eosinophilic droplets in tubular epithelial cells.

In the recent past, inhabitants of Minimata—a Japanese fishing village—suffered from a mysterious neurologic disorder that was traced to the consumption of fish from a coastal area contaminated by mercury-bearing industrial wastes. A general alarm followed about tinned fishes, such as tuna, that were derived from related waters. But analyses indicate that with control of the pollution, the hazard has disappeared.

# PHYSICAL AGENTS

The physical agents most often involved in causing injury can be categorized as (1) mechanical, (2) thermal, and (3) electromagnetic. Among these, mechanical violence unleashed by a vehicular accident is obviously the most common cause of damage. Burns continue to be a lamentable source of morbidity and mortality, and nonfatal injury related to radiation is an ever-present hazard in this era of radiotherapy of cancers. Fatalities related to radiation are, however, relatively uncommon, and we can only hope that they will remain so in a peaceful world spared from nuclear weapons.

## MECHANICAL VIOLENCE

The injuries caused by such violence as an automobile accident fall into three categories: (1) soft tissue injuries, (2) bone injuries, and (3) head injuries. The last two categories are considered elsewhere. Soft tissue injury is more the province of the surgeon than the pathologist. However, a few terms should be clarified. An *abrasion* constitutes a loss of the superficial layers or the entire thickness of the epidermis resulting from a shearing force. A *laceration* is a linear or jagged tear resulting from overstretching of the skin and underlying tissues. When caused by a sharp object, such as a scalpel or glass, it is usually called an *incised wound*. A *contusion* is usually inflicted by a blunt force that ruptures subcutaneous vessels and causes interstitial bleeding without disruption of the continuity of the overlying skin. Blunt

force may cause deep-seated lacerations in organs such as the liver or spleen with remarkably little apparent superficial injury to the skin.

## THERMAL BURNS

Burns are particularly tragic causes of morbidity and mortality because they are totally preventable and too often affect children and young adults with "so much life left to live." Those of the surface of the body and those of the respiratory tree have sufficiently different clinical effects to merit separate consideration.

*Surface burns* have significance in direct proportion to their size and depth. At one time, involvement of 50% of the body surface was almost always fatal. However, with the great improvements in therapy, there is almost no upper limit, and victims are now surviving with involvements of 80% or more surface area. Depth of the burn is clinically characterized as either *partial* or *full thickness*.

A *partial-thickness burn* implies loss of up to the entire epidermis but preservation of the dermal appendages from which reepithelialization may occur. Although the wound may expose large areas of the dermis and be followed by considerable inflammatory reaction with sometimes massive exudation of fluids, including plasma proteins, skin grafting is usually not necessary. Secondary infection of the burn wound, an ever-present danger, is discussed below. Partial-thickness burns generally imply a low intensity of heat that induces injury by accelerated metabolism of cells, inactivation of temperature-critical enzymes, and induction of vascular injury from which the exudation occurs. The epidermal cells, down to the dermis, may be totally incinerated, may undergo coagulative necrosis with nuclear pyknosis, or, in the deeper epidermal layers, may disclose evidence of deranged membrane permeability with nuclear and cellular swelling.[92]

*Full-thickness burns*, when large, usually require skin grafting. For wounds of comparable size, full-thickness burns have greater loss of fluid and proteins than partial-thickness burns and are always vulnerable to superimposed infections. In full-thickness burns there is, of course, incineration or coagulation not only of the entire epidermis but also of all adnexal structures. The dermal collagen, if not destroyed, takes on the appearance of a homogeneous gel. The cells in the deeper layers of subcutaneous tissue and even skeletal muscle may undergo coagulative necrosis if they have not been totally incinerated. In the span of hours to a day or two, a well-defined cellular and vascular inflammatory reaction beomes evident in the immediately subjacent preserved tissue, which is far more marked in the full-thickness than in the partial-thickness burn.

*Far more important than the local changes are the potential postburn sequelae.* When more than 20%

of the body surface has been involved, the development of shock (p. 79) is the most immediate threat to life. Although pain and neurogenic mechanisms may play some role, shock is largely caused by the massive outpouring of fluid, electrolytes, and plasma proteins from the denuded wound. Acute gastroduodenal "stress" ulcers may appear within the first or second day and, by bleeding, they compound the loss of blood volume. Thus, the "burn shock" is in reality attributable to hypovolemia. Intravascular hemolysis in the still-functional vessels in the base of the burn wound may aggravate the anemia and lead to hemoglobinuria.

*Secondary infection is a threat in all burns marked by loss of the epidermis.* The wound is generally sterile for approximately 24 hours, but unless vigorous preventive measures are taken promptly, microbial contamination and growth ensues in the rich medium of the exudate and devitalized tissue. It may reach the staggering number of millions of bacteria per square centimeter of wound. Staphylococci and streptococci were once the major offenders, but with present-day antibiotics, coliforms and particularly *Pseudomonas aeruginosa* now predominate as causes of infection.[93] The organisms progressively invade into the deeper layers and are only temporarily slowed in their penetration by the subjacent viable tissues. The growth and death of these gram-negative rods releases products that sometimes lead to *endotoxic shock. P. aeruginosa*, when it penetrates into the viable tissues, has a predilection for invading the walls of blood vessels to thus induce local thromboses that increase the injury, but, even worse, the organism may become disseminated throughout the bloodstream. Devitalization of tissues and exudation are not the only factors potentiating burn wound infection; burned patients are immunologically compromised, a fact that is attributed to either the appearance of an immunosuppressive factor in the blood or to activation of T-suppressor cells.[94] Thus, burn victims with large surface wounds are not only in pain, they are also at risk of the subsequent development of potentially fatal shock or infection.

*Inhalation burn injuries* are in general more serious than surface wounds. Individuals trapped in a burning building, depending on duration of exposure and intensity of heat, may succumb within minutes or, if rescued, suffer thermal injuries at any level of the respiratory tract from the naso-oral cavities to the lungs. The intensity of the heat in a burning room is not generally appreciated; it can reach 2000°C. At this level of heat "flashover" occurs when even so-called noninflammable substances ignite and the entire room becomes an inferno. Death may occur within minutes from hypoxia (as the oxygen is depleted) and the inhalation of superheated gases and fumes. At less extreme levels of heat, burns in the oral cavity may appear analogous to those described on the body surface, ranging up to charring of all surfaces including tongue, epiglottis, and larynx. The inspired heat and fumes may similarly injure the lining of the respiratory passages and the lung parenchyma, and in such circumstance usually causes death within the hour. With less damage, hours to days later an acute respiratory distress syndrome with severe pulmonary transudation and exudation appears (p. 410). Exudative plugging of airways causes focal to massive areas of atelectasis. Secondary infection in the course of a day or two leads to the development of bronchopneumonia. Survival is precarious and depends on intensity and extent of the injury and on prompt and effective therapy.

## ELECTROMAGNETIC (RADIATION) INJURY

Although electrical energy, particularly in the form of lightning, may certainly impair one's "joie de vivre," the resultant injuries are too rare to deserve comment. Radiant energy, on the other hand, even in the absence of nuclear blasts, is an important source of tissue damage. Everyone is exposed to cosmic radiation and sunlight, many to diagnostic x-ray procedures, and a significant number to the radiotherapy of cancers. Radiant energy is therefore a double-edged sword; it provides an invaluable means of clinical diagnosis and sometimes a curative mode of therapy but at the same time it is a potent mutagen and destroyer of cells and, on occasion, of life.

It is not necessary to delve in great detail into the physics of radiation; suffice it that it occurs in two forms: (1) electromagnetic waves (x-rays and gamma rays) and (2) charged particles (alpha, beta—also known as electrons, protons, neutrons, and others). Further details on these types of radiation are available in specialized texts.[95, 96] All forms of radiation exert their effects on cells by transferring energy to molecules and atoms with which they collide. With sufficient energy transfer, electrons are displaced from the atomic nucleus, causing ionization of the atom or molecule. Ionized states are unstable and initiate chain reactions with contiguous elements. However, it is unclear whether the effects of energy are the consequence of direct or indirect actions on critical atoms or molecules. The *direct or target theory* proposes direct interaction with vital molecules and encompasses the possibilities that single or multiple direct hits may be required to ionize them.[97] The most vulnerable intracellular target is DNA, more specifically the linkages and bonds within the molecules, particularly when the cell is in the process of mitosis. However, other molecules, membranes, and enzymes are also damaged by radiation. The *indirect action theory* proposes that radiant energy exerts its effect by producing free "hot" radicals perhaps by radiolysis of cell water (p. 9). These free radicals then interact with critical components of the cell to cause cell damage or death.

## Factors Modifying Effects of Radiation on Cells

Any type of cell in the body can be damaged or killed by a sufficient dose of radiation, depending on many factors:

Dosage
Penetrability
Linear Energy Transfer (LET)
Latency
Rate of Delivery
Cellular Repair
Oxygen Effect
Radiosensitivity of Cells

Other variables being equal, damage is proportional to the dose. Dosage is measured in various units. The *amount delivered in air* to a target is measured in roentgens (R). All of this energy is not absorbed and so *the amount absorbed by the target* is quantitated in rads (r). Air exposed to 1 R of radiation absorbs 0.87 rads. One gray (gy) equals 100 r. The radioactivity of an isotope is measured in curies (Ci) and its half-life. The curie defines the amount of energy released in a finite period of time based on its rate of decay, but the half-life denotes the length of time required for the isotope to have undergone disintegration of one half of its atoms. *Although the effects of all types of radiant energy are qualitatively the same, they differ in their penetrability and intensity of radiation delivery along their paths.* For example, gamma rays have a high velocity and penetrate deeply but dissipate their energy over a long distance. Thus the amount of energy they deliver per unit path length (expressed as the linear energy transfer—LET—value) is smaller than that for alpha particles, which have a lower velocity and larger mass and penetrate less deeply but deliver more energy per unit path length. It follows that for equal radiation dosage, alpha-particulate radiation is more likely to kill cells within its range (have a high relative biologic effectiveness—RBE) than gamma radiation having a low RBE because it is more widely diffused. However, alpha radiation is less likely to reach deep targets. Thus, with equal dosage schedules delivered from external sources to an endometrial cancer, for example, alpha radiation is more likely to cause injury to the skin and superficial tissue in the pathway of the radiation than is gamma radiation.

The effects of radiation may be *latent* (i.e., may not be evident immediately). Witness the radiation-induced cancers that have appeared years, sometimes decades, later in the suvivors of the atomic blasts. This *latency* is poorly understood. Does it imply sequential intracellular interactions eventually extending to some crucial molecule or function, or instead is the first interaction so minor that it exerts a deleterious effect only through potentiating ever more severe dislocations in successive generations of cells?

The *rate of delivery of radiant energy* significantly modifies its effect, especialy when it is delivered in divided doses or fractions, as is the practice in radiotherapy. Although radiant energy is cumulative, cells are able to repair at least some of the sustained damage. The best evidence of the importance of repair is the increased incidence of skin cancers in individuals with the genetic disorder *xeroderma pigmentosum.* These persons lack the requisite enzymes for excising ultraviolet light–induced dimers or possibly other enzymes needed to reunite the severed ends of the DNA molecule, and so, when exposed to sunlight, they sustain cumulative radiation-induced mutations in epidermal cells that lead to skin cancers (p. 227).[98] In the normal individual with intact repair mechanisms, if sufficient time elapses after the initial radiation-induced injury, the cell may have almost completely recovered by the time it receives a second exposure and there would be no cumulative effect. *Divided dosages, then, have cumulative effects only to the extent that recovery in the interval is incomplete.* Radiotherapy of tumors takes advantage of the fact that in general normal cells are more slowly dividing than most cancer cells and thus sustain less injury (discussed below), which is therefore more amenable to repair.

Another variable that modifies the effect of radiation is the oxygenation of cells and tissues ("oxygen effect"). Molecular oxygen has two unpaired electrons that may interact with radiation-induced free radicals to amplify their damaging effect. This oxygen effect is of particular importance in the use of radiation to destroy neoplasms. Often the centers of such neoplasms are poorly vascularized and relatively hypoxic and therefore are less likely to suffer radiation destruction.

The *radiosensitivity of cells and tissues* is determined by the inherent response of the cells to a pulse of radiation, by the kinetics of cellular repair between radiation exposures, and by the proliferative state of the cells. Thus cells vary in their radioresponsiveness. Although there are many potential intracellular targets, DNA is thought to be most vulnerable, especially immediately prior to and during mitotic division. For this reason the induction of *cell necrosis is most closely correlated with the reproductive activity of cells and inversely correlated with their level of specialization.* Unless the dose of radiation has been massive, cells already in mitosis at the time of irradiation complete their division but may suffer mutations rendering them unable to undergo subsequent mitosis. Thus, cancer cells are more vulnerable than normal cells, and rapidly dividing, undifferentiated cancers are generally more responsive to radiotherapy than are slowly growing, well-differentiated cancers. The same principle applies to the various normal cells of the body and their tumors (Table 9–7).

Despite this generalization, there are exceptions. Some lymphocytes such as "memory T cells" are long-lived, but nonetheless all lymphocytes appear

Table 9–7. RADIOSENSITIVITY OF SPECIALIZED CELLS AND THEIR TUMORS*

| Radiosensitivity | Normal Cells | Tumors |
|---|---|---|
| High | Lymphoid, hematopoietic (marrow), germ cells, intestinal epithelium, ovarian follicular cells | Leukemia—lymphoma, seminoma, dysgerminoma, granulosa cell carcinoma |
| Fairly high | Epidermal epithelium, adnexal structures (hair follicles, sebaceous glands), oropharyngeal stratified epithelium, urinary bladder epithelium, esophageal epithelium, gastric gland epithelium, ureteral epithelium | Squamous cell carcinoma of the skin, oropharyngeal, esophageal, cervical and bladder carcinoma, adenocarcinoma of gastric epithelium |
| Medium | Connective tissue, glia, endothelium, growing cartilage or bone | Endothelio- and angiosarcomas, astrocytomas, the vasculature and connective tissue elements of all tumors |
| Fairly low | Mature cartilage or bone cells, mucous or serous gland epithelium, pulmonary epithelium, renal epithelium, hepatic epithelium, pancreatic epithelium, pituitary epithelium, thyroid epithelium, adrenal epithelium, nasopharyngeal nonstratified epithelium | Liposarcoma, chondrosarcoma, osteogenic sarcoma, adenocarcinoma of: breast epithelium hepatic epithelium renal epithelium pancreatic epithelium thyroid epithelium adrenal gland epithelium colon epithelium Squamous cell cancer of the lung |
| Low | Muscle cells, ganglion cells | Rhabdomyosarcoma, leiomyosarcoma, ganglioneuroma |

*Adapted from Rubin, R., and Casarett, G. W.: Clinical Radiation Pathology. Philadelphia, W. B. Saunders Co., 1968, p. 903.

to be exquisitely sensitive to radiation. Moreover, among cancers there is no perfect correspondence between sensitivity to radiation and rate of growth.

**The morphologic changes induced within cells by irradiation are not distinctive or qualitatively different from those encountered with injury caused by other agents (e.g., nitrogen mustard, Myleran).** Both the cytoplasm and the nucleus are affected. The initial response takes the form of cellular swelling, cytoplasmic vacuolization, mitochondrial enlargement, and distortion, disruption, swelling, and fragmentation of the endoplasmic reticulum. However, lysosomes appear to be resistant and sometimes are increased in number.[99] The nuclei swell, become vacuolated, and in severely affected cells undergo pyknosis or karyorrhexis. Disruptions of both the nuclear membrane and the plasma membrane occur in heavily irradiated cells. All manner of chromosomal damage may be seen in cells undergoing division, including deletion, breaks, translocations, interadherence, and fragmentation of chromosomes. Disorderly mitoses, polyploidy, and all manner of aneuploidy may appear. Unquestionably, other, more subtle mutations at the level of individual genes must also be present. **It is this damage to the genetic apparatus of the cell that underlies the lethality, oncogenicity, and mutagenicity of radiation energy**. It might be noted in passing that the cytoplasmic, nuclear, and mitotic changes seen in irradiated cells make them closely resemble cancer cells, a problem that plagues the pathologist when evaluating postirradiation tissue for the possible persistence of tumor cells.

Much of the effect of radiation on both normal and tumorous tissue is mediated by radiation injury of the vasculature. During the immediate postirradiation period blood vessels may show only dilatation, accounting for the erythema of the skin seen so often following radiotherapy. Later (or with more intense exposure), endo-thelial cells undergo swelling, vacuolation, and even destruction. With time, heavily damaged vessels may rupture, thrombose, or undergo progressive fibrosis and narrowing of their lumens (Fig. 9–15). The contiguous connective tissue becomes increasingly sclerotic. In this

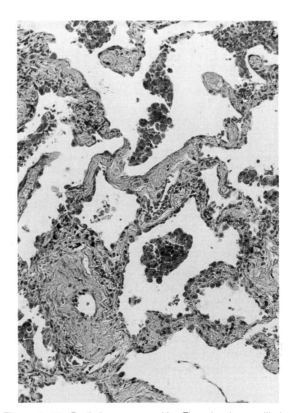

Figure 9–15. Radiation pneumonitis. The alveolar capillaries have been markedly narrowed, some have been obliterated, and the larger vessel (*lower left*) reveals marked fibrous thickening of its wall. Collectively an interstitial fibrosing pneumonitis results.

**Table 9–8.** RADIATION EFFECTS ON
ORGANS AND SYSTEMS

| Organ Affected | Level of Sensitivity | Interval to Appearance |
| --- | --- | --- |
| *Skin* | Moderate | |
| Erythema | | Begins 2 to 3 hours, peaks 2 to 3 weeks |
| Radiodermatitis | | Months |
| Hyperpigmentation | | |
| Depigmentation | | |
| Telangiectasis | | |
| Atrophy | | |
| Epilation | | |
| Ulcerations | | Months to years |
| Squamous cell carcinoma | | Years to decades |
| *Hemolymphoid Systems* | High | |
| Lymphopenia | | Begins in hours |
| Lymph node, splenic shrinkage | | 5 to 10 days |
| Neutropenia | | 5 to 10 days |
| Thrombocytopenia | | 5 to 10 days |
| Anemia | | 3 to 4 weeks |
| *Gonads* | | |
| Ovary—destruction of granulosa cells and ova | High | Beginning 2 to 3 weeks |
| Testis—destruction of spermatogonia, spermatocytes | Moderate | Same |
| *Lungs* | High | |
| Edema | | Days |
| Adult respiratory distress syndrome | | Hours to days |
| Interstitial fibrosis—capillary thromboses | | Beginning 2 to 3 weeks |
| *Gastrointestinal Tract (exposed segments)* | High | |
| Hyperemia | | Days |
| Mucosal ulcerations | | 5 to 10 days |
| Mural fibrosis and narrowing | | Weeks to months |
| *Central Nervous System* | | |
| In adults | Low | Resistant up to heavy exposure |
| In embryo (microcephaly, mental retardation) | Moderate | Postnatal |

way the dependent parenchymal cells are deprived of their nutrition and thus undergo atrophy or die. These changes and the associated parenchymal atrophy are much like those encountered in aging.

### Effects of Radiation on Organ Systems

Certain organs and systems are affected particularly frequently or severely either because of their location or because of their vulnerability to radiation injury. They are listed in Table 9–8 along with some order of magnitude of their radiosensitivity and response time.

### Total Body Radiation

Exposure of large areas of the body to even small doses of irradiation may have devastating effects. Although it is not uncommon to employ in a carefully circumscribed field 4000 rads or more of radiation in the treatment of cancer, total body exposure to as little as 200 to 300 rads may be lethal. An excellent summary of the significance of various levels of whole body exposure is provided in Table 9–9, taken from Warren.[100] These reactions are classically divided into three general patterns: (1) hematopoietic, (2) gastrointestinal, and (3) cerebral.

The *hematopoietic syndrome* may follow low doses of total body irradiation and usually begins with mild gastrointestinal symptoms related to injury to the gut, followed by the changes in the peripheral blood and bone marrow that have been cited earlier.

The *gastrointestinal syndrome* may begin with dosages of 50 to 100 rads but becomes more significant with dosages in the range of 300 to 1000 rads. The manifestations reflect the sensitivity of the gastrointestinal tract to radiation injury.

The *cerebral syndrome*, with convulsions, coma,

**Table 9–9.** EXPECTED SHORT-TERM EFFECTS
FROM ACUTE WHOLE BODY RADIATION*

| Dose in Rads | Probable Effect |
| --- | --- |
| 10 to 50 | No obvious effect except, probably, minor blood changes. |
| 50 to 100 | Vomiting and nausea for about 1 day in 5 to 10% of exposed personnel. Fatigue, but no serious disability. Transient reduction in lymphocytes and neutrophils. |
| 100 to 200 | Vomiting and nausea for about 1 day, followed by other symptoms of radiation sickness in about 25 to 50% of personnel. No deaths anticipated. A reduction of approximately 50% in lymphocytes and neutrophils will occur. |
| 200 to 350 | Vomiting and nausea in nearly all personnel on first day, followed by other symptoms of radiation sickness, e.g., loss of appetite, diarrhea, minor hemorrhage. About 20% die within 2 to 6 weeks after exposure; survivors convalesce for about 3 months, although many have a second wave of symptoms at about 3 weeks. Up to 75% reduction in all circulating blood elements. |
| 350 to 550 | Vomiting and nausea in most personnel on first day, followed by other symptoms of radiation sickness, e.g., fever, hemorrhage, diarrhea, emaciation. About 50% die without 1 month; survivors convalesce for about 6 months. |
| 550 to 750 | Vomiting and nausea (or at least nausea) in all personnel within 4 hours after exposure followed by severe symptoms of radiation sickness, as above. Up to 100% die; few survivors convalesce for about 6 months. |
| 1000 | Vomiting and nausea in all personnel within 1 to 2 hours. All die within days. |
| 5000 | Incapacitation almost immediately (minutes to hours). All personnel will die within 1 week. |

*From Warren, S.: The pathology of ionizing radiation. *In* Bioastronautics Data Book. 2nd Ed. Washington, D.C., NASA, 1973.

and death, appears only with high levels of radiation, usually above 1500 rads.

*Nonfatal whole body irradiation has resulted in a number of late-appearing sequelae in atomic bomb survivors.* These have been movingly detailed by Morgan.[101] Most of the more than 100,000 immediate or early fatalities at Hiroshima and Nagasaki were caused by blast injuries and the ensuing fire storms.[102] Soon thereafter one of the syndromes already described appeared and often caused death within a few days to weeks by overwhelming infection or massive fluid and electrolyte dislocations. Much later a variety of forms of cancer began to appear, depending on age at time of exposure and severity of exposure. For example, at least a 20-fold increased incidence of acute leukemia has occurred in those who were less than 10 years or over 50 years of age at the time of the blasts. The latent period for the appearance of these disorders in children was approximately 5 to 10 years, whereas in adults it was 10 to 20 years. For unknown reasons, acute lymphocytic and acute (as well as chronic) myelogenous leukemia but not chronic lymphocytic leukemia were induced. Those under 10 years of age have experienced an increased risk of breast cancer (in females) and thyroid cancer and possibly lymphoma, multiple myeloma, and cancers of the stomach, esophagus, urinary tract, and salivary glands.[103] When the exposure occurred at the age of 50 years or older, there was a notable increase in the incidence of lung cancer. Besides having these postirradiation oncogenic changes, atomic bomb survivors have also developed lenticular opacities, persistent chromosomal aberrations in lymphocytes, and microencephaly and mental retardation among individuals exposed in utero. There is no evidence to date of genetic mutations being passed from parents to children.[104]

Although it is hoped that we will never again be confronted with total body exposure from atomic bomb blasts, the awesome potential of nuclear power plant accidents, nuclear waste, or even of therapeutic radiation should never be forgotten by the physician. Even such low dosages as 300 to 600 rads employed therapeutically to the head and neck during childhood have been followed in 20 to 40% of individuals by thyroid and brain cancers some decades later.[105] "Be sure that the treatment is not worse than the disease."

## References

1. Barney, G. O.: The Global 2000 Report to the President of the United States: Entering the 21st Century. New York, Pergamon Press, 1980, p. 1.
2. Natusch, D. F., and Wallace, J. R.: Urban aerosol toxicity: The influence of particle size. Science 186:695, 1974.
3. Fielding, J. E.: Smoking: Health effects and control. N. Engl. J. Med. 313:491 (pt. 1), 555 (pt. 2), 1985.
4. U.S. Department of Health, Education, and Welfare: Smoking and Health 1979: A Report to the Surgeon General. No. 79–50066. Rockville, Maryland, Public Health Service, 1979.
5. Sandler, D. P., et al.: Cumulative effects of lifetime passive smoking on cancer risk. Lancet 1:312, 1985.
6. Silverberg, E.: Cancer Statistics 1985. CA 35:19, 1985.
7. Rosenberg, L., et al.: The risk of myocardial infarction after quitting smoking in men under 55 years of age. N. Engl. J. Med. 313:1511, 1985.
8. Green, G. M., et al.: Defense mechanisms of the respiratory membrane. Am. Rev. Respir. Dis. 115:479, 1977.
9. Kleinerman, J., et al.: Pathology standards for coal workers' pneumoconiosis. Arch. Pathol. Lab. Med. 103:375, 1979.
10. Fisher, E. R., et al.: Objective pathological diagnosis of coal workers' pneumoconiosis. J.A.M.A. 245:1829, 1981.
11. Lapp, N. L.: Lung disease secondary to inhalation of nonfibrous minerals. Clin. Chest Med. 2:219, 1981.
12. Seaton, A., et al.: Quartz and pneumoconiosis in coal miners. Lancet 2:1272, 1981.
13. Ames, R. G.: Does coal workers' pneumoconiosis predict to lung cancer? Some evidence from a case-control study. J. Soc. Occup. Med. 33:141, 1983.
14. Schmidt, J. A., et al.: Silica-stimulated monocytes release fibroblast proliferation factors identical to interleukin I. A potential role for interleukin I in the pathogenesis of silicosis. J. Clin. Invest. 73:1462, 1984.
15. Doll, N. J., et al.: Immunopathogenesis of asbestosis, silicosis, and coal workers' pneumoconiosis. Clin. Chest Med. 4:3, 1983.
16. deShazo, R. D.: Current concepts about the pathogenesis of silicosis and asbestosis. J. Allergy Clin. Immunol. 70:41, 1982.
17. Warnock, M. L., et al.: The relation of asbestos burden to asbestosis and lung cancer. Pathol. Annu. 18(Part 2):109, 1983.
18. Varkey, B.: Asbestos exposure. An update on pleuropulmonary hazards. Postgrad. Med. 74:93, 1983.
19. Casey, K. R., et al.: Asbestos-related diseases. Clin. Chest Med. 2:179, 1981.
20. Craighead, J. E., and Mossman, B. T.: The pathogenesis of asbestos-associated diseases. N. Engl. J. Med. 306:1446, 1982.
21. Brody, A. R., et al.: Initial deposition pattern of inhaled minerals and consequent pathogenic events at the alveolar level. Ann. N.Y. Acad. Sci. 428:108, 1984.
22. Kagan, E., et al.: Enhanced release of a chemoattractant for alveolar macrophages after asbestos inhalation. Am. Rev. Respir. Dis. 128:680, 1983.
23. Crouch, E., and Churg, A.: Ferruginous bodies and the histologic evaluation of dust exposure. Am. J. Surg. Pathol. 8:109, 1984.
24. Davies, D.: Asbestos-related diseases without asbestosis. Br. Med. J. 287:164, 1983.
25. Woodworth, C. D., et al.: Squamous metaplasia of the repiratory tract. Possible pathogenic role in asbestos-associated bronchogenic carcinoma. Lab. Invest. 48:578, 1983.
26. Craighead, J. E., et al.: The pathology of asbestos-associated diseases of the lungs and pleural cavities: Diagnostic criteria and proposed grading schema. Arch. Pathol. Lab. Med. 106:544, 1982.
27. Churg, A., and Golden, J.: Current problems in the pathology of asbestos-related disease. Pathol. Annu. 17(Part 2):33, 1982.
28. Wright, J. L., and Churg, A.: Morphology of small-airway lesions in patients with asbestos exposure. Hum. Pathol. 15:68, 1984.
29. Cotes, J. E., et al.: A long-term follow-up of workers exposed to beryllium. Br. J. Indust. Med. 40:13, 1983.
30. Reeves, A. L.: Berylliosis as an autoimmune disease. Ann. Clin. Lab. Sci. 6:256, 1976.
31. Freiman, D. G., and Hardy, H. L.: Beryllium disease. The relation of pulmonary pathology to clinical course and prognosis based on a study of 130 cases from the U.S. Beryllium Case Registry. Hum. Pathol. 1:25, 1970.
32. Constantinidis, K.: Acute and chronic beryllium disease. Br. J. Clin. Pract. 32:127, 1978.

33. Kuschner, M.: The carcinogenicity of beryllium. Environ. Health Perspect. 40:101, 1981.

34. Wagoner, J. K., et al.: Beryllium: An etiologic agent in the induction of lung cancer, non-neoplastic respiratory disease, and heart disease among industrially exposed workers. Environ. Res. 21:15, 1980.

35. Levy, M., et al.: Hospital admissions due to adverse drug reactions. Am. J. Med. Sci. 277:49, 1979.

36. Steel, K., et al.: Iatrogenic illness on a general medical service at a university hospital. N. Engl. J. Med. 304:638, 1981.

37. Martys, C. R.: Adverse reactions to drugs in general practice. Br. Med. J. 2:1194, 1979.

38. Ingelfinger, F. J.: Counting adverse drug reactions that count. N. Engl. J. Med. 294:1003, 1976.

39. Riddell, R. H.: Pathology of drug-induced and toxic diseases. New York, Churchill Livingstone, 1982.

40. Hurwitz, E. S., et al.: Public Health Service Study on Reye's syndrome and medications. Report of the pilot phase. N. Engl. J. Med. 313:849, 1985.

41. Piper, J. M., et al.: Heavy phenacetin use and bladder cancer in women aged 20 to 49 years. N. Engl. J. Med. 313:292, 1985.

42. Shakespeare, W.: Hamlet, Act III, i. 56.

43. Johns, M. W.: Self-poisoning with barbiturates in England and Wales during 1959–74. Br. Med. J. 1:1128, 1977.

44. Morrow, C. P.: The benefits of estrogen to the menopausal woman outweigh the risks of developing endometrial cancer. CA 34:220, 1984.

45. Shapiro, S., et al.: Risk of localized and widespread endometrial cancer in relation to recent and discontinued use of conjugated estrogens. N. Engl. J. Med. 313:969, 1985.

46. Bland, K. I., et al.: The effects of exogenous estrogen replacement therapy of the breast: Breast cancer risk and mammographic parenchymal patterns. Cancer 45:3027, 1980.

47. Hoover, R., et al.: Menopausal estrogens and breast cancer. N. Engl. J. Med. 295:401, 1976.

48. Hoover, R., et al.: Stilboestrol (diethylstilbestrol) and the risk of ovarian cancer. Lancet 2:533, 1977.

49. Stampfer, M. J., et al.: A prospective study of postmenopausal estrogen therapy and coronary heart disease. N. Engl. J. Med. 313:1044, 1985.

50. Wilson, P. W. F., et al.: Postmenopausal estrogen use, cigarette smoking, and cardiovascular morbidity in women over 50: The Framingham Study. N. Engl. J. Med. 313:1038, 1985.

51. Tooke, J. E., and McNicol, G. P.: Thrombotic disorders associated with pregnancy and the pill. Clin. Haematol. 10:613, 1981.

52. Sartwell, P. E., and Stolley, P. D.: Oral contraceptives and vascular disease. Epidemiol. Rev. 4:95, 1982.

53. Stubblefield, P. G.: Oral contraceptives and neoplasia. J. Reprod. Med. 29(Suppl. 7):524, 1984.

54. Vessey, M. P., et al.: Neoplasia of the cervix uteri and contraception: A possible adverse effect of the pill. Lancet 2:930, 1983.

55. Shapiro, S.: Oral contraceptives: Time to take stock. N. Engl. J. Med. 315:450, 1986.

56. Centers for Disease Control (CDC): Long-term oral contraceptive use and the risk of breast cancer. J.A.M.A. 249:1591, 1983.

57. Editorial: Another look at the pill and breast cancer. Lancet 2:985, 1985.

58. Jick, H., et al.: Oral contraceptives and breast cancer. Am. J. Epidemiol. 112:577, 1980.

59. Editorial: Second malignancies in lymphoma patients. Lancet 2:1163, 1985.

60. Calabresi, P.: Leukemia after cytotoxic chemotherapy—A Pyrrhic victory? N. Engl. J. Med. 309:1118, 1983.

61. Greene, M. H., et al.: Acute nonlymphocytic leukemia after therapy with alkylating agents for ovarian cancer. A study of five randomized clinical trials. N. Engl. J. Med. 307:1416, 1982.

62. Murray, B. E., and Moellering, R. C., Jr.: Patterns and mechanisms of antibiotic resistance. Med. Clin. North Am. 62:899, 1978.

63. Bedrossian, C. W., et al.: Azathioprine-associated interstitial pneumonitis. Am. J. Clin. Pathol. 82:148, 1984.

64. Myers, B. D., et al.: Cyclosporine-associated chronic nephropathy. N. Engl. J. Med. 311:699, 1984.

65. Isselbacher, K. J.: Metabolic and hepatic effects of alcohol. N. Engl. J. Med. 296:612, 1977.

66. Edmondson, H. A.: Pathology of alcoholism. Am. J. Clin. Pathol. 74:725, 1980.

67. Fink, R., et al.: Increased free-radical activity in alcoholics. Lancet 2:291, 1985.

68. Lieber, C. S.: To drink (moderately) or not to drink? N. Engl. J. Med. 310:846, 1984.

69. Pollack, E. S., et al.: Prospective study of alcohol consumption and cancer. N. Engl. J. Med. 310:617, 1984.

70. Marmot, M. G., et al.: Alcohol and mortality: A U-shaped curve. Lancet 1:580, 1981.

71. Mahaffey, K. R., et al.: National estimates of blood lead levels: United States, 1976–1980. N. Engl. J. Med. 307:573, 1982.

72. Yule, W., et al.: The relationship between blood lead concentrations, intelligence and attainment in a school population: A pilot study. Dev. Med. Child. Neurol. 23:567, 1981.

73. Walton, K. G., et al.: Effects of $Mn^{2+}$ and other divalent cations on adenylate cyclase activity in rat brain. J. Neurochem. 27:557, 1976.

74. Hartnoll, R., et al.: Estimating the prevalence of opioid dependence. Lancet 1:203, 1985.

75. Johnson, R. B., and Lukash, W. M. (eds.): Summary of Proceedings of the Washington Conference on Medical Complications and Drug Abuse. Am. Med. Assoc. Comm. on Alcoholism and Drug Dependence. Washington, DC, Dec. 7, 1972.

76. Kandel, D. B., and Logan, J. A.: Patterns of drug use from adolescence to young adulthood: 1. Periods of risk for initiation, continued use and discontinuation. Am. J. Public Health 74:660, 1984.

77. Editorial: Epidemiology of drug usage. Lancet 1:147, 1985.

78. Patrick, G. B.: Marijuana and the lung. Postgrad. Med. 67:110, 1980.

79. Relman, A. S.: Marijuana and health. N. Engl. J. Med. 306:603, 1982.

80. Nahas, G. G.: Keep off the Grass: A Scientific Inquiry into the Biological Effects of Marijuana. New York, Pergamon Press, 1979.

81. Ostor, A. G.: The medical complications of narcotic addiction. No. 1. Med. J. Aust. 1:410, 1977.

82. Ostor, A. G.: The medical complications of narcotic addiction. No. 2. Med. J. Aust. 1:448, 1977.

83. Ostor, A.G.: The medical complications of narcotic addiction. No. 3. Med. J. Aust. 1:497, 1977.

84. Landesman, S. H., et al.: Special Report: The AIDS epidemic. N. Engl. J. Med. 312:521, 1985.

85. Kaplan, E. L., et al.: A collaborative study of infective endocarditis in the 1970s. Emphasis on infections in patients who have undergone cardiovascular surgery. Circulation 59:327, 1979.

86. Miller, D. J., et al.: Chronic hepatitis associated with drug abuse: Significance of hepatitis B virus. Yale J. Biol. Med. 52:135, 1979.

87. Cunningham, E. E., et al.: Heroin nephropathy. A clinicopathologic and epidemiologic study. Am. J. Med. 68:47, 1980.

88. Becker, C. E., and Coye, M. J.: Recent advances in occupational cancer. J. Toxicol. Clin. Toxicol. 22:195, 1984.

89. Wynder, E. L., and Gori, G. B.: Contribution of the environment to cancer incidence: An epidemiologic exercise. J. Natl. Cancer Inst. 58:825, 1977.

90. Ernst, P., and Theriault, G.: Known occupational carcinogens and their significance. Can. Med. Assoc. J. 130:863, 1984.

91. Schottenfeld, D., and Haas, J. F.: The workplace as a cause of cancer. Clin. Bull. 8:54, 1978.
92. Cuppage, F. E., et al.: Morphologic changes in rhesus monkey skin after acute burn. Arch. Pathol. 195:402, 1975.
93. Teplitz, C.: Pathology of burns. In Artz, C. P., and Moncrief, J. A. (eds.): The Treatment of Burns. 2nd ed. Philadelphia, W. B. Saunders Co., 1969.
94. Ninnemann, J. L., et al.: Thermal injury–associated immunosuppression: Occurrence and in vitro blocking effect of postrecovery serum. J. Immunol. 122:1736, 1979.
95. Pizzarello, D. J., and Witcofski, R. L.: Basic Radiation Biology. 2nd ed. Philadelphia, Lea & Febiger, 1975.
96. Prasad, K. N.: Human Radiation Biology. Hagerstown, MD, Harper & Row, 1974, p. 58.
97. Hutchinson, F.: The molecular basis for radiation effects on cells. Cancer Res. 26:2045, 1966.
98. Setlow, R. B.: Repair-deficient human disorders and cancer. Nature 271:713, 1978.
99. Ghidoni, J. J.: Light and electron microscopy study of primate liver 36–48 hours after high doses of 32 million electronvolt protons, Lab Invest. 16:268, 1967.
100. Warren S.: The pathology of ionizing radiation. In Bioastronautics Data Book. 2nd ed. Washington, DC, NASA, 1973.
101. Morgan, C.: Hiroshima, Nagasaki and the RERF (Radiation Effects Research Foundation). Am. J. Pathol. 98:843, 1980.
102. Ohkito, T.: Review of thirty years study of Hiroshima and Nagasaki atomic bomb survivors. II. Biological effects. J. Radiat. Res. Supplement:49, 1975.
103. Finch, S. C.: The study of atomic bomb survivors in Japan. Am. J. Med. 66:899, 1979.
104. Wagner, B. M.: Editorial: Genetics and the atomic bombs. Hum. Pathol. 16:101, 1985.
105. Lyon, J. L.: Radiation exposure and cancer. Hosp. Pract. 19:159, 1984.

# II

# 10

# The Vascular System

L. MAXIMILIAN BUJA, M.D.*

Vascular diseases have obvious importance; not only do they weaken vessels and render them vulnerable to rupture, they also narrow and occlude the vascular lumens and so threaten the blood supply to the tissues and organs of the body. The major vascular disorder, atherosclerosis, is the commonest ailment of Western populations. The organ injuries it induces, as for example to the heart and brain, account for about one half of all deaths in the United States and Europe. Varicose veins and venous thromboses (phlebothrombosis) are also extremely common and cause a great deal of disability; the thromboses may, as you already know, give rise to fatal pulmonary emboli. Thus, vascular disorders are responsible for a large portion of clinical practice. Here they will be divided into those affecting arteries and those involving veins, followed by brief treatments of lymphatic diseases and tumors of the vascular system that have essentially similar morphologic patterns whether they arise from arteries, veins, or lymphatics.

# Arterial Diseases

## ARTERIOSCLEROSIS

Arteriosclerosis is the generic term for three patterns of vascular disease, all of which cause thickening and inelasticity of arteries. The dominant pattern is *atherosclerosis*, discussed in detail later. It is marked by the formation of intimal fibrofatty plaques that often have a central grumous core rich in lipid. The Greek stem "athera" means "gruel, or porridge." The second morphologic form of arteriosclerosis is the rather trivial *Mönckeberg's medial calcific sclerosis*, characterized by calcifications in the media of muscular arteries. It is encountered in medium-sized muscular arteries in individuals usually over the age of 50 years. The calcifications take the form of irregular medial plates or discrete transverse rings, which create a nodularity on palpation and are readily visualized radiographically. Occasionally, the calcific deposits undergo ossification. Since these medial lesions do not encroach on the vessel lumen, medial calcific sclerosis is largely of anatomic interest alone.

---

*A. J. Gill Professor of Pathology, University of Texas Health Science Center at Dallas.

However, arteries so affected may also develop atherosclerosis. Disease of small arteries and arterioles is known as *arteriolosclerosis*. Small vessel sclerosis is most often associated with hypertension and diabetes mellitus. There are two anatomic variants, hyaline and hyperplastic, that are related to the cause and rate of progression of disease. Both cause thickening of vessel walls with luminal narrowing and may in the aggregate induce ischemic injury to tissues or organs. Since the lesions are often prominent in the kidneys, where they induce distinctive forms of nephropathy, they are described on page 478. Thus only atherosclerosis requires further consideration here. Indeed, atherosclerosis is so clearly the dominant form of arteriosclerosis that it is often loosely referred to as arteriosclerosis.

## ATHEROSCLEROSIS (AS)

No disease in the United States is responsible for more deaths, has stimulated more research, and has engendered more controversy about approaches to its control than atherosclerosis. It is characterized by the formation of intimal fibrofatty lesions called *atherosclerotic plaques*, which narrow the vascular lumen and are associated with degenerative changes in media and adventitia. Some are largely fibrous plaques; others are soft, fatty and prone to undergo superimposed complications (calcification, ulceration with overlying thrombosis, and intraplaque hemorrhage) that worsen the luminal narrowing or cause total occlusion. The centers of these plaques often contain a grumous, lipid-rich debris containing cholesterol and cholesteryl esters, from which the designation atherosclerosis was derived; the plaques with large lipid-rich cores are called *atheromas*. In practice, the three terms, atherosclerotic or atheromatous plaque, fibrous plaque, and atheroma, are used interchangeably. Beginning with subtle changes in childhood, the asymptomatic vascular involvement tends silently to become more severe with advancing age and usually only becomes clinically apparent in middle to later life, when it causes arterial insufficiency or weakening. *AS has assumed its awesome importance because of its predilection for the coronary arteries, the arterial supply to the brain, and the aorta.* Atheromatous involvement of the coronary arteries underlies the dominant form of heart disease, coronary heart disease (CHD), also known as ischemic heart disease (IHD, p. 316), the most important manifestations of which are myocardial infarction and sudden death (p. 320). IHD alone is the commonest cause of death in atherosclerosis-prone populations. The involvement of the arteries supplying the brain accounts for a large fraction of strokes caused by cerebral ischemia and infarction. Aortic atherosclerosis leads to aneurysms (abnormal dilatations), particularly of the abdominal aorta, that sometimes rupture and cause massive, fatal hemorrhages.

Other, less common consequences of AS are gangrene of the lower leg from atherosclerotic involvement of the iliac, femoral, or popliteal arteries, intracranial hemorrhages secondary to rupture of a weakened artery, and renal ischemia or hypertension incident to atherosclerotic narrowing of the ostia of the renal arteries. Since the vascular involvement itself causes no signs and symptoms, the presence of advanced atherosclerosis in a patient is usually revealed by the appearance of one of these consequences of the disease, principally IHD.

**EPIDEMIOLOGY.** AS is virtually ubiquitous among the populations of North America, Europe, and the Soviet Union. In contrast, as judged by the clinical heart attack rate and extent of disease at autopsy, it is much less prevalent in Central and South America, Africa, Asia, and the Orient.[1, 2] For example, in 1977 the death rate from IHD in Finland was 996.9 per 100,000 population (the highest in the world among nations having reasonably accurate data). In contrast, it was 94.8 in Japan. The United States ranked sixth in 1977, with a mortality rate from IHD of 715.1 per 100,000 population. These striking contrasts are believed to be related largely to environmental rather than genetic influences, although there is some evidence that heredity may play a small role. Persons migrating from countries with a low incidence to those with a high incidence of IHD progressively develop the risk of their adopted land. Although the bases for these striking contrasts are still uncertain, currently favored is the notion that they relate to differing dietary habits and lifestyles, as will become evident later.

During the first half of the twentieth century, there was a steady increase in the recognized incidence of cardiovascular disease, most of which was related to AS. By 1940, IHD was the leading cause of death in the United States, and its frequency continued to increase thereafter. Just as it began to appear that there was no controlling this insidious epidemic, the mortality rate from IHD began to level off, and from 1968 to 1978 it remarkably fell by 26.5% and has continued to decline.[1] The reasons for this welcome trend are still debated, but it appears that the decline has been mediated in large measure by a reduction in AS (primary prevention), perhaps influenced by changes in diet and lifestyles, and by improved therapy for established IHD (secondary prevention).[3, 4] Although death from heart disease in the United States is declining, AS remains the foremost killer of Americans and other economically privileged populations.

Large-scale population-based studies such as the Framingham study (and many more) have identified influences that bear a strong relationship to the probability of having or developing severe AS and IHD; these influences are referred to as "*risk factors.*"[1, 5, 6]

Within vulnerable populations, there are personal characteristics that influence the individual's likelihood of developing AS. *Most important is age.* There is substantial evidence that atheroma formation begins early in life; an autopsy study of young soldiers killed during the Korean War in the early 1950s revealed that 77% already had some coronary artery atherosclerosis, obviously not sufficient to cause IHD.[7] However, only rarely (in predisposed individuals, to be characterized later, who develop so-called premature atherosclerosis) does it cause clinical disease before the age of 35 years in males and 45 years in females. From this point in life, as judged by the mortality rate of IHD, the prevalence of clinically significant AS increases with each decade among both men and women. Some concept of the rate of climb can be gathered from the fact that the death rate from IHD among white males aged 65 to 74 years old is more than 25 times greater than that in the age group 35 to 44 years.

The *sex of the individual* is also a significant determinant. Other factors being equal, males are much more prone to develop AS than are females. At all age groups, the female mortality rates from coronary heart disease are lower than the male rates. Women appear to be relatively sheltered from the ravages of AS during reproductive life except when predisposing influences are present, such as diabetes mellitus, heavy cigarette smoking, or prolonged oral contraceptive intake. As will be seen (p. 320), the male mortality rate from IHD in the middle years of life is many times greater than that of females until advanced age, when the difference lessens.

Certain risk factors are very strongly correlated with AS and IHD and also are amenable to control. These are called *major risk factors*, and include: (1) *hypercholesterolemia*, (2) *hypertension*, (3) *cigarette smoking*, and (4) *diabetes mellitus*.

***Hypercholesterolemia.*** Considerable evidence points to hypercholesterolemia as a major risk factor.[1, 5, 6, 8] It takes many forms: (1) The classic lipid-laden atherosclerotic plaque is rich in cholesterol and cholesterol esters, which tracer studies prove are largely derived from the blood cholesterol. (2) A diet that increases the serum cholesterol level is the classic method of producing atherosclerosis in a number of animals. (3) Disorders predisposing to hypercholesterolemia lead to "premature atherosclerosis" and IHD early in life. For example, genetic disorders of lipid metabolism, such as familial hypercholesterolemia, induce florid atherosclerosis in the first few decades of life and often cause death from coronary heart disease before the age of 20 years. Hypercholesterolemia is also encountered in patients with diabetes mellitus, hypothyroidism, and the nephrotic syndrome (p. 464), and so patients with these conditions are particularly vulnerable to IHD. (4) Population studies demonstrate that the higher the plasma cholesterol level, the greater the risk of developing IHD. For example, there is about a tenfold difference between the incidence or death rates from IHD in middle-aged men in Japan, where

the mean plasma cholesterol levels are quite low, and those for men in Finland, where the levels are high. *There is no single level of plasma cholesterol that identifies those at risk; the higher the level, the greater the risk.* However, there is some evidence that the risk rises significantly once a plateau level of about 200 mg/100 ml is exceeded. In the Framingham study, men and women 35 to 44 years of age with serum cholesterol levels of 265 mg/100 ml or higher had a five times greater risk of developing coronary heart disease than did those with levels below 200 mg/100 ml. The role of elevated levels of the other blood lipid, triglyceride, as a risk for IHD is less clearly defined. However, there is some evidence of increased risk in certain subjects with hypertriglyceridemia (normal range is less than 200 to 250 mg/100 ml, with considerable variation with age and gender).

*There is a large body of evidence that a high dietary intake of cholesterol and saturated fats will raise the plasma cholesterol level.*[1, 5, 6] Contrariwise, a low-fat, low-cholesterol diet with a higher ratio of polyunsaturated to saturated fats will lower the plasma cholesterol level. However, critics have pointed out that dietary lipids have only an indirect effect on the plasma lipid levels, since most of the plasma cholesterol is endogenously synthesized. Furthermore, there has been little direct evidence from controlled clinical trials that dietary modifications reduce the risk of AS and IHD. However, the recently completed Lipid Research Clinics Coronary Primary Prevention Trial has found a significant reduction in cardiovascular mortality associated with reduction in plasma cholesterol in a select population whose hypercholesterolemia was treated with diet and drugs.[9, 10] These results have provided the most conclusive evidence to date that lowering serum cholesterol does decrease the risk for IHD.[9, 10] The American Heart Association recommends a "prudent" diet based on the preponderance of the available evidence.[11] It should be noted that the decline in the incidence of coronary heart disease in the last decade has been associated with a significantly decreased consumption of cholesterol in the United States.

*Low-density–lipoprotein levels in the plasma have the same predictive significance as the levels of cholesterol.*[1] Cholesterol and triglycerides do not circulate in the blood as free lipids but rather occur in the form of lipoprotein complexes.[12, 13] These can be divided on the basis of their density and electrophoretic mobility into lipoprotein families, the major categories of which are (1) chylomicrons; (2) very-low-density lipoproteins (VLDL), also known as pre-beta lipoproteins; (3) low-density or beta lipoproteins (LDL); and (4) high-density or alpha lipoproteins (HDL). The lipids are complexed to carrier apoproteins, of which the major types are designated A, B-48, B-100, C, and E. The apoproteins are responsible for receptor-mediated endocytosis and metabolism of the lipoproteins (Fig. 10–1). The B-100 apolipoprotein appears in LDL. Immunofluorescence methods

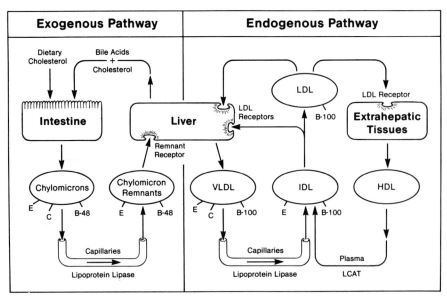

**Figure 10–1.** Pathways for receptor-mediated metabolism of lipoproteins carrying endogenous and exogenous cholesterol. HDL = high-density lipoprotein; LCAT = lecithin:cholesterol D acyltransferase; LDL = low-density lipoprotein; IDL = intermediate-density lipoprotein; VLDL = very-low-density lipoprotein. The distinction between exogenous and endogenous cholesterol applies to the immediate source of the cholesterol in plasma lipoproteins. After the exogenous cholesterol has been delivered to the liver and has been secreted in VLDL, it is considered endogenous cholesterol. Note that HDL is the lipoprotein that removes cholesterol from extrahepatic cells. (From Goldstein, J. L., et al.: Defective lipoprotein receptors and atherosclerosis. N. Engl. J. Med. *309*:288, 1983. Reprinted by permission of The New England Journal of Medicine.)

for identification of apoprotein B-100 thus provide a means of identifying the localization of LDL in tissues. Although all of these lipoproteins contain some cholesterol, the richest content is found in LDL, which is composed of about 50% cholesterol. About 70 to 75% of the total plasma cholesterol is transported in the form of LDL. In contrast, VLDL is composed primarily of triglycerides and contains only about 12% of cholesterol. It is catabolized intravascularly into an intermediate-density lipoprotein (IDL) and ultimately to LDL. *The level of HDL, in contrast, bears an inverse relationship to risk of atherosclerosis and coronary heart disease; the higher the level, the smaller the risk.*[1] Although the relationship between HDL, LDL, and cholesterol is still somewhat uncertain, one of the roles of HDL is the removal of surplus cholesterol from peripheral cells for transport back to the liver. Of interest, the levels of HDL are increased by exercise and moderate intake of alcohol, the former providing a rationale for the joggers of the world and the latter a "modus vivendi" for the sedentary writers of textbooks.

A useful classification of patients with hyperlipidemia is based on the type of lipoprotein involved (Table 10–1). One should note that the classification is a phenotypic rather than an etiologic one and that both acquired and genetic disorders are included. Familial hypercholesterolemia (type IIA) is the most outstanding cause of hypercholesterolemia.[13] This autosomal dominant disorder was described on page 105. Here it suffices to note that this condition, found in 0.1 to 0.5% of the population, is characterized by

a defect affecting the cell membrane receptors for LDL. Normally, receptor binding of LDL is necessary for its transfer into the cell, where it ultimately both suppresses cholesterol synthesis and the formation of LDL receptors. Homozygotes totally lack normal LDL receptors in the common variants of this condition and may develop fivefold elevations of the plasma cholesterol levels; many die of myocardial infarction before the age of 20 years.[14] Heterozygotes have approximately 50% of normal receptors, develop two- to threefold elevations of plasma cholesterol level, and have an increased risk of IHD in middle age. Many of the other forms of hyperlipidemia are also associated with hypercholesterolemia and premature coronary heart disease. Although useful from the viewpoint of classification, phenotyping of lipoprotein patterns is not cost effective for screening of lipoprotein disorders. Important and, in many cases, adequate information can be obtained from a careful personal and family history coupled with measurements of serum levels of total triglycerides and total cholesterol; the latter may be relatively easily fractionated into HDL- and non-HDL cholesterol.

***Hypertension.*** Every major epidemiologic study has documented that *elevation of blood pressure, both systolic and diastolic, imposes an increased risk of AS and IHD.*[1, 6] The risk steadily increases with the severity of the hypertension, and there is no specific level that demarcates "risk" from "no risk." In those under the age of 45 years, hypercholesterolemia appears to be the most important risk factor, whereas hypertension assumes this importance in persons over this age. In the Framingham study, men aged 45 to 62 years old with blood pressures exceeding 160/95 had five times the risk of coronary heart disease of those with blood pressures of 140/90 or less.

*Cigarette Smoking. There is a strong and consistent relationship between cigarette smoking and IHD.*[1, 6] The relationship is strongest in men aged 35 to 55 years old and shows some decrease with advancing years. In one large study, the smoking of one pack of cigarettes daily increased the risk of IHD threefold over the risk of those who never smoked. It should be noted that the risk decreases after cessation of smoking and approaches that of the "never smokers" after several years.

*Diabetes Mellitus.* This metabolic disorder predisposes to the early development of atherosclerosis and to its more rapid progression. It has greater effect in women than in men and increases the risk of an acute coronary event nearly threefold in the former but only about 50% in the latter.[1] In some part, at least, the effects of diabetes are mediated by the elevation of blood lipid levels, characteristic of this condition particularly during periods of poor diabetic control. Other possible mechanisms were discussed on page 92.

*Other Risk Factors.* These are sometimes referred to as "minor" or "soft" factors, since they are controversial and in any event are associated with a less pronounced effect on the risk of developing AS. Included are (1) a lack of regular physical exercise,

(2) a stressful, competitive lifestyle (Type A personality structure), (3) the use of oral contraceptives (p. 266), (4) hyperuricemia, (5) obesity, (6) a high carbohydrate intake, and (7) softness of the drinking water ("The harder the water, the softer the arteries"). The interested reader should consult other sources for more details.[1]

In concluding this analysis of the factors that identify the individual at risk of developing atherosclerosis and IHD, it is important to remember that *any one of the risk factors by itself is not necessary for the development of atherosclerosis; however, when two or more of the major risk factors are present, they multiply the risk, and when all four are present the probability of developing IHD is increased many fold.*[1, 6, 7] Indeed, current theories of causation draw upon the major risk factors. However, it should be pointed out that the established risk factors only partially account for the variation in AS in a population.[15, 16] In other words, we still have much to learn about factors that contribute to the development of AS. Before we can consider the pathogenesis of this condition, as currently understood, it is desirable to have an understanding of its morphology.

**MORPHOLOGY.** Characterization of the lesions of AS is difficult for two reasons: (1) there is still no agreement on the nature of the early lesions, and (2) the morphologic changes evolve over time as they progress from their inception to advanced stages of the disease. Nonetheless, it is widely accepted that the **atherosclerotic**

Table 10–1. THE HYPERLIPOPROTEINEMIAS*

| Type | Familiar Name | Prevalence | Lipoprotein Abnormality | Cholesterol Level | Triglyceride Level | Cause | Coronary Disease Risk |
|---|---|---|---|---|---|---|---|
| Normal | | | None: LDL > HDL > VLDL; chylomicra absent | < 200 to 220 mg per 100 ml | < 200 to 250 mg per 100 ml | Moderation in all things | |
| I | Exogenous or dietary hypertriglyceridemia | Rare | Chylomicra present | + or normal | + + + | Dietary fat not cleared from plasma | |
| IIA | Hypercholesterolemia (familial) | Moderately common | LDL raised | + + | Normal | Hereditary metabolic defect | + + + |
| IIB | Combined hyperlipidemia | Common | LDL and VLDL raised | + to + + | + to + + | Long-term dietary excess ? + hereditary element occasionally | + + + |
| III | Remnant hyperlipidemia | Rare | Broad beta (β-VLDL) present | + + | + + | Hereditary metabolic defect | + + + |
| IV | Endogenous hypertriglyceridemia | Common | VLDL raised | + | + + | Excessive intake of carbohydrates | + + |
| V | Mixed hypertriglyceridemia | Fairly common | Chylomicra present and VLDL raised | + | + + + | ?Metabolic defect | + |

*Modified from Havel, R. J., et al.: Lipoproteins and lipid transport. *In* Bondy, P. K., and Rosenberg, L. E. (eds.): Metabolic control and disease. 8th ed. Philadelphia, W. B. Saunders Co., 1980, pp. 393–494.

**plaque**, including its different morphological variants, is the lesion of established AS.[8] It is also recognized that other arterial lesions, of earlier age of onset than the plaques, may also contribute to atherogenesis.[17, 18] The best characterized and most easily recognized of these lesions is the **fatty streak**.

In the normal muscular artery, the intima is a narrow zone bounded on the luminal surface by a layer of continuous endothelial cells with interdigitated, closely bound cell junctions and on the opposite side by fenestrated internal elastic membrane. The aorta has no internal elastic membrane but has instead multiple layers of elastin fibers that alternate with layers of smooth muscle cells, creating so-called lamellar units. In this vessel the outer boundary of the intima is marked by the most internal elastic layer. In the child the intima is very thin and contains only a scant amount of various components between its inner and outer limits: extracellular connective tissue matrix, an occasional smooth muscle cell (myointimal cell), and infrequent blood-derived mononuclear cells. However, over the course of life, the intima thickens with the accumulation of extracellular matrix components and smooth muscle cells. This process is often exaggerated at points of hemodynamic turbulence, such as at arterial branchings and about the ostia of exiting vessels. Still unanswered is the question of whether this diffuse intimal thickening and accumulation of smooth muscle cells is a normal process of aging or a pathologic change. With these few details of normal vessel structure, we can turn to the fatty streak and then the atherosclerotic plaque.

**Fatty streaks are routinely encountered in infants (often in the first year of life) and young children**. They appear as slightly raised, yellow intimal streaks averaging 2 by 10 mm in size. They occur frequently in the region of the aortic valve ring; the thoracic aorta, particularly in the dorsal aspect of the descending thoracic aorta adjacent to the orifices of the intercostal arteries; and in the abdominal aorta. **At about 10 years of age, fatty streaks also appear in the coronary arteries, most abundantly in the proximal segment of the left coronary artery**. Histologically, all of these lesions contain lipid-laden cells, called "foam cells," which are derived from blood-borne monocytes and smooth muscle cells of the vessel wall (Fig. 10–2).

The role of the fatty streak as a precursor lesion of AS has been a subject of considerable discussion. The lesions differ from atherosclerotic plaques in that, typically, most of the lipid in fatty streaks is intracellular; fibrosis and necrosis are absent, and experimentally these lesions are readily and completely reversible.[8] Fatty streaks are encountered in populations throughout the world, including those that rarely develop progressive AS. On the other hand, the general distribution of fatty streaks and atherosclerotic plaques is similar, although the topographical relationship is not a perfect one.[19] Furthermore, lesions showing transitional features between fatty streaks and plaques have been identified.[8, 20] Thus, it is likely that some fatty streaks, perhaps by virtue of their location and exposure to "risk factors," are destined to develop into atheromatous plaques.

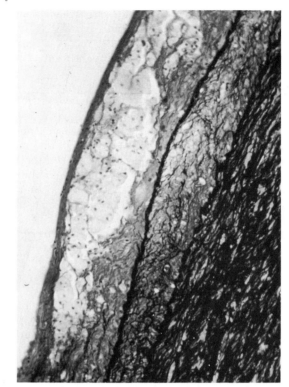

Figure 10–2. A fatty streak in the aorta, composed of intimal lipid-laden cells.

In addition to the fatty streak, two other "early" lesions have been described.[17] One is the gray, gelatinous lesion that appears to represent an area of increased endothelial permeability and intimal edema. Another is the microthrombus. Since these lesions are difficult to identify grossly, their frequency has not been well defined. However, the existence of these lesions has implications regarding the pathogenesis of AS, as discussed below.

The **atherosclerotic plaque** is the hallmark of AS. The plaques are fibrofatty intimal lesions that tend to be ovoid but can be quite irregular in shape. The size of most plaques is on the order of 1 to 3 cm in largest dimension. At autopsy, atherosclerotic plaques appear as elevated lesions in the collapsed arteries; however, under physiological conditions, uncomplicated plaques tend to lie flush with the uninvolved intimal surface owing to injury and loss of elasticity of the underlying media.[21] Even in distended vessels, larger plaques, particularly those with overlying mural thrombi, do project into and narrow the lumen. Some plaques are largely cellular and fibrous, whereas others are particularly rich in lipids. Their gross appearance, therefore, varies from white to yellow-white to yellow.

**There is a tendency for plaques to be located in certain vessels. In descending order of extent and severity of involvement, these are: lower abdominal aorta, coronary arteries, popliteal arteries, descending thoracic aorta, internal carotid arteries, and circle of Willis**.[19] Other medium-sized muscular arteries may also be affected, but the vessels of the upper extremities,

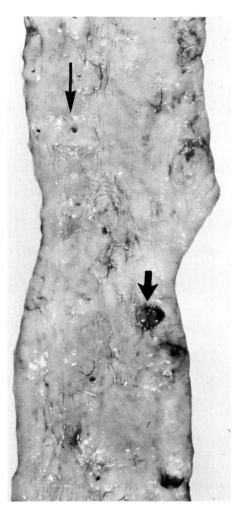

Figure 10–3. Atherosclerosis of the aorta. Virtually the entire intimal surface is involved. Note the well-developed atheroma enclosing the mouth of one of the intercostal arteries (*small arrow*) and the small mural thrombus (*large arrow*).

mesenteric arteries, and renal arteries are usually spared, except at their ostia. The aortic arch also tends to be spared, except when the patient has an underlying syphilitic aortitis. Early in life the plaques are irregularly distributed, with large intervening areas of uninvolved intima. At this stage, most plaques are localized adjacent to points of arterial branching and about the ostia of vessels arising from the aorta (Fig. 10–3). With time and progression, they become more numerous and may, in severe cases, become virtually coalescent in the abdominal aorta. Similarly, they become more numerous in the coronary arteries but are usually most abundant in the first 6 cm of the major left arteries and in the proximal and distal thirds of the right coronary artery. It is likely that hemodynamic factors and structural and, possibly, metabolic characteristics of the vessels play an important role in the propensity for plaque development in certain arteries and in certain regions of these arteries.[22]

Microscopically, **plaques have essentially three components**: (1) **cells, including vascular smooth muscle cells and blood-derived monocytes/macrophages**; (2) **connective tissue fibers and matrix**; and (3) **lipids**.[8] Depending upon the age of the plaques, these three components appear in varying proportions. In some lesions, a large number of smooth muscle cells are present, which together with collagen and elastin fibers create a fibrous plaque; such lesions contain relatively small amounts of lipid. In other lesions, the cellular and matrix elements create a luminal "fibrous cap" overlying a soft grumous center containing a variable mixture of proteoglycans, cellular debris, fibrin and other plasma proteins, and, most importantly, cholesterol (which may form needle-like crystals) and cholesteryl esters (Fig. 10–4). In the margins of this soft center are a few or many lipid-laden foam cells. The foam cells of plaques develop from macrophages that, in turn, are derived primarily from blood monocytes that have infiltrated the arterial wall and from vascular smooth muscle cells that have proliferated in the plaque.[23, 24] The connective tissue components (i.e., proteoglycans, collagen, and elastin) of the plaque are synthesized by the vascular smooth muscle cells. As the plaques enlarge, they cause atrophy and fibrosis of the underlying media, evoke a lymphocytic infiltrate in the contiguous adventitia, and develop vascularization about their margins.[25, 26] Vascularization of plaques results initially from ingrowth of vessels from the vasa vasorum. After mural thrombi form on plaques, the thrombi become organized and incorporated into the plaques; canalization

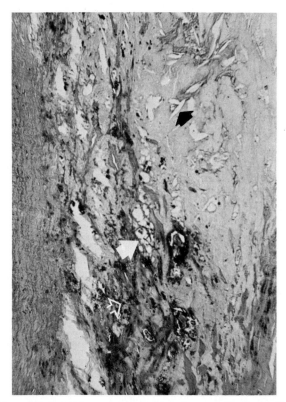

Figure 10–4. A high-power detail of an advanced atherosclerotic plaque. The media is to the left. The pale fibrous atheroma (*upper right*) contains cholesterol clefts (*black arrow*), a few remaining "foam" cells (*white arrow*), and granular black precipitates of calcium (*open arrow*).

of the organizing thrombi is an additional mechanism of vascularization of the plaques.

**The classic lesions described are preceded by earlier changes and are followed by a variety of modifications that significantly alter a lesion's appearance and clinical import**. The earliest change in the development of the atheromatous plaque is shrouded in the mysteries of the origin of AS.[8, 17, 18] However, most would agree that the earliest unmistakable lesion is a focal accumulation in the intima of smooth muscle cells and macrophages with intra- and extracellular lipid deposits. These lesions progress into typical atheromatous plaques, and, by 40 years of age, most individuals in vulnerable populations have multifocal AS of the major arteries. A number of pathways may then be followed. The relationship between lipid-rich and lipid-poor plaques is undoubtedly complex, but at least one method of alteration may be that progressive collagenization converts the fatty atheroma to a fibrous scar, which is seen as a gray-white elevated plaque. Alternatively, **the typical plaque may undergo one of four changes, giving rise to so-called complicated plaques**: (1) in advanced disease, plaques frequently undergo patchy or massive calcification, and arteries may be converted to virtual pipestems; (2) ulceration of the luminal surface and rupture of the plaque may discharge debris into the bloodstream (cholesterol emboli); (3) ulcerated lesions may develop superimposed thrombosis (Fig. 10–5); and (4) hemorrhage in a plaque may result from loss of endothelial integrity (early ulceration), leading to progressive influx of blood from the vessel lumen, or extravasation of blood from intraplaque capillaries that originate from the vascularization process described above. In early ulceration, the hemorrhage under arterial pressure may first expand the plaque and lead to its rupture (see page 318). Plaques may develop the four complications in any combination. It is evident that **ulceration, thrombosis, and major intraplaque hemorrhage have serious consequences in smaller vessels, such as those of the heart and brain, because they may cause total vascular occlusion**. In larger vessels (e.g., the aorta), such complications have little effect on the luminal diameter, but damage to the underlying media may yield an **atherosclerotic aneurysm** (p. 300).

**PATHOGENESIS.** For some time there have been two classic theories of the pathogenesis of AS.[8] The two are not mutually exclusive, but neither singly nor in combination do they encompass all of the relevant observations. The first has been called the "*lipid infiltration*" or "*insudation*" theory. The second theory can be referred to as the "*encrustation*" or "*thrombogenic*" theory. More recently the two theories have been molded together into what is called a "*response or reaction to injury*" hypothesis.[27] First the two classic theories will be briefly described, followed by the "response to injury" hypothesis.

The "*lipid infiltration*" or "*insudation*" theory holds that atherosclerotic plaques develop as a reaction of the vessel wall to increased filtration of plasma proteins and lipids from the blood. It is known that

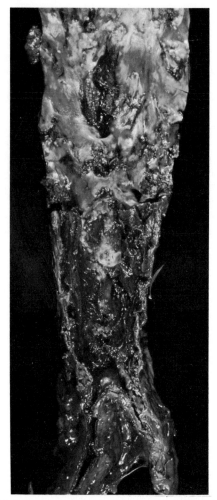

Figure 10–5. Advanced atherosclerosis of the abdominal aorta (iliac bifurcation is at bottom). Many of the ulcerated plaques are covered by mural thrombi.

there is a flux of plasma macromolecules, including plasma proteins and lipoproteins, into and out of the intima. Indeed, there is no blood supply to the intima, since the vasa vasorum or nutrient vessels penetrate from the adventitial surface but terminate within the outer media. Thus, the viability of the intima and internal layers of the media depends on this plasma flux. As originally proposed, this theory does not explain precisely the events responsible for progressive lipid accumulation and leaves unanswered the question of whether the lipid accumulation reflects an increased influx or a decreased egress (or catabolism) of lipoproteins. Potential mechanisms and consequences of altered lipoprotein flux in the arterial wall are discussed below.

The "*encrustation*" or "*thrombogenic*" theory views atherogenesis as the result of repeated episodes of mural thrombosis and organization leading to the progressive buildup of elevated plaques. The lipid content of the atheromas could be derived from the breakdown of platelets, leukocytes, and erythrocytes. However, despite meticulous study, it has not been possible to prove that initial lesions in atherogenesis routinely arise from thrombi. Clearly, thrombosis does occur as a complication of atherosclerotic plaques, and so organization of thrombi is most convincing as a mechanism of plaque progression rather than plaque initiation.

The *"response to injury" hypothesis* of AS is now widely held as most consonant with the large body of accumulated data. This theory states that (1) *atherosclerosis is initiated as a response to various forms of injury to arterial endothelium* and (2) *endothelial injury leads to*: (a) *attachment of monocytes and platelets to the intimal surface*; (b) *proliferation of smooth muscle cells in the arterial intima*; (c) *synthesis by these cells of large amounts of connective tissue matrix, including collagen, elastic fibers, glycosaminoglycans, and proteoglycans*; and (d) *deposition of intracellular and extracellular lipid that eventually results in the formation of a pool of lipid and cell debris in the core of advanced lesions.*[27-29] It should be stressed that endothelial injury can include subtle changes such as increased permeability and altered metabolism or surface properties, and that frank endothelial denudation is not a requirement.[30] Another important factor in lesion progression is the association with repetitive or chronic injury. This feature may be linked to evidence that areas of endothelial regeneration appear particularly prone to atheroma development.[31] There is good evidence that injured endothelium promotes the attachment of monocytes and platelets and secretes growth factors that stimulate the proliferation of smooth muscle cells.[23, 29, 32] Smooth muscle mitogens also are secreted by activated platelets and macrophages. An important class of mitogens from all three sources consists of substances that are chemically related to *platelet-derived growth factor (PDGF)*. Blood monocyte–derived macrophages also infiltrate the intima, where they accumulate lipid to contribute, along with smooth muscle cells, to the foam cell population. A scheme of atherogenesis incorporating these postulates is shown in Figure 10–6.

The mechanisms of lipid accumulation in developing lesions are undoubtedly complex. The normal endothelium permits only a "trickle" of macromolecules, which traverse endothelial cells in micropinocytotic vesicles.[30] Injury to endothelium damages the barrier and permits plasma proteins and lipoproteins to enter more readily. Other factors may include altered arterial wall metabolism of lipoproteins and altered efflux. Localized increases of glycosaminoglycans (the carbohydrate moiety of proteoglycans) or increased amounts of deposited fibrin, or both, might immobilize or bind LDL and increase its concentration within the intima.[18] Another issue is the mechanism for accumulation of lipid intracellularly in plaques. Normal LDL metabolism involves receptor-mediated transport and control of cellular cholesterol levels (Figs. 10–1 and 4–15). Perhaps local alterations of the smooth muscle cells and macrophages or of

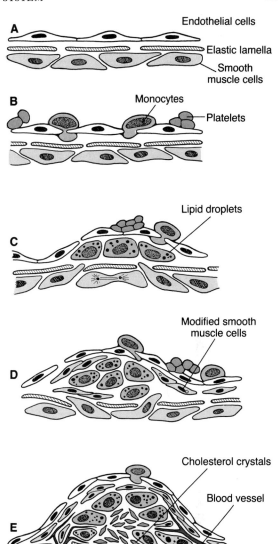

Figure 10–6. Postulated sequence of events in the pathogenesis of atherosclerosis. *A*, Normal vessel wall. *B*, Endothelial cell injury leading to attachment of monocytes and platelets. *C*, Monocytes infiltrate the intima and accumulate lipid. Smooth muscle cells proliferate in response to growth factors secreted by platelets, endothelium, and macrophages. *D*, Smooth muscle cells migrate into the subendothelial space and some of them accumulate lipid droplets. *E*, Foam cell population consisting of lipid-containing monocytes and smooth muscle cells continues to build up. Lipid released from degenerating foam cells accumulates extracellularly as cholesterol crystals.

the LDL molecule, or both, promote receptor-independent, large-scale absorptive endocytosis of the lipid, leading to the formation of foam cells.[20, 33] Regardless of the mechanism of intra- and extracellular lipid accumulation, *the major component of the lipid content of plaques is derived from plasma LDL.*

In a number of experimental settings, perturbation of the vessel wall, including endothelial injury, is followed by the development of intimal lesions.[27, 28] These experimental types of injuries have been mechanical (balloon denudation), hemodynamic (arteriovenous fistula), immunologic (immune complex deposition), physical (irradiation), infectious (viruses), and chemical (homocystine, constituents of cigarette smoke, and hyperlipidemia). In humans, similar phenomena, including the major risk factors (i.e., hypercholesterolemia, cigarette smoking, and hypertension), also have been postulated as initiators of vascular injury. *Hyperlipidemia may exert adverse effects on the vascular wall in a number of ways*: (1) induction of endothelial damage, (2) promotion of attachment and activation of platelets and monocytes, leading to their release of smooth muscle mitogens, (3) increasing the amount of lipid traversing the vessel wall, and (4) directly stimulating smooth muscle cell proliferation by components of hyperlipidemic blood.[27–29] *Hemodynamic factors* also are clearly important in the promotion and localization of atherosclerotic lesions. In arteries with pulsatile flow, there is an expansile stress directed primarily on the media, thereby contributing to medial weakening, and an oblique or shear stress directed primarily on the endothelium.[34] Increased turbulence of blood flow occurs adjacent to branch points in vessels. Some workers attribute the prevalence of plaques in these regions to increased endothelial injury secondary to increased shear stress.[34] Others contend that turbulent flow leads to stagnant pockets of blood in which blood elements collect and microthrombi form with atherogenic consequences.[35, 36] These issues require further clarification. *Remember, however, the salient points that hemodynamic stress contributes to atherogenesis and that this stress is increased by hypertension.*

Although endothelial injury as an initiating event in the response of the vessel wall to injury is an attractive postulate, *an alternative proposal is that smooth muscle proliferation is the primary event and that endothelial injury is a secondary or contributory phenomenon.*[16] Many of the experimental and clinical findings discussed above could be encompassed in this schema. The primacy of smooth muscle proliferation has been given impetus by the report that some plaques appear to be composed of progeny of a single parent cell—i.e., these plaques are monoclonal, as are many neoplasms (see p. 191).[16] This observation raises the possibility that mutagenic agents, such as viruses and carcinogens, could initiate cellular proliferation leading to plaque formation.[16, 37] However, an alternative explanation is that plaques are oligoclonal, composed of a few clones of smooth muscle cells that proliferate in response to a variety of stimuli, including age-related loss of inhibitory substances that participate in normal growth control.[38–40] It is reasonable to conclude that the evidence favoring primary smooth muscle proliferation in AS is currently less well developed than that for primary endothelial injury, although it is clear that both endothelial injury and smooth muscle proliferation are important factors in atherogenesis.

Finally, it is important to realize that the biology of the vessel wall is a dynamic process.[27] Single or short-lived injuries are followed by restoration of the endothelium and smooth muscle. However, repeated or chronic injury will finally result in the development of an atherosclerotic plaque. Even at this stage, the potential for regression exists, as discussed below. It is clear that we are far from having an adequate understanding of the complexities of AS. Increasingly, the conviction grows that atherosclerosis does not have a single cause. Perhaps many combinations of influences lead to a common endpoint, and regrettably most of the influences appear to be too prevalent in many societies.

**CLINICAL CORRELATION.** AS is an insidious disorder. Throughout much of its evolution *the arterial changes develop silently and cannot be detected by ordinary clinical examination. It makes its presence known by (1) predisposing to thrombosis, which may give rise to emboli; (2) causing ischemia of some vital organ, such as the heart, brain, intestines, or kidney, or by inducing gangrene of the lower leg; or (3) weakening an arterial wall, usually the aorta, resulting in an aneurysm.* The importance of these clinical effects was amply documented by some of the data cited earlier in this discussion and by data to be offered in the consideration of IHD (p. 316). Accordingly, there is intense interest in methods to reduce this toll. The therapeutic attack focuses on attempts to slow the progression of atherosclerotic plaques, methods to induce reversal or regression of atherosclerosis, and efforts to prevent the thrombotic complications. All regimens aimed at controlling or reversing atherosclerosis have as their point of departure the assumption that five factors capable of modification are of cardinal importance: diets high in cholesterol and saturated fat, hypercholesterolemia, hypertension, cigarette smoking, and diabetes. There is little dispute about the desirability of controlling hypertension and cigarette smoking. With regard to diabetes, the dominant view is that control of blood sugar retards the progression of atherosclerosis. When we come to the issue of control of the atherosclerosis by modification of the diet and blood lipid levels, opinions differ. Let us look at some of the evidence.

There is considerable experimental documentation in the rhesus monkey and in swine that when atherogenic diets are stopped and the serum cholesterol concentration returns to baseline levels, over the course of 12 to 40 months atherosclerotic lesions become smaller.[8, 41] In such experimental models it is possible to obtain reasonably controlled conditions and morphologic analyses. Numerous studies have been done on human patients, but the data are less reliable because the severity of atherosclerosis can only be measured by means of sequential arteriography.[41] Nonetheless, there are a number of reports suggesting retardation of progression or regression of AS with multiple risk-factor interventions, in particular diet or drugs or ileal bypass procedures to lower the serum cholesterol level. In human studies, it appeared that it was possible only to achieve some slowing of the progression of advanced atheromas in some patients, but not others, and regression was possible only in those patients judged to have "latent atherosclerosis" (i.e., early disease). However, in the recent Lipid Research Clinics Coronary Primary Prevention Trial, a reduction in mortality from cardiovascular disease was achieved with significant lowering of serum cholesterol in high-risk subjects.[9, 10] All of these studies were carried out on adults whose disease must be presumed to be long past the fatty streak stage. As you recall, AS begins early in life and might be considered a pediatric problem. Perhaps control efforts that begin with middle-aged adults, particularly those with clinical disease, amount to locking the barn after the horse has been stolen. Nonetheless, until we learn more about the cause of this insidious killer, efforts aimed at reducing risk factors would appear to be justified.

# VASCULITIS

Any artery or vein may become inflamed by spread of a contiguous inflammatory process, such as a bacterial infection. The resultant vascular lesion is usually localized, but it may provide a focus for dissemination of microbiologic agents via the blood. There are in addition a variety of diseases that are primary in vessels and are characterized by inflammatory and often necrotizing changes in the walls of the vessels themselves; these are referred to as *vasculitis syndromes*. Arteries, veins, or capillaries may be affected randomly in some syndromes, but in others there are particular patterns of involvement. The vasculitis may be the predominant or even the sole manifestation of the disease, as in polyarteritis nodosa (p. 166), or it may be only one component of the condition, as in systemic lupus erythematosus (p. 152). All of these vasculitic syndromes have the potential of inducing tissue ischemia.

The classifications of these vasculitic syndromes frequently engender a sense of hopelessness, not without considerable justification. They are ever changing, always complex, and sometimes contradictory. In some part this derives from the use of varying terminology for the same entity, but in larger part it stems from the tendency of these disorders to overlap and sometimes produce "hybrids" that are difficult to classify. Nonetheless, some order can be made out of the confusion, which now assumes great clinical importance since certain syndromes are potentially lethal but have shown dramatic response to appropriate therapy.

The present discussion will limit itself to the better defined, more common vasculitic syndromes. An overview of their major features is offered in Table 10–2. More comprehensive reviews are available.[42, 43] The syndromes will be divided into four categories:

1. *A polyarteritis nodosa group of systemic necrotizing vasculitides.* The hallmark of these disorders is a necrotizing vasculitis of small and medium-sized muscular arteries, which often leads to microaneurysm formation. Distinctive of this group of conditions is the fact that the vascular lesions are systemic in distribution and therefore involve multiple organ systems, with resulting random widespread ischemic changes.

2. *Hypersensitivity vasculitis.* This category includes a heterogeneous group of syndromes that have in common predominant involvement of small vessels, principally postcapillary venules. Although the skin is usually the dominant site of lesions, producing a palpable purpura, the vascular lesions in some instances are systemic in distribution.

3. *Granulomatous (giant cell) arteritides.* Two entities are included in this group, temporal arteritis and Takayasu's arteritis; both are marked by inflammatory changes in small to large arteries made distinctive by the presence of granulomatous inflammation with giant cells in many instances.

**Table 10–2.** VASCULITIS SYNDROMES

| Syndrome | Vessels Involved | Organ or Tissue Affected | Principal Morphologic Features |
|---|---|---|---|
| Polyarteritis nodosa | Medium and small arteries | GI tract, liver, kidney, pancreas, muscles, other sites. | Acute necrotizing arteritis, all layers with fibrinoid necrosis; neutrophil and eosinophil infiltrate throughout walls with periarterial involvement; later fibrosis |
| Hypersensitivity vasculitis | Arterioles, capillaries, venules | Widespread, but particularly skin, serosal membranes, glomeruli | Fibrinoid necrosis with neutrophil infiltrate |
| Temporal (cranial) arteritis | Large, medium, small arteries | Widespread, predilection for temporal (cranial) arteries | Neutrophil infiltrate with giant cells about fragmented elastica |
| Takayasu's arteritis | Large and medium arteries | Aorta, pulmonary, origins of aortic branches | Adventitial mononuclear infiltrate later involving media and intima |
| Thromboangiitis obliterans | Arteries, veins, and nerves | Upper and lower extremities | Inflammatory thrombosis with extension through vessel wall to involve veins and nerves |

4. *Specific disorders having well-characterized clinico-pathologic features, along with necrotizing vasculitis.* Included here are such entities as Wegener's granulomatosis, systemic lupus erythematosus, rheumatoid arthritis, and thromboangiitis obliterans (Buerger's disease).

There are many other clinical settings associated with vasculitis, such as lymphomas, Hodgkin's disease, multiple myeloma, and ulcerative colitis, in which the vascular lesions are too inconstant to merit further consideration here.

## POLYARTERITIS NODOSA GROUP OF SYSTEMIC NECROTIZING VASCULITIDES

*Polyarteritis nodosa* was already described in some detail on page 166. Here we wish only to relate it to the other vasculitic syndromes and in particular to three closely related entities that fall within this group: (1) allergic granulomatosis; (2) an entity that can only be called "overlap syndrome," which shares features of the others; and (3) infantile polyarteritis nodosa and closely related syndromes. You may recall that classic polyarteritis nodosa is marked by segmental necrotizing vasculitis of small and medium-sized muscular arteries throughout the body. The vascular lesions in the various vessels may be of different stages (i.e., some may be acute whereas others are fibrosing). The arterial supply to any organ or tissue can be affected but the lung is rarely involved, and the vascular lesions may lead to infarcts and also to nodular microaneurysms, which can often be palpated in subcutaneous vessels. Although an immunologic cause is suspected and supported by the finding of immunoglobulins and complement in the vascular lesions of some cases, these may not imply a causal mechanism but merely reflect leakage of plasma proteins. Many patients are hypertensive, and hemodynamic stress has been proposed as an additional potential cause of the vascular lesions. However, chronic hepatitis B antigenemia is a well-recognized precursor of classic polyarteritis nodosa, supporting the belief that at least some cases are caused by immunologic mechanisms.[44]

*Allergic granulomatosis of Churg and Strauss* is marked by vascular lesions that strongly resemble those of classic polyarteritis nodosa. Often there is also involvement of small vessels, such as capillaries and venules, which is not seen in classic polyarteritis nodosa. Lung involvement is always present in this condition; there is almost invariably a background of allergy (particularly severe asthma) as well as granulomatous lesions, sometimes in association with the vascular lesions. Typically these patients have marked peripheral eosinophilia, and eosinophils may also be found in the vascular and granulomatous lesions. There is, then, considerable evidence that allergic granulomatosis is a hypersensitivity disorder.

An additional syndrome within this group is the so-called *overlap syndrome.* As the name implies, it partakes of features of classic polyarteritis nodosa and of allergic granulomatosis. It is a multisystem disease with involvement of vessels ranging from medium-sized arteries to arterioles, capillaries, and venules. Lesions in larger vessels are identical to those of polyarteritis nodosa; those in small vessels are similar to those of allergic granulomatosis. Frequently there is an associated granulomatous reaction. However, an allergic history, peripheral eosinophilia, eosinophilic infiltrates in lesions, and lung involvement may or may not be present.

*Infantile polyarteritis nodosa* is a rare systemic disease of infants and young children that is characterized by vasculitis similar to that observed in adults with polyarteritis nodosa. A closely related entity is known as *mucocutaneous lymph node syndrome* or *Kawasaki's disease.*[45] This entity is characterized by a high incidence (up to 70%) of cardiac involvement, including necrotizing vasculitis of the coronary arteries, which predisposes to thrombosis and aneurysm formation. A viral origin is suspected. The prognosis appears to be better than for adult polyarteritis nodosa, since the majority of the patients recover spontaneously. However, severe coronary involvement can lead to a fatal outcome from coronary thrombosis, coronary rupture, or myocardial infarction.

## HYPERSENSITIVITY VASCULITIDES

Hypersensitivity vasculitis is found in a large and heterogeneous group of syndromes, which is made distinctive by the facts that (1) small vessels, principally postcapillary venules, are affected and (2) most of the vascular lesions occur in the skin and produce a prominent, palpable purpura. However, internal organs and tissues are occasionally affected. There are other distinctive features. In most cases, the vasculitis is mediated by immune complex deposition characteristic of a type III hypersensitivity reaction. Most often a drug such as sulfonamide or penicillin or a microorganism such as beta-hemolytic streptococcus is the causal antigen, although endogenous antigens are sometimes implicated. Hepatitis B antigenemia may also in some instances evoke this form of immune complex vasculitis. The vascular involvement is marked by an infiltration of neutrophils with nuclear debris (leukocytoclasis), fibrinoid necrosis, and extravasation of erythrocytes. Some authors refer to this pattern of vascular involvement as "*leukocytoclastic vasculitis.*"[46] In further contrast to polyarteritis nodosa, the vascular lesions are usually all of the same age, suggesting a brief rather than continuous exposure to immune complexes. This form of disease is usually self-limited, but it can be recurrent or become chronic.

A number of clinical syndromes fall into the category of hypersensitivity vasculitis, including serum sickness, Henoch-Schönlein purpura, and the vasculitis encountered with various forms of malignancy.

A few words about Henoch-Schönlein purpura are in order. In addition to the cutaneous vasculitis and resultant skin purpura, which are usually strangely confined to the lower half of the body, this condition also involves gastrointestinal bleeding, arthralgia, and, more importantly, renal disorders. The kidney changes may take the form of a focal or a diffuse, rapidly progressive glomerulonephritis of immunologic origin. Typically, the glomerular lesions reveal depositis of IgA by immunofluorescence (p. 471).

## GRANULOMATOUS (GIANT CELL) ARTERITIDES

This category includes two reasonably well defined entities: temporal arteritis and Takayasu's arteritis. Some cases lack clear-cut features of either of these two entities and so are merely called granulomatous arteritis.

### Temporal Arteritis (Cranial Arteritis)

Although temporal arteritis characteristically involves branches of the carotid artery, particularly the temporal artery, it is a systemic arteritis that may affect any medium-sized or large artery.[47, 48] The disease is rarely encountered in patients younger than 50 years of age and is more common in women.

**The condition is characterized by a panarteritis that may assume one of three patterns, probably depending on the duration of the involvement.** Classically, all three layers of the arterial wall are involved by granulomatous inflammation (epithelioid macrophages, lymphocytes, prominent multinucleated giant cells), although discrete nodular granulomas are rarely present (Fig. 10–7). In early cases, the media is involved most prominently. Necrosis of smooth muscle cells and destruction of the internal elastic membrane are common findings. Elastic fiber fragments may sometimes be found within the giant cells. Intimal involvement may lead to thrombosis of the vessel lumen. The second pattern can be categorized as a nonspecific inflammatory reaction traversing the entire arterial wall and marked by an infiltration of neutrophils, lymphocytes, and eosinophils. The third pattern is intimal fibrosis, without marked alteration of either the media or internal elastic membrane. The fibrosing reaction may fill the vascular lumen. As mentioned, these three histologic presentations may reflect the natural course of the disease. Initially the media may be affected, but with time the inflammation spreads throughout the arterial wall and the intense infiltrate of inflammatory cells may obscure the granulomatous process. With subsidence of the active process, only intimal fibrosis remains. Giant cells are not necessary for the diagnosis.

The arteritis classically involves long segments of affected vessels. However, on occasion there are "skip lesions," areas of normal vessel interposed between

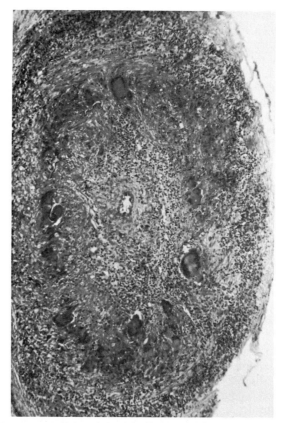

Figure 10–7. Temporal arteritis. The intense inflammatory reaction with numerous giant cells has virtually obliterated the architecture of the arterial wall and caused marked stenosis of the lumen.

segments of active arteritis. In some instances, the affected vessels develop nodular enlargements, which may be palpable in certain locations, such as the temple. Sometimes the overlying skin is red and edematous. Favored sites of involvement include the ophthalmic and posterior ciliary branches of the internal carotid as well as the superficial temporal, occipital, facial, and maxillary branches of the external carotid system. However, in addition, the disease may become systemic and show involvement of mesenteric, femoral, brachial, and axillary arteries; abdominal aorta; and aortic arch. The renal vasculature is rarely involved, serving as a differential feature from polyarteritis nodosa.

The etiology of this disorder is unknown. An autoimmune reaction to elastin fibers has been proposed and is supported by the demonstration in some cases of immunoglobulin deposits close to the disrupted internal elastic membrane. Another theory invokes ultraviolet light damage to elastin, which then induces an immunologic reaction. Both theories are speculative.

The clinical manifestations of temporal arteritis are extremely variable and depend on the site of arterial involvement. Often the disease is heralded by such nonspecific symptoms as weakness, malaise, low-grade fever, and weight loss, suggesting a flu-like syndrome. More specific findings are a headache, which may be nonspecific or quite distinctive, with radiation of the pain to the neck, face, jaws, or tongue. The scalp may become exquisitely sensitive to the slightest pressure. Intermittent claudication of the jaw is a highly characteristic feature. When cranial vessels are principally involved, especially the ophthalmic artery, blurred vision, diplopia, and sudden blindness may develop. Anemia and a high erythrocyte sedimentation rate are also frequently present.

Some patients develop a so-called *polymyalgia rheumatica syndrome* characterized by stiffness, aching, and pain in the muscles of the neck, shoulders, lower back, hip, and thighs.[49] There is still disagreement as to whether this syndrome is a part of temporal arteritis or is instead a separate entity that tends to occur in those with the vascular disease. In recognition of the close relationship between temporal arteritis and polymyalgia rheumatica, some experts refer to them both under the heading of *polymyalgia arteritica.*

Diagnosis may be made by biopsy, but since the process is patchy, a negative biopsy does not rule out temporal arteritis.

Although ischemia may produce disastrous effects, such as sudden blindness, myocardial ischemia, or neurologic derangements, temporal arteritis is, in general, a relatively benign disease that usually follows a chronic course, leading eventually to remission. When serious complications do occur, it is imperative to establish the diagnosis within hours, since prompt therapy typically produces a dramatic reversal of the process. In a small proportion of cases, the disease is fatal.

### Takayasu's Arteritis (Pulseless Disease)

In 1908 Takayasu described a clinical syndrome characterized principally by ocular disturbances and marked weakening of the pulse in the upper extremities. These clinical findings are common manifestations of a form of arteritis known as *Takayasu's arteritis or "pulseless disease".*[50–52] It principally affects young women (the sex ratio is 7 to 1). Most cases demonstrate an *aortic arch syndrome* due to involvement of the origins of the great vessels of the aortic arch. Clinically there is weakening of the pulse in the upper part of the body, often accompanied by hypertension in the lower extremities. Takayasu's arteritis is not the only cause of aortic arch syndrome; other origins include arteriosclerosis, syphilitic aortitis, dissecting aneurysm, connective tissue disorders (including SLE), and temporal arteritis. *Although classic Takayasu's arteritis involves only the aortic arch, in 32% of cases it also affects the remainder of the aorta and its branches, and in 12% it is limited to the descending thoracic and abdominal aorta.*

The etiology of Takayasu's arteritis is unknown. Associations with a positive tuberculin test and pulmonary tuberculosis were reported in patients in a large study in Mexico.[51] However, neither tubercle bacilli nor any other microorganisms have been found in the arterial lesions. Circulating antiartery antibodies have been demonstrated in some cases, but whether these represent cause or effect is unclear. Other findings suggest an immunologic etiology, including hyperglobulinema and occasional positive serological tests for rheumatoid and LE factors. Genetic factors are suggested by the increased incidence of some HLA types (e.g., HLA-B5) in affected individuals and by the occurrence of the disease in monozygotic twins.

The gross changes are usually limited to a marked irregular mural thickening of the aortic arch and the proximal segments of the great vessels, resulting in severe stenosis of the latter structures. In approximately 50% of cases, the pulmonary artery is also involved. Histologically the early changes consist of an adventitial mononuclear infiltrate surrounding the vasa vasorum. These alterations are similar to those of syphilitic aortitis. However, unlike the case with the luetic lesion, a diffuse polymorphonuclear infiltration and later a mononuclear infiltration soon appear in the media. The medial inflammation may exhibit a granulomatous character, including the presence of giant cells, and in these cases the lesion may closely resemble temporal arteritis. In the course of time, the intima becomes markedly sclerotic and thickened, as do the media and adventitia. The fibrosing reaction thickens the wall three- or fourfold and narrows the vascular lumen. Final occlusion of narrowed aortic branches is usually caused by a thrombus, which then undergoes organization. By this time, the inflammatory changes have largely disappeared and are replaced by fibrous scarring of the vessel wall.

About two thirds of patients with Takayasu's arteritis develop nonspecific symptoms, including malaise, low-grade fever, weight loss, and nausea, usually a few weeks before the onset of localizing symptoms. There may also be a variety of cardiopulmonary symptoms, including palpitations and dyspnea. With the narrowing of the mouths of the aortic branches or the development of vessel occlusion, ischemia of the upper body—particularly of the brain—follows and leads to dizziness, syncope, visual disturbances, and paresthesias. As with temporal arteritis, there is usually a very high erythrocyte sedimentation rate, which correlates well with activity of the disease. The diagnosis is confirmed by aortography. The clinical course is variable. Of 84 patients followed from 6 months to 40 years, the condition of 60 remained unchanged, 12 improved, six worsened, and six died from their disease.

## SPECIFIC DISORDERS ASSOCIATED WITH VASCULITIS

There are a number of diseases, most described elsewhere in this text, associated with vasculitis, such as systemic lupus erythematosus, rheumatoid arthritis, acute rheumatic fever, Wegener's granulomatosis, and thromboangiitis obliterans. The vascular lesions in the first three entities are essentially typical of hypersensitivity immune complex–mediated vasculitis, described on page 142. Those in Wegener's granulomatosis (p. 168) have resemblance to the lesions of allergic granulomatosis. Thromboangiitis obliterans has many distinctive features.

### Thromboangiitis Obliterans (Buerger's Disease)

This is a remitting, relapsing, inflammatory arterial disorder characterized by recurrent thrombosis of medium-sized vessels, principally the tibial and radial arteries.[53, 54] *Although it is primarily an arterial disease, adjacent veins and nerves are also involved.* The lesion occurs almost always in cigarette smokers, usually young men between the ages of 25 and 50 years. Only extremely rarely has it been reported in nonsmokers or in women.

There has been controversy in the past as to whether thromboangiitis obliterans is a separate disease. However, many aspects of the disorder—including its predilection for young men, its regular association with smoking, the frequent involvement of small and medium-sized vessels in the arms as well as legs, the absence of generalized atherosclerosis in most cases, and the histologic changes—contrast sharply with the usual features of atheromatous peripheral vascular disease and suggest that thromboangiitis obliterans is a distinct entity.

Strong circumstantial evidence indicates that cigarette smoking has an important role in the pathogenesis of Buerger's disease.[55] Genetic factors are suggested by population differences, since the disease is rare in the U.S. and Europe but more common in Israel, Japan, and India, and by the increased prevalence of HLA-A9 and HLA-B5 in patients with Buerger's disease.[56] Vascular injury in susceptible individuals may involve several potential mechanisms, including direct toxic effects on vessels caused by some tobacco products such as carbon monoxide, enhanced vasoconstriction produced directly and via altered catecholamine levels, impaired oxygen dissociation from hemoglobin (carbon monoxide effect), a hypercoagulable state, and cell-mediated immune hypersensitivity to vascular collagen.[55, 57]

**Almost invariably, thromboangiitis begins in arteries and secondarily extends to affect contiguous veins and nerves.** The affected segment of vessel is firm and indurated. At the site of the lesion, there is a thrombus showing varying stages of organization and recanalization. With light microscopy, the thrombus itself is seen to contain small microabscesses that have a central focus of neutrophils and often a surrounding zone of granulomatous inflammation. The enclosing vessel wall shows a nonspecific inflammatory infiltrate and remarkable preservation of the underlying architecture. With pro-gression, the inflammatory response extends to the tunica adventitia and, in due course, fibrosis and periarterial scarring envelop the adjacent vessels and nerves. **This fibrous encasement of all three structures—artery, vein, and nerve—is an important distinguishing characteristic of thromboangiitis obliterans.**

Often full-blown thromboangiitis obliterans is preceded by recurrent episodes of patchy thrombophlebitis of superficial veins. Eventually, with involvement of the tibial or, less frequently, the radial artery, the characteristic manifestations of ischemia ensue. Typically, in the affected limb there is pain that is precipitated by exercise and eventually even occurs at rest. When first seen by a physician, many of these patients have chronic ulcerations of their toes or feet, and often the disease progresses to gangrene of the lower leg, necessitating amputation. As the underlying thrombus becomes recanalized, total occlusion gives way to partial resumption of blood flow, and the findings abate somewhat, only to recur when a new lesion develops. Cessation of cigarette smoking often brings dramatic relief from further attacks.

## RAYNAUD'S DISEASE

Unlike the vasculitic syndromes, which have well-defined organic lesions, *Raynaud's disease* (as opposed to Raynaud's phenomenon) refers to paroxysmal pallor or cyanosis of acral parts (usually the digits of the hands, sometimes those of the feet, and infrequently the tip of the nose or the ears) caused by intense spasm of local small arteries and arterioles. It is an idiopathic disease, principally of otherwise healthy young women. In contrast, *Raynaud's phenomenon* refers to arterial insufficiency of the acral parts secondary to another disorder—for example, SLE or systemic sclerosis. Although the etiology of Raynaud's disease is unknown, it would appear to be based on an exaggeration of normal central and local vasomotor responses to cold or to emotion. Anatomically, the involved vessels are normal until late in the course, when prolonged vasospasm may cause secondary intimal thickening.

In the classic case, the paroxysms are first noticed in cold weather and may initially be infrequent. The fingers of both hands become virtually white as the arteries constrict, then cyanotic as the blood stagnates in the capillaries distal to the constriction, later hyperemic as normal blood flow resumes when the hands are again warmed. These changes are most pronounced toward the tips of the fingers. The course of Raynaud's disease is variable. Often it remains static for years and constitutes no more than a nuisance for the patient, who must avoid situations likely to precipitate an attack. In some cases, the disorder subsides spontaneously. Occasionally patients develop a progressive disease, having some degree of cyanosis at all times. Eventually trophic changes and ulcerations appear in the skin, and even areas of gangrene may occur at the fingertips.[58]

## ANEURYSMS

Abnormal dilatations of arteries or veins are called aneurysms. They are described here because they are much more frequent and important in arteries, especially in the aorta.[59] They develop wherever there is marked weakening of the wall of a vessel. Any vessel may be affected by a wide variety of disorders, including congenital defects, local infections (mycotic aneurysms), trauma (traumatic aneurysms or arteriovenous aneurysms), or systemic diseases that weaken arterial walls. The principal causes of aortic aneurysms are atherosclerosis, syphilis, and medionecrosis leading to dissecting and nondissecting aneurysms. Congenital defects of the intracranial arteries, termed *berry aneurysms*, are also fairly frequent; they represent an important cause of cerebrovascular accidents (CVA) and, as such, are discussed on page 737.

Some descriptive terms applicable to aneurysms require explanation. *Aneurysms may be characterized grossly as saccular, fusiform, cylindroid, or berry-shaped.* A *saccular lesion* implies a balloon-like dilatation, up to 15 or 20 cm in diameter, that involves a portion of the vessel circumference. The orifice may be small, but often it has the same diameter as the aneurysm itself. Because the blood within such outpouchings is relatively stagnant, saccular aneurysms are usually partially or completely filled with thrombus, which is often laminated. As the thrombus forms and contracts, it may pull away from the aneurysmal wall and fresh blood may seep into this space. Thus, paradoxically, the freshest portion of the thrombus may be adjacent to the vessel wall. This seemingly trivial detail implies that the dilated aneurysmal sac continues to be exposed to the hydrodynamic stress of the blood pressure, making possible continued expansion of the vascular dilatation.

*Fusiform aneurysms* are spindle-shaped dilatations, generally involving the entire circumference of the vessel, that gradually expand and then taper to the diameter of the unaffected vessel. The dilatation is not always completely symmetrical; one aspect may be more affected than another. Mural thrombi may or may not be present.

*Cylindroid lesions* arise abruptly as long, cylinder-like dilatations that subside abruptly. Here again, asymmetry and mural thromboses may be present.

*Berry aneurysms* are readily characterized as small, saccular lesions 0.5 to 2 cm in size and most often encountered in the smaller arteries of the brain, especially the circle of Willis.

With these descriptive terms we can now deal with the three major etiologic forms of aortic aneurysms.

## ATHEROSCLEROTIC ANEURYSM

As the incidence of tertiary cardiovascular syphilis has declined, atherosclerosis has become the most common cause of aortic aneurysms.[59] They are most frequent in males (5:1 ratio) after the fifth decade of life. Although any site in the aorta may be affected, including the thoracic aorta, the great preponderance of these lesions occur in the abdominal aorta, usually below the renal arteries. *Until proved otherwise, an abdominal aneurysm is assumed to be atherosclerotic in origin.* Occasionally, several separate dilatations occur, and not infrequently abdominal aortic lesions are accompanied by additional aneurysms in the iliac arteries.

Atherosclerotic aneurysms take the form of saccular (balloon-like), cylindroid, or fusiform swellings, sometimes up to 15 cm in greatest diameter and of variable length (up to 25 cm) (Fig. 10–8). As would be expected, at these sites there is severe complicated atherosclerosis, which destroys the underlying tunica media and thus produces the weakening of the aortic wall. Mural thrombus frequently is found within the aneurysmal sac. In the saccular forms, the thrombus may completely fill the outpouching up to the level of the surrounding aortic wall. The elon-

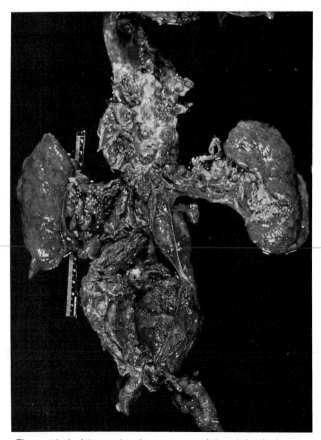

Figure 10–8. Atherosclerotic aneurysm of the abdominal aorta, situated below the renal arteries and above the iliac bifurcation. The atherosclerosis throughout the aorta is far advanced. Some mural thrombus layers the back wall of the aneurysm.

gated fusiform or cylindroid patterns more often have layers of mural thrombus that only partially fill the dilatation.

The clinical consequences of these aneurysms depend principally on their location and size. Occlusion of the iliac, renal, or mesenteric arteries may result either from pressure of the aneurysmal sac or from propagation of the thrombus. The thrombus may embolize. As enlarging pulsatile masses, these aneurysms not only simulate tumors but also progressively erode adjacent structures such as the vertebral bodies. They have been known to erode the wall of the gut or, when they occur in the thorax, the wall of the trachea or esophagus. Rupture is the most feared consequence and is related to the size of the dilatation. In general, when they are less than 6 cm in diameter, these aneurysms rarely rupture, whereas 80% of patients with larger lesions die of rupture within 10 years of their diagnosis. Fortunately, since most such aneurysms occur below the level of the renal arteries, many can be replaced with prosthetic arterial channels with excellent results. The operative mortality before rupture is about 5%; after rupture it rises sharply to 50%.

## SYPHILITIC (LUETIC) AORTITIS AND ANEURYSM

As will be pointed out in the general discussion of syphilis in Chapter 18, the tertiary stage of the disease shows a predilection for the cardiovascular and nervous systems. Fortunately, with better control and treatment of syphilis in its early stages, these involvements are becoming rare. Before discussing the cardiovascular lesion, which is termed *syphilitic (luetic) aortitis*, reference should be made to Chapter 18 for the basic tissue reactions incited by *Treponema pallidum* (i.e., *obliterative endarteritis, perivascular cuffing*, and *gumma formation*).

Although obliterative endarteritis in tertiary syphilis may involve small vessels in any part of the body, it is clinically most devastating when it affects the vasa vasorum of the aorta. Such involvement gives rise to thoracic aortitis, which in turn leads to the aneurysmal dilatation of the aorta and aortic valve ring characteristic of full-blown cardiovascular syphilis. Propensity for involvement of the proximal thoracic aorta may be related to the greater density of vasa vasorum in this region.[22] Since this sequel to infection by *T. pallidum* does not manifest itself until 15 to 20 years later, it is seen most frequently in the age range of 40 to 55 years. Males are involved three times as often as females.

Syphilitic aortitis is almost always confined to the thoracic aorta, usually to the ascending and transverse portions, and rarely extends below the diaphragm.[59] The earliest changes are obliterative endarteritis with perivascular cuffing of the vasa vasorum by plasma cells. The narrowing of these nutrient arteries leads to ischemic destruction of the elastic tissue and muscle of the media and to subsequent development of stellate-shaped fibrous scars in the media and fibrous thickening of the adventitia. With contraction of the irregular medial scars, longitudinal wrinkling or "tree-barking" of the intimal surface ensues. More importantly, the scarring may envelop and narrow the ostia of vessels arising from the aorta, including those of the coronary arteries.

With destruction of the tunica media, the aorta loses its elastic support and tends to become dilated, producing a syphilitic aneurysm (Fig. 10–9). Secondary atherosclerotic involvement of these damaged areas is almost invariable and may contribute to the weakening of the aortic wall. The end result is diffuse involvement by calcified atherosclerotic plaque, which obliterates the intimal "tree-bark" pattern. **Even when these aneurysms are complicated by atherosclerosis, their location in the thorax tends to distinguish them from typical atherosclerotic aneurysms, which rarely affect the aortic arch and never involve the root of the aorta.** Calcification of the ascending aorta on chest x-ray is diagnostic of leutic aortitis. Syphilitic aneurysms are

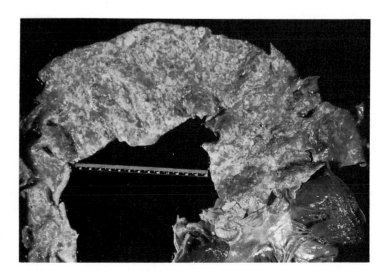

Figure 10–9. Syphilitic aortitis, with superimposed florid atherosclerosis. The heart is seen in the lower right. The lesions begin at the aortic valve and are most marked in the thoracic region, where there is some aneurysmal widening of the aorta.

sometimes enormous, achieving a diameter of 15 to 20 cm. They may contain mural thrombus. When the aneurysmal dilatation includes the aortic valve ring, the valvular commissures are widened and the valve leaflets are stretched, so that their free margins tend to roll and become thickened. Incompetence of the valve results. The increased work of the left ventricle leads to marked, sometimes extraordinary, hypertrophy and dilatation of this chamber, with resultant heart weights of up to 1000 gm. Such hearts are known as "**cor bovinum**."

Syphilitic aortitis with aneurysmal dilatation may give rise to (1) respiratory difficulties as a result of encroachment on the lungs and airways; (2) difficulty in swallowing, owing to compression of the esophagus; (3) persistent brassy cough, from pressure on the recurrent laryngeal nerve; (4) pain, caused by erosion of bone (ribs and vertebral bodies); and (5) cardiac disease. As the aneurysm leads to dilatation of the aortic root, signs of aortic valvular insufficiency develop; these typically include a loud, diastolic murmur and widening of the pulse pressure to produce a bounding pulse (Corrigan's pulse). Most patients with syphilitic aneurysms die of heart failure due to aortic valvular incompetence. Myocardial ischemia (or infarction) from coronary ostial stenosis may contribute to cardiac dysfunction. Other causes of death include rupture of the aneurysm (with fatal hemorrhage) and erosion of vital contiguous structures, such as the bronchi or esophagus, by the expanding pulsatile mass.

## IDIOPATHIC CYSTIC MEDIAL NECROSIS (MEDIONECROSIS) AND RELATED DISSECTING AND NONDISSECTING ANEURYSMS

*Cystic medial necrosis (medionecrosis)* is characterized by multifocal loss of the elastic and muscular tissue of the media of the aortic wall, particularly in the thoracic aorta.[59, 60] Infrequently, other major arteries, including the coronary arteries, are involved. Since acute necrosis and inflammation are not typically observed, the entity is best regarded as a chronic degenerative process. However, the terms cystic medial necrosis and medionecrosis are entrenched in the medical literature. The frequency and severity of medionecrosis increase with age, and medionecrosis of mild degree commonly occurs as an incidental lesion in the absence of clinical disease. *When more severe and extensive, medionecrosis weakens the aortic wall and leads to aneurysm formation. As discussed below, these aneurysms may be dissecting or nondissecting. They typically involve the thoracic aorta and may be associated with aortic valvular incompetence.* In fact, cystic medial necrosis is currently the leading cause of thoracic aortic aneurysms. It should be recalled, however, that the most common type of aneurysm is the atherosclerotic abdominal aortic aneurysm.

Current evidence suggests that medionecrosis results from a metabolic defect in the synthesis of the connective tissue fibers (collagen and elastin) in the tunica media.[61, 62] Another theory (namely, disease of the vasa vasorum) has gained little supportive evidence. Medionecrosis occurs most commonly as a seemingly isolated lesion of variable severity in middle-aged patients, many of whom are hypertensive. In addition, medionecrosis of severe degree is a common manifestation of Marfan's syndrome and related hereditary diseases of connective tissue. It also may develop in the late stages of pregnancy, and it commonly occurs in the proximal aortic segment in patients with coarctation of the aorta. The groups with severe cystic medial necrosis have an increased incidence of thoracic aneurysms. The association with Marfan's syndrome has led to the thesis that medionecrosis represents a congenital defect in connective tissue metabolism. Indeed, it has been suggested that isolated medionecrosis is simply a forme fruste or milder expression of Marfan's syndrome.

On the other hand, some experimental data indicate that medionecrosis can be an acquired metabolic abnormality. Although it is known that turkeys may develop medionecrosis spontaneously, these fowl show an increased frequency of the lesion when treated with estrogens. The increased incidence of dissecting aneurysm in women during pregnancy has been attributed to a "loosening" effect of estrogens on connective tissue. Lesions similar to those of medionecrosis can be produced experimentally by induction of copper deficiency or by administration of beta-aminopropionitrile (*lathyrism*). The lathyrogenic agents block the cross-linkages in collagen and elastin fibers and thus impair their tensile strength. Copper deficiency may affect copper-dependent enzymes in the aortic media. Conceivably, some metabolic error in the formation or maintenance of the connective tissue fibers leads to similar defects in the human disease. Hemodynamic trauma, which is accelerated by hypertension, contributes to the progression and, possibly, the development of cystic medial necrosis in predisposed individuals. The propensity of aneurysms to develop in the thoracic aorta in subjects with cystic medial necrosis is related to a hemodynamic mechanism, namely, the fact that the thoracic aorta is exposed to the maximal energy of the cardiac-generated pulse wave.[63] In summary, the multitude and diversity of etiologic theories emphasize the idiopathic nature of cystic medial necrosis.

The lesion is characterized microscopically by poorly delineated focal defects within the tunica media that are filled with basophilic, metachromatic glycosaminoglycans (ground substance) and are devoid of elastic fibers and smooth muscle cells. The lesions are most pronounced in the outer half of the tunica media, and they focally replace the normal laminar pattern of elastic fibers. Although the lesions are called cystic, the defects are not demarcated by well-defined margins. Typically, there is no inflammatory response to the destructive process. In-

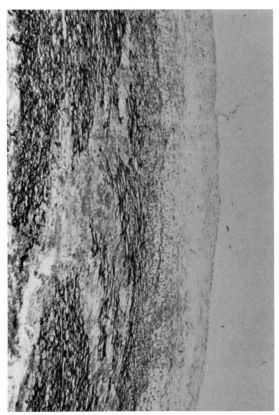

Figure 10–10. Cystic medionecrosis of the aorta. The intima is to the right. An elastic tissue stain accentuates the elastica of the media. The irregular cleft-like areas devoid of elastica represent the foci of medionecrosis. Note the absence of inflammatory reaction.

deed, it can be said in general that these lesions are subtle and rather easily overlooked, unless elastic tissue stains are employed (Fig. 10–10). These preparations generally reveal patchy degeneration of elastic tissue that is more extensive than the more obvious cystic lesions. The amount of atherosclerosis in aortas with cystic medial necrosis is highly variable, and severe cystic medial necrosis can occur in the virtual absence of atherosclerosis. Clearly, cystic medial necrosis is a primary medial disease that develops independently of atherosclerosis. The aorta with cystic medial necrosis may appear grossly normal in mildly affected cases, there may be simple aneurysmal dilatation of the weakened wall, or a dissection may be present.

*Dissecting aneurysm* or *hematoma* is a relatively frequent and major complication of medial degenerative disease.[64–66] This condition is characterized by the longitudinal dissection of blood along a laminar plane within the outer media of the artery until at some point rupture occurs, either internally into the vessel lumen, or, more commonly, externally. In the typical case, there is an intimal tear in the thoracic aorta, which serves as the entry site of the blood. Dissection in an aorta with marked aneurysmal dilatation is the exception rather than the rule, although frequently some widening of the aorta may be detected on chest x-ray. For this reason, the terms

"aortic dissection" or "dissecting hematoma" as well as "dissecting aneurysm" are commonly used.

Dissecting aneurysm occurs most commonly in the 40- to 60-year age group, and it is seen in males two to three times more frequently than in females. However, in younger individuals there is no sex preponderance, owing to the predisposing influences of pregnancy and heritable diseases of connective tissue. An important relationship exists between medial degeneration and hemodynamic forces in the pathogenesis of dissecting aneurysm. In certain predisposed patients with severe cystic medial necrosis, such as those with Marfan's syndrome, dissecting aneurysm typically develops in the presence of normal blood pressure. However, in the absence of hereditary predisposition, a very high percentage of patients with dissecting aneurysm exhibit evidence of significant hypertension.[66] In hypertensives with dissection, medionecrosis may be mild, whereas in normotensives with dissection, medionecrosis is typically severe. Nevertheless, hypertension is a common disease, and only a minority of hypertensive patients develop dissection. These observations suggest that hemodynamic trauma contributes to the development of dissection in individuals predisposed to the event because of significant medial degeneration.

The event responsible for the initiation of dissection has also been a subject of controversy. The most likely mechanism is a sudden tearing of the tunica intima of the weakened arterial wall, which permits blood to enter the tunica media from the lumen and dissect along a laminar plane in the outer media (where degenerative changes are typically most severe). An intimal tear may also lead to a localized transmural perforation rather than dissection. Another theory is that dissection originates from rupture of the vasa vasorum in the diseased area of the media. The former theory is favored since a proximal intimal tear can be identified in virtually all cases in which the vessels are preserved in a state adequate for careful study.

When dissections occur, they usually begin in the ascending portion and extend toward the heart as well as distally along the length of the aorta (Fig. 10–11). Sometimes the proximal dissection extends into and about the coronary arteries. Distortion of the aortic root may cause aortic valvular incompetence. Although the length of the dissection is quite variable, not infrequently the entire aorta is traversed and there is progression into the iliac and femoral arteries. The renal arteries may similarly be involved, sometimes with total compression of their lumina. The intramural hemorrhage usually involves most but not all of the circumference of the vessel. Characteristically, the plane of dissection cleaves the outer third of the tunica media from the inner two thirds. The amount of contained hemorrhage is variable but may be quite massive. In virtually all cases there is a transversely oriented intimal tear through which the hemorrhage penetrates the intima and enters the media. In 90%

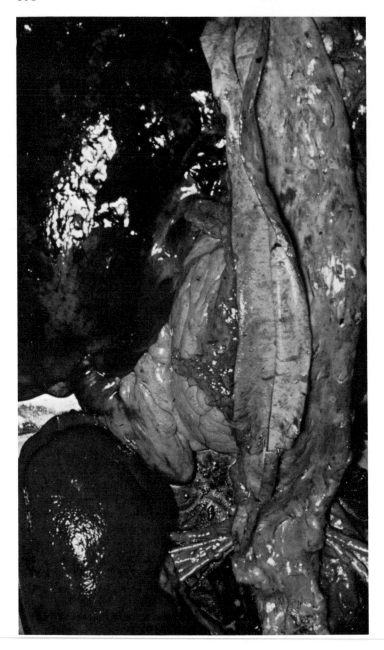

**Figure 10–11.** Dissecting aneurysm of the aorta extending to the level of the renal artery. The cleaved aorta has been folded back on the left, and the contained hemorrhage has been removed.

of cases, the intimal tear is found in the ascending aorta, 5 to 10 cm from the aortic valve. There may also be a distal intimal tear, but this is less frequent. This may result, in blood entering a proximal tear and exiting through the distal tear to create two functioning lumens **(double-barreled aorta).** In these cases, the surface of the false lumen develops a neointima composed of fibrous tissue lined by endothelium. Most patients are not so fortunate, since there is a high incidence of external hemorrhage into the periadventitial tissues or serosal cavities, usually the pericardium. The latter event can occur because the first few centimeters of the great vessels are enclosed within the pericardial sac.

With dissection, there is characteristically sudden onset of excruciating pain, usually beginning in the anterior chest and, in classic cases, radiating to the back and moving downward as the dissection progresses. The intensity of this pain often leads to the misdiagnosis of acute myocardial infarction or of perforated peptic ulcer. The pain is often episodic and recurrent as bouts of advancing dissection occur. A murmur of aortic valvular regurgitation may be present owing to extension of the dissection into the aortic root. As the origins of the aortic branches become involved in the process, a multitude of seemingly bizarre findings evolve. Compression of the small vertebral branches may cause striking sensory and motor changes in the lower half of the body. Involvement of the renal arteries may cause hematuria, flank pain, and oliguria, and sometimes dissection into the walls of the renal artery compresses its

**Figure 10–12.** DeBakey classification of dissections into Types I, II, and III, respectively, from left to right. In the newer classfication, Types I and II are combined into Type A (involving ascending aorta) and Type III is designated Type B, *not* involving ascending aorta. (From Anagnostopoulos, C. E.: Acute Aortic Dissection. Baltimore, University Park Press, 1975.)

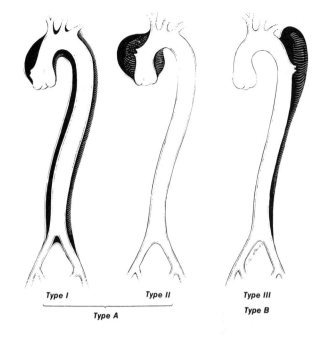

Type I | Type II | Type III

Type A | Type B

lumen and renal infarction results. Rarely, a myocardial infarction results from dissection into and about a coronary artery. Unequal compression of major arteries leading to the limbs may produce sudden changes or inequalities in blood pressures. Radiography may disclose a widened ascending aorta and sometimes a double aortic shadow. Retrograde aortography with contrast medium confirms the diagnosis by revealing changes such as an intimal flap, an abnormally thick aortic wall, or a double-barreled vessel. Diagnostic evidence now can also be obtained by noninvasive techniques such as computerized tomography and magnetic resonance imaging. Rarely, evidence of chronic dissection may be detected in a minimally symptomatic patient.

Dissections have been subclassified clinically into three patterns, now simplified into two (Fig. 10–12).[59, 65] Type A begins in the ascending aorta; Type B spares the ascending aorta but begins distal to the subclavian artery and extends distally into the descending aorta (Fig. 10–12). Without vigorous intervention, a dissecting aneurysm is almost invariably fatal, due to external rupture into the pericardial pleural or pericardial cavities. In the absence of surgical intervention, the mortality rate is higher for Type A than for Type B dissections; Type A is also more common than Type B. Immediate surgical intervention and intensive antihypertensive therapy are used for Type A, but with Type B reliance is more often placed on antihypertensive therapy alone. With this approach, 65 to 75% of all patients with dissections now leave the hospital alive, a remarkable record compared with that of only a relatively few years ago. It has been estimated that about 5% of patients with dissecting aneurysms have the good fortune to develop a second complete channel and thus escape sudden death.

*Of the nondissecting aneurysms associated with cystic medial necrosis, the most distinctive entity is annuloaortic ectasia.* This lesion is caused by severe but localized medionecrosis and is characterized by fusiform aneurysmal dilatation that starts at the aortic valve ring (annulus) and extends upward to involve the ascending aorta.[67] Annuloaortic ectasia creates an hourglass or figure-eight configuration of the heart and ascending aorta that may be recognized on chest x-ray. Such aneurysms frequently produce dilatation of the aortic root and chronic, progressive aortic valvular incompetence. These aneurysms may develop localized dissections or sometimes transmural tears with external rupture.

## ARTERIOVENOUS FISTULA (ANEURYSM)

Abnormal communications between arteries and accompanying veins may arise as developmental defects, from rupture of an arterial aneurysm into the adjacent vein, from penetrating injuries that pierce the walls of both artery and vein and permit an artificial communication, and from inflammatory necrosis of adjacent vessels. The connection between the vessels may be formed by the canalization of a thrombus, or it may be constructed of an aneurysmal sac. When a fistula takes the form of a tangled mass of intercommunicating vessels, it is designated a *cirsoid aneurysm.* The clinical significance of all these fistulae lies not only in their vulnerability to hemorrhage but also in the added burden they may place on the heart by short-circuiting blood from the arterial to the venous system. This last-mentioned consequence may also occur with those arteriovenous communications that are present in the lungs.

# Venous Disorders

Although none of the disorders of veins have the impressive frequency of atherosclerosis, several, such as varicose veins and phlebothrombosis, are extremely common. Varicose veins induce a great deal of discomfort and morbidity but are rarely life-threatening. On the other hand, phlebothrombosis, although somewhat less prevalent, may have lethal consequences. Discussions of these two venous disorders, as well as of the relatively rare involvements of the superior and inferior vena cava, follow.

## VARICOSE VEINS

Varicose veins are abnormally dilated, tortuous veins; this condition is caused by increased intraluminal pressure and, to a lesser extent, by loss of support of the vessel wall. *Although any vein in the body may be affected, the superficial veins of the leg are by far the most frequently involved.* This predilection is due to the high venous pressure in the legs when they are dependent, coupled with the relatively poor tissue support for the superficial, as opposed to the deep, veins. Even in otherwise normal individuals, these factors produce a tendency toward the development of varices with advancing age and its attendant loss of tissue tone, atrophy of muscles, and degenerative changes within the vessel walls followed by sufficient dilatation of veins to render their valves incompetent. Indeed, this disorder is seen in approximately 50% of individuals over the age of 50 years. There exists a familial tendency toward the development of varicose veins relatively early in life. Because of the venous stasis in the lower legs caused by pregnancy, females develop varicose veins more often than do males.

In addition to the usual burdens on the veins of the legs, any condition that compresses or obstructs veins, causing local increases in intraluminal pressure, clearly increases the risk of varix formation distal to the obstruction. Hence, intravascular thrombosis, tumors that impinge on veins, and the wearing of tightly encircling garments or surgical dressings all promote the development of varicosities, in the legs or elsewhere.

Attention should be called to two special sites of varix formation. *Hemorrhoids* result from varicose dilatation of the hemorrhoidal plexus of veins at the anorectal junction. The causative mechanism is presumed to be prolonged pelvic congestion resulting, for example, from repeated pregnancies or chronic constipation and straining at stools. An important cause of hemorrhoids is portal hypertension due usually to cirrhosis of the liver (p. 584).

*The second and more important special site of varicosities is the esophagus,* and this form is encountered virtually only in patients with cirrhosis of the liver and its attendant portal hypertension. Rupture of an esophageal varix may be more serious than the primary liver disease itself (p. 584).

**MORPHOLOGY.** The affected veins are dilated, tortuous and elongated. Characteristically, the dilatation is irregular, with nodular or fusiform distentions and even aneurysmal pouchings. Accompanying this asymmetric dilatation is marked variation in the thickness of the vessel wall. Thinning is seen at the points of maximal dilatation, whereas compensatory hypertrophy of the media and fibrosis of the wall may produce thickening in a neighboring segment. Valvular deformities (thickening, rolling, and shortening of the cusps) are common, as is intraluminal thrombosis. Microscopically, the changes are quite minimal and consist of variations in the thickness of the wall of the vein. Smooth muscle hypertrophy and subintimal fibrosis are apparent in the areas of compensatory hypertrophy. Frequently there is degeneration of the elastic tissue in the major veins and spotty calcifications within the media (**phlebosclerosis**).

**CLINICAL COURSE.** Sometimes distention of the veins in the legs is painful, although most often early varicose veins are asymptomatic. As the valves become incompetent, a vicious circle is established, with the resultant venous stasis further increasing intraluminal pressure. Marked venous congestion with edema may occur. Such edema impairs circulation, rendering the affected tissues extremely vulnerable to injury. In these severe cases, trophic changes, stasis dermatitis, cellulitis, and chronic ulceration are common. *Although varicose veins frequently thrombose, embolization to the lungs is uncommon from the superficial leg veins.* Hemorrhoids, as is well known, not only are uncomfortable but also may be a source of bleeding. Sometimes they thrombose and in this distended state are prone to painful ulceration.

## PHLEBOTHROMBOSIS AND THROMBOPHLEBITIS

These two designations are synonyms for thrombus formation within veins. This condition was described in some detail on page 73. Here we need only recall that the thrombi most often arise in the deep veins of the lower extremities, particularly the muscular veins of the calf. Frequently they are silent clinically but have the distressing potential of giving rise to emboli that lodge in the lungs to produce pulmonary embolism and infarction, which are extremely important causes of morbidity and mortality. You may recall that phlebothrombosis is most often associated with cardiac failure, prolonged bed rest or immobilization of an extremity, postoperative and postpartal states, neoplasia, and any form of severe trauma, particularly extensive burns. In cases of cancer, particularly those primary in the abdominal cavity, the venous thromboses have a tendency to appear spontaneously in one site, only to disappear and be followed by thromboses in other veins, giving rise to the entity referred to as *migratory thrombophlebitis (Trousseau's sign)* (p. 74). Because of the clinical settings in which phlebothrombosis appears, pulmonary embolization often constitutes the final mortal blow to those already gravely ill.

## OBSTRUCTION OF SUPERIOR VENA CAVA (SUPERIOR VENA CAVAL SYNDROME)

This dramatic entity is usually caused by neoplasms that compress or invade the superior vena cava. Most commonly, a primary bronchogenic carcinoma or a mediastinal lymphoma is the underlying lesion. Occasionally, other disorders, such as an aortic aneurysm, may impinge on the superior vena cava. Regardless of the cause, the consequent obstruction produces a distinctive clinical complex, referred to as the *superior vena caval syndrome*. It is manifested by dusky cyanosis and marked dilatation of the veins of the head, neck, and arms. Commonly, the pulmonary vessels are also compressed, and consequently respiratory distress may develop.

## OBSTRUCTION OF INFERIOR VENA CAVA (INFERIOR VENA CAVAL SYNDROME)

This is analogous to the superior vena caval syndrome and may be caused by many of the same processes. Neoplasms may either compress or penetrate the walls of the inferior vena cava. In addition, one of the most common causes of inferior vena caval obstruction is propagation of a thrombus upward from the femoral or iliac veins. Certain neoplasms, particularly hepatocarcinoma and renal cell carcinoma, show a striking tendency to grow within the lumens of the veins, extending ultimately into the inferior vena cava.

As would be anticipated, obstruction to the inferior vena cava induces marked edema of the legs, distention of the superficial collateral veins of the lower abdomen, and, when the renal veins are involved, massive proteinuria.

# Lymphatic Disorders

Disorders of the lymphatic channels fall into two categories: primary diseases, which are extremely uncommon, and secondary processes, which develop in association with inflammations or cancers. In both patterns, there is frequently obstruction to the lymphatic channels followed by lymphedema, entirely analogous to the edema that develops distal to venous obstructions.

## LYMPHEDEMA

Although inflammatory drainage through lymphatics, as frequently occurs with group A beta-hemolytic streptococcal infections, may cause acute lymphangitis marked by redness and dilatation of the lymphatic channels, these changes are usually self-limited and rapidly subside with control of the primary infection. More ominous than the involvement of the lymphatic channels is the extension of the infection to the regional lymph nodes (lymphadenitis, described on p. 48), which may then permit spread of the infection into the major lymphatic ducts and eventually the bloodstream.

Frequently more disabling is the *secondary lymphedema* that may develop from (1) postinflammatory scarring of lymphatic channels, (2) spread of malignant neoplasms with obstruction of either the lymphatic channels or nodes of drainage, (3) radical surgical procedures with excision of regional lymph nodes (as, for example, the removal of axillary nodes in radical mastectomy), (4) postradiation fibrosis, and (5) filariasis.

In contrast, *primary lymphedema* may occur as an isolated congenital defect (*simple congenital lymphedema*), or it may be familial, in which case it is known as *Milroy's disease* or *heredofamilial congenital lymphedema*. Both entities are presumed to be caused by faulty development of lymphatic channels, possibly with poor structural strength, permitting abnormal dilatation and incompetence of the lymphatic valves. Classically, these disorders involve the lower extremities, although they may affect other areas, sometimes in a rather sharply limited, bizarre distribution. Both simple congenital lymphedema and Milroy's disease are present from birth. In contrast, a third form of primary lymphedema, known as *lymphedema praecox*, appears between the ages of 10 and 25 years, usually in females. The etiology is unknown. This disorder begins in one or both feet, and the edema slowly accumulates throughout life, so that the involved extremity may increase to many times its normal size; the process may extend upward to affect the trunk. Although the size of the limb may produce some disability, more serious complications are unusual.

With lymphedema from any cause, the morphologic changes within the lymphatics consist of dilatation distal to the point of obstruction, accompanied by increases of interstitial fluid. Persistence of edema leads to interstitial fibrosis, most evident subcutaneously. The thickened skin assumes the texture of orange peel, a finding termed "peau d'orange." Enlargement of the affected part, brawny induration, infection (cellulitis), and chronic skin ulcers are common sequelae to lymphedema, as they are to varicose veins.

With secondary lymphedema, the clinical picture is usually that of the underlying disorder. Although lymphedema itself is disfiguring and disabling, it is rarely life-threatening. However, persistent ulcers and secondary infection may present serious clinical problems.

# Tumors

Tumors of vessels (blood or lymphatic) run the gamut from the benign lesions that generally reproduce vascular channels to more aggressive tumors that have a larger component of solid masses of endothelial cells sometimes admixed with fibroblasts.[68] The benign lesions reproducing vascular channels are subdivided into capillary and cavernous angiomas. As their cellularity and potential for aggressive behavior increase, the neoplasms are referred to as angioendotheliomas, or, with more extreme anaplasia, angiosarcomas.

Neat as this categorization may be, two complexities remain. The majority of benign angiomas—capillary and cavernous—are present from birth and expand along with the growth of the child, and many spontaneously regress at or before puberty. It may be that trauma during childhood initiates thrombosis, which rapidly spreads throughout the lesions and thus leads to their eventual organization and disappearance. The question arises—are these true neoplasms or merely hamartomatous congenital anomalies? For this reason many pediatricians elect to "watch and wait" with such lesions. The second problematic area is the differentiation of capillary hemangiomas of the skin from vasoproliferative reactive lesions. For example, the *granuloma pyogenicum* represents an exuberant overgrowth of granulation tissue richly larded with vascular channels secondary to some localized infection. Analogously, the exuberant vasoproliferation that occurs at the gingivodental margin in about 10% of pregnant women, sometimes referred to as *pregnancy tumor*, almost always regresses after delivery. Such reactive proliferations are easily mistaken for capillary hemangiomas, but the clinical setting in which they appear and the prominence of inflammatory cells in the granuloma pyogenicum serve as differential features.

With these few introductory remarks, we can turn to some of the more common lesions, which are nonetheless sufficiently trivial or infrequent to merit only brief description.

## ANGIOMAS

Angiomas may be composed of masses of cavernous or capillary-like channels filled with either blood or lymph.

MORPHOLOGY. **Cavernous angiomas** may arise in blood vessels or in lymphatics. The cavernous hemangiomas often occur on the skin and mucosal surfaces of the body but may also arise in viscera, particularly in the liver, spleen, pancreas, and, rarely, the brain. In infants they sometimes constitute large lesions of the skin of the face or scalp, creating so-called "port-wine stains." Cavernous hemangiomas are generally red-blue, compressible, spongy lesions, 2 to 3 cm in diameter, sharply defined at their margins, and composed of large cavernous spaces filled with fluid blood; they sometimes have partially thrombosed channels. In most instances, these cavernous lesions are of little clinical significance and, as mentioned, in children may regress. Those in the brain are most threatening, since they may cause pressure symptoms or rupture.

**Cavernous lymphangiomas** are also known as **cystic hygromas**. These are much more rare than cavernous hemangiomas and are usually located in the neck or axilla or, occasionally, in the retroperitoneum. They tend to be large masses that may produce readily evident deformities in the neck and axilla. Despite their benign nature, they tend to expand by budding-off new channels and so may infiltrate in and about adjacent structures, such as the brachial plexus or vessels in the neck. As can be anticipated, they are composed of lymphatic channels filled with clear lymph fluid. Sometimes the interstitial tissue contains a scant lymphoid infiltrate or occasional islands of fat or muscle. Because of the deformity they induce, they are generally surgically excised but often recur because of technical difficulties in their total extirpation.

**A capillary hemangioma** is an unencapsulated tangle of closely packed capillaries separated by a scant connective tissue stroma. The channels are usually filled with fluid blood. However, thrombosis and fibrous organization within some of the component capillaries is common. The endothelial cells of the lining appear normal. Although any organ or tissue may be involved, capillary hemangiomas usually occur in the skin, subcutaneous tissues, or mucous membranes of the oral cavity and lips. On gross inspection, they appear as bright red to blue lesions, ranging from a few millimeters to several centimeters in diameter. They may be level with the surface of the surrounding tissue, slightly elevated, or—occasionally— even pedunculated. Uncommonly, capillary hemangiomas take the form of large, flat, map-like discolorations covering large areas of the face or upper parts of the body, producing "port-wine stains" analogous to those caused by cavernous hemangiomas.

Capillary hemangiomas, because they are usually located on the skin or mucous membranes, are of significance only because they are vulnerable to traumatic ulceration and bleeding.

## HEMANGIOENDOTHELIOMA AND ANGIOSARCOMA

Both of these neoplasms represent the malignant counterparts of the benign angiomatous lesions. The hemangioendothelioma constitutes an intergrade between the benign hemangiomas and the unmistakably malignant anaplastic angiosarcoma.

In the hemangioendothelioma, vascular channels are usually readily discernible within the masses of proliferating, reasonably well differentiated endothelial cells. In the angiosarcoma, vascular channels may be virtually inapparent. Thus, the angiosarcoma is composed of masses of anaplastic spindle cells with sparsely scattered, poorly formed vascular channels, themselves lined by tumorous endothelial cells. Both patterns of tumors are found in the same locations as their benign counterparts and tend to be larger, more solid, less obviously vascular, and more unmistakably invasive. In some cases the tumor cells contain factor VIII–related antigens, a product of normal endothelium.

The angiosarcomas are of interest because there is now good evidence that chronic exposure to arsenic compounds or polyvinyl chloride (used in plastics industries) predisposes to the development of these neoplasms in the liver.

## GLOMANGIOMA (GLOMUS TUMOR)

This uncommon but curious benign lesion, which arises from the cells of a glomus body, is invariably small, red-blue in color and exquisitely painful to the slightest pressure.

Glomangiomas are most commonly encountered in the distal fingers and toes, especially under the nails. They are supplied with an afferent artery, arteriovenous anastomoses, and efferent veins. Surrounding the anastomoses are the glomus cells, which are apparently specialized pericyte cells resembling epithelial cells. The tumors are small and of the order of 5 mm in diameter. When in the skin, they are slightly elevated, rounded, red-blue, firm nodules. Under the nail, they appear as minute foci of fresh hemorrhage.

They are usually readily excised and cured.

## KAPOSI'S SARCOMA (MULTIPLE IDIOPATHIC HEMORRHAGIC SARCOMATOSIS)

This once-obscure tumor has gained attention as an important complication of AIDS. Its incidence in the United States has risen substantially in association with the AIDS epidemic (see p. 175). In subjects without AIDS, it is uncommon in the United States, usually occurring on the legs of men (male to female ratio 10:1) aged 40 to 70 years. In contrast, it is said to account for about 10% of all cancers in both children and adults in certain parts of Africa. There is strong suspicion of a viral origin for this tumor.

The skin is the major target of the disease. In about 10% of cases visceral lesions are also present. Early cases have been described that show multiple disseminated skin lesions resembling either benign capillary hemangiomas or vascularized chronic inflammatory foci. Over the course of time, repeated biopsies have disclosed a progressive sarcomatous transformation. When fully evolved, red-blue subcutaneous plaques or nodules appear, often with a verrucous surface. Histologically, the following four components are seen: (1) endothelial cell proliferation, either as cellular sheets or as new vessel formations; (2) extravascular hemorrhage with hemosiderin deposition; (3) anaplastic fibroblastic proliferation; and (4) a granulation-like inflammatory reaction.

The clinical course is extremely indolent in sporadic non-African cases, and the patient often dies of unrelated causes, although occasionally lesions are aggressive and assume the characteristics of other sarcomas. In Africans, there tends to be internal (cervical lymph nodes, salivary glands, and intestinal tract) and cutaneous involvement, and the course of the disease is more aggressive and more often fatal. In patients with AIDS, Kaposi's sarcoma is also a more virulent disease.[69] These patients frequently present with disseminated disease, and approximately 40% of patients with AIDS and Kaposi's sarcoma (and often with opportunistic infections) die after one year.

## TELANGIECTASIS

This term refers to focal red-blue lesions created by the abnormal dilatation of preexisting small vessels. As such, telangiectases are not true neoplasms. In many of these lesions, a small, central, dilated vessel can be seen surrounded by radiating fine channels. This is understandably called a spider telangiectasis.

Most commonly, telangiectases are seen in pregnant women and in patients with chronic liver disease. In both instances, it is thought that they are in some way evoked by hyperestrinism, relative or absolute.

Multiple, small, aneurysmal telangiectases distributed over the skin and mucous membranes throughout the body, including the gut, may be transmitted as an autosomal dominant trait. This uncommon disorder is known as *hereditary hemorrhagic telangiectasia (Rendu-Osler-Weber disease).* It is present from birth. Typically, the disease is characterized by recurrent hemorrhages from rupture of the many superficial lesions. These hemorrhages are usually readily controlled and rarely threaten life or reduce longevity.

## References

1. Levy, R. I., and Feinlieb, M.: Risk factors for coronary artery disease and their management. *In* Braunwald, E. (ed.): Heart Disease: A Textbook of Cardiovascular Medicine. 2nd ed. Philadelphia, W. B. Saunders Co., 1984, p. 1205.
2. Tejada, C., et al.: Distribution of coronary and aortic atherosclerosis by geographic location, race, and sex. Lab. Invest. *18*:49, 1968.
3. Goldman, L., and Cook, E. F.: The decline in ischemic heart disease mortality rates. An analysis of the comparative effects of medical interventions and changes in lifestyle. Ann. Intern. Med. *101*:825, 1984.
4. Strong, J. P., and Guzman, M. A.: Decrease in coronary atherosclerosis in New Orleans. Lab. Invest. *43*:297, 1980.
5. Kannel, W. B., et al.: Cholesterol in the prediction of atherosclerotic disease. New perspectives based on the Framingham Study. Ann. Intern. Med. *90*:85, 1979.
6. Pooling Project Research Group: Relationship of blood pressure, serum cholesterol, smoking habits, relative weight and ECG abnormalities to incidence of major coronary events: final report of the Pooling Project. J. Chron. Dis. *31*:201, 1978.
7. Enos, W. F., et al.: Coronary disease among United States soldiers killed in action in Korea. J.A.M.A. *152*:1090, 1953.
8. Wissler, R. W.: Principles of the pathogenesis of atherosclerosis. *In* Braunwald, E. (ed.): Heart Disease: A Textbook of Cardiovascular Medicine. 2nd ed. Philadelphia, W. B. Saunders Co., 1984, p. 1183.
9. Lipid Research Clinics: Coronary Primary Prevention Trial Results: I. Reduction in incidence of coronary heart disease. J.A.M.A. *251*:351, 1984.
10. Lipid Research Clinics: Coronary Primary Prevention Trial Results: II. The relationship of reduction in incidence of coronary heart disease to cholesterol lowering. J.A.M.A. *251*:365, 1984.
11. Gotto, A. M., Jr., et al.: Recommendations for treatment of hyperlipidemia in adults. A joint statement of the Nutrition Committee and the Council on Arteriosclerosis. Circulation *69*:1067A, 1984.
12. Havel, R. J., et al.: Lipoproteins and lipid transport. *In* Bondy, P. K., and Rosenberg, L. E. (eds.): Metabolic Control and Disease. 8th ed. Philadelphia, W. B. Saunders Co., 1980, pp. 393–494.
13. Goldstein, J. L., et al.: Defective lipoprotein receptors and atherosclerosis. N. Engl. J. Med. *309*:288, 1983.
14. Buja, L. M., et al.: Cellular pathology of homozygous familial hypercholesterolemia. Am. J. Pathol. *97*:327, 1979.
15. Solberg, L. A., et al.: Risk factors for coronary and cerebral atherosclerosis in the Oslo Study. *In* Gotto, A. M., Smith, L. C., and Allen, B. (eds.): Atherosclerosis V. New York, Springer-Verlag, 1979, p. 57.
16. Benditt, E. P., and Gown, A. M.: Atheroma: The artery wall and the environment. Int. Rev. Exp. Pathol. *21*:55, 1980.
17. Haust, M. D.: The morphogenesis and fate of potential and early atherosclerotic lesions in man. Hum. Pathol. 2:1, 1971.

18. Smith, E. B.: Molecular interactions in human atherosclerotic plaques. Am. J. Pathol. *86*:665, 1977.
19. Schwartz, C. J., and Mitchell, J. R. A.: The morphology, terminology and pathogenesis of arterial plaques. Postgrad. Med. J. *38*:25, 1962.
20. Small, D. M.: Cellular mechanisms for lipid deposition in atherosclerosis. N. Engl. J. Med. *297*:873, 1977.
21. Crawford, T., and Levene, C. I.: Medial thinning in atheroma. J. Pathol. Bacteriol. *46*:19, 1953.
22. Glagov, S.: Hemodynamic risk factors: mechanical stress, mural architecture, medial nutrition, and vulnerability of arteries to atherosclerosis. *In* Wissler, R. W., and Geer, J. C. (eds.): The Pathogenesis of Atherosclerosis. Baltimore, The Williams & Williams Co., 1972, p. 164.
23. Joris I., et al.: Studies on the pathogenesis of atherosclerosis. I. Adhesion and emigration of mononuclear cells in the aorta of hypercholesterolemic rats. Am. J. Pathol. *113*:341, 1983.
24. Geer, J. C., and Haust, M. D.: Smooth muscle cells in atherosclerosis. Basel, S. Karger, 1972.
25. Crawford, T.: Morphological aspects in the pathogenesis of atherosclerosis. J. Atheroscl. Res. *1*:3, 1961.
26. Barger, A. C., et al.: Hypothesis: Vasa vasorum and neovascularization of human coronary arteries: A possible role in the pathophysiology of atherosclerosis. N. Engl. J. Med. *310*:175, 1984.
27. Ross, R., and Glomset, J. A.: The pathogenesis of atherosclerosis. N. Engl. J. Med. *295*:369, 420, 1976.
28. Ross, R.: The pathogenesis of atherosclerosis—An update. N. Engl. J. Med. *314*:488, 1986.
29. Davies, P. F.: Vascular cell interactions with special reference to the pathogenesis of atherosclerosis. Lab. Invest. *55*:5, 1986.
30. Gimbrone, M. A., Jr.: Vascular endothelium and atherosclerosis. *In* Moore, S. (ed.): Vascular Injury and Atherosclerosis. New York, M. Dekker, Inc., 1981, p. 25.
31. Hajjar, D. P., et al.: Endothelium modifies the altered metabolism of the injured aortic wall. Am. J. Pathol. *102*:28, 1981.
32. DiCorleto, P. E., and de la Motte, C. A.: Characterization of the adhesion of the human monocytic cell line U937 to cultured endothelial cells. J. Clin. Invest. *75*:1153, 1985.
33. Mahley, R. W.: Development of accelerated atherosclerosis: Concepts derived from cell biology and animal model studies. Arch. Pathol. Lab. Med. *107*:393, 1983.
34. Fry, D. L.: Hemodynamic forces in atherogenesis. *In*: Scheinberg, P. (ed.): Cerebrovascular Diseases. New York, Raven Press, 1976, p. 77.
35. Fox, J. A., and Hugh, A. E.: Localization of atheroma: A theory based on boundary layer separation. Br. Heart J. *23*:388, 1966.
36. Muller-Mohnssen, H., et al.: Microthrombus formation in models of coronary arteries caused by stagnation point flow arising at the predilection site of atherosclerosis and thrombosis. *In* Nerem, R. M., and Cornhill, J. F. (eds.): The Role of Fluid Mechanics in Atherogenesis. Columbus, Ohio State University Press, 1978, p. 1–12.
37. Majesky, M. W., et al.: Focal smooth muscle proliferation in the aortic intima produced by an initiation-promotion sequence. Proc. Natl. Acad. Sci. USA *82*:3450, 1985.
38. Thomas, W. A., and Kim, D. N.: Atherosclerosis as a hyperplastic and/or neoplastic process. Lab. Invest. *48*:245, 1983.
39. Martin G. M.: Cellular aging—Clonal senescence. A review (Part I). Am. J. Pathol. *89*:484, 1977.
40. Castellot, J. J., Jr., et al.: Cultured endothelial cells produce a heparinlike inhibitor of smooth muscle cell growth. J. Cell Biol. *90*:372, 1981.
41. Malinow, M. R.: Regression of atherosclerosis in humans: Fact or myth? Circulation *64*:1, 1981.
42. McCluskey, R. T., and Fienberg, O.: Vasculitis in primary vasculitides, granulomatoses, and connective tissue diseases. Hum. Pathol. *14*:305, 1983.
43. Cupps, T. R., and Fauci, A. S.: The vasculitic syndromes. Adv. Intern. Med. *27*:315, 1982.
44. Sergent, J. S., et al.: Vasculitis with hepatitis B antigenemia: Long-term observations in nine patients. Medicine *55*:1, 1976.

45. Melish, M. E.: Kawasaki's syndrome (the mucocutaneous lymph node syndrome). Ann. Rev. Med. 33:569, 1982.

46. Sams, W. M., et al.: Leukocytoclastic vasculitis. Arch. Dermatol. 112:219, 1976.

47. Goodman, B. W., Jr.: Temporal arteritis. Am. J. Med. 67:839, 1979.

48. Bengtsson, B. A., and Malmvall, B. E.: Giant cell arteritis. Acta Med. Scand. (Suppl.) 658:1, 1982.

49. Erlinger, R. E., et al.: Polymyalgia rheumatica and giant cell arteritis. Ann. Rev. Med. 29:15, 1978.

50. Nakao, K., et al.: Takayasu's arteritis. Clinical report of 84 cases and immunological studies of seven cases. Circulation 35:1141, 1967.

51. Lupi-Herrera, E., et al.: Takayasu's arteritis. Study of 107 cases. Am. Heart J. 93:94, 1977.

52. Ishikawa, K.: Natural history and clarification of occlusive thromboaortopathy (Takayasu's disease). Circulation 57:27, 1978.

53. McKusick, V. A., et al.: Buerger's disease: A distinct clinical and pathologic entity. J.A.M.A. 181:5, 1962.

54. Williams, G.: Recent views on Buerger's disease. J. Clin. Pathol, 22:573, 1969.

55. Becker, C., and Dubin, T.: Tobacco allergy and cardiovascular disease. Cardiovasc. Med. 3:851, 1978.

56. McLoughlin, G. A., et al.: Association of HLA-A9 and HLA-B5 with Buerger's disease. Br. Med. J. 2:1165, 1976.

57. Adar, R., et al.: Cellular sensitivity to collagen in thromboangiitis obliterans. N. Engl. J. Med. 308:1113, 1983.

58. Brinstingl, M.: The Raynaud syndrome. In Harcus, A. W., et al. (eds.): Arteries and Veins. Edinburgh, Churchill Livingstone, 1975, p. 32.

59. Slater, E. E., and De Sanctis, R. W.: Diseases of the aorta. In Braunwald, E. (ed.): Heart Disease: A Textbook of Cardiovascular Medicine. 2nd ed. Philadelphia, W. B. Saunders Co., 1984, pp. 1540–1571.

60. Klima, T., et al.: The morphology of ascending aortic aneurysms. Hum. Pathol. 14:810, 1983.

61. Bornstein, P.: The crosslinking of collagen and elastin and its inhibition in osteolathyrism. Am. J. Med. 49:429, 1970.

62. Boucek, R., et al.: The Marfan syndrome: A deficiency in chemically stable collagen cross-links. N. Engl. J. Med. 288:804, 1982.

63. Prokop, E. K., et al.: Hydrodynamic forces in dissection aneurysms. In vitro studies in a Tygon model and in dog aortas. Circ. Res. 27:121, 1970.

64. Hirst, A. E., et al.: Dissecting aneurysms of the aorta. A review of 505 cases. Medicine 37:217, 1958.

65. Anagnostopoulos, C. E.: Acute Aortic Dissections. Baltimore, University Park Press, 1975.

66. Roberts, W. C.: Aortic dissection: Anatomy, consequences and causes. Am. Heart J. 101:195, 1981.

67. Lemon, D. K., and White, C. W.: Anuloaortic ectasia: Angiographic, hemodynamic and clinical comparison with aortic valvular insufficiency. Am. J. Cardiol. 41:482, 1978.

68. Enzinger, F. M., and Weiss, S. W.: Soft Tissue Tumors. St. Louis, C. V. Mosby Co., 1983, pp. 379–501.

69. Volberding, P. A.: Kaposi's sarcoma and the acquired immunodeficiency syndrome. Med. Clin. North Am. 70:665, 1986.

# 11

# The Heart

L. MAXIMILIAN BUJA, M.D.*

CONGESTIVE HEART FAILURE (CHF)
    Left-sided Heart Failure
    Right-sided Heart Failure
ISCHEMIC HEART DISEASE (IHD)–CORONARY HEART DISEASE (CHD)
    Angina Pectoris (AP)
    Sudden Cardiac Death (SCD)
    Myocardial Infarction (MI)
    Chronic Ischemic Heart Disease (CIHD)
HYPERTENSIVE HEART DISEASE
RHEUMATIC HEART DISEASE (RHD)
    Rheumatic Fever (RF)
CONGENITAL HEART DISEASE
    Ventricular Septal Defect (VSD)
    Atrial Septal Defect (ASD)
    Patent Ductus Arteriosus
    Coarctation of the Aorta
    Isolated Pulmonic Stenosis, Isolated Aortic Stenosis
    Anomalies of the Coronary Arteries
    Transposition of the Great Vessels
    Tetralogy of Fallot
INFECTIVE ENDOCARDITIS
COR PULMONALE
PERICARDIAL DISEASE
    Pericarditis
MYOCARDIAL DISEASE
    Cardiomyopathy (CMP)
    Myocarditis
ENDOCARDIAL AND VALVULAR DISEASE
    Calcific Aortic Stenosis
    Calcification of the Mitral Annulus
    Mitral Valve Prolapse (Floppy Valve Syndrome; Barlow's Syndrome)
    Nonbacterial Thrombotic Endocarditis (Marantic Endocarditis)
    Nonbacterial Verrucous Endocarditis (Libman-Sacks Disease)
    Carcinoid Syndrome
    Endocardial Fibroelastosis (EFE)
    Myxoma of the Heart

Heart disease is today the leading cause of morbidity and mortality in industrialized nations. In the United States, cardiac diseases are responsible for almost twice as many deaths as cancer (the second most common cause of mortality), accounting for approximately 37% of all deaths. About 88% of these

deaths are caused by ischemic heart disease (IHD) alone, also commonly referred to as coronary heart disease (CHD). Awesome as these data may be, there is a ray of light. The number of deaths from heart disease has been reported to be declining for almost two decades, a fact largely attributable to a decrease in the mortality caused by IHD.[1]

Although dwarfed by the dominating importance of IHD, five other forms of heart disease collectively account for about 5% of the total cardiac mortality and so warrant separate discussion: hypertensive heart disease (approximately 1 to 2%), rheumatic heart disease (approximately 1%), congenital heart disease (approximately 1%), infective endocarditis (less than 1%), and cor pulmonale (less than 1%). The many other forms of heart disease, then, are responsible for the remaining 7% of deaths of cardiac origin. Emphasis will therefore be placed in this chapter on IHD first, then on the five cardiac disorders mentioned, followed by brief presentations of the other patterns of cardiac involvement under the headings of (1) pericardial disease, (2) myocardial disease, and (3) endocardial and valvular disease.

Death from heart disease is usually a direct result either of disturbances in cardiac rhythm or of progressive weakening of the pump. Frequently, one leads to the other. All the major diseases of the heart to be discussed in this chapter may be associated with various arrhythmias, such as atrial fibrillation, extrasystoles, or life-threatening ventricular tachycardia or fibrillation. Disturbances in cardiac rhythm occur when the normal conduction pathways are interrupted by necrosis, inflammation, or fibrosis, or when some local metabolic derangement produces a focus of electric irritability. As such, arrhythmias, although dramatic, are of little help in identifying the specific pathologic lesion. Similarly, all the major cardiac diseases, when sufficiently severe, may interfere with the capacity of the heart to function as a pump. Through either pathway the clinical syndrome known as congestive heart failure (CHF) may ensue and dominate the clinical picture. Because this ultimate consequence of all major forms of heart disease is a rather complex syndrome with protean effects, we will describe CHF in some detail before discussing each disease separately.

*A. J. Gill Professor of Pathology, University of Texas Health Science Center at Dallas

# CONGESTIVE HEART FAILURE (CHF)

Congestive heart failure refers to a clinical syndrome resulting from deficient cardiac stroke volume, relative to body need, with inability of the cardiac output to keep pace with the venous return.[2] This eventually results in blood damming back into the venous system and concomitant diminished filling of the arterial tree. The fundamental derangement may be impaired myocardial contractility, as with intrinsic myocardial disease, or an increased work load placed upon the heart as with, say, valvular incompetence. Not infrequently, both factors are operative. Compensatory mechanisms—myocardial hypertrophy and dilatation, which promote more forceful contraction—may for a time sustain the cardiac output. These cardiac changes are supported by an increased blood volume through renal retention of salt and water by increased plasma levels of aldosterone and catecholamines. Eventually, however, the compensatory mechanisms cease to be effective and, indeed, come to constitute an added burden on an already overtaxed organ. Myocardial hypertrophy becomes detrimental because of the increased oxygen requirements of the enlarged muscle mass. The heart becomes dilated beyond the point at which adequate myocardial contractile tension can be generated. The additional blood volume produces marked congestion, further stressing the heart. Ultimately, cardiac output must fall.

*The principal morphologic changes, as well as the signs and symptoms that characterize CHF, are pro duced by the secondary effects of the failing circulation upon the various organs supplied by the heart.* Grossly, the heart shows only hypertrophy and dilatation, along with the changes of the underlying disease.

Usually the two sides of the heart do not begin to fail simultaneously. Although the heart is a single organ, to some extent it acts as two distinct anatomic and functional entities. Under various pathologic stresses, one side—or, rarely, even one chamber—may fail before the other, so that from the clinical standpoint left-sided and right-sided failure may occur separately. However, since the vascular system is a closed circuit, failure of one side cannot exist for long without eventually producing excessive strain upon the other, terminating in total heart failure. Nevertheless, the clearest understanding of the pathologic physiology is derived from considering failure of each side separately.

## LEFT-SIDED HEART FAILURE

As will be discussed, left-sided heart failure is most often caused by coronary heart disease, aortic and mitral valvular diseases, and hypertension. Except with narrowing of the mitral valve, the left ventricle is usually dilated, sometimes quite massively. With mitral stenosis, the dilatation is confined to the left atrium. The distant effects of left-sided failure are manifested most prominently in the lungs, although the function of the kidneys and brain may also be markedly impaired.

**LUNGS.** With the progressive damming of blood within the pulmonary circulation, pressure in the pulmonary veins mounts and is ultimately transmitted to the capillaries. The congestion is soon followed by edema, secondary to the raised hydrostatic pressure and dilatation of the septal capillaries and widening of the interendothelial junctions.[3] The lung is particularly vulnerable to the development of edema because its loose honeycomb structure exerts no significant tissue pressure against the escape of fluids.

At first the transudate is limited to perivascular "cuffing." Later, there is thickening of the alveolar walls as fluid accumulates within them. Finally, the transudate overflows into the alveoli **(pulmonary edema)** (Fig. 11–1). Not infrequently, transudate accumulates within the pleural space, producing a gross pleural effusion.[4] Persistent elevation of pulmonary venous pressure with repeated episodes of pulmonary edema leads to changes of **chronic passive congestion** of the lungs.

The edema appears as an intraalveolar granular precipitate, with accompanying widening of the alveolar septa. The congestion causes dilatation of the alveolar capillaries. In the more advanced cases, the capillaries may become tortuous, with small aneurysmal outpouchings, and rhexis may produce small hemorrhages into the

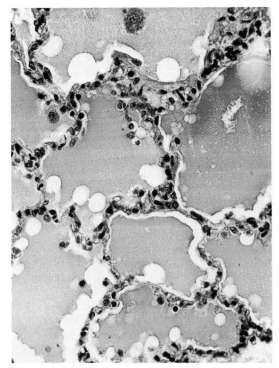

Figure 11–1. The lung in congestive heart failure. The alveolar spaces are filled with a transudate.

alveolar spaces. In these cases, the lining epithelial cells become hypertrophied and cuboidal. As a result of alveolar hemorrhages, hemosiderin-laden macrophages, termed "heart failure cells," appear in the alveolar spaces. The chronic persistence of septal edema often induces fibrosis within the alveolar walls. This fibrosis, together with the accumulation of hemosiderin, is designated "brown induration of the lungs." The weight of each lung is increased up to 700 or 800 gm (normal, 350 to 400 gm). The most severely affected areas, principally the lower lobes, are soggy and subcrepitant. Sectioning of such lungs permits the free escape of a frothy hemorrhagic fluid. All these changes predispose to secondary bacterial invasion, with resultant bronchopneumonia, which in this setting is often referred to as **hypostatic pneumonia.**

These anatomic changes produce striking clinical manifestations. *Dyspnea on exertion* is usually the earliest complaint of patients in left-sided heart failure. Later, shortness of breath is present even at rest. The pathogenesis of this dyspnea is complex and in all likelihood involves hypoxemia of the respiratory center and carotid sinus, reduced lung compliance, and encroachment on the vital capacity of the lungs produced by the congestive vascular distention. Cyanosis may be present because of the impaired oxygenation of the blood, but it is usually minimal in left-sided failure. A characteristic and therefore highly important symptom of left-sided failure is *paroxysmal nocturnal dyspnea*, the sudden onset of respiratory distress that wakens the patient from sleep. The pathogenesis of this phenomenon is not completely understood, but several factors may be operative. With recumbency, there is decreased venous pressure in the dependent portions of the body, hence gradual resorption of tissue fluid and thus an augmented blood volume, which in turn is reflected in an increase in pulmonary congestion. Moreover, there is less functional pulmonary reserve in the recumbent position because the resting position of the diaphragm is higher, encroaching on the vital capacity of the lungs. It is also possible that during sleep depression of the respiratory center reduces ventilation, and simultaneously the lessened irritability of the central nervous system permits the accumulation of edema fluid without evoking such normal defense mechanisms as coughing. As failure becomes more advanced, the patient becomes unable to sleep at all in the recumbent position—i.e., he becomes *orthopneic*—and must prop himself up with pillows. Cough is a common accompaniment of left-sided failure and, in severe cases, may raise frothy, blood-tinged sputum.

In addition to the pulmonary symptoms resulting from pulmonary venous congestion, left-sided heart failure also produces alterations secondary to decreased left ventricular stroke output. Fatigue and diminished exercise capacity are important systemic manifestations of this phenomenon.

**KIDNEYS.** The hemodynamic derangements occurring with left-sided heart failure may markedly affect the kidneys. Decreased cardiac output and effective arterial blood volume lead to alterations in renal blood flow. Activation of the sympathetic nervous system and the renin-angiotensin system induces arteriolar vasoconstriction and shunting of blood away from the peripheral cortex. Thus, the glomerular filtration rate falls and concomitantly proximal tubular reabsorption increases, both leading to retention of salt and water. Teleologically, this may be looked upon as the response of the kidneys to what they interpret as hypovolemia. Salt and water retention is further enhanced by the augmented secretion of adrenal mineralocorticoids, particularly aldosterone. The elaboration of these steroids may represent a nonspecific stress response, as well as a compensatory response to the diminished perfusion of the kidneys. The consequent increase in total blood volume eventually adds considerably to the load upon the heart and contributes to the generalized edema, which develops with advanced (combined left- and right-sided) heart failure. With severe disturbances in renal blood flow, impaired excretion of nitrogenous products may cause azotemia, known as *prerenal azotemia*.

**BRAIN.** Cerebral hypoxia may give rise to many symptoms, such as irritability, loss of attention span, and restlessness, which may even progress to stupor and coma. These symptoms, however, are encountered only in far advanced congestive heart failure.

## RIGHT-SIDED HEART FAILURE

Right-sided heart failure occurs in relatively pure form in only a few diseases. Usually it is combined with left-sided failure because any increase in pressure in the pulmonary circulation incident to left-sided failure must inevitably produce an increased burden on the right side of the heart. The causes of right-sided failure, then, must include all those that create left heart failure, particularly lesions such as mitral stenosis, which produce great increases in the pulmonary pressure.

Fairly *pure* right-sided failure most often occurs with *cor pulmonale*, a right ventricular strain produced by intrinsic disease of the lungs or pulmonary vasculature. In these cases, the right ventricle is burdened by increased resistance within the pulmonary circuit. Dilatation of the heart is confined to the right ventricle and atrium. Other and less common causes of right-sided heart failure include myocardial infarction of the right ventricle and diffuse myocarditis, which appears to affect the right ventricle more often than the left for reasons to be presented later. Rarely, right-sided failure is caused by tricuspid or pulmonic valvular lesions. Clinically, constrictive pericarditis simulates right-sided failure by the damming of blood back into the systemic venous system, although the right ventricle itself may be normal.

The major morphologic and clinical effects of right-sided failure differ from those of left-sided failure in that pulmonary congestion is minimal, whereas engorgement of the systemic and portal systems is more pronounced. It should be remembered, however, that in both instances the twin problems of systemic venous congestion and impaired cardiac output remain qualitatively the same. The major sites affected by right-sided heart failure are the liver, spleen, kidneys, subcutaneous tissues, brain, and entire portal area of venous drainage. In addition, pleural effusions (hydrothorax) and pericardial effusion are likely to occur when combined right- and left-sided heart failure is present.

**LIVER.** The liver is usually slightly increased in size and weight and on sectioning displays a prominent "nutmeg" pattern (Fig. 11–2). This descriptive term refers to congestive red accentuation of the centers of the liver lobules, which are surrounded by the paler, sometimes fatty, peripheral regions. There may be some widening of the space of Disse microscopically, as well as enlargement and congestion of the central veins and central portions of the vascular sinusoids. The increased central venous pressure causes a diminished rate of blood flow through the lobule, leading to chronic oxygen deficiency, particularly for the liver cells in the central region of the

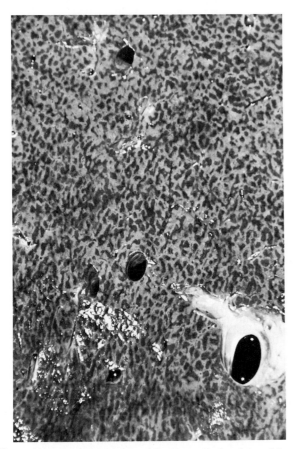

Figure 11–2. A close-up view of the transected surface of the liver with marked chronic passive congestion—the so-called nutmeg pattern.

lobule, which is the last area in the hepatic microcirculation to receive oxygenated blood. The result is ischemic atrophy of the liver cells in the congested central region of the lobule. Together, the changes are called **chronic passive congestion** of the liver. If the congestive failure is severe and rapidly developing, hemorrhage into the space of Disse and acute necrosis of the liver cells may occur, producing **central hemorrhagic necrosis.** This lesion may also occur in severe shock. Thus, central hemorrhagic necrosis may result from severely elevated central venous pressure, diminished arterial perfusion, and, commonly, from both factors. If the patient does not die of the usually severe cardiac failure, in time the central areas become fibrotic, creating so-called **cardiac sclerosis,** also known as **cardiac cirrhosis.**

**SPLEEN.** Splenic congestion produces a large, heavy organ that is tense and cyanotic. On section, blood freely exudes and the tissue collapses, so that the capsule becomes wrinkled. Microscopically, there may be marked sinusoidal dilatation, accompanied by areas of recent hemorrhage and possibly deposits of hemosiderin pigment. With long-standing congestion, the enlarged spleen may achieve weights of 500 to 600 gm (normal, ~ 150 gm) and the edema may produce fibrous thickening of the sinusoidal walls. The areas of previous hemorrhage are now transformed to hemosiderin deposits, to create the firm, meaty organ characteristic of **fibrocongestive splenomegaly.**

**KIDNEYS.** Congestion and hypoxia of the kidneys are more marked with right-sided heart failure than with left, leading to greater fluid retention and more pronounced prerenal azotemia.

**SUBCUTANEOUS TISSUES.** Some degree of peripheral edema of dependent portions of the body occurs regularly. Indeed, ankle edema may be considered a hallmark of CHF. In severe or long-standing cases, edema may be quite massive and generalized, a condition termed **anasarca.** Of probable significance in the perpetuation of edema is the diminished clearing of plasma aldosterone by the congested liver. This contributes to the elevated levels of this hormone.

**BRAIN.** Symptoms essentially identical with those described in left-sided failure may occur, representing venous congestion and hypoxia of the central nervous system.

**PORTAL SYSTEM OF DRAINAGE.** Splenic congestion has already been described. In addition, abnormal accumulations of transudate in the peritoneal cavity may give rise to ascites. Congestion of the gut may cause intestinal disturbances.

In summary, right-sided heart failure presents essentially as a systemic venous congestive syndrome, with hepatic and splenic enlargement, peripheral edema, and ascites. In contrast to left-sided failure, respiratory symptoms may be absent or quite insignificant. *It is to be emphasized at this point that although the consideration of heart failure has been divided into two functional units, in the usual case of frank chronic cardiac decompensation, these early stages have already passed, and the patient presents with the picture of full-blown CHF, encompassing the clinical syndromes of both right- and left-heart failure.*

With this overview of the clinical implications of diseases of the heart, we can turn to consideration of the most important ones.

# ISCHEMIC HEART DISEASE (IHD)—CORONARY HEART DISEASE (CHD)

IHD and CHD are the generic designations for four forms of cardiac disease that result from an imbalance between the myocardial need for oxygen and its supply.[5, 6] In most cases, the imbalance results from insufficient blood flow secondary to complications of atherosclerotic narrowing of the coronary arteries, hence the term "coronary heart disease." The four patterns—(1) angina pectoris, (2) sudden cardiac death, (3) myocardial infarction, and (4) chronic ischemic heart disease—represent a continuum based on the speed of development of the coronary insufficiency and its severity and distribution. These factors determine the outcome of the clinical episode and whether or not there is morphological damage to the myocardium. The first three categories are acute events that are included in the lay rubric, "heart attack."

*Angina pectoris (AP)* is a symptom complex consisting of severe paroxysmal chest pain resulting from transient ischemia.[7] Although hypoxic injury to myocardial cells may be present, it is typically reversible, and, by definition, clinical evidence of infarction does not develop. *Sudden cardiac death (SCD)* is a syndrome in which death occurs rapidly, as fast as a few seconds or minutes, after the onset of symptoms; it is due to an arrhythmia. Although a number of cardiac diseases and noncardiac conditions, including massive pulmonary embolism and intracranial hemorrhage, can be responsible for SCD, the leading cause is IHD. *Myocardial infarction (MI)* is another catastrophic form of IHD, which results usually from sudden and severe inadequacy of the coronary flow. Most often MI is related to a thrombotic occlusion superimposed on underlying severe atherosclerosis of a main coronary arterial trunk. However, in some cases, other mechanisms are involved. Nevertheless, in all cases there are one or more foci of acute myocardial necrosis, either transmural or confined to the subendocardial region. *Chronic ischemic heart disease (CIHD)* is applied to those cases in which episodes of ischemia have resulted in scattered small foci of myocardial scarring and, not infrequently, additional larger areas of scarring from past episodes of acute infarction. Generally, CIHD evolves from slow, progressive narrowing of the coronary arteries, which occurs over a span of years. Obviously there is much overlap among these four patterns. The patient with CIHD is vulnerable to angina and to the

development of an acute MI. By the same token, attacks of angina carry the ominous threat that the ischemia will at some time result in an infarct or sudden cardiac death.

It is impossible to overemphasize the importance of IHD as a cause of mortality and morbidity in affluent societies. Alone it accounts for over one quarter of all deaths in the United States, representing about 550,000 deaths annually. It is estimated that currently there are approximately 7,000,000 patients in the United States who have just had an MI or are recovering from one.[8] Analogous data apply to most countries in northwestern Europe, Canada, Australia, and New Zealand. As mentioned earlier, however, there are some grounds for optimism. The epidemic of ischemic heart disease appears to have begun to wane in the United States, Canada, Australia, and Finland. Between 1972 and 1984, the age-adjusted death rate from ischemic heart disease declined by 33.9% (data from American Heart Association). This is not unreasonably attributed to a decrease in coronary atherosclerosis (see Chapter 10 for further discussion).

**PATHOGENESIS.** Myocardial ischemia exists when there is an imbalance between myocardial oxygen delivery and myocardial oxygen demand. Depending upon the severity, duration, and frequency of the ischemic episodes, any of the four clinical syndromes may result. Elucidation of the pathogenesis of myocardial ischemia has been a difficult problem that has been enveloped in confusion and controversy for many years. In the past decade, new insights have provided a more coherent picture of this complex process. From our current level of understanding, the following concepts have emerged.

Because all four patterns of IHD are usually associated with coronary atherosclerosis, some general comments about the arterial involvement, applicable to all four clinical patterns of disease, are in order.[9]

○ The genesis of coronary atherosclerosis is identical to that of systemic atherosclerosis, already discussed on page 287, and the same "risk factors" apply. However, coronary involvement may be more or less severe than systemic involvement in individual cases.

○ The extent and, surprisingly, the severity of coronary artery atherosclerosis are often much the same in the four clinical patterns of IHD.

○ In fatal IHD, at least one and usually two (or all three) major coronary trunks have more than a 75% reduction of the cross-sectional area (equivalent to a 50% reduction in diameter) of the lumen. This degree of narrowing imposes a greater resistance to flow than that imposed by the more distal arterioles and capillary beds. It follows that lesser degrees of narrowing of the lumens of the major coronary trunks have little or no effect on myocardial perfusion.

○ Frequently several points of stenosis are present in one or more of the major coronary trunks.

○ The most severe atherosclerotic narrowings of the coronary arteries are typically located within the first 2 cm of the left anterior descending and left circumflex arteries and the proximal and distal thirds of the right coronary artery. Occasionally, the left main stem is stenosed prior to its bifurcation.

Although coronary atherosclerosis is the usual subsoil causing myocardial ischemia, a number of mechanisms may more or less acutely reduce myocardial perfusion. Among these, coronary thrombosis superimposed on atherosclerosis is the most ominous, but first we will briefly consider other mechanisms.

Some episodes of acute ischemia are triggered by *increased oxygen demand* in the presence of coronary atherosclerosis. States of physical exertion, excitement, and anxiety can cause ischemia by increasing the major determinants of myocardial oxygen demand—heart rate, myocardial contractility, and blood pressure. Since even in the normal heart myocardial oxygen extraction is near maximal under resting conditions, the only way that the stress-induced increased oxygen demand can be met is by increasing coronary blood flow. Although very severe stenosis is required to reduce resting blood flow through a coronary artery, somewhat less severe stenosis can limit the maximal potential flow through the vessel. Thus, when the stenotic coronary arteries are not capable of delivering the required increment of blood flow during a stressful situation, myocardial ischemia results.

Other mechanisms may unfavorably alter the myocardial demand-supply equation. In patients with coronary atherosclerosis, ischemia may result from the superimposition of any condition that lowers the oxygen-carrying capacity of the blood (e.g., anemia, carbon monoxide poisoning, or a defective oxyhemoglobin dissociation). In addition, hypotensive crises may precipitate myocardial ischemia in patients with coronary atherosclerosis. Typical clinical settings for the latter include surgery and traumatic injury. However, in most patients, these systemic factors are not operative, and the cause of the impaired oxygen delivery lies within the coronary arteries. *Current evidence for the pathogenesis of acute coronary events points to recurrent platelet aggregation, occlusive thrombosis, and, in some cases, coronary arterial spasm, often aided and abetted by degenerative changes in the plaque. In individual patients, these mechanisms may operate singly or in combination to produce ischemia.*

*Coronary arterial spasm* is a paroxysmal, severe, focal or multifocal vasoconstriction of one or more coronary arteries, producing transient occlusion of the vessels.[10, 11] Although the existence of coronary spasm was long suspected, its occurrence was proved only with the advent of coronary angiography. Vasospasm has been shown to be the mechanism responsible for an unusual form of angina pectoris, known as Prinzmetal's angina pectoris (p. 319). In those with coronary arterial spasm, the paroxysmal event is superimosed on fixed atherosclerotic stenosis in about two thirds of cases, but it involves usually patent coronary arteries in the others. Thus, coronary spasm is an attractive explanation for the occurrence of IHD in the small percentage of patients in whom ischemia develops in the absence of significant atherosclerosis. However, coronary vasospasm has been demonstrated at coronary angiography in only about 10% of patients with IHD that have been studied. Thus, the importance of vasospasm as a generally operative mechanism in IHD is uncertain. The cause of vasospasm in predisposed individuals also is unknown, although speculation is centered around altered autonomic neural control of the coronary vasculature, altered contractile function of vascular smooth muscle, and local release of vasoactive chemicals.[12] There have been few anatomic studies of vessels known to be vasospastic during life. One recent study reported increased numbers of mast cells in the artery wall at a site of previous vasospasm, suggesting that vasoactive mediators released from mast cells may be involved.[13]

Another factor in the causation of IHD is *platelet aggregation* leading to formation of platelet *microthrombi* at the site of a stenotic atherosclerotic plaque. Documentation of this relatively subtle phenomenon has been difficult, but several lines of evidence have gradually emerged, which, together, suggest that platelet aggregation is an important mechanism of IHD. In humans, products released during platelet aggregation, including thromboxane, are increased in the coronary circulation during episodes of myocardial ischemia.[14, 15] In patients with fatal IHD, platelet aggregates can be demonstrated, upon careful search, in major coronary arteries and in the coronary microcirculation.[16] Finally, recurrent platelet aggregation has been shown to cause cyclical reductions in coronary blood flow in animals with experimental coronary stenoses.[17] It is likely that platelet aggregation is initiated at the site of a coronary stenosis by local damage or loss of endothelium, possibly induced by hemodynamic trauma or by intrinsic degenerative change in the plaque.[18] One hypothesis for the subsequent development of platelet aggregation involves altered prostaglandin homeostasis, specifically, a shift in the normal balance between endothelium-derived prostacyclin (a platelet antiaggregant and a vasodilator) and platelet-derived thromboxane (a platelet proaggregant and a vasoconstrictor). However, platelet attachment, aggregation, and other interactions with the vessel wall are complex phenomena that are modulated by a number of chemical mediators. In addition to being affected by prostaglandins, platelet aggregation in IHD may be influenced by multiple chemical mediators, such as locally increased concentrations of adenosine diphosphate, serotonin, catecholamines, histamine, and platelet-activating factor. The consequences of platelet microthrombosis include physical narrowing or

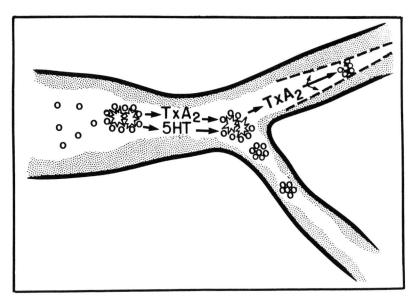

Figure 11–3. Possible mechanisms by which platelet aggregation may decrease coronary blood flow in the patient with ischemic heart disease. Platelet aggregation develops in atherosclerotic coronary arteries at sites of endothelial injury. Aggregating platelets release chemical mediators, including thromboxane A₂ ($TxA_2$) and serotonin (or 5-hydroxytryptamine, 5HT), which cause further platelet aggregation downstream and dynamic alterations in coronary vascular tone. (From Willerson, J. T., et al.: Speculation regarding mechanisms responsible for acute ischemic heart disease syndromes. J. Am. Coll. Cardiol. 8:245, 1986. Reprinted with permission from the American College of Cardiology.)

obstruction of the lumen by the platelet mass at the site of the coronary stenosis as well as vasoconstriction of the adjacent vessel due to release of vasoactive platelet products. Endothelium produces a relaxing factor in addition to prostacyclin, and when endothelium is lost, the vasoconstrictor response of smooth muscle is enhanced. Thus, platelet microthrombosis may induce an element of vasospasm. It is possible that coronary vasospasm and platelet microthrombosis represent a continuum with endothelial injury as a common underlying factor (Fig. 11–3).

Obviously, platelet aggregation on a coronary stenosis is an unstable situation. Detachment of the platelet mass will lead to improved blood flow, which may or may not be followed by a new episode of platelet aggregation. Observations consistent with such episodes have been made in experimental animals and in humans. Although the process may resolve, the other potential outcome is progression to occlusive thrombosis. Clinical evidence in favor of platelet aggregation in the pathogenesis of IHD has come from reports of improved prognosis in patients with certain IHD syndromes following treatment with inhibitors of platelet aggregation such as aspirin and dipyridamole.

*Coronary thrombosis* is of major importance in IHD because it results in rapid and persistent occlusion of a coronary artery and is frequently associated with acute myocardial infarction.[6, 19–24] The probable sequence of events in the formation of some thrombi involves progressive atherosclerosis leading to coronary stenosis, sluggish blood flow, endothelial injury, platelet aggregation, and activation of the coagulation cascade, with an occlusive thrombus as the result. However, in many cases, even more profound changes in the vessel wall lead to coronary thrombosis. Atheromatous plaques with soft necrotic centers and thin fibrous capsules are particularly prone to undergo fissuring, erosion, or ulceration of the

surface. The loss of endothelial integrity can lead to insudation of blood products or actual hemorrhage into the plaque from the luminal surface, followed by an increase in plaque pressure, expansion of the plaque, and, ultimately, its rupture. Cholesterol-rich material is released into the circulation. The flaps of the ruptured plaques can contribute to luminal obstruction. Exposure of the blood to the thrombogenic plaque interior predisposes to thrombus formation. Thus, *most occlusive thrombi form on complicated plaques with fissuring, erosion, ulceration, hemorrhage, or rupture* (Fig. 11–4). These acute changes usually involve large stenotic plaques, but they can occur with plaques that had previously produced minimal stenosis. Once thrombi form, mechanisms are initiated to reestablish the lumen of the occluded artery. These involve activation of the fibrinolytic system, retraction of thrombus from a portion of the vessel wall, and, subsequently, organization of the thrombus. However, the occlusion usually persists for at least several hours.

Other rare causes of coronary arterial insufficiency include coronary embolism; a dissecting aortic aneurysm, which extends back into the walls of the coronary arteries; osteal stenosis in luetic aortitis; direct trauma to the coronary vessels, which causes thrombosis; and a variety of arteritides (polyarteritis nodosa, Kawasaki's disease, and temporal arteritis).

It is important to understand that the consequences of a sudden coronary occlusion can be significantly influenced by several chronic and interacting processes such as the rate of development, the extent and severity of atherosclerosis, and various compensatory mechanisms in the heart. Thus, during the course of slowly progressive atherosclerosis, anastomotic channels can enlarge and mature within the distribution of a single major coronary bed (intracoronary collaterals), between major coronary arteries (intercoronary collaterals), and between coronary and medias-

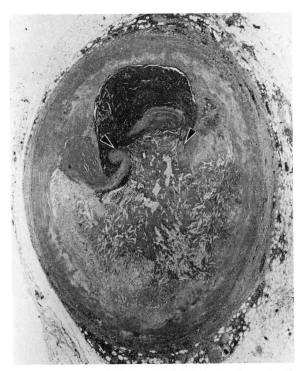

Figure 11–4. Coronary artery with ruptured atherosclerotic plaque and occlusive thrombus. The ruptured plaque has a thin fibrous capsule and a large core of lipid-rich material including slit-like cholesterol crystals. Note the separation of the capsule (*arrowhead*), outward displacement of plaque contents across the rupture site, and communication of plaque contents with the overlying thrombus. (From Buja, L. M., and Willerson, J. T.: Clinicopathologic correlates of acute ischemic heart disease syndromes. Am. J. Cardiol. 47:343, 1981.)

tinal arteries (extracoronary collaterals), thereby establishing a functionally significant collateral circulation. However, the magnitude of this collateral circulation varies significantly from case to case. Therefore, the extent of myocardial damage following an acute coronary occlusion can vary considerably. Finally, the induction of myocardial ischemia may involve an interaction between coronary atherosclerosis and factors that adversely affect the relationship between myocardial demand and supply of oxygen. Thus, myocardial hypertrophy, hypertension, and aortic stenosis can predispose to ischemia with less severe coronary arterial disease. In concluding these general comments, it merits reemphasis that in IHD there is almost always some atherosclerotic involvement of the coronary arteries, but it may be minimal, and, as has already been pointed out, other mechanisms may lead to the critical hypoxia. Against this general background of the causes of IHD we can turn to specific patterns.

## ANGINA PECTORIS (AP)

Angina pectoris is a clinical syndrome characterized by paroxysmal chest pain associated with episodes of transient hypoxic insult to the myocardium that typically fall precariously short of causing myocardial necrosis.[5–7] By definition, clinical evidence of myocardial infarction is not present. The pain is usually substernal or precordial, often radiating to the left shoulder and arm or to the jaw, and it typically lasts for several minutes. The mechanism by which myocardial ischemia causes referred pain has not been resolved. Three distinctive subsets of this condition are now recognized: (1) typical AP, (2) variant angina or Prinzmetal's angina, and (3) unstable angina. *Typical angina* occurs during exertion, when the elevation of heart rate, myocardial contractility, or blood pressure (or all three) increase myocardial oxygen demand, and myocardial ischemia results from an imbalance between demand and the available supply through stenotic coronary arteries. Electrocardiograms reveal ST-segment depression because the ischemic focus appears to be largely limited to the subendocardial region of the left ventricle. The episodes are typically relieved promptly by rest and nitroglycerin. In contrast, *Prinzmetal's variant angina* occurs at rest and therefore is not triggered by increased myocardial demand. Rather, it is related to episodic reduction of the myocardial blood supply, with resultant transmural ischemia and ST-segment elevation in the electrocardiogram. Coronary arterial spasm has been shown to be the cause of this syndrome. Occasionally, patients manifest symptom complexes intermediate between typical and variant angina.

*Unstable angina pectoris* refers to progressive angina, characterized by increasing frequency or duration of episodes, or both, with the angina frequently occurring at rest.[5–7] Severe and prolonged episodes of ischemia are often referred to as "acute coronary insufficiency." In some patients, unstable angina may occur when luminal narrowing reaches a critical point during the final stages of progression of severe multifocal atherosclerosis. However, in most patients other factors are likely involved, since there is not a perfect correlation between IHD and anatomic extent of atherosclerosis. Platelet aggregation and coronary arterial spasm have been implicated in the pathogenesis of unstable angina pectoris, but the exact contribution of these factors in individual patients is often difficult to determine.[18] Although, by definition, clinical evidence of myocardial infarction is not present, fatal cases may exhibit small foci of myocardial necrosis at autopsy.[6] The course of unstable angina pectoris is variable and may include improvement (either spontaneous or with medical treatment), fatal arrhythmia, or progression to myocardial infarction. Angina, whatever the type, constitutes a "red flag" warning of the precariousness of the balance of the myocardial demand and supply; however, episodes of myocardial ischemia can occur without clinically manifest angina pectoris. Diabetic patients are particularly prone to so-called silent myocardial ischemia.

## SUDDEN CARDIAC DEATH (SCD)

Persons suffering SCD from IHD represent those unfortunate individuals who either experience sudden chest pain and die within minutes to hours, typically outside of the hospital, or who collapse on the street or at home and are dead on arrival at the hospital.[25] SCD is responsible for 350,000 deaths per year, representing over half of all IHD deaths. Some subjects may have had previous clinically recognized episodes of IHD, whereas in others SCD may be the first and last manifestation of IHD. Previously, it was widely but incorrectly assumed that acute myocardial infarction was responsible for essentially all cases of SCD in IHD. It is true that *postmortem studies of subjects with SCD show a high incidence of significant coronary artery disease, and some have evidence of old, healed infarcts, but only a small fraction have recent myocardial infarcts or, in most studies, recent occlusive coronary thrombi at autopsy.*[26–29] However, study of SCD is complicated by the fact that MI is not detectable by standard gross and light microscopic techniques for several hours after the onset of irreversible injury, giving rise to the previous assumption about the relationship between MI and SCD. Recently new insights have been provided by the advent of techniques to resuscitate potential SCD victims in the community. Several studies have shown that only a minority of patients who are resuscitated after virtual SCD later have detectable acute MI.[25] For example, in one large study, there were 923 individuals who were unconscious, pulseless, and in ventricular fibrillation when medical assistance arrived.[30] Of the 146 who were successfully resuscitated, only 17% later showed diagnostic evidence of a recent MI on serial electrocardiograms. Thus, there are two subsets of patients within the category of SCD, with the common thread being a fatal arrhythmia, usually ventricular fibrillation. One subset consists of a smaller group of patients who have had a recent MI, most often a subendocardial infarct that is complicated by an arrhythmia, and the other consists of a much larger group who develop an arrhythmia in the absence of an MI. It is likely that most of the latter cases of fatal arrhythmia are triggered by episodes of myocardial ischemia produced in many cases by a coronary event—vasospasm, platelet aggregation, or even thrombosis—and, in some cases, by increased myocardial oxygen demand induced by exertion or some other stress.

It is important to remember that ischemia rapidly induces shifts in potassium, calcium, and sodium between cells and the extracellular fluid, creating the potential for altered electrical activity and, ultimately, ventricular fibrillation, and that these ischemia-induced electrical changes develop during the potentially reversible phase of injury. Another interesting observation in many cases of SCD is that even though confluent myocardial necrosis of an MI is absent, there may be multiple small foci of hypercontraction injury in the myocytes, an alteration that also can be produced by exposure of the heart to excess amount of catecholamines.[27] These observations suggest the possibility that abnormal catecholamine discharge may participate in the process of SCD.[31] Finally, some fatal arrhythmias may develop without new ischemia in a subset of patients with previous myocardial damage. In these patients myocardial fibrosis can lead to aberrant electrical conduction with the potential for the sudden formation of an ectopic, rapidly conducting focus that precipitates ventricular fibrillation. Thus, *patients with IHD may develop SCD from a ventricular arrhythmia induced by ischemia or aberrant conduction, or they may develop an acute MI that secondarily initiates an arrhythmia at any point in the course.* In spite of the evidence indicating that primary SCD and acute MI are separate entities, accurate diagnosis in individual patients is difficult. Furthermore, although some progress has been made, identification of those factors that will predispose a given patient to sudden arrhythmic death remains a major challenge.

## MYOCARDIAL INFARCTION (MI)

Acute ischemic necrosis of an area of myocardium—myocardial infarction—is a dramatic and potentially lethal pattern of IHD and is a major cause of death in industrialized nations. Moreover, sequelae of acute infarcts, which manifest themselves months to years later as chronic ischemic heart disease, account for a major proportion of the remaining deaths caused by IHD. Thus, acute IHD, including sudden cardiac death and documented MI, and its aftereffects account for about 20 to 30% of all deaths in atherosclerosis-prone societies. The critical event that suddenly alters the supply of oxygen to regions of the myocardium in MI involves coronary thrombosis or one of the other pathophysiological factors discussed on page 317.

**EPIDEMIOLOGY.** The prevalence of myocardial infarction in a population, as you would surmise, follows the distribution of severe atherosclerosis. The prevalence of fatal MI rises with age to peak in the 55- to 64-year-old group in males and in the eighth decade in females. However, the disease continues to exact a high toll in the very elderly. Individuals with such predispositions to atherosclerosis as hypertension, diabetes mellitus, and familial hyperlipoproteinemia may suffer an infarct in the early decades of life. *Males are more vulnerable than females, with an overall ratio of 3:1.* This male preponderance is most striking between the ages of 33 and 55 years, with a male-to-female risk in these years of about 6:1. During reproductive life, women, for reasons still unknown, are remarkably spared unless they have an underlying predisposition to atherosclerosis, such as diabetes mellitus. In the later decades, the male preponderance steadily diminishes and approaches

1:1 in extreme old age. The risk factors leading to such a distribution of this disease have already been considered in the earlier discussion of atherosclerosis. In addition to the "big four"—hypertension, hypercholesterolemia, cigarette smoking, and diabetes mellitus—two other influences that bear on myocardial infarction should be brought up here: physical activity and the use of oral contraceptives. However, before discussing these it might be mentioned that there is no substantial evidence of a genetic or familial predisposition, other than that related to such risk factors as hyperlipidemia, hypertension, and diabetes, which do run in families.

There is a widely prevalent opinion that regular strenuous exercise protects against coronary atherosclerosis and myocardial infarction. Witness the epidemic of jogging. Indeed, statistical data drawn from comparisons of postal carriers with postal clerks, farmers and other laborers with the rest of the community, and marathon runners with sedentary individuals all suggest that vigorous exercise reduces the rate of fatal heart attacks.[32] Several studies point out that strenuous physical activity tends to raise the serum level of high-density lipoproteins.[33] Earlier (p. 288) it was pointed out that elevated levels of high-density lipoproteins appear to exert a protective effect against atherogenesis. There is additional evidence that physical conditioning augments the fibrinolytic response and might conceivably constitute an important protective mechanism in the resolution of thrombi within coronary arteries.[34] Despite all these observations, it has been suggested that individuals who engage in strenuous activity tend to have family backgrounds relatively free of MI and so are protected by hereditary and constitutional factors and not by the exercise itself. There is as yet no firm conclusion as to the role of physical activity in protecting against myocardial infarctions,[35] but even sedentary writers of textbooks must concede that the accumulating evidence suggests a beneficial effect.

There is also controversy about the effect of oral contraceptive pills with high estrogen content on the incidence of MI. This issue is discussed in some detail on page 266. It suffices for here to state that the overall risk of developing fatal MI is approximately five times higher among women who use oral contraceptives with a high estrogen content than among those who do not use these "pills," and that *this increased risk largely occurs among a subgroup of women who are also over 35 and smoke.* Although it is expected that the newer "pills" with their reduced estrogen content will substantially reduce the hazard, this remains to be proved.

**PATHOGENESIS.** *It is important at the outset of this consideration to emphasize that acute myocardial infarcts are largely localized to the left ventricle and take one of two forms: (1) a transmural lesion conventionally defined as greater than 2.5 cm in greatest extent that traverses virtually from endocardium into the subepicardial myocardium and (2) a subendocar-* *dial infarct, usually confined to the inner one half to one third of the left ventricular wall. The transmural infarct is more common than the subendocardial lesion.*

The pathogenesis of the transmural infarct has been the subject of controversy in the past, in part because a distinction was not made between SCD and MI. However, *current evidence favors the view that thrombosis superimposed on a complicated stenosing atheroma is the dominant cause of the ischemic necrosis of the dependent myocardium.*[6, 19–24] The stenosis is usually greater than 75% of the cross-sectional lumen of the vessel, and the events that initiate the thrombosis are discussed in detail on page 318. *In this view, the thrombosis is the critical event that causes the MI.* There is indeed much evidence to support such a conception. In many postmortem surveys, occlusive thrombi have been identified in 85 to 95% of acute transmural infarcts.[6, 19–24] Moreover, in most instances, the thrombus was anatomically related to the infarct in such a way as to make it likely that it was the cause of the infarct. In some postmortem studies of fatal IHD, however, the same high incidence of thrombosis has not been found, leading to the suggestion that thrombosis may occur sporadically and as a secondary event in MI.[36, 37] It has been suggested that myocardial necrosis might be triggered directly in the myocardium by factors such as excess neural stimulation and release of catecholamines.[38] Experimentally, myocardial necrosis begins in the subendocardium and proceeds as a "wavefront" into the subepicardium,[39] and, in humans, subendocardial infarction frequently occurs without occlusive coronary thrombosis. Yet there is little direct evidence to support other triggering mechanisms for transmural MI. Furthermore, case selection and classification can influence the results of the postmortem studies. Even if myocardial ischemia can be initiated by other factors, the evidence indicates that occlusive coronary thrombosis is a major factor in the genesis of transmural ischemia and infarction.

Recent studies on living patients have provided strong supportive evidence for the role of thrombosis in transmural MI. In one series, angiography performed within four hours of the onset of symptoms revealed total coronary occlusion in 87% of patients with an acute MI.[40] A thrombus could be withdrawn from the occluded coronary arteries during coronary bypass surgery in the great majority of such cases. In other patients, when the angiography was performed 12 to 24 hours after onset of symptoms, coronary occlusion was found in fewer cases (65%). These angiographic findings have been extensively confirmed.[41, 42] Furthermore, many patients with unstable angina pectoris have angiographic evidence of complicated coronary lesions with features suggestive of plaque erosion and microthrombosis.[43–45] Such lesions may progress to occlusive thrombosis in association with the development of MI. What of the

5 to 15% of patients with transmural MIs that have no demonstrable coronary thrombus? Some of these cases may be caused by coronary spasm, platelet aggregation, or possibly a thrombus that was removed by fibrinolysis or fragmentation. Such phenomena likely account for the findings in the angiographic study cited above. The relationship between coronary artery spasm, platelet aggregation, and occlusive thrombosis were discussed in a previous section.

*The pathogenesis of the subendocardial infarct is multifactorial.*[46] Subendocardial MIs may consist of a single focus of necrosis in the inner half of the left ventricular wall or multiple foci scattered about the circumference of the left ventricle. There is agreement that the left ventricular subendocardium is the cardiac region most susceptible to ischemia, primarily because of a tenuous oxygen supply-demand relationship. There is also general agreement that, *although severe stenosing atherosclerosis is usually present in one or more of the three main coronary trunks, superimposed thromboses and total occlusions are present in only about one third or less of these hearts.*[6, 19–24] In a few cases with occlusive thrombosis, relatively abundant collateral blood flow apparently limits the necrosis to the subendocardium. In other cases, coronary arterial spasm or platelet microthrombosis are responsible. In still others, dynamic factors, such as strenuous exercise, hypertension, congestive heart failure, or hypotension, are superimposed on severe coronary atherosclerosis and result in sufficient impairment of the relationship of myocardial oxygen supply and demand to cause subendocardial necrosis.

**MORPHOLOGY.** Both transmural and subendocardial infarcts are largely limited to the left ventricle. Contiguous involvement of the right ventricle is encountered in up to 20 to 30% of transmural infarcts of the inferoposterior wall and posterior portion of the septum, usually related to severe atherosclerosis of the **right** coronary artery. Contiguous involvement of the left atrium is uncommon. Isolated right ventricular infarcts are only seen when there is marked right ventricular hypertrophy, as may occur in cor pulmonale (p. 338). First the classic transmural infarct will be described, followed by some brief comments about the subendocardial infarct.

As the term implies, the **transmural infarct** extends virtually from the endocardium into the subepicardial myocardium, covering an area ranging from 2.5 cm in diameter to possibly encompassing the entire circumference of the left ventricle. The distribution of the arterial involvement and the resultant areas of infarction are as follows:

| | | |
|---|---|---|
| Left anterior descending coronary artery | 40–50% | Anterior wall of left ventricle; anterior two thirds of interventricular septum |
| Right coronary artery | 30–40% | Posterior (inferior) wall of left ventricle; posterior one third of interventricular septum |
| Left circumflex coronary artery | 15–20% | Lateral wall of left ventricle |

Typically stenosis or thrombosis is generally found in the first 2 cm of the two major divisions of the left coronary artery and the proximal and distal third of the right coronary artery. All infarcts have an irregular perimeter dictated by the pattern of the interdigitating vascular supply.

The gross appearance of the infarct depends upon the duration of survival of the patient following the critical event, but a fairly predictable sequence of changes ensues.[47] **No grossly visible changes are evident in infarcts less than six to 12 hours old.** At this time, a slight pallor may be present. In these recent lesions (three to six hours old), it may be possible to highlight the loss of dehydrogenase activity in the necrotic focus macroscopically by exposing cross sections of the ventricle to triphenyl-tetrazolium chloride, which imparts a red-brown color to the noninfarcted myocardium, leaving the pale, enzyme-depleted infarcted area unstained.[48] By 18 to 24 hours, the pallor even in unstained cross sections is more clearly evident. Between the second and fourth day, the necrotic focus becomes more sharply defined, with a hyperemic border, and the central portion becomes yellow-brown and soft. By the tenth day, the color change is well developed and the infarct is quite yellow and maximally soft, often containing areas of hemorrhage. Thereafter the lesion becomes rimmed by an intensely red, highly vascularized zone of granulation tissue, which is progressively replaced by pale gray scarring over the

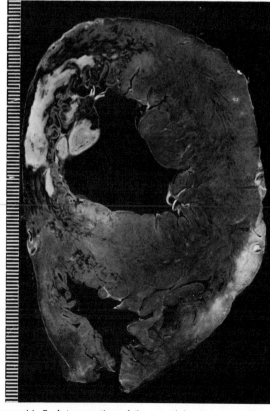

Figure 11–5. A transection of the ventricles to expose the 10- to 14-day-old myocardial infarct seen on the left. The pale, sharply demarcated fatty areas are surrounded by a darker rim of vascularized, fibrous, early repair.

course of time (Fig. 11–5). The ingrowth of the granulation tissue into the necrotic area and the scarring are well advanced by the end of the sixth week, but the time required for total replacement depends, of course, on the size of the original lesion.

A number of ancillary gross changes may appear during the progression of the acute MI. The earliest change is the appearance of a **fibrinous pericarditis,** which may be more or less localized to the area of necrosis or be generalized. Such fibrinous exudation usually resolves, but occasionally it leads to the development of delicate fibrous adhesions, which do not often impair cardiac function. An **intraventricular mural thrombus** may develop in relation to the zone of endocardial damage, providing a potential source of **arterial embolism.** If it is to develop, it usually appears within the first week. **Rupture of the infarct** with cardiac tamponade occurs in 1 to 5% of cases, generally toward the end of the first week or at the beginning of the second, when the lesion is maximally soft.[49] Much later in the course, when the infarct has already undergone fibrous scarring, stretching of the scar may lead to a so-called **ventricular aneurysm.** It may be followed by mural thrombosis within the aneurysmal dilatation.

The histologic progression of events seen in routine tissue stains by light microscopy are those typical of coagulative ischemic necrosis seen in all cells. First these will be briefly reviewed, followed by some details of ultrastructural and histochemical alterations that may aid in the identification of very early infarcts. Stretching and waviness of myocardial fibers at the border of the ischemic area may be evident by light microscopy in some cases within an hour of onset of the infarct.[50, 51] These alterations are nonspecific. The first unmistakable evidence of cell death by light microscopy appears in about four to six hours in the form of cytoplasmic eosinophilic coagulative changes sometimes accompanied by clumping and condensation of the nuclear chromatin. Soon thereafter, some shrinkage of the cells appears, along with intercellular edema and neutrophilic infiltration in the margins of the infarct (Fig. 11–6). Even in transmural infarcts a few layers of subepicardial and subendocardial myofibers are preserved, presumably because of auxiliary epicardial blood supply and transendocardial imbibition. Although myocytes in the infarct center are arrested in a relaxed state, the myocytes at the edges of the infarct receive some marginal perfusion and eventually die in a hypercontracted state, which produces intensely eosinophilic, transverse "contraction bands" in these myocytes. During the subsequent days, the neutrophilic exudation increases, the necrotic fibers become more distinctly coagulated, the nuclei become pyknotic and subsequently disappear, and the cross striations within the fibers become indistinct. Toward the end of the first week, there is progressive removal of the sarcoplasmic carcasses by autolysis, heterolysis, and phagocytosis by infiltrating macrophages. The fibrovascular ingrowth pointed out in the gross description becomes evident in the margins at the end of the first week or in the second week and progressively invades the necrotic lesion as the dead

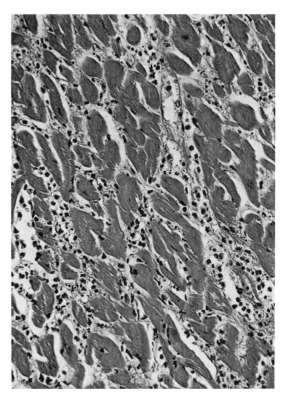

Figure 11–6. A fresh myocardial infarct 48 to 72 hours old. All the fibers have undergone coagulative necrosis, nuclei have disappeared, and there is an interstitial inflammatory reaction with edema and neutrophil infiltration.

cells are removed. Thereafter, collagenous scarring progressively replaces the necrotic cells.

A great deal of attention has been directed toward methods of identifying infarcts within the early hours after their onset.[50, 51] Many patients die after an extremely brief course. Moreover, there is great interest in determining whether the "border zone" of the infarct is sharply defined soon after it occurs.[52, 53] Do dead cells directly abut on healthy cells or instead is there a gradation from living cells to reversibly injured cells to dead cells? If a "twilight zone" does exist, even for a brief time, it might be possible by therapeutic interventions to rescue the cells not yet irreversibly injured and thus reduce the size of the infarct. Regrettably, by 24 hours no injured but viable interface can be found.[39]

The electron microscope and histochemical techniques reveal changes long before they become apparent with the light microscope. Mitochondrial swelling first appears 15 to 20 minutes after the onset of complete ischemia and is followed by the sequence of changes detailed in the earlier consideration of hypoxic injury to cells (p. 7). Mitochondrial matrix densities and sarcolemmal membrane defects are early signs of probable irreversible injury. However, the ultrastructural abnormalities are not generally useful for the identification of hypoxic cell death because often they are obscured by the postmortem artifacts that have appeared between the time of death of the patient and the tissue sampling. Moreover, some period of reversible hypoxic injury may have transpired prior to the death of the cells, which would introduce yet another variable. Ultimately, you may recall, the line between reversible injury and lethal injury is difficult to define with the electron microscope.

Histochemical and biochemical techniques may be more helpful than the electron microscope in identifying early infarcts. The potassium levels of an area of infarction are somewhat reduced within an hour of the death of cells as their membranes become abnormally permeable. Reduced levels of succinic and isocitrate dehydrogenases,[54] cytochrome oxidase, and phosphorylase appear within the lesion in two or three hours after the onset of infarction. Depletion of glycogen, demonstrated by the PAS strain, begins within five minutes after coronary ligation in the experimental animal. In humans, glycogen depletion within an area of infarction is well developed in 30 to 60 minutes.[39] However, all of the methods described for the detection of early infarcts (reviewed in Table 11–1) are fallible. The state of preservation of the tissues following death and the varying rates of loss of enzymes, potassium, and glycogen from specific lesions make recognition of early infarcts difficult and somewhat uncertain.

Turning now to subendocardial infarcts, the light microscopic, ultrastructural, and histochemical changes seen in the cells of transmural infarcts are replicated in the subendocardial lesions. Only the macroscopic appearance and distribution of the lesion differs. Subendocardial infarcts typically appear as one or more areas of necrosis, confined to the inner one third to one half of the left ventricular wall. The lesions may be patchy or confluent, and they may be confined to the distribution of a single coronary artery or encompass a significant segment of the circumference of the left ventricle. After several hours, subendocardial infarcts become grossly visible. They may be pale or hemorrhagic, depending upon the extent of residual blood flow into the infarcted area. The small areas of necrosis undergo more rapid evolution than the larger transmural infarcts and so are replaced by granulation tissue in the course of two to three weeks and then undergo fibrous scarring. Although they may be complicated by mural thrombi overlying the adjacent endocardium, rupture, pericarditis, or ventricular aneurysms rarely appear.

**CLINICAL COURSE.** The onset of an MI is usually sudden and devastating, with intense, crushing substernal or precordial pain, often radiating to the left shoulder, arm, or jaw. The pain is frequently accompanied by sweating, some degree of breathlessness, and marked anxiety. There may be nausea and vomiting. In some individuals this calamitous event is preceded by a period of days to weeks of prodromal symptoms. The most common of these symptoms is undue fatigue, but there may also be a change in the pattern of preexisting angina pectoris or there may be the onset of dyspnea. Occasionally, the clinical manifestations of an acute MI are trivial and passed off by the patient as "indigestion." The onset may also be entirely painless, as is the case in as many as one third of patients.[55]

Patients with a myocardial infarct who survive to reach the hospital follow one of several courses. The outcome may be uneventful, with gradual subsidence

### Table 11–1. SEQUENCE OF CHANGES IN MYOCARDIAL INFARCTION

| Time | Electron Microscope | Histochemistry | Light Microscope | Gross Changes |
|------|---------------------|----------------|------------------|---------------|
| 0–2 hr | Mitochondrial swelling; distortion of cristae; matrix densities; relaxation of myofibrils; margination of nuclear chromatin | ↓ Dehydrogenases<br>↓ Oxidases<br>↓ Phosphorylases<br>↓ Glycogen<br>↓ K and ↑ Na$^+$ and Ca$^{++}$ | ? Waviness of fibers at border | |
| 4–12 hr | Margination of nuclear chromatin | | Beginning coagulation necrosis; edema; hemorrhage; beginning neutrophilic and macrophage infiltrate about dying and dead myofibers | |
| 18–24 hr | | | Continuing coagulation necrosis (pyknosis of nuclei, shrunken eosinophilic cytoplasm); marginal contraction band necrosis | Pallor |
| 24–72 hr | | | Total coagulative necrosis with loss of nuclei; heavy interstitial infiltrate of neutrophils | Pallor, sometimes hyperemia |
| 3–7 days | | | Beginning resorption of myofibers by macrophages; onset of marginal fibrovascular response | Hyperemic border; central yellow-brown softening |
| 10 days | | | Advanced cellular degradation; prominent fibrovascular reaction in margins | Maximally yellow and soft; vascularized margins, red-brown and depressed |
| 7th wk | | | | Scarring complete |

of symptoms and progressive healing, or it may be dominated by one or both of two types of sequelae: electrical derangements or pump failure. Disturbances in rate, rhythm, or conduction occur so commonly that they are virtually an inherent part of the process. Such arrhythmias have been reported in up to 90% of carefully monitored patients.[56] They are most common at the very outset and are almost always responsible for the early deaths. The most frequent arrhythmias are ventricular and atrial extrasystoles, sinus tachycardia, and sinus bradycardia. The most lethal are complete heart block, ventricular fibrillation, and sinus tachycardia. Because these disturbances can often be controlled, the deaths they cause are largely preventable and thus are particularly to be lamented.

With or without arrhythmias, the clinical picture may be dominated by the onset of pump failure, manifested as CHF. Some degree of left ventricular failure is an almost invariable accompaniment of an MI. Even when there are no clinical manifestations, careful studies demonstrate pulmonary vascular congestion and transudation into the interstitial space. In over 60% of patients, CHF is clinically apparent, but this may be very transient. In some patients, however, overt *pulmonary edema* develops, and this considerably worsens the prognosis.

Acute failure of the left ventricle implies not only pulmonary congestion but a diminished cardiac output as well. Commonly, there is some drop in blood pressure. This, too, is often of little consequence. However, when over 40% of the left ventricle is infarcted, a profound drop in cardiac output results, constituting *cardiogenic shock.*[57] This occurs in about 12% of patients. The onset of cardiogenic shock is of particularly grave import, since 80% of patients who develop it do not survive. When pulmonary edema and cardiogenic shock occur concomitantly, the outlook for the patient is bleak indeed.

Among the more typical patients who are followed from the inception of pain, the diagnosis is confirmed by electrocardiogram and enzyme changes. Although the ECG alterations are complex and beyond our scope, they can be briefly characterized with transmural infarcts as, first, elevation of the ST segment within 24 hours, followed by the development of abnormal Q waves and inversion of the T waves. Occasionally, however, depending on the location of the infarct, its size, and the number of electrocardiographic leads examined, ECG changes may be minimal or absent. Elevation of the serum level of isoenzymes, particularly creatine kinase-MB (CK-MB), is present in 80 to 85% of patients.[55] The MB isoenzyme is found in significant amounts only in heart muscle, and elevated levels of this enzyme thus constitute a highly specific and sensitive marker for MI. The mean appearance time of this isoenzyme following the onset of the infarct is about seven hours, and it is eliminated from the serum in about 48 hours. There are five isoenzymes of lactic dehydrogenase (LDH). Normally, serum levels of $LDH_1$ are lower than those of $LDH_2$. The reversal of this ratio is indicative of myocardial necrosis. The level of $LDH_1$ peaks later than CK-MB and so is useful in patients who present more than 48 hours after onset of symptoms. However, determinations of LDH are not as specific as those of CK, and false-positive results are encountered in other conditions (e.g., hemolytic disease and renal cortical necrosis).

The later complications of myocardial infarction include (1) rupture of the infarcted portion of the heart, which occurs most often in the week following infarction, when the ischemic focus is maximally soft. When the rupture communicates with the pericardial sac, tamponade and death follow at once. Rarely, rupture of the interventricular septum produces a left-to-right shunt and severe strain on the right heart. (2) Rupture of a papillary muscle, leading to severe mitral regurgitation with a loud murmur. (3) The development of a ventricular aneurysm at the point of scarring. (4) Various thromboembolic phenomena, which may arise from mural thrombi within the heart or from thrombosis in the deep veins of the legs, which develops during prolonged bed rest.

What can be said of the overall prognosis for the patient with an MI? Recall that sudden coronary death exacts a very high toll of those with IHD, but that many of these deaths cannot truly be attributed to infarction. More properly, they can be referred to as "acute ischemic events." Of patients who reach the hospital alive, about 10% succumb during the first month. The risk of death is greatest at the onset and declines rapidly with each passing day. Critically important in the outlook is the degree of left ventricular dysfunction. During the next six months, there is about a 9% mortality rate, which then drops to an annual rate of 3 to 4% for the subsequent four to five years.[55]

Promising to improve significantly the prognosis in these patients are current acute and long-term interventions. In patients with clinical evidence of an evolving MI, efforts are focused on immediate efforts to relieve pain, stabilize the patient hemodynamically, and, possibly, to reduce the size of the MI or prevent its extension.[8, 58] In experimental models, propranolol, calcium channel antagonists, hyaluronidase, and other modalities appear to reduce the extent of necrosis that develops in the ischemic "bed-at-risk." However, there is little evidence that similar results have been achieved in patients. The presence of a coronary occlusion limits the capacity of these agents to improve the oxygen supply and demand relationship. Recently, a direct and promising approach to relieve acute myocardial ischemia has been instituted in the treatment of transmural MI. This involves coronary thrombolytic therapy using streptokinase or tissue plasminogen–activating factor administered intravenously or via an intracoronary catheter.[41, 42] Reestablishment of coronary blood flow through a previously occluded coronary artery has been demonstrated in a high percentage of patients treated early with coronary thrombolytic therapy. However, the extent of salvage of jeopardized myocardium that can be achieved is still to be determined. It is important to remember that there are significant temporal restraints on all interventions designed to salvage myocardium in patients with evolving MI. Experimentally, transmural myocardial necrosis is completed within three to six hours of coronary occlusion, and so the period of maximum opportunity is limited to a few hours.[39]

A variety of other approaches are now in progress to reduce the awesome mortality from MI. Primary prevention aimed at lowering the incidence of MI by controlling the development of coronary atherosclerosis by modifying risk factors (e.g., hyperlipidemia, hypertension, cigarette smoking) is yielding promising results,[59] as discussed on page 295. Secondary prevention aimed at risk-factor modification in individuals who have had an acute event can be described as possibly beneficial. Other efforts are focused on more direct interventions in patients who are at high risk for the development of an MI, such as those with unstable AP. Medical therapy includes nitrates, calcium channel antagonists, adrenergic blocking drugs, and the antiplatelet agent aspirin. In two large clinical trials, aspirin has reduced the incidence of MI and death in patients presenting with unstable AP.[60] In patients who do not respond to medical therapy, coronary artery bypass surgery is often performed. This procedure involves the bypass of obstructive coronary lesions by the insertion of vascular grafts, derived from saphenous veins or internal mammary arteries, into the distal coronary arteries. The effectiveness of coronary bypass surgery has been the subject of much controversy. Although the procedure clearly relieves symptoms, it has been proved to reduce long-term mortality only in patients with left main coronary stenosis and possibly in those with severe multivessel coronary artery disease.[61] More recently, dilatation of stenotic coronary plaques has been performed in patients with angina by using balloon-tipped angiographic catheters. The long-term patency rate is yet to be determined with this procedure, which is known as percutaneous transluminal coronary angioplasty.[62] The combined use of coronary angioplasty and thrombolytic therapy in patients with early acute MI is also under investigation.

Yet another approach concerns itself with reducing the late post-MI mortality rate. Most of these deaths are attributable to sudden cardiac death from ventricular arrhythmias, recurrent MI, or progressive cardiac failure. Clinical trials have shown a beneficial effect on mortality rate in post-MI patients treated with agents that block the effects of adrenergic stimulation, including propranolol and timolol.[63] Antiplatelet therapy, including aspirin, has been less effective in preventing recurrent IHD in patients who have already sustained an MI than in preventing MI in those presenting with unstable angina pecto-

ris.[60] It is evident that the outcome for the patient following MI will likely change with the many therapeutic interventions under exploration. What effect they will have on the incidence of the disease and its morbidity and mortality, only time will tell. But the total effort currently expended will surely move even a mountain.

## CHRONIC ISCHEMIC HEART DISEASE (CIHD)

CIHD is by far the most common clinical as well as anatomic pattern of IHD and so is the most common of all cardiac diseases. It is also thought to be a major cause of unexplained heart failure, particularly in diabetic patients.[64] As explained earlier (p. 316), it comprises multifocal areas of myocardial atrophy and fibrosis secondary to slowly developing coronary atherosclerosis, sometimes accompanied by the larger scars of past infarcts. In the past this condition had also been called *arteriosclerotic heart disease*. Generally, patients with this form of myocardial damage, if they do not succumb to an intercurrent MI, eventually experience the insidious onset of cardiac decompensation and ultimately fatal CHF. However, the decompensation is generally amenable to therapeutic control for some time. The course of the disease may be very protracted unless, of course, it is punctuated by acute myocardial infarcts.

**MORPHOLOGY.** The pathognomonic anatomic criteria of this entity are atherosclerotic involvement of the coronary arteries and myocardial changes indicative of ischemic damage. The heart size is variable. It may be smaller than normal due to the multifocal scars or larger than normal due to compensatory hypertrophy, particularly in patients with larger infarcts and cardiac dilatation and failure. The coronary atherosclerosis is usually diffuse and responsible for widespread but irregular narrowing of all three major trunks. Total thrombotic occlusions may be present with or without evidence of prior episodes of infarction. As pointed out, collateral circulation or bypass channels may have prevented infarction despite occlusion of a coronary vessel. Within the myocardium there are scattered foci of gray fibrous pallor or larger, obviously fibrotic healed infarcts. In such areas of massive scarring, the wall is reduced in thickness and there is compensatory hypertrophy of the remaining, less involved myocardial wall. The epicardium and endocardium are generally normal in appearance but may have slight pearly opacity due to underlying fibrotic changes. Often there is atrophy of subepicardial fat commensurate with the loss of adipose tissue generally encountered in aged individuals. Valvular changes are inconstant and probably unrelated to the atherosclerotic process. When present, the leaflets of the left side of the heart may show slight fibrous thickening accompanied by some increased coarseness of the chordae tendineae of the mitral valve. Occasionally there is heavy calcification of the mitral annulus behind the valve leaflets and piled-up masses of calcium within

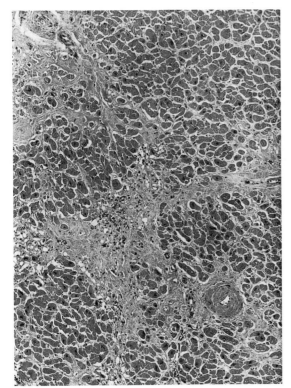

Figure 11–7. Patchy fibrous scarring principally about blood vessels of the myocardium in chronic ischemic heart disease.

the sinuses of the aortic leaflets. These changes are attributable to "wear and tear" over the span of decades rather than to ischemic injury.

**Microscopically, the distinctive features comprise (1) small fibrotic scars, usually about small vessels, and widening of the preexisting fibrous septa** (Fig. 11–7); **(2) isolated empty sheaths of myocardial fibers that have undergone ischemic necrosis with resorption of the sarcoplasm and nucleus (myocytolysis),**[65] and **(3) possibly large areas of scarring in those hearts that have had previous acute myocardial infarcts.** The diagnosis rests, then, on the presence of diffuse atherosclerotic disease and myocardial scarring secondary to ischemia.

**CLINICAL COURSE.** CIHD tends to progress slowly over the course of many years, manifesting itself only during periods of stress, such as with intercurrent infections. Usually it remains largely asymptomatic, and frequently it is discovered only as an incidental finding at autopsy. Eventually, however, if the patient does not succumb from other causes, sustained CHF develops. When scarring involves the cardiac conduction system, various arrhythmias may occur. Concomitant angina pectoris is common. Often, death results from a supervening MI or from a cardiac arrhythmia.

Congestive heart failure caused by CIHD is most often initially left-sided, due to the relatively greater demands on the left ventricle. Moreover, the thinner right ventricle appears to be less vulnerable to coronary arterial narrowing. Perhaps the transmural thebesian system is sufficient to sustain at least partially the thinner muscle mass. Right-sided CHF, however, ultimately follows chronic left-sided failure. Decompensation may develop insidiously or more or less acutely after a precipitating episode, such as pneumonia or an intercurrent MI. At one time, the prognosis after the onset of right-sided decompensation was poor, with survival time of only one to two years. However, with effective therapy, including sodium restriction and the administration of diuretics and digitalis glycosides, patients may survive comfortably for many years. The outlook is relatively better, of course, if there is a precipitating factor that can be modified.

## HYPERTENSIVE HEART DISEASE

This term refers to the secondary effects on the heart of prolonged, sustained systemic hypertension. Remarks here are limited to a brief description of the anatomic effects on the heart, since hypertension in general will be discussed on page 478.

Hypertensive heart disease is characterized anatomically principally by thickening of the left ventricle and an accompanying increase in the weight of the heart. The left ventricular wall may reach a thickness of more than 2.5 cm, and the weight of the heart may be increased to 500 to 700 gm. Thickening occurs inwardly at the expense of the left ventricular chamber and is therefore referred to as **concentric hypertrophy.** With the onset of CHF, however, the heart begins to dilate, and for the first time cardiac enlargement is discernible by chest x-ray or clinical examination. As dilatation progresses, the left ventricular wall becomes progressively stretched and thinned, which may obscure the preexistent thickening. Frequently there is coronary atherosclerosis, predisposed to by the hypertension.

Although the diameter of the individual myofibers is increased, it may be too slight to be evident with the light microscope. The nuclei are sometimes enlarged and may assume bizarre shapes secondary to polyploidy in these hypertrophied but nondividing cells. With the electron microscope, the hypertrophied fibers disclose many changes, including increased numbers and enlargement of mitochondria and increased synthesis of myofibrils.[66]

It should be emphasized that *the anatomic diagnosis of hypertensive heart disease can be made only in the absence of other lesions (e.g., valvular), which themselves can lead to increased cardiac work load, with consequent myocardial hypertrophy.* Even then, there must also be a history of hypertension or the presence of typical hypertensive vascular changes to establish the diagnosis since the cardiomyopathies, too, may produce cardiac enlargement without apparent cause.

# RHEUMATIC HEART DISEASE (RHD)

## RHEUMATIC FEVER (RF)

*Rheumatic fever is a systemic, nonsuppurative, inflammatory disease, often recurrent, which is most likely related to prior infection with group A beta-hemolytic streptococci. Although the pathogenesis is not completely clear, the disease probably represents an immune reaction in some way induced by the streptococcus.*[67, 68] The joints, heart, skin, serosa, blood vessels, and lungs are predominantly affected, in variable combinations. Although the joints are the single most frequent site of involvement and initially of most distress to the patients, *the importance of rheumatic fever derives entirely from its capacity to cause severe damage to the heart.* Its effects on other parts of the body are nearly always benign and transient.

Although rheumatic fever may occur at any age, 90% of patients have their first attack between the ages of five and 15 years. It is infrequent under the age of four years.[69] Males and females are affected equally. The incidence is higher among the poor, a fact that seems to be most strongly correlated with overcrowded living conditions and epidemics of streptococcal sore throats. Undoubtedly, limited access to adequate medical care of streptococcal infections also plays some role. The incidence, morbidity, and death rate from RF and its sequela, *rheumatic heart disease* (RHD), have declined dramatically in the United States. The mortality rate from RF and RHD between 1940 and 1944 was 21 per 100,000 population. This rate fell to six per 100,000 in 1975, where it has remained to the present time, according to the most recent data available. This gratifying improvement can largely be attributed to the antibiotic treatment and prophylaxis of streptococcal infections. Improved socioeconomic conditions and changes in the inherent virulence of the streptococcus may also contribute. Nonetheless RF and RHD still account for almost 13,000 deaths annually in the United States—tragically, many in school-age children. In underdeveloped countries, RF and RHD remain a major public health problem.

**ETIOLOGY AND PATHOGENESIS.** Although some details are still lacking, the weight of evidence indicates that RF and its sequela, RHD, result from sensitization to streptococcal antigens and thus usually follow one to four weeks after a streptococcal infection. There has been speculation regarding a role for viruses in RF, but the supporting evidence is equivocal. In the great majority of cases, the inciting infection is a streptococcal pharyngitis ("sore throat"). Many patients are unaware of the antecedent infection and furthermore have negative throat cultures at the time the RF is discovered. Nonetheless, evidence of a prior infection is almost always present. About 95% of patients have elevated titers of anti-streptolysin O (ASO), antistreptokinase, antistreptodornase, or antistreptohyaluronidase when the rheumatic attack is diagnosed. Why certain individuals develop this poststreptococcal complication and others do not is still not clear. As far as we know, any strain of the group A beta-hemolytic streptococci may be implicated, but several factors may be important: the virulence and antigenicity of the streptococcal strain, the magnitude of the immune response of the host, and the persistence of the infecting organism in the pharynx. When the organism is still recoverable after 21 days of treatment of an acute pharyngitis, the attack rate is approximately 3%, whereas those free of organisms at this time have a rate of only 0.3%.[69] Probably related to virulence is the fact that "epidemic sore throat" constitutes a greater risk than the sporadic endemic forms of the disease, which tend to be milder. There does not appear to be genetic predisposition, although clearly more than one member of a family may develop RF, presumably because of spread of the streptococcal infection within the family group.[71] Once the disease is contracted, the risk of recurrence following a new streptococcal infection is as high as 50 to 60%.

Granted that streptococci are involved, how do they induce RF? The lesions of RF are sterile, and so direct bacterial spread is not implicated. Release of toxic products has also been reasonably well ruled out. Most of the evidence favors an autoimmune mechanism based on cross-reactions between cardiac antigens and antibodies evoked by one of the many streptococcal antigens.[67, 68] One implicated antigen is streptococcal M protein. Cross-reactive antibodies can be identified in the sera of patients with acute rheumatic fever. Some bind to cardiac myofibers, skeletal muscle, and smooth muscle cells. Others react with glycoproteins extracted from heart valves. With immunofluorescent techniques, immunoglobulins and complement are found along the sarcolemmal sheaths of cardiac myofibers. However, surprisingly, the active inflammatory foci in hearts referred to as Aschoff bodies seldom contain immunoglobulins or complement. This enigma raises the question, were they once present in these foci at an earlier stage of the disease, or must our present conception of the mechanism of injury be reevaluated? For this reason, attention has turned to the possibility that cell-mediated immunity may be the critical factor, since lymphocytes are found about Aschoff bodies. There are indeed fragmentary data suggesting involvement of T lymphocytes in the pathogenesis of RF.[67, 68] Depressed responsiveness to skin antigens may indicate abnormal T-suppressor–cell function in these patients. T lymphocytes from guinea pigs sensitized to group A streptococcal antigens have been said to be cytotoxic for cultured fetal guinea pig myofibers. However, other studies have failed to confirm these findings, and so it is evident that many details are missing. Nevertheless, we can conclude that RF appears to result from sensitization to streptococcal antigens inducing some form of immunologically mediated tissue injury.

MORPHOLOGY. **The basic and pathognomonic morphologic lesion of rheumatic fever is the Aschoff body.** When it is fully evolved, it comprises a focus of fibrinoid materal surrounded by a characteristic cellular infiltrate. In active rheumatic fever, the Aschoff body is classically found in the heart. Similar lesions, however, may be seen in the synovia of the joints, in and about joint capsules, tendons, and fascia, and, less often, in other connective tissues of the body. The Aschoff body represents a localized area of tissue injury of possible immune origin. Most believe the target of the injury is the collagen, but some still contend that it represents muscle fibers. The development of the Aschoff body proceeds through three phases: the early **exudative phase,** the intermediate **proliferative phase,** and the late **healed phase. Only the proliferative phase is diagnostic.** During the exudative phase, the central focus of injury is surrounded by leukocytes, chiefly neutrophils, with scattered lymphocytes, plasma cells, and histiocytes. The proliferative phase is characterized by a central focus of swollen collagen fibrils, which may be layered with fibrin and plasma proteins enclosed within a rim of inflammatory cells. The cellular zone contains large differentiated mesenchymal cells known as **Anitschkow cells** and occasional multinucleate **Aschoff giant cells,** as well as mononuclear leukocytes and fibroblasts (Fig. 11–8). The Anitschkow cells are known as "caterpillar cells" because the nuclear chromatin is aggregated into the center of the nucleus in the form of a slender, wavy ribbon with innumerable fine, leg-like projections. An abundant basophilic cytoplasm with cytoplasmic processes encloses the nucleus. The origin of these cells is controversial. Most consider them to be altered fibroblasts or macrophages, rather than modified myocytes.[70] The Aschoff giant cells are considerably larger and have one or two nuclei or a folded multilobular nucleus with prominent nucleoli. They probably are derived from the Anitschkow cells. The healed phase of the Aschoff body results from progressive hyalinization and fibrosis of the lesion and is discernible only as a focus of nonspecific scarring. The significance of the Aschoff body is uncertain. Diagnostic Aschoff bodies may be encountered in hearts in the apparent absence of signs of activity of the disease. Either these lesions persist long after clinical signs of activity have abated, or latent activity may be present without producing clinically apparent disease.

*Heart.* Rheumatic heart disease develops with the initial attack of rheumatic fever in about 30% of cases. Usually the cardiac involvement affects all three layers—the pericardium, myocardium, and endocardium—simultaneously. However, the layers may be involved singly or in any combination.

During the acute stage, the **pericarditis** takes the form of a diffuse, nonspecific, fibrinous or serofibrinous inflammation. This is described on page 44.

Myocardial involvement is responsible for most deaths during the **acute** phase of rheumatic fever, and it is largely in the myocardium that the classic Aschoff bodies

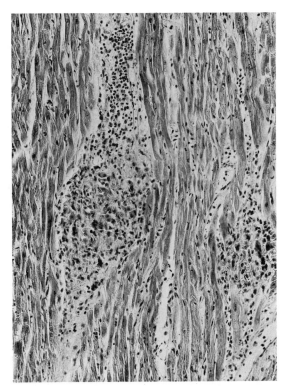

Figure 11–8. Microscopic detail of two Aschoff bodies in the myocardium in acute rheumatic heart disease. The variability in the size of the cells within the foci reflects the mixed composition of fibroblasts, giant cells, and mononuclear leukocytes.

are found. Gross alterations in the myocardium are minimal and are confined usually to a flabby softening and dilatation of the heart. The Aschoff bodies are found principally in the interfascicular fibrous septa, in the perivascular connective tissue, and in the subendothelial region. A histologic diagnosis may be difficult unless Aschoff bodies in the pathognomonic proliferative phase are found.

**Most deaths from rheumatic fever occur long after the acute disease has subsided and result from endocardial involvement, principally of the heart valves.** Although any of the four valves may be affected, the mitral valve alone is affected in nearly 50% of cases, and the mitral and aortic valves are affected together in an approximately equal number of cases. Occasionally a trivalvular pattern occurs, when the tricuspid valve is also affected. It was once thought that isolated aortic valve involvement was fairly common, but it is now believed that such aortic disease is probably only rarely rheumatic in origin.[71] During the early, acute phase of rheumatic fever, the leaflets of the affected valve or valves become red, swollen, and thickened. Later, a row of tiny, 1 to 2 mm, wart-like, rubbery to friable vegetations, called **verrucae,** form along the lines of closure of the valve leaflets on the surface exposed to the forward flow of blood. These vegetations probably result from erosion of the inflamed endocardial surface where the leaflets impinge upon each other. Similar verrucae may occur along the chordae tendineae of the atrioventricular valves. Histologic examination of these lesions may reveal only pre-

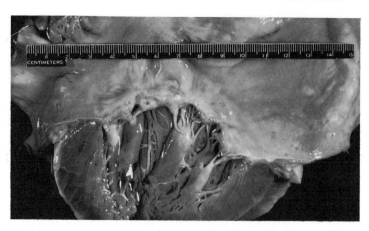

Figure 11–9. Chronic (healed) mitral valvulitis in rheumatic heart disease. The opened valve is markedly thickened, the leaflets have fused, and the chordae tendineae are cord-like and shortened. The left atrium is greatly dilated and shows fibrous thickening of the endocardium as a result of chronic distention.

cipitated fibrinoid material and nonspecific inflammatory cells. However, often the underlying valve has a palisade of altered fibroblasts intermixed with mononuclear white cells, resembling to some extent the Aschoff body. As organization of the endocardial inflammation takes place, the valvular leaflets become thickened, fibrotic, shortened, and blunted. Fibrous bridging across the valvular commissures may produce a rigid "fish-mouth" or "buttonhole" stenotic deformity. However, if commissural fusion is not severe, the predominant lesion is valvular incompetence (insufficiency, regurgitation). The chordae tendineae also become thickened, fused, and shortened (Fig. 11–9). With the passage of time, focal calcifications may develop in the affected valves. Sometimes nodular calcific masses virtually fill the sinuses of Valsalva behind the aortic valve, a pattern characteristic of aortic stenosis from other causes as well. With severe mitral stenosis or incompetence, the left atrium progressively dilates, and often a thrombus forms within the auricular appendage. The mural endocardium may develop plaque-like thickenings, usually of the atria, called **MacCallum's plaques.** Microscopically, these show pooling of ground substance, sometimes accompanied by Aschoff bodies. In time they tend to undergo fibrosis, leaving only a map-like area of endocardial thickening and wrinkling.

***Joints.*** About 75% of patients with rheumatic fever have either joint pains without arthritis (arthralgia) or inflammatory rheumatic arthritis. During the early clinical phases of arthritis, the synovial membranes are thickened, red, and granular, and frequently they are ulcerated. Histologically, increased amounts of ground substance, foci of fibrinoid deposition, and lesions resembling Aschoff bodies have been described in the synovial membranes and occasionally in the joint capsules, tendons, fasciae, and muscle sheaths. These changes are largely reversible, and rheumatic arthritis is classically transient.

***Skin.*** A minority of patients with rheumatic fever have skin lesions, classically either **subcutaneous nodules** or a rash known as **erythema marginatum.** The subcutaneous nodules are most often found overlying the extensor tendons of the extremities, at the wrists, elbows, ankles, and knees. Several or only one of these sites may be involved. The nodules vary in size from 1 to 4

cm in diameter and are sharply circumscribed, freely moveable, painless masses that are often associated with inflammatory hyperemia of the overlying skin. Histologically, they represent large areas of fibrinoid necrosis resembling confluent Aschoff bodies. Erythema marginatum refers to large, macular, map-like lesions that occur chiefly on the trunk and tend to be migratory.

***Other Sites.*** Any of the blood vessels may show foci of acute exudative necrosis accompanied by a polymorphonuclear exudate. These lesions resemble the changes of hypersensitivity angiitis and polyarteritis nodosa. The lungs occasionally show a nonspecific interstitial pneumonitis similar to that of viral pneumonia. Rheumatic vasculitis and pneumonitis are usually inconspicuous components of RF.

**CLINICAL COURSE.** The onset of rheumatic fever may be sudden and stormy, with fever, tachycardia, and painful, swollen joints, or it may be insidious and subtle, manifested only by malaise and low-grade fever. When the disease is preceded by a clinically overt streptococcal infection, this has characteristically subsided before the onset of rheumatic fever. *None of the clinical or laboratory features of rheumatic fever is specific for this disease.* The diagnosis must therefore be based on the presence of a constellation of findings. On this basis, the clinical manifestations of rheumatic fever are divided into "major" and "minor" criteria.[72] It is generally accepted that a diagnosis can be based on the presence of at least two of the major criteria or on one major and two minor criteria. *Major criteria include polyarthritis, carditis, subcutaneous nodules, erythema marginatum, and the presence of the spasmodic involuntary muscle movements termed Sydenham's chorea.* The minor criteria include various indications of a prior streptococcal infection, such as elevated antibody titers to the streptococcal antigens; nonspecific reflections of an inflammatory process, such as leukocytosis, fever, and an elevated erythrocyte sedimentation rate; and indirect suggestions of arthritis or carditis, such as arthralgias or a prolonged PR interval on the electrocardiogram. Because patients with a first attack of rheumatic fever are vulnerable to recurrences, a history of rheumatic fever should be weighed heavily when the diagnosis is entertained.

The younger the patient, the more likely it is that there is involvement of the heart. The presence of carditis is indicated by the development of a heart murmur, as a result of either valvular disease or acute myocarditis with dilatation of the heart. Other manifestations of myocarditis, such as arrhythmias and conduction disturbances, may also be present. The combination of auricular thrombosis and atrial fibrillation predisposes to embolization of fragments of the clot.

The prognosis for survival of the acute attack of rheumatic fever is good. Death occurs in only 1% of cases, usually from fulminant myocarditis. The long-term prognosis depends on the presence and severity of the initial carditis. When there is no carditis during the initial attack, almost all patients remain free of rheumatic heart disease, even over long periods of follow-up. Most deaths occur many years after an initial acute carditis, in the so-called healed phase, and are related to valvular deformities, principally mitral stenosis. During the long phase of compensated heart disease, the heart murmur may be the only indication of cardiac involvement. It was at one time thought that the valves were progressively damaged by the steady continuation of a smoldering rheumatic process. However, it is more likely that progressive valvular disease can be attributed to subclinical exacerbations, as well as to evolving fibrotic reactions and a steadily diminishing tolerance to the hemodynamic derangements. Women show a greater tendency toward progressive valvular scarring than do men and, probably for this reason, they are more vulnerable to long-standing mitral stenosis.

The long-term outlook for patients with cardiac involvement once was poor. However, with antibiotic prophylaxis and successful valvular surgery or prosthetic replacement of damaged valves, the prognosis now is considerably brighter. Without surgery, the 10-year survival rate among patients with mild stenosis of the mitral valve is about 84%. If the initial mitral damage is severe, 10-year survival rate is low. Death from rheumatic heart disease usually results from intractable congestive heart failure. Other frequent causes of death include cerebral embolization, recurrent acute attacks, and pneumonia superimposed on long-standing pulmonary congestion. About 4% of a group of patients with rheumatic heart disease developed infective endocarditis over a 10-year period, and this, too, may be a cause of death.[73]

## CONGENITAL HEART DISEASE

The exact incidence of congenital heart disease is unknown, but it is estimated to be present in nine births per 1000. Since the incidence of rheumatic heart disease has declined in the United States, congenital heart disease is now the most common form of heart disease among infants and children in this country. There are a large number of congenital anomalies of the heart.[74, 75] Almost all of them have in common interference with the normal streamlined flow of blood through the chambers of the heart and the great vessels. The resultant turbulence creates heart murmurs that are usually fairly dramatic. In many cases, blood is short-circuited through defects in the heart or great vessels. This diverts blood either toward the systemic circuit or toward the pulmonary circuit. *When blood is shunted from right to left (i.e., toward the systemic vasculature), without passing through the pulmonary tree, the blood is only partially oxygenated and cyanosis is prominent, usually from birth. In contrast, when the blood is short-circuited from left to right, a larger than normal volume of blood reaches the lungs, and there is initially no cyanosis.* However, the resultant pulmonary hypertension, which is eventually transmitted to the right side of the heart, may cause reversal of the shunt. At this point, late in the course, a cyanotic condition termed *cyanose tardive* or *Eisenmenger's syndrome* develops.

The following list indicates the most important congenital anomalies, their relative frequencies, and whether they are associated with early cyanosis. The frequencies given are necessarily approximate. Individuals with the more serious lesions die relatively early, hence the reported incidences vary markedly from study to study, according to the age range of the patients.

|  | Per Cent |
|---|---|
| A. Congenital anomalies without cyanosis (although there may be cyanose tardive) | |
|    1. Ventricular septal defects | 20–30 |
|    2. Atrial septal defects | 10 |
|    3. Patent ductus arteriosus | 10 |
|    4. Coarctation of the aorta | 7 |
|    5. Isolated pulmonic stenosis | 7 |
|    6. Isolated aortic stenosis | 6 |
|    7. Anomalies of the coronary arteries | ? |
| B. Congenital anomalies with cyanosis | |
|    1. Transposition of the great vessels | 5 |
|    2. Tetralogy of Fallot | 6 |

The etiology of congenital cardiac anomalies is in most cases not clear. Undoubtedly, both environmental and genetic factors contribute.[76] The best documented environmental influences are maternal rubella (German measles) during the first trimester of pregnancy and thalidomide when taken during pregnancy. Rubella may cause any one of a range of malformations, including persistent ductus arteriosus, pulmonary artery hypoplasia, pulmonary valve stenosis, ventricular septal defect, and tetralogy of Fallot. Other infections during pregnancy may also be implicated but are not well-documented cardiac teratogenic influences. That genetic factors may contribute as well is borne out by two lines of evidence: first, the frequent appearance of cardiac abnormalities in abnormal chromosomal syndromes, and second, the tendency for these disorders to run in families. Congenital heart disease is frequently encountered in trisomy 21 (Down's syndrome), trisomy 13, trisomy 18, cri du chat syndrome, Turner's syndrome, and in the multi-X disorders. Family studies show a well-defined increase in the incidence of congenital heart disease in the siblings of affected patients. Surprisingly, the malformations are not always concordant in monozygotic twins and indeed, more often than not, both of a pair of twins do *not* each have cardiac malformations. Nonetheless, there are suggestions that atrial septal defects and ventricular septal defects may be transmitted in a minority of instances by a single gene mutation, possibly dominant in the case of atrial septal defect. Despite these findings, with few exceptions, infants with isolated heart defects have no family history of cardiac malformations.

Most children with congenital heart disease are male. However, specific lesions have a definite sex preponderance; patent ductus arteriosus and atrial septal defect are more common in females, and valvular aortic stenosis, coarctation of the aorta, tetralogy of Fallot, and transposition of the great vessels are more common in males.

## VENTRICULAR SEPTAL DEFECT (VSD)

Ventricular septal defects are located most frequently just below the aortic valve in the region of the membranous ventricular septum *(membranous VSD)*, but they may be more apical in the muscular ventricular septum *(muscular VSD)*. The membranous VSDs result from defective formation of the membranous septal region, which is normally derived from (1) endocardial cushion tissue and (2) the conal ridges of the bulbus cordis. A significant percentage of VSDs present at birth close spontaneously. Persistent VSDs may be minute or as large as several centimeters in diameter. A systolic murmur and systolic thrill along with a diastolic rumbling murmur are typical findings. Depending upon the size of the defect, life expectancy may be normal or materially reduced. Patients with large, uncorrected defects die in infancy. Those with moderate defects may survive until young adulthood. In most cases, surgical correction is possible. Pathophysiologically, the VSD allows shunting of blood during systole from the left ventricle across the defect through the right ventricular outflow tract and pulmonary arteries into the lungs. Areas of endocardial thickening, called jet lesions, may develop in the right ventricle at the point where the jet stream of blood impinges upon the lining of the right ventricular chamber. In response to the left-to-right shunt, there is a compensatory increase in blood volume. In infants with large VSDs, this can lead to left ventricular enlargement and failure. Another consequence is right ventricular enlargement due to increasing pulmonary vascular resistance. Eventually, pulmonary hypertension with pulmonary vascular sclerosis develops and can become sufficiently severe to cause reversal of blood flow through the defect. Congestive heart failure is the most common cause of death, followed by infective endocarditis (p. 335) on the margins of the defect or on the right ventricular jet lesions.

## ATRIAL SEPTAL DEFECT (ASD)

The mature atrial septum has a complex derivation from several embryologic structures: septum primum, septum secundum, sinus venosus, and endocardial cushions. After septum primum is formed, septum secundum grows downward from a superior location and to the right of septum primum; it then partially fuses with septum primum. Two openings normally form in the developing atrial septum. One is the ostum primum, which is located low in the atrial septum in its septum primum portion and just above the atrioventricular valves. This ostium is normally closed by proliferation of endocardial cushion tissue. The endocardial cushions are specialized areas of the fetal heart that contribute to the formation of the membranous ventricular septum and the mitral and tricuspid valves and to the closure of ostium primum in the atrial septum. Failure of closure of the ostium primum results in an *ostium primum ASD*. It is common in Down's syndrome. The second opening (ostium secundum) is located in the superior part of septum primum, in the region that lies opposite to the foramen ovale in septum secundum. This opening normally remains patent during intrauterine life and then becomes closed after birth by a flap-like effect of the fully formed septum primum against septum secundum when pressure in the left atrium becomes higher than the pressure in the right. This is followed by complete fibrous union of the two septa in the first few months after birth. If incomplete fibrous union occurs, there may be a patent foramen ovale that is functionally closed by the normal pressure differential between the two atria. However, if a deficiency of septum primum develops in this area, the result is a hole in the middle of the mature septum, designated an *ostium secundum ASD*. A third type of ASD, known as a *sinus venosus ASD*, is located high in the atrial septum near the entrance of the superior vena cava. This defect is due to abnormal incorporation of the sinus venosus into the developing atria. Defects of this type are sometimes accompanied by anomalous connections of pulmonary veins from the right lung into the superior vena cava or right atrium. Partial or total anomalous pulmonary venous connections also can occur without an ASD.

Ostium secundum ASDs account for approximately 90% of atrial septal defects. ASDs occur in females more frequently than in males. Even though left-to-right shunting occurs, the important distinctions from VSDs are that propulsion of blood into the lungs under high pressure does not occur and significant pulmonary hypertension typically does not develop or does so only very late in the course. Thus, ASDs tend to be relatively benign; survival into middle age is usual. When pulmonary hypertension develops, death may occur from right-sided heart failure or *paradoxical embolism* (a condition in which emboli pass through the defect from the right to the left side of the heart and into the systemic circulation). Infective endocarditis is rare. Surgical correction is commonly successful.

Ostium primum ASDs are frequently associated with a gap or cleft in the anterior mitral leaflet. This combination of anomalies is known as a *partial* or *incomplete atrioventricular canal defect.* It generally has a somewhat less favorable outlook than ordinary ASDs, because some patients with this condition have significant mitral regurgitation. Total failure of ingrowth of endocardial cushion tissue results in a *complete atrioventricular canal defect.* This condition comprises an ostium primum ASD, a contiguous membranous VSD, and a single atrioventricular valve that straddles the large defect in the center of the heart. Although surgical approaches to this condition have been devised, it still has a bad prognosis.

## PATENT DUCTUS ARTERIOSUS

Functional closure of the ductus arteriosus, which joins the pulmonary artery to the aorta just distal to the origin of the innominate, carotid, and subclavian arteries, usually occurs owing to muscular contraction within the first day after birth and is followed by fibrous obliteration within the next few weeks to months. When the ductus remains patent, there is shunting of blood from the aorta to the pulmonary artery. This anomaly occurs most often in females. Although it may exist as a solitary lesion, more often it is associated with other congenital malformations. As will be seen later, the patency of the ductus may be life-saving with these multiple anomalies. Patent ductus arteriosus is commonly associated with intrauterine rubella infection, prematurity, and infantile respiratory distress syndrome.

The morphology of the ductus is quite variable. It may be a distinct vessel, with a length of 1 to 2 cm and a diameter of 1 to 10 mm, that bridges a gap between the aorta and the pulmonary arterial trunk. In other cases, however, the ductus is merely represented by a fenestration between the apposed pulmonary and aortic trunks.

The most striking clinical feature of a persistent ductus arteriosus is a loud, continuous systolic and diastolic murmur, which has been variously described as machinery-like, humming, sawing, and "train-in-tunnel." The amount of the shunt is less than that with large ventricular septal defects. The prognosis is relatively good; average survival is to middle age.

Death usually results from right-sided heart failure or from infective endocarditis. This malformation is readily corrected by surgery.

## COARCTATION OF THE AORTA

This anomaly is of two forms. The preductal or "infantile" form is characterized by severe narrowing of the aorta proximal to the ductus arteriosus, which remains patent, thereby permitting blood to reach the systemic vasculature from the pulmonary artery. It has an equal sex distribution and is often associated with other malformations. Infants with a severe degree of coarctation of the aorta usually die soon after birth, unless surgical repair is accomplished. Preductal coarctation may be an incomplete form of a more severe malformation referred to as *hypoplastic left heart syndrome.* This condition is characterized by: (1) underdevelopment of the left cardiac chambers, (2) atresia or stenosis of one or both of the left-sided valves, and (3) hypoplasia of the proximal aorta. Commonly, there is endocardial fibroelastosis of the left chambers (p. 347). In utero, a patent ductus arteriosus allows blood to reach the aorta from the right heart. However, infants with this condition manifest cardiac failure from birth and die within a few days as the ductus begins to narrow postnatally.

Postductal or "adult" coarctation involves a portion of the aorta distal to the ductus arteriosus. Narrowing involves a much shorter segment, often appearing as a prominent inner ring or an almost complete membrane. The ductus arteriosus is characteristically closed. In nearly 50% of cases of both forms of coarctation, there is a coexistent bicuspid aortic valve. Adult coarctation is somewhat more frequent in males (1.7:1). It commonly occurs in patients with Turner's syndrome. The adult coarctation anomaly may remain asymptomatic. When symptoms occur, they are usually referable to the severe hypertension in the arterial system proximal to the constriction, with concomitant hypotension distal to the narrowing. Dilated and tortuous collateral vessels develop to serve the lower half of the body. Since the narrowing is distal to the left subclavian artery, the most prominent collaterals are the intercostal arteries bilaterally, which, as they enlarge, cause radiographically visible notching of the lower margins of the ribs. A typical clinical feature is a marked difference in the blood pressure in the upper and lower extremities. The markedly elevated pressure in the aorta proximal to the coarctation often leads to aortic medionecrosis and dissecting aneurysm (p. 302). Unless coarctation is surgically corrected, death usually occurs before middle age and is attributable most often to rupture of a dissecting aneurysm in the proximal aorta, bacterial invasion of the aorta at the point of narrowing (endarteritis), cerebral hemorrhage from local hypertension, or left-sided congestive heart failure.

## ISOLATED PULMONIC STENOSIS, ISOLATED AORTIC STENOSIS

These anomalies are being recognized with increasing frequency. Stenotic pulmonic valves are often dome-shaped with a central orifice. Stenotic aortic valves are often bicuspid and, occasionally, unicuspid. The course of both lesions is extremely variable, depending upon the degree of stenosis.

Symptoms of pulmonic stenosis are dyspnea on exertion and fatigability. Formerly, 50% of these patients died in childhood, usually from right-sided heart failure. However, surgical repair is now quite feasible.

Aortic stenosis with a severely deformed valve and a diminutive aortic annulus may present in infancy or childhood. Less severely deformed valves do not give rise to symptoms until later in life (see p. 345). The congenitally anomalous aortic valve becomes increasingly stenotic with time, as a result of severe calcification. Symptoms of significant stenosis are dyspnea, fatigue, and angina pectoris. Eventually, left-sided CHF develops, and from this point the lesion is rapidly fatal unless surgical intervention occurs. Occasionally, aortic stenosis first manifests itself in sudden death.

## ANOMALIES OF THE CORONARY ARTERIES

A variety of possible anomalies of the coronary arteries may occur, including multiple ostia and unusual sites of origin from the aorta. These are usually without functional significance. However, quite rarely, one of the coronary arteries takes its origin from the pulmonary artery rather than from the aorta. Left-to-right shunting of blood occurs from the high-pressure coronary artery into the low-pressure coronary artery, thereby diverting a significant amount of coronary blood flow from the myocardial capillaries. This results in progressive ischemic changes and eventual heart failure. It will be seen that this form of congenital anomaly is sometimes associated with endocardial fibroelastosis.

## TRANSPOSITION OF THE GREAT VESSELS

This is an extremely grave anomaly that affects males more often than females. It is characterized by reversed positions of the aorta and pulmonary artery, with the aorta arising from the right ventricle and the pulmonary artery from the left ventricle. Cyanosis is usually apparent from birth, along with poor feeding and breathlessness. Most of these infants rapidly develop CHF and die. Longer survival is permitted if there are coexistent anomalies, such as septal defects or a patent ductus arteriosus, that allow communication between the pulmonary and the systemic circuits. Surgical correction is difficult and involves rerouting the flow of systemic venous and pulmonary venous blood to the left and right atrium, respectively, or by repositioning the aorta and pulmonary artery.

A variation of this anomaly, termed "corrected transposition of the great vessels," involves transposition of the ventricles as well as of the aorta and pulmonary artery, so that the aorta emerges from a left-sided morphological right ventricle that receives blood from the left atrium and the pulmonary artery emerges from a right-sided morphological left ventricle that receives blood from the right atrium. Thus, since the aorta receives oxygenated blood and the pulmonary artery unoxygenated blood, the circulation is essentially normal and this anomaly by itself is merely a curiosity, save that the left-sided ventricle undergoes hypertrophy. However, other malformations are commonly present, clouding the outlook.

## TETRALOGY OF FALLOT

This is the most common form of cyanotic congenital heart disease that permits survival to adult life. Its components are (1) a ventricular septal defect; (2) a rightward displaced aorta, which overrides the septal defect and receives blood from both the right and left ventricles; (3) pulmonic stenosis; and (4) consequent right ventricular hypertrophy. The disorder probably results from anomalous development of the septum of the conus arteriosus in the embryonic heart, thereby affecting the relative size of the pulmonary outflow tract (infundibulum), pulmonary valve, and pulmonary artery. The course and prognosis of the tetralogy of Fallot vary with the degree of pulmonic stenosis. When this is severe, survival is possible only with a concomitant patent ductus arteriosus, which allows blood to enter the pulmonary vascular bed from the aorta. Most often the lesion is manifest from infancy, with cyanosis, dyspnea, clubbing of the fingers, and poor feeding and development. Often, cyanosis and dyspnea occur in paroxysms, which arise for no apparent reason and are frequently followed by syncope. The unusual patient with mild pulmonary obstruction may not have cyanosis. Unless the condition is corrected surgically, the prognosis is generally poor, although it is somewhat better than in transposition of the great vessels. Most patients without surgical intervention die in childhood or early adulthood; survival to middle age rarely occurs. Death commonly results from intercurrent respiratory infections and sometimes from infective endocarditis. With complete surgical correction, over 90% of the patients can expect long-term survival.

# INFECTIVE ENDOCARDITIS

One of the most serious of all infections, infective endocarditis (IE) is caused by colonization of the heart, usually the valves, by any one of a variety of bacteria or sometimes fungi or rickettsiae. The great majority of these infections are caused by bacteria and hence this condition is often referred to as bacterial endocarditis. *The disease is characterized by the buildup of friable thrombi heavily laden with organisms, creating so-called infective vegetations.* The organisms may become established at a site already damaged by previous heart disease—e.g., healed rheumatic valvular disease, calcific aortic stenosis, aging valvular changes or congenital malformations (principally septal defects and bicuspid aortic valves)—or sometimes immediately following cardiac surgery. But in a substantial number of cases (some say almost 50%), normal hearts are attacked.[77–79] Rheumatic heart disease once accounted for 65% of all cases, but with the decline in the incidence of this disease the other conditions have assumed increased importance. Moreover, cardiac surgery and drug addiction have further altered the profile of predisposing influences. Recent surveys show that infective endocarditis is now principally a disease of individuals over the age of 50 years, whereas formerly, with the dominating importance of rheumatic heart disease, it was largely encountered in younger individuals.[77] Males are affected somewhat more commonly than females.

*From the clinical standpoint, infective endocarditis is sometimes divided into acute and subacute forms (also known as acute and subacute bacterial endocarditis).* In the former, the infectious process is usually caused by a highly virulent organism and announces itself promptly with high fever and severe constitutional manifestations. The disease usually runs a rapidly progressive course to death within weeks to a few months from overwhelming disseminated infection, embolization, or cardiac decompensation secondary to erosion of valves or chordae tendineae, unless the microbiologic invasion can be controlled by therapy. Subacute endocarditis, on the other hand, is a much more insidious disease, usually caused by organisms of lesser virulence than those encountered in the acute disease. Often it presents as the mysterious onset of low-grade fever, anemia, and debility. Indeed, some of these patients may not have fever, only malaise. The vegetations develop more slowly and are less erosive and so cardiac signs and symptoms may be minimal or not even evident. Untreated, the duration of the disease exceeds three to six months. When fatal, the usual causes of death are valvular dysfunction and congestive heart failure, renal complications, or progressive debility due to the infection. Embolization or metastatic foci of infection in other organs is less common. The anatomic findings tend to reflect the nature of the organism

and the duration of the clinical course, and no single feature clearly separates acute from subacute endocarditis. Moreover, many cases pursue a clinical course that is intermediate between the acute and subacute patterns just described. In the last analysis, as with all infections, infective endocarditis must be viewed as a host-parasite interaction. The severity and outcome of the clinical infection will ultimately depend on the ability of the host to resist, the virulence of the infecting organism, and the vulnerability of the organism to antibiotic control.

**ETIOLOGY AND PATHOGENESIS.** In general, subacute endocarditis occurs in vulnerable hosts—i.e., those with preexisting heart conditions—whereas a considerable proportion of patients with acute endocarditis have previously normal hearts. Thus, the pathogeneses of these two forms of the disease differ.

*Four factors have been identified as having importance in the development of subacute endocarditis:* (1) disturbances in blood flow that induce jet effects and zones of turbulence, (2) the formation of sterile platelet-fibrin deposits, (3) the seeding of these deposits by blood-borne organisms, and (4) agglutinating antibodies creating clumps of organisms.[81, 82] Jet streams and turbulence favor the deposit of sterile thrombi at sites where they impinge, particularly in the "low-pressure sinks" in the eddy currents about their periphery. Such phenomena also favor the settling out of clumps of bacteria on the small thrombi. Thus, in mitral stenosis and insufficiency, as in rheumatic heart disease, the infected blood from the left ventricle regurgitating into the lower pressure atrium favors the deposition of both blood elements and bacteria on the atrial surface of the damaged valves close to the margins of the regurgitant orifice. With aortic stenosis, the ventricular surface of the stenotic orifice becomes the "low-pressure sink" during diastole. A similar explanation obtains for the localization of infective vegetations about the margins of interventricular septal defects and regurgitant bicuspid aortic valves. It may also explain why interatrial septal defects in the low-pressure atria are rarely complicated by infective endocarditis. The agglutinating antibodies, by creating larger clumps of organisms, predispose to the settling out of a bacteria-laden nidus. Obviously, blood-borne organisms are requisite. In the subacute form of endocarditis, only rarely is there a clinically significant infection elsewhere in the body. More commonly, the bacteremia has such banal origins as microtrauma to the gingiva, intestinal mucosa, or lining of the urogenital tract. In those with cardiac abnormalities, this endogenous flora assumes pathogenetic significance. Thus, dental surgery, catheterization of the urinary bladder, and even minor surgical procedures may assume great importance in patients with preexisting heart disease or valvular prostheses incident to cardiac surgery and often call for prophylactic antibiotic coverage prior to the procedure.

While the precise spectrum of organisms isolated from patients with subacute endocarditis differs from one series to the next, overall, about 50% of cases are caused by *Streptococcus viridans*. Other streptococcal species, including enterococci, account for about 15%, and gram-negative bacilli for about 10%, but at one time or another, virtually every other known organism, including those of remarkably low virulence (e.g., *A. aerogenes, Serratia*, diphtheroids, and *Staphylococcus epidermidis*, to mention only a few) as well as fungi (*Candida, Actinomyces, Aspergillus, Mucor*, and others) and rickettsiae have been isolated from sporadic cases.

*Acute infective endocarditis has a clinical expression and bacterial flora quite distinct from that of subacute endocarditis.* In over half of the cases, it develops in previously normal hearts. In acute endocarditis, the organisms or their toxins damage the surface of the heart valve and predispose to the formation of thrombi, which rapidly become infected with organisms. As in subacute endocarditis, this process develops along the valve margin. The causative agent in about 50% of the cases is *S. aureus*, and many of these cases are resistant to a large variety of antibiotics. Streptococci are implicated in about 35%.[83] Frequently, there is a well-defined infection elsewhere in the body that provides the source of the bacteremia. Any other organisms in the particularly vulnerable host—e.g., the chronic alcoholic, the immunosuppressed patient, one that has a chronic underlying debilitating condition, or an individual receiving cancer chemotherapy—may initiate an acute fulminating endocarditis. Particular attention should be paid to the growing role of parenteral drug addiction in acute endocarditis. In these individuals, there is usually no preexisting heart disease, the most frequent infecting agent is *S. aureus*, and in over half of the cases, the vegetations involve the tricuspid valve alone, a rare localization in the nonaddict population. Also implicated in drug addicts are *Candida, S. epidermidis* and *Streptococcus viridans*, as well as other organisms. Another important clinical

setting for acute IE is its development as a complication of cardiac surgery, particularly in patients receiving prosthetic heart valves. With previous cardiac surgery and emplacement of "foreign" prostheses, the causative organisms are generally those found in the air or on the skin and run the gamut from highly virulent *Staphylococcus aureus* to the innocent, normal flora of the skin such as *S. epidermidis*, diphtheroids, and aerobic gram-negative bacilli. The widespread use of antibacterial prophylaxis before, during, and after the surgery may account for the fact that *Candida* and *Aspergillus*, resistant to usual antibacterial agents, are now responsible for almost 15% of cases of infective carditis in postcardiotomy patients.

It should be noted that in all series of reported cases, there is a small number (5 to 10%) of patients from whom no organism can be isolated clinically and, less frequently, even at autopsy. The interpretation of such negative results is obscure. Conceivably, the infective agent was eradicated by antibiotic therapy. Alternatively, viruses or anaerobic organisms difficult to isolate might be involved. It hardly needs pointing out that such cases constitute serious clinical dilemmas. The major clinical finding on which the diagnosis rests is lacking, and there are no guideposts for the selection of the most appropriate antibiotic therapy.

**MORPHOLOGY.** The anatomic changes of acute and subacute endocarditis are more alike than dissimilar.[84] In both, the basic lesion consists of friable, rather bulky masses of thrombus containing the causative organism hanging from the leaflets of the affected valves or attached at the site of the congenital defect or prosthetic valve (Fig. 11–10). These vegetations may be as large as several centimeters in diameter and occur singly or in groups in haphazard fashion. Almost always, the vegetations of infective endocarditis, whether acute or subacute, are considerably bulkier than those encountered in other forms of vegetative endocarditis (acute rheumatic, Libman-Sacks, marantic). The location of the vegetations

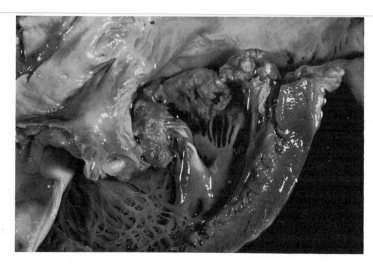

Figure 11–10. Infective (bacterial) endocarditis of the mitral valve (streptococcal). The thickened chordae tendineae suggest a preexistent rheumatic disease. The vegetations engulf the mitral leaflets.

is dictated by the nature of the preexisting heart disease when such is present. Overall, the aortic valve alone or the mitral valve alone is the site affected in approximately 80 to 90% of cases. Right-sided valves are infrequently involved save in drug addicts, among whom only the tricuspid valve is affected in more than half the cases. Only infrequently is more than one valve involved.

Histologically, irregular, amorphous tangled masses of fibrin strands, platelets, and blood cell debris, along with the masses of bacteria or other microorganisms, constitute the vegetation. In subacute endocarditis, there tends to be less tissue destruction and a chronic inflammatory response, including granulation tissue formation and vascularization of the valve. In acute endocarditis, tissue destruction is greater and the inflammatory response variable in degree and suppurative in type. The bacteria may be extremely difficult to identify and often are deeply buried within the vegetation, a situation that explains the difficulty in controlling these infections by antibiotic therapy once they are well developed. It should be emphasized that an essential feature of the morphologic examination is the culture of ground-up samples of the fresh vegetation.

A number of sequelae may ensue. Sometimes the valvular infection, particularly in acute endocarditis caused by virulent organisms, perforates the underlying valve leaflet or erodes the chordae tendineae. In a growing number of cases, control of the infection leads to healing with progressive organization, fibrosis, and calcification of the vegetations. Dissemination of the organisms and fragments of the vegetations through the blood produces small hemorrhages and abscesses in any tissue or organ of the body, particularly in the kidneys. Such systemic complications are more typical of acute endocarditis. In subacute endocarditis, emboli are less extensive and tend to produce larger, bland infarcts. At one time, about a third of patients developed, in addition to renal abscesses or infarcts, one of several forms of glomerular involvement—i.e., focal glomerulitis (formerly called focal embolic glomerulonephritis) or diffuse proliferative glomerulonephritis, both of which are thought to represent immune complex disease. Perhaps more prompt and effective control of the infection by antibiotic therapy has reduced the frequency of these forms of renal disease to the present incidence of only about 15% of cases.[85]

**CLINICAL COURSE.** Although classically fever and a changing cardiac murmur have been said to be the two cardinal manifestations of infective endocarditis, one or both may be deceptively absent in as many as 10 to 20% of cases of the subacute form of the disease. Subacute endocarditis may indeed be insidious in onset and often relatively mild in nature, presenting only slight to moderate fever, fatigue, hematuria, progressive microcytic hypochromic anemia, and weight loss. Shaking chills are quite uncommon, and the white blood cell count may only be mildly elevated, the effect of a relative neutrophilia. Somewhat immature cells of the granulocyte series (shift to the left) are often present. Classically, splenomegaly and linear (splinter) hemorrhages in the nail beds may appear. Sometimes present are such unusual manifestations as arthralgia, backache, or signs of meningitis or encephalitis. When a murmur is present it may be related to the preexisting cardiac disease and may not change in character, as do those related to the buildup and fragmentation of vegetations. However, in some cases the murmur may indeed change from day to day, pointing strongly to the appropriate diagnosis. Important for the diagnosis are positive blood cultures, splinter nail bed hemorrhages, and signs and symptoms relating to embolic infarctions of organs (e.g., in the spleen or kidneys). In most cases of the subacute disease, there are high titers of agglutinating, complement-fixing, and opsonizing antibodies specific for the invading organism.

Acute endocarditis typically presents more dramatic findings, with the sudden onset of high fever, shaking chills, splinter hemorrhages, splenomegaly, petechial and pustular skin lesions, and rapidly progressive anemia and hematuria. Embolic infarction of various organs is more characteristic of the acute disease than of the subacute form of endocarditis. Murmurs may again be absent, particularly when the tricuspid valve alone is involved, but when present, they often change in character as the vegetations build up and fragment. Generally, there is little difficulty in obtaining positive results from a blood culture in these cases.

Before the antibiotic era, infective endocarditis was almost always fatal. Currently, the overall mortality rate stands at about 30 to 35%. The subacute form of the disease, especially when caused by streptococci, is curable in 90 to 95% of patients when detected early and effectively treated. Acute endocarditis, particularly when caused by antibiotic-resistant *S. aureus*, is still a most serious form of infection, with a fatality rate in the range of 60 to 80%. Fungal endocarditis poses a special problem, particularly when encountered in young narcotic addicts or in severely predisposed (e.g., immunosuppressed) patients.

The major cause of death in all patients is cardiac failure, usually secondary to damage to valvular function, erosion of a valve, or rupture of a chorda tendineae. Other potential causes include embolic infarction of the heart or brain, uncontrolled sepsis, arrhythmias related to the involvement of the conduction system, and rupture of a mycotic aneurysm caused by seeding of a large artery with blood-borne organisms. Less frequently, the demise is related to dehiscence of a prosthetic valve that had become the site of an infective endocarditis, to cardiac surgery when an attempt is made to excise the infected valve and replace it with an artificial valve, or to renal failure. With the present-day armamentarium of highly potent antibiotics, the challenge for the future is the prompt recognition of these too often fatal infections.

# COR PULMONALE

*Cor pulmonale is defined as right ventricular hypertrophy, with or without CHF, caused by pulmonary hypertension from primary disease within the lung substance or within its vessels.* It is an important cause of death in these disorders.[86]

*Nearly any long-standing lung disease* may lead to cor pulmonale, including chronic obstructive pulmonary disease (chronic bronchitis and primary emphysema), the pneumoconioses, idiopathic interstitial fibrosis, and bronchiectasis. These entities produce pulmonary hypertension, in part simply through destruction of portions of the pulmonary vascular bed, which results in increased flow through the remaining vessels, and in part through the vasoconstrictive effects of hypoxemia and respiratory acidosis.

*Abnormalities of the pulmonary vasculature* constitute a second and more direct cause of pulmonary hypertension. Paramount in this category are multiple or large pulmonary emboli. Intrinsic pulmonary vascular disease is a less frequent cause of pulmonary hypertension. Most often such intrinsic disease is caused by an idiopathic disorder known as *primary pulmonary vascular sclerosis* (p. 410).[87] Rarely, it represents pulmonary involvement by one of the systemic disorders such as systemic sclerosis or Wegener's granulomatosis.

Uncommonly, cor pulmonale is caused by *skeletal or neuromuscular derangements* that interfere with normal ventilation (e.g., severe kyphoscoliosis, poliomyelitis, the muscular dystrophies, and the Pickwickian syndrome). Presumably these act through pulmonary vasoconstriction induced by the hypoxemia and hypercapnia that they produce.

It is apparent that the common denominator in all the previously mentioned disorders is pulmonary hypertension. In general, cor pulmonale is asymptomatic until right-sided congestive heart failure ensues. Until then, the picture is usually dominated by the primary disorder.

The morphologic changes associated with cor pulmonale are entirely analogous to those of hypertensive heart disease, with the right ventricle rather than the left ventricle being primarily affected. The right ventricle may thicken up to 1.5 cm, and thus it may achieve virtually the same dimensions as the left ventricle (Fig. 11–11).

It should be noted in passing that right ventricular hypertrophy often develops secondary to left-sided CHF. Cardiac congenital malformations may produce left-to-right shunts and consequent hypertrophy of the right ventricle. Such changes are not included within the present definition of cor pulmonale.

# PERICARDIAL DISEASE

The pericardium may be involved in a variety of hemodynamic, inflammatory, neoplastic, and congenital disorders. Pericardial disease is manifested by accumulation of fluid, termed *pericardial effusion*, inflammation (i.e., *pericarditis*), or both components.[88] The hemodynamic involvements take the form of collections of serous edema fluid (*hydropericardium*), such as may occur in CHF or in the systemic edema associated with advanced renal or liver disease. An accumulation of blood in the pericardial sac (*hemopericardium*) is usually secondary to rupture of an acute MI or dissection of the aorta back into the pericardial sac or, more rarely, from penetrating or nonpenetrating chest trauma. But whatever its origin, intrapericardial hemorrhage often causes fatal *cardiac tamponade*. The congenital anomalies, such as total absence of the pericardium or partial defects, are rarely the cause of clinical disease. The pericardium may be involved in the spread of cancers that are primary elsewhere, but neoplasms arising initially in the pericardium are rare—indeed, exotic.

## PERICARDITIS

The most important involvements of the pericardium are inflammatory—pericarditis—and have a di-

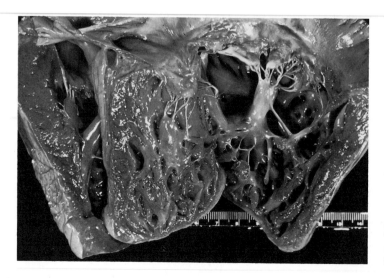

Figure 11–11. Cor pulmonale. The right ventricle and tricuspid valve have been opened to expose the thickened wall and trabeculae carneae. Compare with the thickness of the wall of the left ventricle, seen on the extreme left.

**Table 11–2.** ETIOLOGY OF PERICARDITIS

Infectious
    Viral
    Bacterial
    Tuberculous
    Fungal
    Others
Metabolic disorders
    Uremic
    Cholesterol
    Myxedema
Neoplastic
Related to myocardial infarction
Traumatic
Hypersensitivity or autoimmunity
    Rheumatic fever
    Systemic lupus erythematosus
    Rheumatoid arthritis
    Scleroderma
    Postmyocardial infarction
    Drug-induced
Postpericardiotomy or thoracotomy
Postradiation
Idiopathic

versity of origins. In most instances, the pericarditis is secondary to disease elsewhere in the body, as, for example, spread of a pulmonary infection into the pericardial sac or as one component of a systemic disease, such as systemic lupus erythematosus. However, occasionally pericarditis occurs as a primary disorder. The classification of the causes of pericarditis is provided in Table 11–2. Because it is often difficult to be certain of the etiology in a particular case, and because the idiopathic variety is perhaps the most common type, an alternative classification divides these involvements into *acute, subacute,* and *chronic* forms. There is virtue to this approach since, as will be seen, the clinical manifestations of these various stages of inflammatory involvement are distinctive. However, the overlap is great. An anatomic system of classification is also widely used, based on the character of the inflammatory exudate. Thus, pericarditis may be divided into (1) *serous,* (2) *serofibrinous,* (3) *fibrinous,* (4) *suppurative,* and (5) *hemorrhagic.* There is, as we shall see, some correlation between these anatomic patterns and the causation of pericarditis. Moreover, there are wide differences in the natural history of these divisions. For example, serous pericarditis usually resolves without residuals, whereas fibrinous and, more particularly, suppurative forms may lead to fibrous organization and the development of chronic pericarditis, which can be extremely disabling. However, in many instances, the type of inflammatory exudate is more a function of the severity of injury than of the etiology.

**PATHOGENESIS.** As is clear from the etiologic classification, in some instances, such as in SLE or rheumatic fever, the pericarditis is a relatively minor aspect of a systemic disease and is referred to as *secondary.* Comments here are limited to those involvements in which the pericarditis is a dominant feature of the clinical picture. *The great majority of*

*such significant inflammations are of microbiologic origin.*

*Viruses* are gaining increasing importance as causes of primary pericarditis. Indeed, some workers believe that viruses cause most, if not all, cases of acute "idiopathic" pericarditis. Among known cases of viral pericarditis, those caused by the Coxsackie B viruses, influenza A and B viruses, some of the echo viruses, and the Epstein-Barr virus (in association with mononucleosis) are particularly important. The pathogenesis of viral pericarditis is not clear. Frequently, it follows an acute upper respiratory infection, but whether or not the causative viruses then spread to the pericardium is not known. There is some support for the view that many viruses do not directly invade pericardial tissue but rather in some way incite a hypersensitivity phenomenon that in turn involves the pericardium.

*Bacteria* may reach the pericardium either by direct spread from contiguous structures, such as the lung or pleura, or by hematogenous or lymphatic seeding. In recent years, bacterial pericarditis has markedly declined in incidence, although staphylococcal and tuberculous causations remain important. Among children, especially, staphylococcal pericarditis is relatively frequent and is almost always associated with either pneumonia or osteomyelitis.[89] Obviously, whether septic pericardial involvement dominates the clinical picture or is a small part of it is variable.

As bacterial pericarditis has declined in importance, fungi and protozoa have taken on new importance as causes of pericardial disease. Very often there is an associated myocarditis. *Coccidioides immitis, Histoplasma capsulatum,* and *Candida albicans* among the fungi, and *Toxoplasma gondii* among the protozoa may produce apparently primary pericardial involvement and should be suspected in cases of idiopathic pericarditis.

Among the *metabolic* pericarditides, that resulting from uremia occurs most frequently, as is mentioned on page 458. A rare form of metabolic pericarditis, of unknown etiology, is termed "cholesterol pericarditis" because of the presence of cholesterol crystals in the intrapericardial fluid. Myxedema, too, causes pericardial effusion, but this is noninflammatory; hence, it does not represent a true pericarditis.

Primary tumors of the pericardium are extremely rare. *Neoplastic pericarditis,* then, almost always stems from direct or metastatic spread of tumors arising outside the pericardial sac. Most often, direct spread is from mediastinal lymphomas or from bronchogenic or esophageal carcinomas. Although metastases from any cancer in the body may involve the pericardium, such spread is in general an infrequent occurrence.

The pericarditis accompanying acute myocardial infarction is described on page 323.

*Traumatic pericarditis* is a relatively common sequela to nonpenetrating chest trauma. It reflects either mild contusions to the epicardial surface of the heart or the presence of blood in the pericardial sac, which evokes a reparative response, just as it does in the pleural or peritoneal cavities. Infrequently, penetrating chest wounds introduce bacteria directly into the pericardial cavity, producing a suppurative pericarditis.

The pericardium, like the other serosal membranes, is peculiarly vulnerable to *hypersensitivity states*. The major immune diseases are discussed in Chapter 5 and, in the case of rheumatic fever, in this chapter. Suffice it here to describe briefly the postcardiotomy, postmyocardial infarction (post-MI), and posttraumatic syndromes, all of which are presumed to be based on an immune mechanism.[90] All are characterized by pericarditis, usually with a significant collection of fluid in the pericardial sac, and are often accompanied by pleuritis and, less frequently, by pneumonitis. *Postcardiotomy pericarditis* develops in some patients two to five weeks after any heart surgery involving wide incision of the pericardium. A small number of patients develop a similar syndrome two to five weeks following MI or trauma to the pericardium. Clinically, these three entities are virtually identical, manifesting themselves as fever and chest pain, which subside either spontaneously or with anti-inflammatory drugs. All have a marked tendency to recur periodically, sometimes for months or even years. *It must be remembered that in all three cases, the initial inciting event—namely, cardiotomy, MI, or pericardial trauma—is itself often associated with an immediate, transient pericarditis, which should not be confused with the later-developing immune syndrome.* In most cases, these patients have high serum titers of autoantibodies to heart tissue. It has been suggested that antigens released from damaged myocardial tissue evoke the formation of antibodies and that the inflammation is mediated by soluble antigen-antibody complexes.

The largest single category of pericarditis is *idiopathic*. However, with improved diagnostic measures, particularly for the isolation of viruses, fewer cases are now being assigned to the idiopathic group. Undoubtedly many cases of idiopathic pericarditis are in reality of viral origin; possibly the Coxsackie viruses are most important. It should be remembered that viral and immune causes are not mutually exclusive, since it is suspected that viral pericarditis does not always represent direct invasion by the organisms.

**MORPHOLOGY.** The various etiologies are expressed in a variety of morphologic patterns. The term "acute pericarditis" usually refers to a **serous, fibrinous**, or **serofibrinous** inflammation. It is characterized by a small intrapericardial exudative effusion, usually not greater than 200 ml, containing gray-yellow strands or clumps of fibrin. Frequently a fine granular precipitate of fibrin is deposited on the serosal surfaces. This may cause adherence of the two layers of the pericardium, described as "bread and butter" pericarditis because the shaggy pericardial surfaces resemble lavishly buttered slices of bread when separated (see Fig. 2–12, p. 44). Such a condition is encountered in rheumatic fever, MI, and sometimes in the immune and viral forms of pericarditis. Microscopically, the subserosal inflammation is nonspecific and consists of both polymorphonuclear and mononuclear leukocytes. A **suppurative** effusion almost always denotes the presence of bacteria or fungi. With neoplastic involvement, the exudate is usually **hemorrhagic** and often contains malignant cells shed from the tumor. Tuberculosis evokes a **caseous** exudate.

Occasionally large amounts of pericardial effusion may accumulate. When the volume is massive (sometimes over a liter) or when the accumulation is rapid, diastolic filling may be impaired, a condition known as **cardiac tamponade**. Such large effusions are particularly likely with the more subacute to chronic processes, such as tuberculous, neoplastic, or immune pericarditis.

The late sequelae of these acute involvements are somewhat dependent on the severity of the reaction and on the specific etiology. In general, the serous and fibrinous patterns resolve completely. Infrequently, organization of fibrinous exudate yields delicate, bridging fibrous strands or shiny opaque thickenings of the pericardial surfaces, but neither change is of much clinical consequence. The suppurative bacterial and caseous tuberculous reactions are more grave. Although these, too, may resolve, more often they lead to fibrous obliteration of the pericardial cavity and adherence of the parietal pericardium to surrounding structures. This pattern of scarring is termed **adhesive mediastinopericarditis** and produces severe cardiac strain, since with each systolic contraction the heart works not only against the parietal pericardium but also against the attached surrounding structures. Diffuse organization within the pericardial sac may create the entity known as **chronic constrictive pericarditis**.[91] This is characterized by encasement of the heart within a dense fibrous scar, which although not attached to surrounding structures, cannot expand adequately during diastole and thus interferes with cardiac function. The fibrosis may constrict the venae cavae as they enter the heart, leading to hepatosplenomegaly and ascites. This pattern of scarring is probably most common with tuberculous pericarditis, although it is also known to occur relatively rapidly a few months after some cases of acute idiopathic pericarditis. In about 50% of cases, the fibrous enclosure becomes calcified. When this calcification is diffuse, it produces the appearance of a plaster mold encasing the heart, known as **concretio cordis**.

**CLINICAL COURSE.** Much of the clinical picture has already been described in discussing the various etiologies as well as the pattern of scarring. With acute fibrinous pericarditis, the principal symptom is the acute onset of chest pain, although the pain may be minimal or absent in up to 50% of cases. Usually there is associated malaise and fever. The pain may be very similar to that of angina pectoris or MI but tends to be distinguishable in having a pleuritic component as a result of a commonly associated pleuritis. The pain is often intensified by body movements and relieved by sitting or leaning forward. The presence of a pericardial friction rub is pathognomonic, but it may be very evanescent. In most cases, the process subsides spontaneously within a few weeks, but it tends to recur.

Principal among the complications of pericarditis are the accumulations of large effusions with resultant tamponade, embarrassment of the venous return to the heart, and the development of chronic adhesive or constrictive pericarditis.

# MYOCARDIAL DISEASE

Myocardial disease is a prominent feature of many of the cardiac disorders already discussed (e.g., ischemic, hypertensive, rheumatic, and congenital heart diseases and cor pulmonale). There remains a miscellany of myocardial involvements, best considered under two broad headings: (1) *myocarditis* and (2) *cardiomyopathies (CMP)*. Myocarditis is typically of acute onset, is often associated with a febrile reaction, tends to pursue a course of varying length, and may be a fatal illness, but in many instances, if not in most, the disease remits with or without therapy and in such cases may leave few if any significant residuals. Anatomically, this pattern of disease is characterized by an inflammatory reaction with necrosis of isolated cells or small groups of myocardial fibers. In contrast, the CMPs are extremely varied in nature and although some may be of relatively acute onset, more often they are insidious in development and run a protracted course; frequently they are fatal. Although a variety of anatomic myocardial alterations may be present, generally there are few if any inflammatory changes. However, there is overlap between the two groups because some cases of myocarditis progress to cardiomyopathy.

## CARDIOMYOPATHY (CMP)

One must be aware of the various clinical uses of the term CMP. It is broadly applied to any cardiac disorder in which the signs and symptoms result entirely or predominantly from myocardial dysfunction. An etiologic classification divides the various entities into primary and secondary forms. *Primary or idiopathic CMP* is a disorder of heart muscle of unknown cause or association that develops in the absence of ischemic, hypertensive, congenital, valvular, and other forms of heart disease.[92-94] *Secondary CMPs* are heart muscle diseases that have a known cause or occur as part of a well-defined systemic illness. Etiologic categories include alcoholism, viral infections, hypersensitivity and connective tissue diseases, neuromuscular diseases (certain muscular dystrophies, Friedreich's ataxia), metabolic disorders (hyperthyroidism, hypothyroidism, beriberi, hemochromatosis), amyloidosis, certain glycogen and lipid

storage diseases, and drug and chemical toxicities. Some authors also include in this category cases of heart disease in which severe myocardial dysfunction dominates the clinical picture—hence, the categorization of end-stage chronic IHD as ischemic CMP. Because of the difficulty in establishing the cause of many cases of CMP, a practical method of classifying the CMPs based on their clinical and pathological features is frequently employed as follows (Fig. 11–12):

*Congestive or dilated CMP:* Characterized by dilatation and hypertrophy of both ventricular cavities and poor systolic function.

*Hypertrophic CMP:* Characterized by a massive increase in ventricular muscle mass, small ventricular cavities, and hypercontracting left ventricle. Subaortic stenosis with outflow obstruction may or may not be present.

*Restrictive and obliterative CMP:* Two designations variously employed for those forms of CMP characterized by restriction of ventricular filling.

The two main types are congestive (dilated) and hypertrophic CMP.

*Congestive CMP is characterized by moderate to marked increase in heart weight and a more or less symmetrical, moderate to marked dilatation of the four cardiac chambers so that the ventricular walls are of normal or reduced thickness, despite the increase in weight.* About 75% of these patients have left ventricular thrombi at postmortem examination;

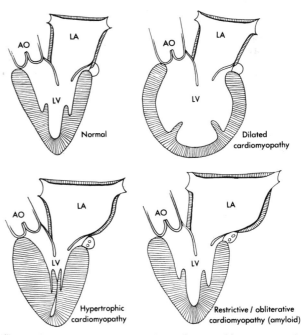

Figure 11–12. Various types of cardiomyopathies compared with normal heart. In the dilated or congestive type, the largest circumference of the left ventricle is not at its base but midway between the apex and base. In the hypertrophic type, the left ventricular cavity is small, and in the restrictive-obliterative variety, as in amyloidosis, the left ventricular cavity is of normal size. (From Roberts, W. C., and Ferrans, V. J.: Pathologic anatomy of the cardiomyopathies. Hum. Pathol. 6:289, 1975.)

thrombi are also frequent in the atrial appendages. Histologically, diffuse interstitial fibrosis is frequently found, but usually there is no evidence of inflammation. Electron microscopy has not identified any specific alterations, only changes of hypertrophy and myofibrillar and mitochondrial damage of variable degree. The cardiac valves are unaffected, and it should be noted that there is usually only mild to moderate coronary atherosclerosis. This last point is of importance in differentiating idiopathic congestive or dilated CMP from chronic ischemic heart disease.

The origins of this condition are obscure. In some studies, many patients have had a history of alcoholism, raising the possibility that congestive CMP is an end stage of *alcoholic CMP*. Alcoholic cardiomyopathy is generally accepted as a cause of CMP, but dissenting opinions persist.[96] It is pointed out that alcohol, by lowering the resistance of the individual, could potentiate the development of myocarditis or possibly predispose to nutritional deficiencies with the induction of beriberi heart disease (p. 245). Moreover, there are no specific histologic, ultrastructural, or histochemical features of alcohol toxicity. Nonetheless, there is an increased frequency of congestive cardiomyopathy in patients having a history of heavy alcohol intake. There is also evidence that alcohol can depress cardiac function. In other patients with congestive CMP, the heart failure presents late in pregnancy or during the first five months after delivery, giving rise to the sometimes used designation *peripartum CMP*. Whether the association with pregnancy is more than coincidental is unknown. Occasionally, the heart failure is preceded by an upper respiratory infection, suggesting a possible infective origin. There is also evidence that some cases of myocarditis of probable viral origin progress to chronic CMP. Thus prior *viral infection* may be a cause of congestive CMP. However, viral particles have not been observed in CMP specimens, nor has any microbiologic agent been identified at the time of necropsy. An *autoimmune* or *immunologic reaction* has also been proposed, perhaps triggered by a previous viral infection, and there is experimental evidence for this concept. Some patients may previously have been hypertensive, but in most there is no documented history of significant elevations of blood pressure. Infrequently, there is a familial predisposition, but, confusingly, two members of the same family may have different forms of CMP. We must leave it that the etiology of this condition is unknown and could possibly represent the end point of a variety of forms of myocardial damage.

Most patients with congestive or dilated CMP are middle-aged. The condition usually presents with the mysterious onset of cardiac failure, which in some cases is rapidly progressive, leading to death over the span of months. As might be anticipated, with a dilated heart there are often murmurs of mitral and tricuspid regurgitation. The diagnosis requires the ruling out of other better defined causes of cardiac decompensation. Conventional therapy is often ineffective, and patients with end-stage dilated CMP constitute a major group currently being treated with cardiac transplantation. The other major group of candidates for the procedure are those with end-stage chronic IHD.

*Hypertrophic CMP exists in two clinical forms: with functional subaortic stenosis and obstruction to the aortic outflow tract, and without obstructive manifestations.* In the past this form of cardiomyopathy was also called idiopathic hypertrophic subaortic stenosis (IHSS), hypertrophic obstructive cardiomyopathy, or asymmetrical septal hypertrophy (ASH). However, these older designations are best avoided since the cardiac changes are not always obstructive and the hypertrophy is not always subaortic or asymmetric.

The anatomic features of hypertrophic CMP are (1) disproportional hypertrophy of the ventricular septum (95%); (2) disorientation and disorganization of myocardial fibers in the ventricular septum (100%); (3) small or normal-sized left and right ventricular cavities (90%); (4) mural endocardial thickening in the left ventricular outflow tract (75%); (5) thickened mitral valve (75%); (6) dilated atria (100%); and (7) abnormal intramural coronary arteries (50%).[93]

Two features are particularly striking in this form of CMP. The ventricular septum is strikingly hypertrophied, usually much more so than the ventricular free wall, averaging 3 cm in thickness in a series of patients. The other distinctive feature is disorganization of myocardial fibers along with disarray of myofibrils and myofilaments within individual cells. The usual parallel array of fibers, fibrils, and filaments is replaced by an extraordinary disarray sometimes accompanied by bizarre shapes to the fibers. Grotesquely shaped nuclei and intracellular accumulation of glycogen may also be present.[97] Although these histologic and ultrastructural details are striking, they are not specific for hypertrophic CMP and are sometimes encountered in other forms of cardiac hypertrophy, but to a lesser extent. The disorganization of myocardial fibers is either confined to or most extensive in the ventricular septum. Whether or not these bizarre myocardial fibers are present in the ventricular free wall, the wall is often thickened, but not to the same degree as the septum. The distribution of the left ventricular free wall thickening has been accorded functional significance. According to Roberts, **in patients with the obstructive pattern of disease, the portion of the left ventricular free wall directly behind the posterior mitral leaflet represents the thickest portion. In the nonobstructive pattern, however, the ventricular free wall behind the posterior mitral leaflet is not thickened.** This anatomic detail may correlate with the functional studies indicating that obstruction to left ventricular outflow is related to displacement of the mitral valve so that the anterior leaflet approaches the septum during systole in a "pinchcock" fashion, inducing outflow obstruction. At the same time, mitral regurgitation may appear, possibly because conformational changes in the papillary muscles may prevent closure of the valves during systole.

The striking septal and cardiac hypertrophy in this form of CMP has a genetic basis in most cases. There is a high incidence of familial involvement and an autosomal dominant inheritance pattern. Echocardiographic visualization of asymmetric septal hypertrophy and abnormal mitral valve motion in asymptomatic relatives of index cases has provided strong evidence in this regard.[98] There also are occasionally sporadic, apparently acquired cases of CMP with features similar to that of inherited hypertrophic CMP. The basic pathophysiological alterations in hypertrophic CMP are increased resistance to diastolic filling and hypercontractile systolic function of the left ventricle. The current thinking is that abnormal cardiac function, usually having a genetic basis, leads to progressive disarray of myofibers and cardiac hypertrophy.

The natural history of this disease is quite variable. Some patients do not have obstruction. Even in those with obstructive features, as the disease progresses, there may be impairment of systolic contractile function and, surprisingly, lessening or disappearance of outflow tract obstruction. More often, in both patterns, there is eventually heart failure. Three serious complications may appear: (a) atrial fibrillation often associated with mural thrombosis and systemic embolism, (b) the development of infective endocarditis on the abnormal mitral valve, and (c) sudden death without premonitory signs and symptoms. It is important to note that the outflow tract obstruction sometimes submitted to surgical correction is now thought to be less important than the reduction in end-diastolic volume.

*Restrictive CMP* results from amyloidosis and other infiltrative disorders such as leukemia and glycogenoses (Pompe's disease) or it may occur on an idiopathic basis. *Obliterative CMP* has been used to describe endomyocardial fibrosis, encountered in the tropics, and a similar condition associated with eosinophilia that is encountered in temperate zones. This last-mentioned variant is sometimes referred to as Löffler's fibroplastic parietal endocarditis. Characteristic of all of these conditions is stiffness and reduced compliance of the ventricular walls or restriction of the left ventricular cavity.[93] Clinically, these CMPs can mimic constrictive pericarditis.

## MYOCARDITIS

The term "myocarditis" refers to myocardial involvements marked by inflammatory changes. Although the commonest causes are microbiologic infections, myocarditis may also be induced by hypersensitivity reactions, radiation therapy, and any chemical or physical agent or drug that induces acute myocardial fiber necrosis and secondary inflammatory changes. In most instances, the myocarditis is only one component of a generalized disease, as, for example, in acute rheumatic fever or cytomegalovirus infection. However, in some instances it may occur as an isolated disorder or at least be the dominating feature of the systemic disease, in which case it is sometimes referred to as *primary myocarditis* to differentiate it from the more common secondary involvements.

The major causes of myocarditis are presented in Table 11–3. This listing is by no means all-inclusive. Depending on the diagnostic criteria employed, myocarditis has been reported to be present in from 1 to 9% of routine autopsies. Even at the lower limit, many of the cases represent incidental and chance morphologic findings that may not have been associated with significant clinical findings during life.[99] Further comments will be restricted to the more common and clinically important forms of myocarditis and to the few having distinctive anatomic changes.

*Viral myocarditis* is by far the most common clinical pattern of myocarditis and the one that most often presents as a primary infection.[100, 101] It is characterized by an interstitial edema and mononuclear infiltrate. There may or may not be myofiber necroses (Fig. 11–13). The Coxsackie group of viruses, principally Coxsackie B, are most often implicated. In an earlier discussion, it was noted that viral infection, particularly by Coxsackie B, may underlie many cases of "idiopathic" congestive CMP. The question has been raised whether such infections may initiate immunologic damage to the myocardium, possibly involving antimyocardial antibodies and cytotoxic cells, and leading eventually to changes later identified as congestive CMP.

When Coxsackie myocarditis appears in children

### Table 11–3. MAJOR CAUSES OF MYOCARDITIS

| | |
|---|---|
| **Viruses and chlamydiae** | **Protozoa** |
| Coxsackie B and A | *Trypanosoma cruzi* (Chagas' |
| Echo | disease) |
| Influenza | Toxoplasmosis |
| Infectious mononucleosis | Amebiasis |
| Poliomyelitis | |
| Mumps | **Parasites** |
| Measles | Trichinosis |
| Chicken pox | |
| Smallpox | **Hypersensitivity** |
| Psittacosis | Rheumatic fever |
| Lymphogranuloma | Dermatomyositis |
| venereum | Scleroderma |
| Herpes simplex | Rheumatoid arthritis |
| Cytomegalovirus | Postviral |
| Hepatitis virus | Autoimmune |
| German measles | |
| Rabies | **Trauma** |
| Yellow fever | |
| | **Idiopathic** |
| **Bacteria** | Fiedler's (giant cell) myocarditis |
| Infective endocarditis | |
| Septicemia | |
| Diphtheria (exotoxic) | |
| Syphilis | |
| *Borrelia recurrentis* | |

and young adults, it is often symptomatic. It affects males twice as often as females. Often there is a history of an upper respiratory tract infection, followed by a latent period of several days. Among adults, the disease is usually associated with pericarditis and often is a relatively benign, self-limited process. However, in the debilitated or immunosuppressed adult, the infection may be far more severe and, indeed, sudden death in young adults may occasionally be caused by Coxsackie myocarditis. Coxsackie B myocarditis acquired in intrauterine or neonatal life is more likely to be a rapidly fatal disease than the disease acquired in adulthood.

Many other viruses may also cause myocarditis (particularly the agents of poliomyelitis and German measles). The former in the vulnerable individual is capable of causing severe disseminated myocardial necroses and sudden death. *Rubella is particularly important when the infection is contracted in utero, during the first trimester of pregnancy.* In this stage of embryogenesis, the rubella virus frequently induces cardiac as well as other defects, most important among which are cataracts, deafness, persistent ductus arteriosus, pulmonary artery hypoplasia, pulmonary valve stenosis, aortic stenosis, ventricular septal defect, and tetralogy of Fallot. It might be pointed out that there is evidence that maternal and then fetal infection with Coxsackie B virus may also produce congenital heart disease.

*Bacterial myocarditis* is rare in comparison with the viral forms. It is principally encountered as a grave complication of infective endocarditis or some other form of bacteremia. Diphtheritic myocarditis is more properly referred to as toxic myocarditis, since the myocardial damage results from the systemic dissemination of exotoxin. The toxin inhibits polypeptide chain elongation and also interferes with the fatty acid transport function of carnitine in myocardial fibers, and so protein synthesis is impaired and triglycerides accumulate in injured myocardial cells.

*Protozoal infections* also cause myocarditis. *Toxoplasma gondii* is recognized as a cause of sporadic cases of myocarditis or pericarditis, which occur as part of a clinically apparent or subclinical systemic infection. In *Chagas' disease,* caused by *Trypanosoma cruzi,* the myocardial involvement is the most important aspect in most patients. Up to half of the population in endemic areas of South America is infected. About 10% of these patients die during the acute phase. In other cases, the disease appears to subside, followed by a latent period of 10 to 20 years before the chronic phase of the myocarditis becomes manifest. A still larger group of patients develops the chronic phase of the disease without a history of an antecedent acute infection. In one endemic area, Chagas' disease has been reported as causing about 25% of all deaths in persons between the ages of 25 and 44 years.[102]

*Idiopathic myocarditis* refers to those sporadic cases of myocarditis that occur without discernible cause in previously healthy individuals. A rapidly fatal form of idiopathic myocarditis is known as *Fiedler's myocarditis* or more recently as *giant cell myocarditis.* This type affects males more frequently than females, with a peak incidence in the third decade. Commonly, there is a concurrent or previous respiratory infection. Myocardial failure is intractable and death usually ensues within weeks. It is likely that Fiedler's myocarditis is not a specific entity and that it represents more severe involvement by any of a number of unknown etiologic agents. It is thought that as routine diagnostic procedures for viral infections become more widespread, much of what has heretofore been called idiopathic myocarditis will emerge as viral myocarditis.

**MORPHOLOGY.** Most of the myocarditides produce essentially similar anatomic changes, which will be described here as characteristic of the group as a whole. Minor variations in the morphologic picture depend on the etiologic agent. Sometimes the heart appears grossly normal; however, more often it is dilated. Although all chambers of the heart may be affected, the right side is generally more dilated and flabby. The myocardium often discloses areas of pallor or yellowish mottling. Cardiac hypertrophy is only present in subacute or chronic cases.

Histologically, there is always some inflammatory infiltrate, usually associated with some edema. The nature of the infiltrate is highly variable. In the more acute processes, such as those caused by direct bacterial invasion or the fulminant forms of Chagas' disease, it may be composed chiefly of polymorphonuclear leukocytes. In other cases, principally those of viral origin, there may be a predominantly mononuclear inflammatory response (Fig. 11–13). Occasionally, there are large numbers of eosinophils and granulomatous formations

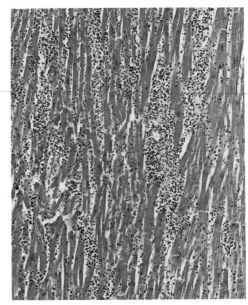

**Figure 11–13.** Viral myocarditis. A heavy interstitial infiltration of lymphocytes separates many of the myocardial fibers.

with giant cells, particularly in certain patterns of **Fiedler's (giant cell) myocarditis**. When involvement is more chronic, such as with long-standing Chagas' disease and with toxoplasmic myocarditis, a fibrous reaction may be seen. Although the myofibers themselves often appear normal, in many of the myocarditides degenerative changes of varying intensity are often seen, including cellular swelling, fatty change, and sometimes actual necrosis. The extent of the myofiber injury correlates better with the severity of the attack than with the specific etiology. Similarly, the intensity of the inflammatory infiltrate versus the amount of fibrous scarring is a function of the chronicity of the disease.

**CLINICAL COURSE.** The clinical picture of myocarditis is extremely variable. In many cases, it is asymptomatic or overshadowed by a systemic disorder. Transient ECG abnormalities may be the only indication of its presence. Acute *symptomatic* myocarditis often manifests itself as malaise, dyspnea, and low-grade fever, with tachycardia more marked than the fever alone would warrant. A gallop rhythm is usually present, and there may be a murmur of mitral or tricuspid insufficiency as the weakened ventricular walls yield and the heart dilates. Conduction defects are common, most often taking the form of varying degrees of atrioventricular block. Other arrhythmias may also occur. With advanced disease, CHF involving both ventricles ensues. This is most often manifested clinically as failure of the right side of the heart, since the symptoms of full-blown left-sided heart failure are dependent to some extent on a relatively healthy right ventricle. In most cases, myocarditis is transient, and the symptoms subside after one to two months. A five-year follow-up study of a number of these patients, however, showed that 25% had persistent symptoms, usually precordial pain and fatigue; 20% had cardiomegaly as seen by chest x-ray; and 19% had abnormal electrocardiograms at rest.[103] Currently, there is widespread clinical interest in the use of myocardial biopsy procedures to evaluate patients with heart failure or arrhythmias of obscure etiology.[104] The purpose is to identify patients with myocarditis who can be treated with corticosteroids and other anti-inflammatory drugs, with the goal of preventing the development of CMP. The rationale is based on the previously stated hypothesis that many of these cases progress from myocarditis to CMP because of virus-induced immunological mechanisms.[101] Confirmation of this approach requires further evaluation.

# ENDOCARDIAL AND VALVULAR DISEASE

The endocardium and valves are involved in a number of cardiac diseases (Table 11–4), including some already discussed in this chapter—e.g., rheumatic heart disease and congenital heart disease.[71] In addition, as indicated on pages 301 and 302, diseases

Table 11–4. MAJOR ETIOLOGIES OF ACQUIRED VALVULAR HEART DISEASE

| Mitral Valve Disease | Aortic Valve Disease |
|---|---|
| *Mitral Stenosis* | *Aortic Stenosis* |
| Rheumatic heart disease | Calcification of congenitally deformed (usually bicuspid) valve |
| | Senile calcific aortic stenosis |
| | Rheumatic heart disease |
| *Mitral Regurgitation* | *Aortic Regurgitation* |
| Abnormalities of leaflets and commissures | Intrinsic valvular disease |
| Rheumatic heart disease | Rheumatic heart disease |
| Infective endocarditis | Infective endocarditis |
| Floppy mitral valve | Aortic disease |
| Abnormalities of tensor apparatus | Cystic medial necrosis |
| Rupture of papillary muscle | Syphilitic aortitis |
| Papillary muscle dysfunction (fibrosis) | Ankylosing spondylitis |
| Rupture of chordae tendineae | Rheumatoid arthritis |
| Abnormalities of left ventricular cavity and/or annulus | Marfan's syndrome |
| LV enlargement (myocarditis, congestive cardiomyopathy) | |
| Calcification of mitral ring | |

of the proximal aorta, notably cystic medial necrosis and luetic aortitis, can give rise to aortic valvular insufficiency and cardiomegaly. A few additional entities remain to be discussed.

## CALCIFIC AORTIC STENOSIS

Aortic stenosis may be encountered in healed rheumatic heart disease or possibly in healed infective endocarditis. A key feature of postinflammatory aortic stenosis is prominent commissural fusion along with fibrosis and calcification of the cusps. In the case of *rheumatic aortic stenosis*, evidence of mitral valve involvement is typically present. However, evidence of an inflammatory origin can be identified in fewer than 10% of patients with calcific aortic stenosis.[71] Nevertheless, by age 55 years, about 5% of individuals have significant calcium deposits in the aortic valve, and this frequency increases 1% per year thereafter. Occasionally, the calcification and associated fibrosis become sufficiently well developed to produce aortic stenosis. Most of the cases in this age range appear to occur as a consequence of cumulative wear and tear on valves rendered vulnerable by a major *congenital defect*, usually a *congenital bicuspid valve* (see p. 334). The process is characterized by progressive fibrosis and calcification with minimal commissural fusion. However, in individuals approximately 65 years or older, so-called *senile calcific aortic stenosis* may develop with a three-cusped aortic valve (Fig. 11–14). In the latter cases,

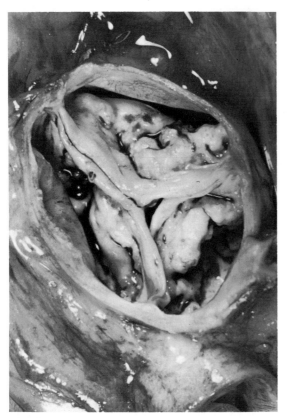

Figure 11–14. Calcific aortic stenosis. A view looking down on the markedly deformed unopened valve with thickened cusps and calcific masses within the sinuses of Valsalva.

slight inequality of cuspal size has been proposed as a predisposing factor. There is no substantial proof for a viral or other infectious or inflammatory etiology for most cases. Regardless of cause, the obstructive stenosis often induces marked left ventricular concentric hypertrophy. Deficient cerebral blood flow may cause faintness, dizziness, syncope, or even epileptiform seizures, and deficient coronary blood flow may result in angina pectoris or congestive heart failure. Some symptomatic individuals are vulnerable to sudden death.

## CALCIFICATION OF THE MITRAL ANNULUS

This lesion has some analogy to calcific aortic stenosis, just described. However, *the calcification is generally limited to the annular ring of the mitral valve; the leaflets are not calcified but only slightly fibrous and thickened.* Thus, the calcific changes may induce beading at the base of the mitral leaflets but rarely functionally significant stenosis. These mitral changes, like those in most cases of calcific aortic stenosis, are attributed to aging and "wear and tear."[105]

## MITRAL VALVE PROLAPSE (FLOPPY VALVE SYNDROME; BARLOW'S SYNDROME)

*In this condition, one or both mitral valve leaflets prolapse backward or balloon into the left atrium during left ventricular systole.*[106] The sudden tightening of the elongated chordae tendineae produces a midsystolic click on auscultation and sometimes a late systolic murmur of mitral regurgitation. Occasionally, there is only the late systolic murmur without the click. Mitral valve prolapse is surprisingly common and has been reported in between 5 and 10% of the general population. Although both sexes are affected, 20- to 30-year-old females have the highest incidence of this condition.

Morphologically, the involved leaflets are voluminous, thickened, and elongated, having a parachute-like appearance, with the dome projecting into the atrium.[107] The chordae are elongated, thickened, or thinned and sometimes ruptured. The leaflets themselves may have fissures and sometimes small attached thrombi, most often in the sulcus between the valve leaflet and the atrial walls. Microscopically, there is replacement of the central fibrous structure of the leaflet by loose, myxomatous tissue rich in metachromatic ground substance. The posterior leaflet is always involved, the anterior leaflet less frequently. Rarely, the tricuspid valve is also affected.

The origin of these changes is unclear. Some consider them a forme fruste of Marfan's syndrome (p. 105), and indeed some cases (10 to 15%) are familial, with autosomal dominant inheritance. However, the majority are sporadic and nonfamilial and have none of the skeletal features of Marfan's syndrome. About 80% of the cases have abnormal left ventricular function, possibly related to autonomic nervous system dysfunction, suggesting that the prolapse may be secondary to the ventricular dysfunction.[108] All of these theories must at the present time be considered speculative.

In most cases the floppy mitral valve is merely an interesting auscultatory clinical finding and without significance. However, it has been associated with bizarre chest pains, various arrhythmias, thrombi causing cerebral ischemic events,[109] and even sudden death in young individuals. Rarely, the abnormal valves provide a soil for the development of infective endocarditis.

## NONBACTERIAL THROMBOTIC ENDOCARDITIS (MARANTIC ENDOCARDITIS)

This disorder is characterized by the deposition of small masses of fibrin and other blood elements upon the valve leaflets, usually but not necessarily in the left side of the heart. In contrast to infective endocarditis, the vegetations are sterile and tend to be small (about 1 to 5 mm in diameter). Moreover, they may occur singly or multiply in random locations along the lines of closure of the leaflets. This distribution differentiates them somewhat from acute rheumatic endocarditis, characterized by numerous minute vegetations dotting the lines of closure of affected valves. Only the verrucous endocarditis associated with systemic lupus erythematosus creates a close morphologic parallel.

The term "marantic," derived from marasmus, implies that these lesions are associated with debilitation. Indeed, there is a well-defined association with metastatic cancer.[110] However, they may occur in young individuals, even children, and sometimes in patients who are well nourished and distinctly not marantic.[111] They are occasionally found in patients with venous thromboses or pulmonary embolization, suggesting that the valvular vegetations are another manifestation of a hypercoagulable state. It is generally thought that the vegetations develop preterminally but there are many instances to document that this "inconsequential" condition may have clinical consequences.[112] Fragmentation or dislodgement of the vegetations has given rise to emboli to the brain, kidneys, lungs, and elsewhere to produce significant clinical morbidity or even mortality. They may also have importance as an antecedent to the development of infective endocarditis (p. 335).

## NONBACTERIAL VERRUCOUS ENDOCARDITIS (LIBMAN-SACKS DISEASE)

Nonbacterial verrucous endocarditis refers to the valvular lesions associated with systemic lupus erythematosus (SLE), and reference should be made to the discussion of this disorder on page 152.

## CARCINOID SYNDROME

The carcinoid syndrome is characterized by transient paroxysms of hypotension, cyanosis, bronchoconstriction, and diarrhea in patients with argentaffin tumors. Often there are associated lesions of the valves of the right side of the heart, producing murmurs. This interesting syndrome is discussed on page 538.

## ENDOCARDIAL FIBROELASTOSIS (EFE)

EFE is an uncommon heart disease of obscure etiology that is characterized by patchy or diffuse fibroelastic thickening of the endocardium. It is likely that this entity represents the final outcome of a variety of forms of cardiac damage.[75, 113] The peak incidence of clinical presentation is in the first two years of life. About one third of cases are associated with congenital malformations of the heart—hypoplastic left heart syndrome, aortic stenosis, mitral stenosis, coarctation of the aorta, and anomalous origin of the left coronary artery from the aorta. These cases, which are sometimes referred to as secondary EFE, typically present in early infancy. In hearts with anomalies it is proposed that deranged intrauterine hemodynamics produce hypodeveloped, small cardiac chambers and consequent endocardial stress injuries, which lead to the striking fibroelastosis. Intrauterine hypoxia also may play a role, particularly in cases associated with anomalous coronary arteries. Most cases of EFE occur in hearts without other malformations and are sometimes referred to as primary EFE. They typically present with cardiac dilatation and failure. The etiology and pathogenesis of primary EFE are unknown, but the current favored theory of causation of most cases is an intrauterine viral infection involving both the endocardium and adjacent myocardium, which in time induces the characteristic scarring. A number of viruses have been implicated, including mumps and the Coxsackie B group. Occasionally, identical involvement has been reported in twins, triplets, and siblings, but the pattern of transmission is uncertain

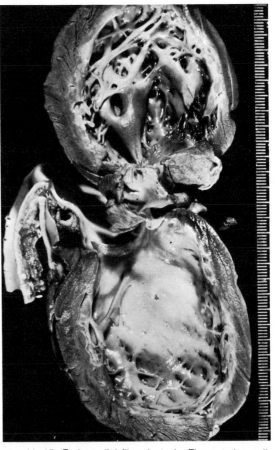

Figure 11–15. Endocardial fibroelastosis. The anterior wall of the left ventricle has been lifted to expose the white, opaque, fibrous endocardial layer, which can be seen covering the entire surface of the chamber. The fibrosis extends superficially into the adjacent myocardium.

and both autosomal dominant and autosomal recessive inheritance have been proposed.[114]

Endocardial fibroelastosis appears as a diffuse or patchy, pearly-white thickening of the mural endocardium, predominantly of the left ventricle (Fig. 11–15). However, the left atrium, right ventricle, and right atrium, in this order of frequency, may also be involved. The endocardial lining may attain a depth up to 10 times normal. Mural thrombi sometimes overlie these fibrous areas. In many cases, the endocardial fibrosis extends into the mitral and aortic valves, which thus become thickened and stenotic. In most cases without other cardiac malformations, the heart is enlarged and dilated. Histologically, there is a marked increase of collagenous and elastic fibers on the endocardial surface, which may extend into the myocardium. The fibers generally run parallel to the surface. Occasionally, scattered lymphocytes and focal necroses in the underlying myocardium may be seen.

The significance of this lesion depends upon the extent of involvement. When focal, it may have no functional importance and permit normal longevity. When severe, however, it produces intractable CHF. This may be especially fulminant in infants and may lead to death within hours of the first noticeable manifestations. Unless there are concomitant congenital anomalies or markedly fibrotic valves, a heart murmur is not usually present until the heart has begun to dilate. About 50% of these patients do not respond to treatment, and death follows.

## MYXOMA OF THE HEART

This benign tumor is the most common neoplasm of the heart and the only one to occur sufficiently frequently to warrant description in this chapter. However, it remains one of the least common causes of heart murmur. Myxomas most often develop between the ages of 30 and 60 years and affect women twice as often as men.[115]

Myxomas appear as globular or polypoid masses arising from the endocardial surface and projecting into the cardiac chambers. Ninety per cent occur within the atria, most often on the left. Some are sessile, but many are attached by a slender stalk, permitting them to move freely in the blood, sometimes to act as ball-valve obstructions to the heart valves, most often the mitral. They are usually covered by a thin, glistening endothelial layer and have a semitranslucent, yellow-gray, gelatinous transected surface. Microscopically, they are composed of an abundant acellular ground substance in which are found widely separated polyhedral or stellate cells resembling fibroblasts or myxoma cells. Scattered within the ground substance are occasional smooth muscle cells, multinucleate giant cells, lymphocytes, plasma cells, pigmented macrophages, and extracellular hemosiderin. Vessels of varying size are also present, some well developed, others having large, cavernous lumens.

The vascular components and the variety of cell types led to the suggestion that these lesions are actually organizing thrombi. However, most observers consider them to be true neoplasms. This view is supported by electron microscopic evidence that the lesions arise from multipotential mesenchymal cells capable of differentiating along the cell lines mentioned.[116]

## References

1. Goldman, L., and Cook, E. F.: The decline in ischemic heart disease mortality rates. An analysis of the comparative effects of medical interventions and changes in lifestyle. Ann. Intern. Med. 101:825, 1984.
2. Braunwald, E.: Pathophysiology of heart failure and Clinical manifestations of heart failure. In Braunwald, E. (ed.): Heart Disease. A Textbook of Cardiovascular Medicine. 2nd ed. Philadelphia, W. B. Saunders Co., 1984, p. 447 and p. 488.
3. Teplitz, C.: Pulmonary cellular and interstitial edema. In Fishman, A. P., and Renkin, E. M. (eds.): Pulmonary Edema. American Physiologic Society (Clinical Physiology Series). Baltimore, Williams & Wilkins, 1979, p. 97.
4. Wiener-Kronish, J. P., et al.: Relationship of pleural effusions to pulmonary hemodynamics in patients with congestive heart failure. Am. Rev. Respir. Dis. 132:1253, 1985.
5. Willerson, J. T., Hillis, L. D., and Buja, L. M.: Ischemic Heart Disease: Clinical and Pathophysiological Aspects. New York, Raven Press, 1982.
6. Buja, L. M., and Willerson, J. T.: Clinicopathologic correlates of acute ischemic heart disease syndromes. Am. J. Cardiol. 47:343, 1981.
7. Buja, L. M., and Willerson, J. T.: Pathophysiology of angina pectoris and acute ischemic heart disease. Cardiovasc. Rev. Rep. 4:1553, 1983.
8. Braunwald, E.: Treatment of the patient after myocardial infarction. N. Engl. J. Med. 302:290, 1980.
9. Roberts, C. S., and Roberts, W. C.: Cross-sectional area of the proximal portions of the three major epicardial coronary arteries in 98 necropsy patients with different coronary events: Relationship to heart weight, age and sex. Circulation 62:953, 1980.
10. Hillis, L. D., and Braunwald, E.: Coronary-artery spasm. N. Engl. J. Med. 299:695, 1978.
11. Buja, L. M., et al.: The role of coronary arterial spasm in ischemic heart disease. Arch. Pathol. Lab. Med. 105:221, 1981.
12. Shepherd, J. T., and Vanhoutte, P. M.: Spasm of the coronary arteries: Causes and consequences (the scientist's viewpoint). Mayo Clin. Proc. 60:33, 1985.
13. Forman, M. B., et al.: Increased adventitial mast cells in a patient with coronary spasm. N. Engl. J. Med. 313:1138, 1985.
14. Hirsh, P. D., et al.: Release of prostaglandins and thromboxane into the coronary circulation in patients with ischemic heart disease. N. Engl. J. Med. 304:685, 1981.
15. Fitzgerald, D. J., et al.: Platelet activation in unstable coronary disease. N. Engl. J. Med. 315:983, 1986.
16. Davies, M. J., et al.: Intramyocardial platelet aggregation in patients with unstable angina suffering sudden ischemic cardiac death. Circulation 73:418, 1986.
17. Bush, L. R., et al.: Effects of the selective thromboxane synthetase inhibitor, dazoxiben, on variations in cyclic blood flow in stenosed canine coronary arteries. Circulation 69:1161, 1984.
18. Willerson, J. T., et al.: Speculation regarding mechanisms responsible for acute ischemic heart disease syndromes. J. Am. Col. Cardiol. 8:245, 1986.

19. Davies, M. J., et al.: Pathology of acute myocardial infarction with particular reference to occlusive coronary thrombi. Br. Heart J. 38:659, 1976.

20. Ridolfi, R. L., and Hutchins, G. M.: The relationship between coronary artery lesions and myocardial infarcts: Ulceration of atherosclerotic plaques precipitating coronary thrombosis. Am. Heart J. 93:468, 1977.

21. Horie, T., et al.: Coronary thrombosis in pathogenesis of acute myocardial infarction: Histopathological study of coronary arteries in 108 necropsied cases using serial section. Br. Heart J. 40:153, 1978.

22. Davies, M. J., et al.: The relation of coronary thrombosis to ischemic myocardial necrosis. J. Pathol. 172:99, 1979.

23. Falk, E.: Plaque rupture with severe pre-existing stenosis precipitating coronary thrombosis: Characteristics of coronary atherosclerotic plaques underlying fatal occlusive thrombi. Br. Heart J. 50:127, 1983.

24. Fuster, V., et al.: Role of platelets and thrombosis in coronary atherosclerotic disease and sudden death. J. Am. Col. Cardiol. 5(Suppl.):175B, 1985.

25. Cobb, L. A., et al.: Sudden cardiac death. Mod. Concepts Cardiovasc. Dis. 49:31, 1980.

26. Reichenbach, D. D., et al.: Pathology of the heart in sudden cardiac death. Am. J. Cardiol. 39:865, 1977.

27. Baroldi, G., et al.: Sudden coronary death. A postmortem study in 208 selected cases compared to 97 "control" subjects. Am. Heart J. 98:20, 1979.

28. Warnes, C. A., and Roberts, W. C.: Sudden coronary death: Comparison of patients with to those without coronary thrombus at necropsy. Am. J. Cardiol. 54:1206, 1984.

29. Davies, M. J., and Thomas, A.: Thrombosis and acute coronary artery lesions in sudden cardiac ischemic death. N. Engl. J. Med. 310:1137, 1984.

30. Baum, R. S., et al.: Survival after resuscitation from out-of-hospital ventricular fibrillation. Circulation 50:1231, 1974.

31. Eliot, R. S., and Buell, J. C.: Role of emotions and stress in the genesis of sudden death. J. Am. Col. Cardiol. 5(Suppl.):95B, 1985.

32. Paffenbarger, R. S., Jr.: Physical activity and fatal heart attack—Protection or selection? In Amsterdam, E., Wilmore, J. H., and DeMaria, A. N. (eds.): Cardiovascular Health and Disease. New York, York Medical Books, 1977, p. 35.

33. Hartung, G. H., et al.: Relation of diet to high-density lipoprotein cholesterol in middle-aged marathon runners, joggers and inactive men. N. Engl. J. Med. 302:357, 1980.

34. Williams, R. S., et al.: Physical conditioning augments the fibrinolytic response to venous occlusion in healthy adults. N. Engl. J. Med. 302:987, 1980.

35. Rennie, D., and Hollenberg, N. K.: Cardiomythology and marathons. N. Engl. J. Med. 301:103, 1979.

36. Roberts, W. C.: Coronary thrombosis and fatal myocardial ischemia. Circulation 49:1, 1974.

37. Silver, M. D., et al.: The relationship between acute occlusive coronary thrombi and myocardial infarction studied in 100 consecutive patients. Circulation 61:219, 1980.

38. Hellstrom, H. R.: Evidence in favor of the vasospastic cause of coronary artery thrombosis. Am. Heart J. 97:449, 1979.

39. Reimer, K. A., and Jennings, R. B.: The "wavefront phenomenon" of myocardial ischemic cell death. II. Transmural progression of necrosis within the framework of ischemic bed size (myocardium at risk) and collateral blood flow. Lab. Invest. 40:633, 1979.

40. DeWood, M. A., et al.: Prevalence of total coronary occlusion during the early hours of transmural myocardial infarction. N. Engl. J. Med. 303:897, 1980.

41. Rentrop, K. P., et al.: Effects of intracoronary streptokinase and intracoronary nitroglycerin infusion on coronary angiographic patterns and mortality in patients with acute myocardial infarction. N. Engl. J. Med. 311:1457, 1984.

42. TIMI Study Group: The thrombolysis in myocardial infarction (TIMI) trial. Phase I findings. N. Engl. J. Med. 312:932, 1985.

43. Neill, W. A., et al.: Acute coronary insufficiency—coronary

occlusion after intermittent ischemic attacks. N. Engl. J. Med. 302:1157, 1980.

44. Ambrose, J. A., et al.: Coronary angiographic morphology in myocardial infarction: A link between the pathogenesis of unstable angina and myocardial infarction. J. Am. Col. Cardiol. 6:1233, 1985.

45. Wilson, R. R., et al.: Quantitative angiographic morphology of coronary stenoses leading to myocardial infarction or unstable angina. Circulation 73:286, 1986.

46. Geer, J. C., et al.: Subendocardial ischemic myocardial lesions associated with severe coronary atherosclerosis. Am. J. Pathol. 98:663, 1980.

47. Mallory, G. K., et al.: The speed of healing of myocardial infarction. Am. Heart J. 18:747, 1939.

48. Lie, J. T., et al.: Macroscopic enzyme-mapping verification of large homogeneous experimental infarcts of predictable size and location in dogs. J. Thorac. Cardiovasc. Surg. 69:599, 1975.

49. Bates, R. J., et al.: Cardiac rupture—Challenge in diagnosis and management. Am. J. Cardiol. 40:429, 1977.

50. Bouchardy, B., and Majno, G.: Histopathology of early myocardial infarcts. Am. J. Pathol. 74:301, 1974.

51. Sakurai, I.: Pathology of acute ischemic myocardium: Special reference to (1) evaluation of morphological methods for detection of early myocardial infarcts and (II) lipid metabolism in infarcted myocardium. Acta Pathol. Jpn. 27:587, 1977.

52. Janse, M. J., et al.: The "border zone" in myocardial ischemia—An electrophysiological metabolic and histochemical correlation in the pig heart. Circ. Res. 44:576, 1979.

53. Factor, S. M., et al.: The histologic border zone of acute myocardial infarction—Island or peninsulas? Am. J. Pathol. 92:111, 1978.

54. Morales, A. R., and Fine, G.: Early human myocardial infarction—A histochemical study. Arch. Pathol. 82:9, 1966.

55. Lester, R. M., and Wagner, G. S.: Acute myocardial infarction. Med. Clin. North Am. 63:3, 1979.

56. Bigger, J. T., Jr., et al.: Ventricular arrhythmias in ischemic heart disease: Mechanism, prevalence, significance, and management. Prog. Cardiovasc. Dis. 19:255, 1977.

57. Page, D. L., et al.: Myocardial changes associated with cardiogenic shock. N. Engl. J. Med. 285:133, 1971.

58. Rude, R. E., et al.: Efforts to limit the size of myocardial infarcts. Ann. Intern. Med. 95:736, 1981.

59. World Health Organization European Collaborative Group: European collaborative trial of multifactorial prevention of coronary heart disease: Final report on the 6-year results. Lancet 1:869, 1986.

60. Harker, L. A.: Clinical trials evaluating platelet-modifying drugs in patients with atherosclerotic cardiovascular disease and thrombosis. Circulation 73:206, 1986.

61. Braunwald, E.: Effects of coronary-artery bypass grafting on survival: Implications of the randomized coronary-artery surgery study. N. Engl. J. Med. 309:1181, 1983.

62. Leimgruber, P. P., et al.: Influences of intimal dissection on restenosis after successful coronary angioplasty. Circulation 72:530, 1985.

63. Willerson, J. T., and Buja, L. M.: Short- and long-term influence of beta-adrenergic antagonists after acute myocardial infarction. Am. J. Cardiol. 54(Suppl. E):16E, 1984.

64. Boucher, C. A., et al.: Cardiomyopathic syndrome caused by coronary artery disease. III. Prospective clinicopathological study of its prevalence among patients with clinically unexplained chronic heart failure. Br. Heart J. 41:613, 1979.

65. Schlesinger, M. J., and Reiner, L.: Focal myocytolysis of the heart. Am. J. Pathol. 31:443, 1955.

66. Maron, B. J., and Ferrans, V. J.: Ultrastructural features of hypertrophied human ventricular myocardium. Prog. Cardiovasc. Dis. 31:207, 1978.

67. Kaplan, M. H.: Rheumatic fever, rheumatic heart disease and the strep connection: The role of streptococcal antigens cross-reactive with heart tissue. Rev. Infect. Dis. 1:988, 1979.

68. Zabriskie, J. B.: Rheumatic fever: The interplay between host, genetics, and microbe. Circulation 71:1077, 1985.

69. Stollerman, G. H.: A global view of rheumatic fever today. In Russek, H. I.: Cardiovascular Problems: Baltimore, University Park Press, 1976, p. 381.

70. Yang, L. C., et al.: Streptococcal induced cell-mediated destruction of cardiac myofibers in vitro. J. Exp. Med. 146:344, 1977.

71. Roberts, W. C., et al.: Nonrheumatic valvular cardiac disease: A clinicopathologic survey of 27 different conditions causing valvular dysfunction. In Likoff, W. (ed.): Valvular Heart Disease. (Cardiovascular Clinics, Vol. 5, No. 2) Philadelphia, F. A. Davis Co., 1973, p. 333.

72. Jones, T. D.: Diagnosis of rheumatic fever. J.A.M.A. 126:481, 1944.

73. Quinn, E. L.: Bacterial endocarditis. Postgrad. Med. 44:82, 1968.

74. Moller, J. H., Amplatz, K., and Edwards, J. E.: Congenital Heart Disease. Monograph of Universities Associated for Research and Education in Pathology. Kalamazoo, Michigan, Upjohn Co., 1971.

75. Perloff, J. K.: The Clinical Recognition of Congenital Heart Disease. 2nd ed. Philadelphia, W. B. Saunders Co., 1978.

76. Nora, J. J., and Nora, A. H.: The evolution of specific genetic and environmental counseling in congenital heart diseases. Circulation 57:205, 1978.

77. Watanakunakorn, C.: Changing epidemiology and newer aspects of infective endocarditis. Adv. Intern. Med. 22:21, 1977.

78. Editorial: Infective endocarditis. Br. Med. J. 282:677, 1981.

79. von Reyn, C. F., et al.: Infective endocarditis and analysis based on strict case definitions. Ann. Intern. Med. 94:505, 1981.

80. Lowes, J. A., et al.: Ten years of infective endocarditis at St. Bartholomew's Hospital: Analysis of clinical features and treatment in relation to prognosis and mortality. Lancet 1:133, 1980.

81. Weinstein, L., and Schlesinger, J. J.: Pathoanatomic, pathophysiologic and clinical correlations in endocarditis. N. Engl. J. Med. 291:837, 1122, 1974.

82. Durack, D. T., and Beeson, P. B.: Pathogenesis of infective endocarditis. In Rahimtoola, S. H. (ed.): Infective Endocarditis. New York, Grune & Stratton, 1978, p. 1.

83. Kaplan, E. L., et al.: A collaborative study of infective endocarditis in the 1970s. Emphasis on infections in patients who have undergone cardiovascular surgery. Circulation 59:327, 1979.

84. Roberts, W. C.: Characteristics and consequences of infective endocarditis (active or healed or both) learned from morphologic studies. In Rahimtoola, S. H. (ed.): Infective Endocarditis. New York, Grune & Stratton, 1978, p. 55.

85. Pelletier, L. L., Jr., and Petersdorf, R. G.: Infective endocarditis: A review of 125 cases from the University of Washington Hospitals, 1963–72. Medicine 56:287, 1977.

86. Hartman, R. B.: Pulmonary heart disease: Pathophysiology, diagnostic signs and therapy. Postgrad. Med. 66:58, 1979.

87. Wagenvoort, C. A., and Wagenvoort, N.: Primary pulmonary hypertension: A pathologic study of the lung vessels in 156 clinically diagnosed cases. Circulation 42:1163, 1970.

88. Roberts, W. C., and Spray, T. L.: Pericardial heart disease. Curr. Probl. Cardiol. 2:1, 1977.

89. Evans, E.: Symposium on pericarditis: Introduction. Am. J. Cardiol. 7:1, 1961.

90. Engle, M. A., et al.: The postpericardiotomy and similar syndromes. Cardiovasc. Clin. 7:211, 1976.

91. Hancock, E. W.: Constrictive pericarditis: Modern view of diagnosis and management. J. Cardiovasc. Med. 41:367, 1980.

92. Goodwin, J. R., and Oakley, C. M.: The cardiomyopathies. Br. Heart J. 34:545, 1972.

93. Roberts, W. C., and Ferrans, V. J.: Pathologic anatomy of the cardiomyopathies. Hum. Pathol. 6:289, 1975.

94. Olsen, E. G. J.: The pathology of the cardiomyopathies. A critical analysis. Am. Heart J. 98:385, 1979.

95. Cambridge, G.: Antibodies to Coxsackie B viruses in congestive cardiomyopathy. Br. Heart J. 41:692, 1979.

96. Rubin, E.: Alcoholic myopathy in heart and skeletal muscle. N. Engl. J. Med. 5:28, 1979.

97. Maron, B. J., et al.: Quantitative analysis of the distribution of cardiac muscle cell disorganization in the left ventricular wall of patients with hypertrophic cardiomyopathy. Circulation 63:882, 1981.

98. Clark, C. E., et al.: Familial prevalence and genetic transmission of idiopathic hypertrophic subaortic stenosis. N. Engl. J. Med. 289:709, 1973.

99. Wenger, N. K.: Infectious myocarditis. Postgrad. Med. 44:105, 1968.

100. Levine, H. D.: Virus myocarditis: A critique of the literature from clinical, electrocardiographic, and pathologic standpoints. Am. J. Med. Sci. 277:132, 1979.

101. Woodruff, J. F.: Viral myocarditis: A review. Am. J. Pathol. 101:425, 1980.

102. Fejfar, Z.: Cardiomyopathies—An international problem. Cardiologia (Basel)52:9, 1968.

103. Bengtsson, E.: Myocarditis and cardiomyopathy: Clinical aspects. Cardiologia (Basel) 52:97, 1968.

104. Mason, J. W.: Endomyocardial biopsy: The balance of success and failure. Circulation 71:185, 1985.

105. Korn, D., et al.: Massive calcification of the mitral annulus: A clinical pathological study of 14 cases. N. Engl. J. Med. 267:900, 1962.

106. Wigle, E. D., et al.: Mitral value prolapse. Ann. Rev. Med. 27:165, 1976.

107. Davies, M. J., et al.: The floppy mitral valve. Br. Heart J. 40:468, 1978.

108. Gaffney, F. A., et al.: Abnormal cardiovascular regulation in the mitral valve prolapse syndrome. Am. J. Cardiol. 62:316, 1983.

109. Barnett, H. J. M., et al.: Further evidence relating mitral valve prolapse to cerebral ischemic events. N. Engl. J. Med. 302:139, 1980.

110. Rosen, P., and Armstrong, D.: Non-bacterial thrombotic endocarditis in patients with malignant neoplastic diseases. Am. J. Med. 54:23, 1973.

111. Young, R. S. K., and Zalneraitis, E. L.: Marantic endocarditis in children and young adults: Clinical and pathological findings. Stroke 12:635, 1981.

112. Olney, B. A.: The consequences of the inconsequential: marantic (nonbacterial thrombotic) endocarditis. Am. Heart J. 98:513, 1979.

113. Schryer, M. J. P., and Karnauchow, P. N.: Endocardial fibroelastosis: Etiologic and pathogenetic considerations in children. Am. Heart J. 88:557, 1974.

114. Westwood, M., et al.: Heredity in primary endocardial fibroelastosis. Br. Heart J., 37:1077, 1975.

115. Wold, L. E., and Lie, J. T.: Cardiac myxomas. A clinicopathologic profile. Am. J. Pathol. 101:219, 1980.

116. Ferrans, V. J., and Roberts, W. C.: Structural features of cardiac myxomas. Histology, histochemistry and electron microscopy. Hum. Pathol. 4:111, 1973.

# 12

# The Hematopoietic and Lymphoid Systems

**RED CELL DISORDERS**

HEMORRHAGE—BLOOD LOSS ANEMIA

INCREASED RATE OF RED CELL
DESTRUCTION—THE HEMOLYTIC ANEMIAS
    Hereditary Spherocytosis (HS)
    Sickle Cell Anemia (and Other Hemoglobinopathies)
    Thalassemia
    Glucose-6-Phosphate Dehydrogenase (G6PD)
      Deficiency
    Paroxysmal Nocturnal Hemoglobinuria (PNH)
    Immunohemolytic Anemias (Autoimmune Hemolytic
      Anemia)
    Erythroblastosis Fetalis (Hemolytic Disease of the
      Newborn)
    Hemolytic Anemias Resulting from Mechanical Trauma
      to Red Cells
    Malaria

ANEMIAS OF DIMINISHED ERYTHROPOIESIS
    Iron Deficiency Anemia
    Megaloblastic Anemias
        Folate (folic acid) deficiency anemia
        Vitamin $B_{12}$ (cobalamin) deficiency
          anemia—pernicious anemia (PA)
    Aplastic Anemia
    Myelophthisic Anemia

POLYCYTHEMIA

**WHITE CELL DISORDERS**

LYMPHOMAS
    Non-Hodgkin's Lymphoma (NHL)
    Cutaneous T-cell Lymphomas
    Hodgkin's Disease

LEUKEMIAS AND MYELOPROLIFERATIVE DISEASES
    Acute Leukemias
    Chronic Myeloid Leukemia (CML)
    Chronic Lymphocytic Leukemia (CLL)
    Unusual Types of Leukemias and Lymphomas
    Myeloproliferative Disorders
        Polycythemia vera
        Myeloid metaplasia with myelofibrosis

NEUTROPENIA—AGRANULOCYTOSIS

PLASMA CELL DYSCRASIAS AND RELATED
DISORDERS

**THE HEMORRHAGIC DIATHESES**

DISSEMINATED INTRAVASCULAR
COAGULATION (DIC, CONSUMPTION COAGULOPATHY,
DEFIBRINATION SYNDROME)

THROMBOCYTOPENIA
    Idiopathic Thrombocytopenic Purpura (ITP)
    Thrombotic Thrombocytopenic Purpura (TTP)

COAGULATION DISORDERS

    Deficiencies of Factor VIII Complex
      von Willebrand's disease
      Factor VIII deficiency (hemophilia A, classic
        hemophilia)
    Factor IX Deficiency (Hemophilia B, Christmas
      Disease)

**MISCELLANEOUS DISORDERS**

INFECTIOUS MONONUCLEOSIS

CAT-SCRATCH DISEASE

DERMATOPATHIC LYMPHADENITIS (LIPOMELANOTIC
RETICULOENDOTHELIOSIS)

HISTIOCYTOSES
    Histiocytosis X

SPLENOMEGALY

Disorders of the hematopoietic and lymphoid systems encompass a wide range of diseases. They may affect primarily the red cells, the white cells, or the hemostatic mechanisms. *Red cell disorders* are usually reflected in *anemia*. *White cell disorders*, in contrast, most often involve overgrowth, usually malignant. Hemostatic derangements result in *hemorrhagic diatheses*. Finally, a group of *miscellaneous disorders*, some of which prominently involve the spleen, are discussed at the end of the chapter.

# Red Cell Disorders

As mentioned, disorders of the red cells usually result in some form of anemia or, sometimes, in an increase in red cells—erythrocytosis (p. 369). *Anemia* may be considered as a reduction below normal levels of hemoglobin concentration and red cell mass, with consequent impaired delivery of oxygen to the tissues. (Although hemodilution may cause a decrease in hemoglobin and red cell *concentration*, these special cases are not usually associated with impaired oxygenation.) Anemias occur in diverse clinical settings, but it is possible to group them into three major categories on the basis of underlying mechanisms (Table 12–1).

**Table 12–1.** CLASSIFICATION OF
ANEMIA ACCORDING TO MECHANISM
OF PRODUCTION

**I. Blood Loss**
  A. Acute: Trauma
  B. Chronic: Lesions of GI tract, gynecologic disturbances
**II. Increased Rate of Destruction (Hemolytic Anemias)**
  A. Intrinsic (intracorpuscular) abnormalities of red cells
    *Hereditary*
    1. Disorders of red cell membrane cytoskeleton, e.g., spherocytosis, elliptocytosis
    2. Red cell enzyme deficiencies
      a. Glycolytic enzymes: Pyruvate kinase deficiency, hexokinase deficiency
      b. Enzymes of hexose monophosphate shunt: G6PD, glutathione synthetase
    3. Disorders of hemoglobin synthesis
      a. Deficient globin synthesis: Thalassemia syndromes
      b. Structurally abnormal globin synthesis (hemoglobinopathies): Sickle cell anemia, unstable hemoglobins
    *Acquired*
    1. Membrane defect: Paroxysmal nocturnal hemoglobinuria
  B. Extrinsic (extracorpuscular) abnormalities
    1. Antibody mediated
      a. Isohemagglutinins: Transfusion reactions, erythroblastosis fetalis
      b. Autoantibodies: Idiopathic (primary), drug-associated, SLE
    2. Mechanical trauma to red cells
      a. Microangiopathic hemolytic anemias: Thrombotic thrombocytopenic purpura, DIC
      b. Cardiac traumatic hemolytic anemia
    3. Infections: Malaria
**III. Impaired Red Cell Production**
  A. Disturbance of proliferation and differentiation of stem cells: Aplastic anemia, pure red cell aplasia, anemia of renal failure, anemia of endocrine disorders
  B. Disturbance of proliferation and maturation of erythroblasts
    1. Defective DNA synthesis: Deficiency or impaired utilization of vitamin $B_{12}$ and folic acid (megaloblastic anemias)
    2. Defective hemoglobin synthesis
      a. Deficient heme synthesis: Iron deficiency
      b. Deficient globin synthesis: Thalassemias
    3. Unknown or multiple mechanisms: Sideroblastic anemia, anemia of chronic infections, myelophthisic anemias due to marrow infiltrations

# HEMORRHAGE—BLOOD LOSS ANEMIA

With acute blood loss, the immediate threat to the patient is hypovolemia with shock, rather than anemia (see p. 79). If the patient survives, hemodilution begins at once and reaches its full effect within two to three days, unmasking the extent of the red cell loss. Eventually, the red cells are completely replaced, provided that iron stores are sufficient. Although this involves some increased marrow function, it is rarely of a degree to convert areas of inactive fatty marrow into functional marrow. Internal hemorrhages, such as intraperitoneal bleeding, permit total recapture of the iron. On the other hand, with external bleeding, the iron is lost. In these cases,

unless there are adequate iron stores, replacement of the red cells is incomplete and iron deficiency anemia results (see p. 364).

Iron deficiency also results from chronic insidious blood loss. In these cases, iron stores are the limiting factor, since both hemodilution and marrow expansion are well able to keep pace with the slow loss of blood.

# INCREASED RATE OF RED CELL DESTRUCTION—THE HEMOLYTIC ANEMIAS

Shortened survival of red cells may be due either to inherent defects in the erythrocyte (intracorpuscular hemolytic anemia), which are usually inherited, or to external influences (extracorpuscular hemolytic anemia), which are usually acquired. Several examples are listed in Table 12–1.

Before proceeding to discuss the various disorders individually, we will describe certain general features of hemolytic anemias. All hemolytic anemias are characterized by (1) *increased rate of red blood cell destruction* and (2) *retention by the body of the products of red cell destruction, including iron*. Since the iron is conserved and recycled readily, there is little to limit efforts of the marrow to keep pace with the hemolysis. Consequently, these anemias are almost invariably associated with marked hypercellularity within the marrow due to an increase in erythropoiesis. Sometimes there is also extramedullary hematopoiesis in the liver and spleen. *Red cell regeneration is reflected by an increase in the reticulocyte count in peripheral blood.* The destruction of red cells may occur within the vascular compartment (*intravascular hemolysis*) or within the cells of the mononuclear phagocyte, or reticuloendothelial (RE), system (*extravascular hemolysis*).

*Intravascular hemolysis* is seen in red cells subjected to mechanical trauma, hemolytic transfusion reactions, and paroxysmal nocturnal hemoglobinuria. Whatever the cause, intravascular hemolysis results in hemoglobinemia, hemoglobinuria, and hemosiderinuria. Conversion of the heme pigment to bilirubin may lead to jaundice. Massive intravascular hemolysis sometimes leads to acute tubular necrosis (p. 476).

*Extravascular hemolysis* is the more common mode of red cell destruction; it takes place largely within the phagocytic cells of the spleen and liver. The mononuclear phagocyte system removes erythrocytes from the circulation whenever red cells are injured or immunologically altered. Since extreme alterations of shape are required for red cells to successfully navigate the splenic sinusoids, reduction in deformability makes this passage difficult and leads to splenic sequestration, followed by phagocytosis (Fig. 12–1). This is believed to be an important factor in the pathogenesis of red cell destruction in a variety of hemolytic anemias.[1] Extravascular hemolysis is not

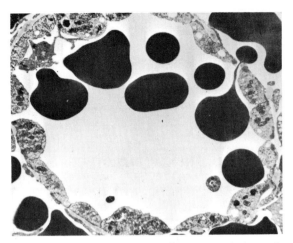

Figure 12–1. Splenic sinus (electron micrograph). An erythrocyte is in the process of squeezing from the cord into the sinus lumen. Note the degree of deformability required for the red cell to pass through the wall of the sinus. (From Enriquez, P., and Neiman, R. S.: The Pathology of the Spleen. A Functional Approach. Chicago, American Society of Clinical Pathologists, © 1976, p. 7. Used by permission.)

associated with hemoglobinemia and hemoglobinuria, but jaundice may result and in long-standing cases lead to gallstone formation. In most forms of hemolytic anemia, there is hyperactivity of the RE system, which results in splenomegaly.

Because the pathways for the excretion of excess iron are limited, there is a tendency in hemolytic anemias for abnormal amounts of iron to accumulate. The iron is deposited in many organs and tissues in the form of *ferritin* and *hemosiderin*, which is generally believed to represent insoluble aggregates of ferritin. Since the hemolytic anemias are the most important cause of widespread hemosiderin deposition (*hemosiderosis*), this iron storage disorder will be discussed in some detail here, but it is also included with other possible causes of systemic iron overload on page 594. The hemosiderin first accumulates within the cells of the mononuclear phagocyte system, where it appears as golden-brown cytoplasmic granules. With the electron microscope, the granules are seen to be bound to membranes within phagosomes. The iron content of hemosiderin is demonstrable by the Prussian blue reaction, in which colorless potassium ferrocyanide applied to the tissue is converted by the iron to blue-black ferric ferrocyanide. *Local hemosiderosis* occurs in a number of situations, such as hematomas and hemorrhagic infarcts, which involve the breakdown of extravasated blood. In fact, it is hemosiderin that accounts for the yellowish discoloration that develops several days after a bruise of the skin. *Systemic hemosiderosis*, however, most often results from hemolytic anemia. The tendency toward hemosiderosis is compounded when red cell transfusions are given, adding to the already increased iron stores. Impaired utilization of iron may also lead to hemosiderosis, as occurs with thalassemia and sideroblastic anemia, both of which

involve a defect in hemoglobin synthesis. Whatever the cause, deposition of hemosiderin in systemic hemosiderosis occurs initially in the mononuclear phagocytes of the liver, bone marrow, spleen, and lymph nodes and in scattered macrophages throughout the body. With progressive accumulation of hemosiderin, parenchymal cells throughout the body (principally in the liver, pancreas, heart, and endocrine organs) become pigmented. Although the excess iron in hemosiderosis generally does not cause functional or morphologic damage to involved organs, the more extreme iron accumulations may lead to a clinical state resembling idiopathic hemochromatosis (p. 594), with associated injury to the liver, pancreas, and other organs as well. However, the severity of iron storage encountered in red cell disorders rarely causes visceral organ injury.

## HEREDITARY SPHEROCYTOSIS (HS)

*This disorder is characterized by an inherited (intrinsic) defect in the red cell membrane that renders the erythrocytes spheroidal, less deformable, and vulnerable to splenic sequestration and destruction.*[2] Hereditary spherocytosis is transmitted as an autosomal dominant trait; however, in 20% of the cases, there is no family history, indicating that the mutation can arise de novo.

**PATHOGENESIS.** Although the exact defect has not yet been clarified, *it is generally accepted that the primary abnormality resides in the proteins that form the skeleton of the red cell membrane.* Three such proteins—spectrin, ankyrin, and protein 4.1 (Fig. 12–2)—form an interlocking but flexible structure on the intracellular face of the cell membrane.[2] Together they are responsible for the normal shape, strength, and flexibility of the red cell. Although a quantitative or qualitative defect in any one of the membrane skeletal proteins could adversely affect the shape of red cells, most available evidence points to defects in spectrin molecules. In some kindreds, the abnormality in spectrin is expressed as reduced binding to protein 4.1 (Fig. 12–2); paradoxically, in other fami-

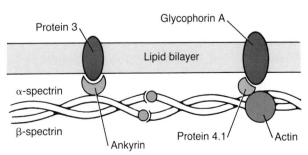

Figure 12–2. Schematic view of the proteins that form the cytoskeleton of the red cell membrane. Spectrin consists of α- and β-chains that lie on the inner surface of the cell membrane and are connected to it through ankyrin, actin, and protein 4.1.

lies the mutant spectrin is tethered very tightly to the cell membrane. Thus HS seems to be genetically heterogeneous. How these various defects contribute to the spheroidal shape and reduced red cell plasticity is not yet clear. According to some, HS erythrocytes have reduced membrane stability and consequently lose membrane fragments as the cells are exposed to shear stresses in circulation. Reduction in the membrane substance (and surface area) forces the cells to assume the smallest possible diameter for a given volume, namely, a sphere.[3]

Regardless of the precise molecular defect in HS, there is no doubt that *the spleen plays a major role in the destruction of spherocytes.* As mentioned earlier, red cells have to undergo extreme degrees of deformation to leave the cords of Billroth and enter the splenic sinusoids. Because of their spheroidal shape and reduced membrane plasticity, spherocytes have great difficulty in leaving the splenic cords. The sequestered abnormal red cells are eventually destroyed by macrophages, which are plentiful in the splenic cords. *The critical role of the spleen in this process is illustrated by the invariably beneficial effect of splenectomy. The red cell defect persists, but the anemia is corrected.*

**MORPHOLOGY.** On smears the red cells lack the central zone of pallor because of their spheroidal shape. Spherocytosis, although distinctive, is not diagnostic since it is also seen in immune hemolytic anemias. To compensate for the excessive red cell destruction, erythropoiesis in the marrow is stimulated. As with other hemolytic anemias, red cell regeneration is reflected by reticulocytosis in the peripheral blood. Splenomegaly is greater in HS than in any other form of hemolytic anemia. Weights are usually between 500 and 1000 gm but may be greater. The enlargement of the spleen results from striking congestion of the cords of Billroth, leaving the splenic sinuses virtually empty. Phagocytized red cells are frequently seen within hypertrophied sinusoidal lining cells or reticular cord cells. In long-standing cases there is prominent systemic hemosiderosis.

The other general features of hemolytic anemias described earlier are present with this disorder. In particular, cholelithiasis occurs in 50 to 85% of these patients.

**CLINICAL COURSE.** Usually, hereditary spherocytosis, despite its congenital nature, does not manifest itself until adult life. In some cases, however, it becomes apparent soon after birth. The severity of the disorder is thus highly variable. Asymptomatic cases occur, as well as those characterized by a profound anemia, but in general, the anemia is moderate. Since the red cells are spheroidal in shape, there is little margin for expansion of red cell volume when cells are exposed to hypotonic salt solution. As a result, *increased osmotic fragility is a characteristic finding that is helpful in diagnosis.* The more or less stable clinical course may be punctuated by two kinds of "crises." A *"hemolytic crisis"* may develop, consisting of a wave of increased hemolysis accompanied

by a transient increase in jaundice, splenomegaly, and anemia. These episodes, often triggered by infection, are usually self-limited. Less commonly, a life-threatening *"aplastic crisis"* associated with complete cessation of marrow function with consequent leukopenia and thrombocytopenia may appear. Transfusions may be necessary to support the patient. HS is cured by splenectomy.

## SICKLE CELL ANEMIA (AND OTHER HEMOGLOBINOPATHIES)

*The hemoglobinopathies are a group of hereditary disorders characterized by the presence of a structurally abnormal hemoglobin.* Over 300 hemoglobins have been discovered, one third of which are associated with significant clinical manifestations. The prototype and most prevalent hemoglobinopathy results from a mutation in the gene coding for the $\beta$-globin chain that causes the formation of the sickle hemoglobin (HbS). The associated disease sickle cell anemia will be discussed here; other hemoglobinopathies are far too infrequent for our consideration, and the interested reader is referred to specialized texts.[4]

Hemoglobin S, like 90% of other abnormal hemoglobins, results from a single amino acid substitution in the globin chain. Hemoglobin, as you may recall, is a tetramer of four globin chains, comprising two pairs of similar chains. In the normal adult, hemoglobin is composed of 96% HbA ($\alpha_2\beta_2$), 3% HbA$_2$ ($\alpha_2\delta_2$), and 1% fetal hemoglobin (HbF, $\alpha_2\gamma_2$). *Substitution of valine for glutamine at the sixth position of the $\beta$ chain produces HbS.* In the homozygote, all of HbA is replaced by HbS, whereas in the heterozygote, only about half is replaced. Thus, this autosomal codominant disease in heterozygotes, called *sickle cell trait,* is mild; those homozygous for HbS suffer full-blown *sickle cell anemia.*

**INCIDENCE.** Approximately 8% of American blacks are heterozygous for HbS. In parts of Africa where malaria is endemic, the gene frequency approaches 30%, attributed to the slight protective effect of HbS against falciparum malaria. In the United States, sickle cell anemia affects approximately one of every 600 blacks; worldwide, sickle cell anemia is the most common form of congenital hemolytic anemia.

**ETIOLOGY AND PATHOGENESIS.** Upon deoxygenation HbS molecules undergo polymerization, a process sometimes called gelation or "crystallization." The change in the physical state of the HbS causes distortion of the red cell, which assumes an elongated crescent or "sickle" shape (Fig. 12–3). A greater degree of hypoxia is required to produce this change in heterozygotes than in homozygotes. Indeed, in homozygotes, even such trivial events as exertion or deep sleep may induce sufficient hypoxia to trigger a sickling crisis. Hemoconcentration such as may be induced by sweating, fever, or use of diuretics may

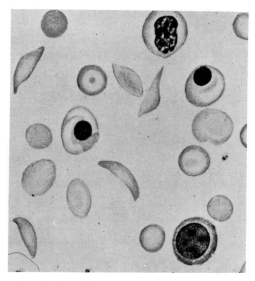

**Figure 12–3.** In vivo sickling in a patient with sickle cell anemia. (From Robbins, S. L., Cotran, R. S., and Kumar, V.: Pathologic Basis of Disease. 3rd ed. Philadelphia, W. B. Saunders Co. 1984, p. 619.)

also provoke sickling by withdrawing water from red cells, thereby increasing intracorpuscular concentration of HbS. With the electron microscope, sickled cells reveal microtubular structures, each tubule con-

sisting of six to eight aggregated HbS molecules.[5] Polymerization of deoxygenated HbS (and therefore sickling) is initially reversible by oxygenation. However, membrane damage occurs with each episode of sickling and eventually the cells accumulate calcium, lose potassium and water, and become irreversibly sickled despite adequate oxygenation.

Two major consequences stem from the sickling of red cells (Fig. 12–4). *Sickled red cells become rigid and therefore susceptible to sequestration and hemolysis within the spleen, as already discussed* (p. 352). Their mean life span is reduced to approximately 20 days. In addition to hemolytic anemia, *sickle cell disease is associated with widespread microvascular obstructions and resulting ischemic damage.* It is generally assumed that occlusion of small blood vessels results from rigidity and "log-jamming" of the sickled cells. However, recent observations suggest that the presence of HbS is associated with several abnormalities in the cell membrane that play a significant role in the pathogenesis of vascular occlusion.[6, 7] These include:

○ Abnormal distribution of charges on the sickle cell surface that increases adherence of cells to endothelium. The adhesion of HbS-containing red cells to vascular endothelium does not require deoxygenation or frank sickling; normal-appearing red cells may adhere and, by impeding the flow of

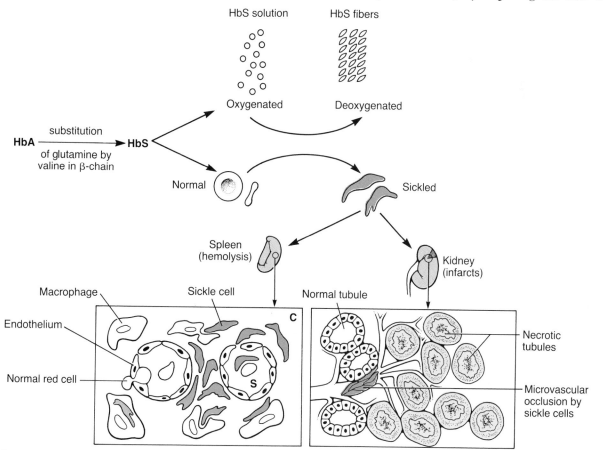

**Figure 12–4.** Pathophysiology and morphologic consequences of sickle cell anemia. Key: S, splenic sinusoids; C, splenic cords.

blood in the microcirculation, cause local anoxia and sickling of red cells. The sickled cells could then contribute to further impairment of blood flow and set up a vicious circle.

Alterations in membrane phospholipids that may activate clotting factors and thus induce a hypercoagulable state.

**MORPHOLOGY.** **The anatomic alterations stem from the following three aspects of the disease: (1) hemolysis with resultant anemia, (2) increased release of hemoglobin with bilirubin formation, and (3) capillary stasis with thrombosis.** When tissue sections are fixed in formalin so that anaerobiosis develops before complete fixation, sickled red cells are evident as bizarre, elongated, spindled, or boat-shaped structures. Both the severe anemia and the vascular stasis lead to hypoxic fatty changes in the heart, liver, and renal tubules. Fatty marrow is activated. The hypercellularity of the marrow occurs principally at the level of the normoblasts. Expansion of marrow may lead to resorption of bone with appositional new bone formation on the external aspect of the skull, leading to the "crew cut" appearance on radiographs. Extramedullary hematopoiesis may appear in the spleen and liver.

In children there is moderate splenomegaly—up to 500 gm—caused by congestion of the red pulp with masses of red cells sickled and jammed together. Eventually this splenic erythrostasis leads to enough hypoxic tissue damage, sometimes with frank infarction, to create a shrunken, fibrotic spleen. This process is termed **autosplenectomy** and is seen in all long-standing adult cases. Ultimately, only a small nubbin of fibrous tissue remains of the spleen.

Vascular congestion, thrombosis, and infarction may affect any organ, including bones, liver, kidney, and retina. Approximately 50% of adult patients develop leg ulcers because of hypoxia of the subcutaneous tissues. Cor pulmonale may result from thromboses in the pulmonary vessels. As with the other hemolytic anemias, hemosiderosis and gallstones are common.

**CLINICAL COURSE.** Homozygous sickle cell disease usually becomes apparent toward the end of the first year of life, as fetal hemoglobin (HbF) is gradually replaced by HbS. The anemia is severe, with hematocrit values ranging between 18 and 30%. The chronic hemolysis is associated with marked reticulocytosis and hyperbilirubinemia. From the time of onset, the process runs an unremitting course, punctuated by sudden episodes of so-called crises. The most serious of these are the *vaso-occlusive, or painful, crises*. The pain is usually localized to the abdomen (sometimes simulating an acute abdomen) or to some portion of the skeletal system. The painful crises are believed to result from microvascular occlusions and associated hypoxic tissue injury. Ischemia of the central nervous system is manifested by headaches, convulsions, or hemiplegia. An *"aplastic crisis"* represents a sudden but usually temporary cessation of bone marrow activity. Reticulocytes dis-

appear from the blood and anemia is worsened. Both types of crises are usually triggered by infections, to which these patients are very susceptible. The basis of increased susceptibility to infections is probably multifactorial. Impaired splenic function due to erythrophagocytosis interferes with bacterial killing. In later stages total splenic fibrosis removes an important biologic filter of blood-borne microorganisms. There are defects in the alternate complement pathway that impair opsonization of encapsulated bacteria such as pneumococci. For reasons not entirely clear, patients with sickle cell disease are particularly predisposed to develop *Salmonella* osteomyelitis.

With the full-blown *sickle cell disease*, at least some sickled erythrocytes can be seen on an ordinary peripheral blood smear. Ultimately, the diagnosis depends on the electrophoretic demonstration of HbS. Prenatal diagnosis of sickle cell anemia can be performed by analyzing the DNA in fetal cells obtained by amniocentesis. The sickle mutation abolishes the recognition site for a restriction endonuclease enzyme, Mst II. When DNA extracted from fetal cells is digested with Mst II, the presence of sickle mutation leads to generation of DNA fragments of abnormal sizes. These can be detected by Southern blot analysis, as described in detail on page 125.

The clinical course of patients with sickle cell anemia is highly variable. As a result of improvements in supportive care, an increasing number of patients are surviving into adulthood. However, many patients still die before the age of 30 years. Sickle cell *trait*, in contrast, generally remains entirely asymptomatic unless unusual circumstances, such as a plane flight in an unpressurized craft, lead to abnormally low oxygen tensions. A variety of antisickling agents have been proposed, but none has stood the test of time. At present the therapeutic approach is largely symptomatic.

## THALASSEMIA

*The thalassemias are a heterogeneous group of genetic disorders of hemoglobin synthesis characterized by a lack of or decreased synthesis of globin chains.* In α-thalassemia, α-globin chain synthesis is reduced, whereas in β-thalassemia, β-globin chain synthesis is either absent (designated $\beta^0$-thalassemia) or markedly deficient ($\beta^+$-thalassemia). Unlike the hemoglobinopathies, which represent qualitative abnormalities, thalassemias result from quantitative abnormalities of globin chain synthesis. The consequences of reduced synthesis of one globin chain derive not only from the low intracellular hemoglobin but also from the relative excess of the other globin chain, as will be discussed later.

Thalassemia is inherited as an autosomal codominant condition. The heterozygous form (*thalassemia minor* or *thalassemia trait*) may be asymptomatic or mildly symptomatic. The homozygous form, called *thalassemia major*, is associated with a severe hemolytic anemia. The mutant genes are particularly common among Mediterranean, African, and Asian populations.

**PATHOGENESIS.** A complex pattern of molecular defects underlying the thalassemias has emerged in recent years. To understand these, we must first review the structure and expression of normal globin genes. Here we will summarize only the salient features; more details are available in several reviews.[8-10] The adult hemoglobin, or HbA, contains two α chains and two β chains (coded by two β-globin genes located on each of the two number 11 chromosomes). In contrast, two pairs of functional α-globin genes are located on each number 16 chromosome. With recombinant DNA techniques it has been possible to clone all the human globin genes, and their nucleotide sequences have been determined. The basic structure of the α- and β-globin genes as well as the steps involved in the biosynthesis of globin chains are similar. These are depicted schematically in Figure 12–5. Each β-globin gene has three coding sequences, or *exons*, that are interrupted by two intervening sequences, or *introns*. Flanking the 5′ extremity of the globin gene are a series of untranslated "*promoter sequences*" that are required for the initiation of β-globin mRNA synthesis.

As with all eukaryotic genes, the biosynthesis of globin chains begins with the transcription of the globin genes within the nucleus (Fig. 12–5). The initial mRNA transcript contains a copy of the entire gene, including all the exons and introns. This large mRNA precursor undergoes several posttranscriptional modifications (processing) before it is converted into mature cytoplasmic mRNA ready for translation, i.e., splicing out the two introns and religating the exons. The mature mRNA so formed leaves the nucleus and becomes associated with ribosomes, on which translation takes place. The pathway of α-globin gene expression is very similar. With this background we can discuss the molecular pathologic changes associated with the two major forms of thalassemia. The β-thalassemias have been more extensively studied, and hence they will be discussed first.

As mentioned earlier, β-thalassemia syndromes can be classified into two categories: (1) β⁰-*thalassemia*, associated with total absence of β-globin chains in the homozygous state, and (2) β⁺-*thalassemia*, characterized by reduced (but detectable) β-globin synthesis in the homozygous state. Sequencing of cloned β-globin genes obtained from thalassemic patients

**Figure 12–5.** The biosynthesis of β-globin is shown schematically. Gene expression begins in the nucleus with transcription of the entire gene, including exons and introns. During posttranscriptional processing, the intron transcripts are removed by "splicing" from the precursor mRNA. The re-ligated mRNA is transported to the cytoplasm, where it is translated to form β-globin. (Modified from illustration by A. D. Iselin in Bank, A.: Genetic disorders of hemoglobin synthesis. Hosp. Pract. 20:109, 1985.)

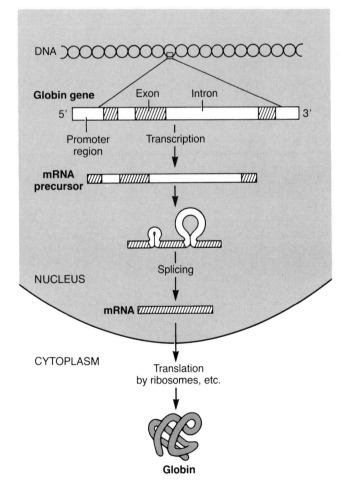

has revealed over 30 different mutations responsible for β⁰- or β⁺-thalassemia. Most of these result from single base changes. As opposed to the case with α-thalassemias, described later, gene deletions rarely underlie β-thalassemias.

Details of these mutations and their effects on β-globin synthesis are beyond our scope, but a few illustrative examples will be cited (Fig. 12–6). The promoter region controls the initiation and rate of transcription, and therefore mutations affecting promoter sequences usually lead to reduced globin gene transcription. Since some β-globin is synthesized, the patients develop β⁺-thalassemia. Mutations in the coding sequences are usually associated with more serious consequences. For example, in some cases a single nucleotide change in one of the exons leads to the formation of a "termination" or "stop" codon, which interrupts translation of β-globin mRNA. Premature termination generates nonfunctional fragments of the β-globin, leading to β⁰-thalassemia. *Mutations that lead to aberrant splicing are the commonest cause of β-thalassemia.* Most of these affect introns, but some have been located within exons. If the mutation alters the normal splice junctions, splicing does not occur and all of the mRNA formed is abnormal. Unspliced mRNA is degraded within the nucleus, and β⁰-thalassemia results. However, some mutations affect the introns at locations away from the normal intron-exon splice junction. These mutations create new sites sensitive to the action of splicing enzymes at abnormal locations—within an intron, for example. Since normal splice sites remain unaffected, both normal and abnormal splicing occur, giving rise to normal as well as abnormal β-globin mRNA. These patients develop β⁺-thalassemia.

*Two factors contribute to the pathogenesis of anemia in β-thalassemia. Reduced synthesis of β-globin leads to inadequate HbA formation, so that the overall hemoglobin concentration per cell is lower and the cells appear hypochromic. Much more important is the hemolytic component of β-thalassemia. This is due not to lack of β-globin but to the relative excess of α-globin chains, whose synthesis remains normal.* Free α chains form insoluble aggregates that precipitate within the erythrocytes (Fig. 12–7). These inclusions damage the cell membranes, reduce their plasticity, and render the red cells susceptible to phagocytosis by the mononuclear phagocyte system (RE cells). Not only are mature red cells susceptible to premature destruction but also a majority of the erythroblasts within the marrow are destroyed, owing to the presence of the inclusions ("*ineffective erythropoiesis*").

The molecular basis of α-thalassemia is quite distinct from that of β-thalassemia. Most importantly, *most of the α-thalassemias are due to deletion of α-globin gene loci.* Since there are four functional α-globin genes, there are four possible severities of α-thalassemia based on loss of one to four α-globin genes from the chromosomes. These cover a wide spectrum of clinical disorders, the severity of which is related to the number of deleted α-globin genes (Table 12–2). On one end, loss of a single α-globin gene is associated with a silent carrier state, whereas deletion of all four α-globin genes is associated with fetal death in utero, since there is virtually no oxygen-carrying capacity. The basis of the hemolysis is similar to that in β-thalassemia. With loss of three α-globin genes, there is relative overproduction of β-globin chains, which form insoluble tetramers within red cells and render the cells vulnerable to phagocytosis and destruction.

**MORPHOLOGY.** Only the morphologic changes in β-thalassemia, which is more common in the United States, will be described. Typically, in thalassemia major the peripheral blood smear shows microcytic, hypochromic red cells. Some red cells have an abnormal distribution of hemoglobin, giving them a target-like appearance (target cells). In addition, there is severe poikilocytosis, anisocytosis, and reticulocytosis. Normoblasts are present in the peripheral blood.

In β-thalassemia major, the anatomic changes are those of all hemolytic anemias, but especially prominent are hyperactivity of the bone marrow and splenomegaly. The marrow is expanded to the fetal level, and thus all the fatty marrow may be reactivated. In the red cell series,

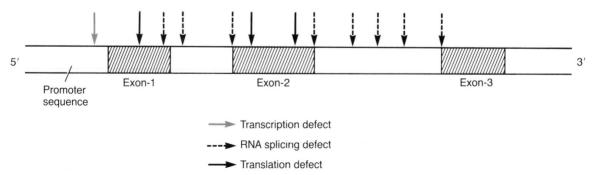

Figure 12–6. Diagrammatic representation of the β-globin gene and some sites where point mutations giving rise to β-thalassemia have been localized. (Modified from Wyngaarden, J. B., and Smith, L. H., Jr.: Cecil Textbook of Medicine. 17th ed. Philadelphia, W. B. Saunders Co., 1985, p. 137.)

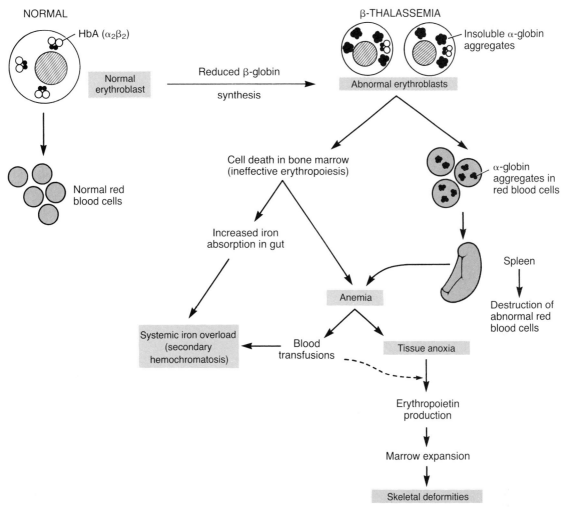

**Figure 12–7.** Pathogenesis of β-thalassemia major. Note that aggregates of excess α-globin are not visible on routine blood smears. Blood transfusions on the one hand correct the anemia and reduce stimulus for erythropoietin secretion and deformities induced by marrow expansion; on the other hand, they add to systemic iron overload.

**Table 12–2.** CLINICAL AND GENETIC CLASSIFICATION OF THALASSEMIAS

| Clinical Nomenclature | Genotype | Disease | Molecular Pathology |
|---|---|---|---|
| *Beta-thalassemia* | | | |
| Thalassemia major | $\beta^0/\beta^0$ or $\beta^+/\beta^+$ | Severe transfusion-requiring anemia | Defects in β-globin mRNA transcription, splicing, or translation; gene deletions are rare |
| Thalassemia minor | $\beta^0/\beta$ or $\beta^+/\beta$ | Asymptomatic with mild or no anemia; red cell abnormalities seen | |
| *Alpha-thalassemia* | | | |
| Silent carrier | $--\alpha/\alpha\alpha$ | Asymptomatic; no red cell abnormality | |
| Alpha-thalassemia trait | $--/\alpha\alpha$ or $\alpha-/\alpha-$ | Asymptomatic; like thalassemia minor | Mainly deletions of α-globin genes |
| HbH disease | $--/-\alpha$ | Severe anemia; tetramers of α-globin (HbH formed in red cells) | |
| Hydrops fetalis | $--/--$ | Lethal in utero | |

there is a striking shift toward primitive forms. Massive erythropoiesis within the bone invades the bony cortex, impairs bone growth, and produces skeletal deformities. Splenomegaly and hepatomegaly result from marked extramedullary hematopoiesis as well as RE cell hyperplasia. Over the span of years, excessive breakdown of red cells and ineffective erythropoiesis result in severe hemosiderosis and, rarely, a form of hemochromatosis (p. 594). The iron overload is due in part to excessive dietary iron absorption that is associated with ineffective erythropoiesis and to the repeated blood transfusions these patients need for survival (Fig. 12–7).

**CLINICAL COURSE.** Thalassemia major manifests itself as soon as HbF is normally replaced by HbA. These children fail to develop normally and are retarded almost from birth. They are sustained only by repeated blood transfusions, which not only improve the anemia but also reduce the skeletal deformities associated with excessive erythropoiesis. With transfusions, survival into the second or third decade is possible, but gradually systemic iron overload develops. Cardiac failure resulting from secondary hemochromatosis is an important cause of death in those who reach adolescence. The average age at death is 17 years.

With thalassemia minor there is usually only a mild microcytic hypochromic anemia, and in general these patients have a normal life expectancy. Since iron deficiency anemia is associated with a similar appearance of red cells, it should be excluded by appropriate laboratory tests, described later in this chapter. The diagnosis of β-thalassemia minor is made by hemoglobin electrophoresis. In addition to reduced amounts of HbA ($\alpha_2\beta_2$), the level of HbA$_2$ ($\alpha_2\delta_2$) is increased. The diagnosis of β-thalassemia major can generally be made on clinical grounds. Hemoglobin electrophoresis shows severe reduction or absence of HbA and increased levels of HbF. The HbA$_2$ levels may be normal or increased.

## GLUCOSE-6-PHOSPHATE DEHYDROGENASE (G6PD) DEFICIENCY

A miscellaneous group of congenital hemolytic anemias is based on enzyme deficiencies within erythrocytes.[11] The prototype and most prevalent of these anemias is caused by a functional deficiency of G6PD. The G6PD gene is located on the X chromosome, and there is considerable polymorphism at this locus. Over 150 G6PD genetic variants, most of which are not associated with disease, have been identified. In the United States, the G6PD A$^-$ variant is associated with hemolytic anemia. It is encountered primarily in blacks. Approximately 10% of the black males in the United States are affected. To explain such a high frequency of a deleterious gene, it has been suggested that some G6PD variants, as in the case of HbS, confer protection against malaria.

*This disorder remains asymptomatic unless the red cells are subjected to oxidant injury by exposure to certain drugs or toxins.* The drugs incriminated include antimalarials (e.g., primaquine), sulfonamides, nitrofurantoin, phenacetin, aspirin (in high doses), and vitamin K derivatives. Infections can also trigger hemolysis, presumably owing to release of free radicals from phagocytic cells. The major effect of these offending agents is to oxidize hemoglobin to methemoglobin and to denature globin chains by oxidation of the sulfhydryl groups. Denatured hemoglobin is precipitated within the red cells in the form of inclusions called *Heinz bodies.* Not only are inclusion-bearing red cells less deformable, their cell membranes are further damaged when splenic phagocytes attempt to "pluck" out the inclusions. All these changes predispose the red cells to becoming trapped in the splenic sinuses and destroyed by the phagocytes. Normally, the hemoglobin is protected from such oxidative injury by reduced glutathione, which itself gets oxidized when exposed to the oxidant drugs and toxins. However, the presence of the G6PD A$^-$ variant is associated with reduced activity of G6PD, which in turn impairs the regeneration of reduced glutathione by the hexose monophosphate shunt.

The drug-induced hemolysis is acute and of variable clinical severity. Typically, the patients develop evidence of intravascular hemolysis after a lag period of two to three days. Since the G6PD gene is located on the X chromosome, all the erythrocytes of affected males are deficient in enzyme activity. However, owing to random inactivation of one X chromosome in women (p. 123), heterozygous females have two distinct populations of red cells—some normal, others deficient in G6PD activity. Indeed, females heterozygous for G6PD enzymes have two populations of all somatic cells. Thus affected males are more vulnerable to oxidant injury, whereas most carrier females are asymptomatic. Only when heterozygous females have a very large proportion of deficient red cells ("unfavorable lyonization") are they susceptible to induced hemolysis. The common type of G6PD deficiency is most marked in older red cells, which therefore are more susceptible to lysis. As the marrow compensates by producing new (young) red cells, hemolysis tends to abate even if drug exposure continues.

## PAROXYSMAL NOCTURNAL HEMOGLOBINURIA (PNH)

This rare disorder of unknown etiology is mentioned here because it is distinctive in that it is the *only form of hemolytic anemia resulting from an acquired intracorpuscular defect.* The basic abnormality seems to be the proliferation of an abnormal clone of myeloid stem cells whose progeny (red cells, granulocytes, and platelets) are inordinately sensitive to the lytic activity of complement. These patients have intravascular hemolysis and a striking predisposition to infections and intravascular thromboses. The nature of the membrane abnormality that renders the cells susceptible to complement is not clearly defined, although several possibilities have been suggested.[12] PNH is presumed to result from a mutational event of unknown etiology that affects the myeloid stem cells.

## IMMUNOHEMOLYTIC ANEMIAS (AUTOIMMUNE HEMOLYTIC ANEMIA)

In these disorders, the hemolytic anemia is caused by the presence of antibodies reactive against normal or altered red cell membranes. In the majority of cases there is no apparent cause for the generation of anti–red cell antibodies, and hence it has been customary to use the designation *autoimmune hemolytic anemias*. However, in recent years several exogenous factors have been recognized that are capable of causing antibody-induced hemolytic anemia, and hence the term *immunohemolytic anemia* is preferred. These anemias are classified on the basis of the nature of the antibody involved and possible predisposing associated factors, presented in simplified form in Table 12–3.

Whatever the cause of antibody formation, the diagnosis of immunohemolytic anemias depends upon the demonstration of anti–red cell antibodies. *The method most commonly used to detect such antibodies is the Coombs' antiglobulin test, which is based upon the capacity of antihuman globulins (prepared in animals) to agglutinate red cells.* A positive test indicates that the patient's red cells are coated with antibody globulins that can react with the antihuman globulin serum. This is called the *direct Coombs' test*. The *indirect Coombs' test* is used to detect antibodies in the patient's serum and involves incubating normal red cells with the patient's serum, followed by a direct Coombs' test on these incubated red cells.[13]

**WARM ANTIBODY IMMUNOHEMOLYTIC ANEMIAS.** These are characterized by the presence of IgG (rarely IgA) antibodies, which are active at 37°C. A great majority of cases (over 60%) are idiopathic

**Table 12–3.** CLASSIFICATION OF AUTOIMMUNE HEMOLYTIC ANEMIAS

**Warm Antibody Type**
    Primary
    Secondary: Lymphomas and leukemias (CLL and non-
             Hodgkin's lymphomas)
             SLE
             Drugs (e.g., α-methyldopa, penicillin, quinidine)

**Cold Antibody Type**
    Acute: Mycoplasma infection, infectious mononucleosis
    Chronic: Idiopathic
             Associated with lymphomas

(primary) and hence belong to the category of autoimmune diseases. As is the case with most forms of autoimmunity, the cause of autoantibody formation is unknown. Factors discussed in the earlier general consideration of autoimmunity (p. 150) may also apply to these cases. Approximately one fourth of the cases are so-called secondary because there is an underlying disease (such as SLE) affecting the immune system or the anemias are induced by drugs. The pathogenesis of hemolysis in most instances involves opsonization of the red cells by the IgG antibodies and subsequent phagocytosis by splenic macrophages. Spheroidal cells resembling those found in hereditary spherocytosis are often found in idiopathic immune hemolytic anemia. Presumably, bits of cell membrane are injured and removed during attempted phagocytosis of antibody-coated cells; this reduces surface area and induces spheroidal conformation. The spherocytes are then sequestered and destroyed in the spleen, as already discussed (p. 354). The mechanisms of hemolysis induced by drugs are varied and in some cases poorly understood.[14] Drugs such as α-methyldopa induce an anemia indistinguishable from the primary idiopathic form of hemolytic anemia. Autoantibodies directed against intrinsic red cell antigens, in particular Rh blood group antigens, are formed. How α-methyldopa induces autoantibody formation is not clear. Drugs such as penicillin are believed to act as haptens. They bind to the red cell membrane, evoking the formation of antidrug antibodies. These antibodies attach to the cell-bound penicillin and predispose the cells to phagocytic destruction, as outlined previously. Yet other drugs, such as quinidine, bind to plasma proteins and evoke an antibody response. Immune complexes composed of protein-bound drug and antibody molecules then become deposited on the red cell membranes and damage the erythrocytes as innocent bystanders.

**COLD ANTIBODY IMMUNOHEMOLYTIC ANEMIAS.** These anemias are characterized by the presence of IgM antibodies, which have enhanced activity at temperatures below 30°C. The hemolytic process occurs because of fixation of complement on IgM-coated red cells. This interaction occurs best in the distal body parts, where the temperature may drop below 30°C. Once the red cells are coated with antibody and complement, they are removed from the circulation by the RE cells, particularly Kupffer cells. Cold agglutinins occur acutely during recovery from mycoplasma pneumonia and infectious mononucleosis. The resulting anemia is mild, transient, and of no clinical import. Chronic cold agglutinin formation and associated hemolytic anemia may also occur in association with lymphoproliferative disorders or as an idiopathic condition. In addition to anemia, Raynaud's phenomenon may occur in these patients owing to agglutination of red cells in the capillaries of exposed parts of the body.

# ERYTHROBLASTOSIS FETALIS (HEMOLYTIC DISEASE OF THE NEWBORN)

*Erythroblastosis fetalis may be defined as an antibody-induced hemolytic disease in the newborn that is caused by blood group incompatibility between mother and fetus.* Obviously, such an incompatibility can occur only when the fetus inherits red cell antigenic determinants from the father that are foreign to the mother. Important in this respect are the ABO and Rh blood group antigens. Although the incidence of hemolytic disease due to Rh incompatibility has declined remarkably in recent years, it is necessary to discuss Rh hemolytic disease in some detail since successful prophylaxis of this disorder has resulted chiefly from an understanding of its pathogenesis.

**ETIOLOGY AND PATHOGENESIS.** The underlying basis of erythroblastosis fetalis is the immunization of the mother by blood group antigens on fetal red cells and the free passage of antibodies from mother through the placenta to the fetus. Fetal red cells may reach the maternal circulation during the last trimester of pregnancy, when the cytotrophoblast is no longer present as a barrier, or during childbirth itself. The mother thus becomes sensitized to the foreign antigen.

Of the numerous antigens included in the Rh system, only the D antigen is the major cause of Rh incompatibility. Red cells bearing the D antigen are known as Rh-positive; those lacking it, as Rh-negative. Several factors influence the immune response to Rh-positive fetal red cells that reach the maternal circulation. *Concurrent ABO incompatibility protects the mother against Rh immunization,* because the fetal red cells are promptly coated by isohemagglutinins and removed from the maternal circulation. Since the antibody response depends upon the *dose of the immunizing antigen,* hemolytic disease develops only when the mother has experienced a significant transplacental bleed, i.e., more than 1 ml of Rh-positive red cells. Transplacental bleeds of this magnitude occur primarily during childbirth. *Prior sensitization is of great importance in the pathogenesis of Rh erythroblastosis.* The intitial exposure to Rh antigen evokes the formation of IgM antibodies, which are relatively harmless since they cannot cross the placenta. It is for this reason that Rh disease is very uncommon with the first pregnancy. Subsequent exposure during the second or third pregnancy generally leads to a brisk IgG antibody response; IgG antibodies can cross the placenta and induce hemolysis of Rh-positive fetal red cells. Appreciation of the role of prior sensitization in the pathogenesis of Rh erythroblastosis has led to its remarkable control in recent years. Currently, Rh-negative mothers are administered anti-D globulin soon after the delivery of an Rh-positive baby. The anti-D antibodies mask the antigenic sites on the fetal red cells that may have leaked into the maternal circulation during childbirth, thus preventing long-lasting sensitization to Rh antigens.

*Although ABO incompatibility occurs in approximately 20 to 25% of pregnancies, only about 10% of infants subsequently born develop hemolytic disease and, in general, the disease is much less severe.* It occurs almost exclusively in infants of group A or B who are born of group O mothers. The normal anti-A and anti-B isohemagglutinins in group O mothers are usually of the IgM type and so do not cross the placenta. However, for reasons not well known, certain group O individuals possess IgG antibodies directed against group A or B antigens (or both) even without prior sensitization. Therefore, the first-born may be affected. Fortunately, even with transplacentally acquired antibodies, lysis of the infant's red cells is minimal. Two factors seem to be responsible for this happy circumstance: neonatal red cells express group A and B antigens poorly, and the widespread presence of these antigens on other tissue cells serves to "soak up" some of the transferred antibodies. There is no effective method of preventing hemolytic disease resulting from ABO incompatibility.

**MORPHOLOGY.** The anatomic findings with erythroblastosis fetalis depend entirely upon the severity of the hemolytic process. Sometimes these infants are stillborn, with marked anemia and manifestations of edema and congestive heart failure **(hydrops fetalis)**. Live-born infants may succumb promptly or within several weeks, unless there is exchange transfusion. Immediate postnatal death is usually caused by severe hemolysis and consequent circulatory failure. In its mildest form, the child may be only slightly anemic and survive without further complications **(congenital anemia of the newborn)**. With more severe hemolysis, the anemia and pallor are accompanied, within several days, by obvious hyperbilirubinemia **(icterus gravis)**. In all forms, the bone marrow is hyperactive and extramedullary hematopoiesis is present in the liver, spleen, and possibly other tissues, such as the kidneys, lungs, and even the heart. The increased hematopoietic activity accounts for the presence in the peripheral circulation of large numbers of immature red cells, including reticulocytes, normoblasts, and erythroblasts (hence the name erythroblastosis fetalis).

When hyperbilirubinemia is marked (usually above 20 mg in full-term infants, often less in premature babies), the central nervous system may be damaged **(kernicterus)**. The circulating unconjugated bilirubin is taken up by the brain tissue, on which it apparently exerts a toxic effect. The brain becomes enlarged and edematous and, when sectioned, has a bright yellow pigmentation of the basal ganglia, thalamus, cerebellum, cerebral gray matter, and spinal cord. This pigmentation is evanescent and fades within 24 hours, despite prompt fixation. It is of interest that adults are protected from this effect of hyperbilirubinemia by the blood-brain barrier.

**CLINICAL COURSE.** As was indicated, the clinical patterns of erythroblastosis fetalis vary from lethal disease (stillborn infants) to the mildest degrees of anemia in otherwise healthy children. Kernicterus may manifest itself by apathy and poor feeding, and later by mental retardation, cerebral irritability, extrapyramidal signs, and cranial nerve palsies. In the most severe form of erythroblastosis fetalis (fetal hydrops), the anemia and kernicterus are accompanied by congestive heart failure and generalized edema.

Since severe erythroblastosis fetalis can be treated, early recognition of the disorder is imperative. That which results from Rh incompatibility may be more or less accurately predicted, since it correlates well with rapidly rising Rh antibody titers in the mother during pregnancy. Amniotic fluid obtained by amniocentesis may show high levels of bilirubin. As might be expected, the result of a direct Coombs' test is positive on fetal cord blood if the red cells have been coated by maternal antibody. Exchange transfusion of the infants is an effective form of therapy. Postnatally, phototherapy is helpful since visible light converts bilirubin to readily excreted dipyrroles. As already discussed, administration of anti-D globulins to the mother can prevent the occurrence of Rh erythroblastosis.

Group ABO erythroblastosis fetalis is more difficult to predict, but it is readily monitored by awareness of the blood incompatibility between mother and father and by hemoglobin and bilirubin determinations on the vulnerable newborn infant.

## HEMOLYTIC ANEMIAS RESULTING FROM MECHANICAL TRAUMA TO RED CELLS

Red blood cells may be disrupted by physical trauma in a variety of circumstances. *Clinically important are the hemolytic anemias associated with insertion of valve prostheses and with narrowing or obstruction of the vasculature.* In the case of prosthetic valves, the red cells are damaged by the shear stresses resulting from the turbulent blood flow and abnormal pressure gradients caused by the artificial cardiac valves. *Microangiopathic hemolytic anemia,* on the other hand, is characterized by mechanical damage to the red cells as they squeeze through abnormally narrowed vessels. Most often the narrowing is caused by widespread deposition of fibrin in the small vessels, in association with disseminated intravascular coagulation (p. 395). Other causes of microangiopathic hemolytic anemia include malignant hypertension, systemic lupus erythematosus, thrombotic thrombocytopenic purpura (TTP), hemolytic uremic syndrome, and disseminated cancer. Most of these disorders are discussed elsewhere in this book. Suffice to say that common to all these disorders is the presence of vascular lesions that predispose the circulating red cells to mechanical injury. The morphologic alterations in the injured red blood cells may be striking. Thus "burr cells," "helmet cells," and "triangle cells" may be seen in the peripheral blood film. It should be pointed out that except for TTP and the related hemolytic uremic syndrome, the extent of hemolysis is not a major clinical problem in most instances.

## MALARIA

It has been estimated that 15 to 20 million persons suffer from this infectious and hemolytic disease; hence, it is one of the most widespread afflictions of mankind. It is endemic in Asia and Africa, but with widespread jet travel, cases are reported from all over the world. The fact that the eradication of malaria is theoretically feasible makes its prevalence even more unfortunate. Malaria is caused by one of four types of protozoa: *Plasmodium vivax* causes benign tertian malaria; *Plasmodium malariae* causes quartan malaria, another benign form; *Plasmodium ovale* causes ovale malaria, a relatively uncommon and benign form similar to vivax malaria; and *Plasmodium falciparum* causes malignant tertian, estivoautumnal, or falciparum malaria, which has a high fatality rate. All are transmitted only by the bite of female *Anopheles* mosquitoes, and humans are the only natural reservoir.

**ETIOLOGY AND PATHOGENESIS.** The life cycle of the plasmodia is a well understood but complex process, which may require review.

Briefly, it consists of two phases: (1) asexual reproduction, or schizogony, which occurs in humans, and (2) sexual reproduction, or sporogony, which occurs in the mosquito. When the parasites are introduced into human blood by the mosquito, they circulate only briefly, then invade the liver cells (exoerythrocytic cycle). This represents the incubation period of malaria. For **P. vivax** and **P. ovale**, it is about 14 days; for **P. malariae**, 24 days; and for **P. falciparum**, 8 to 20 days. Within the liver, the parasites develop into schizonts, which rupture the liver cells and yield free merozoites that in turn enter red cells. During the erythrocytic cycle, further development of the parasites occurs, yielding trophozoites, which are somewhat distinctive for each of the four forms of malaria. Thus, the specific form of malaria can be recognized in appropriately stained thick smears of the peripheral blood. For details on such parasitology, reference should be made to specialized texts. When the trophozoites are fully grown within the red cells, they divide into merozoites, which rupture the erythrocytes and may then reenter other red cells, where they develop into gametocytes that infect the next hungry mosquito.

The distinctive clinical and anatomic features of malaria are related to the following: (1) Showers of new merozoites are released from the red cells at intervals of approximately 48 hours for *P. vivax* and *P. ovale* and 72 hours for *P. malariae.* The recurrent clinical spikes of fever and chills are timed with this release. (2) The parasites destroy large numbers of red cells and thus cause a hemolytic anemia. (3) A characteristic brown malarial pigment, probably a derivative of hemoglobin that is identical to hematin, is released from the ruptured red cells along with the merozoites, discoloring principally the spleen but also the liver, lymph nodes, and bone marrow. (4) Activation of the phagocytic defense mechanisms of the host leads to marked RE hyperplasia throughout the body, reflected in massive splenomegaly. Less frequently, the liver may also be enlarged.

**CLINICAL COURSE.** Benign malaria is characterized by recurrent paroxysms of shaking chills, high fever, and drenching sweats, correlated with the release of merozoites from the ruptured red cells. Occasionally jaundice is evident. There is progressive hepatosplenomegaly, particularly in those long-standing, smoldering cases associated with partial immunity. In the usual course of events, spontaneous recovery ensues or the patient benefits dramatically from antimalarial drugs. For unknown reasons, however, relapses are frequent with *P. vivax* and *P. malariae*. Indeed, about 30% of patients with vivax malaria have relapses, sometimes as long as 30 years after the initial infection. Whether these cases are associated with persistence of exoerythrocytic forms or imply a continuation of the erythrocytic cycles at low levels is not known.

Fatal falciparum malaria is characterized by prominent involvement of the brain. Cerebral blood vessels are full of parasitized red cells and are often occluded by microthrombi. The disease may begin suddenly or slowly, but it is rapidly progressive, with the development of high fever, chills, convulsions, shock, and death, usually within days to weeks. In other cases, falciparum malaria may pursue a more chronic course but may be punctuated at any time by a dramatic complication known as *blackwater fever*. This syndrome is characterized by the sudden onset of severe chills, fever, jaundice, vomiting, and the passage of dark red to black urine. The trigger for this complication is obscure, but it is associated with massive hemolysis, leading to jaundice, hemoglobinemia, and hemoglobinuria. Disseminated intravascular coagulation, to be discussed later, may be a factor in this form of malaria. With appropriate chemotherapy, the prognosis with most forms of malaria is good. However, treatment of falciparum malaria is much more difficult owing to the emergence of drug-resistant strains. Because of the potentially serious consequences of this disease, early diagnosis and treatment are particularly important but are sometimes delayed in nonendemic settings.

# ANEMIAS OF DIMINISHED ERYTHROPOIESIS

In this category are included those anemias caused by an inadequate supply to the bone marrow of some substance necessary for hematopoiesis (nutritional anemias). The most common deficiencies are those of iron, folic acid, or vitamin $B_{12}$. Infrequently, there is a *pyridoxine-responsive anemia* or a *thiamine-dependent anemia*. Another important cause of impaired erythropoiesis is suppression of marrow stem cells, exemplified by aplastic anemia and myelophthisic anemia. In the following section some common examples of anemias resulting from nutritional deficiencies and marrow suppression will be discussed individually.

## IRON DEFICIENCY ANEMIA

It is estimated that 10 to 20% of the population in developed countries and as many as 25 to 50% in developing countries are anemic. Iron deficiency accounts for most of this prevalence.[15] It is without question the commonest form of nutritional deficiency and is most often caused by some combination of inadequate intake, increased requirement, and excessive losses. Thus it is most commonly encountered:

○ in infants, when the dietary intake is likely to be deficient since milk alone does not provide adequate amounts.

○ in adolescents, with their rapid growth and increased requirement for iron.

○ in pregnant women, because of the fetal drain of iron.

○ in the very elderly, with their marginal diets, chronic ailments, and infections.

○ in most alcoholics, with their deficient diets.

*It is a clinical maxim that in the absence of overt causes, iron deficiency anemia in adult males and nonmenstruating women indicates gastrointestinal tract blood loss until otherwise proved.*[16]

Some aspects of normal metabolism of iron are discussed on page 594. There it is indicated that it is a rigorously conserved element in the body; there are regulated mechanisms of absorption, limited pathways of excretion, and modest reserves. As you know, it is necessary for the synthesis of hemoglobin, myoglobin, and a large number of iron-containing enzymes such as the cytochromes and flavoproteins. Indeed, it appears that the major clinical consequences of an inadequate metabolic pool of iron relate to the functional deficiencies of iron-dependent enzymes rather than to low levels of hemoglobin.

The development of the deficient state occurs insidiously. At first there is depletion of the storage iron, which is marked by a decline in serum ferritin and depletion of stainable iron in the bone marrow. There follows a decrease in circulating iron, with a low level of serum iron and a rise in the serum transferrin iron-binding capacity. Ultimately, the inadequacy makes its impact on the hemoglobin, myoglobin, and other iron-containing compounds. With more significant deficits, impaired work performance and brain function and reduced immunologic competence may develop.

**MORPHOLOGY.** Except in unusual circumstances, iron deficiency anemia is relatively mild. The red cells are microcytic and hypochromic, reflecting the reduced mean corpuscular volume (MCV) and mean corpuscular hemoglobin concentration (MCHC). Although the bone marrow is hyperplastic, particularly at the level of the normoblasts, the active marrow is usually only slightly increased in volume. Extramedullary hematopoiesis is uncommon.

The skin and mucous membranes of these patients are pale, and the nails may become spoon-shaped and have longitudinal ridges. In some cases, atrophic glossitis is present, giving the tongue a smooth, glazed appearance. When this is accompanied by dysphagia and esophageal webs, it constitutes the **Plummer-Vinson syndrome** (see p. 507).

**CLINICAL COURSE.** In most instances, iron deficiency anemia is asymptomatic. Nonspecific indications, such as weakness, listlessness, and pallor, may be present in severe cases. Rarely, in the United States and more often in Scandinavia and Great Britain, the *Plummer-Vinson syndrome* occurs. With long-standing severe anemia, thinning, flattening, and eventually "spooning" of the fingernails sometimes appears.

Diagnostic criteria include low hemoglobin concentration, low hematocrit, low mean corpuscular volume, hypochromic microcytic red cells, low serum iron levels, low transferrin saturation, increased total iron-binding capacity, and, ultimately, response to iron therapy.[17] *Individuals frequently die with this form of anemia, but rarely of it.* It is well to remember that in reasonably adequately nourished individuals, microcytic hypochromic anemia is not a disease but rather a symptom of some underlying disorder.

# MEGALOBLASTIC ANEMIAS

There are two principal types of megaloblastic anemia, one caused by a folate deficiency and the other by a lack of vitamin $B_{12}$. The megaloblastic anemias may be caused by a nutritional deficiency of folic acid (folate) or, in many cases, the deficiency reflects impaired absorption, as is the case with vitamin $B_{12}$ (p. 366). Both have in common enlargement of proliferating cells, in particular erythroid precursors that create *megaloblasts* and correspondingly abnormally large red cells (*macrocytes*). Other proliferating cells such as granulocyte precursors are enlarged (*giant metamyelocytes*), yielding enlarged *hypersegmented neutrophils.* Underlying the cellular gigantism, paradoxically, is impairment of DNA synthesis, so that proliferating cells laboriously synthesize DNA and enlarge their nuclei but the ultimate mitotic division is delayed in time. However, synthesis of RNA and cytoplasmic elements proceeds at a normal pace. The nuclei are thus immature, whereas the cytoplasm is fully mature; this is referred to as *nuclear-cytoplasmic asynchrony.* Because of these maturational derangements, there is an accumulation of megaloblasts in the bone marrow, yielding too few

erythrocytes, hence the anemia.[18] Two concomitant additional processes further aggravate the anemia: (1) ineffective erythropoiesis, referring to the predisposition of megaloblasts to undergo autohemolysis, and (2) increased hemolytic destruction of the abnormally large red cells. This increased breakdown of red cells and precursors leads to iron accumulation, mostly in the mononuclear phagocytic cells of the bone marrow.

## Folate (Folic Acid) Deficiency Anemia

Megaloblastic anemia secondary to a lack of folate is not common, but precarious folate levels in the body are surprisingly common: among the economically deprived of all countries who live on marginal diets; among pregnant women, in whom dietary inadequacies combine with increased metabolic requirements; and among alcoholics and drug addicts, with their well-known grossly inadequate diets. Although reserves of this nutrient are relatively modest in the body, a negative balance will not become evident for months unless there is concomitantly an increased demand, as occurs with rapid growth, pregnancy, or chronic disease. Ironically, folate is widely prevalent in nearly all raw foods. However, it is readily destroyed by 10 to 15 minutes of cooking. Thus the best sources of folate in the diet are fresh or fresh-frozen vegetables and fruits eaten either uncooked or lightly cooked. Food folates are predominantly in the polyglutamate form, and most must be split into monoglutamates for absorption. Acidic foods and conjugase inhibitors found in beans and other legumes hamper absorption by inhibiting intestinal conjugases that catalyze the formation of monoglutamates from polyglutamates. Dilantin and a few other drugs also inhibit folate absorption. The principal site of intestinal absorption is the upper third of the small intestine, and so malabsorptive disorders such as celiac disease and tropical sprue, which affect this level of the gut, impair absorption.[16]

The metabolism and physiologic functions of folic acid after absorption are complex. It suffices for our purposes that after absorption, folic acid is transported in the blood mainly as a monoglutamate. Within cells it undergoes conversion to several derivatives, but of principal importance is that it must be reduced to tetrahydrofolate (THF) by a reductase. (This reductase is sensitive to inhibition by folate analogues such as methotrexate, which deprives cells of folate and the capacity to rapidly divide—the basis for the use of folic acid antagonists as antineoplastic agents.) The primary function of THF is as an acceptor and donor of one-carbon units in a variety of steps involved in DNA synthesis. Several one-carbon transfers are critical to the synthesis of purines, thymidylate, and therefore thymine. Thus it should be apparent why a deficiency of folate causes the slow DNA synthesis that accounts for megaloblastic anemia.[19]

**MORPHOLOGY.** The principal anatomic changes are seen in the bone marrow and blood, with secondary alterations referable to the anemia in severe cases. The bone marrow is markedly hypercellular and extends into areas formerly occupied by inactive fatty marrow. The hypercellularity results predominantly from increased numbers of megaloblasts (i.e., abnormal erythroblasts). These cells are larger than normoblasts and have a delicate, finely reticulated nuclear chromatin (suggestive of nuclear immaturity) and an abundant, strikingly basophilic cytoplasm. Normoblasts are, by comparison, few in number, and there is a notable absence of maturing red cells, suggesting a maturation arrest at the megaloblastic level. Analogously, the granulocytic precursors also demonstrate nuclear-cytoplasmic asynchrony, yielding giant metamyelocytes. As mentioned previously, stainable iron is present diffusely throughout the marrow rather than in discrete patches, as in normal bone marrow.

In the peripheral blood, the earliest change is usually the appearance of hypersegmented granulocytes. These appear even before the onset of anemia. Although the normal number of lobes in a granulocyte nucleus is two to three, with the megaloblastic anemias this may be markedly increased, to five or six. Macrocytosis of the red cells may also be present before the development of anemia. Such erythrocytes are oval in shape and are obviously enlarged. Although macrocytes appear hyperchromic because of their large size, in reality the mean corpuscular hemoglobin concentration is normal. Morphologic changes in other systems, especially the gastrointestinal tract, may also occur, giving rise to some of the clinical features discussed next.

**CLINICAL COURSE.** Typically, patients with folate deficiency anemia are rather sick and present a complex clinical picture, since the malnutrition that is responsible for folic acid deficiency produces other deficiencies as well. In most cases, a clearly inadequate diet is discovered by history, and the patient may appear obviously malnourished. The onset of the anemia is insidious and is associated with nonspecific symptoms, such as weakness and easy fatigability. Since the gastrointestinal tract, like the hematopoietic system, is associated with rapid cell turnover, symptoms referable to the alimentary tract are common and often severe. These include sore tongue and cheilosis. It should be stressed that unlike the case with vitamin $B_{12}$ deficiency, neurologic abnormalities do not occur.

The diagnosis of a megaloblastic anemia is readily made from examination of a smear of peripheral blood and the bone marrow. Of importance is the differentiation of the anemia of folate deficiency from that of vitamin $B_{12}$ deficiency; this is best accomplished by assays for serum folate and vitamin $B_{12}$ and red cell folate levels. Rarely, the folate levels are spuriously low, and more sophisticated diagnostic procedures are available, as described by Herbert.[18]

### Vitamin $B_{12}$ (Cobalamin) Deficiency Anemia—Pernicious Anemia (PA)

Inadequate levels of vitamin $B_{12}$, or cobalamin, in the body result in a megaloblastic macrocytic anemia

similar hematologically to that of folate deficiency. However, a deficiency of vitamin $B_{12}$ causes at the same time a demyelinating disorder involving the peripheral nerves and, ultimately and most importantly, the spinal cord. Thus, unlike the case with folate deficiency, the megaloblastic anemia of $B_{12}$ deficiency, when sufficiently prolonged and severe, is marked by neurologic dysfunction (hence the designation "combined systems disease"). The term "pernicious anemia," sometimes called Addisonian pernicious anemia, should be clarified at this point. There are many potential causes for a $B_{12}$ deficiency state, including inadequate diet, increased requirement, and impaired absorption. *Only the vitamin $B_{12}$ deficiency resulting from inadequate gastric production or defective function of intrinsic factor (IF) necessary to absorb $B_{12}$ constitutes pernicious anemia.*

**PATHOGENESIS.** Among the many potential causes of cobalamin deficiency, inadequate diet and malabsorption are the most common and important. A dietary deficiency of cobalamin is virtually limited to strict vegetarians. This nutrient is abundant in all animal foods, including eggs and dairy products. Indeed, bacterial contamination of nonanimal foods and water may provide adequate amounts of $B_{12}$; it is stored in the liver and efficiently reabsorbed from the bile, and so it would require 20 to 30 years to deplete the normal reserves. Moreover, it is resistant to cooking and boiling. A tiny daily supply, therefore, suffices. *Thus, a dietary lack of $B_{12}$ is uncommon; until proven otherwise, a deficiency of this nutrient implies pernicious anemia (PA) secondary to inadequate production or function of IF.* The deranged synthesis of IF appears to be caused by an autoimmune reaction against parietal cells and IF itself, producing gastric mucosal atrophy. It is significant that patients with pernicious anemia also frequently have other autoimmune diseases such as Hashimoto's thyroiditis, Graves' disease, and rheumatoid arthritis. The gastric atrophy rarely develops before the fourth decade of life, and the incidence progressively rises thereafter so that approximately one in 200 individuals over the age of 60 develops PA. The specific autoantibodies and their effects on the gastric mucosa are also discussed on page 514. In brief, there are three types of autoantibodies: (1) those against parietal cells (approximately 85 to 90% of patients); (2) those against intrinsic factor, preventing the binding of vitamin $B_{12}$ (about 75% of patients); and (3) those against IF-$B_{12}$ complexes blocking absorption of $B_{12}$ (about 75% of patients). It should be noted that in a small minority of patients having inadequate production of IF, no autoantibodies can be demonstrated. Perhaps in these patients age-related gastric mucosal atrophy is the root problem. Conversely, low titers of autoantibodies have been identified in elderly individuals who do not have pernicious anemia, suggesting that critical threshold levels are necessary to significantly affect IF production. It might be noted in passing that infrequently juvenile pernicious anemia of unknown cause appears in children who have normal gastric mucosal tissue.[20] Equally rare is vitamin $B_{12}$ deficiency anemia following gastrectomy in which the fundic origin of IF has been removed.

The precise role of IF in the absorption of $B_{12}$ is somewhat complex, but in brief it involves the following steps. With normal levels of gastric acidity, $B_{12}$ is liberated from foods by gastric and intestinal enzymes. The vitamin then attaches to salivary and gastric $B_{12}$-binding proteins (R-binders), but a little is bound directly to IF. The R-$B_{12}$ complexes are broken down in the small intestine when exposed to pancreatic proteases, and the released $B_{12}$ then attaches to IF. In this form the IF-$B_{12}$ complex is resistant to further degradation and passes into the ileum, where it adheres to IF-$B_{12}$ specific brush border receptors on the ileal cells. It is likely, but not certain, that the complex then splits and the $B_{12}$ enters the intestinal mucosal cells. It is then complexed to a $B_{12}$-delivery protein known as transcobalamin II, which delivers it to the liver, bone marrow, and other proliferating cells.

The precise metabolic defects induced by a cobalamin deficiency that eventually lead to a megaloblastic anemia and neuropathy are still somewhat uncertain, and many theories have been offered. Most widely accepted is the view that $B_{12}$ deficiency in effect produces a folate deficiency by blocking utilization of 5-methyl-THF (p. 365). The cellular uptake and retention of 5-methyl-THF is dependent on $B_{12}$ but intestinal absorption is not. Thus, there is a serum "pile-up" of folate (referred to as the "folate trap") but a cellular deprivation and hence the reduced formation of thymidylate, thymine, purines, and, therefore, DNA.[18] Other consequences of a $B_{12}$ deficiency may be direct impairment of synthesis of thymidylate synthetase and, possibly, failure of formation of polyglutamate folate, an important folate coenzyme, but much is controversial.[21] As mentioned earlier, a deficiency of vitamin $B_{12}$ impairs synthesis of myelin and hence a demyelinating neuropathy develops. However, the precise biochemical derangement has not been pinpointed.

**MORPHOLOGY. Pernicious anemia is characterized by changes in the bone marrow, alimentary tract, and nervous system.** The appearance of the bone marrow is similar to that described with folate deficiency anemia. It is soft, red, jelly-like, and extremely hypercellular, with extension into the formerly inactive areas. A maturation arrest at the megaloblastic level is seen, with nests of megaloblasts and relatively few normoblasts and maturing red cells (Fig. 12–8). Diffuse stainable iron is present.

The peripheral blood picture is also closely similar to that of folate deficiency anemia, with macrocytes and hypersegmented granulocytes as the hallmarks. In general, the MCV is perhaps higher than with folate deficiency; it is very rarely normal.

The atrophic gastric mucosa of pernicious anemia will be described on page 515. In addition, atrophic glossitis

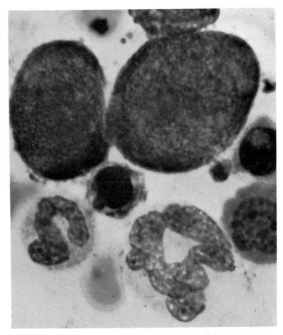

Figure 12–8. A marrow smear from a patient with pernicious anemia. Two megaloblasts are seen above and a "macropoly" (macropolymorphonuclear neutrophil) appears below. (From Robbins, S. L., Cotran, R. S., and Kumar, V.: Pathologic Basis of Disease. 3rd ed. Philadelphia, W. B. Saunders Co., 1984, p. 630.)

may be present in these patients. The tongue is beefy red and slightly swollen and has a glazed appearance. Histologically, there is nonspecific submucosal chronic inflammation, with atrophy of the overlying epidermis and papillae. The neurologic lesions associated with PA comprise, in essence, demyelination of the posterior and lateral columns of the spinal cord, sometimes beginning in the peripheral nerves. In time axonal degeneration may supervene.

An element of hemolysis, discussed earlier, contributes to the hemosiderosis that is frequently seen within the liver, spleen, and bone marrow.

**CLINICAL COURSE.** In general, these patients are less sick than those with folate deficiency anemia. Nonspecific indications of severe anemia include weakness, dyspnea, and syncope. Since most of these patients are elderly, the anemia and hypovolemia (which is present for obscure reasons) often lead to angina pectoris, palpitations, and high output cardiac failure. Gastrointestinal symptoms similar to those described under folate deficiency may also be present. Of particular concern is the appearance of neurologic changes such as symmetric numbness, tingling, and burning in feet or hands followed by unsteadiness of gait and loss of position sense, particularly in the toes. *Although the anemia responds dramatically to vitamin $B_{12}$ therapy, the neurologic manifestations may persist.*

The diagnostic features of PA include (1) low serum vitamin $B_{12}$ levels, (2) normal or elevated serum folate levels, (3) histamine-fast gastric achlorhydria, (4) inability to absorb an oral dose of cobalamin (the Schilling test), (5) moderate to severe megaloblastic anemia, (6) leukopenia with hypersegmented granulocytes, and, most critically, (7) dramatic reticulocytic response (within 2 to 3 days) to the parenteral administration of vitamin $B_{12}$.

It is frequently stated that patients with long-standing pernicious anemia have a three to five times greater risk of gastric carcinoma, but relatively recent studies place the increased risk at a significantly lower level.[22]

## APLASTIC ANEMIA

Suppression of bone marrow function occurs in a variety of clinical forms. Most often there is a failure or suppression of stem cells leading to a hypocellular marrow, anemia, thrombocytopenia, and agranulocytosis (*pancytopenia*). Although all the formed elements are affected, this condition is usually called *aplastic anemia*.[23] In some cases, however, marrow suppression may be selective, affecting erythroid stem cells (*pure red cell aplasia*), granulocytic stem cells (*agranulocytosis*), or megakaryocytes (*thrombocytopenia*). The following discussion will be restricted largely to aplastic anemia, which is the most common expression of marrow failure. Agranulocytosis and thrombocytopenia will be discussed later.

**ETIOLOGY AND PATHOGENESIS.** In over half the cases, aplastic anemia appears without any apparent provoking cause and so is termed *idiopathic*. In other cases, exposure to a known myelotoxic agent can be identified, such as *whole body irradiation* (as may occur with nuclear plant accidents) or use of *myelotoxic drugs*. Drugs and chemicals are the commonest causes of secondary aplastic anemia. With some agents, the marrow damage is predictable, dose-related, and usually reversible. Included in this category are antineoplastic drugs (alkylating agents, antimetabolites), benzene, and chloramphenicol. In other instances marrow toxicity occurs as an apparent "idiosyncratic" or sensitivity reaction to small doses of known myelotoxic drugs (such as chloramphenicol) or following the use of such agents as phenylbutazone, sulfonamides, or methylphenylethylhydantoin, which are not myelotoxic in other individuals.

Recently, a number of cases of aplastic anemia have been reported in patients who have had viral infections.[24] The implicated viruses include EBV, cytomegalovirus, herpes varicella zoster, and hepatitis virus. The disease associated with hepatitis is particularly severe. Marrow aplasia develops insidiously several months after recovery from non-A, non-B hepatitis and follows a relentless course.

The pathogenetic events leading to marrow failure are obscure, even when an etiologic agent can be identified. Recent studies suggest that aplastic anemia is not a single entity but comprises a heterogeneous group of pathogenetically distinct disorders.[25]

It has been postulated that it may result from (1) defective or deficient hematopoietic stem cells, (2) a defect in the bone marrow stroma ("hematopoietic microenvironment") that causes it to be unable to support normal stem cell function, or (3) suppression of marrow stem cells by immunologic mechanisms.[26] Each of these mechanisms is supported by some evidence. Restoration of normal hematopoiesis, in many cases by bone marrow transplantation, suggests that defective stem cells may be the cause of aplasia. In other patients administration of antithymocyte globulin has led to recovery of marrow function, implicating T-suppressor cells as the cause of stem cell failure.[27] It is clear that we are only beginning to unravel the pathogenetic mechanisms in aplastic anemia; much remains to be known.

**MORPHOLOGY.** As was mentioned earlier, the bone marrow typically is hypocellular, with an increase in the amount of fat cells. Small foci of lymphocytes and plasma cells may be seen in the fibrous stoma. Scattered islands of primitive hematopoietic cells are seen in less severe cases. A number of secondary changes may accompany marrow failure. Hepatic fatty change may result from anemia, and thrombocytopenia and granulocytopenia may give rise to hemorrhages and bacterial infections, respectively. Multiple transfusions may cause hemosiderosis.

**CLINICAL COURSE.** Aplastic anemia may occur at any age and in both sexes. Usually the onset is gradual, but in some cases the disorder strikes with suddenness and great severity. The initial manifestations vary somewhat, depending on the cell line predominantly affected. Anemia may cause the progressive onset of weakness, pallor, and dyspnea. Petechiae and ecchymoses may herald thrombocytopenia. Granulocytopenia may manifest itself only by frequent and persistent minor infections or by the sudden onset of chills, fever, and prostration. *Splenomegaly is characteristically absent, and if present the diagnosis of aplastic anemia should be seriously questioned.* Typically, the red cells are normocytic and normochromic, although occasionally slight macrocytosis is present; *reticulocytosis is absent.*

The diagnosis rests upon examination of bone marrow biopsy and peripheral blood. It is important to distinguish aplastic anemia from myelodysplastic syndromes (p. 383). Since pancytopenia is common to both these conditions, their clinical manifestations are often indistinguishable. However, with aplastic anemia the marrow is hypocellular owing to stem cell failure, whereas in myelodysplasia the marrow is populated by abnormal and immature myeloid cells. The prognosis of marrow aplasia is quite unpredictable. As mentioned earlier, withdrawal of toxic drugs may lead to recovery in some cases. The idiopathic form has a poor prognosis. Bone marrow transplantation is an extremely effective form of therapy, especially in young (less than 40 years) patients.[28] Older patients benefit from immunosuppressive therapy with antithymocyte globulin.

## MYELOPHTHISIC ANEMIA

This form of marrow failure is caused by extensive replacement of the marrow by tumor or other lesions. This is most commonly associated with metastatic cancer arising from a primary lesion in the breast, lung, prostate, or thyroid. Multiple myeloma, lymphomas, leukemias, advanced tuberculosis, lipid storage disorders, and osteosclerosis are less commonly implicated. Myelophthisic anemia is also seen with progressive fibrosis of the bone marrow (myelofibrosis), to be discussed later (p. 390). The manifestations of marrow infiltration include anemia and thrombocytopenia. The white cell series is less affected. Characteristically, misshapen and immature red cells are seen in the peripheral blood, along with a slightly elevated white cell count ("leukoerythroblastosis"). The treatment obviously involves the management of the underlying condition.

## POLYCYTHEMIA

Polycythemia, or *erythrocytosis*, as it is sometimes referred to, denotes an increased concentration of red cells, usually with a corresponding increase in hemoglobin level. Such an increase may be *relative*, when there is hemoconcentration due to decreased plasma volume, or *absolute*, when there is an increase in total red cell mass. Relative polycythemia results from any cause of dehydration such as deprivation of

**Table 12–4.** PATHOPHYSIOLOGIC CLASSIFICATION OF POLYCYTHEMIA

**Relative**
Reduced plasma volume (hemoconcentration)

**Absolute**

| | |
|---|---|
| Primary: | Abnormal proliferation of myeloid stem cells, normal or low erythropoietin levels (polycythemia vera) |
| Secondary: | Increased erythropoietin levels |
| | Appropriate: lung disease, high-altitude living, cyanotic heart disease |
| | Inappropriate: erythropoietin-secreting tumors (e.g., renal cell carcinoma, hepatoma, cerebellar hemangioblastoma) |

water, prolonged vomiting, diarrhea, or excessive use of diuretics. It is also associated with an obscure condition of unknown etiology called stress polycythemia or Gaisböck's syndrome. *Absolute polycythemia* is said to be *primary* when the increase in red cell mass results from an intrinsic abnormality of the myeloid stem cells and *secondary* when the red cell progenitors are normal but proliferate in response to increased levels of erythropoietin. Primary polycythemia (polycythemia vera) is one of several expressions of clonal, neoplastic proliferation of myeloid stem cells and is therefore best considered with other myeloproliferative disorders (p. 389). Secondary polycythemias may be caused by an increase in erythropoietin secretion that is physiologically appropriate or by an inappropriate (pathologic) secretion of erythropoietin (Table 12–4).

# White Cell Disorders

The most important of the white cell disorders are the malignant proliferative diseases. This category embraces the *lymphomas*, which are characterized by proliferation of native cells within lymphoid tissue; the *leukemias*, which involve the bone marrow with spillover into the blood; and the *plasma cell dyscrasias*, which are manifested by the expansion of a single clone of antibody-producing cells. There are other, less frequent malignant white cell disorders. Some of these can be considered intergradations of the above-mentioned major entities. For example, Waldenström's macroglobulinemia has features of all three—the lymphomas, the leukemias, and the plasma cell dyscrasias. Malignant diseases of the white cells cause about 9% of all cancer deaths. In children under the age of 15 years, they are responsible for a staggering 48% of deaths from cancer.

## LYMPHOMAS

The lymphomas are basically cancers of lymphoid tissue characterized by the proliferation or accumu-

lation of cells native to lymphoid tissue (i.e., lymphocytes, histiocytes, their precursors, and derivatives). Since the lymphomas share the clinical significance of all malignant diseases, it will be appreciated that the term "lymphoma," while hallowed by long usage, is actually a misnomer. At the outset we should distinguish between Hodgkin's disease (closely related to the lymphomas) and non-Hodgkin's lymphomas (NHL). Although both have their origins in the lymphoid tissues, Hodgkin's disease is set apart by distinctive morphologic features, among them the Reed-Sternberg giant cell, which is seen in all variants of Hodgkin's disease. Therefore we will discuss non-Hodgkin's lymphomas and Hodgkin's disease separately.

## NON-HODGKIN'S LYMPHOMA (NHL)

NHL arises in lymphoid tissue, usually in the lymph nodes (65% of cases), as well as in the lymphoid tissue of parenchymal organs (35%). All variants have the potential for spread into other lymph nodes and into various tissues throughout the body, especially the liver, spleen, and bone marrow. In some cases, bone marrow involvement is followed by a spillover of the proliferating cells into the peripheral blood, creating a leukemia-like picture. Although we speak of NHL as a group, we should recognize that it encompasses a wide spectrum of disorders, differing in patient age at onset, the cells of origin, and response to therapy. It is therefore necessary to classify NHL into various subgroups.

Few areas of pathology have evoked as much controversy and confusion as the classification of NHL. We will not attempt to discuss all the current classifications[29] but will present the modified Rappaport classification in some detail. This classification, which is based entirely on morphologic features, has the merits of providing valuable clinicopathologic correlations, of being reproducible, and of being widely used in the United States. However, as we shall discuss later, the availability of cytochemical, immunologic, and molecular techniques to identify cells has indicated there are several "misnomers" in the Rappaport schema. As a result, several alternative classifications have been proposed that are based on an understanding of the organization and physiology of the immune system. Among these, the one most favored in the United States is the *Lukes-Collins classification*.[30] As classifications began to "proliferate," an international panel of expert "lymphomaniacs" decided to stem the tide by proposing yet another (and possibly the ultimate) classification entitled *Working Formulation for Clinical Usage*.[31] In the following section, details of the Rappaport classification will be presented first; it is followed by comments relating to the Lukes-Collins classification and its comparison with the Rappaport classification. Thereafter, brief comments will be made on the recently proposed working formulation.

### Rappaport Classification

The Rappaport classification is based upon two morphologic features: (a) the growth pattern of the tumor cells as *nodular aggregates or diffuse infiltrations* throughout the node and (b) the cytologic character of the cells as seen with the light microscope. *Nodular (follicular) lymphomas* are characterized by cohesive aggregates of neoplastic cells somewhat resembling germinal centers of lymphoid follicles. Unlike germinal centers, however, the lymphomatous nodules are dispersed throughout the cortex and medulla and are more uniform in size, and usually the cells within the neoplastic nodules are more monotonous than those in normal germinal centers. In the United States, approximately 40% of all NHLs in adults are of the nodular variety. On the basis of cytologic characteristics, nodular lymphomas are divided into three subtypes (Table 12–5). Since the cytologic features of nodular and diffuse lymphomas are very similar, all will be described later. *The nodular lymphomas have distinctive clinical features: (1) they occur predominantly in older individuals (rarely under 20 years of age), (2) they affect males and females equally, and (3) despite the common finding of disseminated disease (involvement of many or all nodes as well as possibly extranodal sites) at the time of diagnosis, they have a much better prognosis than diffuse lymphomas*. In one large series the actuarial survival of untreated patients was 73% at 10 years.[32] Paradoxically, it is virtually impossible to eradicate these indolent tumors. It seems that even with complete drug-induced "clinical" remissions, residual neoplastic cells persist that eventually lead to a relapse. In view of these observations, most authorities believe that until better treatment protocols are devised, a "hands-off" approach is best for the management of these tumors.[33]

*Diffuse lymphomas* are characterized by flooding of the entire lymph node by neoplastic cells, a process that destroys the normal lymph node architecture. With low-power microscopy (best suited for distinguishing the geographic distribution of lymphoma cells; Figs. 12–9 and 12–10), diffuse lymphomas appear as a somewhat homogeneous sea of cells that obscures any distinction between the cortex and medulla. The diffuse lymphomas are more heterogeneous than the nodular lesions.[34] Each of the major cytologic variants (Table 12–5) is associated with somewhat different clinical features and prognosis, as will be discussed shortly.

At the time the Rappaport classification was first presented in 1966, knowledge of lymphocyte subsets with their cytochemical and immunologic markers was in its infancy. *Therefore, the cytologic subdivision of NHL was based entirely on the following two criteria: (1) the apparent similarity of tumor cells to various normal cell types of the lymphoid system*, as a result of which terms such as lymphocytic and histiocytic lymphoma were used to indicate a resemblance to normal lymphocytes and macrophages; and (2) *within a given category, the "degree of differentiation" of cells*, which is evaluated mainly by nuclear

**Table 12–5. RAPPAPORT CLASSIFICATION**

| Nodular (Follicular) Lymphoma | % All Cases | Diffuse Lymphoma | % All Cases |
|---|---|---|---|
| Lymphocytic, poorly differentiated (PDLL) | 24 | Lymphocytic, well differentiated (WDLL) | 5 |
| Mixed lymphocytic-histiocytic | 14 | Lymphocytic, poorly differentiated (PDLL) | 16 |
| Histiocytic | 3 | Lymphoblastic* | |
| | | Histiocytic | 28 |
| | | Mixed lymphocytic-histiocytic | 6 |
| | | Undifferentiated (Burkitt's and non-Burkitt's) | 6 |

*Recent addition to Rappaport classification; previously included in poorly differentiated lymphocytic category. Makes up approximately half of the cases previously included under poorly differentiated diffuse group.

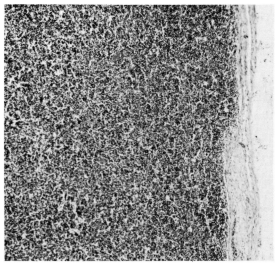

Figure 12–9

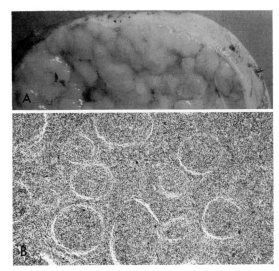

Figure 12–10

**Figure 12–9.** Non-Hodgkin's lymphoma, diffuse pattern of involvement. The capsule of the node is on the right. The architecture of the node is obliterated by the monotonous cells, which have obscured the sinusoids.

**Figure 12–10.** Non-Hodgkin's lymphoma, nodular pattern. *A,* A view of the cut surface of an involved lymph node. *B,* A low-power microscopic view showing the prominent nodules.

and cell size, nuclear configuration, chromatin pattern, and presence or absence of nucleoli. Since it is possible now to identify normal and neoplastic cells of the immune system by a variety of cytochemical and molecular techniques, in the ensuing description we will integrate the Rappaport classification with current information concerning the cell of origin. With this background we can turn to the specific cytologic patterns of lymphomas in the Rappaport classification.

**WELL-DIFFERENTIATED LYMPHOCYTIC LYMPHOMA (WDLL).** In this type, which occurs only in the diffuse pattern, the tumor cells have the appearance of small, round lymphocytes with scant cytoplasm and resemble normal, unstimulated lymphocytes. The nucleus is round and compact, and nucleoli are inconspicuous. Mitotic figures are rare. Closely related to WDLL is chronic lymphocytic leukemia (CLL), which is also characterized by similar small, neoplastic lymphocytes, not only in nodes throughout the body but also in the bone marrow and peripheral blood. Both arise by neoplastic transformation of small B lymphocytes. Histologically, within nodes the two diseases are identical. Their clinical features are also similar.[34] *Both occur primarily in the older age groups; the associated symptoms are mild and prolonged survival is usual.* Generalized or localized lymphadenopathy is the common mode of presentation of WDLL, and involvement of extranodal (parenchymal) sites is rare in this lymphoma.

**POORLY DIFFERENTIATED LYMPHOCYTIC LYMPHOMA (PDLL).** The tumor cells in PDLL consist of atypical B lymphocytes, which may form nodules or diffuse infiltrates.[35] They are slightly larger than those seen in WDLL (but smaller than the nuclei of benign endothelial cells or histiocytes, which are used as a reference when evaluating size). *The nuclei are irregular, with marked indentations in the nuclear membrane and linear infoldings (cleaved nuclei).* The chromatin is coarse and condensed, and mitoses are rare. Some cases of diffuse PDLL are associated with the presence of tumor cells in the peripheral blood (so-called lymphosarcoma cell leukemia), but the frequency of leukemic involvement is much lower than in WDLL.[36]

**HISTIOCYTIC LYMPHOMA (HL).** This type is characterized by the presence of neoplastic cells that are two to three times larger than normal lymphocytes. The tumor cells have vesicular nuclei, which are usually round but sometimes reniform, indented, or lobulated, with one to three nucleoli. The nuclei are larger than those of benign tissue histiocytes. *Although HL can occur in both the nodular and diffuse forms, the latter is much more frequent; indeed, diffuse histiocytic lymphoma is one of the commonest forms of NHL.* Several cytologic subtypes can be recognized among diffuse histiocytic lymphomas, ranging from a monotonous proliferation of large cells to extremely pleomorphic tumors with bizarre cells. A special histologic category associated sometimes with a previous history of an immunologic disorder such as Sjögren's syndrome or with states of immunosuppression (as in renal allograft recipients) has been called *immunoblastic lymphoma. The histiocytic lymphomas have been cited as a prime example of the scientific inaccuracy of the Rappaport classification.* It is now obvious that most tumors classified as HL are not tumors of histiocytes. Immunologic phenotyping has revealed that approximately 60% originate from B cells and 10 to 15% from T cells; in the remaining 25 to 30%, no cell markers can be identified.[37] More recent analyses of DNA extracted from the tumors that did not display T- or B-cell markers has revealed immunoglobulin gene rearrangements, which firmly assigns them to the B-cell lineage.[38] Thus with rare exceptions, so-called HL are now revealed to be made up of activated, enlarged, B- or T-lineage cells. Hence several workers prefer the term *diffuse large cell lymphomas* for this group of tumors. Regardless of what one chooses to call them, these lymphomas are associated with a distinctive clinical presentation. As compared with lymphocytic lymphomas, involvement of extranodal sites is more frequent; indeed, involvement of the gastrointestinal tract, skin, bone, or brain is often the presenting feature. In 50% of the cases, there is involvement of oropharyngeal lymphoid tissue.[39] In the past, these extranodal tumors were called *reticulum cell sarcoma*.

Histiocytic lymphomas are aggressive tumors that until recently were considered incurable. However, with combination chemotherapy, complete remissions can be achieved in up to 80% of the patients, and approximately 40% may remain free of disease for several years. It should be pointed out that despite impressive advances in the accurate identification of the cell of origin in HL, most studies have failed to show any correlation between the cytologic subtype, immunologic phenotype, and response to therapy.[40]

**MIXED LYMPHOCYTIC-HISTIOCYTIC LYMPHOMA.** In this type of lymphoma, cells of the PDLL type as well as the large cell (histiocytic) type are present. In general, a tumor is classified as mixed if the large cells constitute 30 to 50% of the total number of cells. This cytologic pattern is seen in both the nodular and diffuse forms. As in most other cytologic subtypes, the nodular form has better prognosis. However, the relative infrequency of the mixed lymphomas has rendered it difficult to perform careful long-term studies.[41]

**LYMPHOBLASTIC LYMPHOMA.** This is a relatively new addition to the Rappaport classification. Previously, these cases were included under diffuse PDLL, but recent studies indicate that lymphoblastic lymphoma is a distinct clinicopathologic entity, closely related to T-cell acute lymphoblastic leukemia (ALL). The tumor cells in lymphoblastic lymphoma are relatively uniform. In common with the leukemic cells in ALL, the lymphomatous cells have the appearance of immature lymphoblasts, with finely stippled and delicate chromatin. In many but not all cases the nuclear membrane shows deep invagination, imparting a convoluted (lobulated) appearance. Mitoses are relatively frequent. Lymphoblastic lymphoma predominantly affects young males (2:1); most patients are under 20 years of age, although recently some cases affecting adults have been described.[42] *A very characteristic clinical feature is the presence of a prominent mediastinal mass in 50 to 70% of the cases at the time of diagnosis; this suggests a thymic origin.* The disease is rapidly progressive, and early dissemination to the bone marrow and thence into the blood and meninges leads to the evolution of a picture resembling ALL. Until recently, the prognosis of this tumor was grim, but recent attempts to treat this tumor aggressively by utilizing protocols effective in ALL have produced encouraging results in some studies.

**UNDIFFERENTIATED LYMPHOMA.** This type is so termed because the cells do not have any evidence of "maturation" toward lymphocytes or histiocytes. Within this category, *two clinically distinct subgroups have been recognized: the Burkitt's type and non-Burkitt's type.* Histologically, the undifferentiated non-Burkitt's lymphoma is composed of cells that are intermediate in size between PDLL cells and histiocytes. There is considerable nuclear and cellular pleomorphism along with a high mitotic rate. Clinically, these tumors behave as diffuse large cell lymphomas.[34]

The *undifferentiated Burkitt's-type lymphoma* was described initially in Africa, where it is endemic in some parts, but it also occurs sporadically in nonendemic areas. Histologically, the African and the non-endemic American cases of Burkitt's lymphoma are identical. These tumors consist of a diffuse sea of strikingly monotonous cells, which are 10 to 25 μm in diameter with round or oval nuclei containing two to five prominent nucleoli. There is a moderate amount of faintly basophilic or amphophilic cytoplasm, which frequently contains lipid-filled vacuoles. A high mitotic index is very characteristic of this tumor, as is cell death, accounting for the presence of numerous tissue macrophages with ingested nuclear debris. Since these benign macrophages, which are diffusely distributed among the tumor cells, are often surrounded by a clear space, they create a "starry sky" pattern (Fig. 12–11). It should be noted that the "starry sky" appearance can also be seen in other lymphomas (e.g., lymphoblastic type) that have a high mitotic rate. Both the African and non-African cases are found largely in children or young adults. In both forms, the disease rarely arises in the lymph nodes. In African cases, involvement of the maxilla or mandible is the common mode of presentation (Fig. 12–12), whereas abdominal tumors (bowel, retroperitoneum, ovaries) are more common in cases seen in America. Leukemic transformation may occur but is uncommon, especially in the African cases. These tumors respond well to aggressive chemotherapy, and long remissions have been reported. However, in most cases a relapse occurs, and a majority of patients die within five years.

### Lukes-Collins Classification

Unlike the Rappaport classification, which is based purely on morphologic criteria, *in the Lukes-Collins classification, the NHL are classified into T-cell, B-cell, histiocytic, and null cell categories by the use of immunologic and cytochemical markers as adjuncts to morphologic study.* The precise identification of lymphoreticular cells is based largely on several cri-

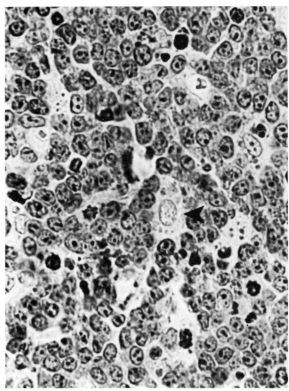

Figure 12–11. Burkitt's lymphoma. Tumor cells have multiple small nucleoli and a high mitotic index. Lack of significant variation in nuclear shape and size lends a monotonous appearance interrupted by pale-staining, benign tissue macrophages (*arrow*), which impart a "starry sky" appearance better appreciated at a lower magnification. (Courtesy of Dr. Jose Hernandez, Department of Pathology, Southwestern Medical School, Dallas, Texas. Reprinted from Robbins, S. L., Cotran, R. S., and Kumar, V.: Pathologic Basis of Disease. 3rd ed. Philadelphia, W. B. Saunders Co., 1984, p. 662.)

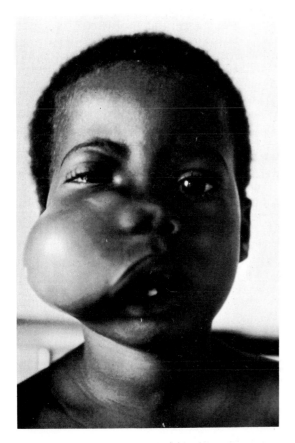

Figure 12–12. Burkitt's lymphoma in a nine-year-old child. The maxillary tumor mass is a characteristic presentation of this disease.

teria, presented in summary form in Tables 5–1 (p. 130) and 12–6.

The Lukes-Collins classification will not be described in detail, but its highlights will be considered insofar as they provide an approach to the newer understanding of the cytologic origins of the NHL. *It has become clear that the great preponderance of NHL, regardless of morphology, arise from B cells.* Since normal B cells have a tendency to form follicles within normal lymph nodes, malignant B cells tend to recapitulate this behavior with nodule formation. Several studies indicate that nodular lymphomas are exclusively composed of B cells.[30, 43] Lukes also pointed out that during differentiation within normal germinal follicles, B cells undergo a series of morphologic changes, characterized by changes in cell and nuclear size and nuclear configuration (clefts or folds); the sequence of changes is small cleaved cell to large cleaved cell to small noncleaved cell to large noncleaved cell. Accordingly, nodular lymphomas that arise from these *follicular center cells (FCC)* may be composed of any one of these differentiation patterns, as though there had been an arrest at a particular stage of transformation. Since a majority of the diffuse lymphomas are made up of cells that are cytologically similar to those seen in nodular lymphomas, *Lukes has further proposed that diffuse lymphomas virtually always arise by extension of nodular patterns.* Indeed, B-cell markers are present on the neoplastic cells in many diffuse lymphomas. However, the distinctly different natural histories of nodular and diffuse lymphomas in patients (cited earlier in the discussion of the Rappaport classification) are not entirely consistent with such a notion. Conceivably, in some cases there is transition from the nodular to the diffuse pattern, but in others the neoplastic B cells might be more aggressive and infiltrate the node diffusely from the outset.

*In contrast with B-cell lymphomas, the frequency of NHL with definite T-cell markers is small (20% versus 65%).* Included among T-cell lymphomas are the lymphomatous disorders of the skin called Sézary syndrome and mycosis fungoides, certain "histiocytic" lymphomas of the Rappaport classification, adult T-cell leukemia-lymphoma associated with human T-cell leukemia virus-I (HTLV-I), and most of the cases of lymphoblastic lymphoma associated with a mediastinal mass. According to Lukes and Collins, *"true" histiocytic lymphomas are very rare, a fact amply documented by cell marker studies.* A third category in the Lukes-Collins classification is the *undefined cell* (U cell) group, which is a heterogeneous group of tumors not classifiable by immunologic and cytochemical techniques. Many of these reveal immunoglobulin gene rearrangements and therefore belong to the B-cell lineage.[38]

### A Working Formulation of NHL for Clinical Usage

In 1982, an international panel of experts suggested a new classification that attempts to assemble the morphologic categories of NHL into three major prognostic groups (Table 12–7). The five-year survival rate for patients with tumors classified as low grade ranges from 50 to 70%; for those with tumors of intermediate grade and high grade, the rates are 35 to 45% and 23 to 32%, respectively. The histologic appearance of tumors within the working formulation may be surmised from the equivalent terms in the Rappaport classification.

**MORPHOLOGY.** The cellular details of the various types of lymphomas have already been presented in the consideration of classification. Further remarks are limited to some of the gross morphologic features.

The fundamental anatomic changes occur first in the lymph nodes. As the disease advances, there is involvement of the liver, spleen, and other viscera. In a large series of cases, the cervical lymph nodes were the initial site of involvement in about 40% of cases and the axillary nodes in 20%. Following them in importance were the inguinal, femoral, iliac, and mediastinal nodes.[44] Unusual patterns of presentation such as primary involvement of the mediastinum, visceral organs, and other extranodal sites have already been mentioned. Grossly, the affected nodes are variably enlarged in all forms, sometimes up to 10 cm in diameter. They vary in consistency from soft to moderately firm, depending on the amount of fibrous tissue present. In the less aggressive processes, the nodes remain discrete and freely moveable, but in other

---

**Table 12–6.** TECHNIQUES USED IN THE DIAGNOSIS OF LYMPHOID NEOPLASMS

| Cell Type | Technique | | |
|---|---|---|---|
| | *Immunologic** | *Molecular†* | *Histochemical* |
| T cells | Monoclonal antibodies (see Table 5–1, p. 130) | T-cell receptor gene rearrangement | — |
| B cells | Cell surface immunoglobulins‡ Monoclonal antibodies | Immunoglobulin gene rearrangements | — |
| Histiocytes | Monoclonal antibodies (HLA-DR⁺, OKM1⁺) | — | Nonspecific esterases |

*Immunologic techniques usually employ indirect immunofluorescence on frozen tissue sections or flow cytometry on cell suspensions.

†Molecular biologic techniques depend on demonstration of T-cell receptor or immunoglobulin gene rearrangements in the DNA extracted from tumor cells.

‡Clonal (neoplastic) proliferation of B cells is indicated by the presence of an immunoglobulin of a single light chain type. Cytoplasmic immunoglobulin, in the absence of surface immunoglobulin, is seen in pre-B cells.

**Table 12–7. A WORKING FORMULATION OF NON-HODGKIN'S LYMPHOMAS FOR CLINICAL USE (EQUIVALENT OR RELATED TERMS OF RAPPAPORT CLASSIFICATION ARE SHOWN)**

| Working Formulation | Rappaport Classification |
|---|---|
| *Low Grade* | |
| A. Small lymphocytic | Lymphocytic, well differentiated |
| B. Follicular, predominantly small cleaved cell | Nodular, poorly differentiated, lymphocytic |
| C. Follicular, mixed small cleaved and large cleaved cell | Nodular, mixed lymphocytic-histiocytic |
| *Intermediate Grade* | |
| D. Follicular, predominantly large cell | Nodular, histiocytic |
| E. Diffuse, small cleaved cell | Diffuse, poorly differentiated, lymphocytic |
| F. Diffuse, mixed large and small cell | Diffuse, mixed lymphocytic-histiocytic |
| G. Diffuse, large cell | Diffuse histiocytic |
| *High Grade* | |
| H. Large cell, immunoblastic | Diffuse histiocytic |
| I. Lymphoblastic | Lymphoblastic lymphoma |
| J. Small noncleaved cell | Undifferentiated, Burkitt's and non-Burkitt's |
| *Miscellaneous* | |

instances, invasion of the capsule and extension into the pericapsular tissues may lead to interadherence and fixation of the nodes, resulting in a matted, irregularly nodular mass of lymphoid tissue. The cut surface in diffuse lymphomas is usually fairly homogeneous, yellow-white to pearl gray. Nodular forms usually reveal vague nodularity, sometimes striking enough to be visible on gross inspection (Fig. 12–10A). Foci of hemorrhage and necrosis are rare but may be present with the more aggressive forms.

**ETIOLOGY AND PATHOGENESIS.** The etiology of malignant lymphomas is as mysterious and puzzling as that of all neoplastic disorders. Because of the accumulating evidence that the etiology and pathogenesis of lymphomas and leukemias involve similar mechanisms, we will discuss them together later in this chapter (p. 386).

**CLINICAL COURSE.** Most patients with lymphoma first present as otherwise healthy individuals with painless enlargement of either a single node or, often, a group of nodes. Occasionally, evidence of extranodal involvement is already present, and symptoms referable to hepatosplenomegaly are the initial complaint in about 25% of patients. Systemic manifestations, including fever, weight loss, weakness, and anemia, may occur but are usually not the presenting features of NHL. The anemia is usually hemolytic, and results are often positive on Coombs' testing. Involvement of the bone marrow varies with the histologic subtype. It ranges from 5 to 15% in patients with diffuse histiocytic lymphoma to over 50% in

those with nodular poorly differentiated lymphoma. The presence of lymphoma cells in the bone marrow is not always accompanied by blood involvement. When leukemic transformation occurs, there is flooding of the blood and bone marrow by the particular lymphomatous cell type. *Histologic examination of the node is required for diagnosis.* Additional studies such as "touch imprints," immunotyping, and cytochemistry require special handling and therefore require that the pathologist be consulted prior to the performance of biopsy. DNA hybridization studies that allow definite assignment to T- or B-cell lineage and aid in the distinction between monoclonal (neoplastic) or polyclonal (reactive) proliferations may be warranted in special cases.[45]

As would be expected, the manifestations of advanced widespread disease are truly protean. Involvement of the gastrointestinal tract may produce diarrhea, sometimes with a full-blown malabsorption syndrome (see p. 532), abdominal pain, or even complete intestinal obstruction. When the bones are involved, multiple osteolytic defects develop, with resultant pain and pathologic fractures. Enlargement of the kidneys may result from direct lymphomatous infiltration or from obstruction to the lower urinary tract by retroperitoneal tumor tissue. Nervous system involvement can create a bewildering array of central and peripheral findings.

A form of clinical staging developed for Hodgkin's disease (Table 12–8) is often used for NHL. However, it is much less useful in NHL since the correlation between the anatomic extent of the disease and the prognosis is less well established. For example, WDLL is generally disseminated when the patient is first seen, but the prognosis in this case is excellent. Furthermore, the pattern of spread of NHL, unlike Hodgkin's disease, is less predictable and hence the utility of clinical staging is diminished.

**Table 12–8. CLINICAL STAGES OF HODGKIN'S AND NON-HODGKIN'S LYMPHOMAS (Ann Arbor Classification)***

| Stage | Distribution of Disease |
|---|---|
| I | Involvement of a single lymph node region (I) or involvement of a single extralymphatic organ or site (I$_E$) |
| II | Involvement of two or more lymph node regions on the same side of the diaphragm alone (II) or with involvement of limited contiguous extralymphatic organ or tissue (II$_E$) |
| III | Involvement of lymph node regions on both sides of the diaphragm (III), which may include the spleen (III$_S$), limited contiguous extralymphatic organ or site (III$_E$), or both (III$_{ES}$) |
| IV | Multiple or disseminated foci of involvement of one or more extralymphatic organs or tissues with or without lymphatic involvement |

*All stages are further divided on the basis of the absence (A) or presence (B) of the following systemic symptoms: significant fever, night sweats, unexplained weight loss of greater than 10% of normal body weight.

From Carbone, P. T., et al.: Symposium (Ann Arbor): Staging in Hodgkin's disease. Cancer Res. *31*:1707, 1971.

## CUTANEOUS T-CELL LYMPHOMAS

Cutaneous T-cell lymphomas include a spectrum of disorders, of which *mycosis fungoides* and *Sézary syndrome* are the best characterized.[46] They are caused by a monoclonal expansion of T-helper lymphocytes (T4+). These closely related lymphoid malignancies that are primary in the skin are far more common than previously suspected. According to some experts, approximately 10,000 new cases are diagnosed every year. *Mycosis fungoides* usually affects males who are 40 to 60 years of age. The lesions begin as poorly defined areas of eczema, followed by formation of plaques and, ultimately, of multiple tumorous nodules. Histologically, there is infiltration of the epidermis and upper dermis by neoplastic T cells that usually have convoluted (cerebriform) nuclei. In most patients, extracutaneous spread to lymph nodes and viscera occurs.

*Sézary syndrome* is a related condition in which skin involvement is associated with generalized exfoliative erythroderma, but the skin lesions rarely lead to tumefaction. Instead, there are atypical lymphocytes in the blood that have the same cerebriform appearance noted in the skin infiltrates of mycosis fungoides. Thus Sézary syndrome may be considered the leukemic variant of cutaneous T-cell lymphoma. With current methods of treatment, the median survival of patients with cutaneous T-cell lymphomas is nine to 10 years.

## HODGKIN'S DISEASE

Hodgkin's disease, like NHL, is a disorder involving primarily the lymphoid tissues.[47] It arises almost invariably in a single node or chain of nodes and spreads characteristically to the anatomically contiguous nodes. Nevertheless, it is separated from NHL for several reasons. First, it is characterized morphologically by the presence of distinctive neoplastic giant cells called Reed-Sternberg (RS) cells, admixed with a variable inflammatory infiltrate. Second, it is often associated with somewhat distinctive clinical features, including systemic manifestations such as fever. Finally, the target cell of neoplastic transformation has yet to be identified with certainty. It accounts for 0.7% of all new cancers in the United States (which amounts to approximately 6900 new cases per year). Although overall it is an uncommon form of cancer, its importance stems from the fact that it is one of the most common forms of malignancy in young adults, with an average age at diagnosis of 32 years. Happily, tremendous progress has been made in the treatment of this disease in the last two decades, and it is now considered to be curable in most cases.

**CLASSIFICATION.** It should be some relief to the student to know that, unlike NHL, there is nearly universal acceptance of a single classification of Hodg-

kin's disease—the Rye classification.[48] Basically, there are four subtypes: (1) *lymphocyte predominance*, (2) *mixed cellularity*, (3) *lymphocyte depletion*, and (4) *nodular sclerosis*. Before delineating them, however, we should describe the common denominator among all—the RS cell—and the method used to characterize the extent of the disease in a patient—namely, the staging system.

The sine qua non for the histologic diagnosis of Hodgkin's disease is the **Reed-Sternberg cell** (RS cell) (Fig. 12–13). However, although necessary, it is not specific for Hodgkin's disease, since it is sometimes found in infectious mononucleosis, mycosis fungoides, and, occasionally, in non-Hodgkin's lymphomas, as well as in other settings.[49] The RS cell has abundant, usually slightly eosinophilic cytoplasm and ranges in size from 15 to 45 μm in diameter. It is distinguished principally either by having a multilobate nucleus or by being multinucleate with large, round, prominent nucleoli. **Particularly characteristic are two mirror-image nuclei, each containing a large ("inclusion-like") acidophilic nucleolus surrounded by a distinctive clear zone; together they impart an owl-eyed appearance. The nuclear membrane is distinct. Other abnormal cells, possibly representing variant RS cells, may also be present in Hodgkin's disease.**

The staging of Hodgkin's disease (Table 12–8) is of great clinical importance, since the course, choice of therapy, and prognosis are all intimately related to the distribution of the disease. Staging involves not only a careful physical examination but also several investigative procedures, including lymphangiography, chest x-ray, biopsy of the liver and bone marrow, scan of liver and

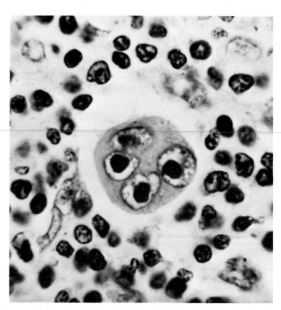

Figure 12–13. Reed-Sternberg cell. (From Neiman, R. S.: Current problems in histopathologic diagnosis and classification of Hodgkin's disease. *In* Sommers and Rosen (eds.): Pathology Annual. Vol. 13, Part 2. East Norwalk, CT, Appleton-Century-Crofts, 1978, p. 289.)

spleen, and computed tomography. In selected cases a laparotomy, which allows direct visualization of the intraabdominal nodes, liver biopsy, and removal of the spleen, is part of the staging protocol. It will become apparent that the more aggressive the variant of the disease, the greater the probability that it will be in a more advanced stage at the time of diagnosis.

With this background we can turn to the morphologic classification of Hodgkin's disease into its subgroups and point out some of the salient clinical features of each.[50] Later the manifestations common to all will be presented. The essential morphologic feature that serves to differentiate three subgroups (lymphocytic predominance, mixed cellularity, and lymphocytic depletion) is the frequency of the neoplastic elements (RS cells) relative to the reactive elements, represented by small lymphocytes. The extent of spread and the prognosis of Hodgkin's disease appear to be directly related to the ratio of RS cells to lymphocytes. The fourth subgroup, nodular sclerosis, appears to represent a special expression of the disease and has distinctive clinicopathologic features. The relative frequency of the four histologic subtypes may be gleaned from Table 12–9.

***Lymphocyte-Predominance Hodgkin's Disease.*** This subgroup is characterized by a large number of mature lymphocytes admixed with a variable number of benign histiocytes (Fig. 12–14). The cells may diffusely flood the lymph nodes and obliterate the normal architecture or may occur within poorly defined nodular areas. Typical RS cells are widely scattered and extremely difficult to find, although variants that have smaller nucleoli may be numerous. Other cells, such as eosinophils, neutrophils, and plasma cells, are scanty or absent, and there is little evidence of necrosis or fibrosis. A majority of patients are males, usually under 35 years of age, and they present with limited disease (Table 12–9). The prognosis is excellent.

***Mixed-Cellularity Hodgkin's Disease.*** This form occupies an intermediate clinical position between the lymphocyte-predominance and the lymphocyte-depletion patterns. Typical RS cells are plentiful, but there are fewer lymphocytes than in lymphocyte-predominance disease. The involvement of the lymph nodes is almost always diffuse. This pattern of Hodgkin's disease is rendered distinctive by its heterogeneous cellular infiltrate, which includes eosinophils, plasma cells, and benign histiocytes. Small areas of necrosis and fibrosis may be present, but they are usually not as prominent as in the lymphocyte-depletion type. The mixed-cellularity form of Hodgkin's disease is also more common in males.

Although the disease may be diagnosed in any of the clinical stages, as compared with the lymphocyte-predominance pattern, more patients present with disseminated disease, and these patients more often have systemic manifestations (Table 12–9).

***Lymphocyte-Depletion Hodgkin's Disease.*** This pattern is characterized by a paucity of lymphocytes and a relative abundance of RS cells or their pleomorphic variants. It presents in two morphologic forms, the so-called **diffuse fibrosis** and the **reticular variants**. In the former, the node is hypocellular and is replaced largely by a proteinaceous fibrillar material that represents a disorderly nonbirefringent connective tissue. Pleomorphic

**Table 12–9.** PERCENTAGE OF PATIENTS IN EACH PATHOLOGIC STAGE ACCORDING TO HISTOLOGIC SUBTYPE*

| Histologic Subtype | Number of Patients | Pathologic Stage (%) | | |
| --- | --- | --- | --- | --- |
| | | *I and* II | III | IV |
| Lymphocyte predominance | 55 | 76 | 22 | 2 |
| Mixed cellularity | 215 | 44 | 47 | 9 |
| Lymphocyte depletion | 21 | 19 | 62 | 19 |
| Nodular sclerosis | 628 | 60 | 35 | 5 |

*From Desforges, J. F., et al.: Hodgkin's disease. N. Engl. J. Med. *301*:1212, 1979. Reprinted by permission of the New England Journal of Medicine.

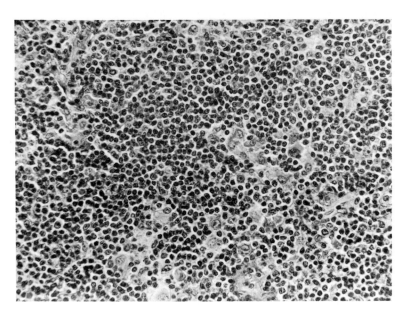

Figure 12–14. Lymphocyte-predominance Hodgkin's disease. (From Neiman, R. S.: Current problems in histopathologic diagnosis and classification of Hodgkin's disese. *In* Sommers and Rosen (eds.): Pathology Annual. Vol. 13, Part 2. East Norwalk, CT, Appleton-Century-Crofts, 1978, p. 289.)

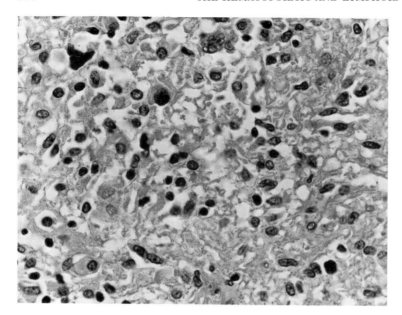

Figure 12–15. Lymph node in diffuse fibrosis Hodgkin's disease. All cellular elements are greatly diminished, and granular, proteinaceous interstitial material is prominent. A few highly atypical polyploid cells that lack the cytologic features of Reed-Sternberg cells are present. (From Neiman, R. S.: Current problems in histopathologic diagnosis and classification of Hodgkin's disease. *In* Sommers and Rosen (eds.): Pathology Annual. Vol. 13, Part 2. East Norwalk, CT, Appleton-Century-Crofts, 1978, p. 289.)

histiocytes, a few typical and atypical RS cells, and some lymphocytes are scattered within the fibrillar material (Fig. 12–15). The reticular variant is much more cellular and is composed of highly anaplastic, large, pleomorphic cells that resemble RS cells. Only a few typical RS cells can be recognized. A majority of patients with the lymphocyte-depletion pattern are older, have disseminated involvement (Table 12–9), present with systemic manifestations, and have an aggressive form of the disease.

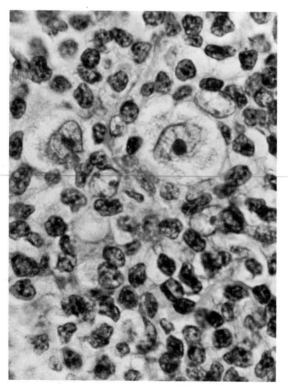

Figure 12–16. Hodgkin's disease, nodular sclerosing pattern. The distinctive "lacunar cell," so called because the cell appears to lie within a cleared space, is apparent.

**Nodular-Sclerosis Hodgkin's Disease.** This pattern is distinct from the other three forms, both clinically and histologically. It is characterized morphologically by two features: (1) the presence of a particular variant of the RS cell, the **lacunar cell** (Fig. 12–16). This cell is large and has a single hyperlobated nucleus with multiple small nucleoli and an abundant, pale-staining cytoplasm with well-defined borders. In formalin-fixed tissue, the cytoplasm of these cells often retracts, giving rise to the appearance of cells lying in clear spaces or "lacunae."(2) The other feature seen in most cases is the presence of collagen bands that divide the lymphoid tissue into circumscribed nodules (Fig. 12–17). The fibrosis may be scant or abundant, and the cellular infiltrate may show varying proportions of lymphocytes and lacunar cells. Classic RS cells are infrequent. In instances in which collagen bands are scanty, the diagnosis may rest with the identification of lacunar cells. Clinically, nodular-sclerosis Hodgkin's disease has several distinctive features: it is the only form more common in women, and it has a striking propensity to involve the lower cervical, supraclavicular, and mediastinal lymph nodes. Most of the patients are adolescents or young adults, and they have an excellent prognosis, especially when seen in clinical Stages I and II.

It is apparent that Hodgkin's disease spans a wide range of histologic patterns and that certain forms, with their characteristic fibrosis, eosinophils, neutrophils, and plasma cells, come deceptively close to simulating an inflammatory reactive process. **The diagnosis, then, of Hodgkin's disease rests solely on the unmistakable identification of the Reed-Sternberg cells in most variants and of the lacunar cells in the nodular-sclerosis pattern.**

In all forms, involvement of the spleen, liver, bone marrow, and other organs and tissues may appear in due course and take the form of irregular, tumor-like nodules of tissue resembling that present in the nodes. At times the spleen is greatly enlarged and the liver is moderately

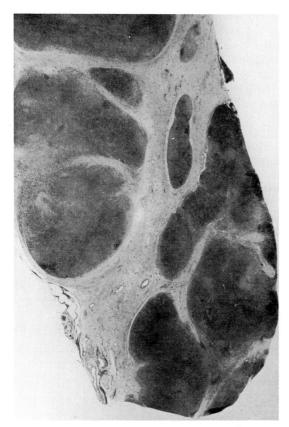

Figure 12-17. Hodgkin's disease, nodular sclerosing pattern. The low-power view shows the division of the nodes into well-defined nodules by wide, fibrous trabeculae.

enlarged by these nodular masses. At other times, the involvement is more subtle and becomes evident only on microscopic examination.

**ETIOLOGY AND PATHOGENESIS.** The origins of Hodgkin's disease are unknown. In the past it was believed that Hodgkin's disease was an unusual inflammatory reaction (possibly to an infectious agent) that behaved like a neoplasm. However, it is now widely accepted that Hodgkin's disease is a neoplastic disorder and that the RS cells represent the transformed cells. But the origin of RS cells remains an enigma. They do not bear surface markers of T cells or B cells. Unlike monocytes, they lack complement and Fc receptors. Some investigators have established from patients with Hodgkin's disease cell lines that seem to be derived from RS cells.[51] These cultured RS-like cells seem to share surface antigens with a very small population of "dendritic" cells in the parafollicular areas of the lymph node. Could these be the class II HLA antigen–positive dendritic cells (p. 133) that are active in antigen presentation to T cells? Reduced antigen-presenting capacity associated with neoplastic transformation of "dendritic" cells may explain the impairment of T-cell immunity so commonly observed in Hodgkin's disease.

Nevertheless, at present these suggestions regarding the origin of RS cells must be considered tentative until more definitive evidence is obtained.

Given that RS cells represent the malignant component of Hodgkin's disease, what causes the neoplastic transformation? For years an infective etiology of Hodgkin's disease has been suspected. Some reports have linked infection with Epstein-Barr virus (EBV) to Hodgkin's disease. However, the absence of EBV nucleic acid sequences in cultured RS cells does not support a role of EBV in the causation of Hodgkin's disease. Interest in the infective etiology of Hodgkin's disease has nevertheless been sustained by reports that suggested a "clustering" of Hodgkin's disease among certain high school students.[52] Other studies, however, have failed to confirm the suggested horizontal spread of Hodgkin's disease.[53] The issue of an infectious origin therefore remains unresolved.

**CLINICAL COURSE.** Hodgkin's disease, like non-Hodgkin's lymphomas, usually presents with a painless enlargement of lymph nodes. Although a definitive distinction between Hodgkin's and non-Hodgkin's lymphomas can be made only by examination of a lymph node biopsy, several clinical features favor the diagnosis of Hodgkin's disease (Table 12–10). Younger patients, with the more favorable histologic types, tend to present in clinical Stages I or II (Table 12–9) and are usually free of systemic manifestations. Patients with disseminated disease (Stages III and IV) are more likely to present with systemic complaints such as fever, unexplained weight loss, pruritus, and anemia. As mentioned earlier (p. 377), these patients generally have the histologically less favorable variants. The outlook following aggressive radiotherapy and chemotherapy for patients with this disease, including those with disseminated disease, is changing rapidly. With current modalities of therapy the histologic picture has very little impact on the prognosis; instead, the clinical stage appears to be the important prognostic indicator. The five-year survival rate of patients with Stages I-A and II-A is close to 100%. Even with advanced disease (Stages IV-A and IV-B) 50% five-year disease-free survival can be achieved. However, the recent therapeutic advances have also brought new problems. Long-term survivors of combined chemotherapy-radiotherapy protocols are at greatly increased risk of devel-

**Table 12–10. CLINICAL DIFFERENCES BETWEEN HODGKIN'S AND NON-HODGKIN'S LYMPHOMAS**

| Hodgkin's Disease | Non-Hodgkin's Lymphoma |
|---|---|
| More often localized to a single axial group of nodes (cervical, mediastinal, para-aortic) | More frequent involvement of multiple peripheral nodes |
| Orderly spread by contiguity | Noncontiguous spread |
| Mesenteric nodes and Waldeyer's ring rarely involved | Waldeyer's ring and mesenteric nodes commonly involved |
| Extranodal involvement uncommon | Extranodal involvement common |

oping acute leukemia or a form of non-Hodgkin's lymphoma.[47]

# LEUKEMIAS AND MYELOPROLIFERATIVE DISEASES

*The leukemias are malignant neoplasms of the hematopoietic stem cells, characterized by diffuse replacement of the bone marrow by neoplastic cells.* In most cases, the leukemic cells spill over into the blood, where they may be seen in large numbers. These cells may also infiltrate the liver, spleen, lymph nodes, and other tissues throughout the body. Although the presence of excessive numbers of abnormal cells in the peripheral blood is the most dramatic manifestation of leukemia, it should be remembered that the leukemias are primary disorders of the bone marrow. Indeed, some patients with a diffusely infiltrated bone marrow may present with leukopenia rather than leukocytosis.

**CLASSIFICATION.** Traditionally, leukemias are classified on the basis of the cell type involved and the state of maturity of the leukemic cells. Thus *acute leukemias* are characterized by the presence of very immature cells (called blasts) and by a rapidly fatal course in untreated patients. On the other hand, *chronic leukemias* are associated, at least initially, with well-differentiated (mature) leukocytes and with a relatively indolent course. Two major variants of acute and chronic leukemias are recognized: *lymphocytic* and *myelocytic* (myelogenous). Thus, a simple

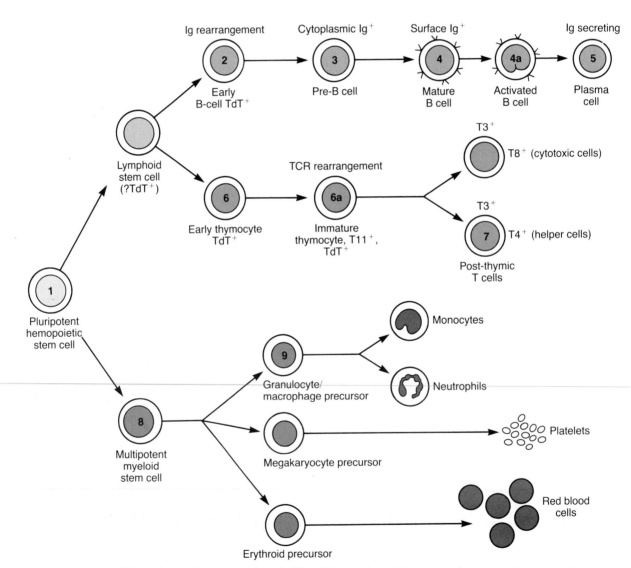

Figure 12–18. A simplified scheme of hematopoietic cell differentiation and possible origins of various leukemias and lymphomas. TdT = terminal deoxynucleotidyl transferase; TCR = T cell receptor. Chronic myeloproliferative syndromes = 8, possibly 1; null cell acute lymphoblastic leukemia (ALL) = 2; pre-B cell ALL = 3; B-cell chronic lymphocytic leukemia (CLL) and well differentiated lymphocytic lymphoma (WDLL) = 4; B-cell non-Hodgkin's lymphomas, 2 to 4a; multiple myeloma = 5; T-cell ALL and lymphoblastic lymphoma = 6 or 6a; cutaneous T-cell lymphoma, adult T-cell leukemia = 7; acute myelocytic leukemia (AML) = 8 or 9.

classification would have four patterns of leukemia: acute lymphocytic leukemia (ALL), chronic lymphocytic leukemia (CLL), acute myelocytic (myeloblastic) leukemia (AML), and chronic myelocytic leukemia (CML). This simple and time-honored classification raises several difficulties when dealing with "chronic leukemias." Acute leukemias, despite differences in their cell of origin, share important morphologic and clinical features. They are associated with replacement of normal marrow elements by a sea of proliferating "blast cells" that do not seem to undergo normal maturation. Consequently, there is a loss of mature myeloid elements such as red cells, granulocytes, and platelets, and hence clinical features of acute leukemias are dominated by anemia, infections, and hemorrhages. In contrast, the grouping together of chronic lymphocytic and myelogenous leukemias is problematic. A characteristic shared by these two disorders is that they are not rapidly fatal, but the clinical and morphologic features that seem to unite the acute leukemias are lacking. Furthermore, this traditional grouping of chronic leukemias has become less tenable with recent advances in our knowledge of the origins of chronic myelogenous leukemia and related disorders. *It is now widely accepted that CML, polycythemia vera, essential thrombocythemia, and myeloid metaplasia represent clonal neoplastic proliferations of the multipotent myeloid stem cells* (Fig. 12–18). If the erythrocytic precursors dominate, the resulting clinical disorder is classified as *polycythemia vera*; on the other hand, the dominance of granulocytic series is manifested as *CML*. It seems that the term *chronic myeloproliferative disorders*, coined by Dameshek almost 40 years ago, best describes these neoplasms of the myeloid stem cell. Although the individual chronic myeloproliferative disorders have distinctive clinical features, interconversions and overlaps between some members of this group are well known and further attest to their relatedness. For example, a patient may present initially with polycythemia vera, but over the years this disorder may "convert" to myeloid metaplasia with myelofibrosis.

In analogy with chronic myeloproliferative disorders, it is possible to segregate chronic lymphoproliferative disorders. This group would include *chronic lymphatic leukemia* and *hairy cell leukemia*, both representing neoplastic proliferations of lymphoid cells, most often of B-cell lineage. It will be apparent that as proliferative disorders of lymphoid cells, they are related to the non-Hodgkin's lymphomas already discussed. Indeed, as already mentioned, there is very little clinical or anatomic difference between CLL and well-differentiated lymphocytic lymphomas.

It should be obvious from the foregoing discussion that the heterogeneity of leukemias defies a rational classification that is scientifically accurate as well as clinically useful. In the ensuing discussion we will therefore follow the traditional, but admittedly im-

perfect, practice of segregating the acute and chronic leukemias from the chronic myeloproliferative disorders such as polycythemia vera and myeloid metaplasia.

Our discussion will focus initially on the distinctive pathophysiologic and clinical features of different forms of leukemias; it will be followed by the description of morphologic changes that are common to most leukemias, and, finally, a discussion of the etiology and pathogenesis of leukemias and lymphomas.

**INCIDENCE.** In the United States, leukemias ranked seventh as a cause of cancer death in 1985. Acute leukemia is the leading cause of cancer death in children under 15 years of age; in this age group it accounts for nearly 50% of all cancers. ALL is the most frequent leukemia in childhood, with a peak incidence between two and four years of age. AML dominates between 15 and 39 years of age, whereas most cases of CML are encountered between 30 and 50 years of age. CLL is a disorder of older people (median age 60 years). There is a slight male preponderance in all forms of leukemias.

## ACUTE LEUKEMIAS

As with all leukemias, the acute ones have their origin in neoplastic monoclonal proliferation of hematopoietic stem cells. Acute leukemias are characterized by a paucity of mature cells and an accumulation of leukocyte precursors (leukemic blasts).

**PATHOPHYSIOLOGY.** Morphologic and cell kinetic studies have indicated that in acute leukemias there is a block in differentiation of leukemic stem cells and that the leukemic blasts have a prolonged rather than shortened generation time. *Thus the accumulation of leukemic blasts in acute leukemia results from a failure of maturation into functional end cells rather than rapid proliferation of the transformed cells.* As the leukemic blasts accumulate in the marrow, they suppress normal hematopoietic stem cells by mysterious mechanisms. A simple hypothesis based on "crowding out" by the malignant cells seems unlikely. Suppression of normal hematopoietic stem cells in acute leukemia has two important clinical implications: (1) the major manifestations result from the paucity of normal red cells, white cells, and platelets, and (2) therapeutically the aim is to reduce the population of the leukemic clone enough to allow recovery of normal stem cells, which because of their faster proliferative rate may overtake the few surviving leukemic stem cells.

**CLASSIFICATION.** Leukemic transformation may affect any stage during the differentiation of pluripotent hematopoietic stem cells (Fig. 12–18). Involvement of the lymphoid series gives rise to ALL, whereas neoplastic transformation of myeloid progenitor cells is expressed in the form of AML.

ALL has been further subdivided by morphologic and immunologic criteria. Three morphologic subtypes designated L1, L2, and L3 have been defined in the French-American-British (FAB) classification of acute leukemias.[54] In practice, ALLs are more commonly classified on the basis of cell markers[55]:

○ In 10 to 12% of patients, the leukemic blasts possess T cell markers such as T11. They also contain the enzyme terminal deoxynucleotidyl transferase (TdT), a marker of primitive lymphoid cells.

○ In less than 2% of the patients, blasts have surface immunoglobulin, a marker of mature B cells.

○ Approximately 75% of the patients do not have surface Ig or T-cell antigens on their neoplastic cells. The leukemic cells in this non-T, non-B group do, however, possess the common acute lymphoblastic leukemia antigen (CALLA). They are TdT-positive.

○ In the remaining 10 to 12% of cases the lymphoblasts are negative for T-cell, B-cell, and CALLA antigens. They may be TdT-positive or TdT-negative.

Recent evidence suggests that most, if not all, of the non-T, non-B acute lymphoblastic leukemias (CALLA-positive or CALLA-negative) are derived from cells committed to the B-cell lineage. Some of them have cytoplasmic Ig (pre-B cells), whereas others show evidence of immunoglobulin gene rearrangements.[56]

Acute myeloblastic leukemias are also of diverse origins. Some arise by the transformation of the multipotent myeloid stem cells, as evidenced by the presence of common cytogenetic abnormalities in granulocytic as well as erythroid precursors, even though myeloblasts commonly dominate the blood and bone marrow. In others the common granulo-cyte-monocyte precursor is involved, giving rise to a myelomonocytic disease. In the widely used FAB classification (Table 12–11), AML is divided into seven categories.[54, 57] This scheme takes into account both the degree of maturation (M1 to M3) and the predominant line of differentiation of leukemic stem cells (M4 to M7).

**CLINICAL FEATURES.** The clinical manifestations of acute and chronic leukemias differ considerably. The acute forms have an abrupt, stormy onset, whereas the chronic leukemias start insidiously. The dominant clinical features of acute leukemias result from depression of normal marrow function and include (1) fever, usually reflecting an infection; (2) easy fatigability due to anemia; and (3) bleeding, secondary to thrombocytopenia. Manifestations of organ infiltration such as hepatosplenomegaly and lymphadenopathy are common in ALL. As discussed earlier (p. 372), a mediastinal mass (reflecting the involvement of the thymus) is frequently seen in ALL of T-cell origin. Infiltration of bones is common in the acute leukemias and is manifested by tenderness. Neurologic symptoms result from direct infiltration as well as intracerebral hemorrhages related to thrombocytopenia. In acute promyelocytic leukemia, disseminated intravascular coagulation (DIC) triggered by the release of thromboplastic substances contained within the abnormal granules may lead to widespread hemorrhages.

Both forms of acute leukemia are characterized by distinctive laboratory findings. Anemia is almost always present. The white count in about half the patients is less than 10,000 cells per mm³ of blood, whereas in about 20% it is elevated above 100,000 cells per mm³. In the rest it ranges between 10,000 and 100,000 cells per mm³. Much more important is the finding of immature white cells, including "blast" forms, in the circulating blood and the bone marrow, where they make up 60 to 100% of all the cells. The platelet count is almost always depressed and in a great majority of cases is less than 100,000 per mm³.

The prognosis for the two forms of acute leukemias is best considered individually since they differ so much. With modern chemotherapy (which includes prophylactic kill of leukemic cells that may find a sanctuary in the CNS) over 90% of children with ALL achieve complete remission and more than 50% are alive five years later. The prognosis is influenced by age and phenotype of leukemic cells. Patients between two and 10 years of age with CALLA-positive cells fare the best. Adults, or children with immunologically defined T-cell disease, fare much less well.[58] The prognosis with acute myelogenous leukemia is at best dismal. Although 60 to 80% of the patients achieve clinical remission with intensive chemotherapy, long-term disease-free survival can be expected only in 10 to 15%. In view of such a grim prognosis, bone marrow transplantation has been attempted in some centers. Early results are promising, but more data are needed.[59] It is being increas-

**Table 12–11.** FRENCH-AMERICAN-BRITISH (FAB) CLASSIFICATION OF ACUTE MYELOBLASTIC LEUKEMIAS

| | |
|---|---|
| M1 | Myeloblastic leukemia without maturation—cells are dominantly blasts without Auer rods or granules. |
| M2 | Myeloblastic leukemia with maturation—many blasts, but some maturation to promyelocytes or beyond. |
| M3 | Hypergranular promyelocytic leukemia—mostly promyelocytes with cytoplasm packed with peroxidase-positive granules. Many Auer rods. |
| M4 | Myelomonocytic leukemia—both myeloid and monocytic differentiation. Myeloid element resembles that of M2. |
| M5 | Monocytic leukemia—both "monoblasts" and monocytes, the former having large round nuclei with lacy chromatin and prominent nucleoli. Diagnosis must be confirmed by fluoride-inhibited esterase reaction. |
| M6 | Erythroleukemia—erythropoietic elements make up more than 50% of cells in marrow and have bizarre multilobate nuclei. May also be present in circulating blood, along with an admixture of myeloblasts and promyelocytes. |
| M7 | Acute megakaryocytic leukemia—30% or more of bone marrow leukemic cells identified as being of megakaryocytic lineage, or megakaryoblasts in peripheral blood, or both. |

ingly recognized that AML is a biologically hetero-geneous group, and future studies are aimed at separating subgroups with differing natural histories. It is already evident that the presence of certain cytogenetic abnormalities significantly influences the likelihood of achieving complete remissions.[60] The morphologic changes of acute leukemias are presented later, along with other forms of leukemias.

Before we leave the subject of acute leukemia, brief mention should be made of a group of related disorders collectively called "myelodysplastic syndromes."[61] The myelodysplastic marrow is cellular but is populated by aberrant cells such as megaloblastoid erythroid precursors, bizarre-looking blasts, and agranular megakaryocytes. Since normal cell maturation fails to occur, the patients present with pancytopenia. Cytogenetic studies reveal that up to 40% of the patients have a chromosomally abnormal clone of cells in the marrow.[62] About one third of these patients develop acute myelogenous leukemia; the remainder are constantly threatened by infections, anemia, and hemorrhages due to lack of differentiated myeloid cells. In this respect, these diseases resemble aplastic anemias, from which they must be distinguished by an examination of bone marrow. Because of their proclivity to transform into frank AML, the term "preleukemia" has been used in the past to describe these disorders.

## CHRONIC MYELOID LEUKEMIA (CML)

As mentioned earlier, CML is one of the four chronic myeloproliferative disorders. Unlike other myeloproliferative disorders, however, CML is associated with the presence of a unique chromosomal abnormality, the Ph[1] (Philadelphia) chromosome. *In approximately 90% of patients with CML, the Ph[1] chromosome, usually representing a reciprocal translocation from the long arm of chromosome 22 to another chromosome (usually the long arm of chromosome 9), can be identified in all the dividing progeny of multipotent myeloid stem cells (i.e., granulocytic, erythroid, and megakaryocytic precursors). This finding is firm evidence for the clonal origin of CML from the myeloid stem cells.* The significance of the Ph[1] chromosome and other translocations in our understanding of the pathogenesis of hematopoietic neoplasia is discussed in a later section.

**PATHOPHYSIOLOGY.** Although CML originates in the multipotent myeloid stem cells, granulocyte precursors constitute the dominant cell line. *Unlike the case in acute leukemias, there is no block in the maturation of leukemic stem cells*, as evidenced by the vast number of mature cells in the peripheral blood. Cell kinetic and in vitro culture techniques reveal that there is a 10- to 20-fold increase in the mass of granulocytic precursors in the bone marrow and spleen but that they do not divide more rapidly than normal stem cells. The basis of the increased myeloid stem cell mass in CML seems to lie in a failure of stem cells to respond to physiologic signals that regulate their proliferation.

**CLINICAL FEATURES.** The onset of CML is usually slow, and the initial symptoms may be nonspecific (e.g., easy fatigability, weakness, and weight loss). Sometimes the first symptom is a dragging sensation in the abdomen caused by the extreme splenomegaly that is characteristic of this condition.[63] The laboratory findings are extremely important in making the diagnosis. Usually, there is a marked elevation of the leukocyte count, commonly exceeding 100,000 cells per mm[3]. The circulating cells are predominantly neutrophils and metamyelocytes, although some myeloblasts may also be present. Since CML originates from the myeloid stem cell, it is not surprising that up to 50% of patients have thrombocytosis. *A characteristic finding in CML is the almost total lack of alkaline phosphatase in granulocytes. This serves to distinguish CML from a leukemoid reaction, which is also associated with a striking elevation of the granulocytic count* in response to infection, stress, chronic inflammation, and certain neoplasms. Other features that help to differentiate leukemoid reactions from CML are the presence of Ph[1] chromosome and increased numbers of basophils in the peripheral blood, both of which are quite typical of CML. The course of CML is one of slow progression, and even without treatment permits survival of two to three years. After a variable (and unpredictable) period, approximately 50% of patients enter an "accelerated phase," during which there is a gradual failure of response to treatment, increasing anemia and thrombocytopenia, acquisition of additional cytogenetic abnormalities, and, finally, transformation into a picture resembling acute leukemia ("blast crisis"). In the remaining 50%, blast crises occur abruptly without an intermediate accelerated phase. It is of interest to note that in 25% of patients, the blasts contain the enzyme TdT, a marker of primitive lymphoid cells. The lymphoblasts belong to the B-cell lineage, as evidenced by the presence of immunoglobulin gene rearrangements. This observation suggests that in CML the target cell for transformation may be the pluripotent stem cell capable of both lymphoid and myeloid differentiation (Fig. 12–18). The treatment of CML is unsatisfactory. Although it is possible to induce remissions with chemotherapy, the median survival (three to four years) is unaltered. The small number of CML patients who lack the Ph[1] chromosome seem to fare worse. Current efforts are directed toward "curing" CML with a continuation of chemotherapy and bone marrow transplantation.[64]

## CHRONIC LYMPHOCYTIC LEUKEMIA (CLL)

CLL is the most indolent of all leukemias, and, as mentioned earlier, it shows considerable overlap with

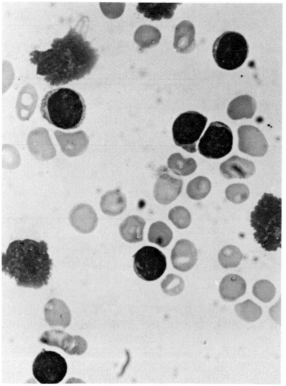

Figure 12–19. Peripheral blood smear from a patient with chronic lymphatic leukemia. Most leukemic cells have the appearance of unstimulated small or medium-sized lymphocytes. Owing to excessive fragility, the neoplastic lymphocytes are often damaged, giving rise to several "smudge" cells. (Courtesy of Dr. Jose Hernandez, Department of Pathology, Southwestern Medical School, Dallas, Texas. Reprinted from Robbins, S. L., Cotran, R. S., and Kumar, V.: Pathologic Basis of Disease. 3rd ed. Philadelphia, W. B. Saunders Co., 1984, p. 677.)

well-differentiated lymphocytic lymphoma. Like most other lymphoid malignancies, CLL is a neoplastic disorder of B cells. The transformed B cells in CLL show the following characteristics:

○ They possess surface immunoglobulin (IgM and IgD), and therefore, unlike the B cells in most cases of ALL, they have the phenotype of mature B cells.

○ They express either the λ or κ light chain, indicating monoclonality.

○ They are long lived but unable to differentiate into antibody-secreting plasma cells.

○ Only a small fraction are proliferating at any given time.

*Thus CLL is characterized by the accumulation of long-lived, nonfunctional B lymphocytes that infiltrate the bone marrow, blood, lymph nodes, and other tissues.*[65] T-cell CLL is uncommon and seems to be a heterogeneous entity since, until recently, the adult T cell leukemia-lymphoma associated with HTLV-I infection (p. 389) was not segregated from chronic T-cell CLL.

**CLINICAL FEATURES.** Patients with CLL are often asymptomatic. When symptoms are present, they are nonspecific and include easy fatigability, loss of weight, and anorexia. Since the leukemic B cells are nonfunctional, these patients often have hypogammaglobulinemia and increased susceptibility to bacterial infections. Generalized lymphadenopathy and hepatosplenomegaly are present in 50 to 60% of the cases. Total leukocyte count may be increased only slightly or may reach 200,000 per mm³. In all cases there is absolute lymphocytosis of small, mature-looking lymphocytes. Only a small fraction of lymphocytes are large ones with indented nuclei and nucleoli. Smudge cells (crushed nuclei of lymphocytes) are commonly seen in peripheral smears (Fig. 12–19). The course and prognosis of CLL are extremely variable. Many patients live for over ten years after diagnosis and die of unrelated causes. The median survival is four to six years. Unlike CML, transformation to acute leukemia with blast crisis is rare.

## MORPHOLOGY OF ALL LEUKEMIAS

There are two aspects to the morphologic feature of leukemias: (1) the specific cytologic details of the leukemic cells seen in peripheral blood smears and bone marrow aspirates and (2) the tissue changes produced by infiltrations of leukemic cells. The cytologic features are specific for each form of leukemia and are covered extensively in texts of hematology. Here we will consider them briefly; they will be followed by a description of the tissue alterations.

Acute leukemias are usually dominated by the presence of leukemic blasts. These cells are large and have high nuclear-cytoplasmic ratios, variable numbers of nucleoli, and deeply basophilic cytoplasm. Myeloblasts in some cases have distinctive intracytoplasmic rod-like structures that stain red in Wright's or Giemsa preparations **(Auer rods).** These are abnormal lysosomal structures considered pathognomonic of myeloblasts. Distinction between various kinds of blasts is based on cytologic and immunocytochemical features. Chronic leukemias are characterized by the presence of more mature forms of white cells in the marrow and peripheral blood as already discussed.

The tissue alterations produced by various leukemias are often similar and may be separated into primary changes, attributed directly to the abnormal overgrowth or accumulation of white cells, and secondary changes, caused both by the destructive effects of masses of these cells and by their relative ineffectiveness in protecting against infection.

**Although the leukemic cells may infiltrate any tissue or organ of the body, the most striking changes are seen in the bone marrow, spleen, lymph nodes, and liver.** In the full-blown case, the **bone marrow** develops a muddy, red-brown to gray-white color as the normal marrow is diffusely replaced by masses of white cells (Fig. 12–20). Sometimes these infiltrates extend into previously fatty marrow and encroach upon and erode the cancellous and cortical bone.

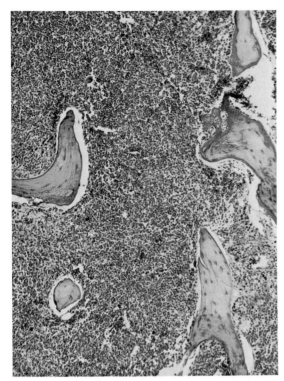

Figure 12–20. Myelogenous leukemia. Low-power view of bone marrow documents the flooding by leukemic cells.

Massive **splenomegaly** is characteristic of CML. Splenic weights of 5000 gm or more are not unusual. Such spleens may virtually fill the abdominal cavity and extend into the pelvis. With CLL, enlargement of the spleen is less striking, and the weight of the spleen rarely exceeds 2500 gm. The acute forms of leukemia produce only moderate splenomegaly, usually between 500 and 1000 gm. On sectioning, the parenchyma is firm and muddy gray in color. When the splenomegaly is massive, as is most characteristic of CML, numerous areas of pale infarction may appear throughout the substance. In minimally enlarged spleens, the histologic appearance may be of focal leukemic infiltrates, with a background of fairly well-preserved normal architecture. In the lymphocytic forms, the white pulp is primarily involved. With more severe involvement the infiltrates become more diffuse. Ultimately, the underlying architecture is obliterated and replaced by a sea of homogeneous leukemic cells.

Whereas splenomegaly is more prominent with myelogenous than with lymphocytic leukemia, extreme **lymph node enlargement** is more characteristic of the lymphocytic forms (Fig. 12–21). Nevertheless, some degree of lymph node involvement is commonly present with all forms of leukemia. The affected nodes remain discrete, rubbery, and homogeneous. The cut section is soft and gray-white and tends to bulge above the level of the capsule. On histologic examination, severely involved nodes are seen to be diffusely flooded by the neoplastic cells. The underlying architecture is obliterated, and sometimes the leukemic cells invade the capsule of the

node and flood out into the surrounding tissues. With CLL, the histologic picture is identical to that of a well-differentiated lymphocytic lymphoma. With minimal involvement in the myelogenous leukemias, the underlying architecture may be largely preserved.

**Enlargement of the liver** is somewhat more prominent with lymphocytic than with myelogenous leukemia. Histologically, the lymphocytic infiltrates are characteristically confined to the portal areas, whereas infiltrates of myelogenous leukemia are not well defined and are present within the sinusoids throughout the lobule.

In addition to the principal sites of involvement, other tissues and organs may be affected. Leukemic infiltrates are frequently found in the kidneys, where they begin as small perivascular aggregates that progressively diffuse throughout the stroma. Similar changes may occur in the adrenals, thyroid, myocardium, testes, and, indeed, any tissue. Of particular importance is the infiltration of the central nervous system by leukemic cells. This occurs most commonly in ALL. Protected by the blood-brain barrier from the effects of cytotoxic drugs, cells in the CNS may survive to eventually initiate a relapse unless prophylactic radiation or intrathecal chemotherapy is administered. **Infiltrates in the gingiva are particularly characteristic of monocytic leukemia.** Patients with

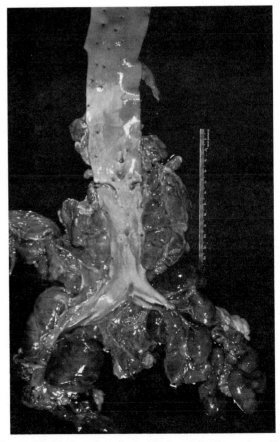

Figure 12–21. Lymphocytic leukemia; periaortic and periliac lymph nodes. The marked lymphadenopathy compresses the vessels.

this disorder have swelling and hypertrophy of the gingival margins, often with secondary infections.

The **secondary changes of all forms of leukemia** derive in large part from the pancytopenia that results from inhibition of normal hematopoiesis by leukemic cells. Anemia and thrombocytopenia are characteristic, especially of acute leukemia. Many times, the bleeding diathesis caused by the thrombocytopenia is the most striking clinical and anatomic feature of the disease. Petechiae and ecchymoses are seen in the skin. Hemorrhages also occur into the serosal linings of the body cavities and into the serosal coverings of the viscera, particularly of the heart and lungs. Mucosal hemorrhages into the gingivae and urinary tract are common. Intraparenchymal hematomas may develop, most frequently in the brain.

Although the total white blood cell count is usually markedly elevated, the defensive capacity of these abnormal cells is considerably less than normal. This is especially true of the acute forms. There is, then, a **functional** leukopenia with a resultant increased susceptibility to bacterial infection. These infections are particularly common in the oral cavity, skin, lungs, kidneys, urinary bladder, and colon, and they are often caused by "opportunists" such as fungi, *Pseudomonas,* and commensals.

## ETIOLOGY AND PATHOGENESIS OF LEUKEMIAS AND LYMPHOMAS

As with all other cancers, the pathogenesis of neoplastic transformation of lympho-hematopoietic cells is shrouded in mystery. However, in recent years there has been much excitement in this area of investigation, stemming from the convergence of research on *oncogenes, chromosomal abnormalities, and oncogenic viruses.*[64, 66, 67] Much of the evidence implicating alterations in structure and function of cellular oncogenes (c-oncs) in the origin of cancer was discussed in Chapter 6, therefore only a brief recapitulation, as it relates to neoplasms of the hematopoietic system, will be offered here. This will be followed by a discussion of the role of viruses in the pathogenesis of leukemias and lymphomas.

Omitting much detail, it can be stated that *c-oncs,* present in all normal eukaryotic cells, play an important role in regulating their growth and differentiation. In many leukemias and lymphomas, karyotypic changes (usually translocations) shift the cellular on-cogenes to new locations within the genome. Such chromosomal rearrangements may alter the function or structure of oncogenes in one of several ways:

○ The translocation may place the oncogene next to a transcriptionally active area, which may lead to overexpression of the c-onc product.

○ During translocation, subtle mutations may be induced in the c-onc, leading to the transcription of a qualitatively different gene product.

○ The c-onc may fuse with another cellular gene normally located at the site to which it is translocated, resulting in the formation of a fusion gene. Such a hybrid gene may code for a new protein that affects cell growth (p. 209).

In any event, overexpression or alteration of the oncogene product, brought about by one or more of the mechanisms listed above, somehow deranges growth regulation so as to produce a cell that is autonomous (p. 209). This schema of the pathogenesis of leukemias and lymphomas is supported by the following observations:

○ With high-resolution banding techniques nonrandom chromosomal abnormalities, most commonly reciprocal translocation, are noted in approximately 60% of all leukemias and lymphomas (Table 12–12).[68]

○ In many instances *c-oncs* have been located at or near the breakpoint that are involved in the translocations (Table 12–12).

○ In translocations associated with leukemias and lymphomas of the B-cell lineage, one of the two breakpoints almost always involves chromosome 14, particularly band q32, which contains the immunoglobulin heavy chain locus (IgH). In contrast, the breakpoint in several T-cell lymphomas involves band q11 on chromosome 14, where the T-cell receptor α-chain gene is located.[69] Since the IgH gene in B cells and the T-cell receptor gene in T cells are normally "turned on," it seems that translocations associated with B- or T-cell tumors uniquely involve those portions of the genome that are transcriptionally active in these cell types. Thus there is the potential for affecting the expression of a normal or mutated c-onc that may come to lie next to these active sites.

The two most extensively investigated transloca-

**Table 12–12.** LEUKEMIAS AND LYMPHOMAS WITH APPARENTLY BALANCED TRANSLOCATIONS AND ASSOCIATED ONCOGENES

| Disease | Translocations | Frequency (%) | Oncogene |
|---|---|---|---|
| *Leukemias* | | | |
| CML | t(9;22) (q34;q11) | >90 | c-abl 9q34 |
| AML (M2) | t(8;21) (q22;q22) | 13 | c-mos 8q22 |
| AML (M3) | t(15;17) (q22;q11) | >90 | c-fes 15q24 |
| AML (M5) | t(9;11) (p22;q23) | 22 | None known |
| ALL | t(9;22) (q34;q11) | 18 | c-abl 9q34 |
| ALL (B cell) | t(8;14) (q24;q32) | >90 | c-myc 8q24 |
| *Lymphomas* | | | |
| Burkitt's | t(8;14) (q24;q32) | >90 | c-myc 8q24 |
| Nodular (non-Hodgkin's) | t(14;18) (q32;q21) | 50 | None known |

tions associated with hematologic malignancies, t(8;14) in Burkitt's lymphoma and t(9;22) in CML, were discussed in Chapter 6. Here we would like to point out that in addition to translocations, certain nonrandom deletions and trisomies have also been found in leukemias and lymphomas. For example, deletions involving long arms of chromosomes 5 and 11 are noted in marrow cells of patients with myelodysplastic syndromes and AML (M4, FAB group), respectively, whereas trisomy 21 is found in T-cell CLL.[70] These alterations are mentioned to emphasize the point that oncogene activation may occur by mechanisms other than translocations. Conceivably, absence of a balancing allele may lead to overexpression of certain oncogenes.

Although much has been learned about the mechanisms by which products of normal or mutated oncogenes may transform cells (p. 209), the agents that *initiate* such disturbances (e.g., translocations) are largely unknown. As with many other cancers, *ionizing radiations* and *chemicals* have been implicated as mutagenic agents that "pull the trigger." There is also suspicion that viruses are somehow involved, since virally induced leukemias and lymphomas are well known in laboratory animals. Although several viruses have been implicated in the causation of human cancer (p. 205), two deserve special mention in the context of leukemias and lymphomas—EBV and the human T-cell leukemia virus.

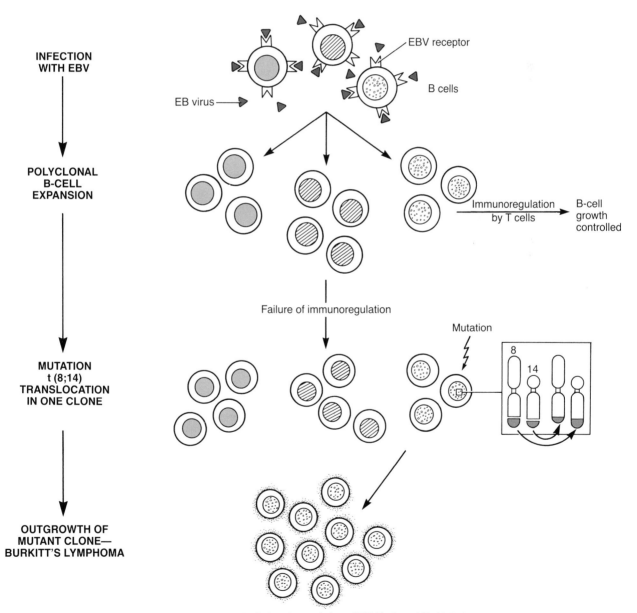

Figure 12–22. A scheme depicting the evolution of EBV-induced Burkitt's lymphoma.

There is a substantial body of evidence linking EBV to the African Burkitt's lymphoma.[70A] As was discussed previously, this tumor is almost always associated with the t(8;14) translocation, a change that may be critical to lymphomagenesis. What role then does the virus play in the pathogenesis of Burkitt's lymphoma? It is postulated that initially EBV acts as a B-cell mitogen and initiates a polyclonal B-cell proliferation (Fig. 12–22). In most individuals the lymphoproliferation is arrested and either there is no disease or a self-limited episode of infectious mononucleosis (p. 400). However, in some individuals, presumably those with some overt or subtle immunologic defect, chronic polyclonal B-cell proliferation continues. The rapidly proliferating cells are at greatly enhanced risk of acquiring cytogenetic aberrations such as the t(8;14) translocation. This translocation may confer growth advantage on the affected cell owing to activation of the c-myc oncogene, thus leading to the emergence of a monoclonal B-cell neoplasm (Fig. 12–22). *According to this view, then, EBV itself is not directly oncogenic, but by acting as a polyclonal B-cell mitogen, it sets the stage for the acquisition of the t(8;14) translocation, which ultimately releases the cells from normal growth regulation.*

Although EBV is associated with only a few lymphomas, it has been postulated that the pathogenesis of other lymphoid malignancies may also involve a similar evolution from polyclonal to monoclonal proliferations.[71] This view has gained some credence from the observation that *the risk of developing malignant lymphomas is higher in those who are subjected to persistent antigenic stimulation, especially in association with defective immunoregulation.* Individuals in such high-risk categories include patients with the X-linked lymphoproliferative syndrome (p. 218), recipients of renal allografts, and patients with autoimmune diseases such as Sjögren's syndrome and AIDS.

We come next to the possible role of retroviruses in human leukemias. Although type C RNA viruses are known to cause leukemias and lymphomas in experimental animals, it is only recently that a retrovirus has been strongly linked to the causation of human leukemia. This virus has been designated human T-cell leukemia virus type I (HTLV-I) owing to its association with certain forms of T-cell leukemias and lymphomas.[72] The evidence implicating HTLV-I in the causation of adult T cell leukemia-lymphoma (ATL) may be summarized as follows:

○ HTLV-I has been repeatedly isolated from neoplastic T cells of patients with ATL.
○ HTLV-I proviral sequences can be detected in the DNA of leukemic T cells but not in DNA of non-neoplastic B cells of the same patient, indicating that the virus is acquired by infection and not transmitted in the germ line.
○ Cultured neoplastic T cells from leukemic patients

release type C virus (HTLV-I) that can immortalize normal cord blood T cells in vitro.
○ Antibodies against HTLV-I are found in over 90% of the patients with ATL.

This disease is endemic in Southern Japan and some Caribbean countries. Sporadic cases of ATL that are positive for HTLV-I have been reported in the United States, Israel, and South America. Viral isolates from patients in these diverse geographic regions show highly conserved nucleotide sequences, suggesting that the same or closely related viruses are responsible for ATL all over the world. Approximately 40% of healthy relatives of ATL patients in endemic areas have anti-HTLV-I antibodies, suggesting that as with other viruses (e.g., EBV) all who get infected do not develop the disease.

Despite the impressive evidence linking HTLV-I with ATL, the molecular mechanisms of neoplastic transformation are still obscure. As was discussed earlier (p. 204), *animal retroviruses transform cells by one of two mechanisms.* Some retroviruses (so-called acute leukemia viruses) contain an oncogene (v-onc) that transforms the host cells after integration of the virus into the genome. Other viruses (so-called chronic leukemia viruses) lack v-oncs but apparently enhance expression of c-oncs by integration at specific sites adjacent to the c-oncs (see Fig. 6–17). HTLV-I does not seem to utilize either of these two mechanisms. Its genome lacks any known v-onc, and analysis of leukemic T cells does not reveal any specific site of HTLV-I integration. Molecular analysis of HTLV-I DNA does reveal a region not found in the genomes of animal retroviruses. This mysterious region, called pX, is believed to be somehow responsible for the transforming activity of HTLV-I, but much remains to be known.[73] In closing this discussion it should be mentioned that in a recent report from Japan, breaks (translocations, deletions, inversions) involving chromosome 14 band 11q were noted in 11 out of 11 patients with ATL.[74] Recall that a transcriptionally active T-cell receptor gene is located at this site. So we are left with the sobering thought that shuffling of normal cellular genes may be a common event in the pathogenesis of several hematopoietic malignancies.

## UNUSUAL TYPES OF LEUKEMIAS AND LYMPHOMAS

**HAIRY CELL LEUKEMIA.** This uncommon form of chronic leukemia is distinguished by the presence of leukemic cells that have fine "hair-like" cytoplasmic projections, best recognized under the phase contrast microscope but also visible in routine blood smears. This disease evoked much interest because hairy cells seem to express cell surface markers of T cells, B cells, and monocytes; therefore, their origin remained mysterious. However, recent studies leave little doubt that despite their somewhat unusual phenotype, hairy cells rearrange and express immunoglobulin genes, which firmly assigns them to the B-cell lineage.[75] Once again recent advances in molecular biology have proved useful in the study of a lymphoid malignancy. For routine diagnosis, however, the practicing pathologist need not enroll in a course of recombinant DNA technology! Mercifully, there is a cytochemical feature that is quite characteristic of hairy cells—the presence of tartrate-resistant acid phosphatase.

Hairy cell leukemia occurs mainly in older males and *its manifestations result largely from infiltration of bone marrow, liver, and spleen. Splenomegaly,* often massive, is the most common and sometimes the only abnormal physical finding. *Hepatomegaly* is less common and not as marked, and lymphadenopathy is distinctly rare. *Pancytopenia,* resulting from marrow failure and splenic sequestration, is seen in over half the cases. *Leukocytosis* is not a common feature, being present in only 25% of patients. Hairy cells can be identified in the peripheral blood smear in most cases. The course of this disease is chronic, and the median survival is four years. Splenectomy is of benefit in approximately two thirds of the patients. Recently α-interferon has proven to be effective in this disease. It may be noted that this is the first disorder (albeit uncommon) in which interferon treatment has passed muster, and therefore α-interferon has been officially approved for treatment of hairy cell leukemia in the United States.

**ADULT T-CELL LEUKEMIA-LYMPHOMA.** This uncommon T-cell neoplasm has gained much prominence owing to its association with human T-cell leukemia virus, already discussed (p. 388). Most of the initial cases were described from the southern part of Japan, where it is endemic, but similar cases have now been found in the West Indies and sporadically in several other countries, including the United States. *Characteristic clinical features of adult T-cell leukemia include generalized lymphadenopathy, hepatosplenomegaly, frequent skin involvement, severe hypercalcemia, and a poor prognosis.*[76] The tumor cells are T4-positive, since HTLV-I, like HTLV-III, is tropic for T-helper cells (p. 176). However, whereas the latter destroys T-helper cells and produces immunodeficiency, HTLV-I causes neoplastic transformation of T4+ cells.

## MYELOPROLIFERATIVE DISORDERS

The concept that myeloproliferative disorders result from clonal neoplastic proliferations of the multipotent myeloid stem cells has already been discussed (p. 381). It was mentioned in our earlier presentation that four disorders—chronic myeloid leukemia, polycythemia vera, myeloid metaplasia with myelofibrosis, and essential thrombocythemia—are included in this group. CML was discussed along with other leukemias. Of the remaining three, only polycythemia vera and myeloid metaplasia with myelofibrosis will be presented here. Essential thrombocythemia occurs too infrequently to merit further discussion.

### Polycythemia Vera

As with all myeloproliferative disorders, polycythemia vera is associated with excessive proliferation of erythroid, granulocytic, and megakaryocytic elements, all derived from a single neoplastic stem cell. However, *in polycythemia vera the erythroid precursors dominate and hence there is an absolute increase in red cell mass.* This should be contrasted with relative polycythemia, resulting from hemoconcentration (p. 369). Furthermore, unlike other forms of absolute polycythemia that result from an increased secretion of erythropoietin, polycythemia vera is associated with low or virtually undetectable erythropoietin levels. It seems that the neoplastic erythroid stem cells have an intrinsic membrane defect that renders them exquisitely sensitive to low levels of erythropoietin.[77]

**MORPHOLOGY.** The major anatomic changes stem from the increase in blood volume and viscosity brought about by the erythrocytosis. Plethoric congestion of all tissues and organs is characteristic of polycythemia vera. The liver is enlarged and frequently contains foci of myeloid metaplasia. The spleen is also slightly enlarged, up to 250 to 300 gm, and quite firm. The splenic sinuses are packed with red cells, as are all the vessels within the spleen. Occasionally, hematopoiesis can be seen within the red pulp. The major blood vessels are uniformly distended with thick, usually incompletely oxygenated blood.

**Consequent to the increased viscosity and vascular stasis, thromboses and infarctions are common; they affect most often the heart, spleen, and kidneys.** Hemorrhages occur in about a third of these patients, probably due to excessive distention of blood vessels and abnormal platelet function. They usually affect the gastrointestinal tract, oropharynx, or brain. Although these hemorrhages are said on occasion to be spontaneous, more often they follow some minor trauma or surgical procedure. Peptic ulceration has been described in about a fifth of these patients.

The basic changes occur in the bone marrow, which is markedly hypercellular.[78] The erythron is markedly enlarged as the fatty marrow is replaced by dark red, succulent, active marrow. Histologically, striking proliferation of all the erythroid forms is seen, particularly the normoblasts. In addition, megakaryocytic hyperplasia is also prominent. There is usually some concomitant increase in granulocytic elements. If the disease changes its course, the marrow reflects the alterations and may become leukemic or fibrotic, as discussed below.

**CLINICAL COURSE.** Polycythemia vera appears insidiously, usually in late middle age (40 to 60 years).

Males are affected somewhat more often than females, and whites are more vulnerable than blacks. Patients with polycythemia vera classically are plethoric and often somewhat cyanotic. There may be an intense pruritus. Other complaints are referable to the thrombotic and hemorrhagic tendencies and to hypertension. Headache, dizziness, gastrointestinal symptoms, hematemesis, and melena are common. Splenic or renal infarction may produce abdominal pain. Hypertension and the increased blood viscosity may lead to heart failure. Due to the high cell turnover, symptomatic gout is seen in 5 to 10% of cases, although many more have hyperuricemia.

The diagnosis is usually made in the laboratory. Red cells counts range from 6,000,000 to 10,000,000 per mm³, with corresponding elevations in hemoglobin and hematocrit values. Since there is hyperproliferation of granulocytic precursors as well as megakaryocytes in the bone marrow, the white cell count may be as high as 80,000 per mm³, and platelet count is often greater than 400,000 per mm³. Classically, granulocyte alkaline phosphatase levels are above normal. About 30% of patients die from some thrombotic complication, affecting usually the brain or heart. An additional 10 to 15% die from some hemorrhagic complication. In patients who receive no treatment, death resulting from these vascular episodes occurs within months after diagnosis. However, if the red cell mass can be maintained near normal by phlebotomies, median survival of 10 years can be achieved.

Prolonged survival with treatment has revealed that the *natural history of polycythemia vera involves a gradual transition to a "spent phase," during which clinical and anatomic features of myeloid metaplasia with myelofibrosis develop.* Approximately 15 to 20% of patients undergo such a transformation after an average period of 10 years. This transition is brought about by creeping fibrosis in the bone marrow (myelofibrosis) and a shift of hematopoiesis to the spleen, which enlarges markedly. It is ironic that these patients, who may once have had to undergo repeated therapeutic phlebotomies, now require blood transfusions to correct their anemia. This is perhaps the most striking example of conversion of one myeloproliferative disorder to another. As with CML (another myeloproliferative disease), certain patients with polycythemia vera develop a terminal acute myeloblastic leukemia. However, the incidence of this transition is much lower than in CML. It is estimated to be about 2% in patients who are treated with phlebotomy alone[78] and about 15% in those who receive myelosuppressive treatment with chlorambucil or marrow irradiation with radioactive phosphorus. Presumably, the increase is related to the mutagenic effects of these therapeutic agents.

### Myeloid Metaplasia with Myelofibrosis

In this chronic myeloproliferative disorder the proliferation of the neoplastic myeloid stem cells occurs principally in the spleen (*myeloid metaplasia*) and, in the fully developed syndrome, the bone marrow is hypocellular and fibrotic (*myelofibrosis*). Sometimes polycythemia vera and, less often, CML "burn out," as it were, and terminate in a myelofibrotic pattern. In many patients, however, extramedullary hematopoiesis in the spleen and marrow fibrosis arise insidiously without an identifiable preceding syndrome; hence the term *agnogenic (idiopathic) myeloid metaplasia* is sometimes used to describe this condition.

*The cause of marrow fibrosis, which is characteristic of myeloid metaplasia, is not clear.* Studies with G6PD isoenzymes indicate that the fibroblasts that replace the marrow do not belong to the neoplastic hematopoietic clone. No toxic cause for marrow destruction and subsequent scarring can be demonstrated, a feature that distinguishes this condition from myelophthisic anemias with extramedullary hematopoiesis, in which there are obvious mechanisms of marrow destruction such as metastatic tumors. It has been suggested that *marrow fibroblasts are stimulated to proliferate owing to an inappropriate release of platelet-derived growth factor and transforming growth factor B (also contained within platelets).*[79] Functional and morphologic abnormalities of platelets are seen in myeloid metaplasia with myelofibrosis, and the two growth factors mentioned above are known to be mitogenic for fibroblasts. According to this view, the proliferation of neoplastic stem cells begins within the marrow and there is subsequent seeding of the spleen and other organs such as the liver. As the disease progresses, marrow fibrosis occurs secondary to the elaboration of fibroblast growth factors mentioned above. By the time the patient comes to clinical attention, fibroblasts have already taken over the marrow, and the spleen remains the major site of myeloproliferation. This scheme is supported by the occasional finding of hypercellular bone marrow with prominent megakaryocytes early during the course of this disease.

**MORPHOLOGY.** The principal site of the extramedullary hematopoiesis is the **spleen**, which is usually markedly enlarged, sometimes up to 4000 gm in weight. On section, it is firm, red to gray, and not dissimilar to spleens seen with myelogenous leukemia. As with CML, multiple subcapsular infarcts may be present. Histologically, however, the distinction is apparent. There is preservation of the native architecture, as well as orderly hematopoiesis, with relatively normal proportions of maturing red cells, white cells, and platelets. Megakaryocytes are usually prominent owing to their large size and nuclear morphology. Occasionally, however, disproportional activity of any one of the three major cell lines is seen.

The **liver** may be moderately enlarged, with foci of extramedullary hematopoiesis. The **lymph nodes** are only rarely the site of blood cell formation and are usually not enlarged. This is an important differential feature, since some degree of lymphadenopathy would be expected with the leukemias.

As was mentioned, the bone marrow in a typical case

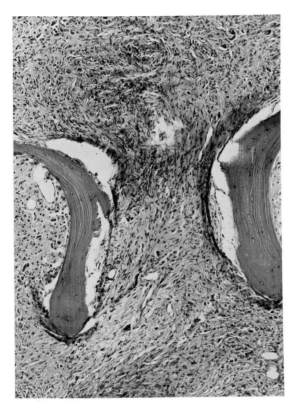

Figure 12–23. Myelofibrosis. The marrow cavity is virtually replaced by fibrous tissue, totally obliterating the normal hematopoietic elements.

is hypocellular and shows diffuse fibrosis (Fig. 12–23). However, the marrow is hypercellular in early cases, with equal representation of the three major cell lines. Megakaryocytes are often prominent and may show dysplastic changes.

**CLINICAL COURSE.** As was mentioned, myeloid metaplasia may begin with a blood picture suggestive of polycythemia vera or myelogenous leukemia, or it may arise as an apparently primary disease. Most patients have moderate to severe anemia. The white cell count may be normal, reduced, or markedly elevated. Early in the course of the disease the platelet count is normal or elevated, but eventually patients develop thrombocytopenia. The peripheral blood smear is markedly abnormal. Red cell abnormalities include the presence of immature forms and bizarre shapes (poikilocytes, teardrop cells). Immature white cells (myelocytes and metamyelocytes) are also seen in the peripheral blood. Platelets are often abnormal in size and shape and defective in function. In some cases, the clinical and blood picture may resemble chronic myelogenous leukemia (CML), but the leukocyte alkaline phosphatase level is normal and Ph[1] chromosome is absent, providing important differentials from CML. Owing to high cell turnover, hyperuricemia and gout may complicate the picture. The outcome of myeloid metaplasia is variable. There is constant threat of infections, as well as thrombotic and hemorrhagic episodes due to platelet abnormal-

ities. Splenic infarctions are therefore common. Up to 10% of cases eventually develop a blast crisis resembling AML. The median survival time overall is four to five years.

# NEUTROPENIA— AGRANULOCYTOSIS

A reduction in the number of granulocytes in the blood is known as neutropenia or sometimes as agranulocytosis when it is severe. It is a serious disorder because it is associated with increased susceptibility to infections, which are too often fatal.

**ETIOLOGY.** Agranulocytosis occurs in a wide variety of clinical settings. It may be a manifestation of generalized marrow failure, such as occurs in aplastic anemia and acute leukemia, or it may occur as an isolated disorder. Drug-induced injury is perhaps the commonest cause of isolated agranulocytosis (p. 263). Like aplastic anemia, it is predictably produced by certain drugs, especially cancer chemotherapy agents; in other cases it occurs as an idiosyncratic reaction to some drugs. Included in the latter category are chlorpromazine, aminopyrine, sulfonamides, and chloramphenicol. In some cases, there is no known predisposing agent (idiopathic agranulocytosis).

Increasing evidence suggests that immunologic mechanisms play a role in the pathogenesis of drug-induced and idiopathic agranulocytosis. Drugs such as aminopyrine may act as haptens and lead to the production of antineutrophil antibodies. Several recent reports indicate that severe neutropenia may occur in association with abnormal, possibly neoplastic, proliferation of T8[+] cells. Apparently, in these patients the T8[+] cells act as suppressors of granulocytic precursors in the bone marrow.[80]

**MORPHOLOGY.** The bone marrow may be hypercellular, but more often it is hypocellular, especially in drug-induced injury. There is a selective reduction in the granulocytic precursors. Infections anywhere in the body are a characteristic feature of agranulocytosis, but ulcerating necrotizing lesions of the gingiva, oral mucosa, and pharynx are particularly common. The infections are characterized by abundant microbial growth, often in colonies, without significant leukocytic response. An absolute neutrophil count below 500 per mm³ is life-threatening since seemingly trivial infections do not remain localized, and death results from overwhelming septicemia.

# PLASMA CELL DYSCRASIAS AND RELATED DISORDERS

The plasma cell dyscrasias are a group of disorders that have in common the *expansion of a single clone of immunoglobulin-secreting cells and a resultant increase in serum levels of a single homogeneous immunoglobin or its fragments.* The homogeneous immunoglobulin identified in the blood is often referred to as an *M component.*[81] Since a common feature of the various plasma cell dyscrasias is the presence in the serum of excessive amounts of immunoglobulins, these disorders have also been called *monoclonal gammopathies, dysproteinemias,* and *paraproteinemias.* In almost all cases, these dyscrasias behave as malignant diseases, although occasionally M components are seen in otherwise normal elderly individuals (as monoclonal gammopathy of undetermined significance). Collectively, these disorders account for about 15% of deaths from malignant white cell disease; they are most common in middle-aged to elderly individuals.

The plasma cell dyscrasias can be divided into five major disorders: (1) multiple myeloma and its variants, (2) Waldenström's macroglobulinemia, (3) heavy-chain disease, (4) primary or immunocyte-associated amyloidosis, and (5) monoclonal gammopathy of undetermined significance. Each of these disorders will be briefly characterized before the morphologic features of all are presented.

**MULTIPLE MYELOMA AND ITS VARIANTS.** Multiple myeloma is by far the most common of the plasma cell dyscrasias.[82] *It is a clonal proliferation of neoplastic plasma cells in the bone marrow that is usually associated with multifocal lytic lesions throughout the skeletal system.* In approximately 60% of patients the M component is IgG; in 20 to 25%, IgA; and, rarely, IgM, IgD, or IgE. In the remaining 15 to 20% of cases, the plasma cells produce *only* κ or λ light chains, which, because of their low molecular weight, are readily excreted in urine, where they are termed *Bence Jones proteins.* In these patients, Bence Jones proteinuria without serum M component is present (*light-chain disease*). However, in up to 80% of patients the malignant plasma cells synthesize both complete immunoglobulin molecules as well as excess light chains, and therefore both Bence Jones proteins and serum M components are present.

Several variants of multiple myeloma have been described,[81] of which only two are sufficiently distinctive to merit brief description. (1) *Localized plasmacytoma* refers to the presence of a single lesion in the skeleton or in the soft tissues. Solitary skeletal myeloma tends to occur in the same locations as multiple myeloma, whereas the extraosseous lesions usually form tumorous masses in the upper respiratory tract (sinuses, nasopharynx, larynx). Modest elevations in the levels of M protein are demonstrable in approximately 25% of these patients. Those with solitary skeletal myelomas usually have occult lesions elsewhere. The patients may remain stable for several years, but after a lapse of 10 to 20 years, most develop disseminated disease. However, extraosseous (soft tissue) plasmacytomas rarely disseminate. They represent limited disease that can be readily cured by local resection. (2) *Plasma cell leukemia* is so defined because more than 20% of the cells in the peripheral blood are plasma cells. This disorder may occur as a terminal leukemic phase of a previously diagnosed multiple myeloma. However, in up to 75% of cases the leukemia occurs before multiple myeloma is diagnosed.[81] This variant has a rapidly progressive course and a median survival rate of two months.

**WALDENSTRÖM'S MACROGLOBULINEMIA.** *This disease is best regarded as a hybrid of well-differentiated lymphocytic lymphoma (WDLL), or, conceivably, chronic lymphocytic leukemia (CLL), and multiple myeloma.* All of these conditions are basically neoplasms of B cells that are distinguished by arrests at particular stages of differentiation. At one end of the spectrum are WDLL and CLL, in which the malignant B lymphocytes are arrested at a stage prior to acquisition of secretory capacity; at the other end is multiple myeloma, in which the neoplastic B cells are fully differentiated into immunoglobulin-secreting plasma cells. In between is Waldenström's macroglobulinemia, which involves B cells that are sufficiently differentiated to secrete immunoglobulins but not enough to look like plasma cells. Interestingly, the morphologic and clinical features of Waldenström's macroglobulinemia overlap those of both WDLL and myeloma. Like myeloma, there is an M component, which in the great majority of cases is due to the production of monoclonal IgM immunoglobulin. However, unlike myeloma (but resembling leukemia-lymphoma), the neoplastic B lymphocytes diffusely infiltrate the lymphoid organs, including bone marrow, lymph nodes, and spleen.

**HEAVY-CHAIN DISEASE.** This is an extremely rare plasma cell dyscrasia in which *only heavy chains are produced.* They may be of the IgG, IgA, or IgM class. Except for the presence of an M component, the disease often mimics a lymphoma-leukemia, and in this respect it resembles Waldenström's macroglobulinemia. However, the precise characteristics depend to some extent on which heavy chain is involved. With IgG heavy-chain disease, there is diffuse lymphadenopathy and hepatosplenomegaly. IgA heavy-chain disease shows a predilection for the lymphoid tissues that are normally the site of IgA synthesis, such as the small intestine and respiratory tract. A small proportion of patients with chronic lymphocytic leukemia secrete IgM heavy chains and hence have concurrent heavy-chain disease.

**PRIMARY OR IMMUNOCYTE-ASSOCIATED AMYLOIDOSIS.** It may be recalled that monoclonal proliferation of plasma cells, with excessive production of light chains, underlies this form of amyloidosis (p. 169). The amyloid deposits (AL type) consist of partially degraded light chains.

**MONOCLONAL GAMMOPATHY OF UNDETERMINED SIGNIFICANCE.** M proteins can be detected in the serum of 1 to 3% of asymptomatic, healthy individuals over the age of 50. *To this dysproteinosis without any associated disease, the term monoclonal gammopathy of undetermined significance (MGUS) is applied.* Previously, this condition was referred to as benign monoclonal gammopathy, but this term is misleading because approximately 20% of patients with MGUS develop a well-defined plasma cell dyscrasia (myeloma, Waldenström's macroglobulinemia, or amyloidosis) over a period of 10 to 15 years.[83] The diagnosis of MGUS should be made with caution and after careful exclusion of all other specific forms of monoclonal gammopathies. In general, patients with MGUS have less than 3 gm/dl of monoclonal protein and no Bence Jones proteinuria.

**ETIOLOGY AND PATHOGENESIS.** As was already pointed out, this group of disorders results from monoclonal proliferation of B cells in various stages of differentiation. The factors responsible for "turning on" a B-cell clone remain mysterious. It is postulated that prolonged antigenic stimulation may be the initial step in the pathogenesis of the plasma cell dyscrasias. This then provides the opportunity for spontaneous mutation, which might result in the neoplastic growth of the affected clone of B cells. As with many other B cell tumors, karyotypic abnormalities involving chromosome 14 band q32 have been detected in myeloma cells. Although the specific translocations are different from the t(8;14) commonly found in Burkitt's lymphoma and B-cell ALL, they may be significant in the pathogenesis of multiple myeloma. Thus, according to this hypothesis, multiple myeloma requires two "hits" for its evolution—a prolonged antigenic stimulus and a mutation (see also p. 388).

**MORPHOLOGY.** Despite the abundance of abnormal biochemical findings, the ultimate diagnosis of multiple myeloma rests on the morphologic identification of abnormal skeletal aggregates of plasma cells (Fig. 12–24), which may constitute 15 to 90% of the cells in the bone marrow. In many instances, the neoplastic cells are normal-appearing, mature plasma cells, but sometimes more immature forms are found that may even resemble lymphocytes. It may be difficult to identify the neoplastic nature of the well-differentiated plasma cell lesions from the cytologic features of the individual cells; more important is their abnormal aggregation or evidence of their destructive potential in the form of infiltration, invasion, and erosion. However, sometimes multinucleated plasma cells are seen in lesions that essentially constitute cancerous giant cells. Electron microscopy has confirmed that the plasma cells have the classic abundant endoplasmic reticulum responsible for the characteristic basophilia and pyroninophilia of the plasma cell cytoplasm. The protein products within the endoplasmic cisternae of these tumor cells have been proved to be immunoglobulin. With the light microscope, aggregates of immunoglobulins may appear as acidophilic intracytoplasmic inclusions called **Russell bodies.**

**Multiple myeloma presents most often as multifocal destructive bone lesions throughout the skeletal system.** Although any bone may be affected, the following distribution was found in a large series of cases: vertebral column, 66%; ribs, 44%; skull, 41%; pelvis, 28%; femur, 24%; clavicle, 10%; and scapula, 10%. These focal lesions generally begin in the medullary cavity, erode the cancellous bone, and progressively destroy the cortical bone. The bone resorption results from the secretion of an osteoclast-activating factor by myeloma cells. Pathologic fractures are often produced by the plasma cell lesions; they are most common in the vertebral column but may affect any of the numerous bones suffering erosion and destruction of their cortical substances. On section, the bony defects are typically filled with soft, red, gelatinous tissue. In approximately 70% of the patients, the lesions appear radiographically as punched-out defects, usually ranging from 1 to 4 cm in diameter (Fig. 12–25). In about 10% of the cases only diffuse demineralization is evident. With progressive disease, plasma cell infiltrations of soft tissues may be encountered in the spleen, liver, kidneys, lungs, and lymph nodes, or more widely.

Renal involvement, generally called **myeloma nephrosis,** is one of the more distinctive features of multiple myeloma. Grossly, the kidneys may be normal in size or color, slightly enlarged and pale, or shrunken and pale because of interstitial scarring. The most characteristic features are microscopic. Interstitial infiltrates of abnormal plasma cells may be encountered. Even in the absence of these, proteinaceous casts are prominent in the tubules and collecting ducts. Most of these casts are made up of Bence Jones proteins, but they may also contain Tamm-

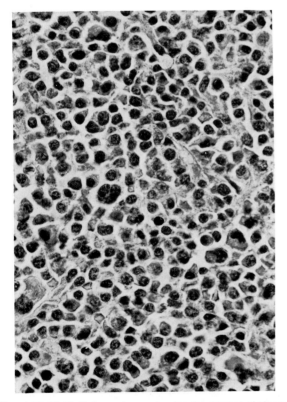

Figure 12–24. Multiple myeloma, showing the masses of plasma cells. The cells are mostly mature but some show anaplasia and are forming tumor giant cells. (From Robbins, S. L., Cotran, R. S., and Kumar, V.: Pathologic Basis of Disease. 3rd ed. Philadelphia, W. B. Saunders Co., 1984, p. 690.)

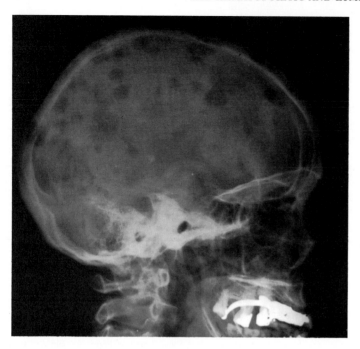

**Figure 12–25.** Multiple myeloma of the skull (x-ray, lateral view). The sharply punched-out bone defects are most obvious in the calvarium.

Horsfall protein and albumin. Some casts have tinctorial properties of amyloid. This is not surprising in view of the fact that AL amyloid is derived from Bence Jones proteins. The casts are usually surrounded by multinucleate giant cells derived either from fusion of infiltrating macrophages or the renal tubular epithelial cells.[84] Very often the cells lining tubules containing casts become necrotic or atrophied. It is believed that free light chains (Bence Jones proteins), which are filtered by the glomerulus and then reabsorbed by the tubular cells, are toxic to the tubular cells.[85] Metastatic calcification may be encountered within the kidney because of the hypercalcemia that frequently accompanies multiple myeloma. When complicated by amyloidosis, typical glomerular lesions associated with renal amyloidosis are present.

In contrast with multiple myeloma, Waldenström's macroglobulinemia and heavy-chain disease are not associated with lytic skeletal lesions. Instead, the neoplastic cells diffusely infiltrate the bone marrow, lymph nodes, spleen, and sometimes the liver. Infiltrations of other organs have also been reported. The cellular infiltrate consists of lymphocytes, plasma cells, lymphocytoid plasma cells, and several other hybrid forms. The remaining forms of plasma cell dyscrasias have either already been described (e.g., primary amyloidosis, p. 169) or are too rare for further description.

**CLINICAL COURSE.** The clinical manifestations of the plasma cell dyscrasias are varied. *They result from the destructive or otherwise damaging effect of the infiltrating neoplastic cells in various tissues and from the effects of the abnormal immunoglobulins secreted by the tumors.* In multiple myeloma, the pathologic effects of tumorous masses of plasma cells predominate, whereas in Waldenström's macroglob-

ulinemia, most of the signs and symptoms result from the IgM macroglobulins in the serum.

Generally, *multiple myeloma becomes evident by the progressive development of bone pain, referable to the skeletal lesions.* Commonly associated are anemia due to bone marrow replacement and a predisposition to infections. Vulnerability to bacterial infections is a serious clinical problem and the most common cause of death. Common infecting organisms include *Staphylococcus aureus, Streptococcus pneumoniae,* and *Haemophilus influenzae.* Many factors are involved in the predilection to infections in multiple myeloma. Deficiency of normal immunoglobulins and an impaired capacity to respond to antigenic challenge are well documented. The latter is caused by poorly defined suppressive influences that prevent immunoglobulin secretion by non-neoplastic B cells.[82] Renal insufficiency develops in approximately 50% of patients and is second only to infections as a cause of death. Hypercalcemia with nephrocalcinosis and direct renal tubular toxicity of Bence Jones proteins seem to be the most important factors that contribute to renal disease. The increase in serum calcium occurs owing to resorption of bones under the influence of osteoclast-activating factor. Amyloidosis develops in about 5 to 10% of patients with multiple myeloma.

The diagnosis of multiple myeloma can be readily made by the characteristic focal, punched-out radiologic defects in the bone, especially when these are present in the vertebrae or calvarium. Electrophoresis of the serum and urine is an important diagnostic tool in suspected cases. *In 99% of cases a monoclonal spike of complete immunoglobulin or immunoglobulin light chain can be detected in the serum or urine, or in both*. In the remaining 1% of cases monoclonal immunoglobulins can be found within the plasma cell masses but not in the serum or urine. Such cases are sometimes called "nonsecretory myelomas."

In Waldenström's macroglobulinemia, most clinical features can be traced to the presence of IgM globulins. Owing to their large molecular weight and high concentration, the viscosity of the serum is markedly increased, resulting in the *hyperviscosity syndrome* (vascular dilatations and hemorrhages in the retina, confusion, and transient paresis). A bleeding tendency may result from the formation of complexes between IgM globulins and the clotting factors, as well as by interference with platelet aggregation. In some cases the abnormal globulins precipitate at low temperatures (less than 37°C), giving rise to symptoms of *cryoglobulinemia*. These include Raynaud's phenomenon, cold urticaria, and ulcers of the exposed parts such as fingers. Cryoglobulinemia and bleeding disorders may also be seen in multiple myeloma, although less frequently. *The diagnosis of Waldenström's macroglobulinemia depends upon the clinical features (lymphadenopathy, hepatosplenomegaly, and associated symptoms), the presence of an infiltrate in the bone marrow, and a monoclonal IgM peak in the serum.*

# The Hemorrhagic Diatheses

These disorders are characterized by spontaneous bleeding or excessive bleeding following trauma. Such abnormal hemorrhage may have as its cause:
1. Increased fragility of the vessels
2. Inadequacy of hemostatic responses
   a. Platelet deficiency or dysfunction
   b. Derangement in the clotting mechanism

*Increased fragility of the vessels* occurs with severe *vitamin C deficiency (scurvy)* (p. 247) as well as with a large number of infectious and hypersensitivity *vasculitides*. These include meningococcemia, infective endocarditis, the rickettsial diseases, typhoid, and Henoch-Schönlein purpura. Some of these conditions are discussed in other chapters; others are beyond the scope of this book. *A hemorrhagic diathesis purely on the basis of vascular fragility is characterized by (1) the apparently spontaneous appearance of petechiae and ecchymoses in the skin and mucous membranes (probably on the basis of minor trauma) and (2) a normal platelet count, bleeding time, and coagulation time.*

*Deficiencies of platelets (thrombocytopenia)* are important causes of hemorrhagic disorders. These may occur in a variety of clinical settings to be discussed later. Here we would like to point out that there are disorders in which platelet function is impaired, *despite a normal platelet count*. Such qualitative defects are seen in uremia, after aspirin ingestion, in von Willebrand's disease, and in a variety of rare inherited disorders. *Thrombocytopenia and platelet dysfunction are similar to increased vascular fragility in that petechiae and ecchymoses are present, as well as easy bruising, nosebleeds, excessive bleeding from minor trauma, and menorrhagia. Similarly, the coagulation time is normal. However, in contrast to the vascular disorders, the bleeding time is prolonged.*

A bleeding diathesis based purely on a *derangement in the intricate clotting mechanism* differs in several respects from those resulting from defects in the vessel walls or in platelets. *The coagulation time is usually prolonged, whereas the bleeding time is normal. Petechiae and ecchymoses, as well as other evidence of bleeding from very minor surface trauma, are usually absent.* However, massive hemorrhage may follow operative and dental procedures and severe trauma. Moreover, hemorrhages into areas of the body subject to trauma, such as the joints of the lower extremities, are characteristic. In this category is a group of *congenital coagulation disorders*.

One of the most complex of the bleeding diatheses, *disseminated intravascular coagulation* (DIC, below), involves consumption of both platelets and the clotting factors, hence it presents laboratory and clinical features of both thrombocytopenia and a coagulation disorder. *von Willebrand's disease* also involves derangements in both modalities.

In this section the following hemorrhagic disorders will be discussed in this order:
1. DIC—consumption of fibrinogen and platelets
2. Thrombocytopenia—deficiency of platelets
3. Coagulation disorders—deficiency in clotting factors

## DISSEMINATED INTRAVASCULAR COAGULATION (DIC, CONSUMPTION COAGULOPATHY, DEFIBRINATION SYNDROME)

Disseminated intravascular coagulation is an acute, subacute, or chronic thrombohemorrhagic disorder that occurs as a secondary complication in a variety of diseases. It is characterized by activation of the coagulation sequence that leads to fibrin deposition throughout the microcirculation. As a consequence of the widespread thromboses, there is consumption of platelets and coagulation factors and, secondarily, activation of fibrinolysis. Thus DIC may give rise either to tissue hypoxia and microinfarcts caused by myriad microthrombi or to a bleeding disorder re-

### Table 12–13. CLINICAL DISORDERS ASSOCIATED WITH DIC

**Obstetric Complications**
  Abruptio placentae
  Retained dead fetus
  Septic abortion
  Amniotic fluid embolism
  Toxemia

**Infections**
  Gram-negative sepsis
  Meningococcemia
  Malaria

**Neoplasms**
  Carcinomas of pancreas, prostate, lung, and stomach
  Acute promyelocytic leukemia

**Massive Tissue Injury**
  Trauma
  Burns
  Extensive surgery

**Miscellaneous**
  Intravascular hemolysis due to incompatible blood transfusion, shock, vasculitis, liver disease

lated to depletion of the elements required for hemostasis (hence the term *consumption coagulopathy*), or to both derangements. This entity is probably a more important cause of pathologic bleeding than all the congenital coagulation disorders, which will be discussed later.

**ETIOLOGY AND PATHOGENESIS.** Before presenting the specific disorders associated with DIC, we shall discuss in a general way the pathogenetic mechanisms by which intravascular clotting can occur. Reference to the earlier comments on normal blood coagulation (p. 68) may be helpful at this point. It suffices here to recall that clotting may be initiated by either of two pathways: the *extrinsic pathway*, which is triggered by the release of tissue factor ("tissue thromboplastin") into the circulation, and the *intrinsic pathway*, which involves the activation within the blood of factor XII by surface contact, collagen, or other negatively charged substances. Both pathways lead to the generation of thrombin. *Clot-inhibiting influences* include the rapid clearance of activated clotting factors (factors X and XI) by the RE system or by the liver and activation of fibrinolysis. From this brief review, we can deduce that intravascular coagulation may result from any of the following:

○ Release of tissue factor into the circulation (extrinsic pathway)
○ Activation of the intrinsic pathway
○ Stasis
○ Defective clearing of activated clotting factors (derangements of the MPS or liver)
○ Defective fibrinolysis (rare)

In actual clinical practice, DIC probably most often results from activation of either the extrinsic or intrinsic coagulation system; the other influences listed are only of occasional importance. How is such abnormal initiation of clotting triggered?

*The simplest mechanism involves the release of tissue factor into the circulation*—for example, from the placenta in obstetric complications, from the cytoplasmic granules in the leukemic cells of acute promyelocytic leukemia, or from neoplastic cells in mucin-secreting adenocarcinomas. Carcinomas may also release other thromboplastic substances such as proteolytic enzymes, mucin, and other undefined tumor products. In still other cases the *coagulation*

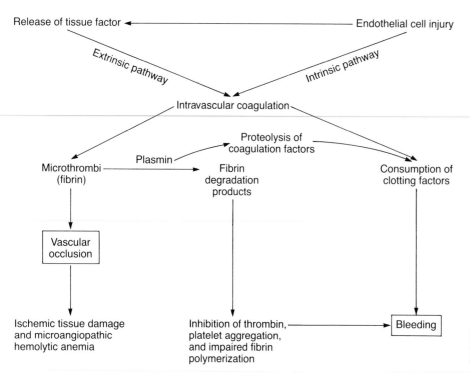

Figure 12–26. Pathophysiology of disseminated intravascular coagulation (DIC).

*may be activated by widespread injury to the endothelial cells,* such as occurs with deposition of antigen-antibody complexes, temperature extremes, vasculitis, or endotoxic damage by microorganisms. Endothelial injury triggers both the extrinsic and intrinsic pathways by releasing tissue factor and initiating activation of factor XII. Simultaneously, exposure of subendothelial collagen causes platelet aggregation. It should be apparent that injury to the endothelium can initiate intravascular coagulation in many ways. As discussed in Chapter 3 (p. 80, Fig. 3–17) endothelial injury is an important consequence of endotoxemia, and, not surprisingly, DIC is a frequent complication of gram-negative sepsis. Several additional disorders associated with DIC are listed in Table 12–13. Of these, DIC is most likely to follow *sepsis, obstetric complications, malignancy,* and *major trauma.* The initiating factors in these conditions are multiple and often interrelated. For example, in obstetric conditions, tissue factor derived from the placenta, retained dead fetus, or amniotic fluid may enter the circulation. However, shock, hypoxia, and acidosis often coexist and may cause widespread endothelial injury. Supervening infections may complicate the problem further.

Whatever the pathogenetic mechanism, DIC has two consequences: (1) There is widespread fibrin deposition within the microcirculation. This leads to ischemia in the more severely affected or more vulnerable organs and to hemolysis as the red blood cells become traumatized while passing through the fibrin strands (*microangiopathic hemolytic anemia*). (2) A bleeding diathesis ensues as the platelets and clotting factors are consumed. This is further aggravated as the extensive clotting activates plasminogen. Plasmin can not only cleave fibrin (fibrinolysis) but also digest factors V and VIII, thereby reducing their concentration further. In addition, fibrinolysis leads to the formation of fibrin degradation products, which themselves have an inhibitory effect on platelet aggregation, have antithrombin activity, and impair fibrin polymerization, all of which contribute to the hemostatic failure (Fig. 12–26).

**MORPHOLOGY.** The anatomic changes of DIC are related, on the one hand, to the widespread fibrin deposition and, on the other, to hemorrhage.

The microthrombi are found principally in the arterioles and capillaries of the kidneys, adrenals, brain, and heart. However, no organ is spared, and the lungs, liver, and gastrointestinal mucosa may also be prominently involved. The glomeruli contain small fibrin thrombi, which may evoke only a reactive swelling of the endothelial cells or may be surrounded by a florid focal glomerulitis. The resultant ischemia leads to microinfarcts within the renal cortex. In severe cases, the ischemia may even extend to destroy the entire cortex (**bilateral renal cortical necrosis**—see p. 478). Involvement of the adrenal glands reproduces the picture of the **Waterhouse-Friderichsen syndrome** (see p. 696). Microinfarcts are also commonly encountered in the brain, surrounded by microscopic or gross foci of hemorrhage. These may give rise to bizarre neurologic signs. Similar changes are seen in the heart and often in the anterior pituitary. It has been suggested that DIC may contribute to **Sheehan's postpartum pituitary necrosis** (see p. 676).

When the underlying disorder is toxemia of pregnancy, the placenta is the site of capillary thromboses and, occasionally, florid degeneration of the vessel walls. In addition, as many as 100% of the villi are devoid of syncytiotrophoblast, as opposed to about 33% of the villi in a normal placenta at term.

The bleeding tendency associated with DIC is manifested not only by larger than expected hemorrhages near foci of infarction but also by diffuse petechiae and ecchymoses, which may be found on the skin, serosal linings of the body cavities, epicardium, endocardium, lungs, and the mucosal lining of the urinary tract.

**CLINICAL COURSE.** The clinical picture is an apparent paradox, with a bleeding tendency in the face of evidence of widespread coagulation. It is almost impossible to detail all the potential clinical manifestations. In general, acute DIC (for example, that associated with obstetric complications) is dominated by a bleeding diathesis, whereas chronic DIC (such as may occur in a patient with cancer) tends to present with thrombotic complications. Typically, the abnormal clotting occurs only in the microcirculation, although large vessels are involved occasionally. The manifestations may be minimal, or there may be shock with acute renal failure, dyspnea, cyanosis, convulsions, and coma. Hypotension is characteristic. Most often, attention is called to the presence of a bleeding diathesis by prolonged and copious postpartum bleeding or by the presence of petechiae and ecchymoses on the skin. These may be the only manifestations, or there may be severe hemorrhage into the gut or urinary tract.

The prognosis with DIC is highly variable and depends on the underlying disorder as well as on the degree of intravascular clotting, the activity of the mononuclear phagocyte system, and the amount of fibrinolysis. In some cases, it can be life-threatening; in others, it can be treated with anticoagulants such as heparin or coagulants contained in fresh frozen plasma. The underlying disorder must be treated simultaneously to prevent progressive derangement of hemostasis.

# THROMBOCYTOPENIA

*Thrombocytopenia is characterized by spontaneous bleeding, a prolonged bleeding time, and a normal coagulation time.* A platelet count of 100,000 per mm³ or less is generally considered to constitute thrombocytopenia, although spontaneous bleeding does not become evident until the count falls below 20,000 per mm³. Platelet counts in the range of 20,000 to 50,000 may lead to posttraumatic bleeding. *The drop in platelets may occur because of either (1) decreased production or (2) excessive destruction.* A decrease in the production of platelets is associated with various forms of marrow failure or injury; these include idiopathic aplastic anemias, drug-induced marrow failure, and marrow infiltration by tumors. In all of these settings the cytopenia is associated with a decrease in marrow megakaryocytes. On the other hand, excessive destruction or peripheral consumption of platelets is characterized by a normal or an increased number of megakaryocytes in the marrow. Accelerated destruction of platelets is often related to antiplatelet antibodies. These may be associated with well-known autoimmune diseases such as SLE or appear as an apparently isolated derangement (*idiopathic thrombocytopenic purpura*). Some of the drug-induced thrombocytopenias are also suspected to be immunologically mediated. Excessive destruction of platelets is in some cases mediated by nonimmunologic means. As mentioned earlier, excessive utilization of platelets occurs in DIC. Other nonimmunologic causes include prosthetic heart valves and the rare disorder called *thrombotic thrombocytopenic purpura* (TTP), to be described later.

Whatever its pathogenetic mechanism, thrombocytopenia is associated with bleeding from small blood vessels. Petechiae or, sometimes, large ecchymoses are commonly found in the skin and mucous membranes of the gastrointestinal and urinary tracts, but no site is immune. Bleeding into the central nervous system constitutes a major hazard in patients with markedly depressed platelet counts.

## IDIOPATHIC THROMBOCYTOPENIC PURPURA (ITP)

A disorder of autoimmune origin, ITP most often occurs as an apparently isolated derangement but sometimes as a first manifestation of SLE. Although an acute form has been described in children, most of the patients are adult females between the ages of 20 and 40 years.[86]

An antiplatelet IgG reactive with a cell surface glycoprotein has been identified in the serum of a majority of patients with ITP. By specialized techniques immunoglobulins can also be demonstrated bound to the surface of platelets. The spleen plays an important role in the pathogenesis of this disorder. It is the major site of production of the antiplatelet antibody and destruction of the IgG-coated platelets. In over two thirds of patients, splenectomy is followed by return of normal platelet counts and complete remission of the disease. The spleen usually appears remarkably normal, with only minimal, if any, enlargement. Such splenomegaly as may be present is attributable to congestion of the sinusoids and enlargement of the lymphoid follicles, which have prominent germinal centers. Histologically, the marrow may appear normal but usually reveals increased numbers of megakaryocytes, many of which

have only a single nucleus and are thought to be young. A similar marrow picture is noted in most forms of thrombocytopenias resulting from accelerated platelet destruction. The importance of marrow examination is to rule out thrombocytopenias resulting from marrow failure. Indeed, significant findings are confined mostly to the secondary hemorrhages. Hemorrhages may be seen dispersed throughout the body, particularly in the serosal and mucosal linings.

## THROMBOTIC THROMBOCYTOPENIC PURPURA (TTP)

*Thrombotic thrombocytopenic purpura* is a rare disorder of obscure origin. It is characterized by widespread microthrombi in the arterioles, capillaries, and venules of all organs; thrombocytopenia; and hemolytic anemia. The microthrombi are composed primarily of loose aggregates of platelets that become consolidated and are eventually replaced by fibrin. The clinical manifestations result largely from the ischemia of various organs, particularly the central nervous system (transient neurologic deficits) and the kidneys. In addition, the microcirculatory lesions cause microangiopathic hemolytic anemia because of fragmentation of red cells (p. 363). The cause of TTP is unknown; it could be the result of immunologically mediated endothelial injury, but firm evidence is lacking. Alternatively, it has been proposed that the primary defect is formation of platelet aggregates in the circulation that then lodge in the microvasculature.[87] Despite similarities with DIC, the two conditions are thought to be separate and distinct.

# COAGULATION DISORDERS

These disorders result from either congenital or acquired deficiencies of the clotting factors. The latter, which are much more common and relatively straightforward, will be considered first.

*Acquired coagulation disorders are usually associated with deficiencies of multiple clotting factors.* As discussed in an earlier chapter (p. 243), vitamin K deficiency may be associated with a severe coagulation defect, since this nutrient is essential for the synthesis of prothrombin and clotting factors VII, IX, and X. The liver is the site of synthesis of several coagulation factors; thus, parenchymal diseases of the liver are probably the commonest cause of hemorrhagic diatheses. In addition, several liver diseases are associated with complex derangements of platelet function and fibrinogen metabolism, all of which contribute to the coagulopathy in liver disease.[88]

*Hereditary deficiencies* have been identified for each of the coagulation factors that characteristically occurs singly. Hemophilia, the most common form, is transmitted as an X-linked recessive disorder, whereas most others are autosomal disorders. Most of these conditions are rare; only von Willebrand's disease, hemophilia, and Christmas disease are important enough to warrant further consideration.

## DEFICIENCIES OF FACTOR VIII COMPLEX

Hemophilia and von Willebrand's disease, two of the most common inherited disorders of bleeding, are caused by qualitative or quantitative defects involving factor VIII. Before we can discuss these disorders it is essential to review the structure and function of factor VIII.[89, 90]

*Plasma factor VIII is a complex made up of two separate proteins that can be distinguished by functional, biochemical, and immunologic criteria.* One component, which is required for the activation of factor X in the intrinsic coagulation pathway, is called *factor VIII procoagulant protein,* or *factor VIII C* (Fig. 12–27). Deficiency of factor VIII C gives rise to classic hemophilia (hemophilia A). Through noncovalent bonds, factor VIII C is linked to a much larger protein called the *von Willebrand's factor* (vWF). The latter, which forms approximately 99% of the factor VIII complex, is not a discrete protein but exists in the form of a series of multimers that range in size from $4 \times 10^5$ to $20 \times 10^6$ daltons. *The most important function of vWF in vivo is to facilitate the adhesion of platelets to subendothelial collagen.* Thus vWF is crucial to the normal process of hemostasis

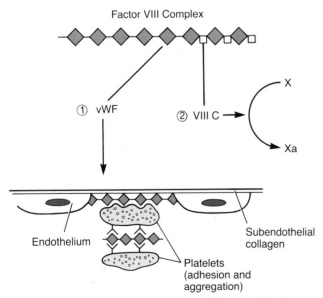

Figure 12–27. The subunit structure and function of the factor VIII complex. (1) von Willebrand's factor (vWF) causes adhesion of platelets to subendothelial collagen and favors platelet aggregation. These two functions (adhesion and aggregation) are mediated by two distinct receptors for vWF on the platelets. (2) Factor VIII procoagulant protein (factor VIII C) takes part in the activation of factor X.

(p. 68), and its absence in von Willebrand's disease leads to a bleeding diathesis. von Willebrand's factor can be assayed by immunologic techniques or by the so-called *ristocetin aggregation test.* Ristocetin (once used as an antibiotic) binds to platelets in vitro and activates vWF receptors on their surface. This leads to platelet aggregation if vWF is available to "bridge" the platelets (Fig. 12–27). Thus ristocetin-induced platelet aggregation can be used as a bioassay for vWF.

The two components of factor VIII complex are coded by separate genes and are synthesized by different cells. The vWF is produced by endothelial cells and megakaryocytes. It can be demonstrated in platelet granules. The site where factor VIII C is synthesized is not entirely clear, but the liver seems to be the favored organ. To summarize, *the two components of factor VIII complex, synthesized separately, come together and circulate in the plasma as a unit that serves to promote clotting as well as platelet–vessel wall interactions necessary to ensure hemostasis.* With this background we can discuss the diseases resulting from deficiencies of factor VIII complex.

### von Willebrand's Disease

*von Willebrand's disease* is characterized clinically by spontaneous bleeding from mucous membranes, excessive bleeding from wounds, menorrhagia, and a prolonged bleeding time in the presence of *a normal platelet count.* In most cases it is transmitted as an autosomal dominant disorder, but several rare autosomal recessive variants have been identified.[89] Its precise incidence is difficult to estimate because in many instances the clinical manifestations are mild and the diagnosis requires sophisticated tests; thus the condition may pass unrecognized.

Without delving into great complexities, we can state that the *classic and most common variant of von Willebrand's disease is characterized by a reduced quantity of circulating vWF.* The synthesis of vWF is not impaired, but the release of vWF multimers is inhibited by some unknown mechanism. Quite unexpectedly, levels of factor VIII C, the procoagulant component of factor VIII, are also reduced. Even more curious is the observation that infusion of factor VIII C–deficient (hemophilic) plasma causes an increase in the level of procoagulant activity. There is no satisfactory explanation for these findings, but it is suggested that vWF either protects factor VIII C from degradation by acting as a "carrier," or in some way influences its synthesis or release. *To summarize, patients with von Willebrand's disease have a compound defect involving platelet function and the coagulation pathway.* However, except in the most severely affected (e.g., homozygous patients), effects of factor VIII C deficiency such as bleeding into the joints, which characterize hemophilia, are uncommon.

### Factor VIII Deficiency (Hemophilia A, Classic Hemophilia)

This disease is caused by a reduced amount or activity of factor VIII C. It is inherited as an X-linked recessive trait, and thus it occurs in males or in homozygous females. However, excessive bleeding has been described in heterozygous females, presumably due to extremely "unfavorable lyonization" (inactivation of the normal X chromosome in most of the cells). The clinical syndrome develops only in the presence of severe deficiency. Mild or moderate degrees of deficiency occur but are asymptomatic, although posttraumatic bleeding may be somewhat excessive. The variable degrees of deficiency in the level of factor VIII procoagulant are best explained by assuming that more than one type of mutation is involved. To add to the complexities, in about 10% of patients with hemophilia, levels of factor VIII C appear normal by immunoassay but the coagulant activity detected by bioassay is low. It is likely that in these patients a mutation causes the synthesis of an antigenically normal but nonfunctional protein. In any event, in all symptomatic cases there is a tendency toward massive hemorrhage following trauma or operative procedures. In addition, "spontaneous" hemorrhages are frequently encountered in regions of the body normally subject to trauma, particularly the joints, where they are known as hemarthroses. Recurrent bleeding into the joints leads to progressive deformities that may be crippling. *Petechiae and ecchymoses are characteristically absent. Although coagulation time is prolonged, bleeding time is normal.* At one time, about 50% of severely affected patients died before the age of five years. However, the recent use of factor VIII concentrates has substantially improved the prognosis.

Replacement therapy, however, is not an unalloyed blessing. It carries with it the risk of transmission of viral hepatitis and AIDS. As discussed in Chapter 5, the prevalence of AIDS in hemophiliacs is about 1%. Many more have antibodies against HTLV-III, indicating exposure to the AIDS virus. Although the gene for factor VIII C has been cloned, genetically engineered factor is not yet available for replacement therapy. A more immediate use of the cloned factor VIII C gene is for detection of carriers and for prenatal diagnosis of hemophilia.[91]

### FACTOR IX DEFICIENCY (HEMOPHILIA B, CHRISTMAS DISEASE)

Severe factor IX deficiency is a disorder that is clinically indistinguishable from hemophilia A. Moreover, it is also inherited as an X-linked recessive trait and may occur asymptomatically or with associated hemorrhage. In about 14% of these patients, factor IX is present but nonfunctional. *The coagulation time is prolonged; bleeding time is normal.* Identification of Christmas disease (named after the first patient with this condition and not the holy day) is only possible by assay of the factor levels.

# Miscellaneous Disorders

## INFECTIOUS MONONUCLEOSIS (IM)

In the Western world, IM is an acute, self-limited disease of adolescents and young adults (it delights in college students) that is caused by the B lymphocytotropic Epstein-Barr virus (EBV), a member of the herpes family. The infection is characterized mainly by fever, sore throat, generalized lymphadenitis, peripheral lymphocytosis with at least 10% atypical lymphocytes, and serologic titers confirmatory of EBV infection. In passing it should be noted that the cytomegalovirus may induce a similar syndrome that can be differentiated only by serologic methods. IM and its causal agent, EBV, are of great interest on several scores:

○ The acute febrile illness is virtually limited to countries with high living standards; in developing countries, acute symptomatic disease is rare, but almost 100% of children by the age of three have serologic evidence of prior EBV infection.

○ Symptomatic IM is almost always a relatively benign disease that runs its course in four to six weeks, but rarely, and usually in individuals having some immunologic deficit, the disease runs amok and either flares into a fatal (polyclonal) lymphoproliferative syndrome or leads to a lymphoma.

○ The EBV has been closely linked to the causation of endemic Burkitt's lymphoma in specific areas of Africa and New Guinea and to nasopharyngeal carcinoma in particular areas of Asia and Africa.

Many of these intriguing points can now be explained.[92]

**EPIDEMIOLOGY AND IMMUNOLOGY.** The EBV is ubiquitous in all human populations. Where economic deprivation results in inadequate living standards, infection early in life is near universal with EBV. At this age symptomatic disease is uncommon, and despite the fact that infected hosts develop an immunologic response (described below), more than half of the population continues to be viral shedders, explaining the dissemination of infection. In contrast, in developed countries enjoying better standards of hygiene, infection is usually delayed until adolescence or young adulthood. Perhaps better standards of health and less underlying intercurrent chronic disease permit a more effective immunologic response to the EBV and so only about 20% of healthy seropositive individuals shed the virus. Concomitantly, only about 50% of those exposed acquire the infection. Transmission to a seronegative "kissing cousin" usually involves direct intimate oral contact. In some unknown manner the virus initially penetrates nasopharyngeal epithelial cells and persists as a subclinical productive infection in the oropharyngeal region (perhaps in the parotid glands). Thus the agent is shed in the saliva. Simultaneously, it spreads to underlying oropharyngeal lymphoid tissue and, more specifically, to B lymphocytes, all of which have receptors for EBV.[93] Within B cells the infection becomes latent as the viral DNA is incorporated within the cellular genome and the cells undergo lymphoblastoid transformation and acquire the capacity for unlimited replication (i.e., are "immortalized"). These virally infected cells are then disseminated in the circulation. In time they evoke an immune response that is both humoral and cellular. Antibodies are elaborated against a number of viral-directed antigens, some of which are membrane associated. For unknown reasons an agglutinin to red cells of sheep and horses also appears, providing the basis for the well-known heterophil (Paul-Bunnell) reaction that is widely available diagnostically as the Monospot test. Although these agglutinins are not as specific for EBV as the antibodies directed against viral antigens, they are nonetheless a highly reliable clinical indicator of IM.

Immunocompetent cells also participate in the immune response to EBV. In addition to NK cells, cytotoxic T cells appear to be targeted on the viral-directed membrane antigens of the B cells. It is these sensitized T cells that make up the largest proportion of atypical lymphocytes in the circulation. It is significant to note that in otherwise healthy individuals the fully developed humoral and cellular responses to EBV act as brakes on viral shedding and limit the number of B cells in the blood and nodes rather than eliminate them. As will be seen, impaired immunity in the host can have disastrous consequences.

**MORPHOLOGY.** The major alterations involve the blood, lymph nodes, spleen, liver, central nervous system, and, occasionally, other organs. The **peripheral blood** shows an absolute lymphocytosis with a total white cell count between 12,000 and 18,000 per mm³, over 60% of which are lymphocytes. Many of these are large, **atypical lymphocytes,** 12 to 16 μm in diameter, characterized by an abundant cytoplasm containing multiple clear vacuolations and an oval, indented, or folded nucleus. These atypical lymphocytes, most of which bear T-cell markers, are usually sufficiently distinctive to permit the diagnosis from examination of a peripheral blood smear.

The **lymph nodes** are typically discrete and enlarged throughout the body, principally in the posterior cervical, axillary, and groin regions. Histologically, the lymphoid tissue is flooded by atypical lymphocytes, which occupy the paracortical (T-cell) areas. There is in addition some B-cell reaction, with enlargement of follicles. Although the underlying architecture is usually preserved, it may be blurred by intense lymphoproliferation. Occasionally cells resembling Reed-Sternberg cells (p. 376) may also be found in the nodes. Together these features sometimes make it difficult to distinguish the nodal morphology from that seen in malignant lymphomas, particularly Hodgkin's disease. Differentiation then depends on recognition of the atypical lymphocytes. Similar changes commonly occur in the tonsils and lymphoid tissue of the oropharynx.

The **spleen** is enlarged in most cases, weighing between 300 and 500 gm. It is usually soft and fleshy, with a hyperemic cut surface. The histologic changes are analogous to those of the lymph nodes, showing a heavy infiltration of atypical lymphocytes, which may result either in prominence of the splenic follicles or in some blurring of the architecture. These spleens are especially vulnerable to rupture, possibly in part resulting from infiltration of the trabeculae and capsule by the lymphocytes.

**Liver** function is almost always transiently impaired to some degree, although hepatomegaly is at most moderate. Histologically, atypical lymphocytes are seen in the portal areas and sinusoids, and scattered, isolated cells or foci of parenchymal necrosis filled with lymphocytes may be present. This histologic picture may be difficult to distinguish from that seen in viral hepatitis.

The **central nervous system** may show congestion, edema, and perivascular mononuclear infiltrates in the leptomeninges. Myelin degeneration and destruction of axis cylinders have been described in the peripheral nerves.

**CLINICAL COURSE.** Although classically IM presents with fever, sore throat, lymphadenitis, and the other features mentioned earlier, quite often it is more aberrant in behavior. It may present with little or no fever and only malaise, fatigue, and lymphadenopathy, raising the spectre of leukemia-lymphoma; as a fever of unknown origin without significant lymphadenopathy or other localized findings; as hepatitis that is difficult to differentiate from one of the hepatotropic viral syndromes; or as a febrile rash resembling rubella. *Ultimately, the diagnosis depends on the following (in increasing order of specificity): (1) lymphocytosis with the characteristic atypical lymphocytes in the peripheral blood, (2) a positive heterophil reaction, and (3) specific antibodies for EBV antigens (viral capsid antigens, early antigens, or Epstein-Barr nuclear antigen).*[94] In the great majority of patients, IM resolves within four to six weeks, but sometimes the fatigue lasts longer. However, uncommonly, one or more complications may supervene. They may involve virtually any organ or system in the body. Perhaps most common is marked hepatic dysfunction with jaundice, elevated hepatic enzyme levels, disturbed appetite, and, rarely, even liver failure. Other complications involve the nervous system, kidneys, bone marrow, lungs, eyes, heart, and spleen (splenic rupture has been fatal).[95] A more serious complication in those suffering from some form of immunodeficiency or receiving immunosuppressive therapy (perhaps posttransplant) is that the proliferative lymphoid responses may run amok, leading to a fatal disorder resembling polyclonal B-cell lymphoma. True monoclonal B-cell lymphomas have also appeared; sometimes they have been preceded by polyclonal lymphoproliferation. These unfortunate consequences were described in a family suffering from an X-linked recessive T-cell defect, and so the condition has been designated Duncan disease or XLP syndrome.[96]

In closing it should be recalled that the Burkitt's B-cell lymphomas endemic in Africa almost always bear evidence of EBV infection as well as a translocation of a *c-myc* oncogene from chromosome 8 to a site usually on chromosome 14, close to an immunoglobulin gene (p. 209). Analogously, as mentioned earlier, DNA for EBV has been observed in the cells of nasopharyngeal carcinoma, but whether it alone is oncogenic remains unknown.[92] It is apparent that the expressions of EBV infection range from the uncomfortable to the grave.

## CAT-SCRATCH DISEASE

This is a benign condition characterized usually by a regional lymphadenitis that occurs after a cat scratch or other puncture. In the usual case, the local injury is trivial, although sometimes it is followed by the development of an erythematous papule or pustule at the site of trauma. Two or three weeks later, but occasionally after a delay of several months, the regional nodes of drainage become painfully enlarged, tense, and red. They may reach a size of 8 to 10 cm in diameter, although usually the enlargement is less marked. In about 50% of cases, the nodes become suppurative, soft, and fluctuant. The histologic reaction is fairly distinctive and can be characterized as "granulomatous abscess formation." When it is full-blown, the lesion consists of an irregular, stellate, round or ovoid abscess containing central debris with fragmented granulocyte nuclei. This focus is enclosed within a rim of mononuclear phagocytic cells and fibroblasts, sometimes including giant cells of the foreign body or Langhans' type. Plasma cells and lymphocytes frequently surround these granulomas. Infrequently, cat-scratch disease presents as an encephalitis, osteomyelitis, thrombocytopenic purpura, or oculoglandular syndrome.[97]

It is almost (but not completely) certain that cat-scratch disease is of bacterial origin. In 1983 gram-negative pleomorphic bacilli were identified by a specific (Warthin-Starry) silver stain within the lesions of involved lymph nodes.[98] These organisms have since been identified in the preponderance of cases but to date have not been grown in culture or transmitted to laboratory animals.[99] Thus, the putative culprit has not yet been fingerprinted or identified by name.

## DERMATOPATHIC LYMPHADENITIS (LIPOMELANOTIC RETICULOENDOTHELIOSIS)

"Dermatopathic lymphadenitis" refers to a distinctive chronic lymphadenitis that affects the lymph nodes draining the sites of chronic dermatologic diseases. It is commonly associated with eczema, psoriasis, exfoliative dermatitis, neurodermatitis, and seborrheic dermatitis. The nodes are usually moderately enlarged and characterized by the following: (1) hyperplasia of the germinal follicles, (2) hyperplasia of the sinusoidal lining cells, (3) accumulation of melanin and, less prominently, of hemosiderin by the phagocytes within the nodes, and (4) the appearance of finely divided lipid granules in these phagocytic cells. The pathogenesis of these changes appears to lie in the persistent drainage to the involved nodes of melanin pigment and fatty debris from the skin lesion. The condition is of little significance, except for its possible confusion with a lymphoproliferative disorder.

## HISTIOCYTOSES

The term "histiocytoses" is an umbrella designation for a large collection of widely varying disorders only having in common lesions marked by aggregation of histiocytes. In some of these conditions the histiocytes represent a reaction of the mononuclear phagocyte system to some "foreign" agent or substance as, for example, in tuberculosis, leprosy, malaria, and the various storage disorders (e.g., Niemann-Pick and Gaucher's diseases). At the other end of the spectrum of the histiocytoses are those that represent overt cancerous conditions such as the rare histiocytic lymphoma. Between these two extremes lie a small cluster of related syndromes of obscure etiology that are collectively referred to as histiocytosis X. It is to these that our attention is now directed, but briefly because of their relative rarity.

### HISTIOCYTOSIS X

At one time histiocytosis X was subdivided into three clinicopathologic subsets: Letterer-Siwe disease, Hand-Schüller-Christian disease, and eosinophilic granuloma. However, there is so much overlap between these subsets it is currently recommended that they be referred to respectively as acute disseminated, chronic progressive, and benign, usually localized, histiocytosis.[100] Although their origins are unknown, all variants of histiocytosis X are marked by proliferation of histiocytes that are closely related to antigen-presenting dendritic Langerhans' cells of marrow origin that are normally found in the epidermis. To acknowledge their differences from normal histiocytes, they are called HX cells. Distinctive of these cells are rod-shaped organelles that have the appearance of "short zippers" (i.e., parallel, tightly applied membranes separated by dense, periodic, transverse striations) that are called LC (Langerhans' cells) granules or Birbeck granules. Thus the syndromes of histiocytosis X are sometimes referred to as Langerhans' cell histiocytoses.[101] On the grounds that the proliferative reaction may reflect a defect in T-cell function, administration of thymic extract has been of benefit in some cases.

*Acute disseminated histiocytosis (Letterer-Siwe disease)* mostly occurs before age two but infrequently may involve adults. The dominant clinical feature is cutaneous lesions that resemble a seborrheic eruption secondary to infiltrations of HX cells over the front and back of the trunk, and the scalp. Most of those affected have concomitant hepatosplenomegaly, lymphadenopathy, pulmonary lesions, and, eventually, destructive osteolytic bone lesions. Extensive infiltration of the marrow often leads to anemia, thrombocytopenia, and predisposition to recurrent infections. The course is usually rapidly fatal, but occasionally it is benign with spontaneous resolution. Although there is no understanding of this range of behavior, in general the prognosis is better in children over three years with limited visceral involvement.

In all sites of involvement, there is a proliferation of HX cells that look much like the histiocytes or macrophages seen in inflammatory reactions. Ultrastructurally, however, these cells reveal the LC or Birbeck granules previously described as well as other distinguishing immunologic and enzymic markers.[102]

*Chronic progressive histiocytosis (Hand-Schüller-Christian disease)* usually begins between the second and sixth years of life and almost always before age 30. *It is characterized principally by bone lesions (particularly in the calvarium and base of the skull), diabetes insipidus, and exophthalmos (in a few cases).* Cutaneous lesions less florid than those in the acute disseminated disease appear in about a third of patients. Less frequently there is pulmonary involvement, hepatosplenomegaly, and lymphadenopathy. Depending on age and extent of dissemination, the course may be more or less benign. Overall, older patients have a long survival and even in the absence of therapy about half die of unrelated causes.

The proliferative reaction of HX cells in this clinical pattern is often admixed with lymphocytes and occasional eosinophils, and the histiocytic forms often are lipid-laden and sometimes enlarged and multinucleated to thus impart a xanthomatous appearance. Occasionally, the lesions have an abundance of eosinophils, and under these circumstances the involvement may be referred to as *multifocal eosinophilic granuloma*, which merges with the localized pattern to be described next.

*The benign localized form of histiocytosis X (eosinophilic granuloma)* usually presents as a unifocal involvement, most often of the skeletal system but rarely of the skin or other soft tissues. The bones affected in decreasing order of frequency are cranial vault, ribs, vertebral column, pelvis, scapulae, and long bones. Deep structures such as the lymph nodes, lungs, liver, and spleen are rarely affected. The prognosis with chemotherapy, curettage, or radiation is excellent, and few patients die of their disease.

As the older name for this variant implies, the lesions are granulomatous and made up of a mixed population of lipid-laden HX cells, usual macrophages, sometimes lipid-laden lymphocytes, and often sheets of eosinophils. The histologic picture has a distinctly inflammatory look, but to date no etiologic agent has been identified.

## SPLENOMEGALY

The spleen is frequently involved in a wide variety of systemic diseases. In virtually all cases, the splenic changes are secondary to disease that is primary elsewhere, and in almost all instances the presentation of the splenic lesion is enlargement. Excessive destruction by the spleen of red cells, leukocytes, and platelets may ensue. Evaluation of splenomegaly is a common clinical problem. It is considerably aided by a knowledge of the usual limits of splenic enlargement caused by the disorders being considered. Obviously, it would be erroneous to attribute enlargement of the spleen into the pelvis to vitamin $B_{12}$ deficiency and equally erroneous to accept as classic a case of chronic myeloid leukemia unless there is significant splenomegaly. As an aid to diagnosis, then, we present the following list of disorders, classified according to the degree of splenomegaly characteristically produced:

A. Massive Splenomegaly (over 1000 gm)
   1. Chronic myeloproliferative disorders (chronic myeloid leukemia, myeloid metaplasia with myelofibrosis)
   2. Chronic lymphocytic leukemia (less massive)
   3. Hairy cell leukemia
   4. Lymphomas
   5. Malaria
   6. Gaucher's disease
   7. Primary tumors of the spleen (rare)
B. Moderate Splenomegaly (500 to 1000 gm)
   1. Chronic congestive splenomegaly (portal hypertension or splenic vein obstruction)

2. Acute leukemias (inconstant)
3. Hereditary spherocytosis
4. Thalassemia major
5. Autoimmune hemolytic anemia
6. Amyloidosis
7. Niemann-Pick disease
8. Histiocytosis X
9. Chronic splenitis (especially with infective endocarditis)
10. Tuberculosis, sarcoidosis, typhoid
11. Metastatic carcinoma or sarcoma
C. Mild Splenomegaly (under 500 gm)
    1. Acute splenitis
    2. Acute splenic congestion
    3. Infectious mononucleosis
    4. Miscellaneous acute febrile disorders, including septicemia, SLE, and intraabdominal infections

The microscopic changes associated with most of the previously mentioned diseases need not be described here since they have been discussed in the relevant sections of this and other chapters.

As mentioned earlier, an enlarged spleen may remove excessive amounts of one or more of the formed elements of blood, resulting in anemia, leukopenia, or thrombocytopenia. This is referred to as *hypersplenism* and may be associated with many of the diseases of the spleen listed previously. In some cases, however, hypersplenism is associated with an apparently normal spleen, without any known cause for splenic hyperfunction. These cases are labeled *primary hypersplenism.*

The splenic white pulp, where various lymphocytes and macrophages reside, is a part of the lymphoid system. The white pulp, therefore, is involved in the same disease processes that affect the lymphoid tissues elsewhere in the body. It also reacts to immunologic stimuli, much in the same manner as lymph nodes. Thus, in several forms of autoimmune disease (such as SLE, rheumatoid arthritis, and ITP) and in certain systemic infections, the splenic lymphoid follicles show features of activation, such as enlarged germinal centers with transformed lymphocytes and maturing plasma cells. On the other hand, several primary immunodeficiency disorders are associated with hypoplasia of the white pulp. As might be expected, neoplastic disorders of the lymphoid tissue (lymphomas) may cause expansion of the splenic white pulp along the distinctive patterns already discussed.

## References

1. Mohandas, N., et al.: Red blood cell deformability and hemolytic anemias. Semin. Hematol. 16:95, 1979.
2. Becker, P. S., and Lux, S. E.: Hereditary spherocytosis and related disorders. Clin. Hematol. 14:15, 1985.
3. Palek, J.: Hereditary elliptocytosis and related disorders. Clin. Hematol. 14:45, 1985.
4. Bunn, H. F., and Forget, B. G.: Hemoglobin: Molecular, Genetic and Clinical Aspects. Philadelphia, W. B. Saunders Co., 1986, p. 381.
5. Dean, J., and Schechter, A. N.: Sickle cell anemia: Molecular and cellular basis of therapeutic approaches. N. Engl. J. Med. 299:752, 1978.
6. Hebbel, R. P., et al.: The adhesive sickle erythrocyte: Cause and consequences of abnormal interactions with endothelium monocytes/macrophages and model membranes. Clin. Hematol. 14:141, 1985.
7. Embury, S. H.: The clinical pathophysiology of sickle cell disease. Ann. Rev. Med. 37:361, 1986.
8. Bunn, H. F., and Forget, B. G.: Hemoglobin: Molecular, Genetic and Clinical Aspects. Philadelphia, W. B. Saunders Co., 1986, p. 226.
9. Bank, A.: Genetic disorders of hemoglobin synthesis. Hosp. Pract. 20(9):109, 1985.
10. Orkin, S., et al.: Polymorphism and molecular pathology of human beta-globin gene. Prog. Hematol. 13:49, 1983.
11. Valentine, W. N., et al.: Hemolytic anemias and erythrocyte enzymopathies. Ann. Intern. Med. 103:245, 1985.
12. Rosse, W. F., and Parker, C. J.: Paroxysmal nocturnal hemoglobinuria. Clin. Hematol. 14:105, 1985.
13. Rosse, W. F.: Autoimmune hemolytic anemia. Hosp. Pract. 20(8):105, 1985.
14. Petz, L. D.: Drug-induced hemolysis. N. Engl. J. Med. 313:510, 1985.
15. Scrimshaw, N. S.: Iron deficiency and its functional consequences. Compr. Ther. 11:40, 1985.
16. Herbert, V.: The nutritional anemias. Hosp. Pract. 15:65, 1980.
17. Reeves, J. D., et al.: Iron deficiency in health and disease. Adv. Pediatr. 30:281, 1983.
18. Herbert, V.: Biology of disease. Megaloblastic anemias. Lab. Invest. 52:3, 1985.
19. Herbert, V., and Colman, N.: Hematological aspects of folate deficiency. In Botez, M. I., and Reynolds, E. H. (eds.): Folic Acid in Neurology, Psychiatry, and Internal Medicine. New York, Raven Press, 1979, p. 63.
20. Levine, J. S., and Allen, R. H.: Intrinsic factor within parietal cells of patients with juvenile pernicious anemia. Gastroenterology 88:1132, 1985.
21. Muir, M., and Chanarin, I.: Separation of cobalamin analogues in human sera binding to intrinsic factor and R-type vitamin B$_{12}$ binders. Br. J. Haematol. 54:613, 1983.
22. Eriksson, S., et al.: Pernicious anemia as a risk factor in gastric cancer. The extent of the problem. Acta Med. Scand. 210:481, 1981.
23. Rappaport, J. M., and Nathan, D. G.: Acquired aplastic anemia. Pathophysiology and treatment. Adv. Intern. Med. 27:547, 1982.
24. Young, N. S., and Mortimer, P. P.: Viruses and bone marrow failure. Blood 63:729, 1984.
25. Thomas, E. D., and Storb, R.: Acquired aplastic anemia: Progress and perplexity. Blood 64:325, 1984.
26. Zoumbos, N. C., et al.: Circulating activated suppressor lymphocytes in aplastic anemia. N. Engl. J. Med. 312:257, 1985.
27. Champlin, R., et al.: Antithymocyte globulin treatment in patients with aplastic anemia. A prospective randomized trial. N. Engl. J. Med. 308:113, 1983.
28. Ansetti, C., et al.: Marrow transplantation in severe aplastic anemia. Ann. Intern. Med. 104:461, 1986.
29. Jaffe, E. S.: An overview of the classifications of non-Hodgkin's lymphomas. In Jaffe, E. S. (ed.): Surgical Pathology of Lymph Nodes and Related Organs. Philadelphia, W. B. Saunders Co., 1985, p. 135.
30. Lukes, R. J., et al.: Immunologic approach to non-Hodgkin's lymphomas and related leukemias. Analysis of the results of multiparameter studies of 425 cases. Semin. Hematol. 15:322, 1978.
31. National Cancer Institute: Sponsored study of classifications of non-Hodgkin's lymphomas. Summary and description of

Working Formulation for Clinical Usage. Cancer 49:2112, 1982.

32. Horning, S. J., and Rosenberg, S. A.: The natural history of low-grade non-Hodgkin's lymphomas. N. Engl. J. Med. 311:1471, 1984.

33. Gaynor, E. R., and Ultmann, J. E.: Non-Hodgkin's lymphomas: Management strategies. N. Engl. J. Med., 311:1506, 1984.

34. Mann, R. B., et al.: Malignant lymphomas—A conceptual understanding of morphologic diversity. Am. J. Pathol. 94:105, 1979.

35. Aisenberg, A. C.: Cell lineage in lymphoproliferative disease. Am. J. Med. 74:679, 1983.

36. Mintzer, D., and Hauptman, S. P.: Lymphosarcoma cell leukemia and other non-Hodgkin's lymphomas in leukemic phase. Am. J. Med. 75:110, 1983.

37. Doggett, R. S., et al.: The immunologic classification of 95 nodal and extranodal diffuse large cell lymphomas in 89 patients. Am. J. Pathol. 115:245, 1984.

38. Cleary, M. L., et al.: Most null large cell lymphomas are B lineage neoplasms. Lab. Invest. 53:521, 1985.

39. Chabner, B. A., et al.: Sequential nonsurgical and surgical staging of non-Hodgkin's lymphoma. Ann. Intern. Med. 85:149, 1976.

40. Winter, J. N., et al.: Phenotypic analysis in diffuse, large cell lymphoma. Clinical and histologic association. Am. J. Clin. Pathol. 85:425, 1986.

41. Nathwani, B. N., et al.: Non-Hodgkin's lymphomas. A clinicopathologic study comparing two classifications. Cancer 41:303, 1978.

42. Nathwani, B. N., et al.: Lymphoblastic lymphoma. A clinicopathologic study of 95 patients. Cancer 48:2347, 1981.

43. Aisenberg, A. C., et al.: Cell surface phenotype in lymphoproliferative disease. Am. J. Med. 68:206, 1980.

44. Banfi, A., et al.: Preferential sites of involvement and spread in malignant lymphomas. Eur. J. Cancer 4:319, 1968.

45. Weiss, L. M., et al.: Clonal T-cell populations in angioimmunoblastic lymphadenopathy and angioimmunoblastic lymphadenopathy like lymphoma. Am. J. Pathol. 122:392, 1986.

46. Knobler, R. M., and Edelson, R. L.: Cutaneous T cell lymphoma. Med. Clin. North Am. 70:109, 1986.

47. Portlock, C. S.: Hodgkin's disease. Med. Clin. North Am. 68:729, 1984.

48. Lukes, R. J., et al.: Report of the nomenclature committee. Cancer Res. 26:1311, 1966.

49. Tindle, B. H., et al.: "Reed-Sternberg cells" in infectious mononucleosis? Am. J. Clin. Pathol. 58:607, 1972.

50. Grogan, T. M.: Hodgkin's disease. In Jaffe, E. S. (ed.): Surgical Pathology of Lymph Nodes and Related Organs. Philadelphia, W. B. Saunders Co., 1985, p. 86.

51. Diehl, V., et al.: Characteristics of Hodgkin's disease derived cell lines. Cancer Treat. Rep. 66:615, 1982.

52. Vianna, N. J., and Polan, A. K.: Epidemiologic evidence for transmission of Hodgkin's disease. N. Engl. J. Med. 289:499, 1973.

53. Gutensohn, N., and Cole, P.: Epidemiology of Hodgkin's disease. Semin. Oncol. 7:92, 1980.

54. Bennett, J. M., et al.: Proposals for the classification of the acute leukemias. French-American-British (FAB) Cooperative Group. Br. J. Haematol. 33:451, 1976.

55. Jacobs, A. D., and Gale, R. P.: Recent advances in the biology and treatment of acute lymphoblastic leukemia in adults. N. Engl. J. Med. 311:1219, 1984.

56. Waldman, T. A.: Advances in diagnosis of hematologic malignancies. Hosp. Pract. 21:69, 1986.

57. Bennett, J. M., et al.: Criteria for the diagnosis of acute leukemia of the megakaryocyte lineage (M7). A report of the French-American-British Cooperative groups. Ann. Intern. Med. 103:460, 1985.

58. Mayer, J: Acute lymphoblastic leukemia in adults. Ann. Intern. Med. 101:552, 1984.

59. Champlin, R. E., et al.: Treatment of acute myelogenous leukemia. Ann. Intern. Med. 102:285, 1985.

60. Freireich, E. J.: Adult acute leukemia. Hosp. Pract. 21:91, 1986.

61. Degnan, R., et al.: Dysmyelopoietic syndrome: Current concepts. Am. J. Med. 76:122, 1984.

62. Knapp, R. H., et al.: Cytogenetic studies in 174 consecutive patients with preleukemic or myelodysplastic syndromes. Mayo Clin. Proc. 60:507, 1985.

63. Spiers, A. S. D.: Chronic granulocytic leukemia. Med. Clin. North Am. 68:713, 1984.

64. Champlin, R., et al.: Chronic leukemias: Oncogenes, chromosomes, and advances in therapy. Ann. Intern. Med. 104:671, 1986.

65. Rai, K., et al.: Chronic lymphocytic leukemia. Med. Clin. North Am. 68:697, 1984.

66. Brodeur, G. M.: Molecular correlates of cytogenetic abnormalities in human cancer cells: Implications for oncogene activation. Prog. Hematol. 14:229, 1986.

67. Gordon, H.: Oncogenes. Mayo Clin. Proc. 60:697, 1985.

68. Yunis, J. J.: Clinical significance of high resolution chromosomes in the study of acute leukemias and non-Hodgkin's lymphomas. In Fairbanks, V. F. (ed.): Current Hematology and Oncology. Vol 3. Chicago, Year Book Medical Publishers, 1984, p. 353.

69. Baer, R., et al.: Fusion of an immunoglobulin variable region gene and a T-cell receptor constant region gene in the chromosome 14 inversion associated with T cell tumors. Cell 43:705, 1985.

70. Dewald, G. W., et al.: Chromosome abnormalities in malignant hematologic disorders. Mayo Clin. Proc. 60:675, 1985.

70A. Pearson, G. R.: Recent advances in research on the Epstein-Barr virus and associated diseases. In Fairbanks, V. F. (ed.): Current Hematology and Oncology. Vol. 4. Chicago, Year Book Medical Publishers, 1986, p. 123.

71. Louie, S., et al.: Immunodeficiency and the pathogenesis of non-Hodgkin's lymphoma. Semin. Oncol. 7:267, 1980.

72. Shaw, G. M., et al.: Human T cell leukemia virus: Its discovery and role in leukemogenesis and immunosuppression. Adv. Intern. Med. 30:1, 1984.

73. Felber, B. K., et al.: The pX protein of HTLV-I is a transcriptional activator of its long terminal repeats. Science 229:675, 1985.

74. Sadmori, N., et al.: Abnormalities of chromosome 14 band 14 q11 in Japanese patients with adult T-cell leukemia. Cancer Genet. Cytogenet. 17:279, 1985.

75. Korsmeyer, S. J., et al.: Cellular origin of hairy cell leukemia: Malignant B cells that express receptors for T cell growth factor. Semin. Oncol. 11:394, 1984.

76. Blayney, D. W., et al.: The human T-cell leukemia/lymphoma virus, lymphoma, lytic bone lesions, and hypercalcemia. Ann. Intern. Med. 98:144, 1983.

77. Ash, R. C., et al.: In vitro studies of human pluripotent hematopoietic progenitors in polycythemia vera. Direct evidence of stem cell involvement. J. Clin. Invest. 69:1112, 1982.

78. Ellis, J. T., et al.: Studies of the bone marrow in polycythemia vera and evolution of myelofibrosis and second malignancies. Semin. Hematol. 23:144, 1986.

79. Annotation. Fibrosis of the marrow: Content and causes. Br. J. Haematol. 59:1, 1985.

80. McKenna, R., et al.: Granulated T lymphocytosis with neutropenia: Malignant or benign chronic lymphoproliferative disorder? Blood 66:259, 1985.

81. Kyle, R. A.: Diagnosis and management of multiple myeloma and related disorders. Prog. Hematol. 14:257, 1986.

82. Oken, M. M.: Multiple myeloma. Med. Clin. North Am. 68:757, 1984.

83. Durie, B. G. M.: Recent advances in multiple myeloma and the related monoclonal gammopathies. In Fairbanks, V. F. (ed.): Current Hematology and Oncology. Vol 3. Chicago, Year Book Medical Publishers, 1984, p. 239.

84. Heptinstall, R. H.: Pathology of the Kidney. 3rd ed. Boston, Little, Brown & Co., 1983, p. 993.

85. McIntyre, O. R.: Current concepts in cancer. Multiple myeloma. N. Engl. J. Med. 301:193, 1979.

86. Karpatkin, S.: Autoimmune thrombocytopenic purpura. Semin. Hematol. 22:260, 1985.

87. Kelton, J. G., et al.: Detection of a platelet-agglutinating factor in thrombotic thrombocytopenic purpura. Ann. Intern. Med. 101:598, 1984.

88. Kumar, R., and Deykin, D.: Pathogenesis and practical management of coagulopathy of liver disease. In Davidson, C. S. (ed.): Problems in Liver Disease. New York, Stratton Intercontinental Medical Book Corp., 1979, p. 66.

89. Ruggeri, Z. M., and Zimmerman, T. S.: Platelets and von Willebrand's disease. Semin. Hematol. 22:203, 1985.

90. Moroose, R., and Hoyer, L. W.: von Willebrand factor and platelet function. Ann. Rev. Med. 37:157, 1986.

91. Oberle, I., et al.: Genetic screening for hemophilia A (classic hemophilia) with a polymorphic DNA probe. N. Engl. J. Med. 312:682, 1985.

92. Epstein, M. A., and Morgan, A. J.: Clinical consequences of Epstein-Barr virus infection and possible control by an antiviral vaccine. Clin. Exp. Immunol. 53:257, 1983.

93. Wolf, H., and Seibl, R.: Benign and malignant disease caused by EBV. J. Invest. Dermatol. (Suppl. 1) 83:88, 1984.

94. Sullivan, J. L.: Epstein-Barr virus and the X-linked lymphoproliferative syndrome. Adv. Pediatr. 30:365, 1983.

95. Murray, B. J.: Medical complications of infectious mononucleosis. Am. Fam. Physician 30:195, 1984.

96. Purtilo, D. T., et al.: Epstein-Barr virus-induced diseases in boys with the X-linked proliferative syndrome (XLP). Am. J. Med. 73:49, 1982.

97. Carithers, H. A.: Cat-scratch disease associated with an osteolytic lesion. Am. J. Dis. Child. 137:968, 1983.

98. Wear, D. J., et al.: Cat-scratch disease: A bacterial infection. Science 221:1403, 1983.

99. Miller-Catchpole, R., et al.: Cat-scratch disease. Identification of bacteria in seven cases of lymphadenitis. Am. J. Surg. Pathol. 10:276, 1986.

100. Gianotte, F., and Caputo, R.: Histiocytic syndromes: A review. J. Am. Acad. Dermatol. 13:383, 1985.

101. Basset, F., et al.: The histiocytoses. Pathol. Annu. (Part 2):27, 1983.

102. Burgdorf, W. H. C.: Malignant histiocytic infiltrates. In Murphy, G. F., and Mihm, M. C., Jr. (eds.): Lymphoproliferative Disorders of the Skin. London, Butterworth's, 1986, p. 217.

# 13

# The Respiratory System

The lungs are the most used and abused organs in the body. Besides constantly exchanging carbon dioxide for life-giving oxygen, they must at the same time not only cope with hundreds of air pollutants (including, inconsiderately, tobacco smoke) but also fend off countless airborne allergens, viruses, bacteria, and other microbes. No small wonder that the lungs are so often injured. Respiratory infections are more frequent than infections of any other organ, particularly in individuals predisposed by debilitating disease. Lung cancer kills more people in Western populations than does any other form of malignancy. Mention has already been made of the many forms of dust-induced pneumoconiosis (p. 254) and the pulmonary consequences of smoking (p. 253). When the heart fails, the lungs become secondarily burdened with excess blood volumes (p. 313). Lung pathology thus looms large.

Only the primary lung diseases that are encountered with reasonable frequency in general medical practice and not discussed elsewhere will be discussed in some detail here. Some of the less common entities will be treated briefly at the end of the chapter.

## PULMONARY EMBOLISM, INFARCTION, AND HEMORRHAGE

The clinical importance of pulmonary embolism cannot be overstated—it is estimated to be the sole cause of death annually of about 100,000 patients in the United States and a major contributing cause in an equal number of deaths. Thus, in this country it is the number three killer (preceded only by heart disease and cancer). The origins of pulmonary embolism were discussed on page 75, but the following points should be emphasized. (1) *Occlusions of the pulmonary arteries by blood clots are almost always embolic, arising from thrombi usually in the deep veins of the legs.* Secondary thrombosis may then build up about the emboli. (2) *Thrombi in the leg veins* are extremely common; depending on the vigor with which they are sought, *they are found in 10 to 65% of autopsies of hospitalized patients.*[1] (3) *Venous thrombosis and pulmonary embolism are particularly common in the following clinical settings—prolonged bed rest; immobilization of an extremity; congestive heart failure; following burns, multiple fractures, and any form of severe trauma; during and after parturition; with disseminated cancer and in women who have taken oral contraceptive pills containing high levels of estrogen such as were used in the past. (4) These thrombi are unsuspected, as is the subsequent pulmonary embolism in most cases. (5) Death may follow a large embolic event within seconds to hours before the diagnosis can be established and before infarction necrosis can develop. (6) When less large, they may not be fatal and may or may not cause infarction, as will be explained.*

MORPHOLOGY. To be emphasized, **embolism is not synonymous with infarction. The consequences of a pulmonary embolism depend on (1) the size of the embolic mass; (2) the related size of the occluded artery; and (3) the state of the general and pulmonary circulations.** Large, often coiled emboli may occlude the main pulmonary outflow tract, impact astride the bifurcation (**saddle embolus**), or lodge in one of the main pulmonary arteries. Death usually follows so suddenly from hypoxemia or acute dilatation of the right heart (acute cor pulmonale) that there is no time for morphologic alterations in the lung parenchyma. **Smaller emboli impact in more peripheral arteries, and with adequate cardiovascular circulation, the bronchial arteries may suffice to sustain the vitality of the lung parenchyma but the alveolar spaces often fill with blood to produce a pulmonary hemorrhage. With inadequate cardiovascular circulation, as in congestive heart disease, the pulmonary arterial occlusion would lead to infarction.** Thus, infarctions tend to be more common in the elderly, who are more likely to suffer from cardiac insufficiency. **The more peripheral the embolic occlusion, the more likely infarction.**[2]

Infarcts of the lungs have an apex pointing toward the hilus of the lung and a roughly pyramidal shape extending always to the pleural surface. Often there is a fibrinous exudate over the affected pleura. As discussed earlier on page 77, they are classically hemorrhagic at least at the outset and appear as raised red-blue consolidations (Fig. 13–1). Sometimes the occluded vessel can be identified near the apex. In the course of a few days, as the red cells lyse, the color fades slightly and eventually becomes red-brown as hemosiderin replaces the hemoglobin. If the patient survives, the infarcted area is eventually converted into a contracted gray-white, sometimes hemosiderin-pigmented scar. Often multiple emboli and infarcts are present, sometimes of different ages. The individual with a single embolic event has a 30% chance of one or more subsequent embolisms. Moreover, a single large embolus may fragment and induce multiple infarcts. **The hallmark of pulmonary infarction is ischemic necrosis of the lung substance, including alveolar walls, bronchioles, and blood vessels. It is this ischemic necrosis that differentiates the pulmonary infarct from pulmonary hemorrhage (having preservation of the vitality of the native architecture).** More-

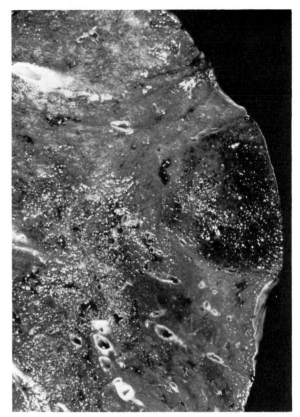

Figure 13–1. A relatively recent, small, roughly wedge-shaped hemorrhagic pulmonary infarct (*right*).

over, the pulmonary hemorrhage is not necessarily peripheral in location (Fig. 13–2).

An infected embolus or infarction of an already infected segment of the lung leads to a **septic infarct** which in time may be converted into an abscess.

CLINICAL COURSE. The clinical consequences of a pulmonary embolus or multiple emboli depend on (a) the amount of the total pulmonary arterial supply occluded—a function of the size and number of obstructed arteries; (b) the general status of the cardiovascular circulation; (c) prompt diagnosis and effectiveness of therapy; and (d) the institution of measures to prevent subsequent embolism (anticoagulation, insertion of a lower vena caval "umbrella" screen, ligation of the inferior vena cava). Based on these variables, the following syndromes may be encountered.

○ *Sudden death with massive pulmonary embolism* (occlusion of the blood supply to four out of the five pulmonary lobes). This is one of the few causes of instantaneous death.

○ *Sudden chest pain, syncope, and dyspnea with occlusion of large lobar vessels.* This syndrome may closely mimic myocardial infarction, and differential diagnosis may require such tests as perfusion lung scan and pulmonary angiography. The patient may or may not survive, depending on the

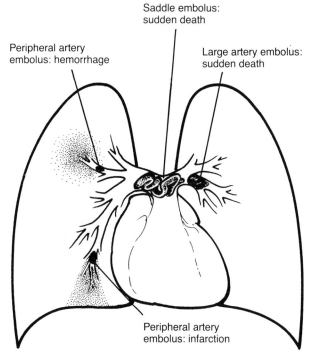

Saddle embolus:
sudden death

Peripheral artery
embolus: hemorrhage

Large artery embolus:
sudden death

Peripheral artery
embolus: infarction

**Figure 13–2.** Diagram representing patterns of pulmonary emboli. The two large central emboli cause sudden death but do not induce infarction. The peripheral arterial embolus at the base causes infarction, whereas the analogous small embolus in a younger patient causes only hemorrhage.

preexisting lung function and cardiovascular circulation. Thus most deaths occur in those over the age of 50. The dyspnea is related to some loss of functioning pulmonary parenchyma but also to vasoconstrictive neuronal reflexes or vasoconstrictor agents. Moreover, hemodynamic compromise is induced by the increased strain on the right heart. If the patient can be kept alive during the immediate postembolic period, the arterial obstruction may rapidly or slowly abate. The embolus may fragment and the small segments be driven out to the periphery, where they may cause small infarcts or be without effect. Alternatively, there may be slower restitution of flow induced first by clot contraction followed by progressive fibrinolysis.[3] To augment this process, fibrinolytic agents are administered to enhance the lysis of the clot.[4] With these, total resolution may occur in hours to days. When not totally resolved, the residual blood clot will become organized into an intimal fibrous plaque that in time may be converted into an atheroma or sometimes into fibrous webs bridging the vascular lumen.

○ *Smaller emboli may be totally asymptomatic, produce an episode of chest pain, cough, and hemoptysis (if there has been only pulmonary hemorrhage), or with infarction may cause chest pain, pleuritic pain, cough, hemoptysis, and possibly mild dyspnea.* Obviously much depends on the number of emboli and the prior cardiopulmonary status of the patient. Typically the infarcts are readily visualized on chest radiograph. Here again, the emboli may resolve or undergo organization. *Multiple small pulmonary emboli compatible with survival may cause pulmonary hypertension and eventually chronic cor pulmonale.*

The recognition of pulmonary embolism and appropriate therapeutic measures materially influence the outcome, as is well shown in Figure 13–3. New fibrinolytic agents promise even better results.[5]

**Figure 13–3.** Diagrammatic representation of the estimated total annual incidence of patients with symptomatic pulmonary emboli in the United States (*top box*). The outcome in each category (number of patients and percentage) is shown in descending order. (From Bell, W. R. and Simon, T. L.: Current status of pulmonary thromboembolic disease. Pathophysiology, diagnosis, prevention and treatment. Am. Heart J. *103*:239, 1982.)

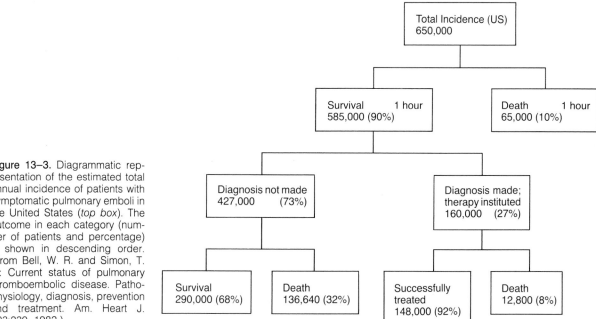

Total Incidence (US)
650,000

Survival        1 hour
585,000 (90%)

Death        1 hour
65,000 (10%)

Diagnosis not made
427,000        (73%)

Diagnosis made;
therapy instituted
160,000        (27%)

Survival
290,000 (68%)

Death
136,640 (32%)

Successfully
treated
148,000 (92%)

Death
12,800 (8%)

# PULMONARY VASCULAR SCLEROSIS

This term refers to the vascular changes associated with pulmonary hypertension. In most instances, plausible pathophysiologic mechanisms can be identified to explain the pulmonary hypertension and so the vascular alterations are referred to as *secondary pulmonary vascular sclerosis.* In about 1% of instances, the basis for the rise in pulmonary blood pressure is obscure, and the vascular lesions are called *primary pulmonary vascular sclerosis.*

*Secondary pulmonary vascular sclerosis* will develop whenever there is some basis for increased resistance to flow in the pulmonary arterial bed or when there is protracted volume overload. The principal conditions associated with secondary pulmonary vascular sclerosis and some of the speculations related to the primary form are given in Table 13–1.

The vascular alterations in all forms of pulmonary sclerosis (primary and secondary) involve the entire arterial tree down to the level of the capillaries, but the nature of the vascular change varies with the size of the vessel (Fig. 13–4). (1) **In the main arteries, the lesions take the form of atheromas** similar to those in systemic atherosclerosis but rarely as severe. (2) In **medium-sized arteries intimal thickening and neomuscularization develops.** (3) **Smaller arteries and arterioles** develop the most striking changes with intimal

thickening, **medial hypertrophy, and reduplication of the internal and external elastic membranes.** In such vessels, the wall thickness may exceed the lumen, which is sometimes narrowed to the point of near obliteration. The severity of all these alterations appears to be a function of the level of elevation of the pulmonary arterial pressure; the alterations are best developed in the primary form. (4) A distinctive arteriolar change (**plexiform lesion**) consists of intraluminal angiomatous tufts that may fuse to form webs that bridge the vascular lumen. This pattern of alterations is thought by some to be diagnostic of primary hypertension.[6]

*Secondary pulmonary vascular sclerosis* may develop at any age. The clinical features reflect in general the underlying disease, usually pulmonary or cardiac, with accentuation of respiratory insufficiency and right-heart strain. *Primary pulmonary vascular sclerosis,* on the other hand, is almost always encountered in young individuals, more commonly women, and is marked by fatigue, syncope (particularly on exercise), dyspnea on exertion, and sometimes chest pain.[7] These patients eventually develop severe respiratory insufficiency and sometimes cyanosis. In this form of the condition, death usually results from right-heart failure, usually within a few years of the diagnosis. Some amelioration of the respiratory distress can be achieved by vasodilators, but the ultimate outcome can at best only be delayed.

---

**Table 13–1. CLASSIFICATION OF CAUSES OF PULMONARY VASCULAR SCLEROSIS**

**Secondary Pulmonary Vascular Sclerosis**
  ***Increased Resistance***
    *Obstructive Conditions*
      Multiple pulmonary emboli
      Large pulmonary surgical resections
      Mitral stenosis
      Pulmonary veno-occlusive disease
    *Arterial Narrowing*
      Scleroderma
      Wegener's granulomatosis
    *Chronic Hypoxia with Vasoconstriction*
      Chronic obstructive pulmonary disease
      Chronic interstitial pneumonitis
      Pneumoconiosis
      Residence at high altitude
  ***Increased Volume Flow***
    *Congenital Heart Disease*
      Atrial septal defect
      Ventricular septal defect
      Tetralogy of Fallot
      Transposition of the great vessels
**Primary Pulmonary Vascular Sclerosis** (unknown origin—many theories)
    Abnormal pulmonary arterial reactivity to neurohumoral constrictor influences—supportive evidence, concurrence of Raynaud's phenomenon.
    Some form of immune-mediated collagen vascular disease.
    Exposure to agents causing chronic vasoconstriction, e.g., drugs, "Bush Tea" derived from crotalaria.
    Endothelial injury (of unknown cause) followed by prolonged vasoconstriction possibly related to elaboration of prostaglandins.

---

# ADULT RESPIRATORY DISTRESS SYNDROME (ARDS)

ARDS is a form of diffuse pulmonary disease that complicates the course of many varied clinical conditions, some of which are not pulmonary disorders. It is therefore not a primary disease. *Basically, it comprises severe widespread increased alveolar capillary permeability, secondary to injury to the alveolar lining epithelium and capillary endothelium. It leads first to the accumulation of a protein-rich edematous fluid within the alveolar septal walls, followed by escape of the fluid into the alveolar spaces. Coagulation of the exudative fluid containing fibrin and cell debris produces hyaline membranes lining the alveolar walls.* As a consequence there is marked impairment of gas exchange, causing severe dyspnea, tachypnea, marked hypoxemia with cyanosis (which is refractory to oxygen therapy), and diffuse bilateral pulmonary infiltrates on radiograph.[8] Although the acute changes are reversible, in some instances they are followed by interstitial fibrosis inducing decreased lung compliance.

The principal conditions associated with ARDS are presented in Table 13–2. With these many associations ARDS has come to be known by several different terms, including *"shock lung," "traumatic wet lung,"* and *"pump lung,"* but perhaps most useful because it best characterizes the lesion is the term *"diffuse alveolar damage"* (DAD).

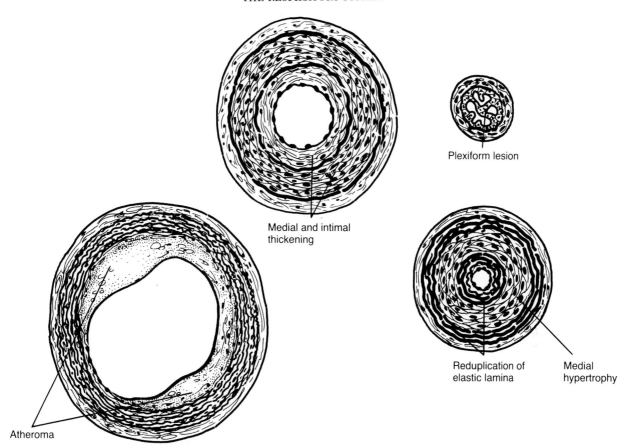

Plexiform lesion

Medial and intimal
thickening

Reduplication of
elastic lamina

Medial
hypertrophy

Atheroma

**Figure 13–4.** Diagrammatic representation of patterns of pulmonary vascular sclerosis, based on the size of affected vessels. Atheroma formation is virtually limited to large vessels; medial and intimal thickening with reduplication of elastica is seen in medium-sized and somewhat smaller arteries, and the plexiform lesion occurs in very small arteries and arterioles.

**Table 13–2.** CAUSES OF ARDS*

| | |
|---|---|
| **Shock** | **Hematologic Disorders** |
| All forms | Disseminated |
| **Infection** | intravascular |
| Gram-negative sepsis | coagulation |
| Diffuse pneumonia | Thrombotic |
| (viral, bacterial, or | thrombocytopenic |
| fungal) | purpura |
| **Trauma** | Multiple transfusions |
| Lung contusion | **Metabolic Disorders** |
| Nonthoracic trauma | Pancreatitis |
| Head injury | Uremia |
| **Inhaled Irritants** | **Miscellaneous** |
| Oxygen toxicity | Cardiopulmonary bypass |
| Smoke | Eclampsia |
| Irritant gases | Fat embolism |
| **Liquid Aspiration** | Amniotic and air |
| Gastric juice | embolism |
| Near-drowning | High altitude |
| **Drug Overdose or** | Radiation pneumonitis |
| **Sensitivity** | |
| Heroin | |
| Barbiturates | |
| Acetylsalicylic acid | |
| Paraquat | |
| Bleomysin | |

*Modified from Hasleton, P. S.: Adult respiratory distress syndrome—A review. Histopathology 7:307, 1983.

**PATHOGENESIS.** With its diverse origins, a single pathogenetic mechanism for the increased capillary permeability in ARDS is most unlikely. Some conditions may primarily damage the alveolar epithelium; in others the endothelium may be the primary target, but ultimately both are involved. In a few settings there appear to be plausible explanations for the damage (e.g., aspiration of gastric contents, near-drowning, inhalation of irritant gases or smoke). Analogously, oxygen toxicity encountered with exposure to high concentrations (70 to 100%) of oxygen may induce injury by the formation of oxygen-derived free radicals (superoxide, singlet oxygen). But these few examples shed no light on most conditions that are sometimes complicated by ARDS. Three hypothetical, possibly interrelated, mechanisms have been invoked to explain these enigmas.[9]

○ Neutrophil-related injury

○ Formation of arachidonic acid metabolites

○ Activation of the coagulation-fibrinolytic sequences
  *Neutrophil-related injury* is currently a favored thesis.[10] It is proposed that in many different settings neutrophils accumulate in the lungs and initiate a train of events depicted in Figure 13–5. The stimulus

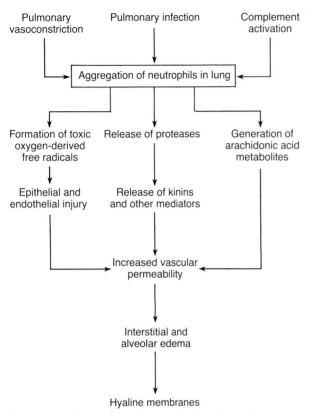

Figure 13–5. Postulated pathogenesis of adult respiratory distress syndrome (ARDS).

nopeptides, and platelet aggregation might contribute to activation of the arachidonic acid pathways and thus potentiate the alveolar injury in ARDS.

In sum, it seems likely that several mechanisms of initiating the pathogenetic sequence are possible and that in some settings all pathways participate to amplify the DAD.[13]

**MORPHOLOGY.** The anatomic changes are remarkably constant, whatever the precipitating condition. The lungs are heavy, dark red to blue, and have focal areas of atelectasis. Often they have a solid, fleshy consistency. Histologically, **the changes begin with capillary congestion and interstitial edema within the alveolar septa, which widens them.** At this time, the electron microscope will disclose injury to type I pneumonocytes and endothelial cells. As the process progresses, the protein-rich edema fluid leaks into the alveolar spaces. Often the alveolar fluid contains red cells, neutrophils, and macrophages. **Accumulation and coagulation of fibrinogen together with cell debris produces hyaline membranes lining the alveolar septa** (Fig. 13–6). Although these changes are reversible, with chronicity there is proliferation of type II pneumonocytes (type I cannot replicate), creating a cuboidal lining to the alveolar spaces; at the same time, the intraseptal edema undergoes fibrosis to thus produce a fibrosing interstitial pneu-

for PMN accumulation might be pulmonary vasoconstriction with exaggeration of normal sequestration; pulmonary infection; activation of complement; or formation of leukotrienes from arachidonic acid. Thereon release of neutrophil proteases and formation of oxygen-derived free radicals mediate the alveolar damage and augment the arachidonic acid cascades.[11] Furthermore, once the injury begins it is autocatalytic with increased accumulation of neutrophils and, in this manner, the downward spiral gains speed.

*Arachidonic acid derivatives* offer an alternative mechanism. ARDS has been observed in neutropenic patients in whom the disease developed in the absence of neutrophils in the lungs.[12] The release of prostaglandins, thromboxane, and leukotrienes from macrophages, platelets, and pulmonary endothelium could well account for all of the features of ARDS. The arachidonic acid derivatives cause pulmonary vasoconstriction, increase vascular permeability, and enhance adherence of such neutrophils as may be present. The secondary release of mediators from platelets, macrophages, and neutrophils might then make their contributions, augmenting the pulmonary injury.

*Activation of the coagulation sequence and fibrinolysis* might underlie ARDS in such settings as DIC, thrombotic thrombocytopenic purpura, lung contusion, endotoxemia, and possibly other clinical disorders. Thereafter complement activation, fibri-

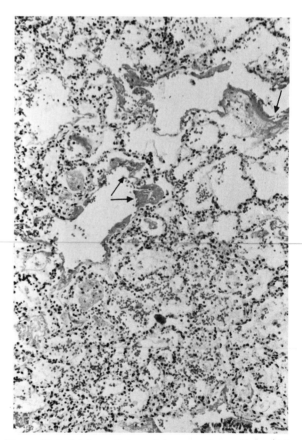

Figure 13–6. Adult respiratory distress syndrome. Some of the alveoli are collapsed, others distended. Many contain proteinaceous debris, desquamated cells, and, here and there, hyaline membranes (*arrows*).

monitis.[8] In fatal cases, bronchopneumonia may supervene.

ARDS is a feared complication because it makes an already serious clinical condition worse. During the acute phase the interposition of edema fluid hampers alveolar-capillary gas exchange and thus renders these individuals hypoxemic. This is worsened by reduction in lung total volume and reduced compliance. Thus these patients often require supportive, positive-end-expiratory-pressure (PEEP) therapy, but care must be taken not to add an element of oxygen toxicity. With this approach, the mortality (often precipitated by the development of bronchopneumonia), which once was about 70%, has now been reduced to 20%. Should the patients survive the acute phase, they are at risk of developing interstitial fibrosis, which can make respiratory cripples of them and ultimately cause death from chronic cor pulmonale.

## NEONATAL RESPIRATORY DISTRESS SYNDROME (HYALINE MEMBRANE DISEASE)

There are many causes of respiratory distress in the newborn, including (1) excessive sedation of the mother, (2) fetal head injury during delivery, (3) asphyxial aspiration of blood clot or amniotic fluid, and (4) intrauterine hypoxia due to coiling of the umbilical cord about the neck. But far more common and ominous is the so-called *neonatal respiratory distress syndrome* (NRDS), also known as *hyaline membrane disease* (HMD) because of the prominence of these membranes in the lungs of infants dying of this condition. Although with the other causes of respiratory distress the newborn may be apneic or hypoxic from the moment of birth, *in HMD the infant appears normal at birth but within minutes to a few hours, a labored, grunting respiration appears, which progressively worsens* and, unless controlled by therapy, causes death. Indeed, HMD accounts for about 20% of all deaths in the first 28 days of life.

*HMD (NRDS) is basically a disease of premature infants*, encountered in 10 to 16% of those weighing less than 2500 gm at birth.[14] Most affected infants weigh 1000 to 1500 gm. *Other contributing influences are diabetes in the mother, caesarian section before the onset of labor, and prenatal asphyxia.*[15] Males are at greater risk than females.

The pathophysiology of this condition is better presented after the morphology.

On gross examination, the lungs are firmer and heavier than normal and are a mottled, red-purple color. Histologically, there are alternating areas of atelectasis and hyperinflation. However, when lung sections are taken immediately after death rather than after a lag of several hours, the lungs are much more evenly aerated.[16] Congestion of the alveolar capillaries is marked. **The most distinctive morphologic feature is the hyaline membrane, which is seen in both the collapsed and the aerated air space.** These changes are highly reminiscent of those in the adult respiratory distress syndrome (see Fig. 13–6). Sometimes the hyaline membrane appears as a thin, acidophilic, amorphous coagulum lining the alveolus; in other instances, it almost fills the air space. Embedded within the hyaline membrane or lying within the alveoli are disintegrating necrotic cells and occasional squamous cells of amniotic origin. Finely granular edema fluid is often present within the alveoli, and red cell extravasation may be seen within the interstitium, as well as in the air spaces.

*In these infants, two basic defects have been identified that explain most of the anatomic findings: (1) a deficiency of pulmonary surfactant and (2) increased pulmonary epithelial permeability.*

The *deficiency of pulmonary surfactant* is attributable in most instances to the immaturity of the lungs in the preterm infant. In utero, the pulmonary air spaces are of course filled with fluid into which, as term is approached, surfactant is secreted by type II pneumonocytes. This pulmonary fluid ebbs and flows into the amniotic fluid as the fetus matures. Surfactant reduces the surface tension in air-fluid interfaces and thus the tendency after birth for alveoli to collapse on expiration. Among the surfactants elaborated, dipalmitoylphosphatidylcholine (DPPC) is most active. Synthesis of surfactant increases throughout fetal development and becomes maximal at 34 to 36 weeks, thus providing for the normal transition of the liquid-lung to the stable air-lung. With a deficiency of surfactant, the newborn has difficulty inflating its lungs and they tend to collapse on expiration, so that subsequent breaths are as difficult as the first. Vaginal delivery further facilitates emptying of the fluid from the fetal lungs by producing chest wall compression and may in some obscure manner enhance secretion of surfactant, explaining why caesarian delivery constitutes a predisposing influence for HMD.

Although surfactant deficiency can explain the atelectasis and congestion seen in these lungs, *increased pulmonary epithelial permeability* has been invoked to account for the protein-rich edema fluid in the alveolar spaces and, most notably, the hyaline membranes.[17] The mechanisms underlying this epithelial change are not clear but could involve mechanical disruption or release of chemical mediators (including arachidonic acid derivatives) followed by recruitment of white cells with their injurious enzymes or free radicals.

The most effective method of reducing the morbidity and mortality from HMD is prevention—notably prevention of premature delivery until the maturing lung is capable of synthesis of adequate surfactant. Reasonably reliable estimates of fetal pulmonary maturity can be achieved by measuring the concentration of surfactants within amniotic fluid obtained by amniocentesis. Although many biochemical precursors can be measured, the most reliable test is the lecithin-to-sphingomyelin ratio (L/S). Lecithin is phosphatidylcholine; its level rises sharply at 34 to 36 weeks of gestation, whereas the level of sphingomyelin either does not change or falls. An L/S ratio of approximately 2 indicates fetal pulmonary maturity, 1.2 indicates a possible risk of HMD, and less than 1 a definite risk. When the tests indicate pulmonary immaturity, efforts are made to delay preterm delivery. The mortality rate varies widely, depending on the birth weight and level of pulmonary immaturity and on the effectiveness of therapy in staving off fatal hypoxemia long enough for the "wee-one" to get its "surfactant motors" running.

## ATELECTASIS

Atelectasis refers either to incomplete expansion of the lungs at birth (*atelectasis neonatorum*) or to collapse of previously fully aerated alveoli, usually in the adult (*acquired atelectasis*).

### Atelectasis Neonatorum

This form may be further subdivided into *primary* and *secondary* patterns. *Primary atelectasis neonatorum* implies that respiration has never been fully established. It is most common in premature infants whose respiratory centers in the brain are not mature and whose respiratory motions are feeble. Precipitating factors include any obstetric complication leading to intrauterine hypoxia during delivery.

The lungs at autopsy are collapsed, red-blue, noncrepitant, flabby, and rubbery. Characteristically, these lungs fail to float when immersed in water. Histologically, the alveoli resemble the native fetal lung, with uniformly small alveolar spaces, surrounded by thick septal walls, which have a crumpled appearance. A prominent cuboidal epithelium lines the alveolar spaces, and often there is a granular, proteinaceous precipitate mixed with amniotic debris within the air spaces.

*Secondary atelectasis neonatorum* represents the form encountered in the neonatal respiratory distress syndrome, discussed earlier.

### Acquired Atelectasis

Atelectasis in the adult always implies some intrathoracic disorder causing collapse of previously expanded airspaces. Thus, it has been divided into *absorption, compression, contraction,* and *patchy atelectasis* (Fig. 13–7). These terms merely allude to the underlying mechanism causing the lung collapse or to the distribution of the changes.

*Absorption atelectasis* occurs whenever an airway is fully obstructed so that air cannot enter the distal parenchyma. The air already present is gradually absorbed into the blood, with collapse of the alveoli.

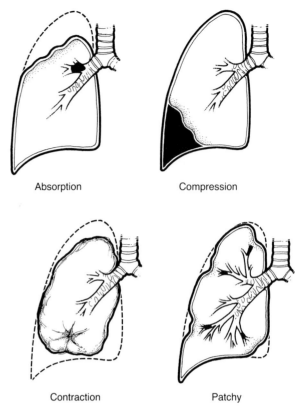

Figure 13–7. Illustration of the various forms of atelectasis in the adult. See text for details.

Depending on the level of airway obstruction, an entire lung, a complete lobe, or a patchy segment may be involved. The most frequent cause of absorption collapse is obstruction of a bronchus by a mucus plug. This frequently occurs postoperatively. Bronchial asthma, bronchiectasis, and acute and chronic bronchitis may also lead to obstruction by mucopurulent plugs. Sometimes obstruction is caused by the aspiration of foreign bodies or blood clots, particularly in children or during oral surgery or anesthesia. Airways may also be obstructed by tumors, especially bronchogenic carcinoma; by enlarged lymph nodes (as from tuberculosis, for example), and by vascular aneurysms.

*Compression atelectasis* most often is associated with accumulations of fluid, blood, or air within the pleural cavity, which mechanically cause collapse of the adjacent lung. This is a frequent occurrence with a pleural effusion from any cause but is perhaps most commonly associated with hydrothorax from congestive heart failure. Pneumothorax (p. 452) also leads to compression atelectasis. In bedridden patients and in patients with ascites, basal atelectasis results from the elevated position of the diaphragms.

*Contraction atelectasis* occurs when fibrotic changes in the lung or pleura hamper expansion and increase the recoil during expiration.

*Patchy atelectasis* comprises multiple small areas of collapsed lung, as occurs with multiple bronchiolar obstructions from secretions or exudate or in both the adult and neonatal respiratory distress syndromes.

In a small number of cases, the atelectasis of uncertain pathogenesis follows injury to the chest wall.

With massive collapse, or with a large pneumothorax, the entire lung may be folded against the mediastinum, leaving an unoccupied pleural space. Usually, however, collapse does not involve the whole lung and is not complete. With absorption collapse, especially, there is some collateral aeration through the pores of Kohn and some edema fluid is present. Compression atelectasis caused by pleural effusion or elevated diaphragms is usually basal and bilateral. The collapsed lung parenchyma is shrunken below the level of the surrounding lung substance and is red-blue, rubbery, and subcrepitant, with a wrinkled overlying pleura. Histologically, the collapsed alveoli are slit-like. Congestion and dilatation of the septal vasculature are usually present as a result of loss of the compressive force of the air. Compensatory overinflation of the unaffected lung parenchyma usually develops.

Acquired atelectasis may be either acute or chronic. Usually that caused by mucus plugs occurs relatively acutely, manifested by the sudden onset of dyspnea. Indeed, the development of acute respiratory distress within 48 hours of a surgical procedure is almost always diagnostic of atelectasis. It is important that atelectasis be diagnosed early and that there be prompt reexpansion of the involved lung, because the collapsed parenchyma is extremely vulnerable to superimposed infection. Persistent atelectasis of a segment of the lung may be an important clue to the presence of a silent bronchogenic carcinoma.

## SUDDEN INFANT DEATH SYNDROME (SIDS)

This particularly tragic calamity, sometimes referred to as *"cot death"* is taken up here because current evidence favors some form of respiratory dysfunction as its primary cause in most instances.[18] Often these infants have from birth irregularities of the respiratory rhythm with apneic spells and sometimes "near-miss" hypoxia that either spontaneously resolves or may require resuscitation. These abnormal breathing patterns are indicative of high risk.

SIDS can be defined as *the sudden unexpected death of an infant between one week and one year of age (most often between one and four months) which remains unexplained, despite a thorough post mortem examination.* Usually the death occurs during sleep and without apparent struggle. Unhappily, SIDS is not a rare event, occurring in the United States in about 2 per 1000 live births. Higher rates are encountered in many developing countries. Not all deaths in this age group are due to SIDS, because about one half are birth determined or the conse-

quence of accident or acquired disease.[19] Nonetheless, cot death is the single most common cause of infant death.

Intensive epidemiologic studies have identified many factors relating to both mother and infant that are associated with an increased risk of SIDS (Table 13–3).[20]

Anatomic studies of these victims have yielded a variety of findings, usually subtle, of uncertain significance and inconstant (i.e., not present in all cases). But by definition an overt cause of death such as bronchopneumonia or a lethal malformation is lacking. The inconstancy of the findings is not surprising because many derangements could lead to this unfortunate consequence. In about two thirds of the cases, subtle alterations have been identified in the structures controlling respiratory and cardiac rhythm (brain stem, carotid bodies, vagus nerves) and in tissues sensitive to chronic hypoxemia (brain, lungs, periadrenal brown fat, adrenal medulla); examples are subtle gliosis in the brain stem in proximity to medullary centers or abnormally small carotid body chemoreceptors or lesions in the coronary branches supplying the conduction system. The changes could well have led to or be secondary to chronic hypoxia. So, the possibility exists that they are not the basic defects. Right ventricular hypertrophy and excessive muscularization of the small pulmonary arteries have also been described; they are possibly related to alveolar hypoxia and pulmonary vasconstriction.[21] Airway blockage has also been implicated, such as might occur with a particularly large tongue that might recess during sleep, a hypermobile mandible that might prolapse during deep sleep, or laryngeal mucous gland hyperplasia that could contribute to excessive secretions. It is evident that straws are being clutched.

In about a third of SIDS cases mechanisms other than those relating to the cardiopulmonary systems have been implicated. Principal among these is infection. Most deaths occur during the winter months and therefore upper respiratory viral infections are suspect. Recently attention has been drawn to unsuspected intestinal infections of *Clostridium botulinum* as a potential cause of death.[22] Overheating caused by excessive clothing or wrapping has also

**Table 13–3. FACTORS ASSOCIATED WITH SIDS**

| Maternal | Infant |
|---|---|
| Young (less than 20 years of age) | Prematurity |
| Unmarried | Low birth weight |
| Short intergestational intervals | Male sex |
| Low socioeconomic group | Product of a multiple birth |
| Smoking | Not the first sibling |
| Drug abuse | SIDS in a prior sibling |
| Risk greater for American blacks than whites (? socioeconomic) | |

been implicated. The litany of speculative hypotheses could be continued, but it suffices that satisfactory explanations are usually lacking to explain these unexplained deaths.

# CHRONIC OBSTRUCTIVE PULMONARY DISEASE (COPD)

Several anatomically distinct diseases of the lung produce remarkably similar respiratory difficulties—chronic airflow limitation, mainly increased resistance to expiratory airflow. Principal among these disorders are *chronic bronchitis and, especially, bronchiolitis* with involvement of the small ramifications less than 2 mm in diameter (*small airway disease*) and *emphysema*, characterized by abnormal enlargement of the airspaces distal to the terminal bronchioles and damage to alveolar septa.[23] Bronchitis and bronchiolitis increase resistance to airflow, because inflammation and secretions narrow the airways, whereas in emphysema damage to the septal walls not only reduces the elastic recoil of the lung but also is often accompanied by small airway disease. It is so often difficult clinically (if not impossible) to differentiate these conditions and, moreover, they so often appear concurrently that clinicians refer to them collectively as COPD, or COLD (Chronic Obstructive Lung Disease). Some authorities also include asthma and bronchiectasis within the category of COPD. *Asthma*, as will become evident, is usually characterized by spasmodic attacks of airflow obstruction, but it sometimes causes persistent airflow limitation in the condition known as chronic asthmatic bronchitis, which has features of both asthma and chronic bronchitis. *Bronchiectasis*, a form of severe infective destruction of the bronchi and larger bronchioles, is infrequently responsible for COPD, and only when very generalized.

Several qualifications need emphasis at this time. "Pure" emphysema (in the absence of airways disease) may or may not cause COPD, depending on its severity. The same might be said about "pure" bronchitis—bronchiolitis. Both patterns of disease are largely caused by cigarette smoking. Not surprisingly, then, the two conditions frequently coexist, and in this circumstance COPD is highly likely. Some concept of these inter-relationships is offered in Figure 13–8. Thus, although emphysema and chronic bronchitis may occur in relatively "pure" forms without causing COPD, their coexistence is almost certain to produce it.

From what has been said about the role of cigarette smoking, it will come as no surprise that the incidence of COPD has increased dramatically in the recent past. Indeed, COPD causes more morbidity and loss of time from the workplace than any other clinical disorder except heart disease. It may convert its victims into respiratory cripples and annually causes 10,000 to 20,000 deaths in the U.S.

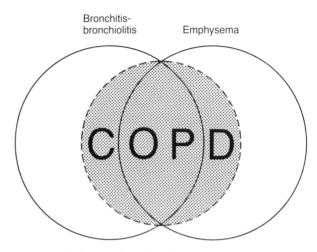

Figure 13–8. Interrelationships of bronchitis-bronchiolitis and emphysema in the production of chronic obstructive pulmonary disease (COPD). Note that when both conditions are present, the occurrence of COPD is virtually invariable. Less often, one or the other disorder alone induces COPD.

## CHRONIC BRONCHITIS (INCLUDING SMALL AIRWAY DISEASE)

Involvement of the pulmonary airways may affect principally the larger bronchi or the small bronchioles less than 2 mm in diameter, but frequently all levels are affected simultaneously. Some degree of irritation of the larger airways is so universal among cigarette smokers and urban dwellers in this era of air pollution that it is difficult to delimit it morphologically from significant bronchitis. Thus a clinical definition is employed, namely, *chronic bronchitis is present when there is a persistent productive cough for at least three consecutive months in at least two consecutive years.* Further subclassification may be employed, such as "simple chronic bronchitis," "chronic mucopurulent bronchitis" when there is presumably superimposed infection, and "chronic asthmatic bronchitis" when the basic disorder is complicated by attacks of bronchospasm. Ultimately, all are merely variations on a theme. When the involvement is restricted to the larger airways, there is usually no chronic airflow limitation at least at the outset, but when it is accompanied by bronchiolitis ("small airway disease") or emphysema, COPD is most likely.[24] Indeed, isolated severe chronic bronchiolitis in the absence of a coexistent chronic bronchitis or emphysema is extremely uncommon.

**PATHOGENESIS.** The distinctive clinical feature of chronic bronchitis-bronchiolitis is hypersecretion of mucus. *The single most important causative factor is cigarette smoking, although other air pollutants, such as sulfur dioxide and nitrogen dioxide, may contribute.*[25] These irritants directly or through neurohumoral pathways induce hypersecretion of the bronchial mucous glands, followed by gland hyperplasia and metaplastic formation of mucin-secreting goblet cells in the surface epithelium of both the large and small airways.[26] The secretion, when copious, contributes to airflow limitation in the larger airways. In the small airways it is even more obstructive because coexistent emphysema often causes loss of tissue support and changes in intra-alveolar intrabronchiolar air pressures, narrowing the finer airways and compounding the limitation of airflow. Microbial infection is often present, but it plays a secondary role. A host of organisms have been isolated from these patients, but the two commonest offenders are *Klebsiella* species and coagulase-positive staphylococci.[27] Viral agents such as adenovirus and respiratory syncytial rhinovirus are sometimes also identified.

**MORPHOLOGY.** Grossly, the mucosal lining of the larger airways is usually hyperemic, swollen, and boggy. Frequently it is covered by a layer of mucinous to mucopurulent secretions. The smaller bronchi and bronchioles may also be filled with similar secretion. Histologically, **the diagnostic features of chronic bronchitis in the major airways, including the trachea, is enlargement of the mucus-secreting glands.** This enlargement is attributable to both hyperactivity and hyperplasia of the glandular epithelium. The magnitude of the increase in size is assessed by the Reid Index—the ratio of the thickness of the submucosal gland layer to that of the bronchial wall. With clinically significant chronic bronchitis, the ratio usually exceeds 1:2. Concomitantly, there is often an increased number of goblet cells in the lining epithelium and loss of ciliated epithelial cells. One of the feared consequences of habitual cigarette smoking and protracted chronic bronchitis is the development of squamous metaplastic and dysplastic changes in the lining epithelial cells; these are important precursors to bronchogenic carcinoma. An inflammatory infiltrate is frequently present in the bronchial mucosa, largely mononuclear in the absence of infection, admixed with neutrophils when there is concomitant microbial infection, and containing eosinophils when there is an allergic component. **Chronic bronchiolitis** is marked by the metaplastic appearance of goblet cells in the lining epithelium. Concomitant inflammation and fibrosis of the walls narrows the lumens and sometimes causes complete obliteration (**bronchiolitis fibrosa obliterans**). These morphologic changes, particularly in the small airways, could well explain chronic airflow limitation.[28]

**CLINICAL COURSE.** The role that diseases of both the large and the smaller airways play in the production of COPD has already been pointed out. It should be reemphasized that it is the "small airway disease" that is mainly responsible for the airflow limitation. Bronchitis alone may be present for some time without causing ventilatory dysfunction; however, it is responsible for a prominent cough and the production of sputum. When dyspnea, hypoxemia, and hypercapnea appear, inadequate oxygenation of the blood may induce cyanosis. Chronic hypoxemia may also lead to persistent pulmonary vasoconstriction and ultimately to *cor pulmonale*. The combination of cyanosis and right-heart failure with its asso-ciated peripheral edema has led to these patients being termed "blue bloaters," in contrast to the emphysematous "pink puffers." However, these classic prototypes are uncommon and so these ungracious terms should be discarded. An even more feared consequence of chronic bronchitis with squamous metaplasia is bronchogenic carcinoma. Thus the very common chronic bronchitis and bronchiolitis are not trivial conditions.

## EMPHYSEMA

*Emphysema is defined as abnormal enlargement of the air spaces of the lung, accompanied by destruction of their walls.*[29] Some experts would broaden the definition to include enlargement of air spaces, whether or not accompanied by destructive changes in their walls. But this conception is not widely held, and so enlargement of air spaces, unaccompanied by destruction, is generally referred to as *overinflation* or *hyperinflation*.

Traditionally, four subvarieties of emphysema have been segregated based on the precise location of the pulmonary changes within the acinus, the unit of lung structure distal to the terminal bronchioles, where gas is exchanged (as is depicted in Figure 13–9A).[30] Reference to this figure will make the following characterizations more intelligible.

*Centrilobular emphysema* involves the *proximal acinus (i.e., the respiratory bronchioles)*, sparing, as depicted, in the early stages the more distal air spaces (Fig. 13–9B). However, with progression, dilatation and destruction of the walls of contiguous distal alveoli may occur. Typically, the changes are more common and more severe in the upper than in the lower zones of the lobes. This form of emphysema is predominantly a disease of cigarette smokers, is more common in males, and is rarely encountered in nonsmokers.

*Panacinar emphysema*, as the name indicates, involves more or less the entire acinus with *progressive enlargement of alveoli and alveolar ducts* and loss of distinction between the alveolar ducts and alveoli (Fig. 13–9C). With progression and destruction of alveolar walls, there is "simplification" of the lung architecture. When the process is diffuse, it is usually most marked at the lobar bases. This form of emphysema is more common in elderly women and is the pattern encountered in association with a genetic deficiency of alpha-1-antitrypsin (protease) inhibitor (discussed later). Although cigarette smoking may contribute to the genesis of this form of emphysema, the association is much less strong than with the centrilobular variant.

*Paraseptal or subpleural emphysema* is generally limited in distribution to subpleural zones and along the interlobar septa. It is marked by *involvement dominantly of the distal acinus* (namely, the alveoli) and only sometimes of the alveolar ducts. This variant

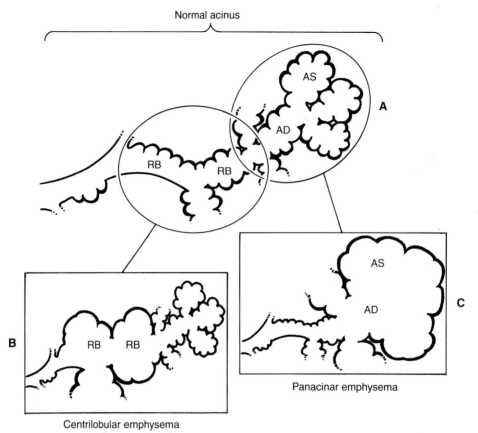

Figure 13–9. *A*, Diagram of normal structures within the acinus, the fundamental unit of the lung. *B*, Centrilobular emphysema with dilatation that principally affects the respiratory bronchioles, at least at the outset. *C*, Panacinar emphysema with initial distention of the peripheral structures (i.e., alveolus and alveolar duct); the disease later extends to affect the respiratory bronchioles. (Key: RB = respiratory bronchiole; AD = alveolar duct; AS = alveolus.)

is generally of limited extent, does not except in rare instances significantly compromise lung function, but is the form that occasionally leads to large bullous blebs directly beneath the pleura and sometimes to pneumothorax in young adults.

*Irregular emphysema* is better characterized as *emphysema associated with lung scarring*. The acinus is irregularly involved and often the scarring is incorporated into the walls of the enlarged air spaces. This pattern of emphysema is generally of limited extent and therefore usually has little impact on respiratory function. However, with widespread pulmonary scarring such as may occur with tuberculosis or pneumoconiosis, irregular emphysema may be widespread and impair lung function.

Despite these seemingly clear-cut differences, there is still some doubt about the separation of centrilobular emphysema from the panacinar form. Although with mild involvement "pure" prototypes can be identified, as centrilobular disease progresses it tends to become panacinar, indeed these "hybrid" patterns are the rule in patients dying of their disease. However, lest the islands become submerged in a sea of confusing detail, we shall continue to differentiate centrilobular from panacinar emphysema. These more common types of emphysema when well

advanced cause COPD because the damage to the walls of the air spaces reduces the elastic recoil of the lungs. The close relationship between emphysema and disease of the airways (bronchitis and small airway disease), particularly with the centrilobular variant, has already been pointed out (p. 416). Indeed, narrowing of the small distal airways is an almost invariable finding in patients with centrilobular emphysema. Both are strongly associated with cigarette smoking. It is still not clear whether involvement of the airways contributes significantly to the genesis of centrilobular emphysema or, conversely, whether the chronic airflow obstruction of emphysema may interfere with airway function and predispose to the bronchitis and bronchiolitis. The following remarks will be largely limited to centrilobular and panacinar emphysema.

First, however, several inappropriate usages of the term emphysema require clarification.[31] *Compensatory emphysema* is a misnomer applied to the alveolar dilatation that follows collapse or loss of lung substance elsewhere, as, for example, the enlargement of remaining lobes following a lobectomy. Because there is no destruction of septal walls, the process is appropriately called *compensatory hyperinflation*. *Senile emphysema* refers to the extremely common increased volume of the lungs so often found in the aged. It is probably the consequence of skeletal changes that increase the anteroposterior diameter of the chest (barrel chest). With such expansion of the chest cage, the lungs expand to fill the pleural cavities. Because there is no septal wall destruction associated with the process, it is better referred to as *senile hyperinflation*. *Bullous emphysema* is not a specific morphologic pattern of the disease. A bulla is an emphysematous space more than 1 cm in diameter. Subpleural bullae may appear in any one of the four well-defined forms of emphysema when severe but are particularly common with the paraseptal form.

*Interstitial emphysema* is an unusual condition that sometimes follows and must be differentiated from pulmonary emphysema. It refers to the accumulation of air in the interstitial tissues. Typically it begins with the entrance of air into the septa of the lung, which may then dissect its way back to the hilus to reach the mediastinum and thence possibly the subcutaneous tissues of the chest, neck, and body. Usually interstitial emphysema is initiated by an alveolar tear in pulmonary emphysema. With inspiration and expansion of the lungs, air enters the interstitium but does not escape as the lungs deflate during expiration. In this manner, air is essentially pumped into the interstitium. In many cases, the initiation of this process can be attributed to a sudden episode of coughing, such as may occur with bronchitis, whooping cough, or aspiration of a foreign body. Instrumentation of the airways, artificial resuscitation, and positive pressure therapy are additional antecedents. Infrequently, a rib fracture or a chest wound that punctures the lung may be followed by this bizarre complication. The condition is generally self-limited, because a blood clot seals the tear or wound in the lung and the escaped air is slowly resorbed.

**INCIDENCE.** Data on the prevalence of centrilobular or panacinar emphysema are remarkably variable, largely because of difficulties in establishing limits on the amount of expansion in air spaces and alteration in septa required to be called "abnormal enlargement" and "destruction," respectively.[32] In one postmortem series some degree of the panacinar or centrilobular emphysema was seen in 50% of patients and was thought to cause either significant disability or death in almost 10% of these cases.[33] Both variants have been increasing in frequency, attributable to the growing use of cigarettes (up to the recent past) and the worsening of environmental air pollution. Indeed, COPD (largely attributable to emphysema) has become so common that it is second only to heart disease as a cause of morbidity and loss of time from the workplace, and the deaths it causes now outnumber those resulting from bronchogenic carcinoma.[34] The centrilobular form is much more common than the panacinar variant, because of its closer association with cigarette smoking and other environmental air

pollutants (oxides of nitrogen and sulfur). Progressively worsening over the span of years to decades, severe emphysema is largely a disease of middle to late adult life.

**PATHOGENESIS.** Any theory of causation of emphysema must explain two central facts: (1) the basis for the injury to the walls of the air spaces and (2) the strong association between cigarette smoking and emphysema, particularly the centrilobular variant. Although uncertainties persist, interest is focused on the following possibilities, principally the first.[35]

○ *Elastase-antielastase imbalance*
○ *Injury to the alveolar epithelium*
○ *Impairment of connective tissue synthesis*

An elastase-antielastase imbalance nicely fits many observations but still must be firmly established.[36] The strongest support comes from the *well-established association of emphysema (usually panacinar) with an hereditary deficiency of alpha-1-antitrypsin (antiprotease)*, which is also an antielastase. The normal individual possesses in the blood a potent inhibitor of proteinases encoded by an autosomal gene on chromosome 14 expressed codominantly. A large number of variants producing somewhat modified proteins having variable levels of antiproteinase activity have been identified in these proteinase-inhibitor (Pi) genes.[36a] The normal Pi allele is M, and the normal homozygote is therefore MM, which has the highest serum antiproteinase level. The M heterozygote has intermediate levels depending on the product of the other Pi allele. The Z allele yields the lowest level of antiproteinase and, as expected, the Pi ZZ homozygote is most deficient in proteinase inhibitor. Among Pi ZZ homozygotes, nearly all who smoke cigarettes develop severe emphysema, usually panacinar, but only about two thirds of nonsmokers develop the disease. However, in the perspective of all cases of emphysema, a genetic deficiency of alpha-1-antiprotease accounts for only a small fraction because a marked hereditary deficiency is rare.

In most cases *the elastase-antielastase imbalance is attributed to increased levels of elastase activity in the lungs, possibly accompanied by some inhibition of antielastase*. The source of the elastase is still not firmly established, but is generally attributed to smoke-induced increased recruitment to the lungs of both neutrophils, rich in elastase and other catabolic enzymes, and monocyte-macrophages, which have lower levels of elastase. Indeed, smokers have a much greater increase in both macrophages and neutrophils in their lungs, as compared with the lungs of nonsmokers. Although macrophages predominate, they may in turn release neutrophil chemoattractants. *Moreover, most important, cigarette smoke has been documented to rapidly inactivate alpha-1-antiproteinase because of its content of oxidants.*[37] Whatever causes the imbalance, elevated levels of elastin-degradation products have been identified in smokers. Unfortunately, this attractive chain of evidence has some weak links. To name only one, it is not always possible to document a loss of elastin biochemically in emphysematous human lungs. Retreat has been made to the explanation of rapid resynthesis of physicochemically abnormal elastin.

Although elastase-antielastase imbalance commands center stage, brief mention should be made of other less favored theories. *The alveolar damage might start with injury to the lining epithelium,* followed by degradation of elastin and possibly other connective tissue components of the septal walls. Cigarette smoke contains many toxic substances, including free radicals. Conceivably, then, the disruption of the integrity of the lining epithelium and exposure of elastin and collagen to injury might be the primary cause of alveolar damage in emphysema (Fig. 13–10). Other more tentative speculations such as impaired collagen synthesis might be offered, but in the last analysis none adequately copes with the presumed anatomic differences in the distribution of centrilobular and panacinar emphysema within the acinus.

**MORPHOLOGY.** Although it is possible to suspect the existence of emphysema from gross inspection of the lungs, especially when severe, confirmation of the diagnosis requires 2 mm giant slices (Gough sections) of inflated lung tissue, which will reveal the loci of abnormal dilatation on microscopic examination. The principal diagnostic features are:

1. Abnormal enlargement of airspaces.
2. Thinning and destruction of septal walls or sometimes only widening of interalveolar fenestrae.

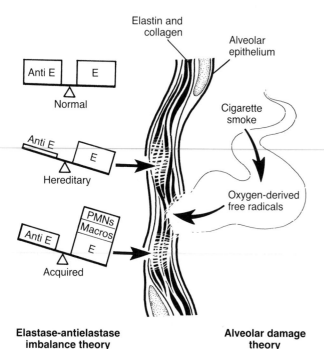

Elastin and collagen

Alveolar epithelium

Anti E | E

Normal

Cigarette smoke

Anti E | E

Hereditary

Oxygen-derived free radicals

PMNs Macros

Anti E | E

Acquired

**Elastase-antielastase imbalance theory**　　　　　**Alveolar damage theory**

Figure 13–10. Schema of the two major potential pathways of alveolar wall damage—excess of elastase relative to antielastase and direct damage by toxic metabolites.

3. Compression of the septal capillaries and, sometimes, the small airways.
4. Accumulation of carbon pigment–laden macrophages, particularly about the small airways in smokers.
5. Bronchiolitis involving the terminal and respiratory bronchioles, particularly in centrilobular emphysema.

As already emphasized, the dominant location of these changes within the acinus serves to differentiate one form of emphysema from another (p. 417). However, in the usual case of a patient dying of the disease, the centrilobular and panacinar variants merge. The paraseptal and irregular variants, when not advanced, can usually be identified by the location of the changes within the lungs.

A few macroscopic features not mentioned earlier merit comment. In **centrilobular emphysema** the upper zones of the lobes are first affected; sometimes a rim of subpleural lung parenchyma is spared. The lungs may not appear particularly voluminous or pale, but these changes develop with more advanced disease. The emphysema is focal and located centrally in the acinus (Fig. 13–11A). Focal carbon pigmentation and pigmentation of the tracheobronchial nodes is usually prominent because of the strong association with cigarette smoking. **Panacinar emphysema** when mild is restricted to the lower zones of the lungs, particularly in elderly patients. This localized form may be difficult to recognize grossly. However, when severe and generalized, as in alpha-1-antiproteinase deficiency, the lungs become extremely voluminous, pale, and pillowy. Often at autopsy they overlap and hide the heart. The emphysematous distention is diffuse (panacinar) (Fig. 13–11B). **Paraseptal or subpleural emphysema** may limit its changes to the development of large bullous airspaces, sometimes many centimeters in diameter and located just below the pleura. They tend to be more frequent in apical locations. **Irregular emphysema,** because of its association with lung scarring, rarely induces increase in lung volume.

**CLINICAL COURSE.** Both centrilobular and panacinar emphysema produce COPD when well advanced. However, less severe involvements may be asymptomatic. There is in general a correlation between the severity of the functional impairment and the severity of the pulmonary disease, but other variables contribute to the airflow limitation, as will be pointed out. Typically, the first symptom is the insidious onset of dyspnea, which becomes steadily more severe as the disease progresses. Often the patients have a wheezing respiration with prolonged expiration and have to squeeze the air out of their lungs with each expiratory effort because the elastic recoil is diminished. Sometimes these patients overventilate—hence the term "pink puffers"—inaccurate and tasteless, as pointed out earlier (p. 417). Cough and expectoration may or may not be present, depending on the coexistence of chronic bronchitis and disease of the small airways. Indeed, some patients with apparently severe emphysematous involvement of the lungs may be remarkably free of symptoms if

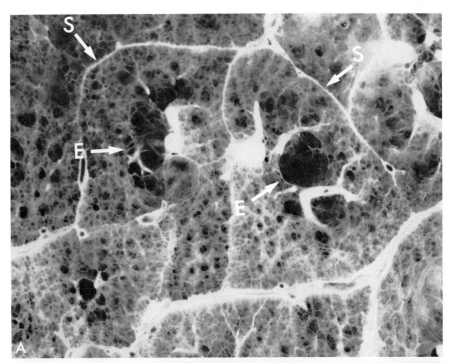

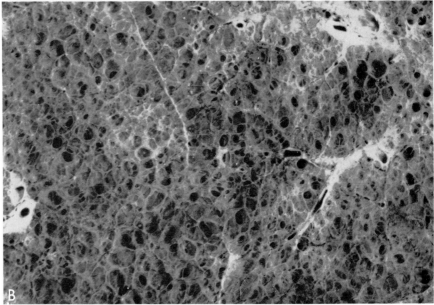

**Figure 13–11.** *A*, Centrilobular emphysema (magnification × 5). The pulmonary arteries contain a mass of injected barium gelatin. The emphysematous foci (*E*) abut blood vessels and are removed from the septa (*S*) where the alveolar spaces cluster. *B*, Panacinar emphysema (× 5) involving the entire pulmonary architecture. Compare with *A*. (From Bates, D. V., et al.: Respiratory Function in Disease. 2nd ed. Philadelphia, W. B. Saunders Co., 1971.)

there is little or no involvement of the bronchi and bronchioles. Thus, although both emphysema in fairly pure form and bronchitis, including bronchiolitis, in fairly pure form may induce COPD, it may not appear until both types of involvement are present. Spirometric studies are usually necessary to determine how much of the chronic airflow limitation is related to involvement of bronchi and bronchioles or to abnormalities of the air spaces. Chest films may show hyperlucency of the lung fields and low, flattened diaphragms, but such findings are also produced by hyperinflation (especially in the elderly) and so are not diagnostic of emphysema. With progression of the disease, the respiratory problems worsen, cyanosis may appear, and weight loss may be so severe as to mimic malignant cachexia.

The immediate cause of death with this disease may be:

○ Relentlessly progressive hypoxemia with hypoxic brain damage.
○ Respiratory acidosis and coma.
○ A superimposed pulmonary infection.
○ Right-sided heart failure (chronic cor pulmonale).
○ Sudden worsening of the hypoxemia secondary to pneumothorax from massive collapse of the lungs.

## BRONCHIAL ASTHMA

*Asthma is characterized by an exaggerated bronchoconstrictor response to many stimuli inducing paroxysmal, mainly expiratory, airflow limitation, marked dyspnea, and wheezing.* Typically the attacks remit spontaneously or with therapy and are interspersed by symptom-free intervals of variable length (days to months). Rarely the attack fails to remit (*status asthmaticus*) and may prove fatal. Asthma is a common condition afflicting about 5% of the U.S. population; in many instances it appears in the first two decades of life. However, a significant number of patients are first diagnosed after 30 years of age.

**CLASSIFICATION.** Based on the stimuli that provoke the asthmatic attacks, two interrelated categories have been segregated: (1) *immunologic extrinsic asthma* and (2) *nonimmunologic intrinsic asthma*. The extrinsic pattern accounts for less than 10% of all cases, is usually seen in childhood, and in general is less severe and more readily managed than the intrinsic type. Most patients with extrinsic asthma are atopic and have a well-defined family history of various forms of allergy and, possibly, bronchial asthma. Intrinsic asthma may occur at any age, tends to be more frequently recurrent and severe, and more often leads to status asthmaticus. However, many patients have features of both.

**PATHOGENESIS.** Although much has been learned about the pathways inducing the bronchoconstrictive attacks, there are still many holes in our knowledge. In greatly simplified terms, two major interrelated pathways are involved (Fig. 13–12).[38]

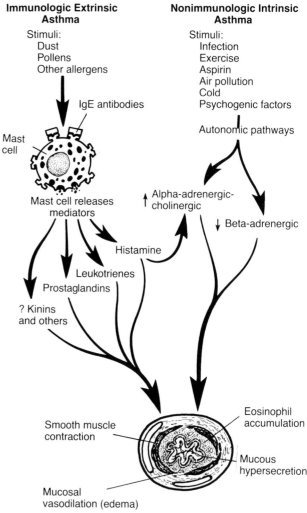

Figure 13–12. Proposed pathogenic pathways of extrinsic and intrinsic asthma.

○ Allergen interaction with specific IgE antibodies bound to mast cells, from which chemical mediators are released.
○ Autonomic hyperreactivity or imbalance leading to neurologic constriction of airways.

*Immunologic extrinsic asthma* is an IgE-mediated type I hypersensitivity disease. It occurs in individuals who are atopic and form IgE antibody on exposure to common allergens. These antibodies are bound to mast cells (and possibly basophils) within the tracheobronchial mucosa. The sensitized cells on subsequent exposure to the allergen promptly release preformed histamine and simultaneously initiate the formation of other mediators, among which prostaglandin $PGD_2$ and the leukotriene $LTD_4$ are the most important. The latter is a thousandfold more potent bronchoconstrictor than histamine.[39] But other arachidonic acid derivatives are also released, including $LTB_4$ (a potent chemoattractant) and thromboxane $A_2$ (activator and aggregator of platelets). In this manner mast cells, all forms of white cells, and platelets participate in the bronchial allergic reaction. These cells then initiate the release of more primary and secondary mediators such as serotonin and, possibly, kinins. The various mediators also interact to amplify their effects.

*Nonimmunologic intrinsic asthma* is postulated to result from some abnormality of the parasympathetic control of airway function. Airway smooth muscle, submucosal glands, and capillaries are regulated by the autonomic nervous system; cholinergic and alpha-adrenergic stimulation causes bronchoconstriction and mucosal secretion, whereas beta-adrenergic stimulation does the reverse. Thus, increased alpha-adrenergic responsiveness or an increase in number of alpha-receptors in the bronchial mucosal cells could account for many of the features of asthma.[40] Alternatively, some interference with the counter-vailing beta-adrenergic pathway might also lead to bronchoconstriction. It is theorized that exposure to cold temperature, increased ventilation with exercise, air pollution, and other nonimmunogenic stimuli provoke cholinergic and alpha-adrenergic vagal efferents, which leads to the characteristic changes in asthma. Attractive as this concept may be, it is not certain that autonomic abnormalities are a primary mechanism.[38]

There are many interactions between the two basic pathogenetic pathways, since many asthmatics react to both allergic and nonallergic stimuli. Histamine released from mast cells may initiate vagal activity. Moreover, both mast cells and basophils possess membrane receptors, which are responsive to autonomic drugs. For example, beta-adrenergic agonists such as epinephrine inhibit the release of mast cell mediators, whereas cholinergic and alpha-adrenergic agonists enhance mediator release. As another example of the relatedness of both forms of asthma, occasional nonallergic individuals develop asthmatic attacks following ingestion of aspirin. Although aspirin is considered to be a nonimmunogenic stimulus producing intrinsic asthma, the effects of this agent are likely to be mediated through arachidonic acid pathways by inhibiting cyclooxygenase and thereby augmenting the formation, via lipoxygenase, of leukotriene mediators. Suffice it that asthma refuses to comply with neat pathogenetic theories.

**MORPHOLOGY.** The chief gross features of advanced asthma are (1) mucus plugs in the bronchi; (2) overinflation of the lungs, but no significant emphysema; and (3) occasional areas of bronchiectasis, particularly in **aspergillosis-related cases.** The airways are frequently plugged with mucus, which may contain desquamated cells. The mucin often contains a seroproteinaceous component arising from the intense inflammatory reaction in the submucosa. The walls of the bronchi may appear slightly thicker than usual. When frank suppurative exudate is present in the lumens, superimposed infection and bronchitis must have supervened.

Histologically, **there is hyperplasia of the mucous glands, an increase in the thickness of the bronchial smooth muscle, and hypertrophy and hyperplasia of mucosal goblet cells.** Areas of denudation of the respiratory epithelium are often found, in addition to subepithelial edema. A moderate increase of inflammatory lymphocytes and particularly eosinophils is present in this edematous mucosa. The plugs within the airways contain (1) whorls of shed epithelium and proteinaceous secretion giving rise to so-called **Curschmann's spirals,** (2) numerous eosinophils with **Charcot-Leyden crystals,** (3) free-lying Charcot-Leyden crystals released from disintegrated eosinophils, and (4) cellular debris. Superimposed bacterial infection may transform the anatomic changes to those of bronchitis.

**CLINICAL COURSE.** On the basis of the anatomic changes, one can anticipate that an asthma attack is characterized by severe dyspnea with wheezing. Because the tracheobronchial tree widens and lengthens during inspiration, the chief difficulty is with expiration. The victim labors to get air into the lungs and then cannot get it out, so that there is progressive hyperinflation of the lungs with air trapped distal to the mucus plugs. The result is characteristic prolonged, wheezing expirations.

In the usual case, attacks last from one to several hours and subside either spontaneously or with therapy, usually by bronchodilators. Intervals between attacks are characteristically free from respiratory difficulty, but persistent, subtle respiratory deficits can be detected by spirometric methods. Helpful in the clinical diagnosis is the finding of eosinophils, Curschmann's spirals, and Charcot-Leyden crystals in the sputum. It is the intermittent nature of bronchial obstruction and the fact that destructive emphysema rarely occurs with uncomplicated asthma that distinguishes asthma from the chronic obstructive pulmonary disease of emphysema. Occasionally, a severe paroxysm occurs that does not respond to therapy and persists for days and even weeks (*status asthmaticus*). In these circumstances, the ventilatory function may be so impaired as to result in severe cyanosis and even death. However, in most cases, the disease is more disabling than lethal. When death occurs, it is typically from superimposed infection or from respiratory failure during status asthmaticus.

## BRONCHIECTASIS

*Bronchiectasis is a chronic, necrotizing infection that either causes or follows abnormal dilatation of the bronchi.* Clinically, it is characterized by cough, fever, and copious foul-smelling purulent sputum. It occurs at any age in both sexes and is frequent in children. In the present era of effective antibacterial therapies, the development of bronchiectasis usually implies some underlying disorder that either impairs the normal physiology of the airways or renders the patient particularly vulnerable to infections. The conditions most commonly predisposing to bronchiectasis in developed nations are presented in Table 13–4. In developing countries, the order of importance of the associated conditions is reversed, and most cases of bronchiectasis follow suppurative pneumonias, tuberculosis, and viral childhood diseases.

**PATHOGENESIS.** *Central to the causation of bronchiectasis are two processes:* (1) *obstruction or abnormal dilatation of bronchi and* (2) *chronic persistent infection.* Which of these processes comes first is not clear, but they are closely interrelated. With obstruction or dilatation of bronchi, normal clearance mechanisms are hampered and so secondary infection soon follows; conversely, chronic infection will in time cause damage to bronchial walls, leading to weakening and dilatation. For example, obstruction such as is encountered with a bronchogenic carcinoma or foreign body not only impairs clearance of secretions but, as the air is resorbed from the dependent lung parenchyma, the loss of support of the occluded airways potentiates dilatation. Although these changes are reversible to a point, superimposed infection damages the wall, and the accumulated exudation further distends the airways to lead to irreversible dilatation. Conversely, a persistent necrotizing inflammation in the bronchi or bronchioles may cause obstructive secretions, inflammation throughout the wall (with peribronchial fibrosis and scarring traction on the walls), and, eventually, the train of events described.

In the usual case, a mixed flora can be cultured from the involved bronchi, including staphylococci, streptococci, pneumococci, enteric organisms, anaer-

obic and microaerophilic bacteria, and frequently, particularly in children, *Haemophilus influenzae* and *Pseudomonas aeruginosa*. Which of these are primary pathogens and which are merely secondary saprophytic invaders is unclear.

**MORPHOLOGY.** The involvement may be unilateral or bilateral. The lower lobes—especially the left lower lobe—are most vulnerable, but the right middle lobe and the lingula are also frequently affected. The most severe involvements are found in the smaller bronchi and bronchioles. These airways are dilated, sometimes up to four times normal size, and so they often can be followed almost out to the pleural surface. The dilated segments may be long and tube-like (**cylindroid**), or they may be **fusiform** or **saccular** in shape. The anatomic changes are best brought out by sectioning the lung at right angles to the long axis of the affected airways. The cut surface of the lung may show an almost cystic pattern created by the widely dilated bronchioles and compression of the intervening lung parenchyma. The lumens of the affected bronchi are characteristically filled with a suppurative, yellow-green, sometimes hemorrhagic exudate that, when removed, exposes a red-green or black, necrotic, edematous, frequently ulcerated mucosa. When the infection extends to the pleura, as it often does, it evokes a fibrinous or suppurative pleuritis.

The histologic findings vary with the activity and chronicity of the disease. In the full-blown, active case, there is an intense acute and chronic inflammatory exudate within the walls of the affected airways that is associated with desquamation of the lining epithelium and extensive areas of necrotizing ulceration. There may be squamous metaplasia of the remaining epithelium. In some instances, the necrosis extends down to the smooth muscle and may even completely destroy the wall, so that the infective process is in direct continuity with the lung parenchyma, creating a lung abscess. In the more chronic cases, fibrosis of the bronchial wall and peribronchial fibrosis develop.

When healing occurs, there may be complete regeneration of the lining epithelium. However, dilatation and scarring usually persist.

**CLINICAL COURSE.** In the Western world in the preantibiotic era, bronchiectasis was most common in the early decades of life when it followed some severe form of necrotizing or interstitial pneumonia; it sometimes occurred as a complication of a childhood infection such as whooping cough, measles, or influenza. The appearance of bronchiectasis was marked by a chronic productive cough, copious amounts of foul-smelling, sometimes bloody, sputum, and a predisposition to recurrent parenchymal infections. Extension of the bronchiectasis sometimes led to lung abscesses. Emaciation, clubbing of the digits, secondary amyloidosis, and a shortened life span were typical consequences. This pattern of the disease is still prevalent in populations having little available medical care. Currently, with effective antibacterial therapy in more favored countries, the manifestations

---

### Table 13–4. PREDISPOSITIONS TO BRONCHIECTASIS

| Major Conditions | Pathogenesis |
|---|---|
| **In Developed Countries** | |
| Bronchial obstruction—tumor, foreign body, mucus impaction | Impaired drainage of bronchial secretions |
| Cystic fibrosis | Hyperviscosity of mucus secretions and superimposed infection with *Staphylococcus aureus* and *Pseudomonas aeruginosa* |
| Immunodeficiency state | Predisposition to infection |
| Immotile cilia syndrome (including Kartagener's syndrome—dextrocardia [situs inversus], male infertility, sinusitis, and bronchiectasis) | Impaired ciliary activity (loss of dynein arms) predisposes to immotile sperm and impaired mucociliary clearance of sinuses and bronchial passages; migration defects in embryo produce malformations |
| **In Developing Countries** | |
| Postsuppurative pneumonias | Residual infection |
| Pulmonary tuberculosis | Scarring and cavitation with secondary necrotizing infection |
| Complication of measles, pertussis, and influenza | Residual pulmonary interstitial fibrosis with impaired airway physiology |

tend to be less severe but still include productive cough, hemoptysis, and predisposition to infections in the involved segments of lung. The cough tends to be worse when the patient is recumbent because of pooling of the inflammatory exudate. Infrequent today are secondary lung abscesses, clubbing, and amyloidosis. Moreover, effective medical therapy, respiratory hygiene (e.g., postural drainage), and surgical resection have materially prolonged life expectancy in most cases in which the predisposing influence can be controlled. However, in those with some underlying childhood disorder such as cystic fibrosis, severe immunodeficiency, or immotile cilia, death from progressive infection may occur before the age of 30.

# INTERSTITIAL (RESTRICTIVE) LUNG DISEASE (ILD)

*ILD is the generic term applied to any disorder characterized mainly by injury to alveolar walls.* The process begins as an interstitial inflammation affecting mainly the septae (interstitial alveolitis).[41] Activated immunocompetent cells then accumulate in the alveolar walls and appear to mediate the damage. At the outset, there is edematous widening of the alveolar walls accompanied by an infiltrate of lymphocytes and monocyte-macrophages. At this time the lining epithelial cells (mostly type I) are injured or become necrotic. They are then replaced by proliferating type II cells, which create a cuboidal epithelial lining that is ill-suited to gas exchange. Alveolar endothelial cells are also injured, which accounts for the exudation of fluid into the interstitium. However, in general the alveolar spaces are remarkably clear albeit reduced in size. Rarely the air spaces may become partially or completely clogged with macrophages; such changes have been accorded a special niche—*desquamative interstitial pneumonia.* In other instances the air spaces may become filled with a lipoproteinaceous debris (*alveolar proteinosis*), but these variations on the basic theme are the exception. *The most feared consequence of ILD is fibrous thickening of the alveolar walls, permanently impairing respiratory function and distorting the lung architecture. Concomitantly, the finer vasculature is narrowed, contributing to pulmonary hypertension. The widening of the alveolar walls and contraction of the fibrous tissue reduces the size of the air spaces and the lung becomes less compliant; thus gas exchange is impaired. Hence ILD comprises restrictive lung disease inasmuch as it "stiffens" the lung and reduces vital and total lung capacity.*

Well over 100 agents (e.g., drugs, radiation, airborne dusts) are known to have the potential of causing ILD. Most of these identified causes have received comment elsewhere. There are also approximately 35 to 40 disorders of unknown cause that are marked principally by interstitial lung involvement.[42]

The more common of these entities are cited in Table 13–5.

The major interstitial lung diseases of unknown cause are sarcoidosis and idiopathic pulmonary fibrosis. These are described in subsequent sections, and capsule characterizations of a few of the other distinctive entities follow.

## SARCOIDOSIS (BOECK'S SARCOID)

*Sarcoidosis is a multisystem disorder of unknown etiology characterized by the formation of noncaseating granulomas* (Fig. 13–13). It is included here because the lungs are a favored site of involvement and because *sarcoidosis also produces a diffuse interstitial alveolitis, thus making it a form of infiltrative restrictive disease. Other characteristic features are bilateral hilar lymphadenopathy and involvement of the skin and eyes. Active disease is also marked by hypercalciuria, usually with hypercalcemia, hypergammaglobulinemia, an elevated serum level of angiotensin-converting enzyme, and a positive Kveim-Siltzback skin test to a saline suspension of human sarcoid tissue (in 80% of patients).*[43]

Sarcoidosis has been identified with varying frequency in almost all countries. For example, it is common in Scandinavia but rare in Asia. Whether these differences are valid or merely reflect case-finding is not clear. The disease is also common in the United States and in Caribbean countries, and in these locales, blacks are more commonly affected than whites and tend to have more chronic disease. There are hints of genetic predisposition but no clear proof.[44] The disease first appears most often in adults under the age of 40. Women in reproductive life are especially vulnerable.

**ETIOLOGY AND PATHOGENESIS.** *The sine qua non of sarcoidosis—the noncaseating granuloma—points strongly to a cell-mediated immunologic reaction to some antigenic stimulus. However, the identity of the antigen remains unknown.* A host of microbial agents have been suspected (especially atypical mycobac-

**Table 13–5.** SOME INTERSTITIAL LUNG DISEASES OF UNKNOWN CAUSE

Sarcoidosis
Idiopathic pulmonary fibrosis (Hamman-Rich syndrome)
ILD in systemic "connective tissue" disorders
    Systemic sclerosis
    Rheumatoid arthritis
    Systemic lupus erythematosus
    Mixed connective tissue disease
Goodpasture's syndrome
Idiopathic pulmonary hemosiderosis
ILD with pulmonary vasculitis
    Wegener's granulomatosis
    Hypersensitivity vasculitis
    Systemic vasculitides
Pulmonary eosinophilia
Histiocytosis X

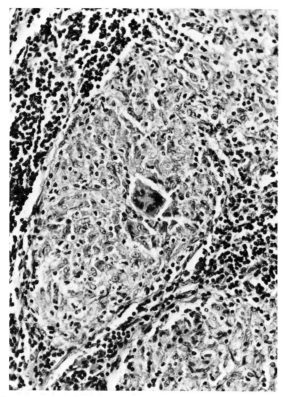

Figure 13–13. Sarcoidosis. The characteristic noncaseating granuloma contains several central giant cells.

teria) but none proved. When all else fails, a lurking virus is suspected, but to date it still lurks.[45] Other possible causes include pine pollen or resin, clay dust, beryllium, and zirconium, to name only a few, but none are established. Until more etiologic evidence is discovered, *it seems best to consider sarcoidosis as a particular response to varied antigens in immunologically predisposed individuals.*

Patients with active sarcoidosis have a great many abnormal immunologic findings, notably:

○ Complete or partial cutaneous anergy to common challenge antigens, suggesting depressed cell-mediated immunity.

○ The number of T4-helper cells in the circulation is depressed but increased at sites of active disease and in bronchoalveolar lavage.

○ T8-suppressor cells in the circulation are increased relative to the T4 cells.

○ B cells are normal or increased in number in the circulation.

○ B cells are hyperreactive with polyclonal hypergammaglobulinemia.

○ Circulating immune complexes are often present.

The explanation of the apparent paradox of cutaneous anergy (implying some defect in T-cell function) in patients with well-formed granuloma formations (requiring T-cell function) awaited the observations that the ratio of T-helper cells to T-suppressor cells within the granulomas (and bronchoalveolar lavages) differs markedly from that in the circulation.[46] In the circulation the suppressor cells are increased in number relative to the helper T cells, but the reverse occurs within granulomas. It is proposed that at sites of antigen localization, macrophages release interleukin 1, activating T cells that release interleukin 2, which induces an expansion of T4-helper cells relative to the T8-suppressor cells. T4 lymphocytes then secrete lymphokines such as migration inhibition factor, augmenting the accumulation of monocyte-macrophages. Activation of the macrophages then gives rise to epithelioid cells, and some coalesce into giant cells. In this manner the noncaseating granuloma of sarcoidosis, the histologic hallmark, evolves. Simultaneously, the lymphokines derived from T4-helper cells induce polyclonal B-cell stimulation, which leads to hypergammaglobulinemia and, together with the inciting antigen, the formation of immune complexes. An overview of this thesis is offered in Figure 13–14. Several additional details should be noted. (1) The tissue injury causing the alveolitis and interstitial fibrosis is mediated by macrophage-derived lysosomal enzymes and oxygen-derived free radicals, and the subsequent fibrosis may at least in part be attributed to macrophage-derived

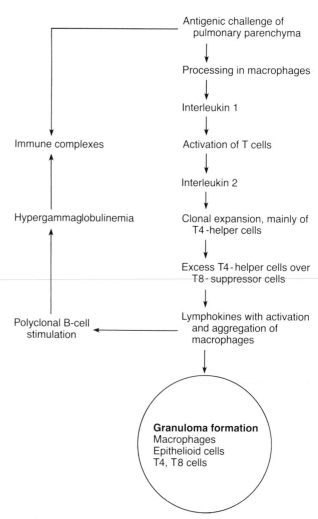

Figure 13–14. Immune changes that occur in sarcoidosis.

growth factor acting on fibroblasts.[47] (2) The granulomas elaborate angiotensin-converting enzyme, accounting for the increased serum levels. (3) The cutaneous anergy is poorly understood but could be caused by the elaboration of serum factors inhibitory to T cells or, more likely, to "redistribution" of T4-helper cells, by which they accumulate in affected tissue sites and are reduced in number in the circulation. This would explain the increase of T8-suppressor cells in the circulation relative to the T4 cells to thus yield cutaneous anergy.[48]

**MORPHOLOGY.** The noncaseating granulomas may be found in almost any organ or tissue of the body, most regularly in lymph nodes, particularly those in the hilar regions of the lung.[49] In most organs the granulomas are randomly scattered, solitary lesions, but they may be clustered and coalescent. Not always do they evoke clinical signs or symptoms, particularly when present in organs of the reticuloendothelial system. **The characteristic granuloma consists of a noncaseating, sharply circumscribed focal collection of large epithelioid cells, often punctuated by multinucleated giant cells and surrounded by a rim of lymphocytes and other mononuclear cells.** Rarely there is some central necrosis, but it is more coagulative than caseous. The giant cells and epithelioid cells may contain inclusion bodies of two types—**Schaumann (conchoid) bodies** ranging up to 100 μm in diameter, representing concentrically laminated basophilic inclusions containing calcium and iron salts, and **asteroid bodies**, which are star-shaped, refractile, acidophilic structures often found within giant cells and composed, apparently, of products of lipoprotein metabolism (Fig. 13–15). As the disease becomes chronic, fibrosis begins in the periphery of the granuloma and may eventually replace it, particularly in the lungs. Although the granulomas are distinctive, they are *not* diagnostic because they can be found in many other disorders, including tuberculosis, leprosy, fungal infections, berylliosis, and others. Moreover, neither the Schaumann body nor the asteroid is exclusive to sarcoidosis.

**Lung involvement** is not only common, it is sometimes severe. Some 20 to 25% of all patients with sarcoidosis develop significant permanent respiratory dysfunction. It has three distinctive components: (1) noncaseating granulomas, (2) a nonspecific lymphocyte-macrophage interstitial alveolitis, and (3) in the late stages, varying degrees of interstitial fibrosis.[50] The granulomas tend to be located in the interstitium and about bronchi and blood vessels. Sometimes they produce endobronchial projections. They may vary in age; some are cellular, others are partially fibrosed, and still others are almost totally fibrosed and hyalinized, contributing to the overall interstitial fibrosis. The alveolitis is widespread and causes some widening of the septal walls. With chronic disease a diffuse interstitial fibrosis develops, which distorts the underlying pulmonary architecture and in some cases produces honeycombing of the lung. As with the granulomas, the alveolitis in some areas may be quite cellular while other areas are largely fibrosed. The overall severity of the

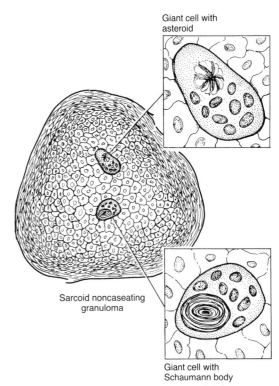

Figure 13–15. Sarcoidosis. A schematic representation of a noncaseating sarcoid granuloma. Asteroid and Schaumann bodies in giant cells are shown in insets.

alveolitis may not necessarily be concordant with the number of granulomas.

**Skin lesions** of sarcoidosis take the form of discrete subcutaneous nodules; focal, slightly elevated erythematous plaques; or red, scaling, flat lesions. Similar changes may appear on the mucous membranes of the oral cavity, larynx, and upper respiratory tract. In all instances, the lesions are characterized by noncaseating granulomas, sometimes deeply situated and typical of **erythema nodosum.**

**Eye involvement** (bilateral or unilateral) appears as iritis, iridocyclitis, or in the posterior uveal tract as choroiditis or retinitis; it may also affect the optic nerve. In all locations, the lesions are marked by noncaseating granulomas that are replaced later by fibrous scars. Such late sequelae may cause considerable loss of vision or even total blindness when they occur bilaterally.

Although many other organs may be affected, note should be made of the major salivary glands, particularly the parotids, because their involvement together with the uveitis form the **Mikulicz's syndrome.** Bone lesions, usually in the short bones of the hands and feet, can be identified by x-ray in 5 to 10% of patients. The numerous granulomas in the marrow cavity may create focal areas of bone resorption or impart a diffuse reticulated, roentgenographic pattern throughout the marrow cavity, widening of the bony shafts, and new bone formation on the outer surfaces. Sarcoid granulomas are also found in the spleen, liver, heart, kidneys, central nervous system, and endocrine glands, particularly in the pituitary.

**CLINICAL COURSE.** Because of the involvement of many systems, it can be anticipated that the clinical manifestations of sarcoidosis are protean. In about 75% of cases, the disease is entirely asymptomatic and is found only incidentally in a biopsy sample of a lymph node or bone marrow or at autopsy. Sometimes it is called to attention by the chance discovery on chest x-ray of bilateral prominent hilar adenopathy ("potato nodes"). Pulmonary parenchymal changes may yield patchy x-ray densities, attributable to either active alveolitis or pulmonary fibrosis. As pointed out earlier, a significant number of patients have impaired pulmonary function, and about 5 to 10% die of the pulmonary involvement. In still other instances, loss of lacrimation, impairment of vision, or enlargement of the salivary glands brings the condition to attention. With sufficiently widespread involvement, active disease may be accompanied by vague constitutional signs and symptoms, including fever, weakness, and weight loss.

Regrettably, there are no diagnostic clinical features of sarcoidosis. Supporting the diagnosis are the following findings: (a) hypergammaglobulinemia, (b) circulating immune complexes, (c) hypercalcemia and hypercalciuria, (d) elevated levels of angiotensin-converting enzyme in the serum, and (e) cutaneous anergy to various common antigens (e.g., tuberculin). None of these features is invariably present, but when present in combination they are highly suggestive in the appropriate clinical setting. Ultimately, recourse must be made to biopsy (usually bone marrow, liver, lymph node) to document the presence of noncaseating granulomas, which are consistent with but not diagnostic of sarcoidosis.

The clinical course of sarcoidosis depends greatly on its manner of presentation. Usually in those under 30, the onset is quite acute, with fever and malaise, hilar adenopathy without parenchymal lung involvement, erythema nodosum of the skin, and high serum levels of angiotensin-converting enzyme. Such patients respond well to corticosteroids and frequently have permanent remissions. In contrast, sarcoidosis in those over the age of 40 often has an insidious onset, with overt lesions in the lungs, involvement of the posterior uveal tract, and sometimes bony changes, parotid enlargement, and renal stones due to protracted hypercalciuria. Such patients respond less well to corticosteroids and often pursue a remitting, relapsing, slowly progressive course. Overall, about 3 to 5% of patients die of their disease, usually from pulmonary fibrosis and cardiac failure incident to cor pulmonale, or from involvement of the central nervous system.

## IDIOPATHIC PULMONARY FIBROSIS (IPF)

This designation refers to a specific disorder characterized by a distinctive combination of clinical, functional, and morphologic features that set it apart from other forms of interstitial lung disease. IPF, also called the *Hamman-Rich syndrome*, is almost as common as sarcoidosis, occurs somewhat more often in males, and is usually, but not always, seen in the fifth and sixth decades of life. The first manifestation of this disorder is usually the appearance of dyspnea, with or without a cough, on exertion; this symptom often follows an illness of apparent viral origin. Typically, the auscultatory findings are unimpressive. Chest films may disclose a more or less diffuse reticulonodular pattern tending to be more prominent at the bases. With these findings it might be anticipated that the disease would run a benign, self-limited course, but idiopathic pulmonary fibrosis behaves otherwise and usually follows a progressive downhill course to death within 3 to 5 years.[51]

The first morphologic changes constitute a patchy edematous thickening of the alveolar walls accompanied by an infiltrate of macrophages, neutrophils, and smaller numbers of lymphocytes. These changes have given rise to the synonym for this condition—**cryptogenic fibrosing alveolitis.** With progression, type 1 pneumonocytes undergo regressive changes that are followed by proliferation of type 2 cells. At about this stage the interstitial edema fluid begins to be replaced by a mixed population of fibroblasts, smooth muscle cells, and myofibroblasts. Continuation of this organization leads to increased deposition of collagen fibers, particularly of type 1, with progressive collagenous fibrosis of septal walls and loss of capillaries. In time the fibrous reaction extends about and into the walls of small airways and arteries (Fig. 13–16). Hence there is considerable disorganization of the native architecture, diminution in the size of the air spaces, impedence to vascular flow, and increased consistence and stiffening of the pulmonary parenchyma.

Although most patients with IPF exhibit the morphologic changes just described, there are rare instances in which the interstitial pneumonitis is accompanied by the accumulation of large numbers of pulmonary alveolar macrophages within the air spaces. When first described, this variant was called **desquamative interstitial pneumonitis** (DIP), but according to current thinking, DIP is probably an early phase of IPF. Thus the more typical pattern of IPF which lacks the desquamative component is sometimes termed **usual interstitial pneumonitis** to add to the welter of confusing synonyms and terms.

As is obvious from its name, the origin of this condition is unknown. Indeed, there may be multiple etiologies, because IPF could result from any poorly controlled inflammatory reaction, whatever the cause.[52] The following process is postulated: a pulmonary challenge stimulates lung B lymphocytes to elaborate immunoglobulins. Together with the inciting antigens, these immunoglobulins form immune complexes within the lung that are phagocytosed by and activate macrophages, which secrete neutrophil chemotactic factor. Thereafter, neutrophils are recruited to the lung, and it is the release of their proteases and oxidants that induces the injury to the

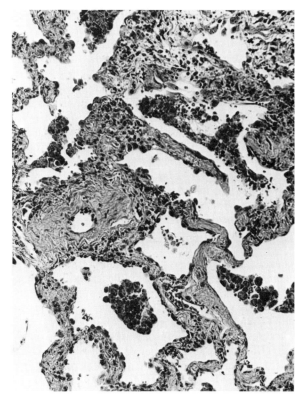

Figure 13–16. Interstitial lung disease. The changes have progressed to fibrosis of the widened alveolar walls and marked perivascular fibrosis, which narrows the lumen.

interstitial tissue and epithelial cells of the alveolar walls (Fig. 13–17).[53]

As has been pointed out, IPF is a most serious disorder. It usually pursues a slow but steady downhill course that is marked by progressive loss of functioning pulmonary parenchyma, worsening dysp-nea, and increasing hypoxemia. The disorder ultimately leads to respiratory failure, typically about five years after onset, although some patients may live longer. Moreover, these patients have an increased incidence of myocardial infarction, pulmonary embolism, and bronchogenic carcinoma.

## GOODPASTURE'S SYNDROME

In this unusual syndrome, necrotizing hemorrhagic interstitial pneumonitis and proliferative, usually rapidly progressive, glomerulonephritis occurs almost concurrently. *Both the pulmonary and renal involvements are caused by circulating antibodies that are cross-reactive with the basement membranes of the alveolar walls and of the glomeruli.*[54] The fact that the pulmonary changes almost always precede the renal abnormalities by one to two weeks suggests that the initial immunologic reaction begins in the lungs. The stimulus initiating the formation of these antibodies against "self" is unknown. Two possible mechanisms have been suggested: (1) an exogenous agent (e.g., influenza virus or some pulmonary toxin) damages the alveolar walls and initiates the formation of antibodies to alveolar basement membranes, or (2) there is some abnormality in the normal breakdown and resynthesis of basement membrane, leading to immunogenic abnormal residues.

The renal changes are described on page 469. The lungs basically have a **patchy but widespread interstitial, sometimes necrotizing alveolitis, accompanied by recent and old intra-alveolar hemorrhages (i.e., fresh red cells and hemosiderin-laden alveolar macrophages).** In time septal wall fibrosis may develop, sometimes marked by hemosiderin deposition. There is

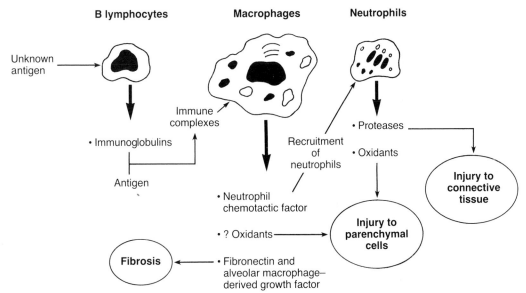

Figure 13–17. Current concepts of the pathogenesis of idiopathic pulmonary fibrosis. Pivotal is the formation of immune complexes by the inciting antigen. (Modified from Crystal, R. G., et al.: Interstitial lung diseases of unknown cause. Disorders characterized by chronic inflammation of the lower respiratory tree. N. Engl. J. Med. *310*:161, 1984.)

no evidence of injury to vessels larger than capillaries. The hemorrhages may be sufficiently large to be macroscopically visible as areas of red or rust-colored consolidation. Immunofluorescent techniques reveal linear deposits of IgG that are sometimes accompanied by complement and that occur along the alveolar and glomerular basement membranes.

Typically the disease presents in young males (male to female ratio is 9:1) who have at first hemoptysis, x-ray evidence of pulmonary infiltration or consolidation, and anemia; soon thereafter, (within a few weeks), glomerular injury with proteinuria, hematuria, and azotemia occur. The loss of blood leads to the anemia. Up to the recent past, most patients died of progressive renal failure, but early diagnosis before the renal disease has become marked and the use of plasmaphoresis, immunosuppression, or large doses of corticosteroids have achieved considerable prolongation of life (even though renal dialysis is sometimes required).[55]

## IDIOPATHIC PULMONARY HEMOSIDEROSIS

This entity, along with Goodpasture's syndrome and vasculitis-associated pulmonary hemorrhage, completes the triad of "pulmonary hemorrhage syndromes." In contrast to Goodpasture's syndrome, idiopathic pulmonary hemosiderosis has no renal involvement or basement membrane antibodies, occurs in younger adults and children, has no male preponderance, and is of variable severity that ranges from mild to progressive disease. Most patients have recurrent episodes of mild to moderate hemoptysis with intervals free of manifestations for variable lengths of time. The blood loss often produces anemia. Usually these patients have a normal longevity, but sometimes the condition is more aggressive; it infrequently proves fatal with the initial hemorrhagic episode.

Morphologically, the lung generally reveals a mild to moderate mononuclear fibrosing interstitial pneumonitis, sometimes containing hemosiderin-laden macrophages in the septal walls, that is accompanied by alveoli filled with preserved red cells or pigment-laden macrophages. Shedding of type 1 alveolar epithelial cells and proliferation of type 2 cells can often be seen along thickened septa, but these changes are probably epiphenomena.[56]

The clinical diagnosis can often be established by the episodes of hemoptysis or by the identification of hemosiderin-laden macrophages in the sputum. The etiology and pathogenesis of this condition are entirely obscure, but vague hypotheses have been made about inhaled toxins, viral infections, or pulmonary hypersensitivity reactions to various antigens, even possibly to those in food.[54]

# PULMONARY INFECTIONS

Despite potent antibiotics, lung infections remain a major cause of death. The normally sterile lower respiratory tract has at one time or another been invaded by every known microbiologic agent. Bacteria, particularly certain species, and viruses lead this parade. Bacterial invaders typically cause intraalveolar exudation resulting in consolidation (solidification) of the pulmonary parenchyma, referred to as pneumonia. Certain organisms tend to cause bronchopneumonia marked by patchy or lobular involvement, usually as an extension of bronchiolitis into the air spaces. Other bacteria tend to induce confluent, sometimes total lobar consolidation—lobar pneumonia. However, the same organism may produce bronchopneumonia on one occasion and lobar pneumonia on another. Moreover, bronchopneumonia can become confluent and induce almost total lobar consolidation, or lobar pneumonia may not involve an entire lobe. Ultimately, the terms "bronchopneumonia " and "lobar pneumonia " merely give some indication of the anatomic distribution of the infection, but there is much overlap. More significant is the total amount of involvement and, especially, the identity of the specific invader and its vulnerability to particular antibiotics.

In contrast to the changes in bacterial pneumonia, viruses and mycoplasma tend to evoke essentially interstitial inflammation, which properly should be referred to as "pneumonitis." However, long usage has sanctified the terms "viral" and "mycoplasmal pneumonia." Pneumonic infections with these agents are rarely fatal, but they predispose to severe superimposed bacterial infections, which too often cause death. In the influenza pandemic of 1915 to 1918, most of the deaths were caused by secondary pulmonary bacterial infections.

Host resistance is of especial importance in pulmonary infections. The very elderly, immunocompromised, or debilitated host is likely to develop extensive severe lung infections. Indeed, organisms of low virulence, including "opportunists" incapable of producing disease in the otherwise normal individual, may cause fatal infections. The patient with AIDS (p. 175) or other immunodeficiency syndromes often becomes a victim to Pneumocystis carinii or Monilia organisms rarely encountered in otherwise normal hosts. Thus in the present era of organ transplantation involving immunosuppression and of anticancer drugs that depress bone marrow and immune function, pulmonary infections, often caused by opportunists, have become major causes of death in predisposed individuals.

## LOBAR PNEUMONIA

Involvement of an entire lobe or a large portion of it is usually caused by a virulent organism. Approximately 90% of these cases are caused by pneumococci, most commonly types 1, 3, 7, or 2. However, in a significant few cases, the causative agent is *Klebsiella pneumoniae* (Friedländer's bacillus) or *Staphylococcus aureus*. Occasionally the streptococci, *Haemophilus influenzae*, or some of the other gram-negative organisms (e.g., *Pseudomonas, Proteus*) are responsible for this pattern of pneumonia, especially in the predisposed host. The general morphology of lobar pneumonia will be presented, followed by a short clinical discussion of each of the principal etiologic types.

**MORPHOLOGY.** Four anatomic stages of lobar pneumonia have classically been described: congestion, red hepatization, gray hepatization, and resolution. Effective therapy frequently telescopes or halts progression of the course of the disease, so that at autopsy the anatomic changes do not conform to the older, classic stages.

The first stage, that of **congestion**, consists of rapid proliferation of the bacteria, with vascular engorgement and serous exudation. Thus the affected lobe or lobes are heavy, red, and boggy. The alveolar spaces contain proteinaceous edema fluid, scattered neutrophils, and numerous bacteria. The alveolar architecture is readily apparent.

The stage of **red hepatization** ensues as the air spaces fill up with a fibrinosuppurative exudate imparting a congested liver-like consolidation to the lung tissue. The alveolar spaces are packed with neutrophils, extravasated red cells, and precipitated fibrin. Fibrin strands may stream from one alveolus though the pores of Kohn into adjacent alveoli, thus obscuring the underlying pulmonary architecture. An overlying fibrinous or fibrinosuppurative pleuritis is almost invariably present.

The stage of **gray hepatization** (consolidation) involves the progressive disintegration of leukocytes and red cells along with the continued accumulation of fibrin within the alveoli. The fibrin now appears clumped and amorphous, and classically it contracts to yield a clear zone adjacent to the alveolar walls, disclosing the preserved native architecture. The pulmonary parenchyma is dry and liver-like except with infections caused by type-3 pneumococci and *Klebsiella,* which produce a thick mucinous exudation that clings to instruments. With all causal agents, the pleural reaction at this stage is most intense.

The final stage, that of **resolution**, follows in uncomplicated cases. The consolidative exudate within the alveolar spaces is enzymatically digested and is either resorbed or removed by coughing. The lung parenchyma again becomes boggy and wet until it is restored to its normal state. The pleural reaction may similarly resolve or undergo organization, leaving fibrous thickenings or permanent adhesions.

This process may involve one or several lobes unilaterally or bilaterally. With pneumococcal pneumonia, the lower lobes, on either or both sides, are typically involved (Fig. 13–18). Pneumonia caused by ***Klebsiella pneumoniae*** involves only the right lung in 75% of cases[57] and usually begins as a lobular process, affecting most

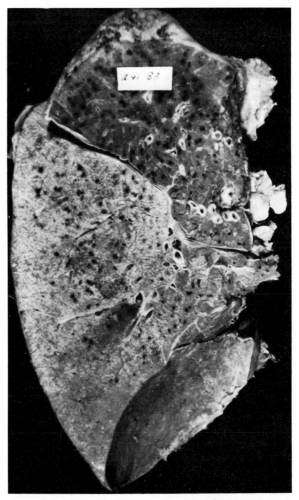

Figure 13–18. Lobar pneumonia. The lower lobe is uniformly consolidated, whereas the upper lobe is relatively unaffected. Note the "plaster-cast" impression of the dome of the diaphragm, preserved in the bottom of the lower lobe, and the fibrinous exudate (pleuritis) layering this diaphragmatic surface.

often the posterior segment of the upper lobe, ultimately extending to include the entire lobe.

This classic evolution may be complicated in the following ways: (1) tissue destruction and necrosis may lead to **abscess formation** within the otherwise solidified lung substance, particularly common in infections with type-3 pneumococci, *Klebsiella*, and staphylococci; (2) suppurative material may accumulate in the pleural cavity, producing an **empyema;** (3) **organization of the exudate** may convert areas of the lung into solid fibrous tissue, and (4) **bacteremic dissemination** may lead to meningitis, arthritis, or infective endocarditis.

**CLINICAL COURSE.** *Pneumococcal pneumonia* usually occurs in otherwise healthy adults between the ages of 30 and 50 years, although type 3 is more common in elderly individuals and in those already debilitated. Characteristically, the onset is sudden, marked by malaise; violent, shaking chills; and high fever. The accompanying cough is at first dry or productive of only thin watery sputum; with the stage of red hepatization, the sputum becomes thick, purulent, and hemorrhagic, known as "rusty sputum." Type-3 pneumococcus typically produces a tenacious mucinous sputum. The pleuritis manifests itself by pleuritic pain and a friction rub; often there is a pleural effusion. Blood cultures are positive in about 65% of cases before antibiotic treatment is instituted.[57] With therapy, the prognosis is excellent. However, complications may occur, such as meningitis, arthritis, or infective endocarditis. Later, residuals such as incomplete resolution or empyema may be seen. Abscesses are rare, except with type-3 pneumococci.

*Klebsiella pneumonia* occurs in a slightly older age group than does pneumococcal pneumonia, and is more frequent among debilitated and malnourished individuals, particularly chronic alcoholics. The onset is similar to that of pneumococcal pneumonia, although prostration may be more severe. The sputum is characteristically extremely thick and gelatinous, so that the patient may have difficulty in bringing it up. Even with treatment this type of pneumonia has a considerably greater mortality than does pneumococcal pneumonia, and complete resolution is less frequent. Abscesses are common, as are areas of fibrosis and bronchiectasis.

*Staphylococcal* or *Pseudomonas pneumonia* is gaining increasing importance, particularly as the most frequent form of pneumonia complicating influenza and as a common occurrence in debilitated hospitalized patients. Most often, it takes the form of a bronchopneumonia with multiple abscess formation, but occasionally it presents as a lobar pneumonia, particularly in infants.

Critical to the management of all forms is identification of the causal agent and its antibiotic sensitivity. With appropriate therapy, less than 10% of patients succumb, usually those severely predisposed to the disease.

## BRONCHOPNEUMONIA (LOBULAR PNEUMONIA)

This patchy pneumonic consolidation usually follows a bronchitis or bronchiolitis. It is a threat chiefly to the vulnerable—infants, the aged, and those suffering from chronic debilitating illness or immunosuppression. Whooping cough and measles are important antecedents in children; in the adult, influenza, chronic bronchitis, alcoholism, malnutrition, and carcinomatosis are all predisposing conditions. The patient with pulmonary edema from cardiac failure is particularly vulnerable.

Although almost any organism may cause bronchopneumonia, frequent offenders are staphylococci, streptococci, *H. influenzae*, *Proteus* species, and *Pseudomonas aeruginosa*. It is evident that many of these organisms may also produce lobar pneumonia. With increasing frequency today, such "opportunists" as *Monilia*, *Pneumocystis carinii*, and *Serratia mar-*

*cescens* cause bronchopneumonia as the terminal event in the immunoincompetent and in those already mortally ill (e.g., afflicted with some form of cancer).

A special type of bronchopneumonia occurs in patients who have aspirated their gastric contents either while unconscious or during repeated vomiting accompanied by a depressed cough reflex. The resultant pneumonia is partly chemical, owing to the extremely irritating effects of the gastric acid, and partly bacterial. Here the key role is played by a mixed flora of anaerobic and microaerophilic organisms normally present in the oral cavity.[58] This type of pneumonia may be extremely fulminant and is a frequent cause of death in patients predisposed to aspiration.

**MORPHOLOGY.** Bronchopneumonia is characterized by foci of inflammatory consolidation distributed patchily throughout one or several lobes. It is frequently bilateral and basal because of the tendency for secretions to gravitate into the lower lobes. Well-developed lesions are slightly elevated, dry, granular, gray-red to yellow, and poorly delimited at their margins. They vary in size up to 3 to 4 cm in diameter. Confluence of these foci occurs in the more florid instances, producing the appearance of total lobular consolidation. Focal areas of necrosis (abscesses) may appear within the areas of involvement.

The lung substance immediately surrounding areas of consolidation is usually slightly hyperemic and edematous, but the large intervening areas are generally normal. A fibrinous or suppurative pleuritis will develop if the inflammatory focus is in contact with the pleura; however, this is not common. With subsidence, the consolidation may resolve if there has been no abscess formation, or it may become organized, leaving residual foci of fibrosis.

Histologically, the reaction comprises a suppurative exudate that fills the bronchi, bronchioles, and adjacent alveolar spaces (Fig. 13–19). Neutrophils are dominant in this exudation, and usually only small amounts of fibrin are present. As expected, the abscesses are marked by necrosis of the underlying architecture.

Particularly in infancy but occasionally in adulthood, the bronchopneumonia usually caused by *E. coli* may remain interstitial, within the alveolar septa, and produce an inflammatory reaction confined to the alveolar walls with little exudate in the air spaces.

**CLINICAL COURSE.** The clinical picture of bronchopneumonia is seldom as well defined as that of lobar pneumonia, largely because it is frequently overshadowed by the predisposing condition. Moreover, the many etiologic agents for this disease have a considerable range of virulence, and patients vary in vulnerability. In general, the onset is insidious, often appearing as a nonspecific worsening of the patient's prior condition, with low-grade fever and cough productive of purulent sputum. Respiratory difficulty is typically not prominent. The course is irregular, but resolution usually occurs if treatment is appropriate and the patient is not severely debilitated.

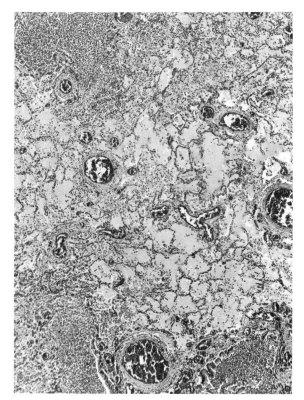

Figure 13–19. Bronchopneumonia. The low-power view reveals two foci of pneumonic consolidation on the left. At the lower right, a bronchus is filled with exudate. The intervening alveoli contain edema fluid and occasional white cells. There is an overall intense vascular congestion.

Complications are more frequent than with pneumococcal pneumonia; abscess formation is especially common.

## LEGIONNAIRES' DISEASE

Legionnaires' disease is basically a form of bronchopneumonia caused by the difficult-to-isolate, gram-negative bacillus *Legionella pneumophila*, one of a group of closely related *Legionella* species. Perhaps because of host or strain differences, the same agent may also cause a flu-like syndrome called *Pontiac fever*. Legionnaires' disease received its colorful name by being recognized first after an epidemic of pneumonia, frequently fatal, among delegates to an American Legion convention in a hotel in Philadelphia. The spread of infection was traced to a contaminated water-cooled air-conditioning system. It has since become evident that legionnaires' disease occurs endemically and sporadically and is a frequent cause of severe pneumonia requiring hospitalization.[59] *L. pneumophila* is also frequently involved in hospital-acquired respiratory infections.

The organism is almost ubiquitous in water, particularly standing, tepid, or warm water. It has been isolated from fresh and salt bodies of water, in water heating and cooling systems, and from both cold and hot tap water; it also survives happily at temperatures below 60°C. Person-to-person spread has not been documented. Legionnaires' disease is unusual in children; it is more common in the elderly and in those with some predisposing condition such as cardiac, renal, immunologic, or hematologic disease.[60] Inhalation of airborne contaminated droplets is the likely mode of spread.

The lung changes may take the form of an apparently patchy bronchopneumonia or sometimes almost complete consolidation of one or more lobes. The affected areas are red or gray, solidified, and sometimes punctuated by microabscesses. Pleural effusions, serous or serosanguineous, are frequently present in fatal cases, but frank empyema is rare.[61] Microscopically, the alveolar spaces in the consolidated areas are filled with an inflammatory exudate composed of neutrophils and macrophages. Often there are areas of necrosis of the native architecture, which creates abscesses that are usually small. Organisms cannot be visualized by routine stains but can be identified in profusion both within phagocytes as well as extracellularly by using immunochemical stains or the Dieterle silver stain.[62]

In the typical patient with legionnaires' disease, about two to 10 days after infection there is a gradual onset of malaise, weakness, lethargy, fever, and a dry cough. Depending on the severity of the disease, these nonspecific complaints are followed by recurring chills, dyspnea, pleuritic pain, and the raising of blood-streaked sputum. Many other manifestations may appear including disturbances of the central nervous system, abdominal pain, arthralgias, and striking elevation of the temperature, sometimes over 104°F. Chest radiographs will usually disclose areas of consolidation, but specific diagnosis rests with identification of the organism, by special stains or by immunochemical methods, in sputum or exudate obtained by transbronchial or percutaneous direct aspiration. The disease can also be diagnosed by a rising titer of serum antibodies, but unfortunately they do not reach diagnostically helpful levels until weeks after acquisition of the infection, too late to be of much aid in the clinical diagnosis of the acute disease.

## PNEUMOCYSTIS PNEUMONIA

*Pneumocystis carinii* is an opportunist that is currently a major cause of pneumonia, often fatal, in debilitated patients and those with AIDS or other forms of immunodeficiency. The airborne infection, at the outset, involves random patchy foci of the lungs but may in very vulnerable hosts spread widely throughout the lungs, producing a macroscopic appearance resembling that of the adult respiratory distress syndrome (p. 410). Microscopically, in the areas of involvement the alveoli are filled with a foamy protein-rich amphophilic fluid (in H and E stains), and the septal walls are thickened, edematous, and infiltrated by mononuclear inflammatory cells, principally plasma cells. The causal agent only becomes apparent in silver stains, which reveal within the alveolar fluid cup- or boat-shaped cyst forms (4 to 6 μm) having central dark dots. In most instances pneumocystic infections are fatal or contribute significantly to the demise of the mortally sick patient. Whether milder infections in less severely immunodeficient individuals are reversible and compatible with survival is not known.

## LUNG ABSCESS

Lung abscess refers to a localized area of suppurative necrosis within the pulmonary parenchyma. They occur at any age and in either sex. The causative organism may be introduced into the lung by any of the following mechanisms: (1) *Aspiration of infective material*, which may arise in carious teeth or infected sinuses or tonsils and which is particularly likely during oral surgery, anesthesia, coma, alcoholic intoxication, and in debilitated patients with depressed cough reflexes. Aspiration of gastric contents may also lead to lung abscesses. (2) As a *complication of pneumonia*. As was mentioned earlier, abscess formation is an occasional complication of pneumonia, particularly that caused by *Staphylococcus aureus, Klebsiella pneumoniae, Legionella pneumophila*, and type 3 pneumococcus. Mycotic infections and bronchiectasis may also lead to lung abscesses. (3) *Bronchial obstruction*. This is particularly likely with bronchogenic carcinoma obstructing a bronchus or bronchiole. Impaired drainage, distal atelectasis, and aspiration of blood and tumor fragments all contribute to the development of sepsis. Even more commonly, the abscess forms within an excavated necrotic portion of the tumor itself. (4) *Septic embolism*, from septic thrombophlebitis or from infective endocarditis of the right side of the heart. (5) *Bacteremic seeding* of the lung. Infrequent causes of a lung abscess include trauma, with direct introduction of bacteria by penetration of the lung; transdiaphragmatic spread from the peritoneum (e.g., from an amoebic hepatic abscess); and infected hydatid cysts. When all these pathogenetic pathways are excluded, there is still a large number of cases of mysterious origin, referred to as "primary cryptogenic lung abscesses."

The most commonly isolated aerobic organisms are *Staphylococcus aureus*, beta-hemolytic streptococci, the pneumococci, and many different gram-negative organisms.[63] Often there is a mixed infection. *Anaerobic bacteria are also present in almost all cases, sometimes in vast numbers.*[64] They have been the *exclusive* isolates in many cases of primary lung abscess. The most frequently encountered anaerobes are commensals normally found in the oral cavity; they are principally species of *Bacteroides, Fusobac-*

*terium, Peptococcus*, and microaerophilic streptococci.

**MORPHOLOGY.** Abscesses vary in diameter from a few millimeters to large cavities of 5 to 6 cm. The localization and number of abscesses are in large part dependent upon their mode of development. Pulmonary abscesses resulting from the aspiration of infective material are much more common on the right side (more vertical airways) than on the left, and most often are single. Within the right lung, the most frequent locations for solitary pulmonary abscesses are in the subapical and axillary portions of the upper lobe and in the apical portion of the lower lobe. These locations reflect the likely course of aspirated material when the patient is recumbent. Abscesses that develop in the course of pneumonia or bronchiectasis are commonly multiple, basal, and diffusely scattered. Septic emboli and pyemic abscesses, by the haphazard nature of their genesis, are commonly multiple and may affect any region of the lungs.

Pulmonary abscesses differ from those in solid organs such as the liver or kidney. As the focus of suppuration enlarges it almost inevitably ruptures into airways. Thus, the contained exudate may be partially drained, producing an air-fluid level on radiographic examination. Moreover, superimposed infections, often with saprophytic organisms, almost always develop. The proteolytic digestion of the exudate favors the growth of all organisms, and thus lung abscesses may expand rapidly into a multilocular cavity with poor margination. The buildup of edema in the area of the abscess may compress the blood supply, adding an element of ischemic necrosis to the preexisting infection—**gangrene of the lung.** Occasionally, abscesses rupture into the pleural cavity and produce bronchopleural fistulas, the consequence of which is pneumothorax or empyema.

Histologically, there is typically suppuration with massed preserved and necrotic neutrophils in the center of the lesion; the area is enclosed within a wall having variable amounts of fibrous scarring and mononuclear infiltration (lymphocytes, plasma cells, macrophages), depending on the chronicity of the lesion.

**CLINICAL COURSE.** The manifestations of a lung abscess are much like those of bronchiectasis. There is a prominent cough that usually yields copious amounts of foul-smelling purulent or sanguineous sputum. Occasionally gross hemoptysis occurs. Characteristically, changes in position evoke paroxysms of coughing caused by the sudden drainage from the abscess. However, if there is no avenue for drainage—or, sometimes, early in the course—sputum may be minimal. Along with the cough there is spiking fever and malaise, and, if the abscess extends to the overlying pleura, there may be pleuritic pain. Dyspnea is characteristically absent. Clubbing of the fingers may become apparent within a few weeks. With chronicity, weight loss and anemia ensue. Chest x-rays show an air-fluid level if there is communication with an airway; otherwise the density is homogeneous. Because cavitation of a neoplasm may also result in an air-fluid level, and because infective abscesses are found in 10 to 15% of patients with bronchogenic carcinoma, it is necessary to rule out an underlying carcinoma.

The course of these lesions is highly variable, depending on their pathogenesis and etiology and on such factors as spontaneous drainage and chronicity prior to diagnosis. When discovered early, most abscesses are eliminated by appropriate antibiotic therapy. Surgical resection or drainage may be necessary in some cases.[65] Overall, the mortality rate is in the range of 10%. Secondary amyloidosis develops infrequently in chronic cases.

## VIRAL AND MYCOPLASMAL PNEUMONIA (PRIMARY ATYPICAL PNEUMONIA)

*In pulmonary infections caused by either viruses or mycoplasma, the inflammatory reaction is largely confined to the interstitium of the alveolar septa and pulmonary parenchyma.* Thus these inflammations actually represent forms of pneumonitis, but long usage has sanctified the designation "pneumonia." Because they lack the characteristic intraalveolar exudation and consolidation seen with bacterial invasion, they are sometimes referred to by the curious name "primary atypical pneumonia." Even more strange, one or the other of these agents can be identified in only about half of the cases; in the remainder, despite the characteristic anatomic changes, the origin of infection remains undetermined. Among the disorders of known etiology, the largest fraction is caused by *Mycoplasma pneumoniae.*[66] Mycoplasma infections are particularly common among children and young adults and occur sporadically, peaking in spring and late summer. However, they may occur as local epidemics in closed communities (schools, military camps, prisons). Viral lower respiratory infections may occur at any age, and in adults they are most often produced by the influenza viruses A, B, and C. Less common offenders are parainfluenza and respiratory syncytial viruses, the latter especially in infants and children. A number of other viruses are sometimes implicated, including those causing measles and chicken pox.

Any one of the agents mentioned may cause an upper or lower respiratory infection. Much depends on the resistance of the host, and so viral and mycoplasmal diseases range from mild to severe. More serious lower respiratory tract infection is favored by old age, infancy, malnourishment, alcoholism, immunosuppression, and debilitation. It is no surprise, then, that viruses and mycoplasma are frequently involved in outbreaks of infection in hospitals. Both categories of agents, particularly viruses, derive their principal importance from their creating a predisposition to secondary bacterial invasion; combined infections are responsible for the alarming mortality rate of 20 to 30%.[67] It is theorized that primary viral infections impair the bactericidal competence of neutrophils and macrophages.[68]

**MORPHOLOGY.** Regardless of etiology, the morphologic patterns are similar. The process may be patchy, or it may involve whole lobes bilaterally or unilaterally. The affected areas are red-blue, congested, and subcrepitant. The weight of the lungs is only moderately increased, in the range of 800 gm each. Because most of the reaction is interstitial, little of the inflammatory exudate escapes on sectioning of the lung. There may be a slight oozing of red, frothy fluid. In contrast to lobar pneumonia, consolidation does not occur. With the light microscope, **the inflammatory reaction is seen to be confined within the walls of the alveoli** (Fig. 13–20). **The alveolar spaces themselves are remarkably free of exudate** but may contain a proteinaceous fluid and occasional mononuclear cells. The septa are widened and edematous; they usually contain a mononuclear inflammatory infiltrate of lymphocytes, histiocytes, and occasionally, plasma cells. In very acute cases, neutrophils may also be present. Sometimes **transudation of fibrin through the walls of severely affected alveolar septa produces a pink hyaline membrane lining the alveolar wall.** In fulminant cases of influenza pneumonia, fibrin thrombi are found within the alveolar capillaries in areas of necro-

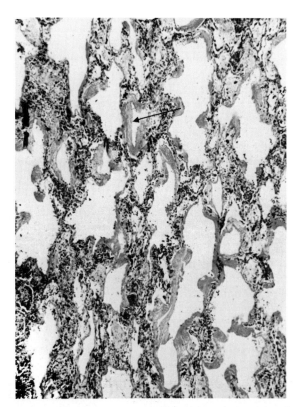

Figure 13–20. Viral pneumonia. The thickened alveolar walls are heavily infiltrated with mononuclear leukocytes. Coagulation of protein-rich intra-alveolar exudate has formed hyaline membranes (*arrow*).

sis of the alveolar walls. In less severe, uncomplicated cases, subsidence of the disease is followed by reconstitution of the native architecture. Often, however, superimposed bacterial infection occurs, resulting in a mixed histologic picture.

CLINICAL COURSE. The clinical course is extremely varied, even among cases caused by the same etiologic agent.[69] Often, primary atypical pneumonia masquerades as a severe upper respiratory infection or "chest cold," and presumably many of these go undiagnosed. In contrast, some cases are fulminant and cause death within 48 hours. The onset is usually that of an acute, nonspecific febrile illness, characterized by fever, headache, and malaise. Only later do localizing symptoms appear. Typically there is a hacking cough, which, in contrast to that of the bacterial pneumonias, tends to be unproductive of sputum. This is because the inflammatory reaction is largely interstitial. Chest x-rays usually reveal transient, ill-defined patches, mainly in the lower lobes. Physical findings are characteristically minimal. Because the edema and exudation are both in a strategic position to cause an alveolocapillary block, there may be respiratory distress seemingly out of proportion to the physical and radiologic findings.

Isolation of the causal agent, even when present, is difficult and takes so long that it is minimally useful in the management of the acute disease. Cold agglutinins are found in elevated titer in about 50 to 70% of cases caused by M. pneumoniae. This test is often used to differentiate the viral atypical pneumonias from those caused by M. pneumoniae. However, elevated cold agglutinins are also present in 20% of adenovirus infections.

The prognosis in uncomplicated cases is good, generally, with complete recovery as the rule. The most serious involvements occur among the infirm and the elderly and are caused by influenza viruses, particularly when complicated by bacterial superinfection.

## LIPID PNEUMONIA

Aspiration of oils may lead to patchy or diffuse consolidation of the lungs, hence the designation "lipid pneumonia." This nonmicrobial lesion occurs most commonly in the aged, in whom there is impairment of the swallowing reflex, in infants, and in adults following the protracted use of oily laxatives or nose drops. Rarely, lipid pneumonia follows the diagnostic use of nonirritating radiopaque oils in x-ray evaluation of the respiratory tree. In general, the more unsaturated the oil, the greater its irritant effect. This lesion is an uncommon cause of clinical disease, and it is usually discovered as an incidental finding on autopsy.

Grossly, foci of lipid pneumonia are gray to yellow, fairly sharply demarcated, and slightly elevated above the surrounding lung surface. The size varies, often from 1 to 3 cm in diameter. Because the texture of these lesions is firm and granular, they may be confused with tuberculous or neoplastic involvements. Histologically, early lipid pneumonia is characterized by the phagocytosis of emulsified oil in the alveoli by macrophages. Many macrophages thus accumulate in the alveoli. These phagocytes become distended by large, spherical, intracytoplasmic vacuoles or by multiple vacuoles. Several such macrophages may coalesce to form giant cells. The alveolar septa characteristically show marked congestion and some widening but remarkably little leukocytic reaction. With progression of the lesion, fibroblasts migrate into the alveoli to organize the phagocytic exudate. Sometimes the actively growing fibroblastic tissue and foreign body multinucleate giant cells form granulomas that resemble those of tuberculosis or sarcoidosis. Although there may be some resorption of oil with resolution of the exudate, permanent fibrous scarring usually ensues.

## CYTOMEGALIC INCLUSION DISEASE (CID)

*This disorder, caused by the cytomegalovirus (CMV), is characterized morphologically by gigantism of isolated cells and their nuclei, which often contain distinctive intranuclear inclusions.* Many organs may be affected in CID, and so inclusion of this infection in a chapter on the lung is admittedly arbitrary. In various surveys around the world, from 50 to 100% of adults were found to have CMV-specific antibody. Exposure to the agent is therefore nearly universal. This dissemination can be attributed largely to the many pathways of spread of the virus. Following an infection, the agent is present in the blood, urine, vaginal secretions, breast milk, semen, tears, saliva, and stool. Infection may be acquired at any time during life, but there are three peak periods: (1) prenatal infection of the fetus when the mother has an active primary or secondary (reactivated) disease; (2) during the first year of life after loss of maternal antibodies, by transmission of the virus through cervical or vaginal secretions at birth or through breast milk in mothers having active infections; (3) childhood or adult infections acquired through the respiratory, fecal-oral, blood transfusion, organ graft, or possibly venereal routes.

The CMV is an avirulent organism. Factors such as age when infected, host resistance, prior exposure, and immunity all modify the consequences of viral exposure, which range from asymptomatic infection in the otherwise normal school-age child or adult to severe, sometimes fatal multisystem disease in the infant or vulnerable host.

*Neonatal infection* may be asymptomatic (90%), cause mild self-limited disease, or take the form of severe multisystem disease (classic CID).[70]

In the classic severe neonatal disease, the organs most often affected, in order of frequency, are the salivary glands, kidneys, liver, lungs, pancreas, thyroid, adrenals, and brain. Grossly, the anatomic changes are minimal, consisting chiefly of slight enlargement of the involved organs, particularly the liver and spleen. The brain is often smaller than normal (microcephaly) and may show foci of calcification. Histologically, the characteristic cellular changes can be appreciated. In the glandular organs, it is the parenchymal epithelial cells that are affected; in the brain, the neurons; in the lungs, the alveolar lining cells; and in the kidneys, the tubular epithelial cells. Random cells are involved and are strikingly enlarged, often to a diameter of 40 μm, have hyperchromatic, enlarged nuclei, and show cellular and nuclear polymorphism. Prominent intranuclear basophilic inclusions spanning half the nuclear diameter are usually set off from the nuclear membrane by a clear halo (Fig. 13–21). Within the cytoplasm of these cells, smaller basophilic inclusions may also be seen. An interstitial pneumonitis may be present, as well as focal necroses within the liver and adrenals. The affected ganglion cells within the brain are often surrounded by a glial reaction, sometimes with calcification.

Clinically, these infants are profoundly ill and manifest jaundice, hepatosplenomegaly, anemia, and

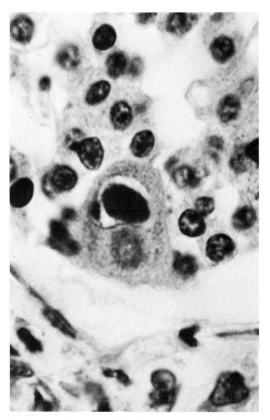

**Figure 13–21.** Cytomegalic inclusion disease. The markedly enlarged cell in the pancreatic islet has a prominent nuclear inclusion surrounded by a cleared halo. There are basophilic cytoplasmic inclusions as well.

a bleeding diathesis from thrombocytopenia. Such findings closely mimic erythroblastosis fetalis. Those infants who survive usually bear permanent residual effects, including mental retardation and various neurologic impairments.[71]

However, the congenital infection is not always devastating and may take the form of an interstitial pneumonitis, hepatitis, encephalitis, or hematologic disorder. Most infants with this milder form of CID recover, although a few may later show mental retardation. Moreover, a rare, totally asymptomatic infection may be followed months to years later by neurologic sequelae.

*Postnatal CMV infection* is equally variable in severity but is usually asymptomatic owing to higher levels of immunity. Only rarely it is severe and multisystemic. After the first year of life otherwise normal hosts almost never develop severe multisystem disease. Probably less than 1% ever develop any type of clinical manifestations, which most often conform to a mononucleosis-like syndrome (p. 400). This pattern of disease is especially associated with a large dose of virus (for example, from multiple transfusions of infected units of blood). Uncommonly, the syndrome takes the form of an interstitial pneumonitis, hepatitis, gastrointestinal ulcerative disease, or an anemia or thrombocytopenia.

By contrast, immunocompromised or debilitated hosts, particularly seriously ill transplant recipients, are more likely to suffer the full blast of the virus or at least one of the intermediate levels of severity described. An overview of the many outcomes of infection is offered in Figure 13–22. It should be evident that the CMV is a proverbial bully; it only becomes nasty with those unable to defend themselves—the newborn, the aged, and the sick.

## TUBERCULOSIS (TB)

Tuberculosis is a communicable chronic granulomatous disease caused by *Mycobacterium tuberculosis*. It usually involves the lungs but may affect any organ or tissue in the body. Typically *the centers of the granulomas undergo caseous necrosis to create "soft tubercles."* Among the medically and economically deprived throughout the world, tuberculosis remains a leading cause of death. In the United States the death rate from it has decreased since the turn of the century from 200 to about two deaths per 100,000 persons. Similar declines have occurred in other industrialized nations. These dramatic results can be attributed to many factors (discussed later), but among them control of spread of infection must be accorded primacy. It is important at this point that *infection* be differentiated from *disease*. Although other routes may be involved, most infections are acquired by direct person-to-person transmission of airborne droplets of organisms from an active case

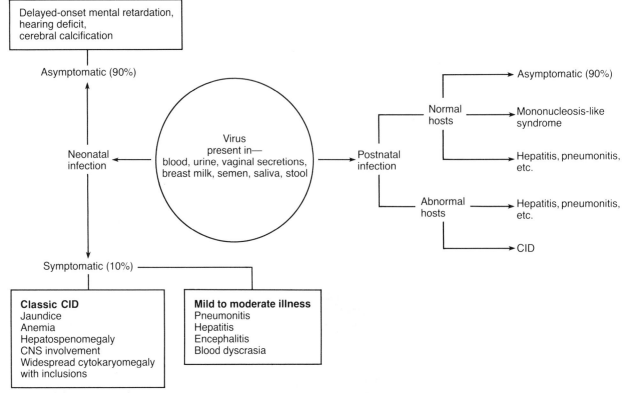

Figure 13–22. Cytomegalic inclusion disease. Possible outcomes of an infection are based on individual's age.

to a susceptible host. Clinically, overt pulmonary disease may or may not develop. Indeed, *in most persons an asymptomatic focus of pulmonary infection appears that is self-limited* and leads only to a tell-tale tiny fibrocalcific marker at the site of the infection. It is important to emphasize that viable organisms may remain dormant in such loci for decades and possibly for the life of the host. *Such individuals are infected but do not have active disease* and so cannot transmit organisms to others. Yet when their defenses are lowered, the infection may "reactivate" to produce communicable and potentially life threatening disease. *Infection, whether active or inactive, can be detected by the tuberculin (Mantoux) test*, which reveals the development of skin sensitivity to tuberculoprotein. About two to four weeks after the infection has begun, an intracutaneous injection of 0.1 ml of purified protein derivative (PPD) will induce a visible and palpable induration (at least 5 mm in diameter) in 48 hours. Sometimes, more or less PPD is required. A positive tuberculin test is generally taken to mean the presence of cell-mediated hypersensitivity to tubercular antigens. However, the possibility has been raised that a positive reaction requires that viable organisms persist in the latent focus of infection.[72] It is well recognized, however, that *false-negative reactions may be produced by viral infections, sarcoidosis, malnutrition, Hodgkin's disease, immunosuppression, and notably overwhelming active tuberculous diseases.* False-positive reactions may result from infection by atypical mycobacteria.[73]

About 80% of the population in South India (and many other Asian and African countries) are tuberculin-positive.[74] In the United States, 5 to 10% of the population (roughly 15 million) reacted positively to tuberculin, but there were less than 25,000 active cases reported in 1983.[75] Thus only a small fraction of those contracting an infection develop active disease.

*Tuberculosis flourishes whenever there is poverty, crowding, and chronic debilitating illness. Similarly, the elderly with their weakened defenses become vulnerable.* A recent study points out the high incidence of infection among the residents of nursing homes.[76] Thus certain segments of all populations continue to show a high incidence of the disease. In the United States, American blacks, Indians, Eskimos, and Hispanics have higher attack rates than other segments of the population. Whether this is all socioeconomic in origin or in part racial is unknown. Genetic resistance can be documented among laboratory animals; witness the vulnerability of the long-suffering guinea pig and the high resistance of the rat. Certain conditions also increase the risk—diabetes mellitus, Hodgkin's disease, chronic lung disease (particularly silicosis), malnutrition, alcoholism, and immunosuppression (e.g., chronic administration of steroids).

At one time the brunt of active disease was borne

mainly by children and young adults, but less than 5% of schoolchildren in the United States now react to tuberculin. The peak morbidity and mortality has shifted to those between 50 and 60 years old who acquired the infection "in the good old days" when tuberculosis was widespread. Their infections became reactivated when immunity and resistance dwindled.[77] However, disease in the young is a still a harsh reality among the underprivileged of all countries.

**ETIOLOGY.** The mycobacteria consist of a large group of slender rods that are acid-fast—i.e., have a sufficient content of complex lipids so that once the Ziehl-Neelsen (carbol fuschsin) stain is taken up, they resist decolorization. *M. tuberculosis hominis* is responsible for most cases of tuberculosis. Its reservoir of infection is generally active pulmonary disease in humans. Transmission is usually direct, by inhalation of airborne organisms, and depends on the concentration of organisms in the coughed-up aerosol and the closeness and duration of contact with the active case. Oropharyngeal and intestinal tuberculosis contracted by drinking milk contaminated with *M. bovis* is now rare in developed nations but still prevalent in countries having tuberculous dairy cows and unpasteurized milk. Both *M. hominis* and *M. bovis* species are obligate aerobes whose slow growth is retarded by a pH lower than 6.5 and by long-chain fatty acids, hence the tendency for tubercle bacilli to disappear within the centers of large caseating lesions where anaerobiosis, a falling pH, and increased levels of fatty acids are found.

**PATHOGENESIS.** Three considerations are involved in the pathogenesis of tuberculosis: (1) the basis of the virulence of the organism, (2) the significance of the development of sensitivity and immunity or resistance to the organism, and (3) the pathogenesis of the caseation necrosis.

*The virulence of the tubercle bacillus* is not related to any known endotoxin or exotoxin. The ability of *M. tuberculosis* to induce disease in experimental animals appears to be related to mycosides in the lipid fraction of the bacteria. One derivative of the mycosides called "cord factor" (because it is responsible for the serpentine, cord-like growth of *M. tuberculosis* in vitro) is highly toxic to mice. It may also serve as an adjuvant and so enhance the antigenicity of tuberculoproteins.

*The development of hypersensitivity to the tubercle bacillus is central to its destructiveness to tissues and probably also to the emergence of resistance to the organisms.* On first exposure to the organisms or in nonreactors, the initial inflammatory response is entirely nonspecific, resembling the reaction to any form of bacterial invasion. *Within two or three weeks coincident with the appearance of delayed hypersensitivity, the reaction becomes granulomatous and the centers often become caseous to form the typical tubercles.* The sequence of events appears to be (1) presentation of antigen to T cells by macrophages

that have engulfed organisms, (2) sensitization of T cells, (3) release of lymphokines such as factors chemotactic to monocytes and macrophages and migration inhibition factor, and (4) aggregation of macrophages and lymphocytes at sites of implantation to form granulomas. Concomitantly, the T cells activate the macrophages by enhancing their phagocytic and bactericidal capacities, possibly by the release of yet another lymphokine, gamma interferon.[78] Thus it is apparent that *the development of hypersensitivity is requisite for granuloma formation and for enhanced resistance to the organisms.* Whether sensitivity and resistance are separate but concurrent functions or are interdependent is uncertain.

As mentioned, *typical granulomas in tuberculosis have central caseation (soft tubercles), although sometimes for obscure reasons there is no caseation (hard tubercles).* What induces the caseation remains a mystery. There are only a few hints. The aggregated macrophages in the granuloma are characteristically transformed to *epithelioid cells*, which have highly ruffled interdigitating cell membranes, numerous mitochondria, well-developed endoplasmic reticulum, and large Golgi complexes. This ultrastructure would appear to be more appropriate for secretory function than for phagocytosis. Could the secretion be catabolic enzymes responsible for caseation?

In summary, the appearance of hypersensitivity signals the acquisition of immunity and resistance to the organism. But at the same time, hypersensitivity is accompanied by the caseating destructive response to the tubercle bacillus. Thus, the sensitized host more rapidly mobilizes a defensive reaction but suffers enhanced necrosis of tissues. Whether the resistive or destructive forces will be ascendent determines whether the primary focus of infection will remain localized and disseminated organisms will be destroyed (or at least kept in check) or disabling disease will appear. Despite having somewhat opposing effects, clinical experience indicates hypersensitivity and immunity tend to block spread and dissemination of primary infections and thus on balance favor the host. Some concept of these interrelationships is offered in Figure 13–23.

The previous considerations have long raised questions about the desirability of inducing hypersensitivity and immunity in nonexposed individuals by the injection of a vaccine of attenuated nonvirulent tubercle bacilli (BCG—Bacille Calmette Guérin). Despite intensive study of the problem and wide use around the world, it is still not clear whether BCG vaccination is an effective method of reducing the prevalence of disease.[79] It is not used very much in the U.S. because by converting the individual to a tuberculin reactor, it abolishes the use of the Mantoux test for finding cases of tuberculosis.

### Primary Tuberculosis

*Primary tuberculosis is the form of disease that develops in a previously unexposed and therefore*

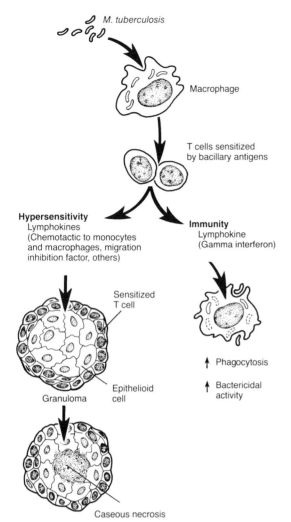

Figure 13–23. Tuberculosis—the dual consequences of the emergence of macrophage activation and sensitization.

mal lesion and the nodal involvement is referred to as the Ghon complex (Fig. 13–24). In most cases the lung and nodal involvement is unilateral, but rarely bilateral or multiple Ghon foci or complexes are encountered. In most cases, the Ghon complex in time undergoes progressive fibrosis and often calcification.

Histologically, **the sites of active involvement are marked by a characteristic granulomatous inflammatory reaction forming both caseating and noncaseating tubercles** (Fig. 13–25). Individual tubercules are of microscopic size, and it is only when multiple granulomas coalesce that they become macroscopically visible. In the immune host, the granulomas or collection of granulomas are enclosed within a fibroblastic rim punctuated by numerous lymphocytes. Multinuclear giant cells typically of Langhans' type are present in the margins of the granulomas. In the more vulnerable host, the fibroblastic walling-off is less well developed and the lymphocytic infiltrate somewhat more sparse. Recall that **many other conditions may produce granulomatous reactions, sometimes with central apparent caseation necrosis** (p. 46). **Thus to establish the diagnosis of tuberculosis, the organisms must be identified in the tissues, either with appropriate stains or by culture methods.**

Primary tuberculosis is usually asymptomatic. Indeed, its existence is only recognized by a positive Mantoux test or the characteristic foci of calcification

*nonsensitized individual. Elderly individuals may lose their sensitivity to the tubercle bacillus and so once again may develop primary tuberculosis. In contrast, the disease that follows reinfection of a sensitized host or (more likely) reactivation of a primary infection is called secondary or postprimary tuberculosis.* With primary tuberculosis, the source of the organism must always be exogenous; only about 5% of those newly infected develop significant disease.

In countries where bovine tuberculosis and infected milk have almost disappeared, primary tuberculosis almost always begins in the lungs. Typically, the inhaled bacilli implant in the distal air spaces of the lower part of the upper lobe or the upper part of the lower lobe, usually close to the pleura. As sensitization develops, a 1- to 1.5-cm area of gray-white inflammatory consolidation emerges—**the Ghon focus.** In most cases the center of this focus undergoes caseation necrosis. Tubercle bacilli, either free or within phagocytes, drain to the regional nodes to there initiate gray-white foci of consolidation, which often caseate. The **combination of the parenchy-**

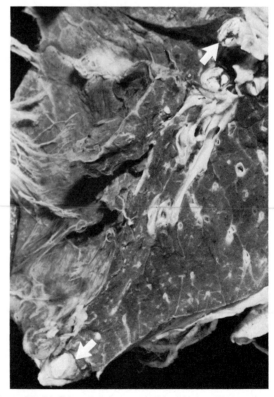

Figure 13–24. Primary pulmonary tuberculosis—Ghon complex. The parenchymal focus is present in the lower left subpleural location (*arrow*). Lymph nodes with caseation are visible in the upper right (*arrow*).

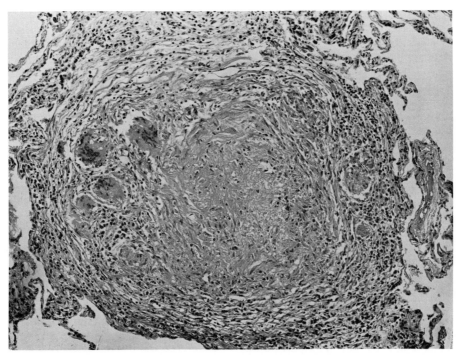

Figure 13–25. A characteristic tubercle in detail illustrates central granular caseation and both epithelioid and giant cells. (From Robbins, S. L., Cotran, R. S., and Kumar, V.: Pathologic Basis of Disease. 3rd ed. Philadelphia, W. B. Saunders Co., 1984, p. 741.)

in the chest radiograph. Uncommonly, primary pulmonary tuberculosis comes to attention when there is fever and pleurisy with effusion. This pattern of disease is usually readily amenable to therapeutic control. The chief significance of primary tuberculosis is (1) it induces hypersensitivity and increased resistance, (2) the foci of scarring may harbor viable bacilli for years and perhaps for life and thus may become reactivated, and (3) the disease may, uncommonly, extend without interruption into so-called progressive primary tuberculosis. The primary focus enlarges, caseates, and cavitates, sometimes to spread through the airways or lymphatics to multiple sites within the lung or even to cause multiple patchy white areas of cheesy consolidation that may cavitate. Infrequently the spread may lead to almost total consolidation of one or more lobes (pneumonia alba). These ramifications are analogous to those that follow secondary tuberculosis and so are described later.

## Secondary Tuberculosis (Reactivation, Postprimary Tuberculosis)

*Secondary tuberculosis is the pattern of disease that arises in a previously sensitized host.* Usually it results from reactivation of dormant primary lesions many decades later. Occasionally it results from exogenous reinfection because of waning of the protection afforded by the primary disease or because of a large inoculum of virulent bacilli. Whatever the source of the organisms, only a few patients (under 5%) with primary disease develop secondary tuberculosis.

*Secondary pulmonary tuberculosis is almost always localized to the apices of one or both upper lobes.* The lesions rarely involve the lower lobes. The reason for this usual apical localization is obscure. Because of the preexistence of hypersensitivity, the bacilli excite a prompt and marked tissue response that tends to wall off the focus. As a result of this localization, the regional lymph nodes are less prominently involved early in the developing disease. On the other hand, cavitation occurs readily with the secondary form, resulting in bronchogenic dissemination. Indeed, *cavitation is almost inevitable in neglected secondary tuberculosis.* Erosion into an airway creates what is known as "open tuberculosis" because the patient now raises infective sputum.

**MORPHOLOGY. The initial lesion is usually a small focus of consolidation, less than 2 cm in diameter, located within 1 to 2 cm of the apical pleura.** Such foci are fairly sharply circumscribed, firm, gray-white to yellow areas that have a greater or lesser component of central caseation and peripheral fibrous induration. The regional lymph nodes soon develop foci of similar tuberculous activity. In favorable cases, the initial parenchymal focus develops a small area of caseation necrosis that does not cavitate because it fails to communicate with a bronchus or bronchiole. The subsequent course may be one of progressive fibrous encapsulation, leaving only fibrocalcific scars that depress and pucker the pleural surface and cause focal pleural adhesions. Sometimes these fibrocalcific scars become secondarily blackened by anthracotic pigment. In many instances, a dense, collagenous, fibrous wall may totally enclose inspissated, caseous debris that never resolves and calcifies as a granular lesion at postmortem examination. Histologically, the active lesions show characteristic coalescent tubercles, usually with some central caseation. Although tubercle bacilli can be demonstrated by appropriate methods in the early exudative and caseous phases, it is usually impossible to find them in the late fibrocalcific stages. However, it cannot be assumed that their absence in histologic sections implies their total destruction, because in many of these instances the presence of the organism can be demonstrated by inoculation into the unfortunate guinea pig.

Although localized apical secondary pulmonary tuberculosis may either spontaneously or following therapy undergo **fibrocalcific arrest**, depending on host-invader factors, the disease may progress and extend along many pathways.

(1) **Cavitary pulmonary tuberculosis** may ensue. The primary apical lesion enlarges with expansion of the area of caseation until it almost fills the apex. Erosion into a bronchus evacuates the caseous center, creating a ragged, irregular cavity lined by caseous material that is poorly walled off by fibrous tissue (Fig. 13–26). Erosion of blood vessels accounts for the hemoptysis these patients frequently have. The infection may spread more widely from direct expansion of the apical lesion but more often by dissemination through airways and lymphatic channels or by miliary dissemination through the vascular system either to the lungs alone or throughout the body. Systemic miliary tuberculosis is discussed later. **Pulmonary miliary disease** occurs when organisms drain through lymphatics into the main lymphatic ducts, thus reaching the venous return to the right heart and then the pulmonary arteries. The individual lesions are microscopic or visible (2 mm) foci of yellow-white consolidation spattered through the lung parenchyma. In the vulnerable host, this miliary distribution may expand and coalesce to yield almost total consolidation of large regions or even whole lobes of the lung (**pneumonia alba**). With chronicity, the secondary scarring may distort the pulmonary architecture almost beyond recognition. With progressive pulmonary tuberculosis, the pleural cavity is invariably involved, and, depending upon the chronicity of the disease, serous pleural effusions, frank tuberculous empyema, or obliterative fibrous pleuritis, sometimes massive, may develop.

(2) **Endobronchial, endotracheal, and laryngeal tuberculosis** may develop when infective material is spread either through lymphatic channels or by being coughed up. The mucosal linings may be studded with minute granulomatous lesions that sometimes only become apparent on microscopic examination.

(3) **Systemic miliary tuberculosis** ensues when infective foci in the lungs seed the pulmonary venous return to the heart; the infection subsequently disseminates through the systemic arterial system. Almost every organ in the body may be seeded, but the lesions may not be visible to the naked eye. When lesions are sufficiently advanced, they may yield coalescent granulomas apparent as 1- to 2-mm, yellow-white foci. For poorly understood reasons, miliary tuberculosis is most prominent in the liver, bone marrow (sites amenable to diagnostic biopsy), spleen, adrenals, meninges, kidneys, fallopian tubes, and epididymides. In contrast, certain organs, including striated muscle, heart, pancreas, stomach, thyroid, and testes, are seldom involved.

(4) **Isolated-organ tuberculosis** may appear in any one of the organs or tissues affected by miliary dissemination. Why a single isolated organ such as the meninges (tuberculous meningitis), kidneys (renal tuberculosis), adrenals (formerly an important cause of Addison's disease), bones (osteomyelitis), and fallopian tubes (salpingitis) are favored localizations and why only one of these sites suffers progressive tuberculous disease in the face of widespread dissemination is totally mysterious.

(5) **Intestinal tuberculosis** should be briefly mentioned. In years past, it was contracted by drinking contaminated milk and was fairly common as the primary focus of tuberculosis. Indeed, often it was preceded by tuberculous involvement of the oropharyngeal lymphoid tissue with spread to the lymph nodes in the neck (scrofula). In developed countries intestinal tuberculosis is currently more often a complication of protracted advanced secondary tuberculosis, secondary to the swallowing of coughed-up infective material. Typically, the

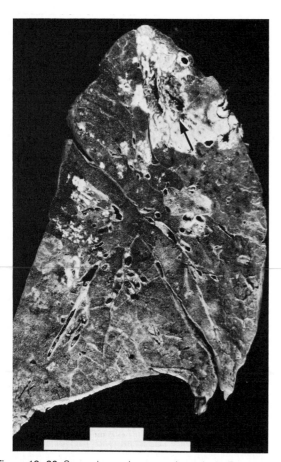

Figure 13–26. Secondary pulmonary tuberculosis. The cut section of the lung discloses massive caseation and cavitation (*arrow*) in the apex. Scattered foci of caseation as well as areas of pneumonic consolidation are present in both lobes.

organisms are trapped in the mucosal lymphoid aggregations of the small and large bowel; these undergo inflammatory enlargement with ulceration of the overlying mucosa, particularly in the ileum.

The many patterns of secondary tuberculosis are seen in Figure 13–27.

**CLINICAL COURSE.** Secondary tuberculosis may be asymptomatic. When manifestations appear they are insidious in onset; there is gradual development of both systemic and localizing symptoms. The basis for systemic symptoms is not clear, but they often appear early in the course and include malaise, anorexia, weight loss, and fever. Commonly the fever is low-grade and remittent (appearing late each afternoon and then subsiding), and night sweats occur. With

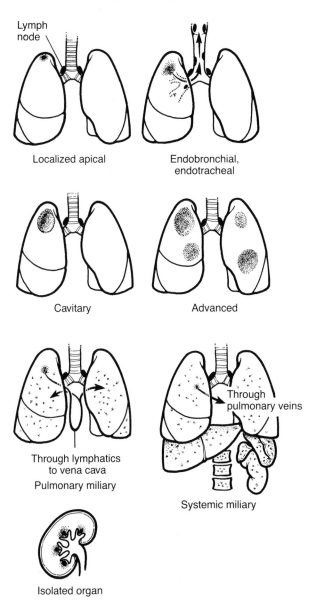

Lymph node

Localized apical

Endobronchial, endotracheal

Cavitary

Advanced

Through lymphatics to vena cava
Pulmonary miliary

Through pulmonary veins

Systemic miliary

Isolated organ

Figure 13–27. Diagrammatic representation of the many patterns of secondary tuberculosis, ranging from initial apical localization to miliary dissemination to isolated involvement of an organ (kidney).

progressive pulmonary involvement, localizing symptoms appear. One of the earliest of these symptoms is a cough that gradually becomes more distressing and yields increasing amounts of sputum, at first mucoid and later purulent. When cavitation is present, the sputum contains tubercle bacilli. Some degree of hemoptysis is present in about half of all cases of pulmonary tuberculosis. Pleuritic pain may also be the first manifestation of the disease, resulting either from spontaneous pneumothorax or from extension of the infection to the pleural surfaces. The diagnosis of pulmonary tuberculosis should be entertained whenever there is chronic cough along with constitutional symptoms, or when hemoptysis or spontaneous pneumothorax occurs. The diagnosis is based in part on the history and the physical and radiologic findings of consolidation or cavitation in the apices of the lungs. Ultimately, however, tubercle bacilli must be identified. Acid-fast smears of the sputum, cultures, and animal inoculation should be done. When sputum is unobtainable, gastric washings should be similarly examined. Currently, chemotherapy is usually effective except in advanced cases.

Miliary tuberculosis is often difficult to diagnose. It may appear as sudden worsening of known pulmonary disease. More often it appears in elderly individuals as a "fever of unknown origin" in the absence of apparent active pulmonary disease. Often the diagnosis rests with the identification of tubercles in bone-marrow or liver biopsies.

The prognosis is generally good with infections localized to the lungs, except when they are caused by drug-resistant strains or occur in the very aged, debilitated, or immunosuppressed individual who is at risk of developing miliary tuberculosis. Amyloidosis may appear in persistent cases, adding another potential cause of death.

## THE DEEP MYCOSES

Many pathogenic fungi limit their activities to the skin. Those that also involve the deeper structures, most frequently the lungs, are of greater importance. In many instances, the guilty fungi are saprophytes that become opportunistic pathogens only under special circumstances, such as chronic illness, cancer chemotherapy or total body irradiation, prolonged treatment with broad-spectrum antibiotics, or immunosuppressive treatment. The pattern of disease produced by the deep mycoses is extremely variable. Clinically, it ranges from an acute pneumonitis to a smoldering, chronic process resembling tuberculosis. In general, the fungi are weak pathogens, produce no toxins, and cause tissue damage primarily by a hypersensitivity reaction in the host to the parasitic proteins. This is particularly true of *Histoplasma capsulatum*, *Coccidioides immitis*, and *Blastomyces dermatitidis*. Only the more important fungi that may involve the lung are described here briefly.

## Candidiasis (Moniliasis)

*Candida albicans* is the most frequent cause of disease among the fungi. It is a normal inhabitant of the oral cavity, gastrointestinal tract, and vagina in many individuals. Under appropriate circumstances, such as lowered resistance and immunity, this organism may cause bothersome but not serious superficial inflammation to fatal blood-borne systemic infection.[80]

**The most common pattern of candidiasis takes the form of a superficial infection on mucosal surfaces of the oral cavity (thrush), or vagina.** Florid proliferation of the fungi creates gray-white, dirty-looking superficial membranes formed by matted organisms and inflammatory debris. Deep to the surface there is mucosal hyperemia and a superficial inflammatory reaction. This form of candidiasis is seen in the newborn, diabetic, debilitated patients, or those receiving broad-spectrum antibiotics that destroy the competing normal bacterial flora. Occasionally, vaginal candidiasis develops in otherwise normal women; it occurs more often in pregnant women and in those who take oral contraceptives. A more erosive chronic mucocutaneous candidiasis occurs particularly in the esophagus in the mortally ill or in association with any hematologic or T-cell derangement that markedly impairs the inflammatory-immune response.

**Invasive candidiasis** implies blood-borne dissemination of organisms to various tissues or organs. Common patterns are (1) renal involvement (abscesses), (2) vegetative endocarditis (often of the right-sided valves in drug addicts), (3) hepatic lesions (abscesses) and (4) pulmonary lesions (large or small irregular or cannonball abscesses, sometimes hemorrhagic, owing to vascular invasion).

Invasive candidiasis is seen only in the context of some serious predisposing condition that cripples the inflammatory-immune response of the host (e.g., marrow ablation in the treatment of leukemia or profound immunosuppression, such as is used to reverse transplant rejection). With systemic dissemination the outlook is grave.

## Actinomycosis and Nocardiosis

The agents causing actinomycosis (*Actinomyces israelii*) and nocardiosis (*Nocardia asteroides*) are now classified as bacteria but are considered here among the fungi because of long precedent. *Actinomyces israelii* is anaerobic or microaerophilic and is a normal inhabitant of the oral cavity. It becomes pathogenic whenever there is devitalization of tissues and sepsis, providing foci of reduced oxygen tension. Thus, actinomycosis may develop following intraoral infection or dental surgery or may become implanted in the lung or gastrointestinal tract, superimposed on an antecedent disorder (e.g., lung abscess, ulceroinflammatory disease of the gut) that provides a favorable environment for its growth. Thus, *there are three classical clinical patterns of actinomycosis, which are not mutually exclusive: (1) cervicofacial, (2) thoracic, and (3) abdominal.*

The *Nocardia* organisms are aerobic and are not normal inhabitants of the oral cavity. They are usually acid-fast, whereas the actinomycetes are weakly and inconstantly acid-fast. Clinically, nocardial infections usually take the form of an acute bronchopneumonia with abscess formation, although they may occasionally simulate tuberculosis. Sometimes there is an associated empyema.

The gross appearance of the lesions caused by both organisms is essentially that of intense suppuration with abscess formation. Typically within the suppurative exudate, **the actinomycetes grow in colony formation, comprising a tangled mass of threads surrounded by radiating, sometimes terminally clubbed organisms.** These colonies are grossly visible as yellow to gray "sulfur granules." *Nocardia* rarely grows in colony formation but more often occurs in branching filaments. Typical of both organisms is great chronicity, burrowing spread of the infection, and, sometimes, penetrating sinus tracts. Thus, lesions in the lung resemble a pyogenic bronchopneumonia with abscess formation. Over the span of time, the abscesses are enclosed within an abundant fibroblastic reaction, but sometimes fistulous sinus tracts develop into the pleural cavities or even through the chest wall. A similar sequence occurs wherever the organisms become implanted.

The diagnosis must be suspected in any persistent suppurative chronic infection with abscess formation. It can be confirmed by isolation of the causative agents or by identification of the colony formations within the inflammatory exudate in actinomycosis.

## Histoplasmosis

Infection caused by *Histoplasma capsulatum* mimics tuberculosis in many ways. It usually begins with a primary pulmonary infection that is localized in nature and frequently asymptomatic; it may then progress to more extensive pulmonary involvement, sometimes cavitary; and, in predisposed individuals, it may disseminate in a miliary pattern. However, as judged by the histoplasmin skin test (analogous to the tuberculin test), only a small fraction of infections give rise to symptomatic disease. Histoplasmosis is endemic in the Ohio and central Mississippi River Valleys and along the Appalachian Mountains in the southeastern United States. Warm, moist soil, enriched by droppings from bats and birds, provides the optimal medium for the growth of the mycelial form, which produces terminal infectious spores. When airborne and inhaled, the spores germinate into the parasitic yeast form in the lungs. In most normal adults in endemic areas, the infection is asymptomatic and takes the form of a peripheral pulmonary lesion associated with hilar lymphadenopathy, recapitulating the Ghon complex of tuberculosis.

Such infection may undergo fibrosis and calcification and only be discovered by radiography in the individual with a positive histoplasmin skin test who is tuberculin-negative. In children or adults with lowered resistance or defective immune responses, this primary complex may be followed by secondary extending, sometimes cavitating, pulmonary infection, leading in some instances to lymphohematogenous dissemination and extrapulmonary disease.[81]

Histoplasmosis is best remembered as a reticuloendothelial disorder. The **round to oval yeast forms, 2 to 5 μm in diameter,** are typically found within macrophages and reticuloendothelial cells, accounting for the frequently used designation "cytomycosis." The primary, solitary pulmonary nodule comprises at first an aggregation of macrophages stuffed with organisms, located usually in a lower lobe, associated with a similar lesion in the regional lymph nodes. These lesions form small granulomas complete with Langhans' giant cells that may in the course of time develop central necrosis and later undergo fibrosis or calcification. The similarity to tuberculosis is obvious, and differentiation requires identification of the yeast forms (best seen with PAS or silver stains). In the vulnerable host upper lobe chronic cavitary disease develops, recapitulating the secondary form of tuberculosis. Histologically, in the margins of the cavity, there are coalescent granulomas with central necrosis. Depending on the host-invader balance, the infection may extend to involve large areas of the lung. Occasionally, usually in infants or immunocompromised adults, histoplasmosis flares into disseminated disease throughout the body (analogous to miliary tuberculosis). Because the T-cell response is inadequate, there is no granuloma formation, but instead the entire reticuloendothelial system becomes overloaded with phagocytized yeast forms and undergoes reactive proliferation, forming small aggregations of phagocytic cells in the organ. As a consequence, there is hepatosplenomegaly, diffuse lymphadenopathy, and multiple ulcerative lesions within the lymphoid tissue of the gastrointestinal tract. In some instances, the dissemination appears to localize principally in certain sites, producing, for example, massive destruction of the adrenals or involvement of the brain and meninges.

The clinical manifestations of histoplasmosis are almost indistinguishable from those of tuberculosis.[82] The infection may be asymptomatic, or it may cause only vague manifestations such as fever, malaise, and myalgias; it can be readily mistaken for "flu," but with more extensive pulmonary involvement, cough, hemoptysis, and even dyspnea and chest pain may appear. Disseminated disease is a hectic, febrile illness that may show hepatosplenomegaly, anemia, leukopenia, thrombocytopenia, and manifestations relating to principal sites of localization. Although the histoplasmin skin test and elevated serum antibody titers reveal exposure to the organism, they do not differentiate present from past disease. The diagnosis of active infection is best made by sputum culture or direct visualization of the organism in lesions and the reticuloendothelial system, usually accomplished by needle biopsies of the bone marrow or liver.

### Coccidioidomycosis

At the risk of being accused of unseemly familiarity with this condition, "cocci," as we shall call it, is caused by *Coccidioides immitis*. It is endemic in the Southwest and Far West of the United States, particularly in the San Joaquin Valley, where it is known as "valley fever."[82] Here almost 80% of the population are coccidioidin-positive (analogous to the tuberculin test). *"Cocci," like histoplasmosis and tuberculosis, takes the forms of (1) an asymptomatic pulmonary infection in 60% of exposed individuals, (2) progressive pulmonary disease, or (3) miliary disease.*

The primary pulmonary form results in a small focus of consolidation in the middle or lower lung fields. Spread to the hilar lymph nodes replicates the Ghon complex of tuberculosis. The sites of infection are usually marked by granulomas that often have central caseation and giant cells. **Fungi appearing as thick-walled, nonbudding spherules, 20 to 60 μm in diameter (often filled with small endospores),** can be visualized within the necrotic debris or sometimes within macrophages or giant cells. In most instances the lesions heal by progressive fibrosis and calcification and the infection is asymptomatic. In 20 to 50% of patients, the disease is symptomatic with fever, chills, cough, and pleuritic chest pain, mimicking a pneumonia caused by mycoplasma or viruses. Often such individuals have varied sensitivity reactions such as erythema nodosum or erythema multiforme, polyarthritis, pleuritis, and pericarditis.[82] In these cases, the histologic reaction may be granulomatous but may take the form of suppuration in which fungal spherules can be seen. Progressive disease is marked by more disseminated involvement of the lungs and coalescent areas of consolidation. Rarely, in the particularly vulnerable or immunodepressed host, miliary dissemination follows with spread to the skin, bones, adrenals, lymph nodes, spleen, liver, and meninges. Suppuration, rather than granuloma formation, is the rule in such disseminated disease.

The clinical diagnosis can be suspected with a positive coccidioidin skin test, but evidence of current infection requires elevated titers of IgM antibodies, which usually reach diagnostic levels within two weeks.

### Other Fungal Infections

*Blastomycosis* caused by *Blastomyces dermatitidis* is most easily remembered as a twin of coccidioidomycosis. *It may take the form of an asymptomatic primary pulmonary infection, progressive pulmonary disease, or (rarely) disseminated miliary disease.*[82]

Similarly, the histologic changes are most often granulomatous but may be suppurative in the particularly vulnerable host. "Blasto," however, has the following differences from "cocci": (1) *The causative agent is smaller (5 to 25 μm in diameter), round to oval, thickly walled, and reproduces by budding rather than endosporulation;* (2) there is no reliable skin test; (3) dissemination frequently involves the skin in the form of indolent papules or enlarging fungating ulcers; and (4) cutaneous infections frequently induce striking pseudoepitheliomatous hyperplasia, readily mistaken for squamous cell carcinoma.

*Cryptococcosis,* caused by *Cryptococcus neoformans,* rarely occurs in otherwise normal individuals. It almost always represents an opportunistic infection in immunocompromised hosts, particularly those with leukemia, lymphoma, or Hodgkin's disease. The fungus, a 5- to 10-μm yeast, has a thick, gelatinous capsule and reproduces by budding. Most often it localizes in the lungs and then may disseminate to other sites, particularly the meninges. *Sites of involvement are marked by a variable tissue response, which ranges from florid proliferation of gelatinous organisms in the complete absence of an inflammatory cell infiltration in the immunodeficient host to a suppurative or granulomatous reaction in the more reactive host.* The introduction of India ink into exudate or cerebrospinal fluid obtained by tap facilitates visualization of the organisms because the heavy capsules produce clear halos about the fungi.

*Aspergillosis and mucormycosis* are uncommon infections, almost always limited to immunocompromised hosts.[83] *Both diseases are caused by fungi that assume mycelial forms in lesions—in mucormycosis hyphae are nonseptate, right-angle branching, and in aspergillosis there are septate hyphae branching at more acute angles.* Mucormycosis preferentially localizes in the nose (from which it may spread to the sinuses and brain), lungs, and gastrointestinal tract. Aspergilli favor the lung, whence they may disseminate. Both agents usually cause a nondistinctive, suppurative, rarely granulomatous reaction. Mucormycosis has a predilection for invading walls of blood vessels and the aspergillus fungus is notable because its spores may induce a form of allergic asthma and because nonpathogenic strains elaborate aflatoxins implicated in hepatocarcinogenesis (p. 598).

# TUMORS

The majority of tumors in the lungs are metastases. All too frequent are bronchogenic carcinomas. Next in order of frequency are bronchial adenomas (a misnomer for a form of low-grade cancer), followed by bronchioalveolar carcinomas. Far down the line come a miscellany of mesenchymal malignancies (e.g., fibrosarcoma, leiomyosarcoma), and a few benign neoplasms, particularly small (3 to 4 cm), discrete hamartomas composed of mature cartilage sometimes admixed with fat, fibrous tissue, and blood vessels.

## BRONCHOGENIC CARCINOMA

Bronchogenic carcinoma is without challenge the number one cancer-killer in industrialized countries. It has long held this position among males in the U.S., accounting in 1985 for about 35% of their cancer deaths.[84] It just assumed this ranking in 1985 among females, bypassing breast cancer and accounting for about 18% of all cancer deaths. The age-adjusted death rate for bronchogenic carcinoma among the males in the U.S. was five per 100,000 population in 1930; in 1980 it had risen to over 70. The only moderately encouraging note is that the rate of climb among males appears to have slackened in the past few years; this is probably attributable to a reduction in cigarette smoking. The comparable rates for females are three per 100,000 in 1930 and 21 in 1980; although they are substantially lower than those for males, the slope of the climb in females now exceeds that in males.[85] These data become even more awesome in the context of almost all other forms of cancer, whose prevalance has declined over the years, held steady, or at the worst slightly increased. One could hate the bronchogenic carcinoma even more, were it not in large part self-inflicted (i.e., by cigarette smoking).

The peak incidence of this form of neoplasia occurs between the ages of 40 and 70; currently, the male-to-female ratio is about 2:1. Male cigarette smokers are about 10 times more likely to die of bronchogenic carcinoma than nonsmokers.

**ETIOLOGY AND PATHOGENESIS.** The conclusion is inescapable—cigarette smoking is the dominant cause of lung cancer.[86] Although other influences such as air pollution and radiation may augment the effects of cigarette smoking or in some instances be solely responsible, their contribution to the overall problem is small. First, the evidence relating to cigarette smoking will be given, followed by a few brief comments on those less important factors.

*An impressive body of evidence—statistical, clinical and experimental—incriminates cigarette smoking. Statistically* there is a nearly linear correlation between the frequency of lung cancer and the pack-years of cigarette smoking.[87] The increased risk becomes 20 times greater among habitual heavy smokers (40 or more cigarettes a day for a span of years). About 80% of lung cancers occur in current smokers, or those who have recently stopped. Cessation of cigarette smoking for at least 10 years brings the risk down to control levels. Passive smoking (proximity to cigarette smokers) increases the risk, but how much is uncertain. Smoking pipes and cigars also increases the risk, but only modestly. The use of filter cigarettes reduces the risk somewhat, but only in those who have used them exclusively for the last 5 to 10 years.

The *clinical evidence* is largely composed of the documentation of progressive alterations in the lining epithelium of the respiratory tract in habitual cigarette smokers.[88] In essence, there is a linear correlation between the intensity of exposure to cigarette smoke and the appearance of ever more worrisome epithelial changes, beginning with atypical squamous metaplasia, then dysplasia, and ultimately abnormalities approaching carcinoma-in-situ, followed in most instances by "the bad news."

The *experimental evidence*, although mounting with each passing year, lacks one important link—it has not been possible to date to produce lung cancer in an experimental animal by exposing it to cigarette smoke. The few tumors produced resemble bronchioloalveolar carcinomas (p. 450). Nonetheless, cigarette-smoke condensate is a witch's brew of tumorigenic delicacies, such as polycyclic hydrocarbons and other potent mutagens and carcinogens.[89] Despite the lack of an experimental model, the chain of evidence linking cigarette smoking to lung cancer grows ever stronger.

Other influences may act in concert with smoking or may by themselves be responsible for some lung cancers. Environmental and occupational air pollutants undoubtedly can contribute; witness the increased incidence of this form of neoplasia in those mining radioactive ores, in asbestos workers (particularly when coupled with smoking) and in those whose occupations cause exposure to dusts containing arsenic, chromium, uranium, nickel, vinyl chloride, and mustard gas. Heavy smokers exposed to asbestos have an approximately 90 times greater risk of cancer than do nonsmokers not exposed to asbestos. Radiation (miners of radioactive ores, those who construct atomic bombs) has yielded an increased incidence of lung cancer. And, finally, mention should be made that one pattern of lung cancer, adenocarcinoma, often arises in proximity to pulmonary scars. Whether growth factors contributed to the scarring and simultaneously the carcinogenic process, or instead the scarring is secondary to a tumorous desmoplastic reaction, is still in dispute.[90]

**CLASSIFICATION AND MORPHOLOGY.** Bronchogenic carcinomas have been subdivided into histologic categories that also have differing clinical implications.[91] Despite these differences, there are features common to all:

○ They arise in the lining epithelium of major bronchi, usually close to the hilus of the lung.

○ All are associated with cigarette smoking, strongest with squamous cell and small cell carcinomas.

○ All are aggressive, locally invasive, widely metastasizing neoplasms (particularly the small cell variant) with a propensity for spread to the liver, adrenals, brain, and bones, but almost every other organ in the body can be affected.

○ All, especially small cell cancers, have the capacity to

**Table 13–6. SIMPLIFIED HISTOLOGIC CLASSIFICATION OF BRONCHOGENIC CARCINOMA**

I. Squamous cell carcinoma (25 to 30%)
   Well to poorly differentiated
II. Adenocarcinoma—excluding bronchioloalveolar carcinoma (30 to 35%)
   Well to poorly differentiated
III. Small cell carcinoma (20 to 25%)
   Oat Cell (lymphocyte-like)
   Intermediate (polygonal cell)
IV. Large cell carcinoma (10 to 15%)
   Ranging up to giant cell and, rarely, clear cell neoplasms
V. Combined patterns (5 to 10%)
   Varying combinations, but particularly frequent are adenocarcinoma and squamous cell carcinoma; small cell and squamous cell carcinoma

synthesize bioactive products producing paraneoplastic syndromes.

A simplified histologic classification of these neoplasms is offered in Table 13–6.

**Squamous cell carcinomas** are much more common in men than in women; they tend to arise centrally in major bronchi and eventually spread to local hilar nodes, but they disseminate outside of the thorax later than other patterns. More is known about the natural history of squamous cell carcinomas than is known about the development of other variants. They are often preceded for years by atypical metaplasia or dysplasia in the bronchial epithelium, which then transforms to carcinoma-in-situ, a phase that may last for several years. There follows the progressive heaping up of these cells to create small areas (1 to 2 cm in diameter) of thickened, irregularly nodular mucosa. Although asymptomatic to this point and unrevealing on chest x-ray, atypical cells may be identified in cytologic smears of sputum or, better, bronchial aspirations or brushings. Eventually the small neoplasm reaches a symptomatic stage, at which time there is a well-defined tumor mass encroaching on or obstructing the lumen of a major bronchus and producing often distal atelectasis and infection. Simultaneously, the lesion invades into the surrounding pulmonary substance along irregular finger-like insinuations. **By this time there is spread to local nodes in 70 to 90% of patients and to more remote lymph nodes (mediastinum, scalene) in about 50 to 60%** (Fig. 13–28). Distant visceral dissemination follows and is present in at least half of the patients by the time of diagnosis.[92] Histologically, these tumors range from well-differentiated squamous cell neoplasms showing keratin pearls and intercellular bridges to poorly differentiated neoplasms having only some residual squamous cell features and merging with the undifferentiated large cell patterns, to be described (Fig. 13–29). Critical to the proof of the bronchial mucosal origin of advanced lesions is the documentation of in-situ changes at the margins of the overt neoplasm. The collective five-year survival is 5 to 7.5%, intermediate between that for adenocarcinomas and the other more lethal variants.

**Adenocarcinomas** have been increasing in frequency and are now the most common variant of bronchogenic

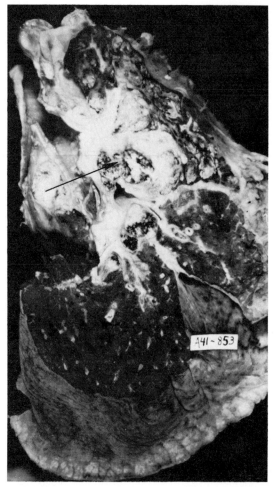

Figure 13–28. Bronchogenic squamous cell carcinoma. The gray-white tumor tissue is seen infiltrating the lung substance. It has encircled and partially replaced two spottily anthracotic lymph nodes (arrow).

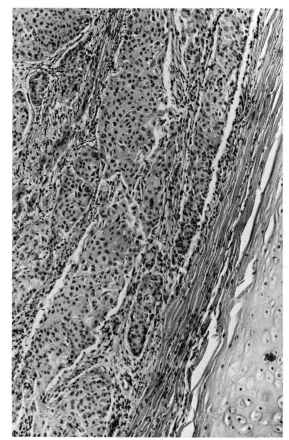

Figure 13–29. Bronchogenic carcinoma, squamous cell type. The bronchial cartilage is seen at the lower right. The neoplasm has replaced the mucosa and is growing into the lumen.

carcinoma. Although some authors include bronchioloalveolar carcinomas within the category of adenocarcinoma, here they are considered separately (p. 450), largely because of their clinical differences. Bronchogenic adenocarcinomas are relatively more frequent in women than are the squamous cell variants. The association with cigarette smoking is less strong than with the squamous cell carcinoma. They may be central lesions like the squamous cell variant, but many are more peripherally located, arising in relation to lung scars. On the whole, these tumors grow slowly and are smaller masses than the other variants. Typically, they are gray-white, firm lesions that infiltrate or destroy the wall of the bronchus of origin and extend into the surrounding substance of the lung. In over half of the cases, overt spread to the hilar lymph nodes is already present at the time of surgical exploration. Histologically, the neoplastic cells are generally cuboidal to columnar, frequently secrete mucin and typically form acinar, tubular, or papillary structures. They tend to metastasize widely at an early stage, particularly to the liver, adrenal glands, central nervous system, and bone; indeed, cerebral metastases are present in about

half of the cases and often call attention to the existence of the pulmonary primary tumor.[93] Nonetheless, the five-year survival is 10 to 12%, the best among all variants of bronchogenic carcinoma.

**Small cell carcinomas (SCC) are rapidly growing lesions that tend to infiltrate widely and disseminate early in their course and so are rarely resectable.** They are therefore almost always treated by combined radiotherapy and chemotherapy, but even with these modalities, the two-year survival has been a dismal 5 to 8%; newer protocols have somewhat improved the outlook.[94] The histogenesis of these neoplasms is still a puzzle. On the one hand, the cells in some of these tumors contain neurosecretory dense-core granules identical to those found in carcinoids, suggesting origin from Kulchitsky cells (belonging to the APUD system). Furthermore, the SCC is the variant most strongly associated with the elaboration of bioactive substances such as hormones inducing paraneoplastic syndromes, further supporting the concept that these neoplasms are APUDomas (p. 536). On the other hand is the evidence that these neoplasms may contain areas of squamous cell and adenocarcinomatous differentiation, suggesting that the cells of origin are the same as those giving rise to all other histologic variants.

Whatever their origins, small cell carcinomas are more common in men than in women and are strongly associated with cigarette smoking. They generally appear as soft-gray, large, centrally located masses with extension into the lung substance and involvement of the **hilar and mediastinal nodes.** Occasionally they take the form of peripheral tumors with extensive paratracheal node involvement. Two histologic patterns can be distinguished. The **oat cell subtype** is composed of small, dark, lymphocyte-like cells (albeit larger than lymphocytes) that have scant cytoplasm and hyperchromatic nuclei, among which mitoses are numerous. Nuclear molding or "smearing" is common. The neoplastic cells often palisade about blood vessels to create pseudorosettes. Occasionally the cells are more spindled or fusiform. Penetration of submucosal vessels is often seen. The **intermediate cell subtype** of SCC is so named because the neoplastic cells are somewhat larger than oat cells but nonetheless smaller than those in large cell carcinomas. Unlike the oat cell variant, intermediate cell neoplasms often have a significant infiltration of lymphocytes and plasma cells and, moreover, the tumor cells tend to nest in cohesive clusters. Despite the fact that a significant number (20 to 40%) of SCC are capable of synthesizing peptide hormones, neurosecretory granules can be visualized in only a few and argyrophilia is usually not demonstrable (p. 538).[95]

**Large cell carcinomas** constitute more or less a wastebasket into which are placed neoplasms that lack cytologic differentiation. The cells are usually anaplastic and have large vesicular nuclei. Sometimes a tumor is composed of wildly anaplastic cells sufficiently large to contain giant cells. These are generally bulky neoplasms, more often peripheral than central, and they have a poor prognosis because of their tendency to spread to distant sites early in their course. Like adenocarcinomas, they have a propensity for the liver, adrenal glands, and brain; over half involve the central nervous system at the time of diagnosis. Occasionally the large tumor cells have cleared cytoplasm, which creates a "clear cell subtype." The five-year survival is 2 to 3%.

**Combined patterns** require no further comment because it has already been made evident that a small but significant fraction of bronchogenic carcinomas reveal more than one, sometimes several, lines of differentiation.

Enough has been said about the tendency of these neoplasms to disseminate in all directions. Involvement of successive chains of nodes about the carina, in the mediastinum, and in the neck (scalene nodes) and clavicular regions eventually appears along with distant metastases, particularly to liver, adrenals, brain, and bone. Biopsy of the scalene or supraclavicular nodes is often performed to establish a diagnosis. These cancers, when sufficiently advanced, often extend into the pericardial or pleural sacs, leading to effusions or inflammations. By progressive encroachment, they may cause the superior vena caval syndrome (p. 307), and apical neoplasms may invade the brachial or sympathetic plexuses to cause severe pain in the distribution of the ulnar nerve or Horner's syndrome (ipsilateral enophthalmus, ptosis,

miosis, and anhidrosis). Such apical neoplasms are sometimes called **"Pancoast's tumors."**

**STAGING.** As with other cancers, TNM categories have been established to indicate the size and spread of the primary neoplasm. Utilizing these, it is possible to create categories expressing the theoretical resectability of the neoplasm. All of the details are beyond our needs, but some concept of the staging system can be derived from the following abbreviated version.[96]

*Occult stage*—No clinical or radiologic evidence of the primary tumor or of spread, but bronchopulmonary secretions contain malignant cells.

*Stage I*—A tumor that is less than 3 cm in greatest diameter, distal to the origin of a lobar bronchus and with or without metastasis to ipsilateral regional nodes, or a larger tumor distal to the carina that invades the visceral pleura but does not have nodal or distant metastases.

*Stage II*—A tumor of any size, distal to the carina, that invades the visceral pleura and extends only to the nodes in the ipsilateral hilar region.

*Stage III*—Any tumor that is more extensive locally or shows metastasis beyond the ipsilateral lymph nodes (e.g., contralateral nodes, mediastinum, liver, brain, and so on).

It is evident that only occult and Stage I tumors offer any real hope of successful resection. With Stage II the issue is clouded, and clearly Stage III tumors can only be palliated with combined radiation and chemotherapy.

**CLINICAL COURSE.** Bronchogenic carcinomas are silent, insidious lesions that more often than not spread beyond resectability while still asymptomatic. Cure by surgical resection is largely limited to the 10 to 15% of neoplasms discovered by chance on x-ray or by cytologic findings. In some instances, chronic cough, expectoration, dyspnea, and wheezing call attention to still localized resectable disease. When hoarseness, chest pain, superior vena caval syndrome, pericardial or pleural effusion, or persistent segmental atelectasis or pneumonitis make their appearance, "the horse is already out of the barn." As noted above, too often attention is drawn to this tumor by symptoms emanating from metastatic spread to the brain (mental or neurologic changes), liver (hepatomegaly), or bones (pain). Although the adrenals may be nearly obliterated by metastatic disease, adrenal insufficiency (Addison's disease) is uncommon because islands of cortical cells, sufficient to maintain adrenal function, usually persist.

For obvious reasons, intensive efforts have been made to discover these tumors at an early stage. Periodic chest x-rays and cytologic screening of sputum can be very rewarding and, as noted, brings to light a small fraction of these neoplasms, but in addition, investigation of mysteriously appearing paraneoplastic syndromes (p. 215) sometimes leads to the discovery of occult lesions. It is variously estimated that about 3 to 10% of all lung cancer patients develop clinically overt paraneoplastic syndromes.[97] The most common are hypercalcemia, Cushing's syndrome (due to increased production of ACTH), diabetes insipidus (due to inappropriate secretion of antidiuretic hormone), and, less frequently, a variety of myopathies, neuropathies, and clubbing of the fingers associated with hypertrophic pulmonary osteoarthropathy. Secretion of calcitonin and other ectopic hormones has also been documented by assays, but these products may not evoke distinctive syndromes. Hypercalcemia is most often encountered with squamous cell neoplasms; the remaining syndromes are much more frequent with small cell neoplasms, but there are many exceptions. The hypercalcemia is related in part to osteolytic bone metastases but more to the elaboration of parathormone (or PTH-like substances) and other calcium-mobilizing products, as discussed on page 216.[98]

The outlook for individuals with particular histologic variants of bronchogenic carcinoma differs, as has previously been noted. Overall, the five-year survival rate at the present time and with the most effective currently available remedies is in the range of 5 to 10%. The ultimate poignancy of these dismal data is that this form of cancer is probably largely preventable.

## BRONCHIOLOALVEOLAR CARCINOMA (BAC)

BAC is a distinctive but controversial adenocarcinoma of the lung that is set apart from bronchogenic adenocarcinomas because (1) *unlike the central location of bronchogenic carcinoma, BAC often takes the form of a peripheral solitary tumor, but some are multicentric;* (2) *the neoplasm does not appear to arise in the major bronchi;* (3) *its histologic appearance differs from the bronchogenic adenocarcinoma;* and (4) *most importantly, it is often curable by resection and so has a distinctly better prognosis.*[99] Not common, BAC represents 2 to 5% of primary lung cancers.

Although there are many variants and intergrades, BAC tends to conform to one of the following two patterns (Fig. 13–30). Less than half of the cases comprise **multifocal mucinous masses** that are sometimes discrete or at other times coalescent (simulating pneumonic consolidation) and are most often confined to a single lobe but sometimes involve multiple lobes and even may occur bilaterally. Histologically, the masses consist of tall columnar cells regularly arrayed along preserved alveolar septa that have abundant intracellular and extracellular mucin and basally located small nuclei. The cytologic appearance is deceptively benign, and mitoses are rare. The other variant is a **localized nonmucinous grayish-white nodule** that is perhaps up to 10 cm in diameter and most often located near the periphery in an upper

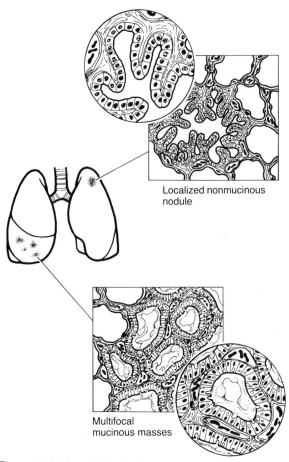

Localized nonmucinous nodule

Multifocal mucinous masses

Figure 13–30. Bronchioloalveolar carcinoma—the two anatomic variants.

lobe. The neoplastic cells usually do not elaborate mucin, are low columnar or cuboidal, and are somewhat irregularly aligned along the tumor's fibrovascular stroma rather than the alveolar septa; papillary configurations are prominent. The nuclei are large, centrally placed, hyperchromatic, and may reveal mitoses.[100] There are many hybrid forms and variations.

Many uncertainties surround BAC. Are the two patterns completely different lesions or merely the extremes of a single spectrum? Is the localized form merely an earlier stage of the multifocal variant? The histologic differences make this seem unlikely. Could the solitary variant represent a metastasis of an occult adenocarcinoma arising elsewhere? The cell of origin is also in dispute. Evidence has been marshalled in support of each of the following cell types: (a) bronchiolar mucin-secreting cells, (b) type 2 pneumonocytes, and (c) nonciliated Clara cells.[101] Indeed, it is highly likely that all three cell types have at one time or another given rise to a tumor. Association with cigarette smoking is less clear-cut than with the classic bronchogenic carcinoma, and questions have been raised about a viral etiology because a remarkably similar lesion of sheep—jaagsiekte disease—has been documented to have a viral origin. Although the condition is transmissible among sheep, spread to humans has never been proved. Despite all the uncertainties one fact stands out: when a solitary focus of tumor is discovered (usually as a chance finding in a chest radiograph), over half of the patients have a 50 to 70% five-year survival rate after resection and many are cured if hilar lymph node involvement is absent.[100] Resection is rarely possible with the multifocal variant, and the lesion is not responsive to radiotherapy or chemotherapy; the five-year survival is about 20 to 25% but still better than that for bronchogenic carcinoma.

## BRONCHIAL CARCINOID

*The older designation, bronchial adenoma, is clearly inappropriate, because these are malignant neoplasms that frequently invade locally but only occasionally metastasize.* The term bronchial carcinoid is also inaccurate, because only 90% of these lesions are argentaffinomas similar to those of the gastrointestinal tract (p. 536). The remaining 10% histologically resemble adenoid cystic salivary gland tumors. Bronchial carcinoids appear at an early age (mean 40 years) and represent about 5% of all pulmonary neoplasms. In happy contrast to bronchogenic carcinomas, they are often resectable and curable.

The carcinoids arise from the Kulchitsky cells in the bronchial mucosa and so are "first cousins" to carcinoids of the intestinal tract (p. 536).[102] These bronchial neoplasms and their intestinal counterparts are APUDomas, which are able to secrete bioactive amines and to produce the carcinoid syndrome.

Most are found in main stem bronchi and produce one of two macroscopic patterns: (1) a polypoid, spherical intraluminal mass or (2) a mucosal plaque with penetration of the bronchial wall to fan out in the peribronchial tissue—the so-called "collar-button lesion." Even these penetrating lesions push into the lung substance along a broad front and are therefore reasonably well demarcated. About 30% of these tumors metastasize to hilar nodes, and a few move to more distant sites (e.g., liver). Histologically, the argentaffinomas, like those in the intestinal tract, are composed of uniform cuboidal cells having regular round nuclei with few mitoses and little or no anaplasia. Occasional tumors are less well differentiated. These cells may be disposed in nests, cords, glandular patterns, or small masses separated by a delicate stroma. Dense-core neurosecretory granules can be visualized by electron microscopy in some. In passing it should be noted that nearly all the same cytologic features are present in some oat cell bronchogenic carcinomas, and so the differentiation of this highly malignant cancer from the much more indolent carcinoid can be difficult.[103] In contrast to mid-gut carcinoids, those of the bronchus (foregut) are rarely argentaffin-positive, but 50 to 75% are argyrophilic and the remainder are nonreactive.

Most bronchial carcinoids are brought to attention because of their interference with airway function and the resulting cough, hemoptysis, and recurrent bronchial and pulmonary infections. Some are asymptomatic and discovered by chance on chest radiographs. Only rarely do they induce the carcinoid syndrome (p. 538). As slowly growing lesions that rarely spread beyond the local hilar nodes, these tumors are amenable to conservative resection. The reported 5- to 10-year survival rate ranges between 50 and 95%, but late recurrences are sometimes encountered.[102]

## MISCELLANEOUS LESIONS

### PLEURAL EFFUSION AND PLEURITIS

The pleural effusion may be a *transudate*, as with congestive heart failure or severe hypoproteinemia. The condition is then termed *hydrothorax*. Hydrothorax from congestive heart failure is probably the most frequent cause of fluid in the pleural cavity. Such fluid is differentiated from an exudate by its clear serous appearance, low specific gravity (below 1.012) and scattered lymphocytes and mesothelial cells but no neutrophils.

Collections of *exudative fluid* in the pleural cavity imply pleuritis which may be sterile and irritative or caused by microbiologic invasion of the pleural cavity. The four principal causes of pleural exudation are (1) cancer—bronchogenic carcinoma, mesothelioma, or metastatic disease to the lung or pleural surface; (2) pulmonary infarction; (3) pneumonia; and (4) viral pleuritis. There are many other, less common causes, such as systemic lupus erythematosus, rheumatoid arthritis, uremia, and post-thoracic surgery. Tuberculosis has become a rare cause of "pleurisy with effusion." Pleuritis, usually without effusion, may be encountered in a host of conditions, notably the pneumoconioses.

Cancer should be suspected as the underlying cause of an exudative effusion in any patient over the age of 40 years, particularly when there is no febrile illness, no pain, and a negative tuberculin test. These effusions characteristically are large and frequently are serosanguineous. Cytologic examination may reveal malignant and inflammatory cells.

The pleural effusion associated with pulmonary infarction frequently is grossly bloody and may contain many inflammatory cells, both polymorphonuclear and mononuclear. The clinical story of sudden dyspnea and pleuritic pain, along with findings consistent with thrombophlebitis, confirms the diagnosis.

Pneumonic effusions are usually associated with pneumococcal pneumonia and either are caused by inflammatory irritation of the visceral pleura without penetration of organisms or are the consequence of bacterial penetration into the pleural cavity. The sterile effusions are usually serous but may be serofibrinous. Those related to direct microbiologic invasion are generally fibrinous or suppurative (empyema). Clinically apparent pneumococcal pneumonia almost always precedes by a few days the accumulation of such effusions.

Whatever the cause, transudates and serous exudates are usually resorbed without residuals if the inciting cause is controlled or remits. Hemorrhagic, fibrinous, and suppurative exudates may lead to fibrous organization yielding adhesions or fibrous pleural thickening and, sometimes, minimal to massive calcifications.

## HEMOTHORAX

The collection of whole blood (in contrast to a hemorrhagic effusion) is almost always a fatal complication of a ruptured intrathoracic aortic aneurysm. It is differentiated from a hemorrhagic effusion by the clotting of the blood.

## CHYLOTHORAX

This refers to a pleural collection of a milky lymphatic fluid containing microglobules of lipid. The total volume of fluid may not be large but chylothorax is always significant because it implies obstruction of the major lymph ducts, usually by an intrathoracic cancer (primary or secondary in the mediastinum, such as lymphoma).

## PNEUMOTHORAX

Pneumothorax refers to the presence of air or other gas in the pleural sac. It may occur in the absence of known pulmonary disease (simple pneumothorax), or it may occur as a result of some thoracic or lung disorder (secondary pneumothorax), such as a fractured rib or emphysema. Pneumothorax as a complication of lung disease occurs with the rupture of any pulmonary lesions situated close to the pleural surface that allows communication between an alveolus or bronchus and the pleural cavity. Inspired air thus gains access to the pleural space through the defect. Such primary lesions include emphysema, lung abscess, tuberculosis, carcinoma, and many other, less common processes. Because these primary diseases are most prevalent in patients over the age of 40 years, it is apparent that this type of pneumothorax tends to occur in the older age group. Mechanical ventilatory assist with high pressures may trigger secondary pneumothorax. In contrast, simple pneumothorax characteristically occurs in young, otherwise healthy adults; the condition is usually seen in males. The cause is unknown; rarely latent tuberculosis is present.

There are several possible complications of pneu-

mothorax. A "ball valve" leak may create a tension pneumothorax that shifts the mediastinum. Compromise of the pulmonary circulation may follow and possibly be fatal. If the leak seals and the lung is not reexpanded within a few weeks (either spontaneously or through medical or surgical intervention), enough scarring may occur so that it can never be fully reexpanded. In these cases, serous fluid collects in the pleural cavity and creates a hydropneumothorax. With prolonged collapse, the lung becomes vulnerable to infection, as does the pleural cavity when communication between it and the lung persists. Empyema is thus an important complication of pneumothorax. Finally, pneumothrorax tends to be recurrent. This is understandable when it complicates other pulmonary disease, because the predisposing conditions remains. What is more surprising and less readily understood is that simple pneumothorax is also recurrent.

## MESOTHELIOMA

It has been traditional to divide mesotheliomas into benign and malignant categories. The concept of a "benign mesothelioma," although firmly fixed in the literature, is regrettable and confusing because in reality it refers to a fibroma that arises in the subpleural connective tissue and protrudes into the pleural space as a 3- to 10-cm pedunculated mass. Although the fibroma is covered by mesothelial cells, they are not the neoplastic element.

In contrast, the diffuse malignant mesothelioma (DMM) is a spreading, invasive cancer composed of mesothelial cells; it most often arises in the pleura but less commonly is primary in the peritoneum and, rarely, elsewhere. Even the pleural lesion is uncommon, but this tumor has assumed great importance because in all but rare instances it is related to occupation and associated with exposure to asbestos air pollution (p. 259).[104] Indeed, about 2 to 3% (some say 10%) of heavily exposed workers develop DMM. In most cases, there is a long latent period (20 to 50 years) between last exposure and the appearance of the neoplasm. However, these neoplasms have appeared in those whose only exposure was living in proximity to an asbestos factory or being a family member of an asbestos worker; it infrequently occurs in individuals having no known exposure. The combination of cigarette smoking and asbestos does not increase the risk, unlike the case with bronchogenic carcinoma (p. 446).

The basis for the carcinogenicity of asbestos is still a mystery.[105] Physical factors seem to be involved because one form of asbestos—crocidilite, which has long, straight fibers (in contrast to the other shorter and curled fibers)—is more carcinogenic than the others. Surprisingly, there is no linear relationship between the body burden of asbestos and frequency of DMM, nor is it possible in most instances to identify either asbestos fibers or asbestos bodies (p. 261) within the neoplasm. Analogously, an individual may develop a mesothelioma without having developed asbestosis.

In the pleural cavity DMM presumably begins in a localized area, evokes an effusion, and in the course of time spreads widely either by contiguous growth or seeding of first the effusion and then the pleural surfaces. At autopsy, the affected lung is typically ensheathed by a yellow-white, firm, sometimes gelatinous layer of tumor that obliterates the pleural space. The neoplasm may directly invade the thoracic wall or the subpleural lung tissue; often it extends into interlobar fissures and sometimes into hilar nodes. Histologically, the neoplastic mesothelial cells conform to one of three patterns: (A) **sarcomatoid**, in which spindled and sometimes fibroblastic-appearing cells grow in nondistinctive sheets; (B) **epithelial**, in which cuboidal cells line tubular and microcystic spaces, into which small papillary buds project; and (C) the most common **biphasic pattern**, having both sarcomatoid and epithelial-like areas. It is evident that the sarcomatoid variant and the epithelial-like variant may be difficult to differentiate from other forms of sarcoma and from metastatic adenocarcinoma, respectively. Features that facilitate differentiation of mesothelioma from metastatic cancers include positive staining of the cells for acid mucopolysaccharide, which is abated by prior treatment with hyaluronidase; strong staining for cytokeratin; long, slender microvilli; and abundant tonofilaments.[106, 107]

These neoplasms tend to remain confined to the thorax but occasionally spread to the liver and other distant sites.

Symptoms of pleural DMM include chest or shoulder pain, recurrent effusions, and at the outset remarkably few manifestations of respiratory dysfunction. However, in time, cough, dyspnea, weight loss, and sometimes finger clubbing and pulmonary osteoarthropathy develop. The diagnosis can usually be established by CT scan, but the possibility that the pleural disease represents metastatic involvement from some other primary tumor must be excluded. Exfoliative cytology is difficult to interpret for reasons already explained. Thus biopsy is frequently necessary. The prognosis is dismal, and few patients survive longer than two years after the diagnosis.[108]

## ACUTE LARYNGITIS

Excessive mucinous secretions and hoarseness may result from allergic reactions of the laryngeal mucosa or more commonly from the irritant effects of air pollutants, notably tobacco smoke. In such instances, it is assumed without proof that microbial agents play little or no role. On the other hand, more significant forms of laryngitis may be induced by many viruses, including influenza A and B, adenoviruses, rhinoviruses, respiratory syncytial virus, and others. These viral invasions may be limited to the larynx but often involve the contiguous pharynx and trachea. In children, influenza A and B viruses and respiratory syncytial virus tend to cause laryngotracheobronchitis, more commonly known as *croup*. Although this pattern of disease may cause disturbing inspiratory stridor and harsh persistent cough, it is generally self-limited. However, in occasional cases the laryngeal inflammatory reaction may sufficiently narrow the airway to lead to respiratory failure. The anatomic changes described in the few fatal cases of croup consist of marked edema and infiltration of mononuclear inflammatory cells into the mucosa. Persistent viral involvement of the upper respiratory tract may of course predispose the patient to secondary bacterial infection. Implicated organisms are staphylococci, streptococci, and, particularly in infants and children, *Haemophilus influenzae*. With superimposed bacterial infection, the inflammatory exudation may change from mucinous to suppurative; superficial ulcerations may appear in severe cases.

*Finally, brief mention should be made of two uncommon but important forms of laryngitis: tuberculous and diphtheritic.* The former is almost always a consequence of protracted active tuberculosis, during which infective sputum is coughed up. Rarely the laryngeal involvement may be one part of miliary tuberculosis. As noted on page 46, diphtheria and diphtheritic membranous laryngitis (sometimes accompanied by tracheobronchitis) have now become rarities. There it was pointed out that after it is inhaled, *Corynebacterium diphtheriae* implants at any location on the mucosa of the upper airways and in the course of a few days elaborates a *powerful exotoxin that causes necrosis of the mucosal epithelium and is accompanied by a dense fibrinosuppurative exudate that creates the classic superficial dirty-gray membrane of diphtheria.* The major hazards of this infection are sloughing and aspiration of the membrane, which causes obstruction of major airways, and absorption of bacterial exotoxins, which produces myocarditis, peripheral neuropathies, and other tissue injuries.

# TUMORS AND TUMOR-LIKE LESIONS OF THE UPPER AIRWAYS

A variety of benign and malignant neoplasms of squamous epithelial and mesenchymal origin may arise in the larynx, but only "polyps," papillomas, and squamous cell carcinomas are sufficiently common to merit citation briefly.

*"Polyps" of the larynx* are smooth hemispheric protrusions (usually less than 0.5 cm in diameter) that are most often located on the true vocal cords. Histologically, they are composed of fibrous tissue that is usually covered by an intact stratified squamous mucosa unless it is ulcerated by the contact

trauma of the other vocal cord or another nodule on it. These lesions occur chiefly in heavy smokers or singers ("*singer's nodes*"), suggesting that they are the result of chronic irritation rather than true neoplasms. The occasional presence of mononuclear white cells within the fibrous stroma and their prominent vascularization support the notion of an inflammatory origin.

*Laryngeal papilloma* is a benign neoplasm usually located on the true vocal cords. It looks like a soft raspberry-like excrescence and is rarely more than 1 cm in diameter. Histologically, it consists of a myriad of slender, finger-like projections supported by central fibrovascular cores and covered by stratified squamous epithelium. The epithelial cells are usually orderly from basal to surface layers and lack anaplasia. When the papilloma is located on the free edge of the vocal cord, trauma may lead to fragmentation of the papillae with hemoptysis, but, more importantly, with exuberant regenerative epithelial activity, the tumor sometimes mimics squamous cell carcinoma. Indeed, instances of carcinomas arising in preexisting papillomas have been reported.

In adults, papillomas usually occur singly, but in children, multiple morphologically similar lesions may appear. The latter have been attributed to human papilloma virus.[109] They almost never become malignant and often spontaneously regress at puberty.

## CARCINOMA OF THE LARYNX

Carcinoma of the larynx is uncommon, representing only 2% of all cancers. It usually develops in smokers over 40 years of age and is more common in males (7:1). Environmental influences, particularly chronic irritation, are probably of great importance in its etiology. Supporting this contention is the fact that neighboring areas of mucosa often show the stratified squamous epithelium to be thickened and hyperkeratotic, with foci of dysplastic epithelial changes. An increased incidence of asbestos exposure has been found in these patients.[110]

About 95% of laryngeal carcinomas are typical squamous cell lesions. Rarely, adenocarcinomas are seen, presumably arising from mucous glands. The tumor usually develops directly on the vocal cords, but it may arise above or below the cords, on the epiglottis or aryepiglottic folds, or in the piriform sinuses. Those confined within the larynx proper are termed intrinsic, whereas those that arise or extend outside the larynx are designated extrinsic. Squamous cell carcinomas of the larynx follow the growth pattern of all squamous cell carcinomas (described on p. 228). They begin as in situ lesions that later appear as pearly gray, wrinkled plaques on the mucosal surface, ultimately ulcerating and fungating. The degree of anaplasia of these laryngeal tumors is markedly variable. Sometimes massive tumor giant cells and multiple bizarre mitotic figures are seen.

Carcinoma of the larynx manifests itself clinically by persistent hoarseness. Later, laryngeal tumors may produce pain, dysphagia, and hemoptysis. Patients with this condition are extremely vulnerable to secondary infection of the ulcerating lesion. With irradiation (sometimes with laryngectomy) the prognosis is relatively good. Five-year survival is over 50%.[111] The usual causes of death are infection of the distal respiratory passages or wide-spread metastases and cachexia.

## NASOPHARYNGEAL CARCINOMA

These rare neoplasms merit comment on two scores: (1) the strong epidemiologic hints linking it to the Epstein-Barr virus (EBV)[112] and (2) the frequency of this form of cancer in Oriental people, raising the possibility of viral transmission. *There are three histologic variants—squamous cell carcinoma, nonkeratinizing carcinoma, and undifferentiated carcinoma*; the last mentioned is the most common and the one most closely linked with the EBV. This neoplasm is characterized by a syncytial pattern of large epithelial cells that have indistinct cell borders and prominent nuclei set against a background of mature lymphocytes.[113] You recall that the EBV is the cause of infectious mononucleosis, marked by viral invasion of and controlled proliferation of lymphocytes; hence the interest in this tumor with its heavy content of lymphocytes, accounting for the often used synonym "*lymphoepithelioma.*"

## References

1. Freiman, D. C., et al.: Frequency of pulmonary thromboembolism in man. N. Engl. J. Med. 272:1278, 1965.
2. Dalen, J. E., et al.: Pulmonary embolism, pulmonary hemorrhage, and pulmonary infarction. N. Engl. J. Med. 296:1431, 1977.
3. Benotti, J. R., and Dalen, J. E.: The natural history of pulmonary embolism. Clin. Chest Med. 5:403, 1984.
4. A National Cooperative Study: The urokinase pulmonary embolism trial. Circulation 47:(Suppl. II):1, 1973.
5. Goldhaber, S. Z.: Acute pulmonary embolism treated with tissue plasminogen activator. Lancet 2:886, 1986.
6. Wagenvoort, C. A., and Wagenvoort, N.: Pathology of pulmonary hypertension. New York, John Wiley & Sons, 1977.
7. Rounds, S., and Hill, N. S.: Pulmonary hypertensive diseases. Chest 85:397, 1984.
8. Hasleton, P. S.: Adult respiratory distress syndrome—A review. Histopathology 7:307, 1983.
9. Stevens, J. H., and Raffin, T. A.: Adult respiratory distress syndrome. I. Aetiology and mechanisms. Postgrad. Med. J. 60:505, 1984.
10. Editorial: Neutrophils and adult respiratory distress syndromes. Lancet 2:790, 1984.
11. Cochrane, C. B., et al.: Pathogenesis of the adult respiratory distress syndrome. Evidence of oxidant activity in bronchoalveolar lavage fluid. J. Clin. Invest. 71:754, 1983.
12. Braude, S.: Adult respiratory distress syndrome after allogeneic bone-marrow transplantation: Evidence for a neutrophil-independent mechanism. Lancet 1:1239, 1985.
13. Editorial: Adult respiratory distress syndrome. Lancet 1:301, 1986.

14. Vidyasager, T., and Bhat, R.: Hyaline membrane disease. Obstet. Gynecol. Annu. 6:223, 1977.

15. Yee, W. F. H., et al.: New concepts in neonatal respiratory distress syndrome. Compr. Ther. 10:55, 1984.

16. Lauweryns, J. M.: Hyaline membrane disease in newborn infants. Hum. Pathol. 1:175, 1970.

17. Jefferies, A. L., et al.: Pulmonary epithelial permeability in hyaline-membrane disease. N. Engl. J. Med. 311:1075, 1984.

18. Krous, H. F.: Sudden infant death syndrome: Pathology and pathophysiology. Pathol. Annu. 19(Pt. 1):1, 1984.

19. Arneil, G. C., et al.: National post-perinatal infant mortality and cot-death study, Scotland 1981–82. Lancet 1:740, 1985.

20. Kelly, D. H., and Shannon, D. C.: Sudden infant death syndrome and near sudden infant death syndrome: A review of the literature, 1964 to 1982. Pediatr. Clin. North Am. 29:1241, 1982.

21. Naeye, R. L., et al.: Cardiac and other abnormalities in the sudden infant death syndrome. Am. J. Pathol. 82:1, 1976.

22. Sonnabend, O. A. R., et al.: Continuous microbiological and pathological study of 70 sudden and unexpected infant deaths: Toxigenic intestinal Clostridium botulinum infection in nine cases of sudden infant death syndrome. Lancet 1:237, 1985.

23. Thurlbeck, W. M.: Chronic airflow obstruction in lung disease. Vol. V. In Bennington, J. L. (ed.): Major Problems in Pathology. Vol. 5. Philadelphia, W. B. Saunders Co., 1976.

24. Fletcher, C. M., and Pride, N. B.: Editorial: Definition of emphysema, chronic bronchitis, asthma and airflow obstruction: 25 years on from the Ciba Symposium. Thorax 39:81, 1984.

25. Holland, W. W.: Evidence for the implication of environmental factors in the aetiology of chronic bronchitis. Z. Erkr. Atmungsorgane 161:130, 1983.

26. Snider, G. L.: Pathogenesis of emphysema and chronic bronchitis. Med. Clin. North Am. 65:647, 1981.

27. Dalvi, S. G., et al.: Chronic bronchitis. I. A bacteriological study of acute exacerbation. J. Postgrad. Med. 29:151, 1983.

28. Cosio, M., et al.: The relations between structural changes and small airways and pulmonary-function tests. N. Engl. J. Med. 298:1277, 1978.

29. American Thoracic Society: Chronic bronchitis, asthma and pulmonary emphysema. A statement by the committee on Diagnostic Standards for Nontuberculous Respiratory Diseases. Am. Rev. Resp. Dis. 85:762, 1962.

30. Snider, G. L.: A perspective on emphysema. Clin. Chest Med. 4:329, 1983.

31. Thurlbeck, W. M.: The pathobiology and epidemiology of human emphysema. J. Toxicol. Environ. Health 13:323, 1984.

32. Thurlbeck, W. M.: Overview of the pathology of pulmonary emphysema in the human. Clin. Chest Med. 4:337, 1983.

33. Thurlbeck, W. M.: The incidence of pulmonary emphysema. Am. Rev. Resp. Dis. 87:206, 1963.

34. Markush, R. E.: National chronic respiratory disease mortality study. I. Prevalence and severity of death from chronic respiratory disease in the United States, 1963. J. Chronic Dis. 21:129, 1968.

35. Hoidal, J. R., and Niewoehner, D. E.: Pathogenesis of emphysema. Chest 83:679, 1983.

36. Snider, G. L.: Two decades of research in the pathogenesis of emphysema. Schweiz. Med. Wochenschr. 114:898, 1984.

36a. Garver, R. I., Jr., et al.: $\alpha_1$-Antitrypsin deficiency and emphysema caused by homozygous inheritance of nonexpressing $\alpha_1$-antitrypsin genes. N. Engl. J. Med. 314:762, 1986.

37. Gadek, J. E., et al.: Cigarette smoking induces functional antiprotease deficiency in the lower respiratory tract of humans. Science 206:1315, 1979.

38. Barnes, P. J.: Pathogenesis of asthma: A review. J. R. Soc. Med. 76:580, 1983.

39. Hardy, C. C., et al.: The bronchoconstrictor effect of inhaled prostaglandin $D_2$ in normal and asthmatic man. N. Engl. J. Med. 311:209, 1984.

40. Black, J. L., et al.: Comparison between airways response to an alpha-adrenoceptor agonist and histamine in asthmatic and non-asthmatic subjects. Br. J. Clin. Pharmacol. 14:464, 1982.

41. Flint, A.: The interstitial lung diseases. A pathologist's view. Clin. Chest Med. 3:491, 1982.

42. Crystal, R. G., et al.: Interstitial lung disease: Current concepts of pathogenesis, staging, and therapy. Am. J. Med. 70:542, 1981.

43. James, D. G., and Neville, E.: Pathobiology of sarcoidosis. Pathobiol. Ann. 7:31, 1977.

44. Kerdel, F. A., and Moschella, S. L.: Sarcoidosis. An updated review. J. Am. Acad. Dermatol. 11:1, 1984.

45. Daniele, R. P.: Sarcoidosis: Diagnosis and management. Hosp. Pract. 18:113, (June) 1983.

46. Rohatgi, P. K., and Goldstein, R. A.: Immunopathogenesis, immunology, and assessment of activity of sarcoidosis. Ann. Allergy 52:316, 1984.

47. Bitterman, P. B., et al.: Alveolar macrophage derived growth factor: A pathogenetic link between alveolitis and interstitial fibrosis in interstitial lung disease. Am. Rev. Resp. Dis. 125(Pt. 2):54, 1982.

48. Hunninghake, G. W., and Crystal, R. G.: Pulmonary sarcoidosis. A disorder mediated by excess helper T-lymphocyte activity at sites of disease activity. N. Engl. J. Med. 305:429, 1981.

49. James, D. G.: Sarcoidosis. Postgrad. Med. J. 60:234, 1984.

50. Thrasher, D. R., and Briggs, D. D., Jr.: Pulmonary sarcoidosis. Clin. Chest. Med. 3:537, 1982.

51. Turner-Warwick, M., et al.: Cryptogenic fibrosing alveolitis: Clinical features and their influence on survival. Thorax 35:171, 1980.

52. Crystal, R. G., et al.: Interstitial lung diseases of unknown cause. Disorders characterized by chronic inflammation of the lower respiratory tract. (Parts I and II.) N. Engl. J. Med. 310:154 and 235, 1985.

53. Snider, G. L.: Interstitial pulmonary fibrosis—which cell is the culprit? Am. Rev. Resp. Dis. 127:535, 1983.

54. Bradley, J. D.: The pulmonary hemorrhage syndromes. Clin. Chest Med. 3:593, 1982.

55. Erickson, S. B., et al.: Use of combined plasmaphoresis and immunosuppression in the treatment of Goodpasture's syndrome. Mayo Clin. Proc. 54:714, 1979.

56. Bailey, P., and Groden, B. M.: Idiopathic pulmonary haemosiderosis: Report of two cases and review of the literature. Postgrad. Med. J. 55:266, 1979.

57. Spencer, H.: Pathology of the Lung. 2nd ed. Oxford, Pergamon Press, 1968.

58. Bartlett, J. G., et al.: The bacteriology of aspiration pneumonia. Am. J. Med. 56:202, 1974.

59. MacFarlane, J. T.: Legionnaires' disease. Practitioner 227:1707, 1983.

60. Edelstein, P. H., and Meyer, R. D.: Legionnaires' disease. A review. Chest 8:114, 1984.

61. Winn, W. C., Jr., and Mayerowitz, R. L.: The pathology of the legionella pneumonias. A review of 74 cases and the literature. Hum. Pathol. 12:401, 1981.

62. Lewin, S., et al.: Legionnaires' disease. Clinical features of 24 cases. Ann. Intern. Med. 89:297, 1978.

63. Rienhoff, H. Y., Jr. (ed.): Lung Abscess. Johns Hopkins Med. J. 150:141, 1982.

64. Johanson, W. G., et al.: Aspiration pneumonia, anaerobic infections, and lung abscess. Med. Clin. North Am. 64:385, 1980.

65. Hagan, J. L., and Hardy, J. D.: Lung abscess revisited. A survey of 184 cases. Ann. Surg. 197:755, 1983.

66. McSherry, J. A.: Mycoplasma pneumoniae infections. Am. Fam. Phys. 27:203, 1983.

67. Glezen, W. P.: Viral pneumonia as a cause and result of hospitalization. J. Infect. Dis. 147:765, 1983.

68. Warr, G. A., and Jakab, G. J.: Pulmonary inflammatory responses during viral pneumonia and secondary bacterial infection. Inflammation 7:93, 1983.

69. Murray, H. W., et al.: The protean manifestations of *Mycoplasma pneumoniae* infection in adults. Am. J. Med. 58:229, 1975.

70. Bhumbra, N. A., and Nankervis, G. A.: Cytomegalovirus infection. Postgrad. Med. 73:62, 1983.

71. Betts, R. F.: Syndromes of cytomegalovirus infection. Adv. Intern. Med. 26:447, 1980.

72. Davidson, P. T.: Tuberculosis. New views of an old disease. N. Engl. J. Med. 312:1514, 1985.

73. Sbarbaro, J. A.: Tuberculosis. Med. Clin. North Am. 64:417, 1980.

74. Pio, A.: Epidemiology of tuberculosis. Minn. Med. 75:507, 1984.

75. Centers for Disease Control: Tuberculosis in the U.S., 1980. Washington, D.C. (DHHS Publ. No. CDC 83-8322), 1983.

76. Stead, W. W., et al.: Tuberculosis as an endemic and nosocomial infection among the elderly in nursing homes. N. Engl. J. Med. 312:1483, 1985.

77. Stead, W. W., and Dutt, A. K.: What's new in tuberculosis? (Editorial) Am. J. Med. 71:1, 1981.

78. Nathan, C. F., et al.: Identification of interferon-gamma as the lymphokine that activates human macrophage oxidative metabolism and antimicrobial activity. J. Exp. Med. 158:670, 1983.

79. Editorial: BCG: Bad news from India. Lancet 1:73, 1980.

80. Drake, T. E., and Marbach, H. I.: Candida and candidiasis. Postgrad. Med. 53:83, 1973.

81. Goodwin, R. A., Jr., and Des Prez, R. M.: Pathogenesis and clinical spectrum with histoplasmosis. South. Med. J. 66:13, 1973.

82. Davies, S. F., and Sarosi, G. A.: Fungal infection of the lung. The big 3—Histoplasmosis, blastomycosis, coccidioidomycosis. Postgrad. Med. 73:242, 1983.

83. Glimp, R. A., and Bayer, A. S.: Fungal infections of the lung. Compr. Ther. 9:49, 1983.

84. Silverberg, E.: Cancer statistics 1985. CA 35:19, 1985

85. Stolley, P. D.: Lung cancer in women—Five years later, situation worse. N. Eng. J. Med. 309:428, 1983.

86. Office on Smoking and Health: The Health Consequences of Smoking: Cancer. A Report of the Surgeon General, Rockville, MD, Public Health Service, United States Department of Health and Human Services, 1982.

87. Frank, A. L.: The epidemiology and etiology of lung cancer. Clin. Chest Med. 3:219, 1982.

88. Auerbach, O.: Changes in bronchial epithelium in relationship to cigarette smoking, 1955–1960 vs. 1970–1977. N. Engl. J. Med. 300:381, 1979.

89. Nakayama, T., et al.: Cigarette smoke induces DNA single-strand breaks in human cells. Nature 314:462, 1985.

90. Madri, J. A., and Carter, D.: Scar cancers of the lung: Origin and significance. Hum. Pathol. 15:625, 1984.

91. Yesner, R., and Carter, D.: Pathology of carcinoma of the lung. Changing patterns. Clin. Chest Med. 3:257, 1982.

92. Yesner, R.: Lung cancer: Histologic factors and five-year survival. *In* Proceedings of the VA Surgical Adjuvant Cancer Chemotherapy Study Group, 1967.

93. Cox, J. D., and Yesner, R. A.: Adenocarcinoma of the lung: Recent results from the Veterans Administration Lung Group. Am. Rev. Resp. Dis. 120:1025, 1979.

94. Carter, D.: Small-cell carcinoma of the lung. Am. J. Surg. Pathol. 7:787, 1983.

95. Yesner, R.: Small cell tumors of the lung. Am. J. Surg. Pathol. 7:775, 1983.

96. Jett, J. R., et al.: Lung cancer: Current concepts and prospects. CA 33:74, 1983.

97. Gropp, C., et al.: Ectopic hormones in lung cancer. Ergeb. Inn. Med. Kinderheilkd. 53:133, 1984.

98. Mundy, G. R., et al.: The hypercalcemia of cancer. Clinical implications and pathogenic mechanisms. N. Engl. J. Med. 310:1718, 1984.

99. Edwards, C. W.: Alveolar carcinoma: A review. Thorax 39:166, 1984.

100. Manning, J. T., Jr., et al.: Bronchioloalveolar carcinoma: The significance of two histopathologic types. Cancer 54:525, 1984.

101. Greenberg, S. D., et al.: Bronchiolo-aveolar carcinoma—Cell of origin. Am. J. Clin. Pathol. 63:153, 1975.

102. Hurt, R., and Bates, M.: Carcinoid tumours of the bronchus: A 33 year experience. Thorax 39:617, 1984.

103. Fisher, E. R., et al.: Comparative histopathologic, histochemical, electron microscopic and tissue culture studies of bronchial carcinoids and oat cell carcinomas of lung. Am. J. Clin. Pathol. 69:165, 1978.

104. Churg, A., and Golden, J.: Current problems in the pathology of asbestos-related disease. Pathol. Annu. 17(Pt. 2):33, 1982.

105. Craighead, J. E., and Mossman, B. T.: The pathogenesis of asbestos-associated diseases. N. Engl. J. Med. 306:1446, 1982.

106. Warhol, M. J., and Corson, J. M.: An ultrastructural comparison of mesotheliomas with adenocarcinomas of the lung and breast. Hum. Pathol. 16:50, 1985.

107. Corson, J. M., and Pinkus, G. S.: Mesothelioma: Profile of keratin proteins and carcinoembryonic antigen. An immunoperoxidase study of 20 cases and comparison with pulmonary adenocarcinomas. Am. J. Pathol. 108:80, 1982.

108. Casey, K. R., et al.: Asbestos-related diseases. Clin. Chest Med. 2:179, 1981.

109. Howley, P. M.: The human papillomaviruses. Arch. Pathol. Lab. Med. 106:429, 1982.

110. Stell, P. M., and McGill, T.: Asbestos and laryngeal carcinoma. Lancet 2:416, 1973.

111. Silverberg, E., and Holleb, A. I.: Cancer statistics, 1975. CA 25:1, 1975.

112. Ringborg, U., et al.: Epstein-Barr virus-specific sero-diagnostic tests in carcinomas of the head and neck. Cancer 52:1237, 1983.

113. Carbone, A., and Micheau, C.: Pitfalls in microscopic diagnosis of undifferentiated carcinoma of nasopharyngeal type (lymphoepithelioma). Cancer 50:1344, 1982.

# 14

# The Kidney and Its Collecting System

RAMZI S. COTRAN, M.D.*

Many students find the kidney and its pathology a difficult subject. Much of the difficulty stems from the rather complex histology of the glomerulus, and for this reason we offer a brief review of the ultrastructure of the normal glomerulus before going on to discuss renal disease.[1]

You will recall that the glomerulus is a vascular-epithelial organ designed for the ultrafiltration of plasma. Except for the stalk containing the afferent and efferent arterioles, the glomerulus is completely enveloped by the cup-shaped *Bowman's capsule*, which is lined by *parietal epithelial cells*. The glomerular capillaries are lined by a unique *fenestrated endothelium*, perforated by pores about 100 nm in diameter and resting on the *basement membrane*. External to the basement membrane are the *visceral epithelial cells (podocytes)*. Each of these cells may be likened to an octopus with only the extended tentacles (*foot processes*) reaching out to contact the basement membrane. In any cross section the foot processes are separated by filtration slits, which are 20 to 50 nm in width. Therefore, in places where an endothelial cell pore is directly apposed to an epithelial cell filtration slit, the only uninterrupted filtration barrier is the glomerular basement membrane. Thus, the structural and functional integrity of the glomerular basement membrane is of great importance. Chemically, it is made up of *collagen type IV*, (which forms up to 50% of its dry weight); several other complex glycoproteins, including *laminin* and acidic sialic acid–rich glycoproteins, which coat endothelial and epithelial cell surfaces; and *polyanionic proteoglycans*, particularly heparan sulfate. The last mentioned, as we shall discuss later, is important in the maintenance of normal glomerular permeability.[2] The entire glomerular tuft is supported by *mesangial cells* lying between the capillaries. Basement membrane–like mesangial matrix forms a meshwork through which the mesangial cells are scattered. These cells of mesenchymal origin are contractile, phagocytic, and capable of laying down both matrix and collagen fibers. Mesangial matrix and glomerular basement membrane develop a rose-purple color with the periodic acid–Schiff (PAS) stain. This property is of

*F. B. Mallory Professor of Pathology, Harvard Medical School, Boston, Massachusetts; Chairman, Department of Pathology, Brigham and Women's Hospital, Boston, Massachusetts.

457

great value in studying these structures with the light microscope. In the ordinary hematoxylin-eosin (H & E) stain, it is almost impossible to discern the glomerular basement membrane, sandwiched as it is between endothelial cells and podocytes. The morphologic details described here are shown schematically in Figure 14–1 and on an electron micrograph in Figure 14–2. With this review of the normal glomerulus, we turn our attention to a few of the general characteristics of renal disease.

Traditionally, diseases of the kidney have been divided into those that affect the four basic morphologic components: glomeruli, tubules, interstitium, and blood vessels. This is generally a useful approach, because the early manifestations of disease affecting each of these components tend to be distinct. Further, some components appear to be more vulnerable to specific forms of renal injury; for example, *glomerular diseases are most often immunologically mediated, whereas tubular and interstitial disorders are more likely to be caused by toxic or infectious agents.* Nevertheless, the anatomic interdependence of structure in the kidney implies that damage to one almost always secondarily affects the others. For example, severe glomerular damage impairs the flow through the peritubular vascular system; conversely, tubular destruction, by increasing intraglomerular pressure, may induce glomerular atrophy. Thus, whatever the

origin, there is a tendency for all forms of chronic renal disease ultimately to destroy all four components of the kidney, culminating in chronic renal failure and what has been called *end-stage contracted kidneys*. The functional reserve of the kidney is large, and much damage may occur before there is evident functional impairment. For these reasons, the early signs and symptoms are particularly important to the clinician, and these are referred to in the discussion of individual diseases.

## RENAL FAILURE

It is appropriate here to discuss the manifestations of renal failure, because this may be the outcome of nearly any serious renal disease. First, the terminology must be clarified. The term *azotemia* refers to the retention of nitrogenous wastes, either through inability of the kidney to excrete them or through their failure to be delivered to the kidneys, as in circulatory failure from any cause. This is reflected in an elevated blood urea nitrogen (BUN) and is usually accompanied by other biochemical abnormalities, such as an elevated creatinine level. When azotemia becomes symptomatic, it is called *uremia*. *Uremia is a complex syndrome characterized by a variable and inconstant group of biochemical and*

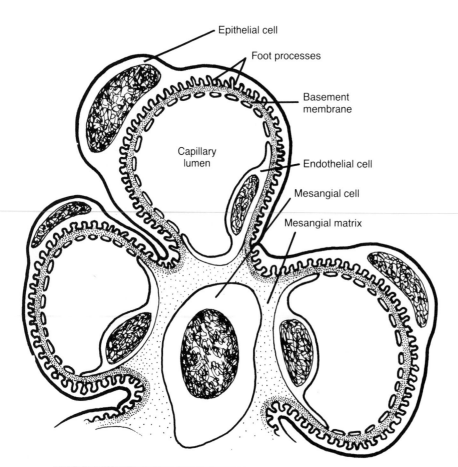

Epithelial cell
Foot processes
Basement membrane
Capillary lumen
Endothelial cell
Mesangial cell
Mesangial matrix

**Figure 14–1.** Schematic representation of a glomerular lobe.

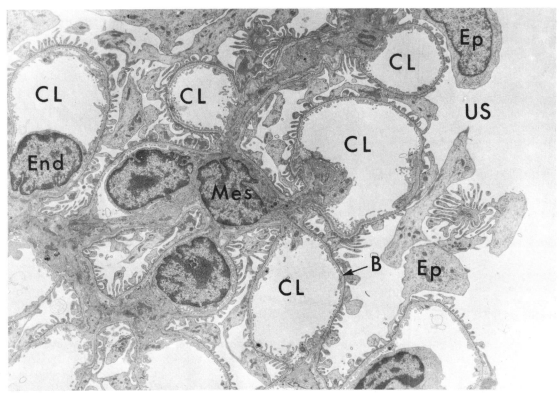

Figure 14–2. Low-power electron micrograph of rat renal glomerulus. CL = capillary lumen; End = endothelium; Mes = mesangium; B = basement membrane; Ep = visceral epithelial cells with foot processes; US = urinary space.

*clinical changes*. These changes are best understood by a consideration of the principal functions of the kidneys: (1) volume regulation, (2) acid-base balance, (3) electrolyte balance, (4) excretion of waste products, and (5) endocrine functions, including the elaboration of renin, erythropoietin, and the active form of vitamin D.

When there is derangement in *volume regulation*, the patient either becomes dehydrated or tends to retain salt and water and becomes edematous. With much chronic renal disease, the former occurs early in the course, when there is impairment of concentrating ability; the latter occurs later, when the glomeruli become hyalinized and plasma can no longer be filtered through to the tubules. Fluid overload may lead to *congestive heart failure* (p. 313), with *pulmonary congestion*. This is particularly likely to occur when there is *hypertension*, which, as we shall see, is a characteristic concomitant of several types of renal disease.

Failure of renal regulation of *acid-base balance* leads to progressive *metabolic acidosis*. The shortness of breath accompanying pulmonary congestion may therefore be compounded by that resulting from acidosis.

Uremia also includes multiple *electrolyte derangements*, the most important of which are *hyperkalemia* and *hypocalcemia*. These may cause both dangerous cardiac arrhythmias and alterations in myocardial contractility. Furthermore, they tend to produce generalized *muscle weakness* and an increase in *neuromuscular excitability*. The last mentioned leads to the muscle twitching and cramping often seen with uremia.

Patients with uremia frequently have *gastrointestinal manifestations*, including nausea, vomiting, anorexia, and, in advanced uremia stomatitis, esophagitis, enteritis, or colitis. Among the most troublesome components of uremia are a range of bone lesions, known collectively as *renal osteodystrophy*. These extend from changes typical of osteomalacia (p. 238) to more advanced alterations known as osteitis fibrosa cystica (p.706). These two patterns are related to disturbances in calcium and bone metabolism. Patients with chronic renal failure have increased serum levels of phosphate and hypocalcemia, in large part attributable to failure of the damaged kidney to synthesize 1,25-dihydroxyvitamin $D_3$, the active form of vitamin D that normally enhances absorption of calcium from the gut.

Uremic patients may also develop a variety of other abnormalities. A diffuse fibrinous *pericarditis* (see p. 338) is present in many patients with uremia. The pericarditis usually is not severe, does not cause pain, and rarely leads to any significant impairment of cardiac function. The *skin* often has a peculiar sallow coloration. This in part results from the accumulation of urinary pigments, principally urochrome, which normally gives urine its characteristic color. The skin color, however, is also materially influenced by a persistent anemia, which is present with renal failure.

The anemia is characteristically normochromic, normocytic, and refractory to any therapy. Although it is considered to be largely the result of impaired renal production of erythropoietin, there is also a shortened life span for the erythrocytes.

Also prominent are disturbances in CNS function resulting from so-called *uremic encephalopathy.* There is usually marked apathy and impaired concentration; later, convulsions, delirium, or coma may develop. Many of the neurologic manifestations are in part referable to the terminal hypertensive crises commonly encountered in these patients. Disturbances in volume regulation that lead to the development of cerebral and generalized edema or dehydration undoubtedly also contribute to the neurologic changes. Often a *peripheral neuropathy* is present, with altered tendon reflexes, muscular weaknesses, and peroneal palsy manifested by foot drop. Occasionally in uremic patients, there is a *hemorrhagic diathesis* accompanied by purpuric manifestations. Although platelets are present in normal numbers, they are qualitatively defective and become relatively ineffective in hemostasis.

This, then, is the syndrome that is termed "uremia." Not all components are present in every patient, and the dominant features may vary from patient to patient. However, it should be emphasized that nearly all the lesions to be discussed may eventually produce uremia. The precise cause, in biochemical terms, of most of the manifestations of uremia is, unfortunately, unknown.

# GLOMERULAR DISEASES

Glomerular diseases constitute some of the major problems encountered in nephrology; indeed, chronic glomerulonephritis is the most common cause of chronic renal failure in humans.

Glomeruli may be injured by a variety of factors and in the course of a number of systemic diseases. Immunologic diseases such as systemic lupus erythematosus (SLE), vascular disorders such as hypertension and polyarteritis nodosa, metabolic diseases such as diabetes mellitus, and some purely hereditary conditions such as Fabry's disease often affect the glomerulus. These are termed *secondary glomerular diseases* to differentiate them from those in which the kidney is the only or predominant organ involved. The latter constitute the various types of *primary glomerulonephritis* (GN) or *glomerulopathy.* Here we shall discuss the various types of primary GN. The glomerular alterations in systemic diseases are covered in other parts of this book.

There are several types of glomerulopathy, but no entirely satisfactory classification is available. Table 14–1 lists the most common forms that have reasonably well defined morphologic and clinical syndromes.

**Table 14–1. GLOMERULAR DISEASES**

**Primary Glomerulonephritis**
  Acute diffuse proliferative glomerulonephritis (GN)
  Rapidly progressive (crescentic) glomerulonephritis
  Membranous glomerulonephritis
  Lipoid nephrosis (minimal change disease)
  Focal segmental glomerulosclerosis
  Membranoproliferative glomerulonephritis
  IgA nephropathy
  Chronic glomerulonephritis
**Secondary (Systemic) Diseases**
  Systemic lupus erythematosus
  Diabetes mellitus
  Amyloidosis
  Goodpasture's syndrome
  Polyarteritis nodosa
  Wegener's granulomatosis
  Henoch-Schönlein purpura
  Bacterial endocarditis
**Hereditary Disorders**
  Alport's syndrome, Fabry's disease

## CLINICAL PATTERNS OF GLOMERULAR DISEASES

The four clinical syndromes we shall consider are (1) *the nephrotic syndrome*, characterized by massive proteinuria, consequent hypoalbuminemia, and generalized edema; (2) *the nephritic syndrome*, characterized by hematuria (with red cell casts in the urine) and a diminished glomerular filtration rate, usually with some degree of consequent oliguria, azotemia, and hypertension; (3) *rapidly progressive glomerulonephritis*, a clinicopathologic syndrome that is distinguished from the acute nephritic syndrome by the presence of profound oliguria and the rapid onset of renal failure; and (4) *the insidious development of uremia* secondary to chronic glomerular disease.

In general, the *nephrotic syndrome* can be correlated with diseases affecting the integrity of the glomerular capillary wall, especially the glomerular basement membrane (GBM). The GBM is the main barrier that normally prevents the passage of protein into the urine. In many cases of the nephrotic syndrome, light microscopy merely shows thickening of the GBM (membranous glomerulonephritis). By electron microscopy and immunofluorescent studies this apparent thickening of the GBM is often seen to be caused by the deposition of immune complexes, usually on the epithelial side. An inflammatory response within the glomerulus may or may not be present. In other cases of the nephrotic syndrome, however, there is no apparent abnormality of the GBM, even on electron microscopy. In such cases biochemical alterations must be present and indeed loss of negatively charged GBM molecules has been detected in some diseases (p. 465). The only constant feature in *all* cases is loss of the foot processes of the visceral epithelial cells (podocytes).

The *nephritic syndrome*, in contrast, is usually caused by those diseases that evoke an inflammatory proliferative response within the glomeruli. The proliferation may involve endothelial, mesangial, or epithelial cells. In some but not all cases there may also be an infiltration of neutrophils within the capillary lumens, in Bowman's space, and sometimes in the periglomerular interstitial tissue.

*Rapidly progressive glomerulonephritis* is a distinctive form of the nephritic syndrome, characterized by increased cellularity in the Bowman's space leading to the formation of crescent-shaped cell masses composed of epithelial cells and macrophages. Although the onset resembles that of an acute nephritic syndrome, there is rapid progression to renal failure within weeks or months.

When glomerular disease leads to the *insidious onset of uremia*, the dominant histologic feature is hyalinization of the glomeruli, and the lesion is termed "chronic glomerulonephritis." Hyalinization is the accumulation within the glomerular tufts of a homogeneous eosinophilic material that resembles GBM substance or mesangial matrix. In the course of hyalinization, the glomerular capillaries are narrowed or obliterated, and the structural detail of the glomeruli is lost.

Having briefly characterized the chief clinical and histologic presentations of glomerular diseases, what can we say of their etiology and pathogenesis? The known causes of glomerular diseases are few; they include sensitivity reactions to a number of microorganisms such as group A streptococci and several drugs, and autoimmune reactions against glomeruli themselves or renal tubular cells. As was stated earlier, glomerular involvement can be an accompaniment of several different systemic disorders, such as diabetes mellitus and SLE. However, in many cases of glomerulonephritis, a precise etiological or inciting agent cannot be found.

# PATHOGENESIS OF PRIMARY GLOMERULAR DISEASES

Although we know little of etiological agents or triggering events, it is clear that immune mechanisms underlie most cases of primary GN and many of the secondary glomerular involvements.[3, 4] Experimentally, GN can be readily induced by classic antigen-antibody reactions, and glomerular deposits of immunoglobulins, often with various components of complement, are found in over 70% of patients with GN. Thus, antibody-mediated mechanisms of damage predominate, and these have received the greatest attention.

Two forms of such antibody-associated injury have been established by experimental work: (1) injury resulting from deposition of *soluble circulating antigen-antibody complexes* in the glomerulus and (2) injury by *antibodies reacting in situ within the glomerulus, either with insoluble fixed (intrinsic) glomerular antigens or with circulating antigens planted within the glomerulus* (Fig. 14–3). These pathways are not mutually exclusive, and in humans both seem to play a role.

## Circulating Immune-Complex Nephritis

The pathogenesis of immune complex diseases (type III hypersensitivity reactions) was discussed in detail in an earlier chapter (p. 140). Here we shall briefly review the salient features that relate to glomerular injury. *With circulating immune complex disease, the glomerulus may be considered an "innocent bystander" because it does not incite the reaction. The antigen is not of glomerular origin.* It may be of endogenous origin, as in the case of the glomerulopathy associated with SLE, or it may be exogenous, as is likely in the glomerulonephritis that follows certain streptococcal infections. Other antigens have recently been implicated, including the surface antigen of the hepatitis B virus (HGsAG), various tumor antigens, *Treponema pallidum*, *Plasmodium falciparum*, and several viruses. Sometimes the inciting antigen is unknown. Whatever the antigen may be, antigen-antibody complexes are formed in the circulation and are then trapped in the glomeruli, where they produce injury, probably in large part through the binding of complement, although complement-independent injury may also occur (see later). The glomerular lesions usually consist of leukocytic infiltration in glomeruli and proliferation of endothelial, mesangial, and epithelial cells. Electron microscopy reveals the immune complexes as electron-dense deposits or clumps that lie either in the mesangium, between the endothelial cells and the GBM (*subendothelial deposits*), or between the outer surface of the GBM and the podocytes (*subepithelial deposits*). Deposits may be located at more than one site in a given case. The presence of immunoglobulins and complement in these deposits can be demonstrated by immunofluorescence microscopy. *When fluoresceinated anti-immunoglobulin or anticomplement antibodies are used, the immune complexes are seen as granular deposits along the basement membrane* (Fig. 14–4A). Once deposited in the kidney, immune complexes may eventually be degraded, mostly by infiltrating monocytes and phagocytic mesangial cells, and the inflammatory changes may then subside. Such a course occurs when the exposure to the inciting antigen is short-lived and limited, as in most cases of poststreptococcal GN. However, if a continuous shower of antigens is provided, repeated cycles of immune complex formation, deposition, and injury may occur, leading to chronic GN. In some cases the source of chronic antigenic exposure is clear, such as in SLE, in which autoimmune injury to the tissues constantly releases nuclear and cytoplasmic antigens. In most cases, however, the antigen is unknown.

## In Situ Immune Complex Nephritis

As noted, antibodies in this form of injury react directly with fixed or planted antigens in the glomer-

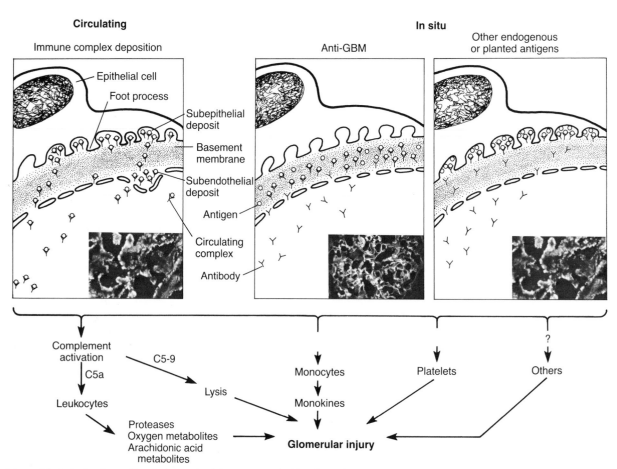

**Circulating**

Immune complex deposition

**In situ**

Anti-GBM

Other endogenous
or planted antigens

Epithelial cell

Foot process

Subepithelial
deposit

Basement
membrane

Subendothelial
deposit

Antigen

Circulating
complex

Antibody

Complement
activation → C5-9 → Lysis

C5a

Leukocytes

Monocytes → Monokines

Platelets

Others

?

Proteases
Oxygen metabolites
Arachidonic acid
metabolites

**Glomerular injury**

Figure 14–3. Antibody-mediated glomerular injury can result either from the deposition of circulating immune complexes (*left panel*) or from in situ formation of complexes (*middle and right panels*). Anti-GBM disease (*middle panel*) is characterized by *linear* immunofluorescence patterns, whereas circulating and other lesions induced in situ develop *granular* patterns. The glomerular injury (*bottom of figure*) results from mediators and toxic products derived from complement, neutrophils, monocytes, platelets, and other factors.

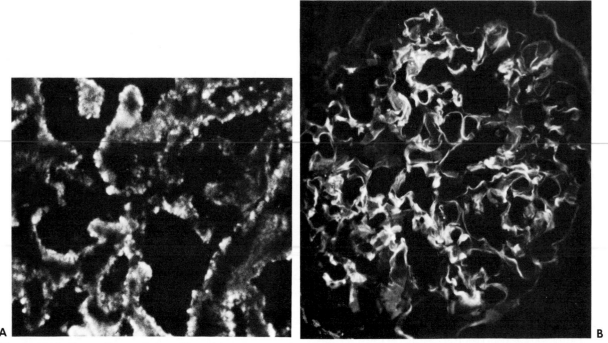

Figure 14–4. Two patterns of deposition of immune complexes as seen by immunofluorescence microscopy. *A, Granular*, characteristic of circulating and in situ immune complex nephritis; *B, Linear*, characteristic of classical anti-GBM disease.

462

ulus. The best-established model is so-called "classic" *anti-glomerular basement membrane (anti-GBM) nephritis* (Fig. 14–3, *middle panel*). *In this type of injury antibodies are directed against fixed antigens in the glomerular basement membrane and reveal a linear pattern of localization by immunofluorescence microscopy.* It has its experimental prototype in the nephritis of rabbits called *Masugi nephritis* or *nephrotoxic serum nephritis.* This is produced by injecting rats with anti-GBM antibodies produced by immunization of rabbits with rat kidney. Although in the experimental model anti-GBM antibodies are produced by injecting "foreign" kidney antigens into an animal, *spontaneous anti-GBM nephritis in humans results from the formation of autoantibodies directed against GBM.* The antibodies directly bind along the GBM to create a "linear pattern," as seen with immunofluorescent techniques, in contrast to the granular pattern described for other forms of antibody-mediated nephritis (Fig. 14–4*B*). Often the anti-GBM antibodies cross-react with other basement membranes, especially those in the lung alveoli, resulting in simultaneous lung and kidney lesions *(Goodpasture's syndrome).* It must be clear that this form of glomerulonephritis is an autoimmune disease. As is true for most autoimmune disorders, we do not know why some individuals develop antibodies against their own tissues. Any one of the several mechanisms discussed earlier (p. 150) in relation to autoimmunity may be involved.

Anti-GBM nephritis accounts for less than 5% of human GN. It is well established as the cause of injury in Goodpasture's syndrome (p. 429). Most instances of anti-GBM nephritis are characterized by very severe glomerular damage and the development of rapidly progressive renal failure.

Although classic anti-GBM disease is the one established form of injury to a glomerular antigen, other fixed antigens have been identified experimentally that initiate in situ immune deposition. Some of these are distributed in a *discontinuous* pattern along the visceral epithelial cell foot processes; thus, the resultant pattern of immune deposition in the glomerulus is *granular* (Fig. 14–3, *right*) rather than diffuse and linear. One of these is the so-called *Heymann* antigen. The Heymann model of rat GN is induced by immunizing animals with preparations of proximal tubular brush border in Freund's adjuvant. The rats develop antibodies to brush border antigens, and a membranous GN (p. 466), closely resembling human membranous GN, develops. This is characterized on immunofluorescence by the deposition of immunoglobulins and complement in a granular (rather than linear) pattern along the GBM. Although it was once thought to be due to trapping of circulating immune complexes, it is now clear that the GN results from the reaction of the anti-brush border antibody with a fixed but discontinuously distributed glycoprotein present on the base of visceral epithelial cells and cross-reactive with brush border antigen.[5]

Antibodies may also react in situ with previously "planted" nonglomerular antigens, which may localize in the kidney by interacting with various intrinsic components of the glomerulus. Planted antigens include cationic molecules that bind to glomerular capillary anionic sites; DNA, which has an affinity for basement membrane components; bacterial products, such as endostreptosin, a protein of group A streptococci (p. 468); large aggregated proteins (e.g., aggregated IgG), which deposit in the mesangium because of their size; and immune complexes themselves, since they continue to have reactive sites for further interactions with free antibody, free antigen, or complement. Most of these planted antigens induce a granular or heterogeneous pattern of immunoglobulin deposition by fluorescence microscopy; this is the pattern found also in circulating immune complex nephritis.

Factors affecting glomerular localization of antigen, antibody, or complexes are legion. The molecular charge and size of these reactants are clearly important. The pattern of localization is also affected by changes in glomerular hemodynamics, mesangial function, and integrity of the charge-selective barrier in the glomerulus. These influences may well explain the variable pattern of immune reactant deposition and histologic change in glomerulonephritis.

Once immune reactants have localized in the glomerulus, how does glomerular damage ensue? One well-established pathway is the *complement-neutrophil–mediated mechanism.* Activation of complement initiates the generation of chemotactic agents (mainly C5a) and the recruitment of neutrophils. The latter release proteases, which cause GBM degradation, as well as oxygen-derived free radicals, which cause cell damage (p. 9). However, this mechanism applies only to some types of GN, since many types show few neutrophils in the damaged glomeruli. Some experimental models suggest complement- but not neutrophil-dependent injury, possibly owing to an effect of the C5–C9 lytic component (membrane-attack complex) of complement. Finally, injury may also occur in the absence of both complement and neutrophils. To explain this, some of the mediator systems reviewed for acute or chronic inflammation have also been invoked in the mediation of glomerular injury in some models; for example, monocyte and platelet factors, arachidonic acid metabolites, and oxygen-derived free radicals all may induce glomerular injury (Fig. 14–3, *bottom*).[6]

We have thus far reviewed in detail antibody-mediated glomerular injury because this mechanism is supported by considerable experimental and clinical evidence. Other mechanisms, however, may play primary or contributory roles in some experimental models and human diseases. The possibility that *delayed-hypersensitivity, cell-mediated* immune reactions participate in glomerular injury is particularly attractive, because it can account for cases of progressive glomerulonephritis in which there are no immune deposits, but the evidence for such reactions is equivocal.[7] *Activation of the alternate complement pathway* occurs in membranoproliferative glomerulonephritis (p. 467) and will be discussed under this entity. *Loss of glomerular polyanions* appears to be critical in the pathogenesis of some diseases associated with the nephrotic syndrome, as discussed on page 463. Finally, there is increasing evidence that *intraglomerular hemodynamic changes*, such as increased glomerular capillary pressures or filtration rates, may induce glomerular injury and progressive glomerulosclerosis (p. 475).

## THE NEPHROTIC SYNDROME

*The nephrotic syndrome refers to a clinical complex comprising the following findings: (1) generalized edema, the most obvious clinical manifestation; (2) massive proteinuria, with the daily loss in the urine of 4 gm or more of protein; (3) hypoalbuminemia, with plasma albumin levels less than 3 gm per 100 ml; and (4) hyperlipidemia and hyperlipiduria.*[8] At the onset there is little or no azotemia, hematuria, or hypertension. The components of the nephrotic syndrome bear a logical relationship to one another. The initial event is a derangement in the capillary wall of the glomeruli, resulting in an increased permeability to the plasma proteins. It will be remembered from the discussion of the normal kidney that the basement membrane acts as the principal barrier through which the glomerular filtrate must pass. Any increased permeability of the GBM, resulting from either structural or physicochemical alterations, allows protein to escape from the plasma into the glomerular filtrate. Massive proteinuria may result. With long-standing or extremely heavy proteinuria, the serum albumin tends to become depleted, resulting in hypoalbuminemia and a reversed albumin-globulin ratio. The generalized edema of the nephrotic syndrome is in turn largely a consequence of the drop in osmotic pressure produced by hypoalbuminemia. As fluid escapes from the vascular tree into the tissues, there is a concomitant drop in plasma volume, with diminished glomerular filtration. Compensatory secretion of aldosterone, along with the reduced GFR, promotes retention of salt and water by the kidneys, thus further aggravating the edema. By repetition of this chain of events, massive amounts of edema (termed *anasarca*) may accumulate. The genesis of the hyperlipidemia is more obscure. Presumably hypoalbuminemia triggers increased synthesis of all forms of plasma proteins, including lipoproteins. Peripheral breakdown of lipoproteins may also be impaired. The hyperlipiduria in turn simply reflects the hyperlipoproteinemia and increased GBM permeability.

The relative frequencies of the several causes of the nephrotic syndrome vary according to age. In children under the age of 15 years, for example, the nephrotic syndrome is almost always caused by a lesion primary to the kidney, whereas among adults it may often be associated with a systemic disease. Table 14–2 represents a composite derived from several studies of the causes of the nephrotic syndrome and is therefore only approximate. As the table indicates, the most frequent *systemic* causes of the nephrotic syndrome are SLE, diabetes, and amyloidosis. The renal lesions produced by these disorders have been described elsewhere in this text. The most important of the *primary* glomerular lesions that characteristically lead to the nephrotic syndrome are *minimal change disease* and *membranous glomerulonephritis*, sometimes called *membranous nephropathy*. The former is most important in children; the latter in adults. Two other primary lesions, *focal glomerulosclerosis* and *membranoproliferative glomerulonephritis*, also produce the nephrotic syndrome. These four lesions will be discussed individually below. The fifth possible primary cause of this syndrome, *proliferative glomerulonephritis (PGN)* will not be considered in this section, because this lesion more frequently presents with the nephritic syndrome.

### Minimal Change Disease (Lipoid Nephrosis)

This relatively benign disorder is the most frequent cause of the nephrotic syndrome in children. *It is characterized by glomeruli that have a normal appearance under the light microscope but disclose diffuse loss of epithelial foot processes when viewed with the electron microscope.* Although it may develop at any age, this disorder is most common in children between two and three years old.

The etiology of lipoid nephrosis is shrouded in mystery. It is unique among primary glomerular diseases in that *there is no evidence for either an immune complex or an anti-GBM pathogenesis.* Several isolated findings have led to the *speculation* that lipoid nephrosis is an immunologic disorder of T-cell dysfunction.

Recent studies have helped to clarify the patho-

**Table 14–2. CAUSES OF NEPHROTIC SYNDROME**

| | Children (Per cent) | Adults (Per cent) |
|---|---|---|
| Primary glomerular diseases | **95** | **60** |
| Minimal change disease (Lipoid nephrosis) | 61 | 9 |
| Focal sclerosis | 10 | 9 |
| Membranous GN | 5 | 25 |
| Membranoproliferative GN | 9 | 4 |
| Other proliferative GN (e.g., focal, pure mesangial, diffuse) | 10 | 13 |
| Associated with systemic disease (most commonly diabetes, SLE, amyloidosis) | **5** | **40** |

genesis of the proteinuria in lipoid nephrosis. It is currently thought that the charge on the GBM is an important factor in governing its permeability.[9] The negatively charged GBM allows greater penetration of neutral and cationic molecules than it does of anionic molecules of the same size. Serum albumin, which is a large anionic molecule, is thus completely excluded from the normal glomerular filtrate. In lipoid nephrosis, reduction in negative charges occurs owing to loss of glomerular polyanions; this in turn permits transmembrane passage of serum albumin, resulting in albuminuria. The cause for loss of polyanions is unknown.

**MORPHOLOGY.** With the light microscope the glomeruli appear nearly normal (Fig. 14–5A). The cells of the proximal convoluted tubules are often heavily laden with lipids, but this is secondary to tubular reabsorption of the lipoproteins passing through the diseased glomeruli. This appearance of the proximal convoluted tubules is the basis for the older term for this disorder, **"lipoid nephrosis."** Even with the electron microscope, the GBM appears normal. The only obvious glomerular abnormality is the uniform and diffuse loss of the foot processes of the podocytes (also called fusion) (Fig. 14–5C). The cytoplasm of the podocytes thus appears smeared over the external aspect of the GBM, obliterating the network

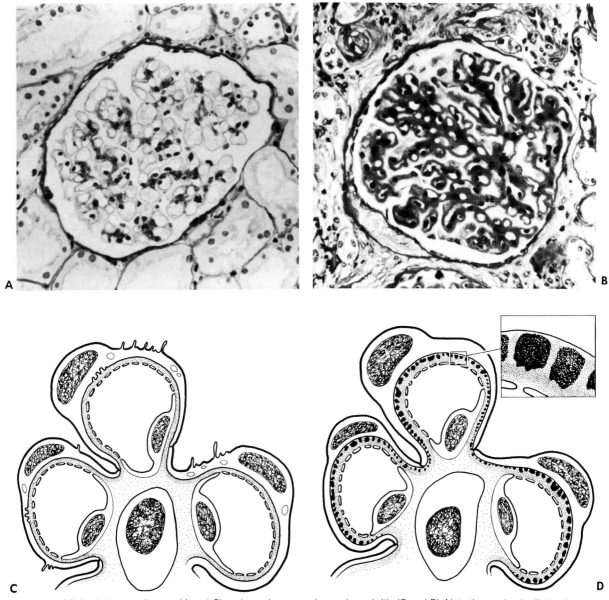

Figure 14–5. Minimal change disease (A and C) and membranous glomerulonephritis (B and D). Note that under the light microscope the glomerulus appears normal, with a thin basement membrane, in minimal change disease (A); compare this with the diffuse thickening of the basement membrane in membranous glomerulonephritis (B). On electron microscopy, minimal change disease exhibits diffuse loss of foot processes of visceral epithelial cells (C), whereas membranous glomerulonephritis (D) is characterized by electron-dense subepithelial deposits.

of arcades between the podocytes and the GBM. The changes in the podocytes are completely reversible after remission of the proteinuria.

**CLINICAL COURSE.** This disease manifests itself by the insidious development of the nephrotic syndrome in an otherwise healthy individual. There is no hypertension, and renal function is preserved in most patients. The protein loss is typically confined only to the smaller serum proteins, chiefly albumin (selective proteinuria). The prognosis in children with this disorder is good. Over 90% of the cases respond to a short course of steroid therapy. However, proteinuria recurs in over two thirds of the initial responders, some of whom become steroid-dependent. A few develop progressive deterioration of renal function. In one large study of biopsy-proved cases followed for up to 10 years,[10] 71% were in complete remission, 22% had persistent disease, and the remaining 7% had died of renal failure. Because of its responsiveness to therapy in children, minimal change disease must be differentiated from the other causes of the nephrotic syndrome in nonresponders. Adults, like children, respond well to steroid therapy, but relapses are more common.

### Membranous Glomerulonephritis (Membranous Nephropathy)

This slowly progressive disease of young adulthood and middle age is characterized morphologically by well-defined alterations in the GBM.[11] The pathogenesis involves the deposition of immune complexes on the epithelial side of the GBM. *Hence, membranous glomerulonephritis is a form of immune complex disease. In most cases the inciting antigen cannot be identified. However, some known antigens are apparently responsible for a few cases.* These include tumor antigens in patients with cancer, hepatitis B surface antigen (HBsAg), DNA antigen-antibody complexes in patients with SLE, and several infectious agents. Drug reactions may evoke a lesion indistinguishable from membranous nephropathy. Offending agents include gold, mercury, and penicillamine. In over 85% of cases the causative agent is unknown (idiopathic membranous glomerulonephritis).

Although immune complexes are readily demonstrated in the glomeruli in this condition, their site of origin is unclear. Circulating immune complexes cannot be identified in over half of the cases, and thus may be formed and deposited in situ (on the GBM). Thus, although membranous glomerulonephritis is spoken of as an immune complex disease, the inciting antigen is often unknown, as are the precise pathogenetic sequence of events.

**MORPHOLOGY.** Seen by light microscopy, the basic change appears to be a diffuse thickening of the GBM (Fig. 14–5B). By electron microscopy, it can be seen that the apparent thickening is caused in part by subepithelial deposits that nestle against the GBM and are separated from each other by small spike-like protrusions of GBM matrix ("spike and dome" pattern) (Fig. 14–5D). As the disease progresses, these "spikes" close over the deposits, thus incorporating them into the GBM. In addition, the podocytes lose their foot processes. The consequent close apposition of the podocytes to the GBM contributes to the appearance of GBM thickening on light microscopy. Later in the disease, the incorporated deposits are catabolized and eventually disappear, leaving for a time cavities within the GBM. These are later filled in with a progressive deposition of GBM matrix. As the disease progresses, the glomeruli become sclerosed and finally become completely hyalinized. Fluorescence microscopy shows typical granular deposition of immunoglobulins and complement along the GBM (Fig. 14–4A).

**CLINICAL COURSE.** The clinical onset of membranous nephropathy is indistinguishable from that of minimal change disease. It is characterized by the insidious development of the nephrotic syndrome, usually without any antecedent illness. However, proteinuria may be present without the full-blown nephrotic syndrome. In contrast to minimal change disease, the proteinuria is usually nonselective. Globulins are lost in the urine, as are the smaller albumin molecules. Membranous GN follows a notoriously indolent course. Overall, about 25% of patients suffer progressive disease terminating in renal failure. Among the remainder, somewhat less than half spontaneously remit, and the others have persistent proteinuria requiring treatment.

### Focal Segmental Glomerulosclerosis

Focal glomerulosclerosis accounts for approximately 10% of all cases of the nephrotic syndrome. *In children it is important to distinguish this cause of the nephrotic syndrome from lipoid nephrosis, because the clinical course is markedly different.* Unlike the case with lipoid nephrosis, patients with this lesion have a higher incidence of hematuria and hypertension, their proteinuria is nonselective, and in general their response to corticosteroid therapy is poor.[12] In one series that included both children and adults, 50% of the patients died within 10 years of diagnosis; of the survivors, most (90%) had persistent urinary abnormalities.[12] Some studies suggest that adults in general fare less well than children.

**MORPHOLOGY.** The disease first affects only some of the glomeruli (thus the term **focal**) and initially only the juxta-medullary glomeruli (Fig. 14–6). With progression, eventually all levels of the cortex are affected. Histologically, **focal glomerulosclerosis** is characterized by sclerosis and hyalinization of some tufts within a glomerulus, sparing the others. Thus, the involvement is both focal and **segmental**. Occasionally glomeruli are completely sclerosed (global sclerosis). In affected glomeruli, immunofluorescent microscopy reveals deposits of immunoglobulins, usually IgM, and complement in the mesan-

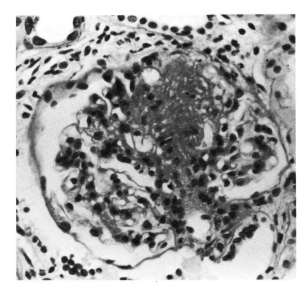

Figure 14–6. Focal segmental sclerosis, high-power view. Only one portion of glomerulus shows an area of sclerosis. There is slight mesangial hyperplasia in the rest of the glomerulus. (From Robbins, S. L., Cotran, R. S., and Kumar, V.: Pathologic Basis of Disease. 3rd ed. Philadelphia, W. B. Saunders Co., 1984, p. 1016.)

gium. Electron microscopy shows increased mesangial matrix in affected glomeruli, along with electron-dense granular deposits in the mesangium. The visceral epithelial cells show "fusion," as in lipoid nephrosis, but are also often focally necrotic.

The pathogenesis of focal glomerulosclerosis is unknown. Some investigators have suggested that focal glomerulosclerosis is a variant, albeit aggressive, of lipoid nephrosis. Others believe it to be a distinct clinicopathologic entity. The lesions do not resemble the classic immune complex nephritides. Undoubtedly, more investigation will be required before any definite conclusions can be reached regarding the pathogenesis of this condition.

### Membranoproliferative Glomerulonephritis (MPGN)

*This type of GN is characterized by basement membrane thickening and cellular proliferation.*[13] When this condition was initially described, persistent hypocomplementemia (low serum complement levels) was considered a characteristic feature. We now know that some patients have normal complement levels during part or all of their illness. Although a nephrotic syndrome is the chief clinical manifestation, some cases may present as acute nephritic syndrome and others may have features of both.

**MORPHOLOGY.** By light microscopy, one can see that the GBM is thickened and there is diffuse proliferation of mesangial cells and an increase in mesangial matrix. The expanding mesangium (cells and matrix) extends into the peripheral capillary loops, causing the basement mem-

brane to be reduplicated (sometimes erroneously referred to as "split"). This distinctive appearance ("tram-track" or "double contour") is best seen with silver methenamine stain. Electron microscopy reveals two morphologic patterns, which form the basis of subdividing MPGN into two major categories. In **type I MPGN**, electron-dense deposits are seen mainly in the subendothelial region. Mesangial cell interposition within the reduplicated basement membrane is also a consistent feature. Immunofluorescence studies show granular deposition of IgG, C3, and early complement components (Clq and C4). In **type II MPGN**, irregular electron-dense material is deposited within the GBM proper, inducing marked irregular thickening, hence the common synonym "dense deposit disease." The "tram-track" appearance is usually present in some capillaries. A diagram contrasting these two patterns is offered in Figure 14–7. In the type II pattern, such deposits are also found in the Bowman's capsule, tubular basement membranes, and peritubular capillaries. Immunofluorescence studies show smooth and granular deposits of C3 in the GBM. On the other hand, IgG and early complement components are often absent.

Different pathogenetic mechanisms are involved in the evolution of type I and type II MPGN disease.[13A] Most cases of type I appear to be caused by a chronic immune complex reaction, but the inciting antigen is not known. The pathogenesis of type II MPGN is less clear. The serum of patients with type II MPGN has a factor called "C3 nephritic factor" ($C_3NeF$),

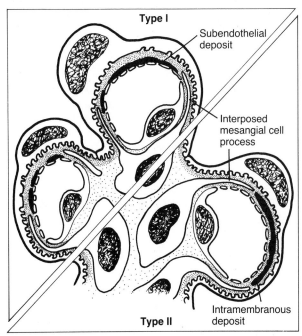

Figure 14–7. Schematic representation of patterns in the two types of membranoproliferative glomerulonephritis, as seen by electron microscopy. In type I, there are *subendothelial deposits*; type II is characterized by *intramembranous dense deposits* (dense deposit disease). In both, mesangial interposition gives the appearance of split basement membranes when viewed in the light microscope.

which can activate the alternate complement pathway. This factor is an immunoglobulin, and because it reacts with a normal plasma protein (C3), it is in a sense an autoantibody. The hypocomplementemia, more marked in type II, is contributed in part by the excessive consumption of C3 and in part by reduced synthesis of C3 by the liver. However, it is still not clear how the complement abnormality induces the glomerular changes.

**CLINICAL COURSE.** The principal mode of presentation is the nephrotic syndrome, although MPGN may begin as acute nephritis or more insidiously as mild proteinuria. The prognosis of MPGN is uniformly poor. In one study, none of the 60 patients followed for one to 20 years showed complete remission. Forty per cent progressed to end stage renal failure, 30% had variable degrees of renal insufficiency, and the remaining 30% had persistent nephrotic syndrome without renal failure. Patients with type II disease have a worse prognosis.

## THE NEPHRITIC SYNDROME

This is a clinical complex, usually of acute onset, characterized by (1) hematuria with red cell and hemoglobin casts in the urine, (2) some degree of oliguria and azotemia, and (3) hypertension. Although there may also be some proteinuria and even edema, these are usually not sufficiently marked to cause the nephrotic syndrome. The lesions that cause this syndrome have in common an inflammatory proliferation of the cells within the glomeruli, often accompanied by a leukocytic infiltrate. This inflammatory reaction injures the capillary walls, permitting the escape of red cells into the urine, and induces hemodynamic changes that lead to a reduction in the glomerular filtration rate. The reduced glomerular filtration rate is manifested clinically by oliguria, reciprocal fluid retention, and azotemia. Hypertension is probably a result of both the fluid retention and some augmented renin release from the ischemic kidneys.

The acute nephritic syndrome may be produced by systemic disorders such as SLE or may be the result of primary glomerular disease. The latter, which is more common, is exemplified by acute diffuse proliferative GN, discussed below.

### Diffuse Proliferative Glomerulonephritis (Diffuse PGN)

This is one of the more frequent of the glomerular disorders and is typically caused by immune complexes. The inciting antigen may be either exogenous or endogenous. The prototype *exogenous pattern* is poststreptococcal GN, whereas that produced by an *endogenous* antigen is *lupus nephritis*, seen in SLE. It is important to remember, however, that diffuse PGN may occur in other clinical settings and may be idiopathic. For example, infections with organisms

other than the streptococci may be associated with diffuse PGN. These include certain staphylococcal infections, as well as a number of common viral diseases such as mumps, measles, chickenpox, and hepatitis B. The lesion may also be associated with infective endocarditis and with a variety of systemic vasculitides, including polyarteritis nodosa, Henoch-Schönlein purpura, and Wegener's granulomatosis. More often, however, these last-named disorders induce a focal GN, to be described later.

The classic case of poststreptococcal GN develops in a child one to four weeks following recovery from a group A streptococcal infection elsewhere in the body.[14] Only certain "nephritogenic" strains of the beta-hemolytic streptococci are capable of evoking glomerular disease. In most cases the initial infection is a pharyngitis or skin infection. There is a general agreement that acute poststreptococcal GN is mediated by deposition of immune complexes. *Typical features of immune complex disease, such as hypocomplementemia and granular deposits of IgG and complement on the GBM, are seen.* Nevertheless, the nature of the pathogenic antigen remains mysterious. Streptococcal antigens, altered GBM, and altered IgG have been implicated at one time or another.

**MORPHOLOGY.** Grossly, the kidneys may appear entirely normal or they may be moderately enlarged. The cortical surface is smooth and free of scarring, as would be anticipated during the acute phase of any inflammation. Fine, punctate petechiae, produced by the acute inflammatory rupture of glomerular capillaries, may be scattered over the cortical surface. With the light microscope, the most characteristic change is a fairly uniform increased cellularity of the glomerular tufts affecting nearly all glomeruli, hence the term **diffuse.** The increased cellularity is caused both by proliferation and swelling of endothelial and mesangial cells and by a variable neutrophilic and monocytic infiltrate. Sometimes there are thrombi within the capillary lumens and necrosis of the capillary walls. In a few cases, there may also be "crescents" (p. 470) inside Bowman's capsule. In general, these are ominous. When they involve most of the glomeruli, the pattern merges with that of rapidly progressive GN, to be discussed. **In the early stages of the disease, the electron microscope shows the immune complexes arrayed as subepithelial "humps" nestled against the GBM** (Fig. 14–8). Immunofluorescent studies reveal IgG and complement within the deposits. These deposits are usually cleared over a period of about 2 months.

**CLINICAL COURSE.** The onset of the kidney disease tends to be abrupt, heralded by malaise, a slight fever, nausea, and the nephritic syndrome. In the usual case, oliguria, azotemia, and hypertension are only mild to moderate. Characteristically, there is gross hematuria, with the urine appearing smoky brown rather than bright red. Some proteinuria is a constant feature of the disease and, as mentioned

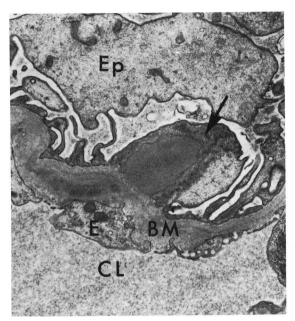

Figure 14–8. Poststreptococcal glomerulonephritis. Electron micrograph shows a hump-shaped, electron-dense deposit (*arrow*) on epithelial side of basement membrane (BM). There is also a dense deposit within BM. CL = capillary lumen; E = endothelium; Ep = epithelium. (From Robbins, S. L., Cotran, R. S., and Kumar, V.: Pathologic Basis of Disease. 3rd ed. Philadelphia, W. B. Saunders Co., 1984, p. 1020.)

earlier, may occasionally be severe enough to produce the nephrotic syndrome. Serum complement levels are low and serum anti-streptolysin O titers elevated.

Oddly enough, the prognosis with such a common disease is in some dispute. Two factors seem to be important: age of the patient and whether the disease is sporadic or part of an epidemic. Nearly all workers agree that complete recovery occurs in most children in epidemic cases. A very few children (2 to 3%) develop rapidly progressive GN or chronic renal disease. The prognosis in sporadic cases is less clear. In adults, 15 to 50% of cases develop chronicity, depending upon the clinical and histologic severity. In contrast, the prevalence of chronicity after sporadic cases of acute GN in children is much lower. The exact figures are difficult to ascertain, because differing criteria for chronicity have been used by various investigators.

The form of PGN caused by endogenous antigens is common in patients with SLE (p. 152). In this setting, serum complement level is low, and DNA antigens and anti-DNA antibodies have been identified in the glomeruli.

The gross and light microscopic changes in the kidneys are identical to those of any other form of diffuse PGN and involve proliferation of the endothelial and mesangial cells. However, with the electron microscope an important difference can be discerned. **You will recall that the immune deposits of poststreptococcal GN are subepithelial. In contrast, those of SLE are principally sub-** **endothelial and mesangial.** Immunofluorescent staining indicates that the deposits in SLE contain complement and a variable profile of immunoglobulins, most notably IgG and IgM, as well as IgA. It should be emphasized that diffuse proliferative GN is only one of several glomerular lesions seen in SLE (see p. 156).

## RAPIDLY PROGRESSIVE GLOMERULONEPHRITIS (RPGN) (CRESCENTIC GN)

Rapidly progressive glomerulonephritis (RPGN) is a distinct clinicopathologic syndrome and not a specific etiologic form of glomerulonephritis. Clinically it is characterized by rapid and progressive loss of renal function, associated with severe oliguria and death from renal failure within weeks to months. Irrespective of the etiology, *the histologic picture is characterized by the presence of crescents in most of the glomeruli (crescentic GN).*[15] These are produced, in part, by marked proliferation of the parietal epithelial cells of Bowman's capsule and in part by infiltration of monocytes and macrophages.

The conditions in which the syndrome of RPGN may occur can be grouped into three categories: (1) postinfectious (poststreptococcal RPGN), (2) GN associated with systemic diseases, and (3) primary or idiopathic RPGN. The first two categories account for about one half of all cases of RPGN. As might be expected from the list of associated conditions (Table 14–3), there is no single pathogenetic mechanism to explain all cases. There is little doubt, however, that in most cases the glomerular injury is immunologically mediated. In association with SLE, in poststreptococcal settings, and in about a third of idiopathic cases, RPGN is mediated by immune complexes.[15]

RPGN associated with Goodpasture's syndrome is a classic example of anti-GBM nephritis (p. 461). In this condition, circulating anti-GBM antibodies can be detected in over 95% of cases by radioimmunoassay.[16] These antibodies cross-react with pulmonary alveolar basement membranes, resulting in the clinical picture of pulmonary hemorrhages associated with renal failure. Cross-reactivity with renal tubular basement membranes is also seen frequently. Linear deposits of IgG, and in many cases C3, can be

**Table 14–3.** RAPIDLY PROGRESSIVE GLOMERULONEPHRITIS (RPGN)

1. Postinfectious RPGN
   Poststreptococcal (1 to 2% of all cases)
2. Associated with systemic diseases
   SLE
   Polyarteritis
   Goodpasture's syndrome
   Wegener's granulomatosis
   Henoch-Schönlein purpura
3. Idiopathic

visualized by immunofluorescence along both the glomerular and alveolar basement membranes. What triggers the formation of anti-basement membrane antibodies is not clear. It should be emphasized that Goodpasture's syndrome is not a common disorder, but it is usually fatal; most patients die of renal failure and some of pulmonary complications.

Idiopathic RPGN accounts for about half of all cases. In a third of these, linear glomerular deposits are found (as in Goodpasture's syndrome) but there is no pulmonary involvement. In another third, as mentioned above, granular glomerular deposits are present and are related to the deposition of immune complexes. But in the last third, there are no immunologic findings. Thus idiopathic RPGN is a "mixed bag."[17]

**MORPHOLOGY.** The kidneys are enlarged and pale, often with petechial hemorrhages on the cortical surfaces. Depending upon the underlying cause, the glomeruli may show focal necrosis (Goodpasture's syndrome), diffuse or focal endothelial proliferation, and mesangial proliferation. However, the histologic picture is dominated by the formation of distinctive crescents (Fig. 14–9). Crescents are formed by proliferation of parietal cells and by migration of monocytes into Bowman's space. The crescents eventually obliterate Bowman's space and compress the glomeruli. Fibrin strands are prominent between the cellular layers in the crescents, and some believe that it is the escape of fibrin into Bowman's space that incites crescent formation. Electron microscopy may, as expected, disclose subepithelial deposits in some cases but in all cases shows distinct ruptures in the GBM.

**CLINICAL COURSE.** The onset of RPGN is much like that of the nephritic syndrome except that the oliguria and azotemia are more pronounced. Ninety per cent of these patients become anephric and require chronic dialysis or transplantation. The prognosis can be roughly related to the number of crescents—patients with crescents in fewer than 80% of the glomeruli have a slightly better prognosis than those with higher percentages of crescents. Plasma exchange is of benefit in some patients, particularly those with Goodpasture's syndrome.

# CHRONIC GLOMERULONEPHRITIS (CHRONIC GN)

Having discussed various forms of glomerular disease, we should now turn to one of their unfortunate outcomes, i.e., chronic glomerulonephritis. It is the most common cause of end stage renal disease presenting as chronic renal failure. Approximately 60% of all patients requiring chronic hemodialysis or renal transplantation have the diagnosis of chronic glomerulonephritis.

By the time chronic GN is discovered, the glomerular changes are so far advanced that it is difficult to discern the nature of the original lesion. It probably represents the end stage of a variety of entities, prominent among which are focal glomerulosclerosis, membranous, and membranoproliferative GN. It has been estimated that perhaps 20% arise with no history of previous renal symptomatic disease. Although chronic GN may develop at any age, it is usually first noted in young and middle-aged adults.

**MORPHOLOGY.** Classically, the kidneys are symmetrically contracted, and their surface is red-brown and diffusely granular, closely resembling advanced benign nephrosclerosis (p. 483).

Microscopically, the feature common to all cases is advanced scarring of the glomeruli and Bowman's spaces, sometimes to the point of complete replacement or "hyalinization" of the glomeruli (Fig. 14–10). This obliteration of the glomeruli is the end point of all cases, and it is impossible to ascertain from such kidneys the nature of the earlier lesion.

The obstruction to blood flow between afferent and efferent arterioles secondary to glomerular damage must of necessity have an impact upon the other elements of the kidney. There is, then, marked interstitial fibrosis, associated with atrophy and replacement of many of the tubules in the cortex. The small and medium-sized arteries are frequently thick-walled, with narrowed lumens, secondary to hypertension and atrophic alterations. Lymphocytic and, rarely, plasma cell infiltrates are present in

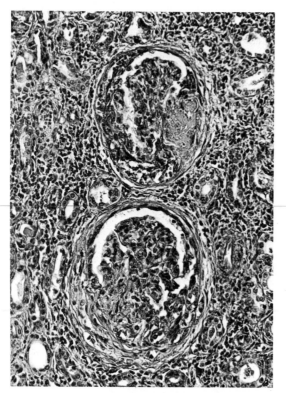

Figure 14–9. Rapidly progressing glomerulonephritis, showing extensive obliteration of the glomerular spaces by masses of epithelial cells admixed with macrophages. The periglomerular interstitial tissue contains a heavy infiltrate of white cells, causing widening of the intertubular spaces.

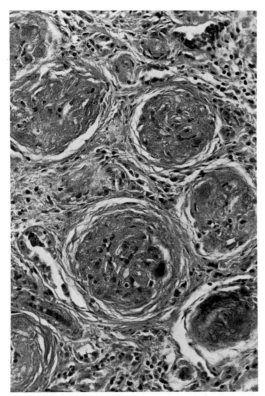

Figure 14–10. Chronic glomerulonephritis. The glomeruli are totally replaced by hyaline connective tissue. (From Robbins, S. L., Cotran, R. S., and Kumar, V.: Pathologic Basis of Disease. 3rd ed. Philadelphia, W. B. Saunders Co., 1984, p. 1020.)

the interstitial tissue. As damage to all structures progresses it may become difficult to ascertain whether the primary lesion was glomerular, vascular, or interstitial. Such markedly damaged kidneys are thus designated "end stage kidneys."

**CLINICAL COURSE.** Most often chronic GN develops insidiously and is discovered only late in its course, after the onset of renal insufficiency. Very frequently, renal disease is first suspected with the discovery of proteinuria, hypertension, or azotemia on routine medical examination. In some patients the course is punctuated by transient episodes of either the nephritic or the nephrotic syndrome. Some of these may seek medical attention for their edema. As the glomeruli become obliterated, the avenue for protein loss is progressively closed and the nephrotic syndrome thus becomes less common with more advanced disease. Some proteinuria, however, is constant in all cases. Hypertension is very common and its effects may dominate the clinical picture. Although microscopic hematuria is usually present, grossly bloody urine is infrequent.

The prognosis is poor, with relentless progression to uremia and death the rule. The rate of progression is extremely variable, however, and 10 years or more may elapse between onset of the first symptoms and death. Renal dialysis, of course, alters this course.

# FOCAL (PROLIFERATIVE) GLOMERULONEPHRITIS

Focal GN is discussed following all other forms of GN, because it may not be associated with any specific clinical presentation. It is a histologic diagnosis based on the presence of proliferative changes that affect only some of the glomeruli (*focal involvement*) and only isolated tufts within the glomerulus (*segmental involvement*). Depending upon the underlying cause, the clinical picture is variable and except in the case of one pattern known as *Berger's disease*, discussed below, there is no typical clinical syndrome associated with focal GN. Many cases of focal GN are secondary to one of a number of systemic diseases. The most frequent of these systemic diseases are *Henoch-Schönlein* purpura in children, SLE, and occasional cases of polyarteritis nodosa in adults. Other causes are infective endocarditis, Wegener's granulomatosis, and the early stages of Goodpasture's syndrome. Like diffuse PGN, this is usually an immune complex disease but differs in that the immune complexes are largely localized to the mesangium of glomeruli.

## IgA Nephropathy (Berger's Disease)

This entity[18] usually affects children and young adults and begins as an episode of gross hematuria occurring within a day or two of a nonspecific upper respiratory infection. Typically, the hematuria lasts for several days, then subsides, only to recur every few months.

*Although the cause of Berger's disease is unknown, the pathogenetic hallmark is the deposition of IgA in the mesangium.* Some have considered Berger's disease to be a variant of Henoch-Schönlein purpura, often characterized by IgA deposition in the mesangium. In contrast to Berger's disease, which is purely a renal disorder, Henoch-Schönlein purpura is a systemic syndrome involving the skin (purpuric rash), gastrointestinal tract (abdominal pain), joints (arthritis), and kidneys (p. 395).

Histologically, the lesions vary considerably. The glomeruli may be normal or may show mesangial widening and segmental proliferation confined to some glomeruli (focal GN); diffuse mesangial proliferation (mesangioproliferative); or rarely, overt crescentic GN. The characteristic immunofluorescent picture is of **mesangial deposition of IgA**, often with C3 and properdin and lesser amounts of IgG or IgM. Early complement components are usually absent. Electron microscopy confirms the presence of electron-dense deposits in the mesangium in most cases.

The pathogenesis is unknown, although there are several clues.[18] Taken together, these clues suggest a primary (probably genetic) abnormality in regulation of IgA production and increased IgA synthesis in response to some environmental agent (? viruses, food proteins). IgA aggregates or complexes are then entrapped in the mesangium, where they activate the alternate complement pathway.

IgA nephropathy is clinically a heterogeneous disease. Although most patients have an initially benign course, the disease appears to be slowly progressive: it is estimated that chronic renal failure develops in more than 50% of cases over a period of 20 years.

# DISEASES AFFECTING TUBULES AND INTERSTITIUM

Most forms of tubular injury also involve the interstitium, hence the two are discussed together. Under this heading we will present diseases characterized by (1) inflammatory involvement of the tubules and interstitium (*interstitial nephritis*), and (2) ischemic or toxic tubular injury, leading to *acute tubular necrosis* and acute renal failure. Although *diffuse cortical necrosis* involves all elements of the renal cortex, it is also presented in this section, because its etiology and clinical manifestations overlap with those of acute tubular necrosis.

## TUBULOINTERSTITIAL NEPHRITIS (TIN)

TIN refers to a group of inflammatory diseases of the kidneys that primarily involve the interstitium and tubules.[19] The glomeruli may be spared altogether or affected only late in the course. In most cases of tubulointerstitial nephritis associated with bacterial infection, the renal pelvis is prominently involved, hence the more descriptive term *pyelonephritis* (pyelo = pelvis). The term *interstitial nephritis* is generally reserved for those cases that are noninfective in origin. These include tubular injury resulting from drugs, metabolic disorders such as hypokalemia, physical injury such as irradiation, and immunologic reactions. On the basis of clinical features and the character of the inflammatory exudate, TIN, regardless of the etiologic agent, can be divided into acute and chronic categories. In the following section we shall present pyelonephritis first, followed by other, less common forms of interstitial nephritis.

### Acute Pyelonephritis

Acute pyelonephritis is a common suppurative inflammation of the kidney and the renal pelvis; it is caused by bacterial infection. It is an important manifestation of urinary tract infection (UTI), which implies involvement of the lower urinary tract (cystitis, prostatitis, urethritis) or the upper urinary tract (pyelonephritis), or both.[20] As we shall discuss, pyelonephritis almost always is associated with infection of the lower urinary tract, although the latter (e.g.,

cystitis) may remain localized without extension to the kidney. Urinary tract infections are extremely common clinical problems; among clinically significant infections, they are second in frequency only to the respiratory infections. Moreover, it seems likely that an additional large number of cases go unrecognized, manifested only by asymptomatic bacteriuria.

**ETIOLOGY AND PATHOGENESIS.** The principal causative organisms are the enteric gram-negative rods. *Escherichia coli* is by far the most common etiologic agent. Other important organisms are species of *Proteus, Klebsiella, Enterobacter,* and *Pseudomonas;* these are usually associated with recurrent infections, especially in patients with urologic manipulations. Staphylococci and *Streptococcus fecalis* may also cause pyelonephritis, but only uncommonly.

There are two routes by which bacteria can reach the kidneys: (1) through the bloodstream (hematogenous) and (2) from the lower urinary tract (ascending infection). Although the *hematogenous route* is the far less common of the two, acute pyelonephritis may result from seeding of the kidneys by bacteria in the course of septicemia or infective endocarditis (Fig. 14–11). *Ascending infection* from the lower urinary tract is clearly the most important route by which the bacteria reach the kidney.[21] The first step in the pathogenesis of ascending infection appears to be colonization of the distal urethra (and the introitus in females) by gram-negative coliform bacteria. From here the organisms must gain access to the bladder, against the flow of urine. This may occur during urethral instrumentation, including catheterization and cystoscopy, which are important predisposing factors in the pathogenesis of UTI. In the absence of instrumentation, UTI most commonly affects females, in whom the short urethra, and perhaps trauma to the urethra during sexual intercourse, facilitates the entry of bacteria into the urinary bladder. Ordinarily, bladder urine is sterile and remains so owing to poorly understood antimicrobial properties of the bladder mucosa (which includes elaboration of IgA), and owing to the flushing action associated with periodic voiding of urine. However, with outflow obstruction or bladder dysfunction, the natural defense mechanisms of the bladder are overwhelmed, setting the stage for UTI. Obstruction at the level of the urinary bladder results in incomplete emptying and increased residual volume of urine. In the presence of stasis, bacteria introduced into the bladder (as may result from catheterization) can multiply in peace, without being unceremoniously flushed out or destroyed by the bladder wall. From the contaminated bladder urine, the bacteria ascend along the ureters to infect the renal pelvis and parenchyma. Accordingly, UTI is particularly frequent among patients with urinary tract obstruction, such as may occur with benign prostatic hypertrophy or in pregnancy.

Although obstruction is an important predisposing factor in the pathogenesis of ascending infection, *it*

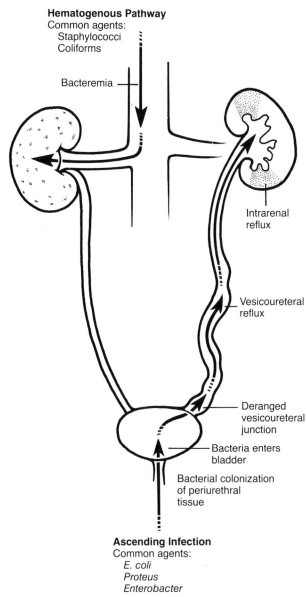

**Figure 14–11.** Schematic representation of pathways of renal infection. *Hematogenous* infection results from bacteremic spread. More common is *ascending infection*, which results from a combination of urinary bladder infection, vesicoureteral reflux, and intrarenal reflux (see text).

ducts at the tips of the papillae (intrarenal reflux). Reflux can be demonstrated radiographically by the voiding cystourethrogram in which the bladder is filled with a radiopaque dye and films are taken during micturition. VUR can be demonstrated in about 50% of infants and children with urinary tract infection.

Besides the various factors already discussed (obstruction, VUR, pregnancy, and instrumentation of the urinary tract), diabetes mellitus is frequently mentioned as an important predisposing influence. There is, however, no clear evidence that diabetics are at greater risk of developing UTI. Nevertheless, it is generally accepted that, when compared with nondiabetics, diabetics tend to have a greater number of serious complications of pyelonephritis, including septicemia, necrotizing papillitis, and recurrence.

**MORPHOLOGY.** One or both kidneys may be involved. The affected kidney or kidneys may be normal in size or enlarged. **Characteristically, discrete, yellowish, raised abscesses are grossly apparent on the renal surface** (Fig. 14–12). They may be widely scattered or

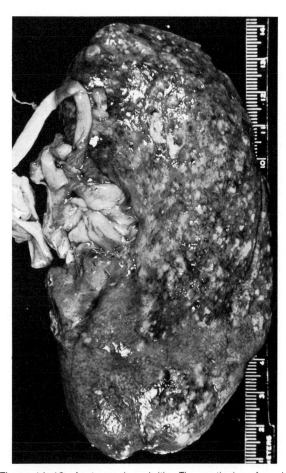

**Figure 14–12.** Acute pyelonephritis. The cortical surface is studded with focal pale abscesses, more numerous in the upper pole and midregion of the kidney; the lower pole is relatively unaffected. Between the abscesses there is dark congestion of the renal surface.

*is incompetence of the vesicoureteral orifice* that allows bacteria to ascend up the ureter into the pelvis. The normal ureteral insertion into the bladder is a competent one-way valve that prevents the retrograde flow of urine, especially during micturition, when the intravesical pressure rises. An incompetent vesicoureteral orifice allows the reflux of bladder urine into the ureters (vesicoureteral reflux, VUR).[22] The effect of VUR is similar to an obstruction in that after voiding there is residual urine in the bladder, which favors bacterial growth. Furthermore, VUR affords a ready mechanism by which the infected bladder urine can be propelled up to the renal pelves and further into the renal parenchyma through some limited to one region of the kidney, or they may coalesce to form a single large area of suppuration.

**The characteristic histologic feature of acute pyelonephritis is suppurative necrosis or abscess formation within the renal substance.** In the early stages, the suppurative infiltrate is limited to the interstitial tissue, but later, abscesses rupture into tubules. Large masses of neutrophils frequently extend within involved nephrons into the collecting ducts, giving rise to the characteristic white cell casts found in the urine. Typically, the glomeruli appear to be resistant to the infection, and often abscesses surround glomeruli without actually invading them.

When the element of obstruction is prominent, particularly when the obstruction is high in the urinary tract, the suppurative exudate may be unable to drain and thus fills the renal pelvis, calyces, and ureter, producing **pyonephrosis.** Not only is the infection, then, more serious, but renal damage from hydronephrosis also occurs (see p. 486).

A second and, fortunately, infrequent special form of pyelonephritic involvement is necrosis of the renal papillae, known as **necrotizing papillitis.** This is particularly common among diabetics who develop acute pyelonephritis and is also seen with the chronic interstitial nephritis associated with analgesic abuse (p. 476). It may also complicate acute pyelonephritis when there is significant urinary tract obstruction. This lesion consists of a combination of ischemic and suppurative necrosis of the tips of the renal pyramids (renal papillae). **The pathognomonic gross feature of necrotizing papillitis is gray-white to yellow necrosis of the apical two thirds of the pyramids.** This is usually sharply defined from the preserved basal portion by a narrow zone of hyperemia. One, several, or all papillae may be affected. Microscopically, the papillary tips show characteristic coagulative necrosis. There is no inflammatory infiltrate within the necrotic tips, and the leukocytic response is limited to the junction between preserved and destroyed tissue.

When the bladder is involved in a urinary tract infection, as it often is, **acute** or **chronic cystitis** results. In long-standing cases associated with obstruction, the bladder may be grossly hypertrophied, with trabeculation of its walls, or it may be thinned and markedly distended from retention of urine. The histologic changes are those expected of a nonspecific acute or chronic inflammation. The inflammatory infiltrate is usually but not necessarily confined to the tunica propria of the mucosa. With chronicity, fibrous thickening and rigidity of the bladder wall commonly develop.

CLINICAL COURSE. When uncomplicated acute pyelonephritis is clinically apparent, the onset is usually sudden, with pain at the costovertebral angle and systemic evidence of infection, such as chills, fever, and malaise. Urinary findings include pyuria and bacteriuria. In addition, there are usually indications of bladder and urethral irritation (i.e., dysuria, frequency, and urgency). Even without antibiotic treatment, the disease tends to be benign and self-limited.

The symptomatic phase of the disease usually lasts no longer than a week, although bacteriuria may persist much longer. In cases involving predisposing influences, the disease may become recurrent or chronic, leading eventually to serious chronic pyelonephritis.

The development of necrotizing papillitis greatly worsens the prognosis. These patients have evidence of overwhelming sepsis and, often, renal failure. Bilateral necrotizing papillitis is usually, but not invariably, fatal.

### Chronic Pyelonephritis (CPN) and Reflux Nephropathy

Chronic pyelonephritis is defined here *as a morphologic entity in which predominantly interstitial scarring of the renal parenchyma is associated with grossly visible scarring and deformity of the pelvicalyceal system.*[21] CPN is an important cause of chronic renal failure and accounts for up to 20% of patients requiring dialysis or transplantation.

CPN can be divided into two forms: chronic obstructive and chronic reflux-associated.

CHRONIC OBSTRUCTIVE PN. We have seen that obstruction predisposes the kidney to infection. Recurrent infections superimposed on diffuse or localized obstructive lesions lead to recurrent bouts of renal inflammation and scarring, which eventually cause CPN. The disease can be bilateral, as with congenital anomalies of the urethra (posterior urethral valves), and result in fatal renal insufficiency unless the anomaly is corrected, or unilateral, such as occurs with calculi and unilateral obstructive anomalies of the ureter.

REFLUX NEPHROPATHY (CHRONIC REFLUX-ASSOCIATED PN). This is by far the more common form of chronic pyelonephritic scarring and results from superimposition of a urinary tract infection on congenital VUR and intrarenal reflux. Reflux may be unilateral or bilateral; thus, the resultant renal damage either may cause scarring and atrophy of one kidney or may involve both and lead to chronic renal insufficiency. Whether VUR causes renal damage in the absence of infection (sterile reflux) is uncertain, because it is difficult clinically to rule out remote infection in a patient first seen with pyelonephritic scarring.

MORPHOLOGY. One or both kidneys may be involved, either diffusely or patchily. **Even when involvement is bilateral, the kidneys are not equally damaged and therefore are not equally contracted. This uneven scarring is useful in differentiating chronic PN from the more symmetrically contracted kidneys, caused by benign nephrosclerosis (p. 483) and chronic GN. The hallmark of CPN is scarring involving the pelvis or calyces, or both, leading to papillary blunting and marked calyceal deformities** (Fig. 14–13).

The microscopic changes are largely nonspecific, and

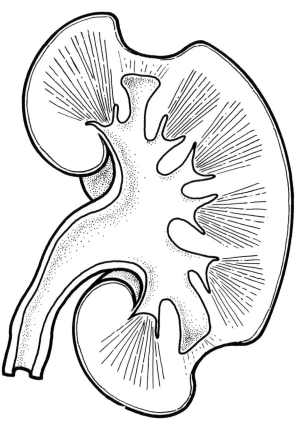

**Figure 14–13.** Typical coarse scars of chronic pyelonephritis associated with vesicoureteral reflux. The scars are usually polar and are associated with underlying blunted calyces.

**CLINICAL COURSE.** Many patients with chronic pyelonephritis come to medical attention relatively late in the course of their disease because of the gradual onset of renal insufficiency or because signs of kidney disease are noticed on routine laboratory tests. Often the renal disease is first heralded by the development of hypertension. Mild proteinuria is typical, but proteinuria sufficient to be associated with the nephrotic syndrome is not common. Pyelograms are characteristic and therefore are important in confirming the diagnosis; they show the affected kidney to be asymmetrically contracted, with some degree of blunting and deformity of the calyceal system (caliectasis). The presence or absence of significant bacteriuria is not particularly helpful diagnostically. Its absence should certainly not rule out chronic pyelonephritis. If the disease is bilateral and progressive, tubular dysfunction occurs with loss of concentrating ability, manifested by polyuria and nocturia.

As noted earlier, some patients with CPN or reflux nephropathy ultimately develop glomerular lesions of *focal segmental glomerulosclerosis.*[23] These are associated with proteinuria and eventually lead to progressive chronic renal failure. Recent experimental studies suggest that such glomerular lesions are caused by adaptive hemodynamic responses in surviving glomeruli after reduction of renal mass by scar tissue.[24] These adaptive responses include glomerular hypertrophy and increases in glomerular filtration rate, glomerular capillary pressure, and plasma flow. Presumably, the increased glomerular capillary pressure eventually causes glomerular injury, increased permeability, proteinuria, and glomerulosclerosis.

### Drug-Induced Interstitial Nephritis

In this era of antibiotics and analgesics, these two groups of drugs have emerged as important causes of renal injury. Two forms of interstitial nephritis caused by drugs are recognized.

**ACUTE DRUG-INDUCED INTERSTITIAL NEPHRITIS.** This is an adverse hypersensitivity reaction to an increasing number of drugs, particularly synthetic penicillins (methicillin), diuretics, and nonsteroidal anti-inflammatory agents.[25] The reactions begin about 15 days after exposure to the drug and consist of fever, eosinophilia, rash, hematuria, mild proteinuria, and eosinophils in the urine. Moderate to severe renal dysfunction may develop but will abate promptly or slowly with discontinuance of the drug. Renal biopsy reveals interstitial edema, mononuclear peritubular infiltrate, and tubular necrosis. Neutrophils and eosinophils may also be seen in the interstitial infiltrate (Fig. 14–14). The presence of (1) eosinophilia, (2) a mononuclear infiltrate, (3) deposits of IgG along tubular basement membranes (seen in some patients), (4) the reported elevation of serum IgE levels, and (5) the latent period all support an immunologic basis for the renal injury. However, which type of hypersensitivity reaction is predomi-

similar alterations may be seen with other disorders, such as analgesic nephropathy (p. 476). The parenchyma shows (1) uneven interstitial fibrosis and an inflammatory infiltrate of lymphocytes, plasma cells, and occasionally neutrophils. (2) Dilatation or contraction of tubules, with atrophy of the lining epithelium. Many of the dilated tubules contain pink to blue glassy-appearing casts known as "colloid casts," which suggest the appearance of thyroid tissue, hence the descriptive term "thyroidization" of the kidney. Often neutrophils are seen within tubules. (3) Concentric fibrosis about the parietal layer of Bowman's capsule, termed periglomerular fibrosis. Glomeruli may appear normal in early cases but eventually undergo hyalinization. (4) In some cases, glomerular lesions, which are indistinguishable morphologically and by immunofluorescence from those present in idiopathic focal glomerulosclerosis (p. 466), are seen. Such cases are often associated with heavy proteinuria, and it is believed that glomerular lesions contribute significantly to the progression of renal failure associated with reflux nephropathy. (5) Chronic inflammatory infiltration and fibrosis involving the calyceal mucosa and wall. (6) Vascular changes similar to those of hyaline or proliferative arteriolosclerosis caused by the frequent association with hypertension.

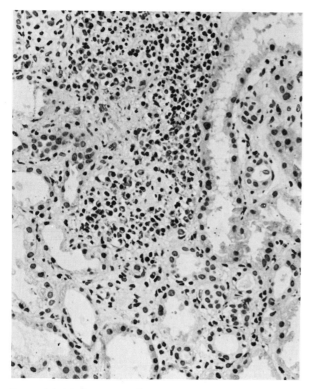

Figure 14–14. Acute drug-induced interstitial nephritis. Note interstitial inflammation and edema. (From Robbins, S. L., Cotran, R. S., and Kumar, V.: Pathologic Basis of Disease. 3rd ed. Philadelphia, W. B. Saunders Co., 1984, p. 1036.)

nantly involved and the nature of the antigenic stimulus remain to be determined.

CHRONIC ANALGESIC NEPHRITIS. *Patients who consume large quantities of analgesics may develop chronic interstitial nephritis often associated with renal papillary necrosis.*[26] Although the renal damage was initially ascribed to phenacetin, most patients who develop this nephropathy consume mixtures containing some combination of phenacetin, aspirin, and acetaminophen. For interstitial nephritis to develop, prolonged exposure to excessive amounts of analgesics is necessary. It has been estimated that consumption of at least 2 to 3 kg of analgesics over a 2- to 3-year period is essential for renal damage to occur. Although phenacetin, aspirin, and acetaminophen each produce lesions experimentally, a mixture of aspirin and phenacetin produces papillary necrosis much more readily and at lower doses. Acetaminophen, a phenacetin metabolite, may injure cells by covalent binding and oxidative damage. The pathogenesis of the renal lesions is not entirely clear. It seems that papillary necrosis is the initial event, and the interstitial nephritis in the overlying renal parenchyma is a secondary phenomenon. Whether the primary renal injury initiated by drugs or their toxic metabolites is damage to the vasa recta or necrosis of tubular epithelial cells, or both, is not known. Aspirin may potentiate the damage by its known ability to inhibit the vasodilatory effects of prostaglandins, thus predisposing the papillae to ischemia.

Initially the necrotic papillae appear yellow, but in advanced cases they have a distinct brownish discoloration. The pigmentation is due to the accumulation of breakdown products of phenacetin and other lipofuscin-like pigments. Later on, the papilla may shrivel, be sloughed off, and drop into the pelvis. Microscopically the papillae show coagulative necrosis associated with loss of cellular detail but preservation of tubular outlines. Foci of dystrophic calcification may occur in the necrotic areas. The cortex drained by the necrotic papillae shows tubular atrophy, interstitial scarring, and inflammation.

Common clinical features of analgesic nephropathy include chronic renal failure, hypertension, and anemia. The last mentioned results in part from damage to red cells by phenacetin metabolites. Cessation of analgesic intake may stabilize or even improve renal function. Another complication of analgesic abuse is the increased incidence of transitional cell carcinoma of the renal pelvis in those patients who survive the renal failure.[27]

## ACUTE TUBULAR NECROSIS (ATN)

*Acute tubular necrosis is a clinicopathologic entity characterized morphologically by destruction of tubular epithelial cells and clinically by acute suppression of renal function.*[28] It is the most common cause of acute renal failure (ARF). In ARF, the 24-hour urinary output abruptly falls to less than 400 ml (oliguria). There are also other causes of ARF; these are (1) severe glomerular diseases such as RPGN, (2) diffuse renal vessel diseases such as polyarteritis nodosa and malignant hypertension, (3) acute papillary necrosis associated with acute pyelonephritis, (4) acute drug-induced interstitial nephritis, and (5) diffuse cortical necrosis. Here we will discuss acute tubular necrosis; diffuse cortical necrosis follows in the next section. The other causes of ARF have been discussed elsewhere in this chapter.

ATN is a reversible renal lesion that arises in a diversity of clinical settings. Most of these, ranging from severe trauma to acute pancreatitis to septicemia, have in common a period of inadequate blood flow to the peripheral organs, usually accompanied by marked hypotension and shock. The pattern of ATN associated with shock is called *ischemic ATN*. Mismatched blood transfusions and other hemolytic crises also produce a picture resembling ischemic ATN. The other pattern, called *nephrotoxic ATN*, is caused by a variety of poisons, including heavy metals (e.g., mercury), organic solvents (e.g., $CCl_4$), and a multitude of drugs such as gentamycin and other antibiotics. Because of the many precipitating factors, ATN occurs quite frequently. Moreover, its reversibility gives it added clinical importance because proper management means the difference between full recovery and certain death.

PATHOGENESIS. The critical event in both ischemic and nephrotoxic ATN is believed to be *tubular dam-*

*age* (Fig. 14–15). Tubular epithelial cells are particularly sensitive to anoxia, and they are also vulnerable to poisoning because they come in contact with toxic chemicals (such as mercury) when these are excreted by the kidney. Although the initial mechanism of tubular injury is different, the subsequent events are probably similar in both forms of ATN. Once tubular injury has occurred, the progression to acute renal failure may follow one of several hypothetic pathways. Tubular damage has been postulated to trigger vasoconstriction of preglomerular arterioles, resulting in a reduced glomerular filtration rate (GFR). This has been ascribed to activation of the renin-angiotensin system, but the exact sequence of events leading to such activation awaits clarification. Damage to the tubules can itself result in oliguria, because tubular debris could block urinary outflow and eventually increase intratubular pressure, thereby decreasing the GFR. Alternatively or additionally, fluid from the damaged tubules could leak into the interstitium, resulting in increased interstitial pressure and col-

lapse of the tubule. Finally, there is some evidence of a direct effect of toxins on the filtration properties of the glomerular capillary wall. Which one of these mechanisms is most important in the onset of the oliguria is controversial. Most investigators agree, however, that mechanical tubular obstruction by necrotic debris and casts is at least an important contributor to the pathogenesis of ARF.

**MORPHOLOGY. Ischemic ATN** is characterized by necrosis of short segments of the tubules. Most of the lesions are seen in the straight portions of the proximal tubule, but no segment of the proximal or distal tubules is spared. Tubular necrosis is often subtle, requiring careful histologic examination; it is usually associated with the difficult-to-discern rupture of the basement membrane **(tubulorrhexis).** A striking additional finding is the presence of proteinaceous casts in the distal tubules and collecting ducts. They consist of Tamm-Horsfall protein (secreted normally by tubular epithelium) along with hemoglobin and other plasma proteins. When crush injuries have produced ATN, the casts are composed of myoglobin. The interstitium usually discloses generalized edema along with an inflammatory infiltrate consisting of polymorphonuclear leukocytes, lymphocytes, and plasma cells. The histologic picture in **toxic ATN** is basically similar, with some differences. Necrosis is most prominent in the proximal tubule, and the tubular basement membranes are generally spared.

If the patient survives for a week, epithelial regeneration becomes apparent in the form of mitotic activity in the persisting tubular epithelial cells. Except where the basement membrane is destroyed, regeneration is total and complete.

**CLINICAL COURSE.** The clinical course of ATN may be divided into four phases. The initial phase, lasting for about 36 hours, is usually dominated by the inciting medical, surgical, or obstetric event in the ischemic form of ATN. The only indication of renal involvement during this initial phase is a decline in urine output with a rise in BUN. At this point, oliguria could be explained on the basis of a transient decrease in blood flow to the kidneys.

The second and most important phase begins anywhere from the second to the sixth day. Urine output falls dramatically, usually to between 50 and 400 ml per day. Sometimes it declines to only a few milliliters per day, but complete anuria is rare. Oliguria may last only a few days, or it may persist as long as 3 weeks. The usual length of this phase is about 10 days. The clinical picture is dominated by the signs and symptoms of uremia and fluid overload. In the absence of careful supportive treatment or dialysis, most patients can be expected to die during this phase. With good care, however, survival is the rule.

The third or diuretic phase is ushered in by a steady increase in urine volume, reaching up to about 3 liters per day over the course of a few days. Because tubular function is still deranged, serious electrolyte imbalances may occur during this phase. There also

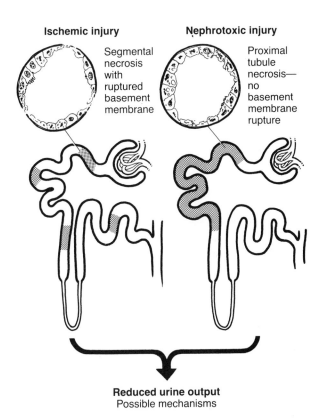

Figure 14–15. Ischemic and nephrotoxic patterns of tubular injury in acute tubular necrosis (see text).

appears to be an increased vulnerability to infections. For these reasons, about 25% of deaths from ATN occur during the diuretic phase.

During the fourth and final phase, there is a progressive return of the patient's well being. Urine volume returns to normal. However, subtle functional impairment of the kidneys, particularly of the tubules, may persist for months. With modern methods of care, patients who do not succumb to the underlying precipitating problem have a 90 to 95% chance of recovering from ATN.

## DIFFUSE CORTICAL NECROSIS

This is an infrequent lesion which in about 50% of cases follows the obstetric emergency of premature separation of the placenta (abruptio placentae). Another 30% of cases occur as a complication of septic shock. At one time, this condition was thought to be invariably fatal, but recently it has been appreciated that patchy involvement of the cortices may occur, and this is compatible with survival.

**PATHOGENESIS.** The morphologic alterations in the kidney suggest that diffuse cortical necrosis results from severe and widespread cortical ischemia. In many instances, renal ischemia is simply the result of generalized hypotension. In addition, however, disseminated intravascular coagulation (DIC) within the interlobular and afferent arterioles is a common component of cortical necrosis. This is most marked when the underlying disorder is an obstetric complication. Local vasoconstriction and intrarenal shunting of blood from the cortex to medulla may also contribute to cortical ischemia. Conceivably, many of these pathogenetic pathways are operative when cortical necrosis follows premature separation of the placenta, which is the most common predisposing cause.

**MORPHOLOGY.** The gross alterations of massive yellowish-white infarction necrosis of the parenchyma are sharply limited to the cortex. The histologic appearance is that of acute ischemic infarction. Rarely, there may be areas of apparently better preserved cortex. At the deeper levels, the areas in contact with the preserved medulla have usually a massive leukocytic infiltration. Intravascular thromboses may be prominent, and occasionally acute necroses of small arterioles and capillaries are present. Hemorrhages occur into the glomeruli, together with precipitation of fibrin.

**CLINICAL COURSE.** The onset of cortical necrosis is similar to that of ATN. Urine output falls, reaching oliguric levels within a day or two. In contrast to ATN, cortical necrosis frequently is characterized by complete anuria. However, more often urine output is in the range of 50 to 100 ml daily. The clinical picture is that of uremia, and unless dialysis is performed, death occurs within days. Occasionally, when the involvement is patchy, renal function returns and the patient survives. In these cases, the kidney is scarred, with areas of necrosis visible on x-ray as spotty calcifications.

# DISEASES INVOLVING BLOOD VESSELS

Nearly all diseases of the kidney involve the renal blood vessels secondarily. Systemic vascular disease such as various forms of arteritis also involve renal blood vessels, and often their effects on the kidney are clinically important. These have been considered in an earlier chapter (p. 295). We will discuss in this chapter hypertension and its effects on renal blood vessels. Although the effects of hypertension are systemic, we have chosen to discuss this entity here owing to the intimate relationship between the kidney and blood pressure.

## HYPERTENSION

Elevated blood pressure is a staggering health problem for three reasons: it is very common, its effects are sometimes devastating, and it remains asymptomatic until late in its course. Its effects are widespread, and no organ is spared. Hypertension has been identified as the single most important risk factor in both coronary heart disease (p. 316) and cerebrovascular accidents (p. 733); it may also lead directly to congestive heart failure (hypertensive heart disease, p. 327) and to renal failure. There is no magic threshold of blood pressure above which an individual is considered hypertensive and below which he or she is safe. Rather, the detrimental effects of blood pressure increase continuously as the pressure increases. Hypertension, then, must be defined somewhat arbitrarily. Most would agree that a sustained diastolic pressure above 90 mm Hg is an essential feature. A sustained systolic pressure above 140 mm Hg also constitutes hypertension, but its clinical consequences differ somewhat from diastolic hypertension. By means of these criteria, the percentage of hypertensive individuals in the general population in one large screening program was 38%.[29] However, most surveys use systolic/diastolic pressures of 160/95 as the dividing line for adults. Even with these values, the prevalence was an alarming 18% in the study already mentioned. The prevalence increases with age, although when present in young adults it tends to be more severe. Blacks are affected about twice as often as whites and apparently are more vulnerable to its complications. Although females are hypertensive more often than males, this sex preponderance is limited to the older age groups, in which the disease is likely to be relatively benign. Under the age of 50 years, hypertension is more common in males.

*About 90% of hypertension is idiopathic and apparently primary (essential hypertension). Of the remaining 10%, most is secondary to renal disease or, less often, to narrowing of the renal artery, usually by an atheromatous plaque (renovascular hypertension).* Only relatively infrequently is secondary hypertension the result of adrenal disorders, such as primary aldosteronism, Cushing's syndrome, and pheochromocytoma. *Both essential and secondary hypertension may be either benign or malignant, according to the clinical course.* In most cases hypertension remains fairly stable over years to decades and, unless a myocardial infarction or cerebrovascular accident supervenes, is compatible with a long life. This form of the disorder is termed *benign hypertension* and produces a renal lesion known as *benign nephrosclerosis.* Although a benign course is most characteristic of idiopathic or essential hypertension, it may also be seen with the secondary disorder. About 5% of hypertensive persons show a rapidly rising blood pressure, which, untreated, leads to death within a year or two. Appropriately enough, this is called *accelerated* or *malignant hypertension,* and the corresponding renal lesion *malignant nephrosclerosis.* The full-blown clinical syndrome of malignant hypertension includes severe hypertension (a diastolic pressure over 120 mm Hg), renal failure, and bilateral retinal hemorrhages and exudates, with or without papilledema. This form of hypertension may develop in previously normotensive individuals, or it may be superimposed upon preexisting benign hypertension, either essential or secondary. In its pure form, malignant hypertension usually affects younger individuals than does benign hypertension. Typically, it develops in the fourth decade.

The morphology and clinical course of the two renal lesions, benign and malignant nephrosclerosis, will be considered separately later (p. 482). First we shall discuss what is known of the etiology and pathogenesis of hypertension in general.

**REGULATION OF NORMAL BLOOD PRESSURE.**[30] Although the cause of most cases of hypertension is unknown, speculations abound and the subject is a source of lively controversy. For our consideration, a reasonable starting point is the well-known observation that arterial pressure is a product of cardiac output and peripheral resistance. These two are in turn affected by a variety of factors, depicted schematically in Figure 14–16. These factors are shown as affecting either vascular resistance or cardiac output, but only to avoid a maze of crisscrossing lines. In reality, most of these factors act at several points; for example, angiotensin not only causes vasoconstriction but also stimulates aldosterone secretion, which in turn affects salt retention and fluid volume. Analogously, salt retention not only increases cardiac output but may also increase peripheral resistance by altering the sensitivity of the vascular smooth muscle to vasoactive stimuli. Such interplays are too numerous to detail, but several examples have been cited to emphasize that in most hypertensive individuals elevation of blood pressure results from an interaction of multiple factors. It is therefore futile to look for a specific or single common biochemical, structural, or hemodynamic defect in all cases of hypertension.

***Role of the Kidney.*** The kidney plays an extremely important role in blood pressure regulation. A variety of factors that influence cardiac output and peripheral resistance are either produced by or act on the kidney. These include the following:

1. *Renin-angiotensin System* (Fig. 14–17). The kidney plays a major role in regulation of normal blood pressure through the elaboration of renin and the subsequent formation of angiotensin II. *Angiotensin II is the major effector molecule of the renin-angiotensin axis.* It alters blood pressure by increasing both peripheral resistance and blood volume. The former effect is achieved largely by its ability to cause vasoconstriction through direct action on vascular smooth muscle; the latter effect is caused by stimu-

Figure 14–16. Blood pressure regulation. (Modified from Kaplan, N. M.: Systemic hypertension: mechanisms and diagnosis. *In* Braunwald, E. (ed.): Heart Disease. 2nd ed. Philadelphia, W. B. Saunders Co., 1984, p. 861.)

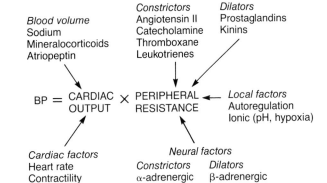

RENIN-ANGIOTENSIN SYSTEM

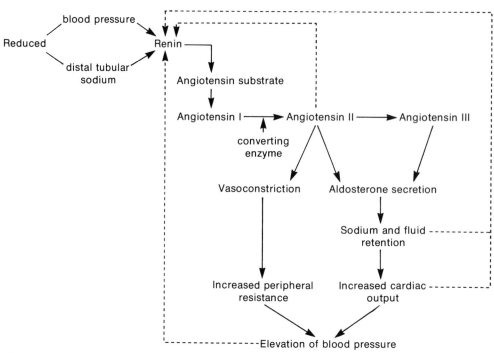

**Figure 14–17.** Role of renin-angiotensin system in regulation of blood pressure. Solid lines represent positive interactions; broken lines show negative interactions or feedback inhibition.

lation of aldosterone secretion, which increases distal tubular reabsorption of sodium and hence water.

2. *Sodium Homeostasis.* You may recall that extracellular fluid volume (and therefore blood volume and cardiac output) is regulated mostly by total body sodium levels. The kidney is intimately involved in the complex process of sodium homeostasis. One mechanism already discussed is the renin-angiotensin system, which, as mentioned, affects distal tubular reabsorption of sodium through the mediation of aldosterone secretion. Two other renal factors have important bearing on sodium homeostasis: *the glomerular filtration rate (GFR)* and GFR-independent natriuretic factors. When blood volume is reduced, the GFR falls; this in turn leads to increased reabsorption of sodium by proximal tubules in an attempt to conserve sodium and expand blood volume. One GFR-independent factor is the newly discovered atrial natriuretic factor or atriopeptin,[31] which is secreted by heart atria in response to volume expansion and inhibits sodium reabsorption at a distal site.

3. *Renal Vasodepressor Substances.* The kidney produces a variety of vasodepressor or antihypertensive substances, which presumably counterbalance the vasopressor effects of angiotensin. The vasodepressor substances include the prostaglandins, a urinary kallikrein-kinin system, and platelet-activating factor (p. 39). Discussion of the complex relationships among various pressor and antipressor mechanisms in the kidney is beyond our scope. Suffice it to say

that fine tuning of the interactions of these mediators is perhaps essential for maintenance of intrarenal blood flow and therefore of systemic arterial pressure.

Against this background of the role of the kidney in the regulation of blood pressure, we can discuss the derangements in homeostasis associated with various clinical forms of hypertension.

### Secondary Hypertension

For the sake of simplicity, we shall start our discussion with secondary hypertension, which, as mentioned earlier, accounts for 10% of all cases of hypertension. By far the commonest causes of secondary hypertension are renal parenchymal diseases and renal artery narrowing. Next in importance are endocrine disorders, among which adrenocortical hyperfunction is a predominant etiologic factor. These will be discussed separately. Use of estrogen-containing oral contraceptives is also a common cause of secondary hypertension, but the elevation in blood pressure is mild and does not constitute in most instances a serious clinical problem.

**RENAL HYPERTENSION.** Because the kidney plays a pivotal role in the maintenance of normal blood pressure, it is not surprising that hypertension is a common accompaniment of several renal diseases. *From the point of view of pathogenesis, two categories of renal hypertension can be recognized—*

those associated with excessive renin secretion (e.g., renovascular hypertension) and those associated with volume excess (e.g., acute glomerulonephritis). In some cases of chronic renal failure, a mixture of both patterns is seen. Experimental models developed by Goldblatt clearly demonstrate these two mechanisms and have greatly helped in our understanding of renal hypertension. Renal ischemia, produced by clamping one renal artery (the so-called Goldblatt kidney) with the other kidney normal, produces hypertension that is mediated by excessive release of renin. It is very likely that a similar mechanism operates in the hypertension associated with renal artery stenosis, such as may be produced by an atheromatous plaque but which in a few cases is caused by fibromuscular hyperplasia of the renal artery.

Renal hypertension is most likely to respond to drugs that interfere with the renin-angiotensin axis.[32] However, the treatment of choice in renal arterial hypertension is reconstruction of the artery. When vascular reconstruction is performed or the affected kidney is removed, blood pressure may return to normal, especially if the hypertension is of recent origin. The procedure is less successful in long-standing hypertension, because the contralateral kidney damaged by the hypertension also begins to release excessive amounts of renin and because other less well understood mechanisms for the perpetuation of hypertension take over.

Activation of the renin-angiotensin system has also been implicated in the pathogenesis of hypertension associated with polyarteritis nodosa, unilateral chronic pyelonephritis, juxtaglomerular cell tumors, malignant hypertension, and chronic renal disease.

**ENDOCRINE CAUSES.** Secondary hypertension caused by adrenal dysfunction usually involves the hypersecretion of one of the mineralocorticoids. Primary aldosteronism (Conn's disease) is the best established of these disorders and is discussed on page 694. Other mineralocorticoids, such as deoxycorticosterone (DOC) and 18-OH-DOC, have also been identified as causes of adrenal hypertension. *Hypertension associated with primary mineralocorticoid excess contrasts with renovascular hypertension in that renin levels are depressed rather than elevated.* This reflects the negative feedback effects of the mineralocorticoids on renin release. Thus, the elevated blood pressure can be considered to reflect hypervolemia rather than vasoconstriction.

Mild secondary hypertension caused by salt retention is common in women who use estrogen-containing oral contraceptives. It is believed that estrogens increase the synthesis of angiotensinogen (angiotensin substrate) by the liver and hence the production of both angiotensin and aldosterone.

## Essential Hypertension

We come now to the vexing problem of the pathogenesis of essential hypertension. At the outset, it is obvious from the term "essential" that the cause is unknown. At the most elemental level, however, it must relate to either a primary increase in cardiac output or an increase in peripheral resistance, and the several theories of the origin of hypertension stress one or the other event.

Those who advocate a *primary increase in cardiac output suggest that the basic nonstructural, genetic defect is reduced renal sodium excretion in the presence of normal arterial pressure* (defective pressure natriuresis). Decreased sodium excretion would lead to an increase in fluid volume and rise in cardiac output. In the face of increasing cardiac output, peripheral vasoconstriction occurs to prevent overperfusion of tissues, which would result from an unchecked increase in cardiac output. This process, called autoregulation, leads to increased peripheral resistance and along with it an elevation of blood pressure.[1] At the higher setting of blood pressure enough additional sodium can be excreted by the kidneys to equal intake and prevent fluid retention. Thus, an altered but steady state of sodium excretion is achieved ("resetting of pressure natriuresis").

*The second hypothesis implicates vasoconstrictive influences as the primary events.* These could be (a) behavioral or neurogenic factors, as shown by the reduction of blood pressure that can be achieved by meditation (the relaxation response); (b) increased release of vasoconstrictor agents (e.g., renin and catecholamines); or (c) a primary increased sensitivity of arterioles, possibly caused by sodium transport defects.

What activates these mechanisms remains even more mysterious. Both heredity and environmental factors have been implicated. When both parents are hypertensive, the children have a greatly increased risk of developing hypertension. Studies on twins and familial aggregations support a role for the genetic constitution in the etiology of hypertension. If heredity is involved, how is the genetic defect manifested? A renal defect relating to sodium reabsorption has been suggested, which could lead to hypertension by the mechanisms described previously. Even if genetic predisposition to hypertension exists, it is likely that environmental factors are also involved in the expression of the genetic abnormalities. The role of environment is illustrated by the lower incidence of hypertension in Chinese people living in their native country as compared with persons of Chinese descent living in the United States. Environmental factors implicated in the causation of hypertension include stress, obesity, smoking, inactivity, and elevated salt intake. Circumstantial evidence linking the level of dietary sodium intake with the prevalence of hypertension in different population groups is impressive. Even among individual patients, such a correlation has been noticed. However, it is also clear that not everyone who ingests large quantities of salt develops hypertension. All of these data are best explained by postulating that only a fraction of human subjects are genetically susceptible to developing hypertension by excessive salt consumption. Support for such a postulate comes from studies in certain inbred strains of rats in which hypertension can be induced by feeding them high-salt diets. It must be stressed in both of the major hypotheses discussed that a high sodium intake augments the hypertension.

Essential hypertension is thus a complex disorder that may have more than one cause. It may be initiated by a disturbance in any of the factors that control normal blood pressure, many of which are environmental (stress, salt intake, estrogens) but act in the genetically predisposed individual. In established hypertension, both increased blood volume and increased peripheral resistance contribute to the increased pressure. Table 14–4 lists the main causes and possible mechanisms of hypertension.

We shall now examine some of the renal vascular disorders associated with hypertension.

## Malignant Hypertension and Malignant Nephrosclerosis

Although the foregoing discussion relating to pathogenesis applies equally to the benign and malignant forms of essential hypertension, the latter is associated with certain other features, which are discussed here.

Malignant hypertension, as pointed out earlier, is far less common than benign hypertension, occurring in only about 5% of patients with elevated blood pressure. It may arise de novo (i.e., without preexisting hypertension) or appear suddenly in an individual with previous mild hypertension. The basis for this turn for the worse in hypertensive subjects is unclear, but the following mechanisms may obtain.

Table 14–4. MAIN CAUSES AND POSSIBLE FACTORS IN THE PATHOGENESIS OF HYPERTENSION

**Essential Hypertension**
  "Genetic" defect in sodium transport and excretion
  Excessive salt intake
  Increased vasoconstrictive influences
    Behavioral, neurogenic, hormonal
**Secondary Hypertension**
  Renal disease
    Increased renin secretion
    Sodium and fluid retention
    Decreased vasodilator (vasodepressor) secretion
  Endocrine causes
    Aldosteronism
    Oral contraceptives
    Pheochromocytoma
    Thyrotoxicosis
  Vascular causes
    Coarctation of the aorta
    Vasculitis
  Neurogenic causes
    Psychogenic
    Increased intracranial pressure

The initial event appears to be some form of vascular damage to the kidneys. This may result from long-standing benign hypertension, with eventual injury to the arteriolar walls, or it may spring from arteritis of some form without elevated blood pressure. In either case, the result is increased permeability of the small vessels to fibrinogen and to other plasma proteins. This is considered by many to be the decisive event in the genesis of malignant hypertension. Once fibrinogen is deposited in the arteriolar walls, the clotting mechanism is activated. Microthrombi thus form in the vessels. The combination of these two changes presents the appearance of fibrinoid necrosis of arterioles and small arteries. This intramural and intravascular clotting, along with a resultant hyperplasia of the intima, causes the lumens of the arterioles to become narrowed and shaggy. Mechanical trauma to red cells coursing through these damaged vessels produces hemolysis and anemia, known as *microangiopathic hemolytic anemia*. With disruption of the red cells, there is further stimulation of the clotting mechanism and some inhibition of fibrinolysis. The vicious circle is now complete, and the deposition of fibrin continues.

The kidneys become markedly ischemic. With severe involvement of the renal afferent arterioles, the renin-angiotensin system receives a powerful stimulus, and indeed *patients with malignant hypertension have markedly elevated levels of plasma renin*. This then sets up a self-perpetuating cycle in which angiotensin II causes intrarenal vasoconstriction and the attendant renal ischemia perpetuates renin secretion. Aldosterone levels are also elevated and salt retention undoubtedly contributes to the elevation of blood pressure. The consequences of the markedly elevated blood pressure on the blood vessels throughout the body is known as malignant arteriolosclerosis. These arteriolar lesions are widespread but particularly prominent in the kidney and produce a form of nephropathy known as *malignant nephrosclerosis (MNS)*.

Grossly, the kidney may be esentially normal in size or slightly shrunken, depending on the duration and severity of the hypertensive disease. Small, pinpoint petechial hemorrhages may appear on the cortical surface from rupture of arterioles or glomerular capillaries, giving the kidney a peculiar "flea-bitten" appearance. When superimposed on preexisting renal disease, the presence of malignant hypertension may be completely undetectable grossly.

The microscopic changes reflect the pathogenetic events discussed earlier. Damage to the small vessels is manifested as **fibrinoid necrosis** of the arterioles. The vessel walls appear to take on a homogeneous, granular eosinophilic appearance masking underlying detail (Fig. 14–18). Also, there is often a sprinkling of inflammatory cells, giving rise to the term **necrotizing arteriolitis**. The inflammation is presumably secondary to vascular damage. A different response is seen in the interlobular arteries and larger arterioles, where the proliferation of

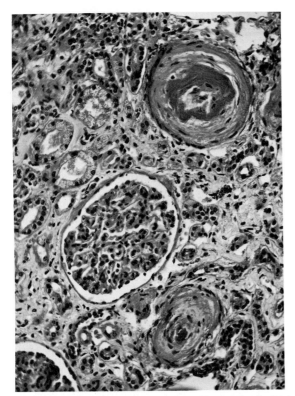

Figure 14–18. Malignant nephrosclerosis. Two markedly thick-ened vessels are seen above and below the glomerulus. The vessel above contains a heavy deposit of fibrinoid and dem-onstrates necrotizing arteriolitis.

intimal cells produces an "onionskin" appearance. This name is derived from the concentric arrangement of cells whose origin is believed to be intimal smooth muscle, although this issue is not fully settled. Thickening and reduplication of the basement membrane also contribute to the concentric lamellar appearance. This lesion, called **hyperplastic arteriolosclerosis**, causes marked narrow-ing of arterioles and small arteries, to the point of total obliteration. Necrotizing arteriolitis may extend to involve the glomeruli (**necrotizing glomerulitis**). Microthrombi may be seen within the glomeruli as well as necrotic arterioles. Rupture of the small vessels and glomerular capillaries is responsible for the petechiae seen on the kidney surface. The tubules show nonspecific changes of ischemia.

The onset of malignant hypertension, whether pri-mary or secondary, is sudden and initially dominated by cerebral and cardiovascular manifestations, al-though it may be ushered in by a transient episode of macroscopic hematuria. Proteinuria becomes pro-nounced, and microscopic hematuria is constant, punctuated by intermittent bouts of gross hematuria. The patient complains of headache, nausea, vomiting, and visual derangements, particularly the develop-ment of scotomata or blurring. Examination of the eye-grounds usually but not invariably reveals hem-orrhages and exudates, and often papilledema is seen. There may be impaired consciousness and even con-

vulsions. Congestive heart failure is frequent, partic-ularly in older patients. Later, renal failure dominates the picture.

Among untreated individuals, most patients die within a year. The cause of death is usually uremia, although occasionally the patient succumbs to a cere-brovascular accident or to heart failure. With treat-ment, the outlook is much better. The 2-year survival rate is about 70%, and 5-year survival about 50%. The chances for long-term survival are largely de-pendent on early treatment, before significant renal insufficiency has developed.

### Benign Nephrosclerosis (BNS)

*Benign nephrosclerosis (BNS), the term used for the kidney of benign hypertension, is always associ-ated with hyaline arteriolosclerosis.* Some degree of BNS, albeit mild, is present at autopsy in many individuals over age 60. The frequency and severity of the lesions are increased in young age groups in association with hypertension and diabetes mellitus.

The kidneys are symmetrically atrophied, each weigh-ing 110 to 130 gm, with a surface of diffuse, fine granu-larity, which resembles grain leather.

Microscopically, the basic anatomic change is thick-ening of the walls of the small arteries and arterioles, known as **hyaline arteriolosclerosis.** This appears as a homogeneous, pink hyaline thickening, at the expense of the vessel lumens, with loss of underlying cellular detail. Electron microscopic studies indicate that the hyaline material arises by intramural deposition of plasma pro-teins and lipids and reduplication of the intimal basement membrane. Similar vascular changes are seen with be-nign hypertension in other organs of the body. The narrowing of the lumens results in a markedly decreased blood flow through the affected vessels, and thus pro-duces ischemia in the organ served. Renal ischemic parenchymal changes, along with the vascular alterations, are necessary for the diagnosis of BNS. All structures of the kidney show ischemic atrophy. The glomeruli develop axial thickening and fibrosis, and sometimes there is fibrotic replacement of Bowman's spaces (Fig. 14–19). In far advanced cases of BNS, the glomerular tufts may become obliterated by this homogeneous hyalinization. Diffuse tubular atrophy and interstitial fibrosis are present. Often there is a scant interstitial lymphocytic infiltrate. The larger blood vessels (i.e., interlobar and arcuate arteries) show reduplication of internal elastic lamina along with fibrous thickening of the media (fibroelastic hyperplasia).

It should be remembered that many renal diseases cause hypertension, which in turn may lead to BNS. Thus, this renal lesion is often seen superimposed on other, primary kidney diseases. In these cases, the his-tologic features may be difficult to interpret.

Because this renal lesion alone rarely causes severe damage to the kidney, it very infrequently leads to uremia and death. Nonetheless, there is usually some

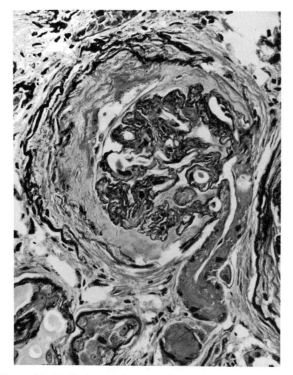

**Figure 14–19.** Benign nephrosclerosis—microscopic detail of a glomerulus and its afferent arteriole, sectioned obliquely. The arteriole has hyaline, thickened walls, and a narrowed lumen. The glomerulus shows diffuse glomerulosclerosis and has marked fibrous thickening of the parietal layer of Bowman's capsule.

functional impairment, such as loss of concentrating ability or a variably diminished glomerular filtration rate. A mild degree of proteinuria is a constant finding. Usually these patients die from hypertensive heart disease or from cerebrovascular accidents, rather than from renal disease.

# CYSTIC DISEASES OF THE KIDNEY

Cystic diseases of the kidney are a heterogeneous group comprising hereditary, developmental but nonhereditary, and acquired disorders.[33] As a group, they are important for several reasons: (1) they are reasonably common and often represent diagnostic problems for clinicians, radiologists, and pathologists; (2) some forms, such as adult polycystic disease, are major causes of chronic renal failure; (3) they can occasionally be confused with malignant tumors. Here we shall briefly mention simple cysts, the most common form, and discuss in some detail adult polycystic kidney disease.

## SIMPLE CYSTS

These generally innocuous lesions occur as multiple or single cystic spaces that vary in diameter over wide limits. Commonly, they are 1 to 5 cm in size; translucent; lined by a gray, glistening, smooth membrane; and filled with clear fluid. Microscopically, these membranes are composed of a single layer of cuboidal or flattened cuboidal epithelium, which, in many instances, may be completely atrophic. These cysts are usually confined to the cortex. Rarely, large massive cysts up to 10 cm in diameter are encountered.

Simple cysts are common postmortem findings without clinical significance. The main importance of cysts lies in their differentiation from kidney tumors, when they are discovered either incidentally or because of hemorrhage and pain during life. Radiologic studies show that, in contrast to renal tumors (p. 487), renal cysts have smooth contours, are almost always avascular, and give fluid rather than solid signals on ultrasound.

## POLYCYSTIC KIDNEY DISEASE

This is a hereditary disease characterized by multiple expanding cysts of *both* kidneys, which ultimately destroy the intervening parenchyma. It is seen in approximately 1 in 400 to 500 autopsies. Often there is accompanying cystic involvement of other organs, principally the liver and pancreas. Two clinical forms are most common: *polycystic disease of the newborn* and *adult polycystic disease*. The former is characterized by the presence of full-blown cysts at birth, many of which are blind pouches into which the glomerular filtrate flows (*closed cysts*). Children with this condition do not survive beyond infancy. At postmortem examination, the kidneys are several times normal size and totally cystic. Inheritance of this form is as an autosomal recessive trait.

The cysts in the adult form, by contrast, are not present at birth and develop slowly throughout subsequent years, rarely producing symptoms before the age of 15 years. Moreover, most of the cysts are in continuity with functioning nephrons (*open cysts*). Inheritance of this form is through a dominant autosomal gene of high penetrance. Adult polycystic disease is a relatively common condition accounting for 6 to 12% of cases of chronic renal failure.

**MORPHOLOGY.** The kidneys in the adult form may achieve enormous sizes, and weights up to 4 kg for each kidney have been recorded (Fig. 14–20). These very large kidneys are readily palpable abdominally as masses extending into the pelvis. On gross examination, the kidney seems to be composed solely of a mass of cysts of varying sizes up to 3 or 4 cm in diameter, with no intervening parenchyma. The cysts are filled with fluid, which may be clear, turbid, or hemorrhagic.

Microscopic examination reveals some normal parenchyma dispersed among the cysts. The cysts themselves may arise at any level of the nephron, from tubules to collecting ducts, and therefore have a variable, often atrophic lining. Occasionally, Bowman's capsules are

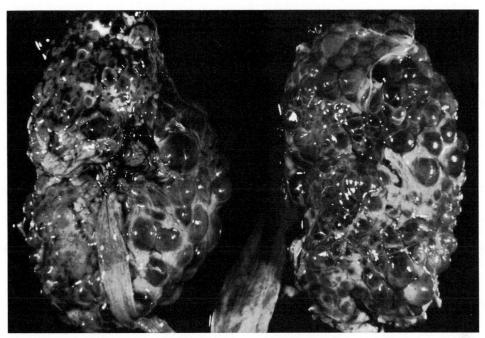

**Figure 14–20.** Polycystic kidney disease in an adult. The kidneys both comprise masses of cysts with no grossly apparent intervening normal parenchyma. The ureters are also malformed and are abnormally dilated.

involved in the cyst formation, and in these cases, glomerular tufts may be seen within the cystic space. The pressure of the expanding cysts leads to ischemic atrophy of the intervening renal substance. Evidence of superimposed hypertension or infection is common.

**CLINICAL COURSE.** Polycystic kidney disease in the adult usually does not produce symptoms until the fourth decade. By this time, the kidneys are quite large. The most common complaint of the patient is flank pain or at least a heavy, dragging sensation. Acute distention of a cyst, either by intracystic hemorrhage or by obstruction, may cause excruciating pain. Sometimes attention is first drawn to the lesion by palpation of an abdominal mass. Intermittent gross hematuria commonly occurs. The most important complications, because of their deleterious effect on already marginal renal function, are hypertension and urinary tract infection. Hypertension of varying severity develops in about 75% of patients. Berry aneurysms of the circle of Willis are present in 10% of patients, and these individuals have a high incidence of subarachnoid hemorrhage. Asymptomatic liver cysts occur in one third of patients.

Although this disease is ultimately fatal, the outlook is in general better than with most chronic renal diseases. The condition tends to be relatively stable and progresses only very slowly. Death usually occurs at about the age of 50 years, but there is wide variation in the course of this renal disorder, and nearly normal life spans are reported. Death usually results from uremia or hypertensive complications.

# URINARY OUTFLOW OBSTRUCTION

Under this heading we discuss two separate but often related entities involving obstruction to the outflow of urine. The first, *urolithiasis*, refers to stone formation within the kidney or collecting system. Most uroliths form within the kidney and produce their most serious consequences when they move into the ureter and cause obstruction. The second entity discussed under this heading is *hydronephrosis*. By definition, this refers to obstruction at some level of the collecting system, with resultant increased pressure within the kidney.

## UROLITHIASIS

*Urolithiasis* refers to calculus formation at any level within the urinary collecting system. Most often calculi arise in the kidney. It is a frequent disorder, as evidenced by the finding of stones in about 1% of all autopsies. Symptomatic urolithiasis is most common in males. A familial tendency toward stone formation has long been recognized.

**ETIOLOGY AND PATHOGENESIS.** About 75% of renal stones are composed of either calcium oxalate or calcium oxalate mixed with calcium phosphate. Another 15% are composed of magnesium ammonium phosphate, and 10% are either uric acid or cystine stones.[34] In all cases, there is an organic matrix of mucoprotein making up about 2.5% of the stone by weight.

The cause of stone formation is often obscure, particularly in the cases of calcium-containing stones. Probably involved is a confluence of predisposing conditions. *The most important is almost certainly an increased urine concentration of the stone's constituents.*

Pak and his colleagues have proposed a classification of urolithiasis on the basis of metabolic and physiologic derangements (Table 14–5). It is seen that over 70% of the patients who develop calcium renal stones have hypercalciuria. Most in this group absorb calcium from the gut in excessive amounts and promptly excrete it in the urine. Some patients have a primary renal defect leading to excessive calcium leakage. Neither of these categories is associated with hypercalcemia. By contrast, patients with primary hyperparathyroidism have hypercalcemia and consequent hypercalciuria. Excessive excretion of uric acid in the urine also favors calcium stone formation; presumably the urates provide a nidus for calcium deposition. Not listed here are conditions in which *hypercalcemia and hypercalciuria* result from obvious predisposing factors like vitamin D intoxication, sarcoidosis, and milk-alkali syndrome.

The causes of the other types of renal stones are better understood. *Magnesium ammonium phosphate stones almost always occur in patients with a persistently alkaline urine owing to recurrent urinary tract infections.* In particular, the urea-splitting bacteria, such as *Proteus vulgaris* and the staphylococci, predispose toward urolithiasis. Moreover, bacteria may serve as particulate nidi for the formation of any kind of stone. In avitaminosis A, desquamated squames from the metaplastic epithelium of the collecting system act as nidi.

#### Table 14–5. CLASSIFICATION OF NEPHROLITHIASIS*

| Group | Primary Metabolic Defect | Per cent Cases |
|---|---|---|
| Absorptive hypercalciuria | Increased intestinal absorption of calcium | 54.3 |
| Renal hypercalciuria | Excessive renal loss of calcium and secondary hyperparathyroidism | 8.3 |
| Primary hyperparathyroidism | Increased PTH secretion | 5.8 |
| Unclassifiable hypercalciuria | — | 5.4 |
| Hyperuricosuric calcium urolithiasis | Excessive uric acid in urine; cause unknown | 8.7 |
| Miscellaneous | Excessive oxalate absorption<br>Uric acid stones associated with idiopathic hyperuricemia<br>Renal tubular acidosis | 6.7 |
| No metabolic abnormality | — | 10.8 |

*From Pak, C. Y. C., et al.: Ambulatory evaluation of nephrolithiasis. Classification, clinical presentation and diagnostic criteria. Am. J. Med. 69:19, 1980.

Gout and diseases involving rapid cell turnover, such as the leukemias, lead to high uric acid levels in the urine and the possibility of *uric acid stones.* About half of the patients with uric acid stones, however, have neither hyperuricemia nor increased urine urate but an unexplained tendency to excrete a persistently acid urine (under pH 5.5) favoring stone formation. *Cystine stones* are almost invariably associated with a genetically determined defect in the renal transport of certain amino acids, including cystine. In contrast to magnesium ammonium phosphate stones, *both uric acid and cystine stones are more likely to form when the urine is relatively acidic.*

In addition to factors already mentioned, such as urine pH and the presence of bacteria, urolithiasis may be influenced by other, less certain factors. Changes in the urinary content of the mucoproteins that form the organic matrix of uroliths may be important. In normal individuals calcium and phosphate are present in the urine in amounts that exceed their solubility product, so it is possible that urolithiasis may result from the lack of influences that normally inhibit precipitation. Inhibitors of crystal formation in urine include pyrophosphate, mucopolysaccharides, and diphosphonates, but no deficiency of any of these substances has been consistently demonstrated in patients with urolithiasis.

**MORPHOLOGY.** Stones are unilateral in about 80% of patients. Common sites of formation are renal pelves, calyces, and the bladder. Often, many stones are found within one kidney. They tend to remain small, having an average diameter of 2 to 3 mm, and may be smooth or jagged. Occasionally, progressive accretion of salts leads to the development of branching structures known as **staghorn calculi,** which create a cast of the renal pelvic and calyceal system. These massive stones are usually composed of magnesium ammonium phosphate.

**CLINICAL COURSE.** Stones may be present without producing either symptoms or significant renal damage. This is particularly true with large stones lodged in the renal pelvis. Smaller stones may pass into the ureter, producing a typical intense pain known as renal or ureteral colic and characterized by paroxysms of flank pain radiating toward the groin. Often at this time there is gross hematuria. The clinical significance of stones lies in their capacity to obstruct urinary flow or to produce sufficient trauma to cause ulceration and bleeding. In either case, they predispose to bacterial infection. Fortunately, in most cases the diagnosis is readily made by pyelography.

### HYDRONEPHROSIS

Hydronephrosis refers to the dilatation of the renal pelvis and calyces, with accompanying atrophy of the parenchyma, caused by obstruction to the outflow of urine. The obstruction may be sudden or insidious, and it may occur at any level of the urinary tract, from the urethra to the renal pelvis. The following list cites the most common causes.

A. Congenital: Atresia of the urethra, valve formations in either ureter or urethra, aberrant renal artery compressing the ureter, renal ptosis with torsion, or kinking of ureter.

B. Acquired:
1. Foreign bodies: Calculi, necrotic papillae.
2. Tumors: Benign prostatic hypertrophy (BPH), carcinoma of the prostate, bladder tumors (papilloma and carcinoma), contiguous malignant disease (retroperitoneal lymphoma, carcinoma of the cervix or uterus).
3. Inflammation: Prostatitis, ureteritis, urethritis, retroperitoneal fibrosis.
4. Neurogenic: Spinal cord damage with paralysis of the bladder.
5. Normal pregnancy: Mild and reversible.

Bilateral hydronephrosis occurs only when the obstruction is below the level of the ureters. If blockage is at the ureters or above, the lesion is unilateral. Sometimes obstruction is complete, allowing no urine to pass; usually it is only partial.

It has been shown that even with complete obstruction, glomerular filtration persists for some time, and the filtrate subsequently diffuses back into the renal interstitium and perirenal spaces, whence it ultimately returns to the lymphatic and venous systems. Because of the continued filtration, the affected calyces and pelvis become dilated, often markedly so. The unusually high pressure thus generated in the renal pelvis, as well as that transmitted back through the collecting ducts, causes compression of the renal vasculature. Both arterial insufficiency and venous stasis result, although the latter is probably more important. The most severe effects are seen in the papillae, because they are subjected to the greatest increases in pressure. Damage becomes progressively less marked toward the cortex. Accordingly, the initial functional disturbances are largely tubular, manifested primarily by impaired concentrating ability. Only later does glomerular filtration begin to diminish. Experimental studies indicate that serious irreversible damage occurs in about 3 weeks with complete obstruction, and in 3 months with incomplete obstruction.[35]

**MORPHOLOGY. Bilateral** hydronephrosis (as well as unilateral hydronephrosis when the other kidney is already damaged or absent) leads to renal failure, and the onset of uremia tends to abort the natural course of the lesion. In contrast, **unilateral** involvements display the full range of morphologic changes, which vary with the degree and the speed of obstruction. With subtotal or intermittent obstruction, the kidney may be massively enlarged (lengths in the range of 20 cm) and the organ may consist almost entirely of the greatly distended pelvicalyceal system. The renal parenchyma itself is compressed and atrophied, with obliteration of the papillae and flattening of the pyramids. On the other hand, **when obstruction is sudden and complete, glomeru-**

**lar filtration is compromised relatively early, and as a consequence, renal function may cease while dilatation is still comparatively slight.** Depending on the level of the obstruction, one or both ureters may also be dilated **(hydroureter).**

Microscopically, the early lesions show tubular dilatation, followed by atrophy and fibrous replacement of the tubular epithelium, with relative sparing of the glomeruli. Eventually, in severe cases, the glomeruli also become atrophic and disappear, converting the entire kidney into a thin shell of fibrous tissue. With sudden and complete obstruction, there may be coagulative necrosis of the renal papillae, similar to the changes of necrotizing papillitis (p. 474). In uncomplicated cases, the accompanying inflammatory reaction is minimal. Complicating pyelonephritis, however, is common.

**CLINICAL COURSE.** *Bilateral* complete obstruction produces anuria, which is soon brought to medical attention. When the obstruction is below the bladder, the dominant symptoms are those of bladder distention. Paradoxically, incomplete bilateral obstruction causes polyuria rather than oliguria, as a result of defects in tubular concentrating mechanisms, and this may obscure the true nature of the disturbance. Unfortunately, *unilateral* hydronephrosis may remain completely silent for long periods of time, unless the other kidney is for some reason nonfunctioning. Often the enlarged kidney is discovered on routine physical examination. Sometimes the basic cause of the hydronephrosis, such as renal calculi or an obstructing tumor, produce symptoms that indirectly draw attention to the hydronephrosis. Removal of obstruction within a few weeks usually permits full return of function. However, with time, the changes become irreversible.

# TUMORS

Many types of benign and malignant tumors occur in the urinary tract. In general, benign tumors such as small (rarely over 2.5 cm in diameter) cortical adenomas or medullary fibromas (interstitial cell tumors) are without clinical significance. The most common malignant tumor of the kidney is the renal cell carcinoma, followed in frequency by Wilms' tumors and by primary tumors of the calyces and pelves. Other types of renal cancer are extremely rare and need not be discussed here. Tumors of the lower urinary tract are about twice as common as renal cell carcinomas, and they are described at the end of this section.

## RENAL CELL CARCINOMA

Renal cell carcinoma is the type of neoplasm usually meant by the term "cancer of the kidney." It represents 80 to 90% of all malignant tumors of the kidney and 2% of all cancers in adults.[36] These lesions

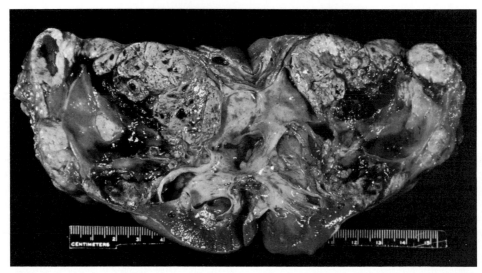

Figure 14–21. Renal cell carcinoma. The kidney has been hemisected to expose the tumor mass, which totally replaces and expands the upper pole of the kidney. Prominently shown are the areas of necrosis, hemorrhage, and cystic softening of the tumor. Only the lower pole of the kidney is recognizable below.

are most common in late middle age, from the fifth to seventh decades, and males are affected twice as often as females. Although no neoplasm has an absolutely predictable course, *the renal cell carcinoma distinguishes itself by being especially variable in its behavior.* Because of a histologic similarity between the cells of this tumor and normal adrenal cells, it was once thought that the renal cell carcinoma arose from adrenal rests within the kidney, hence the well-entrenched misnomer "hypernephroma." It is now clear, however, that these tumors are tubule cell–derived adenocarcinomas.

MORPHOLOGY. These cancers are usually large by the time they are discovered and appear as spherical masses 3 to 15 cm in diameter. They may arise anywhere in the kidney. The cut surface is yellow-gray-white, with prominent areas of cystic softening or of hemorrhage, either fresh or old (Fig. 14–21). The margins of the tumor are well defined. However, at times small processes project into the surrounding parenchyma, and small satellite nodules are found in the surrounding substance, providing clear evidence of the aggressiveness of these lesions. As the tumor enlarges, it may fungate through the walls of the collecting system, extending through the calyces and pelvis as far as the ureter. Even more frequently, the tumor invades the renal vein and grows as a solid column within this vessel, sometimes extending in snake-like fashion as far as the inferior vena cava and even into the right side of the heart. Occasionally there is direct invasion into the perinephric fat and adrenal gland.

Depending on the amount of lipid and glycogen present, the tumor cells may appear almost totally vacuolated or they may be solid. The classic vacuolated (lipid-laden) or **"clear cells"** are demarcated only by their cell membranes; the nuclei are usually pushed basally and are small (Fig. 14–22). At the other extreme are the **solid**

**cells,** resembling the tubular epithelium, which have round, small, regular nuclei enclosed within granular pink cytoplasm. These cells may show great regularity of cytologic detail. Some tumors exhibit marked degrees of anaplasia, with numerous mitotic figures, and giant cells. Between the extremes of clear cells and solid cells, all intergradations may be found. Cellular arrangement, too,

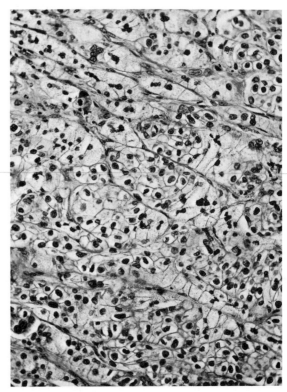

Figure 14–22. A high-power detail of the "clear cell" pattern of a renal cell carcinoma.

varies widely; the cells may form abortive tubules or papillary patterns, or they may cluster in cords or disorganized masses. The stroma is usually scanty but highly vascularized.

**CLINICAL COURSE.** Renal cell carcinomas have several peculiar clinical characteristics that create especially difficult but challenging diagnostic problems. The symptoms vary, but the *most frequent presenting manifestation is hematuria, occurring in over 50% of cases.* Macroscopic hematuria tends to be intermittent and fleeting, superimposed on a steady microscopic hematuria. In other patients, the tumor may declare itself simply by virtue of its size, when it has grown large enough to produce flank pain and a palpable mass. By the time this occurs there may be other extrarenal clues. Among these extrarenal effects are fever and polycythemia, both of which may be associated with a renal cell carcinoma but which, because they are nonspecific, may be misinterpreted for some time before their true significance is appreciated. Fever is present in about 15% of these patients. The basis for this pyrexia is unknown. Polycythemia is an interesting but less frequent accompaniment of renal cell carcinoma, affecting about 5 to 10% of patients with this disease. It is assumed that the polycythemia results from elaboration of erythropoietin by the renal tumor. Uncommonly, these tumors produce a variety of hormone-like substances resulting possibly in hypercalcemia, hypertension, Cushing's syndrome, or feminization or masculinization.

In many patients, the primary tumor remains silent and is discovered only after its metastases have evoked symptoms. This tendency for metastases to be discovered before the primary tumor is one of the common characteristics of renal cell carcinoma. The favored locations for metastases are the lungs and the bones. It must be apparent that renal cell carcinoma presents in many fashions, some quite devious, but *the triad of painless hematuria, longstanding fever, and dull flank pain is pathognomonic.*

CT scanning and sonography are extremely useful diagnostic aids. A characteristic vascular pattern can be seen in nearly all cases on arteriography. The survival rate depends upon the extent and spread of the tumor. In the absence of metastases 70% of patients survive five years, whereas local invasion of perinephric fat or invasion of the renal vein augurs poorly (15 to 20% five-year survival). Nephrectomy is the treatment of choice.

## WILMS' TUMOR

Although Wilms' tumor occurs infrequently in adults, it is the third most common organ cancer in children under the age of 10 years. Unfortunately, it is one of the major cancer-killers in children.[32] These tumors contain a variety of cell and tissue components, all derived from the mesoderm. The vulnera-

bility to Wilms' tumor appears to be inherited and the tumor is sometimes associated with other congenital anomalies.

**MORPHOLOGY.** By the time they are discovered, Wilms' tumors are usually huge spherical masses, dwarfing the kidney. On sectioning, they have a variegated surface, dependent upon the tissue types present. Myxomatous soft fish-flesh areas, solid gray hyaline cartilaginous tissue, and areas of hemorrhagic necrosis are the usual components. The aggressive nature of these neoplasms is manifested by their propensity to rupture through the renal capsule and extend locally into the perirenal tissues. Involvement of the other kidney occurs in about 5% of cases.

Histologically, **the characteristic features are primitive or abortive glomeruli, with poorly formed Bowman's spaces, and abortive tubules, all enclosed in a spindle cell stroma.** In addition, striated muscle, smooth muscle, collagenous fibrous tissue, cartilage, bone, fat cells, and areas of necrotic tissue containing cholesterol crystals and lipid macrophages may all be seen. The most consistent of these various elements are the striated muscle cells. **The histologic diagnosis rests upon identification of the primitive tubules within a spindle cell stroma and the strongly supportive evidence of striated muscle fibers.**

**CLINICAL COURSE.** Patients usually present with complaints referable to the tumor's enormous size. Commonly there is a readily palpable abdominal mass, which may extend across the midline and down into the pelvis. Less often, the patient presents with fever and abdominal pain, with hematuria, or, occasionally, with intestinal obstruction as a result of pressure from the tumor. The outlook for patients with Wilms' tumor is generally very good. Excellent results are obtained with a combination of radiotherapy, nephrectomy, and chemotherapy. Two-year survival rates are as high as 90%, and survival for two years usually implies a cure. These results are all the more remarkable because in many of these patients, pulmonary metastases, present at diagnosis, disappear under the therapeutic regimen.

## TUMORS OF THE URINARY COLLECTING SYSTEM (RENAL CALYCES, PELVIS, URETER, BLADDER, AND URETHRA)

The entire urinary collecting system from renal pelvis to urethra is lined with transitional epithelium, so its epithelial tumors assume similar morphologic patterns. Tumors in the collecting system above the bladder are relatively uncommon; those in the bladder, however, are an even more frequent cause of death than are kidney tumors. Nevertheless, in the individual case, a small lesion in the ureter, for example, may cause urinary outflow obstruction and have greater clinical significance than a much larger mass in the capacious bladder. We shall consider first the range of anatomic patterns principally as they occur in the urinary bladder, followed by their clinical implications.[38]

**MORPHOLOGY.** Tumors arising in the collecting system of the urinary tract range from small benign papillomas to large invasive cancers (Fig. 14–23). The rare benign **papillomas** are small (0.2 to 1.0 cm), frond-like structures, having a delicate fibrovascular axial core covered by multilayered, well-differentiated transitional epithelium. In some of these lesions, the covering epithelium appears as normal as the mucosal surface whence these tumors arise; such lesions are almost invariably noninvasive and benign, and do not recur once removed. Most papillary lesions ranging up to 3 or 4 cm are cancerous. True benign papillomas of the bladder are rare. **Transitional cell carcinomas** range from papillary to flat, noninvasive to invasive, and from extremely well differentiated (Grade I, Fig. 14–24) to highly anaplastic aggressive cancers (Grade III). Grade I carcinomas are rarely invasive but may recur after removal. Whether the regrowth is a true recurrence or a second primary growth is uncertain. Progressive degrees of cellular atypia and anaplasia are encountered in papillary exophytic growths, accompanied by increase in size of the lesion and evidence of invasion of the submucosal or muscular layers. These tumors are unequivocally transitional cell carcinomas, Grade II or Grade III. As these cancers approach the Grade III pattern they tend to be flatter than the less aggressive forms, to cover larger areas of the mucosal surface, to invade more deeply, and to have a shaggier necrotic surface. Occasionally these cancers show foci of squamous cell differentiation, but only 5% of bladder cancers are true **squamous cell carcinomas.** Carcinomas of Grades II and III infiltrate surrounding structures, spread to regional nodes, and on occasion metastasize widely.

In addition to overt carcinoma, an **in situ stage of bladder carcinoma can be recognized,** most frequently in patients with previous or simultaneous papillary or invasive tumors.[39] Indeed, wide areas of atypical hyperplasia and dysplasia are often present. It is now thought

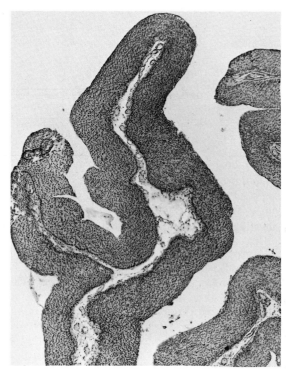

Figure 14–24. A Grade I papillary transitional cell carcinoma of the bladder. The delicate papilla is covered by orderly transitional epithelium.

that these epithelial changes and in situ lesions are caused by the generalized influence of a putative carcinogen on urothelium and that they may be the precursors of invasive carcinomas in some patients. The extent of the "restless epithelium" provides a plausible source for multiple and recurrent lesions. The staging of bladder cancer is exceedingly complex and beyond our scope. Reference may be made to current TNM classifications.[40, 41]

**CLINICAL COURSE.** *Painless hematuria is the dominant clinical presentation of all these tumors.* Because most arise in the bladder we shall consider these first. They affect men about twice as frequently as women, and usually develop between the ages of 50 and 70 years. Although most occur in individuals without a known history of exposure to industrial solvents, bladder tumors are 50 times more frequent in those exposed to beta-naphthylamine (p. 203). Cigarette smoking, chronic cystitis, schistosomiasis of the bladder, and certain drugs (cyclophosphamide) are also believed to induce higher attack rates.

*The clinical significance of bladder tumors depends on several factors: obviously on their benign or malignant nature, on their location within the bladder, and—most important—on the depth of invasion of the lesion.* Except for the clearly benign papillomas, all tend stubbornly to recur after removal and tend to kill by infiltrative obstruction of ureters rather than by metastasis. Lesions that invade the ureteral or urethral orifices cause urinary tract obstruction. In general, with shallow lesions, the prognosis after

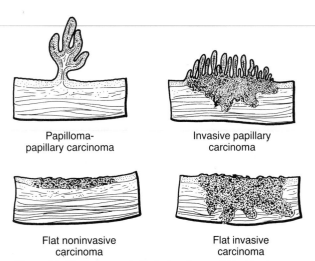

Papilloma-papillary carcinoma

Invasive papillary carcinoma

Flat noninvasive carcinoma

Flat invasive carcinoma

Figure 14–23. Four morphological patterns of bladder tumors.

removal is good, but when deep penetration of the bladder wall has occurred, whatever the histologic pattern, the five-year survival rate is less than 20%. Overall five-year survival is 57%.

Although papillary and cancerous neoplasms of the lining epithelium of the collecting system occur much less frequently in the renal pelvis than in the bladder, they nonetheless make up 5 to 10% of primary renal tumors.[42] Painless hematuria is the most characteristic feature of these lesions, but in their critical location they produce pain in the costovertebral angle as hydronephrosis develops. Infiltration of the walls of the pelvis, calyces, and renal vein worsens the prognosis. Despite removal of the tumor by nephrectomy, fewer than 50% of patients survive for five years. Cancer of the ureter is, fortunately, the rarest of the tumors of the collecting system. Five-year survival is less than 10%.

# References

1. Kanwar, Y. S.: Biophysiology of glomerular filtration and proteinuria. Lab. Invest. 51:7, 1984.
2. Farquhar, M. G., et al.: Role of proteoglycans in glomerular function and pathology. In Robinson, R. (ed.): Nephrology. Vol. 1. New York, Springer-Verlag, 1984, pp. 580–609.
3. Wilson, C. B., and Dixon, F. J.: The renal response to immunological injury. In Brenner, B. M., and Rector, F. C., Jr., (eds.): The Kidney. 3rd ed. Philadelphia, W. B. Saunders Co., 1986, pp. 800–885.
4. Michael, A. F.: Immunologic mechanisms in renal disease. In Robinson, R. (ed.): Nephrology. Vol. 1. New York, Springer-Verlag, 1984, pp. 485–1221.
5. Couser, W. G.: Mechanisms of glomerular injury in immune complex disease. Kidney Int. 28:569, 1985.
6. Adler, S., et al.: Immunologic mechanisms of renal disease. Am. J. Med. Sci. 289:55, 1985.
7. Schreiner, G. F., et al.: Macrophages and cellular immunity in experimental glomerulonephritis. Springer Semin. Immunopathol. 5:351, 1982.
8. Brenner, B. M., and Stein, J. H. (eds.): Nephrotic syndrome. In Contemporary Issues in Nephrology. Vol. 9. New York, Churchill Livingstone, 1982.
9. Cotran, R. S., and Rennke, H. R.: Anionic sites and the mechanisms of proteinuria. N. Engl. J. Med. 309:1050, 1983.
10. Habib, R., and Kleinknecht, C.: The primary nephrotic syndrome of childhood: Classification and clinicopathologic study of 406 cases. Pathol. Annu. 6:417, 1971.
11. Arnaout, M. A., et al.: Membranous glomerulonephritis. In Brenner, B. M., and Stein, J. H. (eds.): Nephrotic Syndrome. Contemporary Issues in Nephrology. Vol. 9. New York, Churchill Livingstone, 1982, pp. 199–236.
12. Goldszer, R. C., et al.: Focal segmental glomerulosclerosis. Annu. Rev. Med. 35:429, 1984.
13. Donadio, J. V., and Holley, K. E.: Membranoproliferative glomerulonephritis. Semin. Nephrol. 2:204, 1982.
14. Glassock, R. J., et al.: Primary glomerular diseases. In Brenner, B. M., and Rector, F. C., Jr. (eds.): The Kidney. 3rd ed. Philadelphia, W. B. Saunders, 1986, pp. 929–1013.
15. Lewis, E. J., and Schwartz, M. M.: Idiopathic crescentic glomerulonephritis. Semin. Nephrol. 2:193, 1982.
16. Briggs, W. A., et al.: Antiglomeruler basement membrane antibody-mediated glomerulonephritis and Goodpasture's syndrome. Medicine 58:348, 1979.
17. Couser, W. G.: Idiopathic rapidly progressive glomerulonephritis. Am. J. Nephrol. 2:57, 1982.
18. Woodruff, A. J., et al.: Mesangial IgA nephritis. Springer Semin. Immunopathol. 5:321, 1982.
19. Cotran, R. S., et al.: Tubulo-interstitial nephropathies. In Brenner, B. M., and Rector, F. C., Jr. (eds.): The Kidney. 3rd ed. Philadelphia, W. B. Saunders Co., 1986, pp. 1143–1173.
20. Tolkoff-Rubin, N. E., and Rubin, R. H.: Urinary tract infection. In Cotran, R. S., et al. (eds.): Tubulo-interstitial Nephropathies. Contemporary Issues in Nephrology. Vol. 10. New York, Churchill Livingstone, 1983, pp. 49–82.
21. Rubin, R., et al.: Urinary tract infection, pyelonephritis, and reflux nephropathy. In Brenner, B. M., and Rector, F. C., Jr. (eds.): The Kidney. 3rd ed. Philadelphia, W. B. Saunders Co., 1986, pp. 1085–1141.
22. Hodson, C. J., and Cotran, R. S.: Vesicoureteral reflux nephropathy and chronic pyelonephritis. In Cotran, R. S., et al. (ed.): Tubulo-interstitial Nephropathies. Contemporary Issues in Nephrology. Vol. 10. New York, Churchill Livingstone, 1983, pp. 83–120.
23. Cotran, R. S.: Glomerulosclerosis in reflux nephropathy. Kidney Int. 21:528, 1982.
24. Brenner, B., et al.: Dietary protein and the progressive nature of renal disease. N. Engl. J. Med. 307:852, 1983.
25. Appel, G. N., and Kunis, C. L.: Acute tubulo-interstitial nephritis. In Cotran, R. S., et al. (eds): Tubulo-interstitial Nephropathies. Contemporary Issues in Nephrology. Vol. 10. New York, Churchill Livingstone, 1983, pp. 151–186.
26. Kincaid-Smith, P.: Analgesic abuse and the kidney. Kidney Int. 17:250, 1980.
27. Bengtsson, U., et al.: Malignancies of the urinary tract and their relation to analgesic abuse. Kidney Int. 13:107, 1978.
28. Brenner, B., and Lazarus, M. (eds.): Acute Renal Failure. Philadelphia, W. B. Saunders Co., 1984.
29. Itskovitz, H. S., et al.: Patterns of blood pressure in Milwaukee. J. A. M. A. 238:864, 1977.
30. Kaplan, N. K.: Systemic hypertension: Mechanisms and diagnosis. In Braunwald, E. (ed.): Heart Disease. 2nd ed. Philadelphia, W. B. Saunders Co., 1984, pp. 849–901.
31. Needleman, P., and Greenwald, J. E.: Atriopeptin: A cardiac hormone intimately involved in fluid, electrolyte, and blood pressure homeostasis. N. Engl. J. Med. 314:828, 1986.
32. Dzau, V. J., et al.: Renovascular hypertension: An update on pathophysiology, diagnosis, and treatment. Am. J. Nephrol. 3:172, 1983.
33. Gardner, K. D.: Cystic diseases of the kidney. In Massry, S. G., and Glassock, R. J. (eds.): Textbook of Nephrology. Baltimore, Williams & Wilkins Co., 1983, pp. 6.160–6.169.
34. Coe, F., et al. (eds.): Nephrolithiasis. Contemporary Issues in Nephrology. Vol. 5. New York, Churchill Livingstone, 1980.
35. Arruda, J. A. L.: Obstructive uropathy. In Cotran, R. S., et al. (eds.): Tubulo-interstitial Nephropathies. Contemporary Issues in Nephrology. Vol. 10. New York, Churchill Livingstone, 1983, pp. 243–274.
36. Garnick, M. B., and Richie, J. P.: Renal neoplasia in the kidney. In Brenner, B. M., and Rector, F. C., Jr. (eds.): The Kidney. 3rd ed. Philadelphia, W. B. Saunders Co., 1986, pp. 1533–1550.
37. D'Angio, G. J., et al.: Wilms' tumor. In Kelalis, P. P., et al. (eds.): Clinical Pediatric Urology. 2nd ed. Philadelphia, W. B. Saunders Co., 1985, p. 1157.
38. Murphy, W. M.: Current topics in the pathology of bladder cancer. Pathol. Annu. 18:1, 1983.
39. Koss, L. G.: Evaluation of patients with cancer in situ of the bladder. Pathol. Annu. 17:353, 1982.
40. McCarron, J. P., et al.: Tumors of the renal pelvis and ureter: Current concepts and management. Semin. Urol. 1:75, 1983.

# 15

# The Oral Cavity and Teeth

## L. R. EVERSOLE, D.D.S., M.S.D., M.A.*

As the portal to the digestive tract, the oral cavity (with its mucous membranes, teeth, and salivary glands) has as its prime function the initiation of foodstuff processing for ultimate absorption and biochemical assimilation. A plethora of disease processes may be encountered here. The mucous membranes are merely an extension of the integument, and although many cutaneous diseases involve the mouth, many other lesions are unique to oral mucosa. Minor salivary glands are ubiquitous in the oral cavity, and inflammatory as well as neoplastic lesions arise in both major and minor glands. The teeth are subject to decay, a bacterial disease, and spread of infection into the pulp and underlying bone is a common problem confronting the dentist. Inflammatory disease of the supporting periodontal tissues is also common. Intraosseous jaw cysts and tumors are en-

countered less frequently. Thus, some lesions of the oral cavity constitute manifestations of a systemic disorder; however, many are local disorders. Our discussion will be limited to those local diseases that are common or potentially life-threatening.

## THE TEETH AND PERIODONTIUM

Humans possess two sets of teeth, the primary deciduous and secondary permanent dentitions. Odontogenesis begins in utero from interactions of the ectodermal and mesodermal germ layers. The coronal portion of the tooth extends through the gingiva and is covered by ectodermally derived enamel, which is generated embryologically by ameloblasts. The enamel coating is extremely hard and durable, being composed of nonvital hydroxyapatite prisms oriented radially. Cusps and recesses with grooves constitute the chewing or occluding surfaces. Underlying the enamel is a thicker layer of mineralized tissue known as dentin. Dentin is traversed by tubules, also radially oriented, that contain viable protoplasmic processes derived from the odontoblasts located in the central pulp, a region composed of areolar fibrous tissue throughout which course neurovascular elements. This dentin layer extends into the tooth root and is covered by a mesodermally derived bone-like layer called cementum. Dense collagen fibers forming the periodontal ligament join the root cementum to the alveolar bone socket.

## DENTAL DECAY (CARIES)

The exposed enamel surfaces of the teeth are subject to accretion of necrotic debris, foodstuff substances, and salivary glycoproteins referred to collectively as *dental plaque*. This tooth-accumulated material contains mono- and oligosaccharides that serve as substrates for microbial growth. Certain bacteria (*Streptococcus mutans* is the predominant organism) enzymatically degrade plaque-associated sugars and cause the production of acid.[1] At low pH, slow, progressive dissolution of enamel mineral ensues, creating a focus of cavitation. These carious lesions have a tendency to affect the pits and fissures on the

---

*Professor and Chairman, Department of Oral Diagnostic Sciences, College of Dentistry, University of Florida, Gainesville, Florida

occluding surfaces as well as the proximal surfaces immediately below the region of contact between juxtaposed teeth.[2] The neck or cervix of the tooth is also subject to caries, particularly among patients with xerostomia secondary to either Sjögren's syndrome or radiation therapy.

Once the zone of demineralized cavitation extends through the full thickness of the enamel layer, other bacterial species assume a pathogenic role and invade the dentinal tubules containing the odontoblastic processes. Dentinal caries is more rapidly progressive, and over time the infectious organisms reach the pulp chamber. If the invading organisms are pyogenic, then an acute inflammatory response will evolve. *Acute pulpitis* is characterized by severe, throbbing pain.

Dental caries is, perhaps, the most common disease to affect mankind. Epidemiologic studies disclose that the prevalence is highest among industrialized societies whose diet includes large amounts of refined carbohydrates. Children are most susceptible.

Clinical and gross pathologic changes in **caries** are characterized by an opaque, chalky change in the enamel, followed by cavitation and brown discoloration (Fig. 15–1). A sharp dental explorer is used to probe the enamel surfaces in the region of pits, fissures, and interproximal surfaces. When the explorer binds or catches in suspected carious foci, the diagnosis is confirmed. Microscopically, decalcified sections disclose the presence of bacteria within the dentinal tubules. Invasion of the pulp results in either acute or chronic inflammation. **Acute pulpitis** is characterized by a focal neutrophilic infiltrate adjacent to the zone of carious exposure. In **chronic pulpitis**, granulation tissue with a mononuclear inflammatory infiltrate is seen microscopically. The inflammatory process compresses the only blood supply to the

pulp through the apical foramen at the root tips (collateral circulation is nonexistent); thus immunologic defense and repair mechanisms are compromised, accounting for the irreversibility of pulpal infection. Ultimately, the pulp tissues undergo necrosis, and infection spreads out through the root canals and into the periodontal tissues.

Dental caries is treated by mechanical débridement of the cavity and subsequent placement of dental restorative materials. A tooth with pulpitis or pulpal necrosis requires root canal therapy or extraction, should it be deemed nonrestorable.

## SPREAD OF ODONTOGENIC INFECTION

When a tooth becomes necrotic due to carious pulp exposure, bacteria escape from the root apices and infect the periodontium. The pathogenic flora is represented by many microbial species; some organisms stimulate an acute response, whereas others provoke chronic inflammation. Acute reactions are generally associated with pain, particularly during chewing or direct percussion of the offending tooth. Once the infection has extended beyond the apex of the tooth, the inflammatory changes follow the path of least resistance and spread locally. Figure 15–2 illustrates the potential routes of spread from both maxillary and mandibular teeth.

Initially, the infection localizes around the root apex. *Periapical infection* may be acute, creating an *apical abscess*, or chronic, a *periapical granuloma*.

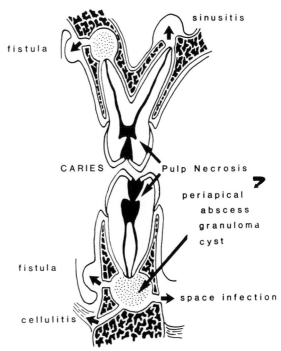

Figure 15–2. When dental caries progresses to pulp necrosis, odontogenic infection may spread orally as a fistula, into the antrum (resulting in sinusitis), into potential tissue spaces, or directly through muscle with resultant cellulitis.

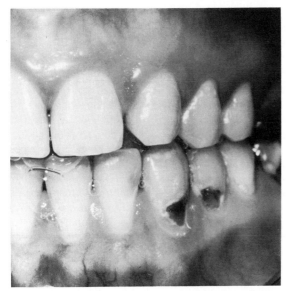

Figure 15–1. Clinical photograph of dental caries above the cervix.

These lesions are identifiable on dental radiographs as radiolucencies around the root apices. Periapical inflammation may stimulate the proliferation of the epithelial rests of Malassez, intraosseous remnants of odontogenesis. The proliferating rests undergo cystic degeneration and evolve into an *apical periodontal cyst*.[3, 4]

Periapical granulomas and cysts are chronic lesions, and pain develops only when the flora changes with an acute exacerbation. Acutely infected periapical lesions may then spread through the alveolar bone into the oral cavity via the gingiva or buccal sulcus as a *fistula or parulis*. Palatal roots on maxillary molars and premolars may drain superiorly into the maxillary sinus. Periapical mandibular infections may drain intraorally as fistulas when the spread of infection progresses above mandibular muscle attachments; if the route of spread lies inferior to the muscle attachments, cellulitis or space infection with facial swelling is the sequela. Space infections are potentially dangerous, since the infection may continue to spread along fascial planes into the parapharyngeal spaces and even into the mediastinum, where edema can lead to acute airway constriction. Occasionally, the inflammatory process remains confined to bone, particularly in the mandible, resulting in osteomyelitis.[5, 6]

Periapical infections are, grossly, grayish, soft tissue nodules or sacs attached to the root tips (Fig. 15–3). Microscopically, apical abscesses show a granulation tissue wall with a centrally located accumulation of pus. Apical granulomas are solid lesions composed of fibrous and granulation tissue infiltrated by mononuclear cells. The apical periodontal cyst is characterized by a lumen filled with exudate and necrotic debris enveloped by a hyperplastic, noncornified, stratified squamous epithelial lining that is supported by a wall of fibrous and granulation tissue.

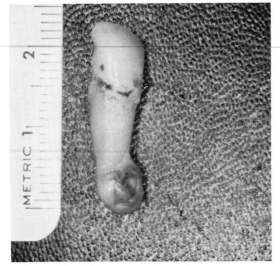

Figure 15–3. Extracted tooth with periapical granuloma attached to root end.

As long as a necrotic tooth or root tip persists, a chronic microbial culture chamber exists, continuing to feed the infectious process. Root canal therapy with débridement and elimination of infected necrotic tissue is the treatment of choice, or extraction can be performed. Space infections and cellulitis usually require antibiotic therapy with incision and drainage, particularly when airway obstruction appears imminent.

## CHRONIC INFLAMMATORY PERIODONTAL DISEASE

Whereas dental caries is more prevalent in younger individuals, chronic periodontal disease is insidious, slowly progressive, and of increasing severity during middle age. Like dental caries, *periodontal disease (pyorrhea)* is extremely common, affecting nearly 90% of the population.[7] The disease begins early in life with gingivitis; however, destruction of the supporting alveolar bone is usually minimal before the age of 20. Although the origin of pyorrhea has not been precisely uncovered, the accumulation of *dental plaque* at and below the gingival attachment to the teeth plays a major role. Plaque-associated microbial antigens elicit a chronic inflammatory reaction in the adjacent gingival tissues, and destructive bacterial enzymes and metabolites are released. Progressive deposition of plaque can serve as a nidus for mineralization, resulting in the formation of *dental calculus*. Calculus is grainy in nature and acts as a mechanical irritant, particularly when it accumulates on root surfaces below the gingival margin. Thus, immunologic, microbial, and mechanical factors appear to participate jointly in the initiation of periodontal inflammation. As the inflammatory changes become more extensive, resorption of the supporting alveolar bone advances and the gingival attachment to the tooth migrates apically to create a *periodontal pocket* with alveolar bone loss. In severe cases, the teeth loosen and exfoliate or require extraction. The disease is insidious, and although gingival swelling, recession, and bleeding are noted, symptoms of pain are rare.

Macroscopically, the gingiva becomes reddened, loses its normal stippling, and may be edematous. A periodontal probe inserted into the gingival sulcus between the tooth and soft tissue will drop into the periodontal pocket. Pocket depths in excess of 3 mm are indicative of disease. Loss of alveolar bone can also be detected radiographically. Microscopically, the periodontal and gingival tissues show aggregates of plasma cells and lymphocytes. Rarely, a focal abscess is encountered, characterized by sheets of neutrophils. In severe alveolar bone loss, granulation tissue with extensive fibrosis is seen.

The loss of supporting soft and hard tissue of the periodontium is essentially irreversible, as reattachment to denuded root surfaces does not occur to any appreciable degree. Therapy is aimed at prevention and arrest of the process by mechanical, surgical, and chemical methods of plaque and calculus removal.

## ORAL SEPSIS AND BACTERIAL ENDOCARDITIS

Oral bacteria, particularly in periapical infections, infections located in the gingival sulcus, or those associated with periodontal disease, can enter the local vessels. Vascular entry is facilitated by mechanical irritation such as brushing the teeth and curettage procedures to remove dental plaque. Tooth extraction, biopsy, and other oral surgical procedures also promote passage of bacteria into blood vessels. A transient bacteremia ensues; in otherwise healthy individuals, these vascular microbial showers are eliminated rapidly by the reticuloendothelial system.

Transient bacteremias are ominous in individuals with any form of cardiac valvular abnormality (congenital or acquired) or certain types of cardiac malformation (ventricular septal defects, patent ductus arteriosus). The bacteria may implant on the abnormal valves or at the developmental defect to produce infective endocarditis, more often the subacute form than the acute (p. 335). *Streptococcus viridans* is the chief culprit.

Oral sepsis and oral surgical procedures culminating in bacteremia cannot be avoided; however, prophylactic antibiotic coverage of patients with cardiac lesions requiring periodontal treatment and oral surgery will usually protect these vulnerable individuals against the potentially lethal consequences of bloodborne organisms.

# DISEASES OF THE MUCOUS MEMBRANES

Whereas the mucosa of the respiratory and digestive tracts is endodermally derived, oral mucosa is an ectodermal derivative. The entire oral mucosa is stratified squamous epithelium that is keratinized in regions bound to bone (i.e., palate and gingiva) and nonkeratinized where the mucosa is supple and movable. Adnexal structures include the major and minor salivary glands, the teeth, and the sebaceous glands of the buccal and lip mucosa. The submucosa is composed of fibrovascular connective tissue with muscle, fat, and bone in the deeper layers.

Disease processes involving the mucosa are usually neoplastic or inflammatory in nature. Among the neoplasms, those of epithelial origin are most frequent. The chief inflammatory lesions include aphthous stomatitis, herpetic stomatitis, lichen planus, and reactive proliferations evoked by irritation.

## BENIGN NEOPLASMS AND REACTIVE LESIONS

A variety of benign epithelial and mesenchymal neoplasms and reactive proliferations arise from oral mucosa. Three are common—papilloma, fibrous hyperplasia, and pyogenic granuloma; others are encountered infrequently. True connective tissue tumors, including lipoma, myoblastoma, angioma, and nerve sheath tumors, are uncommon.

### Papilloma

The squamous papilloma is the most common oral benign epithelial tumor. It may occur at any age and is usually located on the lips, tongue, floor of the mouth, or soft palate. These tumors appear as exophytic projections emanating from either a pedunculated or sessile base.[8] Microscopically there is a thickened parakeratin layer that is superimposed over a papillary spinous layer supported by fibrovascular cores. Some oral papillomas covered by markedly thickened epithelium represent condylomas associated with human papillomavirus; lesions of this nature may be transmitted via oral-genital contact. Papillomas are not premalignant, but surgical excision is recommended.

### Fibrous Hyperplasia

The most common oral swelling is fibrous hyperplasia. The lesion is a reactive proliferation of fibroblasts with abundant collagen fibers that arise in response to chronic irritation. The tongue and buccal mucosa are favored sites, since these tissues are subject to biting. The lesion, also termed *traumatic fibroma*, is a dome-shaped, smooth-surfaced, soft polyp. A similar reactive fibrous growth may arise adjacent to the margins of an ill-fitting denture, creating a bosselated, fissured tumefaction referred to as *epulis fissurata*.[9] These benign hyperplasias are non-neoplastic and slow growing; once they attain a given size, their growth generally ceases. Local excision should be performed because persistent trauma will lead to ulceration.

### Pyogenic Granuloma

Chronic irritation can induce a proliferative granulation tissue response. Lesions of this nature are usually located between teeth, emanating from the gingiva. The term pyogenic granuloma is a misnomer, as pyogenic bacteria are not etiologically involved; rather, a mechanical irritant apparently lodges in the gingival sulcus, and stimulates an overzealous granulation tissue response. Most patients are pregnant women; however, this lesion also occurs in nongravid females as well as in males. The lesion presents as a red, ulcerated, soft mass composed of vascular channels proliferating throughout a delicate fibrous connective tissue matrix, which contains a subacute inflammatory cell infiltrate. Other reactive lesions with a similar clinical appearance may reveal microscopic evidence of calcification (*peripheral ossifying fibroma*) or may exhibit hypercellular fibrovascular connective tissue with interspersed multinucleated giant cells (*peripheral giant cell granuloma* or *epulis*). Giant cell granulomas grow rapidly and, despite their reactive nature, can erode alveolar bone; they fail to resolve spontaneously and require surgical excision.[10]

## LEUKOPLAKIA, ERYTHROPLAKIA, AND CARCINOMA

Oral cancer accounts for about 5% of all malignancies. Men, usually over 50 years of age, are affected more often than women. Squamous cell carcinoma is by far the most common form of cancer; it is followed in frequency by malignancies of the minor salivary glands. Sarcomas of the oral soft tissues are extremely rare.

ETIOLOGY AND PATHOGENESIS. The major etiologic factors associated with oral cancer are tobacco use, alcohol consumption, and, less assuredly, viruses. Both smoking and smokeless tobacco are implicated, as are snuff and, possibly, chewing betel nuts (a common habit in Pakistan and India). Although the majority of patients are smokers and alcohol abusers, about 10% of those with oral cancer deny the use of either tobacco or alcohol; these individuals tend to be older men and women. A viral etiology for oral carcinoma has not been proved; however, antibody titers to herpes simplex virus (HSV) are higher among oral cancer patients than controls.[11] More significantly, RNA complementary to several possibly oncogenic serotypes of human papillomavirus DNA has been identified in some oral squamous cell carcinomas.[12A]

Squamous cell carcinoma may arise *de novo*, yet more often, an evolutionary process akin to that in the uterine cervix is observed. The reader is referred to the chapter on the female genital system for a detailed discussion of precancerous change progressing to invasive carcinoma (p. 639). Precancerous changes in the mouth assume two clinical appearances. *Flat, white plaques that have no identifiable cause other than an association with tobacco use and that fail to rub away are referred to as leukoplakias. Red patches without an associated inflammatory stimulus are called erythroplakias.* Leukoplakia is usually encountered in the buccal vestibule, floor of the mouth, and lateral border of the tongue. At the time of biopsy, 20% of all oral leukoplakias are found to harbor atypical cytologic features indicative of dysplasia, carcinoma-in-situ, or superficially invasive squamous cell carcinoma (described later).[13] When leukoplakia is evaluated according to site, lesions on the floor of the mouth are more serious—40% have cytologic atypia. Over 6% of patients with leukoplakia

devoid of microscopic atypia progress to invasive carcinoma over an average of 8 years, whereas 36% eventually develop cancer if atypia was encountered initially.[14] Erythroplakia is most ominous, showing precancerous or cancerous change in 60 to 90% of the cases.[15]

Invasive squamous cell carcinoma is most often encountered on the lateral border of the tongue and floor of the mouth; it is quite rare on the palate and dorsum of the tongue.[16-18] Invasive islands of tumor metastasize via lymphatics and seed the supraomohyoid and cervical lymph nodes. Hematogenous dissemination is a late sequela and is usually the consequence of nodal metastasis with spread via the thoracic duct into the venous system.

MORPHOLOGY. As noted earlier, leukoplakia appears clinically as a white patch. The surface texture may be smooth but is more commonly fissured or cracked. Microscopically, the epithelium is thickened, showing hyperkeratosis, parakeratosis, acanthosis, or any combination of these. Twenty per cent of lesions have cytologic atypia with hyperchromatism, nuclear pleomorphism, and increased mitotic activity. These changes are temporally progressive. When atypical cells occupy only a portion of the epithelium, it is designated dysplasia; as the cytologic atypia becomes more advanced to the extent that all strata of the epithelium are involved, the lesion is termed carcinoma-in-situ. The next stage involves superficial invasion and separation of tumor islands from the epithelium; the tumor then has metastatic potential (Fig. 15–4). Erythroplakia undergoes a similar progression; however, surface keratosis is lacking and atrophy of the spinous layer is seen.

Invasive squamous cell carcinoma is characterized clinically by an indurated ulcerative lesion. Often the zone of ulceration exhibits a circumferential, rolled border, and the adjacent mucosa may show leukoplakic or erythroplakic margins. When the metastatic cervical nodes have reached sufficient dimensions, they will be palpable, indurated, and fixed (as opposed to movable, supple, and tender when the lymphadenopathy is the result of inflammatory disease).

Microscopically, squamous cell carcinoma shows nests and islands of invasive epithelial cells with variable degrees of differentiation (i.e., keratinization). The connective tissue stroma usually has a mononuclear inflammatory cell infiltrate. The degree of inflammation may be a measure of immunoreactivity to tumor antigens. Some studies indicate a better prognosis in tumors with intense inflammation.

CLINICAL COURSE. Leukoplakia and erythroplakia with cytologic atypia are usually surgically excised; patients so treated have an excellent prognosis. Invasive squamous cell carcinoma has a variable prognosis, depending upon site of origin, extent, differentiation, and microscopic inflammatory infiltration. Combined radiation therapy and surgery is the treatment of choice. Overall, the five-year survival rate of treated patients is 35 to 50%. Complications from

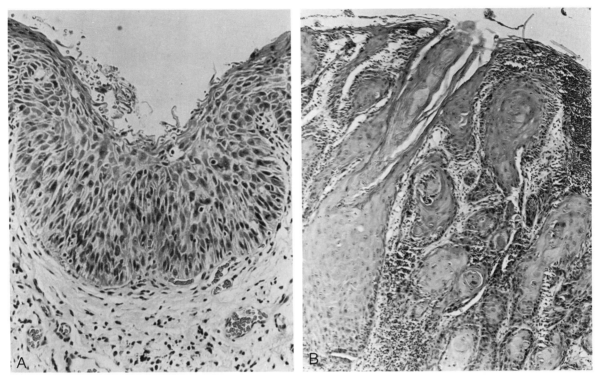

Figure 15–4. *A*, Oral carcinoma-in-situ showing nuclear pleomorphism in all strata of the epithelium. *B*, Oral squamous cell carcinoma. Invasive tumor islands show formation of keratin pearls.

radiation therapy include osteoradionecrosis of the mandible and xerostomia, with a propensity for dental decay (radiation caries).

## ORAL LICHEN PLANUS

Lichen planus is a cutaneous immunopathic disease of unknown etiology although in some instances it can be traced to drug hypersensitivity. Skin lesions and oral lesions may occur simultaneously, but oral lesions alone are very common. Indeed, lichen planus is one of the most common diseases of oral mucosa. Most patients fail to manifest symptoms; however, in approximately one third there is oral burning or sensitivity.

The classic finding is filamentous, thin white lines, called stria of Wickham, that traverse the buccal mucosa and vestibule. The symptomatic erosive form is characterized by white stria superimposed over an erythematous base that shows evidence of erosion and desquamation.[19] Diabetes mellitus or prediabetes is encountered in 20% of patients with oral lichen planus.[20] Microscopically, hyperkeratosis is present, along with basal cell disruption or mucosal erosion. A submucosal zonal lymphocytic infiltrate lies in juxtaposition to the epithelial layer. These changes are indicative of a cell-mediated immune response; however, in most cases, the antigen causing the reaction has not been uncovered.

The disease is chronic, and although the lesions wax and wane, they do not spontaneously resolve. Erosive symptomatic lesions are usually brought under control by application of topical steroids.

## APHTHOUS STOMATITIS

The common *canker sore*, or aphthous stomatitis, is an enigmatic oral disease that at one time or another (usually in early adult life) affects 20% of the population. Suspected in the etiology and pathogenesis of these lesions are mycoplasma and cell-mediated immune reactions.[21]

Clinically, single or multiple round or oval grayish ulcers develop on the lips, buccal mucosa, and tongue. Microscopically, the surface epithelium is denuded and replaced by a fibrinous exudate. The ulcer bed is composed of granulation tissue exhibiting a lymphocytic infiltrate. The ulcers resolve in 10 to 14 days, only to recur at a later date. With advancing age, recurrent episodes become less frequent, and most of the population becomes disease free.

## HERPETIC STOMATITIS

Herpesvirus hominis types I and II infect oral mucosa, but type I is far more prevalent.[22] This DNA virus is both epidermotropic and neurotropic. Less than 1% of the population has had clinically detectable primary infection, yet 95% possess circulating antibodies to herpesvirus type I by age 20. Whether the infection is clinically manifest or subclinical, approximately 15% of the population develops secondary herpes as a consequence of neuronal infection. Herpesvirus is unique in that it may transmigrate across the oral epithelium and be transported axonally to ganglion cell nuclei in the trigeminal tract.[23] The viral genome is then integrated into the DNA of the host ganglion cell, where it remains latent until stimulated by mucosal irritation. In the dormant intracellular integrated state, the virus is sequestered from immunologic defense mechanisms. Once awakened, virions emerge from the ganglion cells and, by retrograde migration down sensory axons, infect the epithelium, usually on the lips.

Herpesviruses produce mucosal vesicular eruptions in both primary and reactivated infections. In the uncommon primary infection the patient suffers malaise, lymphadenopathy, elevated temperature, and vesicular stomatitis. The vesicles classically develop on the gingiva, lips, palate, and tongue. The lesions of secondary or recurrent herpes, evolving from latent ganglionic infection, are more limited, occurring as clustered vesicles on the vermilion borders of the lips or unilaterally on the palatal gingiva. Microscopically, herpetic vesicles are intraepithelial; acantholytic cells contain intranuclear inclusions or the infected cells exhibit nuclear ballooning and degeneration (Fig. 15–5).

Primary herpetic gingivostomatitis runs its course in 10 to 14 days, yet viral shedding takes place for only the first three to four days. Recurrent herpes labialis pursues a similar course, and recurrent episodes become less frequent with advancing age. It is to be noted that clinicians who have not been previously exposed to the virus may contract a herpetic dermatitis of the fingers if they touch active lesions.

# DISEASES OF THE SALIVARY GLANDS

The upper digestive and respiratory passages are replete with serous and mucus-secreting glands that provide saliva and mucus lubrication of the oronasal cavity and larynx. The parotid, submandibular, and sublingual major salivary glands are the chief secretors of saliva; nevertheless, underlying the oral mucous membrane are minor salivary glands located in all areas throughout the mouth except on the dorsum of the tongue. These glands, both major and minor, are subject to developmental, inflammatory, immunopathic, metabolic, degenerative, and neoplastic diseases.

Clinically, salivary disorders are characterized by soft tissue swellings and impaired secretion. In general, bilateral parotid swelling with xerostomia (dry mouth) is indicative of an immunopathic inflammatory disease termed Sjögren's syndrome; this disorder is detailed in the chapter on immunity (p. 165). Neoplasms, characterized by swelling, are most often encountered in the preauricular, parotid region. Most parotid tumors are benign, whereas neoplasms of the sublingual gland are frequently malignant. Oral tumors in minor glands show a 50:50 ratio of being either benign or malignant. The most common nonneoplastic disorders of salivary tissue are mucoceles of minor glands, sialolithiasis, and sialadenitis of the major salivary glands.

## MUCOCELE

Mucoceles occur most frequently in the lower lip. Only rarely are they found in the upper lip, but occasionally they occur in the buccal mucosa, soft palate, and ventral tongue. Young and middle-aged adults are affected most often. Clinically, these lesions are characterized by a fluctuant, soft swelling and a history of trauma to the mucosa (Fig. 15–6). In addition, there is often a history of variation in size; puncture and drainage is generally followed by reappearance.[24]

Mucoceles arise because of trauma, usually lip biting, and severance of the minor salivary gland ducts. The mucous secretion thus extravasates, collecting and pooling in the connective tissues. The resultant lesion appears as a bluish fluid-filled nodule. If the mucous secretions extravasate into deeper tissues, the color is that of the normal mucosa. Excised specimens are cystic with gelatinous mucoid contents. Microscopically, pooled mucin, infiltrated by neutrophils and foam cell histiocytes, can be seen.

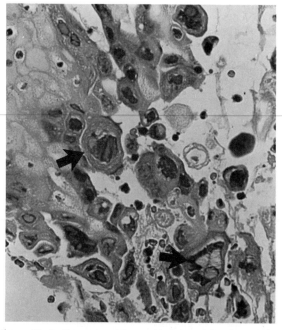

Figure 15–5. Contents of intraepithelial vesicle, the result of stomatitis caused by *Herpesvirus hominis*. Acantholytic epithelial cells reveal nuclear ballooning and degeneration (*arrows*).

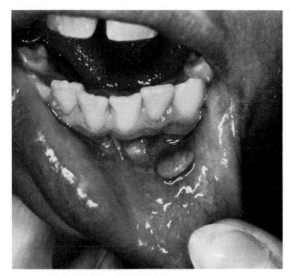

Figure 15–6. A mucocele, typically located on the lower lip.

Grossly, salivary stones appear yellow or white with a grainy surface. They are more often single, yet multiple concretions within extralobular ducts may be encountered. The submandibular gland in long-standing occlusion is firm, lobulated, and fibrotic. Microscopically, salivary stones are acellular, composed of laminated concretions. The associated gland shows acinar degeneration with ductal ectasia, parenchymal fibrosis, and mononuclear inflammatory cell infiltration.

Prolonged occlusion results in loss of function. If stones can be removed early, the gland may remain functional. Chronically diseased nonfunctional glands must be surgically removed, since retrograde acute infectious sialadenitis may develop later, owing to the inability of the gland to flush the ductal system with saliva.

## SIALADENITIS

Inflammation of the major salivary glands may evolve in response to ductal occlusion, viral or bacterial infection, or autoimmune disease. Ductal occlusion has been discussed above, and autoimmune disease (e.g., Sjögren's syndrome) is discussed in the chapter on immune diseases. Mumps is the most common infectious disease of salivary tissue, whereas bacterial parotitis, referred to as "surgical mumps," is relatively uncommon.

Mumps (epidemic parotitis) is a contagious infectious disease most often seen in children. It is caused by a member of the paramyxovirus group.[26] Following a two- to three-month incubation period, unilateral or bilateral parotid enlargement develops and is accompanied by pain, particularly when salivation is stimulated. The swelling is caused by interstitial edema accompanied by a mononuclear inflammatory infiltrate. An exudate may be expressed through the parotid duct. These clinical findings coexist with fever, malaise, and headache. Serum amylase levels are elevated as a consequence of acinar degeneration. Bacterial or suppurative parotitis occurs among elderly patients with a recent history of major thoracic or abdominal surgery.[27] It has also been reported in patients with xerostomia secondary to phenothiazine drug therapy. Presumably, decreased salivation predisposes a patient to retrograde migration of staphylococci and streptococci that acutely infect the parenchyma. Unilateral involvement is the rule, and patients manifest swelling, pain, and a purulent ductal discharge.

Mumps runs its course in 10 to 14 days. Pancreatitis, encephalitis, and orchitis are potential complications. Acute bacterial parotitis can result in parenchymal necrosis and postinfectious fibrosis. Antibiotic therapy, if initiated early, will clear the infection and restore function.

The zone of mucous retention is enveloped by a compressed wall of fibrous or granulation tissue lacking an epithelial lining. The underlying minor glands exhibit acinar degeneration with ductal ectasia, intralobular fibrosis, and mononuclear inflammatory cell infiltration.

Mucoceles rarely resolve spontaneously. They may rupture and collapse; however, recurrence is the rule. Surgical excision, including extirpation of the underlying feeder glands, is the treatment of choice.

## SIALOLITHIASIS

Salivary stones are common; most occur in the submandibular duct. Parotid duct and minor salivary gland duct sialolithiasis occurs far less frequently. Unlike calculus formation within the urinary tract or gallbladder, sialolithiasis does not appear to be correlated with hyperparathyroidism or diet. Nevertheless, the consequences of duct obstruction are similar to those encountered in the kidneys and the liver. Prolonged salivary obstruction can culminate in sclerosing sialadenitis and defective function. Typically, the patient complains of pain, particularly at mealtimes when the gland swells in response to a salivary stimulus (i.e., a thick, juicy steak). X-ray examination will disclose a discrete opacification along the route of the submandibular duct or within the gland proper.[25]

Salivary stones develop when a cluster of desquamated ductal cells enmeshed in glycoproteins forms a nidus within the duct. Laminated concretions of calcium phosphate become deposited, and the stone enlarges circumferentially, eventually culminating in ductal occlusion. Predisposing metabolic or dietary factors have not been uncovered.

## ADENOMAS

Although a wide variety of benign neoplasms arise in both major and minor salivary glands, three types are encountered most often—pleomorphic adenoma or mixed tumor, papillary cystadenoma lymphomatosum (Warthin's tumor), and oncocytoma. The parotid gland is affected more commonly than the other major or intraoral minor glands. Clinically, pleomorphic adenomas of the parotid present as movable preauricular swellings involving the superficial gland; deep localization is uncommon. They are 10 times more common in the parotid than in the submandibular gland, and they represent 70% of all parotid gland salivary tumors. Oral pleomorphic adenomas are found in the palate and buccal mucosa, and account for 50% of all intraoral glandular tumors. The tumor is more common in females than males and tends to occur in the fourth decade of life. Warthin's tumor and oncocytoma are essentially limited to the parotid gland. The former is found predominantly in elderly males. About 15% of the cases are bilateral. Oncocytoma, also a benign tumor, is found primarily in elderly females.

**MORPHOLOGY.** The adenomas are subclassified according to microscopic differences. All are grossly encapsulated, although pleomorphic adenomas may be multinodular. Only Warthin's tumor exhibits large cystic compartments when hemisected. The pleomorphic adenoma may be of ductal myoepithelial origin and, as the name implies, exhibits a wide variety of histomorphologic patterns. Solid sheets or strands of polygonal eosinophilic epithelial cells are intermixed with small duct-like configurations. Interspersed among the epithelial cell nests are spindle-shaped myoepithelial cells and a variety of apparent connective tissues, including myxomatous, adipose, and chondroid elements (Fig. 15–7A). In individual tumors, one or another of these components may predominate.[28] Papillary cystadenoma lymphomatosum is unique, with its multiple, large cystic spaces crowded with papillary projections. These are covered by a regular array of columnar oncocytes, beneath which are sheets of mature lymphocytes admixed with plasma cells sometimes forming germinal centers.[29] Oncocytomas are composed of cords and sheets of large eosinophilic, polygonal epithelial cells (oncocytes) surrounded by a fibrous capsule.[30]

**CLINICAL COURSE.** Warthin's tumor and oncocytoma are easily dissected from the parotid parenchyma, and recurrence is uncommon. In pleomorphic adenomas, cell nests have a tendency to bud from the main tumor mass, accounting for recurrences after enucleation. For this reason, surgical lobectomy is the treatment of choice.[31] Failure to remove these

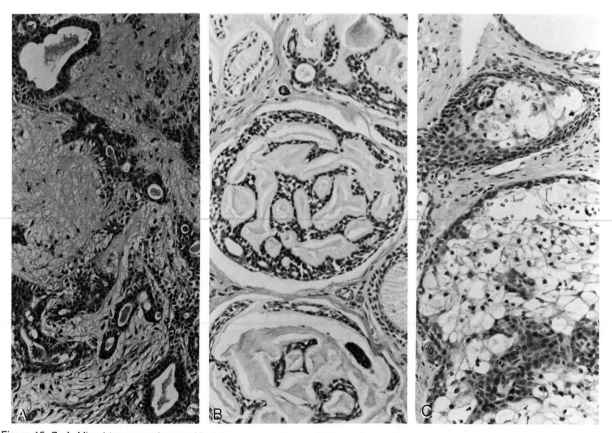

Figure 15–7. *A*, Mixed tumor or pleomorphic adenoma showing ductal formations within a myxomatous stroma. *B*, Adenoid cystic carcinoma with hyperchromatic cells surrounding multicystic foci that have hyalinized contents. *C*, Mucoepidermoid carcinoma composed of squamous, mucous, and clear cells.

tumors surgically results in continued growth; the lesion can reach massive proportions and may encroach upon the seventh cranial nerve and cause facial palsy; however, this clinical finding is more often encountered among the various adenocarcinomas of the parotid gland. Albeit uncommon, a benign pleomorphic adenoma that is recurrent or of long duration may undergo malignant transformation ("carcinoma ex pleomorphic adenoma").[32] Tumors in minor glands show less propensity for recurrence after surgical excision.

## ADENOCARCINOMAS

Malignant glandular lesions are most often encountered in the parotid gland (among the major salivary glands), although the ratio of malignant to benign disease is much greater in tumors of the sublingual gland. Oral tumors of the minor glands show a 50:50 distribution of either benign or malignant disease. Oral adenocarcinomas are most often located in the palate. As with benign adenomas, there is a wide degree of histologic variation among adenocarcinomas of salivary origin. Adenoid cystic carcinoma (cylindroma), mucoepidermoid carcinoma, and acinic cell carcinoma are the more common forms, although the last is rarely found in the oral cavity. Clinically, the adenocarcinomas are firm or indurated masses that tend to become fixed to adjacent tissues. Metastatic spread is usually through lymphatics; however, hematogenous metastasis is observed as well.

**MORPHOLOGY.** Grossly, adenocarcinomas are white and glistening with infiltrating margins. Adenoid cystic carcinoma is composed of solid sheets of monomorphic hyperchromatic cells; mitotic figures are uncommon. The tumor islands show foci of microcyst formation (yielding a so-called Swiss-cheese pattern) surrounded by hyalinized zones of thickened basement membrane (Fig. 15–7B). Microscopic evidence of perineural invasion is a common finding.[33] Mucoepidermoid carcinoma is classified into low, intermediate, and high grades; low-grade tumors show large cystic spaces lined by epidermoid and mucus-secreting cells as well as transitional forms, whereas high-grade lesions are more solid and lack cystic features (Fig. 15–7C).[34] Acinic cell carcinomas are arranged in solid sheets with an organoid pattern. The tumor cells may contain prominent basophilic secretory granules or the cytoplasm may be pale, resembling mucus-secreting cells. None of the salivary malignancies exhibit prominent cytologic atypia with pleomorphism.

**CLINICAL COURSE.** Adenoid cystic carcinoma is a slow-growing, invasive tumor with a tendency to both nodal and hematogenous metastasis. Owing to its tendency for perineural invasion, the tumor may extend well beyond identifiable margins; this accounts for its high rate of recurrence. This slow-growing yet highly malignant tumor has a reported five-year survival rate of 70%; however, the 20-year rate drops to 15%. Low-grade mucoepidermoid tumors metastasize rarely and yield an 85 to 90% five-year survival rate, but the solid high-grade tumors often metastasize to nodes and distant sites, and the outlook for these patients is much more grave. The prognosis for acinic cell carcinoma is good; five-year survival rate is over 80%. Recurrence is common, however, and the 20-year survival drops to 50%.

# DISEASES OF THE JAWS

The most common lesions of the jawbones are the consequence of odontogenic infection, as discussed previously. Somewhat less prevalent are cysts, neoplasms, and reactive lesions that may be of either odontogenic or nonodontogenic origin. The dentigerous cyst is the most frequently encountered noninfectious odontogenic cyst, and, more importantly, the epithelial lining of the cyst may undergo benign neoplastic transformation. Most odontogenic tumors are rare. Nonodontogenic diseases include a variety of benign and malignant proliferations. The benign fibro-osseous diseases of bone are included in this group of nonodontogenic diseases. Only the most common lesions in these categories will be discussed.

## DENTIGEROUS CYST

The crowns of impacted or unerupted teeth are surrounded by the dental follicle, composed of an epithelial layer and an outer zone of areolar fibrous tissue. This epithelial layer is represented by ameloblasts during tooth formation, but it collapses upon completion of amelogenesis; it is then referred to as reduced enamel epithelium. As long as teeth remain embedded within the jawbones, these follicular tissues persist. When the reduced enamel epithelium becomes detached from the coronal enamel, the cells undergo squamous transformation and slowly proliferate, and fluid collects to yield a sac around the crown of the impacted tooth. This *dentigerous cyst* slowly enlarges, acting as an osmotic bag as proteinaceous fluid accumulates. Progressive enlargement causes resorption of the surrounding alveolar bone and creates a pericoronal radiolucency on radiographs. Clinically, symptoms are usually absent, although facial swelling may be seen in large cysts that expand bone. Dentigerous cysts most frequently occur around impacted third molars and maxillary cuspids.

Grossly, a soft tissue sac surrounding the tooth crown is attached to the neck or cervix at the crown-root junction. These cysts can attain a large size. They have a noncornified, stratified squamous epithelial lining, and the lumen often contains eosinophilic amorphous material, sometimes with cholesterol clefts (Fig. 15–8). The follicular fibrous wall is moderately, or occasionally, severely inflamed, and many show associated giant cells.

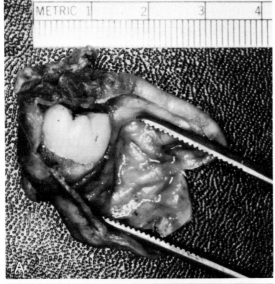

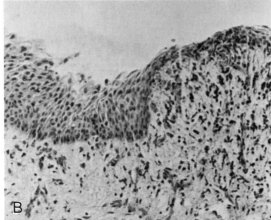

Figure 15–8. *A*, Gross specimen of a pericoronal dentigerous cyst. *B*, Nonkeratinized epithelial lining from a dentigerous cyst.

If left untreated, dentigerous cysts slowly and progressively enlarge and may expand bone. Importantly, as discussed below, keratinizing metaplasia or neoplastic transformation may evolve. The impacted tooth and cystic sac should be surgically enucleated.

## ODONTOGENIC KERATOCYST

Most odontogenic cysts are lined by nonkeratinizing stratified squamous epithelium. A variant is encountered in which keratinizing metaplasia occurs. Cysts of this nature are referred to as *odontogenic keratocysts*, and they may radiographically resemble dentigerous cysts owing to their pericoronal localization; they may also arise between the roots of contiguous teeth. Keratocysts are potentially aggressive and show a tendency for recurrence after surgical enucleation.[35]

Their origin is unknown; odontogenic keratocysts develop without any identifiable stimulus. Whereas most ordinary odontogenic cysts (such as the periapical cyst, associated with necrotic teeth, and the dentigerous cyst) are thought to enlarge passively as a consequence of a transluminal osmotic pressure gradient, the cells lining a keratocyst actively proliferate like a *quasi*-neoplasm.

Grossly, the lumen contains caseous material and the cyst wall is thin. Microscopically, these cysts are lined by a thin, stratified squamous epithelium with multilayered keratin (Fig. 15–9*A*). Basilar epithelial buds extending into the fibrous wall may be encountered with the formation of daughter cysts.

Keratocysts are aggressive and progressively enlarge to expand the cortical plates of bone. They may be loculated, and daughter cysts or pseudopod-like extensions from the main cyst may be left behind after curettage; this accounts for a high rate of recurrence (20% for smaller lesions; over 50% for large loculated cysts). Multiple odontogenic keratocysts of

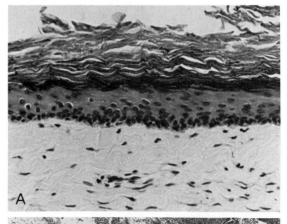

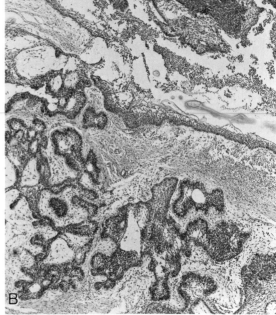

Figure 15–9. *A*, Lining of an odontogenic keratocyst. *B*, Ameloblastoma, arising from an odontogenic cyst, shows neoplastic islands and cords invading the fibrous wall.

the jaws are seen in the *nevoid basal cell carcinoma syndrome,* characterized by a variety of anomalies including, primarily, basal cell tumors of skin, bifid ribs, and calcified falx cerebri.

## ODONTOGENIC TUMORS

Neoplasms and hamartomas arising from odontogenic tissues are relatively rare. The most common is the odontoma, actually a hamartomatous proliferation of ameloblasts, odontoblasts, and cementoblasts. These benign hamartomas are highly differentiated, elaborating all of the hard tissues of teeth, including enamel, dentin, and cementum. The most common odontogenic tumor with aggressive growth potential is the ameloblastoma, which may arise from the enamel epithelium around impacted teeth. Discussion will be restricted to this neoplasm.

The *ameloblastoma* is a benign yet aggressive neoplasm of epithelial odontogenic origin. Two distinct variants with differing pathogenic and behavioral features exist. The *invasive* variant arises from the epithelial rests of Malassez in the periodontal ligament. Tumors of this nature are usually solid.[36] The *cystic* variant arises from the lining of odontogenic cysts.[37]

The invasive ameloblastoma is usually multilobular and expansile. Macroscopically it is solid, white, and glistening. In this variant, islands of neoplastic cells recapitulate the early tooth germ; an outer layer of columnar ameloblasts with nuclei polarized away from the basement membrane envelops an inner sheet of spindled and stellate epithelial cells. In contrast, cystic ameloblastoma is frequently found in conjunction with an impacted tooth and radiographically resembles a dentigerous cyst. The tumor is grossly cystic and shows focal thickening of the cyst wall or luminal excrescences. In these tumors the cells proliferate luminally or murally (into the follicular fibrous wall of the cyst), or both, and have a limited tendency to invade surrounding marrow spaces (Fig. 15–9*B*).

Solid invasive ameloblastoma is seen in adults and may, if left untreated, reach massive dimensions, although metastasis is extremely rare (less than 1%). Recurrence after curettage is high, particularly among maxillary tumors with sinus extension. The cystic variety is less aggressive, remains localized, and tends to occur in teenagers and young adults. Less than 20% recur after enucleation and curettage.

## BENIGN FIBRO-OSSEOUS LESIONS

A variety of benign disease processes of the jawbones share common microscopic features. Normal medullary bone may be replaced by proliferating fibrous tissue, throughout which are dispersed irregular osseous trabeculae. Lesions of this nature are collectively referred to as *benign fibro-osseous le-sions,* which pathogenetically may be inflammatory, neoplastic, or benign dysplastic disease processes of bone. Some of these benign fibro-osseous lesions also contain numerous multinucleated giant cells. Since the microscopic features are similar among these diseases, the definitive diagnosis depends on correlation with radiographic and clinical findings.

### Fibrous Dysplasia and Ossifying Fibroma

Fibrous dysplasia is a benign, non-neoplastic, fibro-osseous disease of bone, whereas ossifying fibroma is neoplastic. These lesions of the jaw occur most frequently during the second and third decades of life, and facial asymmetry with osseous enlargement is common to both. Over 95% of cases of fibrous dysplasia of the jaw are monostotic, whereas the remainder are polyostotic or a facial manifestation of Albright's syndrome (p. 708).

Fibrous dysplasia and ossifying fibroma have similar microscopic features yet differ grossly, clinically, and radiographically. Fibrous dysplasia of the jaws is more often encountered in the maxilla than the mandible, but ossifying fibroma more often affects the mandible. **Fibrous dysplasia** is a diffuse process and, under radiographic examination, is radiopaque and poorly marginated; the maxilla is expanded. **Ossifying fibroma** is a well-defined neoplasm that is radiolucent or radiopaque, depending upon the degree of lesional calcification. Microscopically in both, a cellular, mature, fibrous stroma is seen with irregular osseous trabeculae. The trabeculae fail to show prominent osteoblastic rimming in fibrous dysplasia (Fig. 15–10); this feature may or may not be observed in ossifying fibroma.

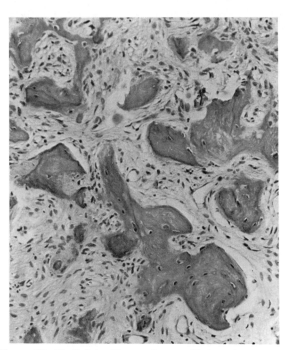

Figure 15–10. Cellular fibrous stroma with irregular osseous trabeculae, as seen in maxillary fibrous dysplasia.

Whenever the diagnosis of fibrous dysplasia is entertained, polyostotic disease must be ruled out. Most instances are monostotic, and the lesion progressively enlarges for three to five years and becomes quiescent once skeletal maturity is attained. The expanded jaw can be surgically sculptured after growth cessation without an attempt to excise the medullary lesional bone. Ossifying fibroma also enlarges slowly; some can become huge. The neoplasm is treated by enucleation and curettage.[38, 39]

### Central Giant Cell Granuloma

The central giant cell granuloma is a reactive intraosseous endosteal proliferation that behaves as a neoplasm. Its etiology is unknown. Giant cell tumors that are associated with hyperparathyroidism appear identical to these granulomas both microscopically and radiographically; however, the vast majority of giant cell lesions of the jaw are isolated entities without associated endocrine disease. Young adults are affected, and the lesions are generally located in the anterior mandible and show a tendency for osseous expansion.[40]

Grossly, giant cell granulomas are spongy, brown, and hemorrhagic. Radiographically, they are multilocular, expansile, radiolucent lesions that tend to separate or resorb contiguous teeth. Microscopically, they are composed of a cellular fibrovascular stroma punctuated by numerous multinucleated giant cells. Osseous trabeculae may be encountered, and hemosiderin pigment is often a prominent feature.

Giant cell granuloma is aggressive and can cause facial deformity. Despite this behavior, recurrence is uncommon after surgical curettage. Once the diagnosis is made, appropriate laboratory tests are necessary to rule out hyperparathyroidism.

### References

1. Fitzgerald, R. J., and Keyes, P. H.: Demonstration of the etiologic role of streptococci in experimental caries in the hamster. J. Am. Dent. Assoc. 61:9, 1960.
2. Losee, F. L.: Dental caries in abutting or bilaterally corresponding tooth surfaces. J. Am. Dent. Assoc. 35:323, 1947.
3. Bhaskar, S. N.: Periapical lesions—Types, incidence, and clinical features. Oral Surg. 21:657, 1966.
4. Lineberg, W. B., Waldron, C. A., and Delanne, G. F.: A clinical, roentgenographic and histopathologic evaluation of periapical lesions. Oral Surg. 17:467, 1972.
5. Kinnmann, J. E. G., and Lee, H. S.: Chronic osteomyelitis of the mandible: Clinical study of thirteen cases. Oral Surg. 25:6, 1968.
6. Shapiro, H. H., et al.: Spread of infection of dental origin. Oral Surg. 3:1407, 1950.
7. Marshall-Day, C. D., Stephens, R. G., and Quigley, L. F., Jr.: Periodontal disease: Prevalence and incidence. J. Periodontol. 26:185, 1955.
8. Abby, L. M., Page, D. G., and Sawyer, D. R.: The clinical and histopathologic features of a series of 464 oral squamous cell papillomas. Oral Surg. 49:419, 1980.
9. Cutright, D. E.: The histopathologic findings in 583 cases of epulis fissuratum. Oral Surg. 37:401, 1974.
10. Eversole, L. R., and Rovin, S.: Reactive lesions of the gingiva. J. Oral Pathol. 1:30, 1972.
11. Shillitoe, E. J., et al.: Immunoglobulin class of antibody to herpes simplex virus in patients with oral cancer. Cancer 51:65, 1983.
12. Eglin, R. P., et al.: Detection of RNA complementary to herpes simplex virus in human oral squamous cell carcinoma. Lancet 2:766, 1983.
12A. Löning, T., et al.: Analysis of oral papillomas, leukoplakias, and invasive carcinomas for human papillomavirus type related DNA. J. Invest. Derm. 84:417, 1985.
13. Waldron, C. A., and Shafer, W. G.: Leukoplakia revisited. A clinicopathologic study of 3256 oral leukoplakias. Cancer 36:1386, 1975.
14. Silverman, S., Jr., et al.: Oral leukoplakia and malignant transformation. A follow-up study of 257 patients. Cancer 53:565, 1984.
15. Shafer, W. G., and Waldron, C. A.: Erythroplakia of the oral cavity. Cancer 36:1021, 1975.
16. Maddox, W. A., Sherlock, E. C., and Evans, W. B.: Cancer of the tongue: Review of thirteen years' experience. Am. Surg. 37:642, 1971.
17. Nakissa, N., Hornback, N. B., Shidnia, H., and Sayoc, E. S.: Carcinoma of the floor of the mouth. Cancer 42:2914, 1978.
18. Cummings, B. J., and Clark, R. M.: Squamous cell carcinoma of the oral cavity. J. Otolaryngol. 11:359, 1984.
19. Andreason, J.: Oral lichen planus. Oral Surg. 25:31, 1968.
20. Howell, F. V., and Rick, G. M.: Oral lichen planus and diabetes: A potential syndrome. J. Calif. Dent. Assoc. 1:58, July 1973.
21. Antoon, J. W., and Miller, R. L.: Aphthous ulcers—A review of the literature on etiology, pathogenesis, diagnosis and treatment. J. Am. Dent. Assoc. 101:803, 1980.
22. Lennette, E. H., and Magoffin, R. L.: Virologic and immunologic aspects of major oral ulcerations. J. Am. Dent. Assoc. 87:1055, 1973.
23. Bastian, F. D., et al.: Herpes virus hominis: Isolation from human trigeminal ganglion. Science 178:306, 1972.
24. Cataldo, E., and Mosadomi, A.: Mucoceles of the oral mucous membrane. Arch. Otolaryngol. 91:360, 1970.
25. Levy, B. M., Remine, W. H., and DeVine, K. D.: Salivary gland calculi: Pain, swelling associated with eating. J.A.M.A. 181:1115, 1962.
26. Elvin-Lewis, M.: Paramyxoviridae. In Schuster, G. S. (ed.): Oral Microbiology and Infectious Diseases. 2nd ed. Baltimore, Williams & Wilkins, 1983, pp. 429–430.
27. Carlson, R. G., and Glas, W. E.: Acute suppurative parotitis: Twenty-eight cases at a county hospital. Arch. Surg. 89:653, 1963.
28. Krolls, S. O., and Boyers, R. C.: Mixed tumors of salivary glands: Long-term follow-up. Cancer 30:276, 1972.
29. Dietert, S. E.: Papillary cystadenoma lymphomatosum (Warthin's tumor) in patients in a general hospital over a 24-year period. Am. J. Clin. Pathol. 63:866, 1975.
30. Eneroth, C. M.: Oncoctyoma of major salivary glands. J. Laryngol. 79:1064, 1965.
31. Clairmont, A. A., Richardson, G. S., and Hanna, D. C.: The pseudocapsule of pleomorphic adenomas (benign mixed tumors). Am. J. Surg. 134:242, 1977.
32. Livolsi, V. A., and Perzin, K. H.: Malignant mixed tumors arising in salivary glands. I. Carcinomas arising in benign mixed tumors. A clinicopathologic study. Cancer 39:2209, 1977.
33. Spiro, R. H., Huvos, A. G., and Strong, E. W.: Adenoid cystic carcinoma of salivary origin. A clinicopathologic study of 242 cases. Am. J. Surg. 128:512, 1974.
34. Spiro, R. H., et al.: Mucoepidermoid carcinoma of salivary gland origin. A clinicopathologic study of 367 cases. Am. J. Surg. 136:461, 1978.

35. Beannon, R. B.: The odontogenic keratocyst: A clinicopathologic study of 312 cases. II. Histologic features. Oral Surg. *43*:233, 1977.

36. Sehdev, M. K., et al.: Ameloblastoma of maxilla and mandible. Cancer *33*:324, 1974.

37. Eversole, L. R., Leider, A. S., and Strub, D.: Radiographic characteristics of cystogenic ameloblastoma. Oral Surg. *57*:572, 1984.

38. Waldron, C. A., and Giansanti, J. S.: Benign fibro-osseous lesions of the jaws: A clinical-radiologic-histologic review of sixty-five cases. I. Fibrous dysplasia of the jaws. Oral Surg. *35*:190, 1973.

39. Eversole, L. R., Leider, A. S., and Nelson, K.: Ossifying fibroma: A clinicopathologic study of sixty-four cases. Oral Surg. *60*:505, 1985.

40. Waldron, C. A., and Shafer, W. G.: The central giant cell reparative granuloma of the jaws. An analysis of 38 cases. Am. J. Clin. Pathol. *45*:437, 1966.

# 16

# The Gastrointestinal Tract

**ESOPHAGUS**
ATRESIA AND STENOSIS
DIVERTICULA
RINGS AND WEBS
ACHALASIA (MEGAESOPHAGUS)
HIATAL HERNIA
ESOPHAGITIS
ESOPHAGEAL VARICES
ESOPHAGEAL LACERATIONS (MALLORY-WEISS
SYNDROME)
CARCINOMA OF THE ESOPHAGUS

**STOMACH**
PYLORIC STENOSIS
GASTRITIS
    Acute (Erosive) Gastritis
    Chronic (Nonerosive) Gastritis
STRESS ULCERS
PEPTIC ULCERS
TUMORS
    Gastric Polyps
    Gastric Carcinoma
    Gastrointestinal Lymphomas

**SMALL INTESTINE**
DIVERTICULA
ISCHEMIC BOWEL DISEASE
    Transmural Intestinal Infarction
    Mucosal and Mural Infarction
INFLAMMATORY DISEASES
    Crohn's Disease (Regional Enteritis)
MALABSORPTION
    Celiac Sprue
    Tropical Sprue
    Disaccharidase Deficiency
    Abetalipoproteinemia
    Whipple's Disease
INTESTINAL OBSTRUCTION
    Hernias
    Intestinal Adhesions
    Intussusception
    Volvulus
TUMORS
    Adenocarcinoma
    Carcinoid (Argentaffinoma, Endocrine Cell Tumor)

**COLON**
HIRSCHSPRUNG'S DISEASE
DIVERTICULAR DISEASE
VASCULAR LESIONS
    Angiodysplasia (Vascular Ectasia)
    Hemorrhoids
ENTEROCOLITIS
    Cholera
    Enteropathogenic *E. coli*
    Shigellosis (Bacillary Dysentery)
    Salmonellosis (Including Typhoid Fever)
    Pseudomembranous Colitis (PMC)
    Amebic Colitis
    Idiopathic Ulcerative Colitis
TUMORS
    Polyps
        Hyperplastic polyps
        Tubular adenoma (pedunculated polyp)
        Villous adenoma
        Tubulovillous adenoma
        Adenoma-carcinoma sequence
    Polyposis Syndromes
        Familial polyposis coli
        Gardner's syndrome
        Turcot's syndrome
        Peutz-Jeghers syndrome
    Carcinoma of the Colorectum

**APPENDIX**
APPENDICITIS
TUMORS (INCLUDING MUCOCELE AND
PSEUDOMYXOMA PERITONEI)

The roster of diseases that affect the alimentary tract is as long as the tract itself. It includes those that are among the most common in clinical practice (peptic ulcer) and some that are too rare for inclusion here. They range in clinical significance from major killers (colorectal cancer) to the lesions that are more annoying than serious (hemorrhoids). In the various segments of the digestive tract that are discussed, only the more common lesions will be considered.

## Esophagus

The many widely differing esophageal lesions are manifested clinically by a remarkably limited range of symptoms, rendering differential diagnosis difficult. Most disorders cause dysphagia (difficulty in swallowing) or "heartburn" (retrosternal pain), or sometimes both. Much less commonly, and mainly with esophageal varices and lacerations, the presentation takes the form of upper gastrointestinal bleeding, which may cause massive vomiting of blood (hematemesis). Obviously, with upper gastrointestinal bleeding, the difficult diagnostic problem arises—is it esophageal or gastric in origin and is the causal lesion likely to be amenable to medical therapy or must emergency surgery be performed? Esophageal disorders are therefore often challenging clinical problems.

## ATRESIA AND STENOSIS

When a segment of the esophagus is congenitally malformed and consists of only a thin, noncanalized cord, the lesion is termed *esophageal atresia*. In about 80 to 90% of cases, the blind lower pouch communicates through a fistulous tract with the trachea or main stem bronchi. Uncommonly, there is a fistulous communication between the upper esophageal pouch and the airways. Such fistulae reflect the common embryologic development of the gut and respiratory tree from a single tube. Atresia is manifested by swallowing difficulties from birth and respiratory difficulties when there is aspiration of food. Surgical intervention is requisite.

*Stenosis* (narrowing of the esophageal lumen) may occur as a developmental defect or may be acquired secondary to (1) inflammatory fibrosis; (2) neoplastic narrowing; (3) collagenization of the esophageal wall, as with systemic scleroderma; or (4) extrinsic compression exerted by some expansile mediastinal tumor or aneurysm. Unlike the case with atresia, stenosis can usually be readily managed with esophageal bougienage (dilatation).

## DIVERTICULA

These relatively innocent lesions are outpouchings (2 to 4 cm in diameter) of the esophageal wall. Some are acquired because of weaknesses or defects in the muscular support of the wall; others are developmental, but, in both instances, exposure to the intraluminal pressure contributes to their expansion. They may occur at any level of the esophagus but tend to appear at one of three locations: (1) at the pharyngoesophageal junction, where defects in the posterior pharyngeal wall permit protrusion of all layers of the esophageal wall (*Zenker's diverticulum*); (2) where the tracheal bifurcation into the main stem bronchi causes slight narrowing of the esophageal lumen, predisposing to increased intraluminal esophageal pressures; and (3) just above the diaphragm, typically in patients with some esophageal motor dysfunction.[1] The important role that an increase in the intraluminal pressure plays in their development is underscored by the association of diverticula with achalasia, esophageal webs, and hiatal hernia, all impairing the ready passage of food. Although diverticula may be asymptomatic, they may induce dysphagia, regurgitation, or a sense of fullness in the neck. Rarely, incarceration of foods leads to inflammation, ulceration, and, even more rarely, perforation.

## RINGS AND WEBS

The terms "rings" and "webs" are both used for ring-like concentric constrictions of the esophagus. Lower esophageal lesions are often called *Schatzki's rings* in token of the radiologist who first described them. Wherever located, some comprise only mucosal folds but others are thicker and also contain submucosa and muscle. For inexplicable reasons numerous authors have labored to segregate rings from webs on the basis of location within the esophagus or the presence or absence of muscle within the constriction, yielding almost as many classifications as there are authors. By whatever name, rings and webs are noteworthy for two reasons. (1) They may produce dysphagia, which may be intermittent as a bolus of food transiently obstructs the lumen of the narrowing. (2) They are sometimes accompanied by atrophic glossitis and iron deficiency anemia, typically in elderly women. *The triad of web, glossitis, and iron deficiency anemia has come to be known as the Plummer-Vinson or Patterson-Brown-Kelly syndrome.* The causal relationship (if any) of these three features is obscure, and, indeed, some experts contend that the concurrence is merely coincidental because of the prevalence of each feature in elderly women.

## ACHALASIA (MEGAESOPHAGUS)

*This uncommon cause of dysphagia represents an esophageal motility disorder that results from a triple defect: (1) ineffectual peristalsis in the lower two thirds of the esophagus, (2) inadequate relaxation of the lower esophageal sphincter (LES) during swallowing, and (3) increased resting pressure of the LES.*[2] With long-standing disease, dilatation of the esophagus (*megaesophagus*) develops.

Esophageal motility is under both neural and humoral control. The former is mediated by the vagus nerves and intrinsic Auerbach's plexus. The humoral mechanisms are poorly understood, but among the many potential mediators, gastrin, acetyl choline, and prostaglandins are thought to be most important. Although uncertainty persists, the weight of evidence points to one or more neural lesions as the cause of achalasia. However, there is great disagreement about the locus and nature of such a lesion. *Most observers point to a decrease in the number of inhibitory ganglion cells in the wall of the body of the esophagus,* but others cite depletion of the ganglion cells in the region of the LES and still others, lesions in the vagal innervation. There is also some question as to whether any or all of the neural changes are primary or secondary.[3] Favoring their primacy is the fact that invasion and destruction of Auerbach's plexus by *Trypanosoma cruzi* in Chagas' disease produces an identical clinical picture of achalasia. But in the other situations, the cause of the neural lesions remains a mystery. Moreover, humoral derangements such as unusual sensitivity of the LES to the constricting effect of gastrin have not been ruled out.[4] Uncertainty abounds.

The body of the esophagus above the level of the lower esophageal sphincter is generally flaccid and often greatly distended. Occasionally, diverticula are present. The wall may be of normal thickness, thickened by hypertrophy, or thinned by dilatation. Most often, ganglion cells of Auerbach's plexus are absent or reduced in number in the lower two thirds of the esophagus and sometimes in the lower esophageal sphincter. Infrequently there is degeneration of the myelin sheaths and breaks in the axons of the intraesophageal ramifications of the vagus nerves.

With long-standing achalasia, stasis of food and secretions occurs proximal to the contracted esophagogastric junction, with consequent superimposed chronic esophagitis. Nonspecific ulceroinflammatory lesions and leukoplakial thickening of the mucosa may therefore be present.

**CLINICAL COURSE.** Although achalasia may manifest itself at any age, it most commonly has its onset between the ages of 21 and 40 years. Males and females are affected equally frequently. The predominant symptom is dysphagia, which often has an abrupt onset during a period of emotional stress. The patient initially complains of a sensation of sticking of food, along with a dull ache beneath the lower sternum. These paroxysms become more frequent,

and eventually regurgitation of undigested food occurs, particularly when the patient is in a horizontal position. Complete obstruction may ensue. Diagnosis can usually be made by fluoroscopy after a swallow of barium. Long-standing achalasia with its chronic mucosal irritation predisposes to the development of carcinoma.

## HIATAL HERNIA

Hiatal hernia refers to an upward herniation of the stomach through the esophageal hiatus, such that a portion of the stomach comes to lie above the diaphragm. Two anatomic variants are recognized, as depicted in Figure 16–1.

In the more common **sliding hiatal hernia**, found in 90% of hernia cases, there is an abnormally short esophagus so that the esophagogastric junction and a bell-shaped portion of the stomach lie above the diaphragm. The less common variant is the **paraesophageal** or **rolling hernia**, characterized by a defect or weakening of the diaphragmatic hiatus such that a portion of the gastric fundus rolls up alongside the esophagus into the thorax. The esophagogastric junction remains in its normal position.

After death, when relaxation of the gastrointestinal tract allows the stomach to slip back into the abdominal cavity, only the largest hiatal hernias are grossly demonstrable. Nor are there diagnostic histologic changes in an uncomplicated hiatal hernia. However, very frequently an associated reflux esophagitis, an esophageal ring or stricture, or, rarely, a "Barrett esophagus" (distal esophagus lined by columnar epithelium, p. 509) may arouse suspicion of an underlying hiatal hernia.

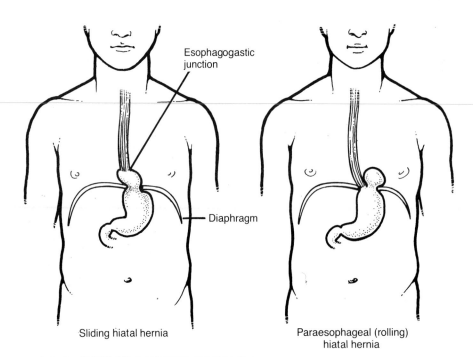

Esophagogastric junction

Diaphragm

Sliding hiatal hernia

Paraesophageal (rolling) hiatal hernia

Figure 16–1. A comparison of the two forms of esophageal diverticula.

The *paraesophageal hernia* produces distinctive symptoms—discomfort associated with a sensation of fullness after eating. Rarely, twisting and strangulation of the herniated pouch produces a major clinical emergency. This type of hernia is generally readily diagnosed by radiologic studies and is a well-defined clinicopathologic entity. By contrast, the symptomatology associated with the *sliding form of hiatal hernia* is inconstant and nondistinctive, comprising only heartburn related to gastroesophageal reflux.[5] Moreover, the criteria for diagnosis of a sliding hiatal hernia are ill defined radiologically, endoscopically, and even anatomically (when muscle tone and pressure relationships disappear). Not surprisingly, then, the reported radiologic incidence of hiatal hernia has ranged between 3 and 75% (with more rigorous criteria, 0.5 to 5%). It is apparent that the diagnosis "hiatal hernia" has been abused or overused, often as a wastebasket for poorly understood complaints. But nonetheless, when present, it often leads to reflux esophagitis and heartburn.

## ESOPHAGITIS

Inflammation of the esophagus, acute or chronic, is a more frequent autopsy diagnosis than a clinical diagnosis because it is usually asymptomatic or develops as a very late change in a terminally ill patient whose defenses are exhausted. Moreover, sometimes it is seen in association with esophageal cancer, and so the inflammatory changes are of little significance. Yet esophagitis in those not mortally ill can be of considerable importance. Not only may it cause swallowing difficulty (dysphagia), the chronic inflammatory changes can also lead to fibrotic narrowing and strictures. Even more important, chronic esophagitis is probably a precursor to cancer.

In Western countries, esophagitis is sometimes idiopathic in origin, but in many instances it can be attributed to one of the influences cited in Table 16–1. Among these, reflux is of particular importance.

**Table 16–1. POSSIBLE ORIGINS OF ESOPHAGITIS**

Recurrent reflux of gastric juice (reflux or peptic esophagitis), in some instances related to hiatal hernia

Alcohol abuse

Heavy smoking

Corrosive agents (accidental or suicidal ingestion); excessively hot liquids (chronic consumption)

Prolonged gastric intubation

Candidiasis; herpesvirus infection

External radiation to the chest

Drugs (KCl; antibiotics, and chemotherapeutic agents)[8]

Uremia

Pemphigus; epidermolysis bullosa

Graft-versus-host disease

The reflux must be chronic and copious (such as may occur with a sliding hiatal hernia) because mild and intermittent reflex is frequent in otherwise normal individuals. The rapidity of clearing the refluxed gastric contents, the adequacy of the lavaging and neutralizing effects of swallowed saliva, and, most importantly, the level of the gastric acidity and peptic activity all condition the impact of the gastric reflux.

Candidal esophagitis usually occurs in debilitated and immunoincompetent patients and those on prolonged regimens of broad-spectrum antibiotics; herpetic esophagitis occurs when the virus is spread by intubation through infected oral territory. Despite all the possible origins mentioned, it is often idiopathic in origin.

In certain regions of China and Northern Iran, chronic esophagitis occurs in more than 80% of the adult population.[6, 7] Reflux alone cannot account for such an extraordinary incidence. Risk factors such as alcohol or tobacco can only play, at most, a small role in these cultures. Vague notions have been entertained of nutritional deficiencies, possibly of vitamins A and C, or excessive consumption of hot or spicy foods, but these are without sound basis. So we must leave it that the origins of esophagitis in these locales remain a mystery.

**MORPHOLOGY.** The anatomic changes of esophagitis depend upon the cause, the duration, and the severity of the process. With reflux esophagitis, the lower third of the esophagus is principally affected. Inflammation induced by a nasogastric tube generally affects the upper two thirds. Analogously, spread of a herpes infection from the oral cavity into the esophagus tends to be limited to the upper levels. Some of the causes mentioned produced distinctive and recognizable lesions, such as the small, raindrop-like vesicles of herpes that, when ruptured, leave round, shallow ulcerations, and the white to gray, patchy encrustations of candidal membranes that later may be sloughed to leave ulcerations. **In most cases, however, the changes are nonspecific and range from hyperemia to mucosal ulcerative lesions during the more acute stages.** Very rarely, deep ulcerations may perforate the esophageal wall. In the chronic stage, progressive fibrous thickening of the esophageal wall appears and may lead to the formation of strictures. The histologic changes can be anticipated largely from the gross features. However, a few special changes must be mentioned. In chronic reflux esophagitis, the squamous epithelium may be replaced by columnar epithelial cells—**Barrett's esophagus.** Most individuals with this lesion have an underlying hiatal hernia.[9] In severe cases, the metaplastic epithelium may extend up to the middle third of the esophagus. Usually one, sometimes several, epithelial types can be identified in the affected mucosa: (1) gastric fundus-like epithelium replete with parietal and chief cells, (2) gastric cardia-like mucosa with no parietal or chief cells, and (3) epithelium similar to that of the small bowel with a villiform surface but containing goblet cells resembling those of the large bowel. Two types of ulcerations may occur in Barrett's esophagus: nonspecific, usually shallow, irregular, acute, or chronic defects, or, less commonly, a typical peptic ulcer (p. 516), usually adjacent to acid-pepsin–secreting mucosa. With chronic esophagitis such as is encountered in China and Iran, the epithelium may become atrophic or hyperkeratotic or, more ominously, dysplastic. The dysplasia is thought to be related to the high incidence of superimposed squamous cell esophageal cancer in China and Iran. There is also an increased risk of adenocarcinoma in Barrett's esophagus, but studies vary (2% to 14%) in the magnitude of the risk.[10]

**CLINICAL COURSE.** The clinical significance of esophagitis is as variable as the putative causes. Less severe involvement may well be asymptomatic, or the lesions may be only an agonal development in an already dying individual. However, the condition may cause distressing substernal pain or it may provoke usually mild bleeding, which when prolonged can cause chronic iron deficiency anemia. Stricture formation may follow chronic esophagitis and may be severe enough to impair the maintenance of adequate nutrition. Heartburn, dysphagia, bleeding, and even perforation are more common and more difficult to control with Barrett's esophagus than with the less severe forms of esophagitis. Most ominously, esophagitis may lead to the development of esophageal carcinoma, particularly when Barrett's changes are present.

## ESOPHAGEAL VARICES

Massive upper gastrointestinal bleeding (usually producing hematemesis) is a fairly frequent and alarming clinical problem.
*The major causes are:*
○ Peptic (gastric or duodenal) ulcer
○ Erosive gastritis
○ Esophageal varices
○ Esophageal laceration

The precise contribution of each to the overall problem varies with the population surveyed, but peptic ulcer would head the list in an unselected population.[11] However, in a series of patients with cirrhosis of the liver and portal hypertension, esophageal varices would vie for first place. Alcoholic cirrhosis is the preponderant cause of esophageal varices in the United States and Europe, but other forms of cirrhosis and other causes of portal hypertension (discussed on p. 583) may be responsible. Here it suffices that, as pressure builds up in the portal system, blood is diverted through the coronary esophageal veins and submucosal plexuses into the azygos veins (p. 584). In time the esophageal submucosal veins progressively dilate, form variceal enlargements, and are at increasing risk of rupturing.

**MORPHOLOGY.** In usual postmortem specimens, esophageal varices may be difficult to demonstrate be-

cause they collapse after transection, when the blood they contain is drained. When not collapsed, they appear as bluish, submucosal, serpentine ridges, running in the long axis of the distal esophagus and bulging into the lumen (Fig. 16–2). Although the overlying mucosa may be normal, it is often eroded and inflamed because of its exposed position, and these secondary changes enhance the likelihood of rupture. If rupture has occurred in the past, thrombosis or marked inflammation may be seen.

**CLINICAL COURSE.** Esophageal varices are characteristically silent until rupture occurs. The ensuing clinical picture is then catastrophic, with the sudden onset of massive, painless hematemesis. Identification of the source of the bleeding and institution of appropriate therapy (conservative measures vs. surgery) are extremely urgent and often difficult.[12] Even with appropriate therapy, the in-hospital mortality for first episodes of variceal hemorrhage is 33 to 50% (several times greater than that for bleeding peptic ulcers). Moreover, there is always the danger of subsequent "bleeds," and an additional third of the patients die within six to eight weeks after the first episode of hemorrhage.

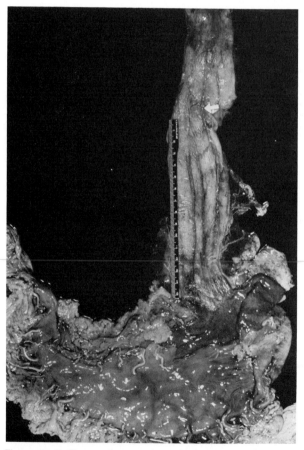

Figure 16–2. Three submucosal veins, rendered prominent by their marked variceal dilatation, are seen in the lower half of the esophagus. The arrow points to one of them.

# ESOPHAGEAL LACERATIONS (MALLORY-WEISS SYNDROME)

Although not as common as esophageal varices, lacerations account for 5 to 15% of all massive bleeding episodes.[13] They are particularly frequent among alcoholics; in most instances an episode of violent retching or vomiting immediately precedes the onset of bleeding. It is assumed that strong antiperistaltic contractions overwhelm the lower esophageal sphincter and the sudden dilatation induces the laceration. However, not all patients are alcoholic, there may not be a history of violent vomiting, and lacerations have followed such varying stresses as coughing, straining, hiccoughing, gastroscopy, cardiopulmonary resuscitation, and childbirth. Concomitant hiatal hernia is reported to be present in 15 to 30% of cases, possibly potentiating the laceration by the inadequacy of the diaphragmatic support of the lower esophagus.

The lacerations lie in the long axis of the gut and range from a few millimeters to several centimeters in length. They may be superficial and involve only the mucosa, but more often the deeper layers are affected as well. Rarely, they extend through the wall. Although the tears in all four patients originally described by Mallory and Weiss were located astride the gastroesophageal junction, in more recent surveys, the gastric wall of the lesser curvature, just below the gastroesophageal junction, emerges as the favored site. Less commonly, the lacerations occur at slightly higher or lower levels. About 15% of patients have more than a single tear. The histologic findings are noncontributory and vary with the duration of the defect and the possible healing and reepithelialization of the lesion.

The hematemesis is usually sudden, massive, and unheralded except for prior vomiting or retching in most cases. Fortunately, the bleeding can usually be managed by medical therapy and only rarely requires surgical intervention. Fatalities are infrequent.[14] Because another bout of bleeding may never occur, it is assumed that lacerations can heal, leaving no residuals.

# CARCINOMA OF THE ESOPHAGUS

Currently esophageal cancer causes about 2% of all cancer deaths. It is therefore a relatively uncommon form of malignancy. In North America, most European countries, Great Britain, and Australia, the incidence of esophageal cancer in white males ranges between two and five per 100,000, and there is a male-female ratio of 3:1. Strangely, in France the incidence in both sexes is nearly three times greater. Even more astounding, the incidence of esophageal cancer in Linxian, China, is over 130 per 100,000, and in the Caspian littoral of Iran there are 114 cases

per 100,000 and females are affected as often as males. Equally baffling are the following findings.[15] Black males in the United States have a roughly four- to fivefold higher incidence than white males, and an analogous discrepancy exists for females. In the Transkei of South Africa, there is an almost 40-fold variation in male mortality from this form of cancer between high-incidence areas in the south and low-incidence areas of the north, yet the distance between these areas could be encompassed within Denmark. Where this cancer is very common, young to middle-aged individuals are affected, but in low-incidence regions, those affected are in the late decades of life. Satisfactory explanations for all these differences are lacking.

**ETIOLOGY AND PATHOGENESIS.** A few observations suggest that environmental influences underlie the epidemiology of this form of cancer. There is a progressive increase in its frequency in those who have migrated from low-incidence to high-incidence areas. Conversely, migration early in life from a high-incidence to a low-incidence area reduces the level of risk, but later in life such a move is without effect. Whatever predisposes an individual to this environmental cancer must exert its effect at an early age. Many influences, some better established than others, are thought to predispose to esophageal carcinoma, as indicated in Table 16–2. Among those mentioned, alcohol abuse, heavy smoking, and esophagitis are most important. The first two, when combined, increase the risk of esophageal cancer as much as 40-fold. Yet neither smoking nor alcohol consumption can be implicated in the high-incidence region of Iran, where the two practices are rare. The effects of dietary carcinogens (such as the nitrosamines), silica dust, and malnutrition are not generally given much credence.[16] There is more convincing epidemiologic evidence that any disorder impairing esophageal structure or function and leading to chronic mucosal injury predisposes an individual to carcinoma, presumably because the reparative-regenerative process provides an optimal environment for the emergence of a neoplasm. In northern Iran and

**Table 16–2.** PREDISPOSING INFLUENCES TO ESOPHAGEAL CANCER

| Established | Questionable |
|---|---|
| Alcohol abuse | Dietary carcinogens |
| Heavy smoking | (nitrosamines, silica dust) |
| Achalasia | Malnutrition |
| Esophageal diverticula | Vitamin deficiencies |
| Esophageal webs (Plummer-Vinson syndrome) | |
| Chronic esophagitis | |
|   With leukoplakia and dysplasia | |
|     (80% of populations in locales | |
|     of northern Iran and China, | |
|     p. 509) | |
|   Reflux esophagitis with Barrett's | |
|     esophagus | |

China, endemic cancer areas, chronic esophagitis is probably the important predisposing influence.[6]

**MORPHOLOGY.** Circumstantial evidence strongly suggests that a long prodrome of mucosal, epithelial alterations (i.e., dysplasia, atypical dysplasia, and finally in-situ carcinoma) precede the appearance of overt neoplasms.[17] In the high-risk locales of China, where cytologic screening is routinely performed, about half of the cases at the time of esophagectomy are intraepithelial neoplasms that occasionally show extension only to the submucosa. Such "early" lesions are rarities in low-incidence locales, where routine cytologic screening is not commonplace. Interestingly, foci of dysplasia are sometimes found at a distance from the cancerous lesion. About 40 to 50% of the invasive cancers are located in the middle third of the esophagus, 35 to 40% in the lower third, and 10 to 15% in the upper third. These may appear as small, gray-white mucosal plaques, but **more often, they encircle the circumference of the esophagus and simultaneously invade the submucosa** (Fig. 16–3). From this point, one of three gross morphologic patterns may evolve: (1) a fungating **polypoid** mass that protrudes into the lumen (60%); (2) a necrotic **ulcerating**

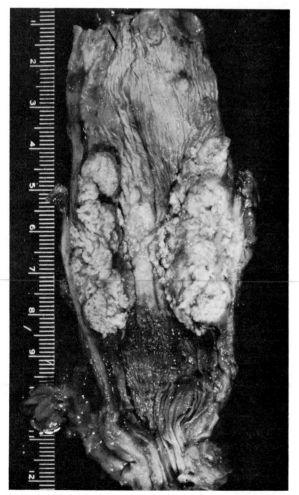

Figure 16–3. Esophageal carcinoma. The polypoid, plaque-like lesion has not encircled the wall; the carcinoma was transected when the esophagus was opened.

lesion that excavates deeply into surrounding structures and may erode into the respiratory tree, aorta, mediastinum, or pericardium (25%); or (3) a **diffuse infiltrative** tumor that causes thickening, rigidity, and narrowing of the lumen with linear irregular ulcerations of the mucosa.

About 90% of the tumors are typical squamous cell carcinomas of varying levels of differentiation. Most of the remainder are adenocarcinomas, beginning either in submucosal glands or in the metaplastic columnar epithelium of Barrett's esophagus. Rare are the small cell undifferentiated cancers, whose origins are apparently neuroendocrine (p. 537).

Classically, esophageal carcinomas tend to spread locally before metastasizing to distant sites. The pattern of spread depends on the location of the lesion. Those of the middle and upper thirds tend to remain confined within the thorax and involve the regional lymph nodes, larynx, trachea, thyroid, and recurrent laryngeal nerves. Such direct spread may give rise to esophagotracheal fistulas. Lesions of the lower third are more likely to involve lymph nodes below the diaphragm and the mediastinal nodes. Distant metastatic spread may involve almost any organ of the body, principally the lungs, liver, and bones.[18]

Many methods of staging this form of cancer have been proposed. All attempt to express the depth of penetration of the esophageal wall and the presence and number of lymph node and organ metastases.[15, 19]

**CLINICAL COURSE.** For some uncertain length of time during their developmental phase, most, perhaps all, esophageal carcinomas are asymptomatic. When symptoms appear, dysphagia is almost always the first manifestation, but characteristically this does not develop until the lesion has spread at least halfway around the circumference of the esophagus. Weight loss is extreme because the effects of the dysphagia are added to the general anorexia that occurs with most malignant tumors. Depending on the exact location of the tumor, other manifestations of esophageal carcinoma include intractable hiccoughs or hoarseness, caused by involvement of the phrenic or recurrent laryngeal nerves, respectively; cough, as a result of invasion of the respiratory tree; and hemorrhage, when a large vessel is eroded. Superimposed infection is frequent. Occasionally, the first indication of the tumor is the dramatic aspiration of food through a tracheoesophageal fistula. Such fistulas are almost always caused by carcinoma of the esophagus, since bronchogenic carcinoma rarely invades the esophagus.

When esophageal carcinomas have reached the stage at which they can be diagnosed by radiographic methods, the results of therapy are most discouraging. The five-year survival rate with radiotherapy or surgical resection or both is about 5 to 10%. The only hope with this form of cancer is much earlier diagnosis by using routine cytologic screening, esophagoscopy, and biopsy in individuals at particular risk. When the lesion is confined to the esophageal wall, the five-year survival rate is 60 to 90%.[20]

# Stomach

Lesions of the stomach are almost as frequent causes of clinical disease as are those of the colon. "Indigestion," some of which arises in bona fide gastritis, is probably more prevalent than the common cold. Peptic ulcers are hallmarks of this stressful, crisis-ridden age. Gastric cancer, although declining remarkably in incidence, remains an important cause of mortality. Thus, diseases of the stomach loom large in clinical practice.

## PYLORIC STENOSIS

Obstructive narrowing of the pyloric lumen is encountered in two clinical settings: (1) as an apparently familial disorder in the newborn and (2) as an acquired or possibly familial condition in adults. Table 16–3 shows the characteristics of both the infantile and adult forms of pyloric stenosis. Although the condition may appear almost at birth, it is not thought to be a congenital malformation. Instead, it is postulated that a hereditary predisposition to pyloric spasm leads to an ulcer in the pyloric channel and subsequent narrowing and hypertrophy.[21] Infants occasionally begin to vomit within the first week of life but more often not until three to four weeks of age. When the lesion is fully developed, hyperactive gastric peristalsis is evident on inspection of the abdomen and a firm ovoid mass is palpable in the upper abdomen. Splitting of the muscularis down to the mucosa usually effects a prompt cure and, in time, disappearance of the muscular hypertrophy. The adult form of the condition could be a late-appearing familial predisposition but is sometimes related to an acquired lesion. Resection of the pylorus may be advisable in adults in order to rule out the possibility of an occult, infiltrative, gastric cancer.

## GASTRITIS

Laymen and physicians alike are guilty of using this term as a "wastebasket" diagnosis for all manner of nonspecific transient complaints—in particular, for any vague epigastric discomfort or vomiting. More rigorously, the designation gastritis should be reserved for several specific derangements that can be diagnosed with certainty only by gastroscopy and biopsy. The two most important categories of gastritis—*acute* (erosive) and *chronic* (nonerosive)—are probably unrelated and have in common only some degree of damage to the gastric mucosa and a variable inflammatory infiltrate.[22] These will be discussed separately.

## ACUTE (EROSIVE) GASTRITIS

This diagnosis is overused and abused because of lack of clear-cut diagnostic criteria, both clinically and anatomically, and because it is so satisfying to clinician and to patient to label any mysterious, transient gastric upset as "acute gastritis." *When the term is correctly applied, it encompasses a spectrum of levels of inflammation embraced by the terms "acute superficial gastritis," "acute hemorrhagic gastritis," and "acute erosive gastritis."* Because of poor lines of demarcation, the term "acute erosive gastritis" is applied increasingly to all variants, albeit in some instances there are no erosions.

**ETIOLOGY AND PATHOGENESIS.** As is so often true, the causation of acute gastritis is unknown, as indeed are the normal defenses of the gastric mucosa against its own aggressive acid-peptic secretion. This much is known—acute gastritis has well-documented associations with the following:

○ Habitual use of nonsteroidal anti-inflammatory drugs, particularly non-enteric-coated aspirin.
○ Chronic alcohol consumption
○ Heavy smoking
○ *Campylobacter* infection
○ Antitumor chemotherapeutic agents
○ Severe stress (e.g., extensive body burns)
○ Trauma or surgery to central nervous system
○ Gastric irradiation
○ Staphylococcal enterotoxic food poisoning

**Table 16–3.** CHARACTERISTICS OF PYLORIC STENOSIS

| Infantile Hypertrophic Pyloric Stenosis | Adult Pyloric Stenosis |
|---|---|
| *Incidence* | *Acquired* |
| Familial? Multifactorial inheritance? | Secondary to stenosing local disease such as pyloric peptic ulcer, |
| One in 300 to 900 live births | gastritis, and gastric cancer |
| Three to four times more common in males | |
| *Pathogenesis* | |
| Hereditary predisposition to pyloric spasm?[221] | |
| *Risk Factors* | *Familial* |
| First-born males of high birth weight who have professional | Late-appearing manifestation of infantile disease; may be related |
| parents | to pyloric spasm |
| High level of concordance in identical twins | |
| *Anatomic Features* | *Anatomic Features* |
| Striking hypertrophy of pyloric muscularis, often associated | Identical to infantile pattern features |
| with mucosal edema | |

With certain of these clinical associations, such as burns or trauma to the CNS, the gastritis tends to be severely erosive, merging into stress ulcerations, but for clarity's sake, stress ulcerations will be treated separately (p. 515). Among associations cited, most clearly and most frequently implicated are nonsteroidal anti-inflammatory drugs, alcohol, and smoking. The worst offender is aspirin. When taken regularly for rheumatoid arthritis (for example), aspirin induces slight occult bleeding from the gastric mucosa in about 70% of patients. Often aspirin is taken as an antidote for alcohol, as indeed for nearly anything, thus exposing the hapless mucosa to a pair of offenders thought by some to potentiate each other.[23] Although oral corticosteroids are thought to contribute to gastric ulceration, their role in gastritis is unclear.

A few insights have been achieved into the mechanisms by which aspirin and other nonsteroidal anti-inflammatory drugs (NSAID), alcohol, and smoking induce acute gastritis. Aspirin in particular is believed to lead to back-diffusion of gastric acid, as is explained on page 519. This in itself is injurious, but in addition, the NSAID inhibit local production of prostaglandins, currently thought to exert a mucosal "cytoprotective" effect.[24] Alcohol and condensate from tobacco smoke may act by local direct cellular injury. Thereafter, transient impairment of acid secretion may permit the growth of microorganisms, and one in particular—*Campylobacter pyloridis*.[25] This bacillus is currently thought to be a major contributor to the development of acute gastritis.[26] However, whether it is a sufficient and necessary ingredient remains to be established.

**MORPHOLOGY.** Acute erosive gastritis may be localized or diffuse. Most often it involves the acid-secreting mucosa of the fundus and body of the stomach. In the milder forms of acute gastritis, there may only be slight hyperemia and edema accompanied by an inflammatory infiltrate of lymphocytes, macrophages, and occasionally neutrophils and eosinophils in the superficial layer of the lamina propria. Sometimes there is focal shedding of the mucosa, which is usually superficial and rarely extends through the mucosal layer. Such changes are but one step removed from stress ulcers and are almost always accompanied by hemorrhages. Between the erosions there may be evidence of regeneration in the form of basophilic, flattened, cuboidal epithelium devoid of mucus secretion.[27] **Acute erosive gastritis is always marked by a prominent inflammatory mucosal infiltrate and by layering of the gastric lining with partially digested blood.**

**CLINICAL COURSE.** Depending on the severity of the lesion, acute gastritis may be entirely asymptomatic; may cause variable degrees of epigastric pain, nausea, and vomiting; or may produce massive hematemesis and melena. Mild cases commonly cause little or no discomfort. Acute gastritis from staphylococcal enterotoxin is associated with the sudden onset (about five hours after eating contaminated food) of intense epigastric distress and vomiting, but it is transient and self-limited. A similar picture following overenthusiastic intake of alcohol is perhaps even more familiar. Habitual use of aspirin rarely causes such a dramatic onset but instead provokes repeated bouts of "heartburn," "sour stomach," and other vague discomforts. Nonetheless, it has been estimated that 25% of all cases of hematemesis and melena in the London area are triggered by aspirin ingestion.[28] Alcohol may without warning cause sudden hemorrhagic erosive gastritis. Although bleeding in these cases may be severe, it usually ceases spontaneously within 36 hours. Because of the relative safety of conservative management, x-ray and gastroscopic confirmation of this cause of hematemesis is important.

## CHRONIC (NONEROSIVE) GASTRITIS

*Chronic gastritis is marked principally by mucosal chronic inflammatory changes and glandular atrophy with metaplasia.* Although usually asymptomatic, it is a significant disorder because of its important relationships to pernicious anemia (p. 366), gastric peptic ulcer, and gastric carcinoma. It may involve the stomach patchily or diffusely, but in some instances it is restricted principally to the fundic gland region (*type A*, or *fundic gastritis*) or to the antral gland region (*type B*, or *antral gastritis*). However, even with these distinctive distributions, whether fundic or antral, there is also often less severe involvement of adjacent zones or even the entire remainder of the stomach. *Whatever the distribution in the stomach, the gastritis can be subclassified into superficial chronic gastritis, atrophic gastritis, and gastric atrophy in order to express the range of severity of the mucosal inflammation and associated glandular changes.* Long-term studies strongly suggest that these levels of severity merely represent stages in the progression or regression of a single underlying condition. Thus, over the span of years, superficial gastritis may be transformed into atrophic gastritis, or, in some instances, the reverse has occurred.[29]

**ETIOLOGY AND PATHOGENESIS.** Chronic gastritis or specific patterns of it are seen particularly in the following clinical settings: (1) in patients with pernicious anemia (PA), (2) in individuals with a gastric ulcer, (3) in association with gastric cancer, (4) in post subtotal gastrectomy stomachs, and (5) in otherwise healthy, aging individuals.

*Earlier it was noted that PA develops because of a lack of intrinsic factor and malabsorption of vitamin $B_{12}$. In these patients there is classically fundal atrophic gastritis or gastric atrophy, type A, which is probably autoimmune in origin.* Three types of autoantibodies have been identified, as detailed on page 366. One is targeted on intrinsic factor (IF), another on IF-$B_{12}$ complexes, and the third on parietal cells (the source of IF). These account for the lack of IF and vitamin $B_{12}$ absorption. The last-mentioned autoantibody is cytotoxic to parietal cells and results in the hypochlorhydria or achlorhydria, characteristic of this form of anemia.[30] However, it should be noted that antibodies against IF and IF complexes cannot be demonstrated in about 25% of patients with PA, and in 10 to 15% of patients, antibodies against parietal cells are not present. Moreover, lower titers of these antibodies are present in many elderly individuals who do not have pernicious anemia.

*Gastric (but not duodenal) peptic ulcers are almost invariably accompanied by chronic antral gastritis.* The gastritis does not appear to be secondary to the ulcer because it may persist after the ulcer is healed, but the role gastritis plays in inducing the ulcer is poorly understood. It is suspected that the influences leading to the gastritis, such as chronic and severe duodenogastric reflux, may in some instances lead eventually to an ulcer. Other etiologies for the antral gastritis have also been raised. The *Campylobacter* bacilli mentioned earlier in association with acute gastritis (p. 513) are often, but not always, seen in the stomachs of patients with antral gastritis and peptic ulceration.[25] The role of chronic aspirin use in the induction of *chronic* antral gastritis is controversial, despite its well-documented association with acute gastritis.

*Subtotal gastrectomy is almost invariably followed by the development of chronic gastritis in the residual stomach.* Although a number of speculations have been offered (such as enterogastric reflux), all are tenuous. The development of chronic gastritis in the stump may well explain the increased incidence of gastric carcinoma, variously cited as up to 15%, in the residual segment of the stomach.

Finally, *there is a clear-cut association between chronic gastritis and aging.* Prevalence data are extremely variable and range from about 15% of the elderly in the United States to about half of the total population over the age of 50 in Japan and Colombia. There is a tendency for the gastritis to be fundal in distribution. In most instances it is superficial, occasionally reaching the severity of atrophic gastritis. Over the span of time, the changes may remain essentially constant, progress in severity, or regress. Often it induces hypochlorhydria or achlorhydria and is accompanied by an iron deficiency anemia. The etiology of the mucosal lesion is obscure, but about half of these patients have antibodies against parietal cell antigens.

**MORPHOLOGY. Superficial gastritis** may involve the entire stomach or only segments of it, as noted previously. It is characterized by increased numbers of lymphocytes and plasma cells; scattered polyps and occasional eosinophils in the lamina propria limited to the foveolae. The surface glandular epithelium is generally unaffected.

**Atrophic gastritis and then gastric atrophy are marked essentially by three features**: (1) The mucosa becomes progressively thinner, revealing more readily the submucosal vasculature, which imparts a red, glazed, shiny surface. (2) The inflammatory infiltrate (previously cited) is more intense, extends through all levels of the lamina propria, and is sometimes accompanied by the appearance of scattered lymphoid aggregates. (3) A variety of epithelial changes appear over time, giving to this condition its major clinical significance. In the fundic variant associated with pernicious anemia, there is typically subtotal to total loss of parietal cells. In all distributions, the surface and pit epithelium may become depleted of mucus as the mildest expression of epithelial change. More striking is intestinal metaplasia, in which the epithelium on the surface or in the pits is transformed into goblet cells resembling those of the intestine. Sometimes apparent villus-like projections appear on the surface, producing more than a passing resemblance to small intestinal mucosa. **With increasing severity, the epithelium on the surface and in the pits may lose its regular columnar arrangement and be replaced by disoriented cells that have nuclei of variable size, shape, and staining and display characteristics of atypical metaplasia to dysplasia.[31]** Such cytologic alterations are thought to lead to gastric carcinoma in some instances. Significantly, individuals with pernicious anemia over the span of decades have a threefold greater risk than controls of developing gastric carcinoma.

**CLINICAL COURSE.** Chronic gastritis seldom produces symptoms. The tendency to use this diagnosis as an explanation of dyspepsia or other vague gastric complaints is regrettable and almost always implies the lack of another diagnosis. However, as has already been made clear, chronic gastritis has important pathogenetic implications. It is basic to the development of pernicious anemia. The atypical metaplasia-dysplasia in long-standing cases predisposes to the development of gastric carcinoma. Much more uncertain is the role of chronic antral gastritis in the development of gastric peptic ulcer (discussed on p. 519).

# STRESS ULCERS

Superficial mucosal erosions in the stomach commonly appear within hours of many forms of acute stress. Usually these lesions are entirely silent, but in about 10% of cases, they bleed (uncommonly massively) and, rarely, one perforates. The clinical settings in which stress ulcers appear include:

○ Severe trauma of any type—when associated with extensive body burns they are called "Curling's ulcers"
○ Major sepsis
○ Traumatic or surgical injury to the central nervous system, or an intracerebral hemorrhage—in this setting they are referred to as "Cushing's ulcers"
○ Significant shock
○ Any serious illness

Whether to call the mucosal lesions induced by nonsteroidal anti-inflammatory drugs (e.g., aspirin), acute erosive gastritis, or drug-induced stress ulcers is a matter of semantics.

The pathogenesis of these lesions is uncertain. Only with Cushing's ulcers is there good evidence for gastric acid–pepsin hypersecretion. With these it is believed that impulses acting through the hypothalamus stimulate autonomic centers and lead to increased production of acid-peptic secretion. In the remaining settings a favored theory proposes splanchnic vasoconstriction. The reduced mucosal perfusion restricts the capacity of the mucosa to secrete adequate amounts of buffering bicarbonate, leading to ulcerations.[32] A variation on this theme focuses on the ischemia-induced oxygen deprivation of mucosal cells.[33] There is also evidence that the ischemia may impair local elaboration of prostaglandins thought to play a mucosal "cytoprotective" role (p. 609). Suffice it that stress ulcerations can be readily induced in experimental animals by several interventions, and that administration of various pharmacologic agents having different actions (such as raising the mucosal pH, increasing prostaglandin levels, and others) all exert protective effects. The plethora of causal and protective approaches suggests that many influences may be ulcerogenic, singly or in combination.

**MORPHOLOGY.** Typically, stress ulcers are small round to ovoid, sometimes irregular, mucosal defects that initially appear in the proximal portion of the gastric mucosa, and when the stress is sufficiently severe, these ulcers extend to the entire stomach. **Individual ulcers rarely exceed 2.5 cm in diameter, usually have a brown base caused by digestion of blood, and, only exceptionally, penetrate more deeply than the muscularis mucosae.** Sometimes the lesions are so numerous they give the appearance of "leopard-spotting" of the mucosa. The histologic findings are essentially those of apparent enzymatic digestion of a mucosal focus. There may be a slight inflammatory infiltrate in the margins as the lesion evolves, but generally there is no significant surrounding hyperemic reaction, and the rugal pattern of the stomach is undisturbed. In some cases, particularly in association with burns and head lesions, stress ulcers extend into the duodenum. For poorly understood reasons, they are much more likely in this location to be deeply penetrating or to perforate. When the precipitating event abates, they usually completely heal, sometimes as rapidly as they develop.

Most often, stress ulcers are totally silent and only come to clinical attention when they cause bleeding. The bleeding is usually mild and requires only simple treatment measures. Infrequently, the bleeding is severe, carrying with it a high mortality rate because of the blood loss in already overtaxed patients. Prophylactic pharmacologic regimens are therefore recommended in situations known to be associated with their development.

# PEPTIC ULCERS

A peptic ulcer can be defined ingloriously as a "mucosal hole" in any portion of the gastrointestinal tract exposed to acid-pepsin secretion—hence the hallowed dictum, "no acid, no ulcer." The definition should be further qualified, as noted in Table 16–4.

*At least 98% of peptic ulcers are located either in the first portion of the duodenum or in the stomach.* About 5% of individuals with gastric ulcers develop duodenal ulcers, but 20% of those with duodenal ulcers develop gastric lesions. Although they may coexist and despite their similar morphology, there is a strong likelihood that duodenal and gastric ulcers have different origins.

**EPIDEMIOLOGY.** The epidemiology of duodenal ulcer is changing rapidly; at one time duodenal ulcers were much more common than gastric, but their incidence and prevalence are now approaching those of gastric ulcers. Today the incidence of duodenal ulcers is about 1.0 to 3.5 cases per thousand males per year.[34] The prevalence of gastric ulcers, however, has remained about the same over the past decades, with an incidence in the United States of about 0.5 per thousand males per year. Only two decades ago, twice as many men as women developed peptic ulcers. Today the ratio appears to be approaching 1.0 for both duodenal and gastric lesions.[35] The changing data on sex ratios reflect a more rapid decrease in ulcer rates for males than for females. In both sexes the peak incidence of the first attack is in the fifth to sixth decades of life, but sometimes it occurs in much younger or older individuals.

*Genetic influences play some role in the predisposition to both forms of ulcer but are more clear-cut with duodenal ulcers.* First-degree relatives of an individual with a duodenal ulcer have a threefold greater risk of developing one. There is a 50% concordance of duodenal ulcers in monozygotic twins but only 14% in dizygotic twins. Individuals in blood group O have a 30% greater chance of developing a duodenal ulcer than those in other blood groups. Analogously, those who fail to secrete blood group

**Table 16–4. DISTINCTIVE FEATURES OF PEPTIC ULCER**

1. Usually occurs singly
2. Tends to be a small mucosal defect (under 4 cm in diameter)
3. Almost always penetrates the muscularis mucosae and may perforate the gastrointestinal wall
4. Is frequently recurrent (although may heal)
5. Is located in the following sites (descending order of frequency):
   (a) Duodenum, first portion
   (b) Stomach, usually antrum
   (c) Within a Barrett's esophagus (p. 509)
   (d) In the margins of a gastroenterostomy (stomal ulcer)
   (e) In the duodenum, stomach, or jejunum in patients with Zollinger-Ellison syndrome (p. 609)
   (f) Within a Meckel's diverticulum that contains ectopic gastric mucosa

**Table 16–5.** FACTORS ASSOCIATED WITH
PEPTIC ULCER

**Duodenal Ulcer**
*Environmental Influences*
  Cigarette smoking
  Aspirin abuse
  Alcohol consumption

*Associated Diseases*
  Cirrhosis of liver
  Pancreatic cancer
  Chronic bronchitis and emphysema
  Renal stones
  ?? Renal failure

*Basic Pathophysiology*
  Mainly, excessive acid-pepsin secretion
  Lowered mucosal resistance may contribute

**Gastric Ulcer**
*Environmental Influences*
  Cigarette smoking
  Aspirin abuse
  Alcohol consumption

*Associated Diseases*
  Chronic bronchitis and emphysema
  Antral gastritis (duodenal ulcer in 20%)

*Basic Pathophysiology*
  Mainly, lowered mucosal resistance
  Acid-pepsin levels normal to low, but some acid requisite

antigens into body fluids such as saliva (an inherited physiologic characteristic) have a 50% increased risk over secretors. The combination of group O and nonsecretor status compounds the risk about 150%. There are in addition several well-defined genetic syndromes predisposing to duodenal ulcer; these include autosomal dominant transmission of excessive secretion of pepsinogen I, which strongly predisposes an individual to duodenal ulceration and hereditary multiple endocrine neoplasia (MEN I; p. 701).

In comparison, it has not been possible to identify genetic subsets that have increased vulnerability to gastric ulcers. Nevertheless, close relatives of a gastric ulcer subject have a two- to threefold greater risk of developing one. There are, then, genetic influences in both forms of ulcer (much stronger with the duodenal), but the differences strongly suggest that the two types of ulcer are not a single disease.

Certain environmental factors and disease states also increase the risk of developing an ulcer. The most important are tabulated in Table 16–5, along with the long-favored concepts of their basic pathophysiology. Among the predisposing influences to both forms of ulceration, cigarette smoking is most clearly documented; the level of risk is linearly correlated with the number of cigarettes smoked daily. Furthermore, smoking retards healing and promotes recurrence.[36] It may stimulate acid secretion but more likely inhibits secretion of pancreatic bicarbonate buffer. The role of alcohol as an ulcerogenic influence is more clearly documented with gastric than with duodenal ulcerations. It is known both to stimulate parietal cell secretion of acid and to be a cause of acute gastritis. Emotional stress has long been suspected to predispose humans to peptic ulcers; witness the time-hallowed cry for mercy— "What are you trying to do, give me an ulcer?" Ulcers can be produced in many laboratory animals by subjecting them to stress such as restraint and forced swimming, but the relevance of emotional stress to humans is unestablished. The claim that coffee drinking is "bad" is also unsubstantiated. Nonsteroidal anti-inflammatory agents such as aspirin have been shown to damage the gastric mucosa and sometimes cause gastritis; they may play some role in gastric ulceration but probably little in duodenal.

**PATHOGENESIS.** As is always the case, there is an inverse relationship between the level of understanding of a disorder and the volumes of writing devoted to hypotheses and speculation about it. This certainly holds for peptic ulcer. Notwithstanding, there has been surprising unanimity about the following beliefs.

1. *Duodenal ulcers arise when the aggressive levels of acid and pepsin overwhelm the defenses, which may be normal or impaired.*

2. *Gastric ulcers are the consequence of weakened defenses even though the aggressive forces are normal or even decreased.*

3. *Thus, all peptic ulcerations arise from an imbalance between the level of aggressive action of acid-pepsin secretion and the normal defenses of the gastroduodenal mucosa (Fig. 16–4).*

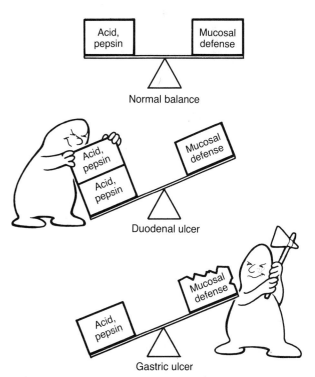

**Figure 16–4.** A schema comparing the theoretic imbalances between acid-pepsin aggression and mucosal defense in duodenal and gastric peptic ulcers.

4. *However, it is simplistic to ascribe to one side or the other of the equation total responsibility for ulceration in either the duodenum or stomach.*

Several derangements have been identified that might alter the balance; some are related to duodenal and others to gastric ulceration, but none except gastric acidity are requisite. It would appear then that there is more than one pathway to the development of a duodenal or a gastric ulcer, and that in the individual only some influences are required, not necessarily all. In this sense there are many different types of ulcers, at least pathogenetically. Indeed, subsets of gastric ulcers have now been delineated. The presumed differing origins of duodenal and gastric ulcers require separate treatment.

**Duodenal Ulcerogenesis.** The favored argument today regarding the origin of a duodenal ulcer can be set forth as shown in Table 16–6.[34, 37] *In essence, an excessive amount of gastric acid and pepsin is emptied into the duodenum because of gastric hypersecretion or rapid emptying time. The hypersecretion is related to an abnormally large total mass of parietal cells in the gastric mucosa (presumably developmental in origin), and perhaps to either increased responsiveness of the parietal cells to secretory stimuli or lack of normal regulatory controls. Increased levels of gastrin or unusual sensitivity of the parietal cells to gastrin stimulation may also be involved.*[38]

Supporting this overall thesis are three well-established lines of evidence: (1) the reduction of acid-pepsin levels by surgical removal of the fundus or by vagotomy, the use of antacids, or regimens of histamine ($H_2$) receptor antagonists (e.g., cimetidine, ranitidine) permit duodenal ulcers to heal and remain healed; (2) patients with the Zollinger-Ellison syndrome (p. 609), who have a gastrinoma or G-cell

**Table 16–6. PHYSIOLOGIC DEFECTS IN PATIENTS WITH DUODENAL ULCER***

Increased number of parietal cells

Increased serum pepsinogen-1 concentration

Increased capacity to secrete acid and pepsin

Increased "drive" to secrete acid and pepsin (increased basal rate)

Increased parietal cell sensitivity to gastrin

Decreased acid-induced inhibition of gastrin release and acid secretion

Increased meal-stimulated gastrin release

Increased duodenal acid and pepsin loads

Increased rate of gastric emptying

*None of these defects occurs in all patients with duodenal ulcer. The individual defects occur in from 20% to 50% of duodenal ulcer patients. Some patients with duodenal ulcer have none of these defects; presumably, they have other defects, probably of mucosal resistance.

From Holt, K. M., and Isenberg, J. I.: Peptic ulcer disease: Physiology and pathophysiology. Hosp. Pract. *20*:101, 1985.

hyperplasia and excessive levels of gastric acidity, characteristically develop a duodenal ulcer, sometimes a gastric ulcer, and sometimes multiple ulcers, even in such aberrant locations as the jejunum; and (3) individuals with total achlorhydria never develop a duodenal ulcer.

Attractive as the preceding construct of duodenal ulcerogenesis may be, every feature of it is open to challenge. Only about one third of patients with duodenal ulceration produce more gastric acid than normal controls, although the mean level for the population with ulcers is above the mean of normals. Many patients with an ulcer have gastric emptying times that are normal or even longer than normal. The parietal cell mass in some normal individuals is greater than that in those with ulcers. In most patients with a duodenal ulcer, there are no excessive basal or food-stimulated levels of gastrin, and the G cells respond normally to inhibitory factors. The litany of refutation could be continued. Recourse has therefore been made to concomitant presumed failure in normal defense mechanisms, at least in some individuals; such failures include deficiencies in mucosal cell renewal, in mucus production, in elaboration of bicarbonate (which serves to neutralize the acidity), and in production of prostaglandin. Among these defenses, particular emphasis is placed on defective bicarbonate secretion (attributed to a raised threshold for secretin release in ulcer patients) and an inadequate production of cytoprotective prostaglandins, particularly $PGE_2$ (p. 39). Perhaps nonsteroidal anti-inflammatory drugs such as aspirin might contribute (more in the gastric mucosa than in the duodenal mucosa) by inhibiting prostaglandin secretion.

What, then, can one cling to, in this welter of theory and contradiction? Only the proposition mentioned earlier—*the causation is multifactorial, and not all causal influences are operative in the individual. In some, hypersecretion of acid and pepsin may be dominant; in other normosecretors, defensive failures may render them vulnerable to even normal levels of acid and pepsin. In other words, there are many pathogenetic subsets of duodenal ulcer.*[39] Still unanswered is the question of why ulcers are discrete, solitary lesions when the entire first portion of the duodenum is exposed to similar conditions. In experimental models, local secretory and motility changes in the duodenum have been observed that might explain the focal nature of the destructive process, but the relevance of these observations to humans has not been established.[40] Obviously, there is still much to be learned.

**Gastric Ulcerogenesis.** Murky as the waters may be about the cause of duodenal ulcers, they are even murkier with respect to gastric ulcers.[41] The problem is made more complex by the recent suggestions that gastric ulcers can be divided into distinctive pathogenetic subsets, one basically related to bile reflux and low levels of gastric acid, and others that demonstrate less reflux but more acid. Despite the putative subsets, the following generalizations can be made about all gastric ulcers (Table 16–7).[42] On average, patients with gastric ulcers have normal or low levels of gastric acid–pepsin secretion, which are possibly related to chronic gastritis. However, these individuals are never completely achlorhydric. Whether these acid levels are spuriously low because of back-diffusion of hydrogen ions is not clear. The gastritis appears to be primary because it may persist after the ulcer heals. Most patients with gastric ulcers have more duodenogastric reflux than normal individuals. The exposure of the gastric mucosa to duodenal contents, particularly bile acids, lysolecithin, and pancreatic secretions, contributes to the gastritis and, in turn, the damaged mucosa permits ulcerogenesis. Still to be evaluated is the role of *Campylobacter* organisms in the possible causation of chronic gastritis and gastric ulcer.[25] No longer considered important is delayed emptying of the stomach, which might expose the mucosa longer to meal-stimulated gastric acid–pepsin and refluxed duodenal contents.

Defects in gastric mucosal resistance are favored mechanisms but have been challenged. Gastric mucosal ischemia is thought to be a major contributor to the development of acute stress ulcers, and it is reasoned by analogy that local areas of ischemia may potentiate solitary peptic ulcers. Repeatedly, some quantitative or qualitative defect in the mucous secretion of the gastric mucosa is raised as a possible contributing mechanism. This theory is supported largely by the beneficial effects of therapeutic regimens that augment secretion of mucus.[43] Presumably, the mucous surface gel aids in the prevention of diffusion of hydrogen ions from the gastric lumen into the mucosa. At the same time, the surface cells elaborate a bicarbonate buffer that is secreted into the mucous gel, further providing a defense mechanism. However, studies to date have not demonstrated convincing evidence of either quantitative or qualitative deficiencies in mucus secretion. As with the duodenal ulcer story, prostaglandin $E_2$ may participate in the mucosal defense. In this connection, aspirin, which is known to cause back-diffusion of hydrogen ions and plays a role in chronic gastritis, may simultaneously inhibit prostaglandin secretion and in this manner may favor gastric ulcerogenesis. Indeed, when chronic antral gastritis is not present, a history of chronic consumption of aspirin can usually be found. Epidemiologic evidence also suggests, as noted earlier (p. 517), a correlation between the intensity and duration of cigarette smoking and the prevalence of gastric ulcers. Analogously, there is an association of adrenocorticosteroid therapy and peptic ulceration.[44] Emotional factors have also been proposed, but the line of evidence is tenuous. Much is speculative, and we must conclude that with gastric ulcers, as with duodenal ulcers, substantial proof of the specific mechanisms leading to their causation is lacking; once again, the likelihood of a multifactorial pathophysiology and multiple subsets must be raised.

**MORPHOLOGY. All peptic ulcers, whether gastric or duodenal, have a basically identical gross appearance. They are round, sharply punched-out holes in the mucosa that penetrate at least into the submucosa and usually into the muscularis.** On occasion they penetrate the wall. Most are 2 to 4 cm in diameter but some are smaller, particularly in the duodenum, and some, usually gastric lesions, are significantly larger. A few unusually large gastric ulcers are sometimes misconstrued to be ulcerative cancers. **In order of frequency, the favored sites for peptic ulcers are the anterior wall of the first portion of the duodenum, the posterior wall of the first portion, and the lesser curvature of the stomach.** The location within the stomach is dictated by the extent of the associated gastritis. Most often, the gastritis involves the entire antrum, and so the ulcer crater is located within the margin of the gastritis closely adjacent to the acid-secreting fundus. Should the gastritis be more extensive, the ulcer will be located more proximally but once again within the zone of gastritis. Occasionally gastric ulcers occur on the greater curvature or anterior or posterior wall, the very same locations where ulcerative cancers are found.

Classically, the margins of the ulcer crater are perpendicular; however, the upstream margin may overhang slightly and the downstream margin may have a slight shelf. **The crater base appears remarkably clean, and the mucosal margins are not elevated, heaped up, or beaded (features of the ulcerative cancer).** On occasion, an eroded vessel can be seen in the base—the origin of the bleeding that may have caused death. With chronicity and underlying scarring, the rugal folds are puckered and appear to radiate out from the crater (Fig. 16–5). In the deeply penetrating ulcer, serosal inflammation may cause adherence to some surrounding viscus, such as the liver or pancreas, and indeed may seal

---

**Table 16–7. PHYSIOLOGIC DEFECTS IN PATIENTS WITH GASTRIC ULCER (NON-DRUG-RELATED)**

Decreased pyloric pressure at rest and in response to acid or fat in duodenum

Increased reflux of duodenal contents (bile and lysolecithin) into stomach, which leads to increased back-diffusion of hydrogen ions into gastric mucosa and acute superficial gastritis

Chronic atrophic gastritis of entire antral mucosa with variable extension into acid-secreting mucosa

Decreased maximal acid output paralleling degree of involvement of acid-secreting mucosa by chronic atrophic gastritis

Occurrence of gastric ulcer in an area of the stomach involved by chronic atrophic gastritis

From Holt, K. M., and Isenberg, J. I.: Peptic ulcer disease: Physiology and pathophysiology. Hosp. Pract. 20:101, 1985.

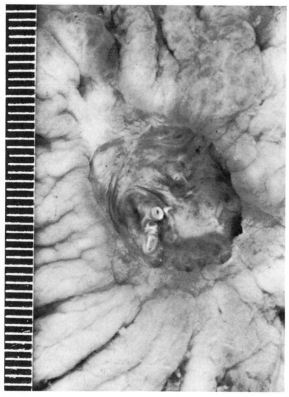

Figure 16–5. A gastric peptic ulcer. The crater has a maximum diameter of about 2 cm, is sharply punched out, and has a deceptively clean base and an eroded, almost transected artery protruding from it. Note the radiating mucosal folds.

the base even with through-and-through penetration (Fig. 16–6). However, "free" perforation into the peritoneal cavity is a well-recognized calamity, more often true of the duodenal than of the gastric lesion.

The histologic appearance varies with the activity, chronicity, and degree of healing. During the active phase, four zones can be distinguished. (1) The base and margins have a thin layer of necrotic fibrinoid debris, underlaid by (2) a zone of active nonspecific inflammatory cell infiltrate with neutrophils predominating, underlaid by (3) active granulation tissue, deep to which is (4) a more solid, fibrous, or collagenous scar that fans out widely toward the serosal surface. The vessel walls within the scarred area are characteristically thickened and occasionally thrombosed, but in some instances they are widely patent, as mentioned. In the gastric lesion, the margins typically show chronic atrophic gastritis (p. 514), and often there is intestinal metaplasia of the glands in the zone of gastritis.

Both gastric and duodenal ulcers may heal, involving filling of the crater with granulation tissue followed by reepithelialization from the margins. Then, over time, differentiation of the newly formed surface layer of cells occurs, which recapitulates, more or less, the normal mucosa, but the underlying scar persists as a permanent residual. In some instances the scarring and consequent ischemia are so marked as to inhibit healing.

**CLINICAL COURSE.** Peptic ulcers are relapsing conditions that tend to recur for the remainder of the patient's life. However, *most patients die with their ulcer or the diathesis for it, rather than of it.* Typically, an active attack is marked by epigastric pain, which is gnawing, burning, or hunger-like. It may be referred to the back (particularly with posterior penetrating lesions) or it may be substernal and be confused with pain of cardiac origin. However, some patients merely have some vague epigastric discomfort or are asymptomatic even with active disease, and the lesion is first brought to attention

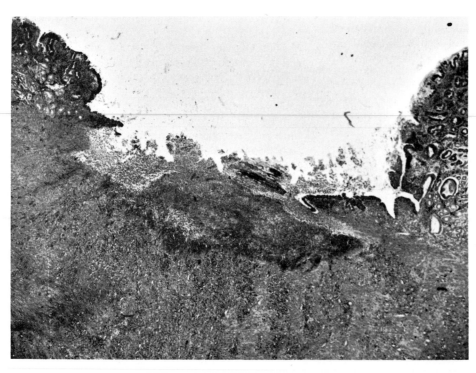

Figure 16–6. A low-power view of a peptic ulcer, illustrating the depth of the lesion.

by a massive bleed or perforation. When pain is present, it may have its onset one to several hours after meals and be relieved by food and antacids. But this "typical" sequence is more often absent than present. The pain may not be relieved by eating, or indeed may be triggered by eating, or it may be sporadic and without relation to food. The old notion that patients with gastric ulcers have different types of pain and pain sequences than those with duodenal ulcers does not stand up to critical analysis. The diagnosis rests ultimately on barium studies and endoscopy of the upper gastrointestinal tract. Determination of the serum level of pepsinogen-1 by radioimmunoassay may provide a clue (when elevated) to a familial pattern of duodenal disease.

The complications of peptic ulcer disease are shown in Table 16–8. *Malignant transformation is unknown with duodenal ulcers and is extremely rare with gastric ulcers.* Much more likely is the misinterpretation of an ulcerative cancer as a benign gastric ulcer that is later discovered to indeed be a cancer.

Distressing as the manifestations of an ulcer may be, the lesion is not often a threat to life. Those with a duodenal ulcer can usually struggle through bouts of active disease under medical regimens with their entrails intact. However, because of the potential of carcinoma masquerading as a benign gastric ulcer, patients with a gastric lesion resistant to medical control may come to surgery.[45]

# TUMORS

A wide variety of mesenchymal neoplasms, such as leiomyomas, leiomyosarcomas, neurofibromas, and lipomas, may arise in the stomach but are all too rare for inclusion here. Also, carcinoids are sometimes primary tumors in the stomach. Because these neoplasms are identical to those of the small intestine, where they are more frequent, they are described in a later section (p. 536). Only polyps, gastric carcinoma, and gastrointestinal lymphomas remain for our present consideration.

**Table 16–8. COMPLICATIONS OF PEPTIC ULCER DISEASE**

**Bleeding**
 Occurs in 25 to 33% of patients
 Most frequent complication; may be massive
 Accounts for about 25% of ulcer deaths
 May be first indication of presence of ulcer

**Perforation**
 Occurs in only 5% of patients
 Accounts for two thirds of all ulcer deaths
 Rarely, is first indication of ulcer

**Obstruction from Edema or Scarring of Pyloric Canal or Duodenum**
 Causes incapacitating, crampy abdominal pain
 Rarely, may lead to total obstruction with intractable vomiting

**Intractable Pain**

**Table 16–9. COMPARISON OF HYPERPLASTIC AND ADENOMATOUS GASTRIC POLYPS**

| Hyperplastic (80%) | Adenomatous (20%) |
|---|---|
| May be single, often multiple | Usually single, but sometimes multiple |
| Soft, pink, nipple-shaped | Have rasberry-like head or appear verrucose and corrugated; may be sessile or pedunculated |
| Usually less than 1 cm in diameter; rarely exceed 2 cm in diameter | May be small, but often exceed 2 cm in diameter |
| Composed of hyperplastic, sometimes cystic, glands lined by normal epithelium resembling that found in surrounding normal gastric pits | Epithelium ranges from well-differentiated, benign-appearing neoplastic cells to poorly differentiated cells with hyperchromatic, overly large nuclei; frequent mitotic figures |
| Intervening stroma usually contains a chronic inflammatory infiltrate | 20 to 25% incidence of malignant transformation[46] |
| Have no malignant potential | |

## GASTRIC POLYPS

The term "polyp" is applied to any nodule or mass that projects above the level of the surrounding mucosa. Occasionally, a lipoma or leiomyoma arising in the wall of the stomach may protrude beneath the mucosa to produce an apparent polypoid lesion. However, *the use of the term "polyp" in the gastrointestinal tract is generally restricted to proliferative and neoplastic lesions arising in the mucosal epithelium.* Gastric polyps are uncommon and are found in 0.4% of routine autopsies, as compared with colonic polyps, which are seen in 25 to 50% of older individuals. *In the stomach, these lesions can be divided into: (1) hyperplastic polyps (80%) and (2) adenomatous polyps (20%).* They are most frequent in the elderly and are associated with achlorhydria and atrophic gastritis; therefore, they are reported in 5% of all patients with pernicious anemia. The essential features of these lesions are given in Table 16–9. From the clinical viewpoint, the likelihood of carcinoma in an adenomatous polyp is correlated with its size and irregularity of contour. Often the stomach harboring a polyp contains a separate carcinoma that may have arisen from a polyp or from an area of chronic atrophic gastritis, which is commonly found in these cases. Multiple polyps are seen in familial polyposis and Peutz-Jeghers and Gardner's syndromes (p. 555).

## GASTRIC CARCINOMA

No longer at the top of the list of cancer-killers in the United States, gastric carcinoma still ranks among the top ten. In contrast to the rates for most forms of cancer, its incidence has declined in the United States from 33 per 100,000 in 1930 to its present level of about six per 100,000. The reasons for this happy trend are mysterious, but the trend is not worldwide. Japan, Chile, Iceland, and Finland have death rates many times those of the low-risk countries.[47] Indeed, in Japan gastric carcinoma is the leading cause of cancer death in males. As will become clear, environmental rather than racial differences are thought to account for these striking differences.

In low-risk countries gastric cancer generally appears in the seventh or eighth decade of life; it is seen only rarely in those under 40 years. The male-female ratio is approximately 1.5:1. In high-risk countries such as Japan, the peak incidence is earlier and there is a stronger male preponderance.

**ETIOLOGY AND PATHOGENESIS.** Arguing strongly for the importance of environmental influences in the initiation of gastric carcinoma is the progressive decline in its incidence in successive generations after migration from high- to low-risk locales (and vice versa). Among the potential environmental influences (Table 16–10), diet has evoked the most interest. Nearly every food known to humans—pickled foods, smoked meat and fish, rice, grain products—has at one time or another been implicated except, fortunately, marshmallows. The favored culprit today is nitrites, which are incorporated into nitrosamines, as detailed on page 251.[48] Correlations have been drawn between gastric carcinoma and the nitrite content of the stomach.[49] Nitrites have long been used as food preservatives, particularly in smoked meats, sausages, frankfurters, and other foods, and widespread use of refrigeration may therefore contribute to the declining incidence of gastric cancer in some countries. Whole milk, fresh fruits, and vegetables (particularly those high in vitamin C) in the diet appear to exert protective effects against this form of neoplasia.[50] It is relevant that vitamin C inhibits the reduction of nitrates to nitrites.

Genetic influences cited in Table 16–10 may also play some role, but only about 4% of patients with a

**Table 16–10.** FACTORS IN GASTRIC CARCINOGENESIS

**Environmental**
Diet
? Nitrites (endogenous and exogenous)
? Low socioeconomic class
? Urban dwelling
? Background irradiation
? Trace elements in soil and water
? Iatrogenic (cimetidine)

**Genetic**
Greater than chance concordance in monozygotic twins
Slightly increased risk in individuals with blood group A
High-incidence families (rare)

**Predisposing Conditions**
Gastric adenomatous polyps
Chronic gastritis, especially in pernicious anemia
Status postgastrectomy

gastric carcinoma have a family history of this form of neoplasia.

*Relative to the clinical conditions predisposing to gastric carcinoma, the least controversial is the association with gastric adenomas,* as has already been discussed on page 521. Chronic gastritis, with its intestinal metaplasia and sometimes dysplasia of mucosal cells, significantly increases the risk of gastric carcinoma.[51] On this account *the atrophic gastritis or gastric atrophy of pernicious anemia is viewed as a precancerous condition,* incurring a threefold increased risk.

*After gastrectomy for benign disease, there is an increased incidence of gastric carcinoma in the remaining stump of the stomach.* Various surveys suggest an incidence of 3%.[52] In some part this association may be related to the frequency of gastritis in the postgastrectomy stump. It is advocated, therefore, that patients with all these conditions repeatedly undergo endoscopy and biopsy to maintain watch for the possible appearance of epithelial dysplasia or "early gastric carcinoma" (as is explained in the following discussion).

**MORPHOLOGY.** The attempt to delineate distinctive clinicomorphologic subsets of gastric carcinoma has led to a proliferation of classifications greater than the proliferative capabilities of the cells being classified. No attempt will be made to delve into all the permutations; remarks will be limited to only the chief categories. Perhaps the most important of these classifications is the division of gastric carcinomas into **early gastric cancer** and **advanced gastric cancer.**

*Concept of Early Gastric Cancer (EGC).* Because of the high mortality from gastric carcinoma, Japanese physicians have recommended gastric endoscopic examinations as a part of routine medical checkups. Many asymptomatic EGCs have thus been discovered. **This term is applied to those cancers that have not invaded the muscularis and are therefore limited to the mucosa and submucosa.**[53] EGC may involve a small area or may sometimes be quite extensive, suggesting the possibility of coalescent multicentric origins. When transected and viewed on profile, an EGC may be mildly elevated, level with the surrounding mucosa, depressed, or even minimally ulcerated (Fig. 16–7). It requires emphasis, **EGC is not synonymous with "in-situ" carcinoma, which implies that the lesion has not even invaded the lamina propria of the mucosa.** Further, EGC may be accompanied by lymph node metastases in a few cases, and in this sense it is not necessarily a disease in its incipient early stage. Nonetheless, it is usually curable by gastric resection and, as will be seen, has a far better prognosis than advanced cancers.[54]

The question arises, is EGC merely a precursor to advanced cancer, discovered at a felicitous stage in its evolution? The most likely answer is "yes." In the experimental animal, gastric cancer induced by chemical carcinogens progresses through EGC to become an advanced lesion. Advanced cancer has followed incomplete

**Early Gastric Cancer**

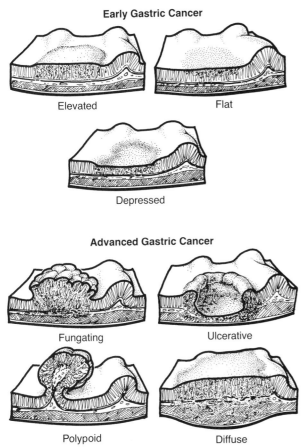

Elevated

Flat

Depressed

**Advanced Gastric Cancer**

Fungating

Ulcerative

Polypoid

Diffuse

Figure 16–7. A representation of the range of macroscopic appearances of "early" and "advanced" gastric carcinoma.

resection of EGC in humans. However, a few observations raise the possibility that EGC may be a different biological entity from the usual advanced carcinoma. The average age of patients with EGC is not significantly younger than those with advanced lesions. Moreover, the presence of lymph node metastases does not seem to affect the outlook.

*Advanced Cancer.* As this term is employed here, it implies that **the neoplasm has extended below the submucosa, infiltrated the muscularis, and perhaps spread more widely.** In the United States, where periodic endoscopic screening of asymptomatic individuals is not practiced, at least 90% of gastric carcinomas, when discovered, would qualify as "advanced." In contrast, in Japan as many as one third of gastric carcinomas constitute EGC. When the site of origin of an invasive lesion can be identified, 50 to 60% arise in the distal pyloroantral segment and only about 15 to 25% are seen more proximally in the cardia. The remainder are diffuse when discovered. They may be located on either curvature or the anterior or posterior walls, or they may involve nearly the entire stomach. Location is of little value in judging whether a lesion is likely to be a cancer or a benign process.[55]

One classification of overt neoplasms divides them on the basis of their gross morphology into (1) fungating, (2) ulcerative, (3) polypoid, and (4) diffusely infiltrative (Fig. 16–7). These terms are merely descriptive; all neoplasms may penetrate to variable depths and appear beneath the serosa as small white, firm nodules, but at the same time they may infiltrate the surrounding wall of the stomach more or less widely. Only two of these patterns require comment. **The ulcerative carcinoma can usually be differentiated from a peptic ulcer on gross inspection.** The cancerous craters are usually (but not always) larger than peptic ulcers, the margins are heaped up and beaded, the base is often shaggy and necrotic, and there is generally overt neoplastic white tissue infiltrating the base and extending laterally into the wall (Fig. 16–8). **In the infiltrative diffuse pattern,** a portion or sometimes the entire stomach wall is thickened (up to 2 cm) but there is no intraluminal mass. The mucosa may have shallow ulcerations, and the underlying wall becomes inelastic, giving rise to the older designations of "linitis plastica," or "leather-bottle" stomach.

Descriptive as the above terms may be, it has been argued that they have little biologic significance because all these lesions pursue a similar course and have the same prognosis, depending on the extent and spread of the lesion. Several other classifications have therefore

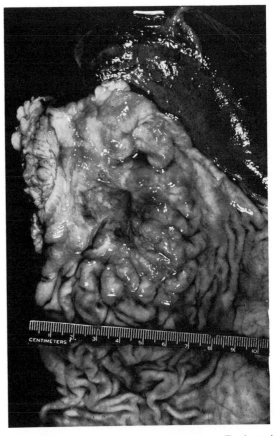

Figure 16–8. Gastric carcinoma, ulcerative pattern. The irregular ulcer crater is situated high in the fundus and has penetrated into the adjacent spleen, which can be seen above it. Note the beaded margins of the ulcer crater and the irregular base.

been proposed. One divides them into (1) **expanding growth patterns,** and (2) **infiltrative growth patterns.**[56] Expanding tumors are characterized by the tendency for cohesive masses of tumor cells to push along a broad front into the stomach wall. It is argued that this pattern of growth tends to be less infiltrative and more amenable to curative resection. In contrast, the infiltrative pattern is marked by strands, nests, and isolated cells that permeate and invade the stomach wall. **Another classification, by Lauren, divides gastric carcinoma into two histologic subsets: (1) diffuse (infiltrative) carcinoma, and (2) intestinal-type carcinoma.**[57] In a general way, the intestinal type conforms to the expanding subset mentioned earlier, since the neoplastic cells have a tendency to reproduce glandular structures interspersed sometimes with papillary formations or solid sheets of cells. The individual cells tend to be columnar in orientation and anaplastic, and sometimes they contain distinct, often multiple, small vacuoles of mucin secretion reminiscent of intestinal-type epithelium. In contrast, the infiltrative neoplasms do not form cohesive masses of cells or epithelium-like cords, and the neoplastic cells are often accompanied by a prominent desmoplastic stroma. Evident within the cells of most of these infiltrative lesions is abundant mucin secretion, sometimes filling the cell and displacing the nucleus to create so-called **signet-ring cells.** For obscure reasons, signet-ring cell carcinomas appear to be occurring more frequently now, particularly in women, accounting at least in part for gastric carcinomas developing almost as often in females as in males (a departure from yesteryear).[58, 59]

One more uncommon but highly interesting form of gastric carcinoma requires mention. It is referred to as "undifferentiated" but is actually thought to be of neuroendocrine origin, derived from enterochromaffin cells found in the gastric mucosa and throughout the gut.[59a] In most of these cancers the cells are small, round to ovoid, and deeply hyperchromatic; they grow in undifferentiated sheets. Rarely, gland formations are produced. Often, the cells contain membrane-bounded cytoplasmic granules that have an affinity for silver salts (argentaffin-positive). Such tumors are now classified as APUDomas (p. 537) and have the capacity to elaborate many different hormones.

Several systems for staging of gastric carcinomas have been devised. One is based on the TNM system; another is basically a surgical system applied after excision of the lesion. Details of these approaches are available in a recent publication.[60]

**CLINICAL COURSE.** Gastric carcinomas usually remain silent until quite late in their course. Even after symptoms arise, they tend to be vague and tolerable to the patient, so that the average lapse of time between their appearance and the patient's seeking medical attention is from six months to one year. By the time the classic syndrome of anorexia, weight loss, and epigastric pain with a palpable mass has developed, the lesion is far advanced. Occult bleeding from the tumor is common and often leads to iron deficiency anemia, but hematemesis and melena from this cause are rare.

Frequently, obvious metastatic disease is the first indication of the gastric carcinoma. Regional lymph nodes and the liver are usually first involved, and the patient may present with hepatomegaly or ascites. Characteristically, there is spread not only to the regional lymph nodes but also to the supraclavicular (*Virchow's*) nodes and scalene nodes. Because these are readily accessible to biopsy, their involvement is of diagnostic importance. Another peculiarity of gastric carcinoma is its tendency toward widespread intraperitoneal seeding. This seeding is most apparent in the pelvis, where a tumor mass in the peritoneal cul-de-sac may be palpable on rectal examination (*rectal shelf*). *A particularly striking mode of spread is to the ovaries, creating large ovarian masses called Krukenberg tumors* (p. 654). Krukenberg tumors may also occur from dissemination of cancers of the pancreas, gallbladder, and other abdominal viscera.

Diagnosis of gastric carcinoma may be made by several different techniques, including barium and computerized tomography studies, gastroscopy, cytologic tests, and scalene node biopsy. Endoscopic biopsy and cytologic examination of gastric secretions are especially important with early lesions and as a routine method of evaluating patients with predisposing disorders, such as atrophic gastritis. When this method is properly performed, more than 90% of cases can be diagnosed.

The overall five-year survival rate with advanced gastric carcinoma in the United States remains as it has for years, in the range of 5 to 15%, because curative resections are only attempted in 35 to 40% of patients. This is in striking contrast to the 80 to 95% five-year survival rates for early gastric carcinoma in Japan.[61] It is obvious that the challenge for the future in low-risk nations is the discovery of gastric cancers while they are curable.

## GASTROINTESTINAL LYMPHOMAS

Lymphomas, usually of the diffuse, non-Hodgkin's types, may arise in any level of the gastrointestinal tract. The stomach and the small intestine are the two most common sites affected, but wherever lymphomas arise, the lesions are much the same and so all are considered here.[62] Lymphomas may also spread to the gastrointestinal tract from other origins. *Unfortunately, the term "primary" is used both for those arising in the gut and for those arising elsewhere when the initial manifestations of the disease are gastrointestinal in nature.* Whatever the definition, primary lymphomas constitute 1 to 4% of all malignant tumors in the alimentary tract, a percentage that is likely to rise as the prevalence of gastric carcinomas falls.

Wherever they arise in the gastrointestinal tract, primary lymphomas take one of three forms: (1) **polypoid masses projecting into the lumen;** (2) **large, elevated plaques often having shaggy necrotic, ulcerated craters;** or (3) **infiltrative neoplasms producing irregular thickening of the wall of the gut.** Any one of these three patterns may occur as a single focus in the gastrointestinal tract, but more often, multiple sites are involved, usually within one segment of the gut. They may be limited to the gut, but more often, they are accompanied by involvement of regional or more disseminated lymph nodes and sometimes of other organs, such as the liver and spleen. **The ulcerative pattern in the stomach or colon may be difficult to distinguish from an ulcerative carcinoma, and the infiltrative pattern in the stomach may cause massive thickening of the rugal folds, producing a close resemblance to infiltrative carcinoma or to the rare hypertrophic gastritis.** In contrast, in the small bowel, the lymphoma tends to be multifocal or sometimes diffusely infiltrative and therefore quite distinctive from other forms of neoplasia. Whatever the distribution, individual lesions are typically soft gray and of fish-flesh consistency and may have areas of necrosis or hemorrhage.

Histologically, lymphomas of the gastrointestinal tract conform to one of the patterns of the non-Hodgkin's lymphomas described in an earlier chapter (p. 369).[63] The most common variant in nearly all analyses is diffuse histiocytic lymphoma (in the Rappaport classification), but immunologic marker studies usually identify it as a large B-cell lymphoma. An unusual type of lymphoma found mainly in the gastrointestinal tract is made of B lymphocytes differentiating toward plasma cells. This is sometimes called plasmacytoid lymphocytic lymphoma. When first recognized in the Middle East, identical neoplasms were referred to as Mediterranean-type lymphomas.[64]

The clinical manifestations of lymphomas are much the same as those produced by carcinomas in comparable segments of the gut and include principally nausea, vomiting, weakness, and weight loss. Colonic lesions sometimes cause abdominal pain or lower abdominal cramps, change in bowel habit, diarrhea, and possibly melena. Diffuse lymphomatous involvement of the small intestine may lead to a malabsorption syndrome (described later). The diagnosis of all lymphomas depends largely on radiologic studies, including CT scan, and on biopsy and endoscopy for gastric and colonic involvements.

The single most important determinant of prognosis is the extent of disease at time of diagnosis. The Ann Arbor staging classification of the lymphomas is used to express the distribution of the disease (p. 375).[62] Overall, the five-year survival rate following surgery, radiation, chemotherapy, or any combination of these therapies is better than that for carcinomas; the range is from an almost 80% five-year survival rate for those with localized disease to an outlook of 12 to 18 months for those with advanced disease.

# Small Intestine

Despite its extended length, the small intestine is curiously far less frequently the seat of disease than the stomach or the colon. Inflammatory diseases and ischemic lesions are more frequent than neoplasms, which are, on the whole, rare, and of which, surprisingly, carcinomas represent only a modest fraction. Malabsorptive syndromes, with various diffuse small intestinal involvements, are also encountered with some frequency.

Before turning to these more significant conditions, a few words about some uncommon developmental lesions are necessary. Anomalous development may result in missing segments or segments that constitute only an unchannelled cord (*atresias*). When a narrow lumen persists, it is called *stenosis*. These may occur singly or at many points at any level of the small intestine, are usually recognized early in life because of signs of obstruction, and are readily managed with surgery. A more frequent anomaly is a rest of *aberrant (heterotopic) pancreatic tissue* (rarely more than 1 to 2 cm in diameter) that is usually located beneath the mucosa, most often in the duodenum. Sometimes a rest protrudes as an apparently sessile nodule into the lumen and may be mistaken for a neoplasm by the radiologist or endoscopist.

## DIVERTICULA

Saccular outpouchings creating diverticula (2 to 3 cm in diameter) are uncommon lesions but are more frequent in the duodenum than in the jejunum or ileum. They tend to be solitary in the duodenum and associated with a healed duodenal ulcer. Multiple saccules, presumably developmental in origin, are more typically found in the jejunum and ileum. Duodenal diverticula may impinge on the pancreatic or common bile ducts, but those in the lower segments assume importance because intestinal stasis within their lumens permits overgrowth of bacteria that use excessive amounts of vitamin $B_{12}$, yielding a syndrome similar to pernicious anemia. Any of these diverticula is subject to inflammation, erosion, and, rarely, perforation when food becomes impacted within it.

*Meckel's diverticulum* is a more important clinical disorder because it occurs in 1 to 2% of the general population.[1] It represents the persistence of a remnant of the omphalomesenteric duct.

These diverticula are usually located within 12 inches of the ileocecal valve, rarely more proximally. They vary from a fibrotic cord to a pouch having a lumen larger than that of the ileum and a length up

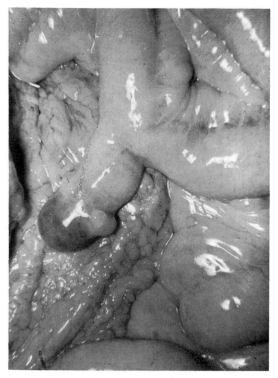

Figure 16–9. Meckel's diverticulitis. The tip of the diverticulum is reddened because of peptic ulceration near a contained rest of gastric epithelium.

to 6 cm. The histologic features of the wall are basically similar to those of the small bowel, but *in about one half of the cases, there are also heterotopic islands of functioning gastric mucosa.* Peptic ulceration in the adjacent mucosa may give rise to symptoms resembling acute appendicitis or to mysterious intestinal bleeding (Fig. 16–9). Infrequently, perforation occurs, or the inflammatory disease causes adhesion to nearby loops of bowel and results in intestinal obstruction. Pancreatic rests may occur in Meckel's diverticula, but they are infrequent.

## ISCHEMIC BOWEL DISEASE

Ischemic lesions of the intestines may be restricted to the small intestine or the colon alone, or they may affect both areas. The localization of the involvement and its distribution (patchy, segmental, or involving long tracts of the intestine) is dependent on many factors, principally, the nature of the arterial supply. The three major supply trunks—celiac, superior, and inferior mesenteric arteries—are richly interconnected by arcades. For example, occlusion of the superior mesenteric artery may in some circumstances produce ischemia not only of much of the small intestine but also of a portion of the large intestine if the other two trunks are already compromised. Obstruction to one (say, by an embolus) may be without

effect if adequate vascular supply is provided by the remaining two. Indeed, if there are no preexisting severe narrowings, one of the three vessels may suffice to maintain the viability of the entire small and large intestine. Other variables include (1) the rate of acquisition of the narrowing or occlusion (slowly developing vascular compromise provides the opportunity for augmentation of the anastomotic collateral flow), (2) the adequacy of the systemic circulation, and (3) the oxygen partial pressure ($Po_2$) of the blood. With all these variables, it should be evident why ischemic lesions may be patchy or large and may affect one or the other level of the bowel or sometimes both regions.

There are numerous causes for vascular compromise of the intestines, as is indicated in Table 16–11.[65] The bowel changes induced by ischemia are the same, whatever the cause. Only these generalizations can be made. The small intestine, which is entirely dependent on the mesenteric blood supply, is more often affected than the colon, which in some areas has additional vascular connections from the posterior abdominal wall. However, the amount of bowel damage for comparable levels of ischemia tends to be greater in the colon because of the rapidity of secondary bacterial invasion there. When the colon is affected, the injury tends to occur in the regions of the splenic flexure and middle portion of the rectum because these areas are watersheds between the superior mesenteric and the inferior mesenteric arteries (for the splenic flexure) and the inferior mesenteric and the hypogastric arteries (for the middle

**Table 16–11. CAUSES OF ISCHEMIC INJURY TO BOWEL**

**30 to 35% of Cases**
*Occlusion of Superior Mesenteric Artery*
  Emboli from left heart
  Thrombi overlying atheromas
  Thrombi secondary to arteritis
  Dissecting aortic aneurysm

**15 to 20% of Cases**
*Occlusion of Inferior Mesenteric Artery*
  As above
  Ligation during replacement of aortic aneurysm with graft
*Mesenteric Venous Occlusion*
  Oral contraceptives
  Cardiac failure
  Polycythemia
  Compression in hernial sacs or by peritoneal adhesions
  Hypercoagulability

**15 to 20% of Cases**
*Nonocclusive Intestinal Ischemia—Low Perfusion States*
  Cardiac failure or shock
    Fibromuscular hyperplasia of end arteries
    ? Digitalis
    ? Norepinephrine

**30 to 35% of Cases**
*Idiopathic (No Occlusion Found)*
  ? Fibrinolytic dissolution of a clot
  ? Fragmentation
  ? Spasm

rectum). The mucosa and submucosa of the intestines are vulnerable to ischemia (the small intestine more so than the large) and may undergo edema and hemorrhagic sloughing; low perfusion states will spare the deeper layers. However, nonocclusive low perfusion, when severe and prolonged, may cause total infarction of the bowel.

In order to express the range of tissue lesions, they have been subdivided into (1) *transmural infarction, embracing the older designation of gangrene of the bowel;* (2) *mural infarction, which shows ischemic injury to mucosa, submucosa, and muscularis but spares the serosa;* and (3) *mucosal infarction, in which only the mucosa and perhaps the submucosa are injured by low perfusion states, usually without a well-defined occlusion.*[66]

## TRANSMURAL INTESTINAL INFARCTION

Also called *"gangrene of the bowel," "mesenteric vascular occlusion"* and, when colonic, *"ischemic colitis,"* this pattern of vascular compromise is an extremely grave clinical emergency. When the clinical setting is appropriate, prompt surgical resection is required. It is usually the consequence of occlusion of one or more large mesenteric vessels and only rarely is seen with low perfusion states. The small bowel is involved more often than the colon, and the mortality rate ranges from about 25% when related to strangulation in a hernial sac or when caused by intestinal adhesions, up to about 75% when caused by mesenteric vascular occlusion, which can be either thrombotic or embolic.[67] The prognosis is heavily dependent on the age of the patient (average age between 60 and 70 years), length of bowel infarcted, and elapsed time before surgical intervention.

Transmural infarction of the bowel may be patchy or may involve a short or long segment, sometimes more than 100 cm of the small bowel. Whether the occlusion is arterial or venous, the infarction always appears hemorrhagic because of the rich anastomotic arcades of the mesenteric arterial supply. Within 18 to 24 hours, the affected area or segment is dusky purple-red with foci of subserosal and submucosal hemorrhage (Fig. 16–10).[68] Later the wall becomes edematous, thickened, and rubbery. With arterial occlusion, the demarcation from adjacent normal bowel is fairly sharply defined. Venous occlusion results in ill-defined margins. The histologic changes are those that would be anticipated: extreme congestion of vessels followed by edema; extravasation of blood into the mucosa, submucosa, and subserosa; and, often, sloughing of the mucosa. Secondary bacterial invasion complicates the changes with the passage of time. A nonspecific acute inflammatory infiltrate will appear at the margins toward the end of the first day. When surgical resection has been delayed longer than 24 hours, a fibrinous peritonitis becomes evident, or sometimes the infarcted bowel perforates. In most instances, the cellular coagulative changes expected in an infarct are not well

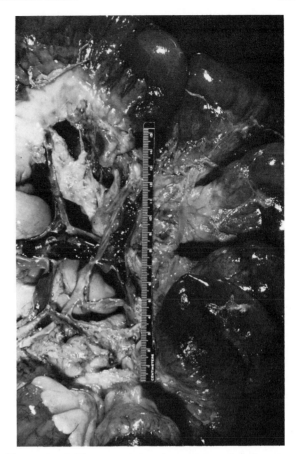

**Figure 16–10.** The mesenteric veins contain a dark thrombus, and the involved loops of small intestine are darkened by the venous infarction.

developed either because the bowel has been resected promptly or the patient has succumbed.

Like other vascular calamities (e.g., dissecting aneurysm) within the abdomen, mesenteric occlusion is often characterized by the sudden onset of excruciating pain in the absence of positive physical findings. There may be associated nausea, vomiting, or bloody diarrhea. At this stage, it may be extremely difficult to distinguish mesenteric vascular occlusion from more common causes of an acute abdomen, especially a perforated peptic ulcer or acute pancreatitis. Some clue to the correct diagnosis may be offered, however, by the strange tendency of vascular calamities to produce *severe* pain significantly before physical findings develop. Selective angiography is helpful in establishing the diagnosis. Unless mesenteric vascular occlusion is recognized and treated early, these patients follow an extremely fulminating course, leading to death within 48 hours from shock, perforation and sepsis, or hemorrhage.

## MUCOSAL AND MURAL INFARCTION

These patterns of ischemic injury have in the past been called *"acute hemorrhagic enteropathy."* Typically, there is less than complete transmural damage related in most instances to hypoperfusion of the bowel secondary to cardiac failure or shock (p. 79). Sometimes these patients have received digitalis and norepinephrine, which are both vasoconstrictors, but how much these agents contribute to the reduced perfusion remains uncertain. Preexisting arterial narrowings, either in the main trunks (atherosclerosis) or in the terminal straight arterial segments just before they enter the intestine (secondary to radiation fibrosis or *fibromuscular hyperplasia*—an entity of unknown etiology), potentiate the damaging effects of low-flow states.

Characteristically, edematous hemorrhagic multifocal lesions are scattered throughout one region or many levels of the small and large intestine. This enigmatic distribution is probably dictated by preexisting, randomly distributed arterial narrowings. Affected foci may or may not be visible from the serosal surface, depending on the severity and depth of the hemorrhagic injury. **By definition, the entire thickness of the bowel and serosal surface is not affected** (Fig. 16–11). When the bowel is opened, hemorrhagic edematous thickening of the mucosa, sometimes with superficial ulcerations, can be seen. The histologic findings range from marked vascular congestion with surrounding edema or hemorrhagic suffusion to hemorrhagic and ischemic necrosis of the inner layers of gut. Inflammatory changes are remarkably scant but may appear with the passage of time; this is perhaps

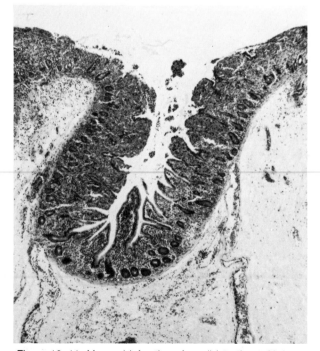

**Figure 16–11.** Mucosal infarction of small intestine, with hemorrhagic suffusion of the lamina propria and superficial sloughing of the surface at upper left. There is marked edema but no hemorrhage in the noninfarcted submucosa. (From Robbins, S. L., Cotran, R. S., and Kumar, V.: Pathologic Basis of Disease. 3rd ed. Philadelphia, W. B. Saunders Co., 1984, p. 833.)

related to bacterial superinfection. In some instances, pseudomembranous inflammation may supervene, particularly in the colon (p. 547).[68]

This pattern of ischemic injury usually presents with abdominal pain, cramps, and bloody diarrhea in a patient who has already been suffering from a myocardial infarct, cardiac failure, or shock. The manifestations must be distinguished from those caused by occlusion of major trunks and transmural infarction, and in many instances mesenteric angiography is required for this differential diagnosis. Mucosal and mural infarction rarely represents a surgical emergency and can be managed by supportive therapy. Indeed, depending on the extent of the infarction, the condition is reversible and there can be complete restoration of the bowel wall. However, resection may be demanded for correction of massive intestinal bleeding in a patient already gravely ill; this procedure carries with it a high mortality rate.

## INFLAMMATORY DISEASES

Abdominal cramps and diarrhea may have noninfectious origins, such as ischemic, uremic, radiation, and cytotoxic drug-induced injury to the bowel. These manifestations are also prominent features of two conditions of obscure origin—Crohn's disease and ulcerative colitis. However, such manifestations are more often caused by enteric infections with viruses, bacteria, or higher parasitic forms. The spectrum of infectious conditions ranges clinically from the more annoying than serious "traveler's diarrhea" to the potentially lethal cholera. Certain agents tend to affect the small intestine more than the colon and others do the converse, but in many instances, both levels of the gut are affected. It seems preferable therefore to treat these entities under the consideration of the colon (p. 540). Only one, Crohn's disease, is more rationally taken up here.

### CROHN'S DISEASE (REGIONAL ENTERITIS)

This chronic relapsing, inflammatory disorder of obscure cause may involve any portion of the gastrointestinal tract from esophagus to anus, but most often the small intestine and colon are affected. *Typically, the inflammatory involvement is sharply segmental.* Early descriptions of this condition emphasized the involvement of the terminal ileum and therefore the disease was called *"terminal or regional ileitis."* However, it was soon appreciated that other levels of the bowel were also frequently affected, *hence the term "regional enteritis."* The small bowel alone, particularly the terminal ileum, is affected in 30 to 35% of cases; disease in the small and large intestines together occurs in 50 to 60% of cases; and in approximately 20% of the cases, the colon alone is involved in the absence of small intestinal lesions.[69] Sometimes there are several diseased segments separated by apparently normal bowel (*skip lesions*). Another characteristic feature is that *the inflammatory reaction always extends through the gut wall into the mesentery, and in 50 to 70% of the cases, it is made distinctive by noncaseating granulomas.* Hence the colonic involvement is designated *"granulomatous colitis"* to differentiate it from the closely related ulcerative colitis.

Although principally a disorder of the alimentary tract, Crohn's disease has caused lesions in the skin, bones, skeletal muscles, synovial tissue, and elsewhere, making clear that this is a systemic disorder. Numerous extraintestinal complications are also seen; they include ankylosing spondylitis, erythema nodosum, myopericarditis, pericholangitis, sclerosing cholangitis, and autoimmune hemolytic anemia, to name a few. These complications appear after the onset of the inflammatory bowel disease and tend to disappear with healing or resection of the intestinal lesions, suggesting some causal association and once again highlighting the systemic nature of Crohn's disease.[70]

There are many similarities between Crohn's disease and ulcerative colitis, and so both are embraced by the term *"inflammatory bowel disease (IBD)."* But there are also some differences. These comparisons are cited in Table 16–12. Further, anatomic differences will emerge in the later discussion. However, in perhaps 10 to 20% of cases, the colitis of Crohn's disease cannot be distinguished either clinically or morphologically from ulcerative colitis.

**EPIDEMIOLOGY.** Although it is worldwide in distribution, there are significant differences in the prevalence of Crohn's disease among nations; incidence rates are around six per 100,000 in some countries (e.g., the United States, England, Scotland, and Scandinavia) and are significantly lower in Japan and the U.S.S.R., for example. The current rates in the high-risk countries reflect a steady increase over the past few decades that may be leveling off.[71] Much of the increase can be attributed to more frequent involvement of the colon than was usual in the past. Interestingly, there has been no comparable rise in the incidence of ulcerative colitis. In the United States, whites are affected more often than blacks (but this may be related in part to availability of medical services), females slightly more often than males, and Jews significantly more often than non-Jews. Most first attacks occur in the second or third decades of life, and there is a small secondary peak for first attacks in the sixth decade.

Many findings point to genetic predisposition; 15 to 40% of first-degree relatives of patients (including monozygotic and dizygotic twins) have inflammatory bowel disease. In unusual instances, five or more persons in the same family are involved. Linkage of a susceptibility gene to the HLA complex has been postulated; in some analyses of affected families, those with the disease share at least one haplotype or, in some instances, both maternal and paternal haplotypes.[72] Further, there is a well-defined association between inflammatory bowel disease and ankylosing spondylitis, the latter strongly linked to HLA-B27. These HLA associations have been interpreted to mean some inherited immunologic susceptibility to Crohn's disease. Nonetheless, no consistent HLA markers for Crohn's disease alone have been identified among all populations.

**ETIOLOGY AND PATHOGENESIS.** The search for the origin of Crohn's disease and ulcerative colitis has revealed many parallels, not the least of which is that both remain of unknown origin. So it is reasonable to consider here the etiology and pathogenesis of both together.

*Much of the epidemiologic data just cited is equally applicable to ulcerative colitis and is compatible with the thesis that both forms of inflammatory bowel disease (IBD) have their origins in genetically determined immunologic susceptibility to some environmental agent or agents.* Thus investigators have searched for a cause in (1) bacteria, (2) viruses, and (3) immunologic abnormalities. Volumes have been written on such studies, but because they are inconclusive, some brevity is justified.

*Bacteriologic observations* have been extensive, but among the many organisms implicated at one time or another, current interest is focused on serotypes of *Escherichia coli*, group D streptococci, *Bac-*

Table 16–12. COMPARISON OF CROHN'S DISEASE AND ULCERATIVE COLITIS

| Characteristic | Crohn's Disease (CD) | Ulcerative Colitis (UC) |
|---|---|---|
| Small intestinal involvement alone | 30–35% | Never |
| Combined small and large intestinal involvement | 50–60% | Only large intestine |
| Large intestinal involvement alone | 20% | Always |
| Extraintestinal complications | Yes | Yes |
| Familial predisposition | Yes | Yes |
| Age, race, sex distribution | Same as UC | Same as CD |
| Causation | Unknown | Unknown |
| Nature of inflammatory reaction | | |
|    Ulcerations | Numerous, linear, penetrating | Coalescent, irregular, rarely penetrating |
|    Transmural fibrosis | + + + + | Rare |
|    Granulomas | + + + | Rare |
| Secondary cancers | + | + + + |

*teroides fragilis, Yersinia enterocolitica, Mycobacterium kansasii,* and chlamydia.[70, 73] The implicating evidence consists largely of the demonstration of elevated titers of agglutinins to particular agents (as, for example, to the O antigens of *E. coli*). However, there is a strong suspicion that the serologic findings are epiphenomena, reflecting some defect in the mucosal barrier, which allows secondary entry of bacteria. In this connection, *colonic mucus in ulcerative colitis is decreased* in quantity and is qualitatively altered. Although in theory these changes could contribute to a loss of barrier function, in Crohn's disease there is hypersecretion of intestinal mucus, which confuses the issue.[74] In sum, there is no strong case for any bacterial agent having an etiologic role.

*Viral agents* were thrust onto the center of the stage with the report some years ago that granulomas could be induced in murine footpads by the injection of cell-free (including bacteria-free) filtrates of Crohn's tissue.[75] In addition, tissue infiltrates from either Crohn's disease or ulcerative colitis, when injected into the peritoneal cavity of rabbits, were reported to cause inflammatory bowel disease, suggesting some organ specificity. Subsequently, "RNA viral agents" were identified in tissue cultures derived from diseased bowel. However, studies by other investigators have failed to confirm these findings and have shown that antigens derived from xenogeneic *normal* tissues will induce inflammatory changes resembling the granulomas of Crohn's disease. Moreover, viral particles cannot be regularly seen in lesions and, when present, could merely be passengers. So the viral search continues, punctuated by interludes of elation in the overall frustration.

*Immunologic abnormalities* relating to humoral mechanisms, cell-mediated immunity, and immunologic deficiencies have been reported by the score, but none has yet proved to be a primary event intrinsic to the development of IBD. A few are of interest. Antibodies to a lipopolysaccharide extract of *E. coli* 014 were identified in some patients that cross-react with antigen in mucus-secreting colonic epithelial cells. Depressed levels of mucosal secretory IgA potentiating bacterial invasion is a seductive but not generally accepted mechanism. Circulating antigen-antibody complexes are present in some patients with IBD; complement activation could provide a mechanism of cell injury. Indeed, the identification of IgG and complement along the basement membrane of colonic epithelium has been reported but has not been confirmed in the general run of cases. Thus immune complexes are not given much credence as primary mediators of the intestinal injury, but they could contribute to the induction of some of the extraintestinal complications mentioned earlier (e.g., spondylitis, erythema nodosum).

The possibility of some cell-mediated mechanism is particularly enticing, especially with Crohn's disease and its associated granulomatous inflammation.

Lymphocytotoxicity, abnormalities of gut-associated lymphoid tissue, and a host of other diverse T-cell changes have briefly held the spotlight and then receded into the background.

Many other putative pathogenetic abnormalities also have been reported. Increased synthesis of prostaglandin $E_2$ has been identified in the bowel wall and contents, as has increased prostaglandin synthetase in the rectal mucosa. Prostaglandins (PGs) are probably mediators of the inflammatory response, so it is not surprising that they are present in increased amounts in IBD. In this regard, suppression of PG synthesis by salicylate derivatives or other inhibitors of the cyclooxygenase pathway are not clinically effective. Emotional stress was once ascribed causal significance, but currently it is thought possibly to contribute to reactivation of the disease, rather than to be a primary mechanism. We conclude where we began. Both forms of IBD are of unknown origin. Indeed, there is no reason a priori not to believe that both diseases may have many possible origins.

**MORPHOLOGY.** The small intestine, particularly the terminal ileum, is involved in about 60% of patients with concurrent colonic involvement half of the time. Sometimes separated, more proximal segments of the small intestine are involved, with or without terminal ileal disease. In about 20% of cases, Crohn's disease is limited to the colon. The colonic involvement (referred to as **"granulomatous colitis"** to differentiate it from ulcerative colitis) most often affects the right colon, sometimes in continuity with ileal involvement, but in a small percentage of cases the disease is restricted to the anorectal area. However, segments of transverse and descending colon and, rarely, even the complete colon may also be affected. In the absence of total colonic involvement, the rectum and rectosigmoid are usually spared, a contrast with ulcerative colitis, in which these segments are almost always involved. **A characteristic feature of the intestinal disease is its segmental nature; affected portions are sharply demarcated from adjacent normal areas.**

The first gross alteration is hyperemia and bogginess, but the wall is neither thickened nor inelastic. Small "aphthoid" mucosal ulcers may appear.[76] **With progression, edema, inflammation, and subsequent fibrosis produce the characteristic rigidity of the involved segments of intestine and cause a "rubber hose" consistency** (Fig. 16–12). The mesentery simultaneously becomes thickened and fibrotic and sometimes appears to creep over the bowel serosa. On cross section of the gut, **the entire thickness of the wall is involved with striking fibrosis**, particularly in the submucosal and subserosal levels. The lumen is markedly narrowed and so permits passage of only a thin stream of barium, giving rise to the "string sign" of Crohn's disease on radiographs. The mucosa itself may appear only hyperemic and edematous or, typically, may be marked by numerous linear ulcers in the long axis of the bowel, creating deep fissures (Fig. 16–13) separated by nodular mucosal thickenings that give a "cobblestone" appearance. Occasion

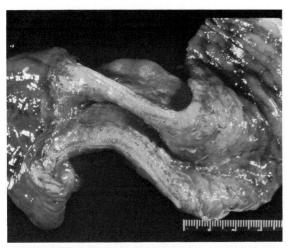

Figure 16–12. Crohn's disease involving a segment of the terminal ileum. Note the sharp borders of the lesion, the markedly thickened wall, and the narrowed lumen.

ally, penetration of the ulcers gives rise to abscesses within the peritoneal cavity or mesenteric fat or to fistulous communications to adherent loops of bowel. The fistulous tracts may penetrate to the skin or through the umbilicus or perineum. The macroscopic colonic changes are similar to those in the small intestines, but the fibrous thickening and stenosis are less pronounced. Anal lesions, when present, take the form mainly of ulcers, with or without fissures or fistulas extending into the perirectal fat and into and about the anus.

The macroscopic features of granulomatous colitis that help to differentiate if from ulcerative colitis are:

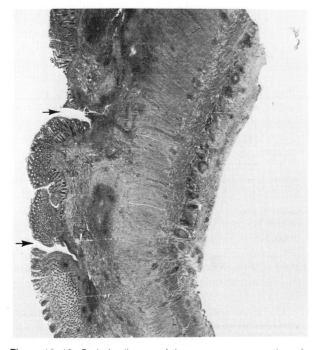

Figure 16–13. Crohn's disease. A low-power cross section of the markedly thickened bowel wall. The serpentine ulcerations are seen in cross section (*arrows*), and the inflammatory reaction produces dark aggregates of white cells in the submucosa and subserosa.

○ Discrete margins of segmental involvement
○ "Skip" lesions
○ Transmural fibrotic thickening of the colonic wall with extension into pericolic and mesenteric tissues
○ Linear ulcerations
○ Absence of "pseudopolyps"
○ Adhesion to and penetrating fissures into adjacent loops of bowel

Nonetheless, as mentioned, in many cases the colitis is indeterminate.

The "classic" histologic features of Crohn's disease are:
○ Nonspecific, suppurative inflammation in base and margin of mucosal ulcers
○ Fibrosing, chronic mononuclear inflammatory infiltrate in deeper layers, particularly marked in the submucosa and subserosa
○ Lymphoid aggregates in all layers of bowel, enclosing (in 60% of cases) noncaseating granulomas (resembling sarcoidosis)
○ Dilation or sclerosis of lymphatic channels
○ Extension of inflammatory fibrosing reaction into mesentery and pericolic fatty tissue

Superimposed on this broad outline are a number of more subtle but highly significant changes. Areas in which small intestinal mucosal villi are thickened, shortened, irregular, and fused are interspersed with areas of total loss of villous architecture. Individual epithelial cells at the tips of microvilli may become necrotic or undergo a variety of inflammatory alterations (to be described). There is hyperplasia of goblet cells and marked increase of mucus secretion, not only in inflammatory zones but also in adjacent uninvolved mucosa.[74] Increased numbers of intact and degranulated mast cells and scattered eosinophils are seen in the lamina propria, suggesting the possibility of an IgE immunologically mediated reaction. Perhaps most important, with long-standing chronic disease, the epithelial surface cells may become dysplastic with loss of columnar orientation, hyperchromatic nuclei, coarse chromatin, and prominent nucleoli. These epithelial changes may be related, as will be noted, to the increased incidence of intestinal carcinoma in these patients.[77]

**CLINICAL COURSE.** The clinical presentation of Crohn's disease is highly variable, depending on the age of the patient, the location and extent of the diseased bowel, and the acuteness of onset of the illness. The dominant manifestations are recurrent episodes of diarrhea, crampy abdominal pain, and fever lasting from days to weeks. These usually begin insidiously, but in some instances, particularly in the young, the onset of pain is so abrupt and the diarrhea so mild (or absent) that abdominal exploration is performed with a diagnosis of appendicitis. Some melena is present in about 50% of cases, but it is usually slight. After the initial attack, the manifestations remit over the span of days to weeks, either spontaneously or with symptomatic therapy. There follows a quiescent interval of weeks to months, or, in 10 to 20% of patients, the symptom-free interval lasts for years. However, the majority of patients have repeated relapses, with the intervals between attacks growing shorter and the crampy pain and diarrhea more pronounced. Intermittent episodes of partial or even complete bowel obstruction may develop.

Additional tribulations sometimes appear. Perianal or perirectal fissures, fistulas, or abscesses develop in a significant number of patients with anorectal involvement during the course of the chronic disease. Manifestations of malabsorption, including steatorrhea, protein wasting, and deficiencies of vitamin $B_{12}$, folic acid, and iron may occur when the disease is extensive in the small bowel. Some of the extragastrointestinal manifestations cited earlier may complicate the course—particularly, arthritis of the large joints, ankylosing spondylitis, erythema nodosum, and any of the other complications previously mentioned.

*The feared consequences of Crohn's disease include intestinal obstruction, perforation with peritonitis or the formation of intraabdominal abscesses, fistula formation between adherent loops of bowel, severe intestinal hemorrhage, toxic dilatation of the colon, and, most of all, carcinoma of the intestines.* The cancers have appeared in the small and the large intestines and sometimes in apparently uninvolved bowel (not seen in ulcerative colitis). In one recent survey, the frequency of gastrointestinal cancer was about 3%; most lesions occurred in colons with granulomatous colitis, but a few were seen in the small intestine. Some of these neoplasms appeared after about 20 years of disease because their incidence increases with duration of Crohn's disease.[78] There was also a suggestion of an increased incidence of extraintestinal cancers and cancers in higher levels of the gut, such as in the esophagus. Noteworthy as these data may be, *the risk of colonic cancer in ulcerative colitis is at least four times greater than it is in Crohn's disease.* This predisposition to intestinal cancer in Crohn's disease underscores the necessity for periodic intestinal biopsy of patients with chronic disease in order to monitor the dysplastic epithelial changes mentioned earlier. Rarely, a patient with long-standing Crohn's disease develops systemic amyloidosis.

## MALABSORPTION

Malabsorption refers to inadequate transport of one or more of the constituents of the normal diet from the intestinal lumen across the intestinal epithelial cells and ultimately into the portal circulation. *It results mainly from three separate malfunctions: (1) maldigestion of ingested foodstuffs, (2) disturbances in the mechanisms responsible for transport of the digested foods across the mucosal barrier, and*

*(3) reduction in the absorptive area of the gut, particularly in the small intestine.*[79] Less commonly it has other origins (cited later). Some malabsorptions are quite specific and affect one type of nutrient (e.g., fats or vitamins), whereas others are more generalized. For example, in celiac sprue there is marked reduction in the total absorptive area of the small intestine and consequent malabsorption of all foodstuffs. In contrast, as was pointed out on page 514, an autoimmune reaction directed against gastric parietal cells and intrinsic factor causes the highly selective malabsorption of vitamin $B_{12}$, inducing pernicious anemia (p. 366). Analogously, biliary tract disease leads particularly to malabsorption of fat (and the fat-soluble vitamins).

The location of the lesion also modifies the nature of the malabsorptive defect. The proximal intestine is the main area for the absorption of iron, calcium, water-soluble vitamins, and the monoglycerides and fatty acids derived from dietary fat. Sugars are principally absorbed in the proximal and middle region of the small intestine, whereas amino acids are absorbed primarily in the middle small intestine but are absorbed to a lesser degree in the upper and lower levels. The ileum is the main absorptive site for vitamin $B_{12}$ and bile salts. Thus, disorders having major impact on one or another level of the small intestine will lead to malabsorption of certain types of nutrients more than others. It is evident, therefore, that malabsorption syndromes come in many shapes and forms, as is shown in Table 16–13.

Despite the many variables, most conditions cited in Table 16–13 evoke remarkably similar manifestations at the outset, including anorexia, weakness, weight loss, muscle wasting, and, with malabsorption of fat, steatorrhea marked by the passage of bulky, greasy, foul-smelling stools. The weight loss occurs despite, usually, an increased appetite. Only later do more specific manifestations become evident relating to the malabsorption of particular nutrients. Thus, with malabsorption of fat, symptoms and signs of a lack of one of the fat-soluble vitamins may become evident.

It is now possible to obtain noninvasively highly satisfactory biopsies of particular levels of small intestine by using special approaches (Rubin tube, Crosby capsule). The histologic findings with some of the syndromes are characteristic and, with a few, diagnostic. In others the changes may be distinctive but not necessarily diagnostic.[80] A capsule characterization of the morphologic abnormalities in some of the malabsorption syndromes is presented in Table 16–14.

The most common disorders giving rise to malabsorption in the United States are celiac sprue, regional enteritis, chronic pancreatitis, and viral enteritis. The last three are described elsewhere, and so only the first and a few other relatively common entities will be treated briefly here.

## Table 16–13. CLASSIFICATION OF MALABSORPTION SYNDROME

I. **Defective intraluminal hydrolysis or solubilization**
  Primary pancreatic insufficiency
  Secondary pancreatic insufficiency
  Deficiency of conjugated bile acids
  Bacterial overgrowth (bile acid deconjugation)
    Blind loops
    Postgastrectomy
II. **Mucosal cell abnormality and inadequate surface**
  Primary mucosal cell disorders
    Disaccharidase deficiency and monosaccharide malabsorption
    Abetalipoproteinemia
    Vitamin $B_{12}$ malabsorption
  Small bowel disease
    Celiac disease
    Whipple's disease
    Amyloidosis
    Small bowel ischemia
    Crohn's disease (granulomatous enteritis)
III. **Lymphatic obstruction**
  Lymphoma
  Tuberculosis and tuberculous lymphadenitis
IV. **Infection**
  Tropical sprue
  Acute infectious enteritis
  Parasitoses
V. **Unexplained**
  Hypogammaglobulinemia
  Carcinoid syndrome
  Hypothyroidism
  Diabetes mellitus
  Mastocytosis
  Hyperthyroidism and hypoadrenocorticism
VI. **Drug-induced malabsorption**
  Cholestyramine
  Colchicine
  Irritant laxatives
  Neomycin
  $p$-aminosalicylic acid
  Phenindione

Modified from Wyngaarden, J. B., and Smith, L. H., Jr. (eds.): Cecil Textbook of Medicine. 16th ed. Philadelphia, W. B. Saunders Co., 1985, p. 722.

## Table 16–14. MALABSORPTION SYNDROMES—ABNORMALITIES IN SMALL INTESTINAL BIOPSIES

**Disorders With Characteristic Findings**

1. *Celiac and tropical sprue:* Blunted or absent villi, abnormal surface epithelium, lengthened crypts, increased mononuclear cell infiltrate in lamina propria
2. *Whipple's disease:* Lamina propria stuffed with glycoprotein-containing macrophages, villous abnormality of variable severity, bacilli demonstrable in macrophages during active disease in ultrathin sections or on electron microscopy
3. *Abetalipoproteinemia:* Mucosal absorptive cells vacuolated by lipid, villous structure normal
4. *Agammaglobulinemia:* Flattened or absent villi, absence of plasma cells, increased lymphocytic infiltrate
5. *Amyloidosis:* Demonstration of amyloid in and about vessels of lamina propria with Congo red staining and birefringence
6. *Regional enteritis:* Noncaseating granulomas
7. *Parasitic infections:* Identification of parasite in biopsy sections— e.g., giardiasis, strongyloidiasis, schistosomiasis, histoplasmosis, cryptosporidiosis
8. *Intestinal lymphoma:* Malignant lymphoid cells in lamina propria, villous abnormality of variable severity
9. *Tuberculosis and tuberculous lymphadenitis:* Chance finding of caseating granuloma or margin of tuberculous ulcer

**Disorders In Which Biopsy May Be Abnormal But Is Not Necessarily Diagnostic**

1. *Folate deficiency:* Shortened villi, megalocytes in blood vessels, decreased mitoses in crypts
2. *Vitamin $B_{12}$ deficiency:* Similar to folate deficiency
3. *Radiation enteritis:* Similar to folate deficiency
4. *Systemic scleroderma:* Increased fibrosis in lamina propria, possible derangement in villous structure

Modified from Robbins, S. L., Cotran, R. S., and Kumar, V.: Pathologic Basis of Disease. 3rd ed. Philadelphia, W. B. Saunders Co., 1984, p. 847.

## CELIAC SPRUE

This major malabsorption syndrome is known by several names—*gluten-sensitive enteropathy, nontropical sprue,* and *adult and childhood celiac disease. The evidence is now convincing that it is caused by some immunologic reaction to gluten, more specifically the alcohol-soluble glycoprotein gliadin, which is found in gluten.* Gliadin is present in wheat, barley, and rye.[81]

The histologic changes in this condition are characteristic but can be mimicked by other malabsorptive states, principally tropical sprue. Normally, in the proximal jejunum (the usual biopsy site) the villi are well developed and have a height relative to crypt depth of 4:1. They are finger- or tongue-shaped, covered by tall columnar epithelial cells with basal nuclei, and have a luminal border of remarkably ordered microvilli. Occasionally, goblet cells

are found among the columnar cells, and widely scattered lymphocytes can be seen between them. The lamina propria normally contains a scattering of plasma cells, lymphocytes, macrophages, and, occasionally, mast cells and eosinophils. As you know, the mitotic activity in this epithelium is normally confined to the crypts, from which the cells then mysteriously slide along the lateral margins of the villi to be desquamated at their tips.

**In celiac disease, damage to the surface epithelium results in more rapid desquamation of cells, leading to progressive shortening of the villi and lengthening of the crypts.** The ratio of villi to crypts may be reduced to 1:1. As the disease advances, the villi may disappear, leaving only a flattened surface punctuated by crypt orifices. The lamina propria accumulates a more marked infiltration of round cells that may also be found between the epithelial cells. Despite the disappearance of the villi, the increased regenerative activity in the crypts maintains a nearly normal mucosal thickness.

In children, removal of gluten from the diet is usually followed in weeks to months by reversion of the mucosa toward normal and, in time, complete restoration of the villi. However, despite avoidance of gluten, histologic normality in adults (and sometimes in children) may not be restored for many months, perhaps never. Nonetheless, avoidance of gluten achieves complete clinical improvement.[82]

*The gliadin-induced mucosal damage is immunologically mediated.*[83] The former theory of direct toxicity of gliadin or of one of its metabolites is now passing into limbo. Genetic influences may underlie this hypersensitivity. Approximately 60 to 90% of those with celiac sprue in the United States test positive for HLA-B8 and 80% are HLA-DW3–positive, whereas the incidence of these antigens in the normal population is in the range of 20 to 25%. Other HLA profiles are seen in other countries. However, whether the immunologic damage is mediated by antibodies or by cells is still uncertain. Increased levels of antigliadin IgA and IgM antibodies can be demonstrated in the inflamed mucosa and in the serum, but it is not clear that they are cytotoxic to mucosal cells or that complement is involved in the cytotoxicity. More recently, attention has turned to the possible role of T cells. Since there is a high proportion of cytotoxic T cells in the inflamed mucosa, they have been proposed as the mediators of the mucosal damage.[84] Furthermore, it is proposed that a gluten antigen activates these cells in patients with celiac sprue.[85] There is then the strong suggestion of deranged immunologic reactivity to gliadin, but the precise nature of the immunologic defect awaits clarification.

Patients with this condition have a markedly increased risk of developing malignant neoplasms, usually lymphomas but occasionally small bowel carcinomas.[86] Rigid adherence to a gluten-free diet will control the malabsorption, but the question persists: Will it reduce the risk of cancer?

## TROPICAL SPRUE

This misleading designation refers to a malabsorptive state that has little in common with nontropical sprue (celiac sprue) except for the similarity of the mucosal changes in the small intestine. It is encountered principally in the Far East, India, and the Caribbean but is disseminated widely by visitors to these locales. The cause of this disorder is still unknown, but it often starts with an acute intestinal infection that is usually bacterial and then, in most instances, dramatically responds to broad-spectrum antimicrobial drugs coupled sometimes with folic acid. There is the suspicion that this is some postinfective state with depleted folic acid reserves. It is hypothesized that *any one of a number of microbial agents may colonize the gut and possibly elaborate enterotoxins or sufficient amounts of toxic bacterial metabolites to induce the histologic changes nearly identical to those seen in celiac disease.* A refinement of this theory proposes that bacterial attachment to the mucosa stimulates the release of enteroglucagon, resulting in small intestinal stasis and further bacterial overgrowth.[87] To avoid confusion in terms, it has been recommended that this entity be called "postinfective tropical malabsorption."

## DISACCHARIDASE DEFICIENCY

A hereditary or acquired deficiency of lactase, sucrase, or maltase leads to an inability to split the respective disaccharide and hence causes a malabsorption of the monosaccharide. The most common is a lactase deficiency manifested by bacterial fermentation of unsplit lactose and the production of lactic and other organic acids in the intestinal lumen. These increase the osmotic load, resulting in diarrhea, crampy abdominal pain, and flatulence. This disorder usually becomes evident with ingestion of milk and milk products. *No specific histologic abnormalities in the intestinal mucosa are evident.* Control of these deficiency states requires elimination of the offending disaccharide from the diet.

## ABETALIPOPROTEINEMIA

This inborn error of metabolism is most consistent with an autosomal recessive disorder. Affected individuals lack apoprotein B in the plasma and have a variety of other abnormalities, including "spiny red cells," lack of beta-lipoproteins, retinitis pigmentosa, and neurologic abnormalities such as ataxia, nystagmus, and motor incoordination. In the absence of apoprotein B, absorbed fat is not incorporated into lipoproteins and hence accumulates within cells as triglycerides. Thus the characteristic histologic finding is the striking *lipid vacuolation of the mucosal epithelium in the small intestine.*

## WHIPPLE'S DISEASE

Whipple's disease is a systemic disorder that involves many organs and tissues throughout the body, including lymph nodes, spleen, heart, liver, kidneys, skeletal muscle, synovial membranes, central nervous system, and, particularly, the small intestine.[88] It usually presents as a malabsorptive syndrome, but it sometimes appears as an obscure form of arthritis, as a neurologic disorder, and in many other guises. Indeed, in some of these unusual presentations, small intestinal lesions may be scant or absent.[89]

An uncommon condition, it merits brief description because of its challenging and frustrating pathogenesis. *All sites of involvement are marked by aggregations of macrophages, which are stuffed with PAS-positive granules that can be resolved as lysosomes filled with bacilliform microorganisms in varying states of degeneration* (Fig. 16–14). Bacillary forms are sometimes seen extracellularly and in the process of being engulfed. The bacilli are on average 0.25 μm wide and 1.5 to 2.5 μm long. Immunohistochem-

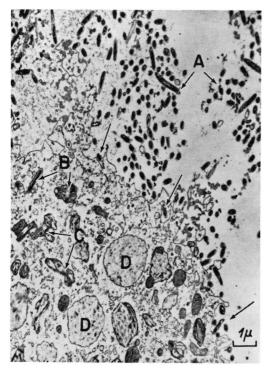

Figure 16–14. Electron micrograph of an involved histiocyte in Whipple's disease. *A* indicates bacilliform bodies outside the cell, and arrows point to loci where the bodies appear to be penetrating cell boundaries. *B* and *C* indicate distorted forms. *D* indicates uninvolved lysosomes. (From Robbins, S. L., Cotran, R. S., and Kumar, V.: Pathologic Basis of Disease. 3rd ed. Philadelphia, W. B. Saunders Co., 1984, p. 850.)

ical studies of the organisms harbored by a number of patients reveal antigenic uniformity among all, suggesting that a single agent is involved. Yet attempts at in-vitro cultivation and identification of the organisms have yielded a host of different agents, among which species of *Corynebacterium* and atypical streptococci predominate.[90] Furthermore, most patients (but not all) respond promptly to antibiotic therapy but not necessarily to the same agent, and sometimes more than one must be employed. There are more riddles. The putative bacteriologic agent does not evoke a characteristic inflammatory reaction other than the aggregation of macrophages.[91] Why are about 90% of the patients middle-aged white men? Why have the data relating to the immunocompetence of these patients been so inconstant and sometimes conflicting? Yes, indeed, a fascinating and frustrating disease!

**In all sites of involvement, the hallmark of this condition is the aggregates of plump macrophages bearing the PAS-positive granules and bacillary bodies.** The organisms are also found extracellularly and trapped in the brush border of the intestinal mucosal cells. In the typical case, the entire small intestine is involved, showing dulling of the serosa and some thickening and induration of the mesentery. When the bowel is opened, the distended mucosal intestinal villi may yield a likeness

to a bear-skin rug. Histologically, the villi are bloated with the macrophages described. The mucosal epithelium is not destroyed but may contain fine cytoplasmic lipid vacuoles, presumably caused by lymphatic obstruction because the lacteals are distended with lipids. Occasionally, rupture of these channels yields lipogranulomas in the lamina propria of the mucosa and in the lymph nodes of drainage. Mucosal thickening and pallor may also be found in the large bowel and stomach but is seen less consistently than the changes in the small intestine. Aggregates of bacilli-bearing macrophages are also found in the draining mesenteric lymph nodes, and, significantly, with antibiotic therapy the bacilli disappear.

Whipple's disease is usually characterized clinically by severe malabsorption, diarrhea and steatorrhea, emaciation, fever, joint pains, and a gray-brown melanin pigmentation of the skin. Diagnosis depends on finding the characteristic macrophages on jejunal biopsy. As mentioned, rare cases have presented as neurologic disorders, diffuse arthritis, or cardiac disease related to valvular or myocardial lesions. Without treatment, these patients usually follow an inexorable downhill course and die within 4 years of the diagnosis. However, antibiotic treatment has resulted in dramatic remissions as well as apparent cures. But in cases with CNS involvement, neurologic symptoms may persist after the gastrointestinal manifestations have cleared.

## INTESTINAL OBSTRUCTION

Many disorders may produce obstruction to the free flow of gastrointestinal contents. Only the most important will be presented here. In one large series of cases, 44% of obstructions were caused by *hernias*, 30% by *adhesions*, 10% by *neoplasms*, 5% by *intussusception*, 4% by *volvulus*, and the remaining 7% by a miscellany of disorders.[92]

### HERNIAS

*Hernia* refers to the protrusion of a serosa-lined pouch through any weakness or defect in the wall of the peritoneal cavity. The principal sites of such weakness are the inguinal and femoral canals, the umbilicus, and old surgical scars. The significance of hernias lies in the propensity for segments of viscera to become trapped in them. Most commonly and of greatest import is entrapment of the small bowel, but the large bowel, omentum, or any other viscus, such as the ovary, may be involved. If the neck of the defect is sufficiently narrow, the venous drainage of the protruding viscus is impaired. The resultant congestion and edema may produce so much swelling that the viscus is permanently trapped or *incarcerated*. Moreover, this swelling may lead to further pressure on the vasculature and may encroach on the arterial supply, thus resulting in ischemic necrosis of the trapped viscus, or a *strangulated hernia*. When the small bowel is involved, the histologic picture is identical to that produced by a mesenteric vascular occlusion (p. 526).

## INTESTINAL ADHESIONS

Fibrous bands may develop from organ to organ or from organ to peritoneal wall in the course of a healing peritonitis or following any abdominal surgery. These adhesions can create closed loops through which other viscera may slide and eventually become trapped, just as in a hernial sac. Partial or complete intestinal obstruction ensues, sometimes with infarction of the involved viscus.

## INTUSSUSCEPTION

In this disorder, one segment of small intestine, constricted by a wave of peristalsis, suddenly invaginates into the immediately distal segment of bowel (Fig. 16–15). Once trapped, the invaginated segment is propelled by peristalsis further into the distal segment, pulling its mesentery along behind it. Intussusception is more common in infants and children than in adults, and in this age group it usually occurs apparently spontaneously in otherwise healthy bowels. In these cases, reduction can frequently be accomplished by the administration of an enema. In adults, however, an intussusception often implies some intraluminal mass or lesion that serves as a point of traction and pulls the base of attachment and segment of gut along with it. Surgical exploration is necessary not only to determine the underlying cause but also to reduce the intussusception. Otherwise,

intestinal obstruction may be followed in time by infarction, as the mesenteric blood supply becomes progressively compressed.

## VOLVULUS

*Volvulus* refers to complete twisting of a loop of bowel about its mesenteric base of attachment. It is seen most commonly in the small intestine, but large redundant loops of sigmoid may be involved. Obstruction and infarction are common in these cases.

## TUMORS

The small intestine is the site of only about 5% of all gastrointestinal neoplasms, which are about equally divided between benign and malignant. The most commonly encountered benign tumors, in descending order of frequency, are (1) leiomyoma, (2) lipoma, (3) adenoma, (4) polyps, (5) angioma, and (6) fibroma.[93] The frequency of the several types of cancer varies among reports; most surveys find the adenocarcinoma to be the commonest, followed in descending order by lymphomas, carcinoids (argentaffinomas), and leiomyosarcomas.[94] More than half of these malignant neoplasms arise in the ileum. The benign tumors, as well as the lymphomas (p. 369) and the leiomyosarcomas, are identical to their counterparts occurring in other sites and require no further comment here. Only the adenocarcinoma and carcinoid will be described here.

### ADENOCARCINOMA

The rarity of adenocarcinomas of the small intestine is a biologic phenomenon of considerable interest in light of the normal rapid replicative turnover of the enormous (90% of the entire gastrointestinal tract) mucosal surface. These tumors are encountered in women slightly more often than in men and generally appear after the age of 40. Typically, these neoplasms grow in a napkin-ring, encircling pattern, but they infrequently occur as intraluminal fungating masses. Some secrete mucin. Because the small intestinal chyme is fluid, these lesions produce obstructive symptoms late and thus are usually diagnosed after they have permeated the bowel wall and spread to regional lymph nodes and to distant sites, particularly the liver and lungs. The 5-year survival rate is a disappointing 15 to 20%.[95]

### CARCINOID (ARGENTAFFINOMA, ENDOCRINE CELL TUMOR)

These neoplasms, when first described, were called "carcinoids" because most, although capable of metastasizing, were slow to spread and slow to kill and

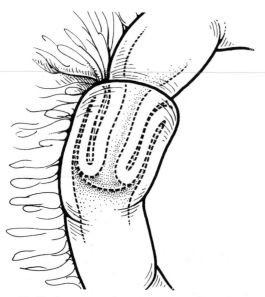

**Figure 16–15.** Intussusception. A segment of small intestine (*above*) has telescoped into the immediately distal segment.

thus were carcinomas in slow motion. Later it became apparent that the cells in many of these neoplasms had an affinity for soluble silver salts, and so they acquired the designation *"argentaffinomas."* The current fashion is to emphasize their ability to secrete bioactive amines and polypeptides by referring to them as *"endocrine tumors."* But old names, like old soldiers, die hard, and so "carcinoids" they remain. They may arise in diverse sites: the respiratory tract, biliary and pancreatic systems, male and female genitourinary tracts, thyroid gland, and breast, but most have origin in the gastrointestinal tract.[96] Wherever they arise, carcinoids have a remarkable anatomic resemblance to each other (as will be detailed), and most are capable of producing one or more of the following amines or polypeptides: 5-hydroxytryptamine (5-HT, serotonin), kinin peptides, histamine, catecholamines, glucagon, gastrin, and others. Whether all of these products are expressions of inherent genetic programs in the endocrine cells or instead are "ectopic" hormones resulting from neo-

plastic alterations of genetic programs is not always clear. Some induce systemic manifestations known as the *carcinoid syndrome.*

Pearse, in the late 1960s, first suggested that such neoplasms were derived from cells of similar embryologic origin that had the common property of being able to synthesize amine and polypeptide products by virtue of Amine Precursor Uptake and Decarboxylation, hence the acronym—APUD system of cells.[97] Because these properties were shared by cells in the adrenal medulla and hypothalamic neurons (releasing hormone-like factors), and for other reasons as well, he further proposed that *all APUD cells were of neuroectodermal origin, more specifically the embryonic epiblast, and thus they were called neuroendocrine cells.* Later it was found that neuroendocrine cells elaborate a neuron-specific enolase, further supporting a neuroectodermal origin.[98] However, this unitary concept has been challenged.[99, 100] Carcinoids arise in the gut from enterochromaffin (Kulchitsky) cells of probable endodermal origin. Carcinoids may

**Table 16–15.** APUDOMAS AND THEIR SECRETORY PRODUCTS

| Site | Neoplasm | Endocrine Secretory Product |
|---|---|---|
| Adenohypophysis | Hyperplasia / Adenoma / Carcinoma | Adrenocorticotropic hormone (ACTH) / Melanocyte-stimulating hormone (MSH) / Growth-stimulating hormone / Prolactin / Gonadotropin |
| Thyroid (C-cell) | Medullary carcinoma | Calcitonin / Prostaglandin / ACTH / MSH / Gastrin / Somatostatin |
| Adrenal medulla | Pheochromocytoma | Dopamine / Norepinephrine / Epinephrine / ACTH / FSH / Insulin / Others |
| Extra-adrenal paraganglia | Chemodectoma / Ganglioneuroma / Neuroblastoma | Dopamine / Norepinephrine / Calcitonin / ACTH |
| Lung | Oat cell carcinoma | ACTH / Antidiuretic hormone / Parathormone / Parathormone-like products / Others |
| Stomach | Gastrinoma | Gastrin / ACTH / Enkephalin |
| Pancreatic islet cells | Glucagonoma / Insulinoma / Somatostatinoma / ? / Gastrinoma / ? / Carcinoid | Glucagon / Insulin / Somatostatin / Pancreatic polypeptide / Gastrin / Vasoactive intestinal peptide / Serotonin / Most other amine and polypeptide hormones |
| Intestine | Carcinoid | Serotonin / Histamine / Most other amine and polypeptide hormones |

Modified from Temple, W. J., Sugarbaker, E. V., and Ketcham, A. S.: The APUD system and its APUDomas. Int. Adv. Surg. Oncol. 4:255, 1981.

also arise in organs of mesodermal origin such as the urogenital tract, which militates against their ectodermal derivation. Despite these uncertainties, the concept of the APUD system is useful to encompass a widely dispersed system of cells sharing the ability to synthesize similar secretory products despite differences in their origins.[101] *Neoplasms, benign or malignant, arising in these cells are called, generically, APUDomas* (including, incongruously, hyperplasias of these cells). A survey of some of the APUDomas and their secretory products is presented in Table 16–15. In this context carcinoids or argentaffinomas of the alimentary tract are APUD *neoplasms* of the diffuse system of endocrine (Kulchitsky) cells found at all levels of the gut.[102]

**MORPHOLOGY.** Carcinoids are distributed as follows:
- Appendix, 35 to 45%
- Small intestine (most located in the ileum), 20 to 30%
- Rectum and rectosigmoid, 12 to 15%
- Colon (except rectum and rectosigmoid), 3 to 7%
- Lungs and bronchi, 10 to 14%
- Esophagus and stomach, 2%, with a scattering in the biliary tract, pancreas, ovary, and other sites

Collectively, gastrointestinal carcinoids are not common and are found in less than 1% of all autopsies. Because appendiceal carcinoids differ in many ways from other intestinal carcinoids, they will be described later. Those **primary in the gut** tend to be small, gray-white to yellow, firm plaques located in the mucosa, often without ulceration of the overlying surfaces. They usually occur as solitary lesions, but multiple discrete tumors are sometimes present, particularly in the small and large intestines. They apparently enlarge very slowly; only rarely do they exceed 4 cm in diameter, and then they may become ulcerated or polypoid. Some lesions appear to be limited to the mucosa and submucosa, but others penetrate the wall and can be seen subserosally. Such obviously advanced tumors, when located in the small intestine, may permeate the contiguous mesentery and, because of their desmoplasia, cause kinking of the affected loop. **Only late in the course of intestinal carcinoids do they involve regional nodes and metastasize to the liver or other sites**. In one study, 58% of primary tumors bigger than 1 cm in diameter had spread to regional nodes and metastasized to the liver. The hepatic metastases tend to take the form of multiple small (1 to 3 cm) implants and do not replicate the massive metastases that are sometimes seen with other forms of cancer. Furthermore, widespread dissemination is uncommon. To be emphasized, therefore, **intestinal and indeed all extraappendiceal carcinoids behave as carcinomas, albeit indolent carcinomas**.

**Appendiceal carcinoids** usually appear as gray to yellow, firm, bulbous swellings in or near the tip of the appendix, obliterating the lumen. Usually the serosal surface appears unaffected grossly, but sometimes subserosal extension is evident. **Spread to regional nodes or elsewhere is the exception**.

Histologically, all carcinoids in all sites of origin are remarkably uniform. The cells are typically cuboidal to polygonal and monotonously similar in size, having uniform, centrally placed round nuclei surrounded by abundant cytoplasm containing granules that are more apparent with special stains. The cells are disposed in trabecular, insular, tubular, acinar, or rosette-like arrangements separated by a framework of connective tissue (Fig. 16–16). **Mitoses and giant cells are rare**. Despite their banal appearance, the tumor cells usually penetrate the submucosa and stream through the muscularis to the serosa, separating muscle bundles. In all sites of penetration and metastatic spread, the histologic details remain unaltered. This infiltrative invasive behavior is seen also with appendiceal carcinoids, although they rarely spread to extraintestinal sites. Occasionally carcinoids are less well differentiated and may display more of the features of anaplasia expected in an invasive neoplasm.

**Cytoplasmic granules are a distinguishing but not invariable feature of carcinoids**. By electron microscopy, the granules are shown to be bounded by membranes, to have a variable electron density of the matrix separated by a halo from the limiting membrane, and to range from 75 to 250 $\mu$m in diameter. Rarely they are much larger. When neoplasms are fixed in chromate solutions, the granules appear yellowish-brown, providing the basis for the designation "enterochromaffin" cells. The granules in most (but not all) carcinoids also have an affinity for silver salts in solution and turn black with deposited silver—hence the designation "argentaffinoma." In some tumors the granules can directly reduce the silver salts (**argentaffin-positive**); in others an exogenous reducing agent is needed (**argyrophil-positive**).

**CLINICAL COURSE.** Nonappendiceal argentaffinomas may appear at any age, but the peak incidence is in the sixth decade. Appendiceal lesions are most often incidental findings in appendectomies; there is a peak incidence in the fourth decade. There is no sex predilection. Tumors of the small and large intestines are usually asymptomatic and discovered only at autopsy. They may, however, come to clinical attention because (1) there is spread to the liver and subsequent hepatomegaly, (2) crampy discomfort or abdominal pain emanating from small intestinal kinking, or (3) they evoke the distinctive carcinoid syndrome.

*Only a few patients with argentaffinomas develop the carcinoid syndrome, characterized in Table 16–16.* Some neoplasms are nonsecretory. Furthermore, the syndrome is encountered with intestinal tumors only when there are fairly extensive metastases to the liver because the bioactive products in the portal flow are immediately inactivated in a single pass through the liver. Primary lesions located outside the portal venous watershed (e.g., carcinoids of the bronchi or ovaries) may induce the carcinoid syndrome even in the absence of hepatic metastases. Rarely, the carcinoid syndrome is encountered with other forms of cancer, such as oat cell bronchogenic carci-

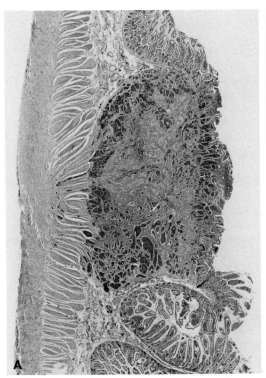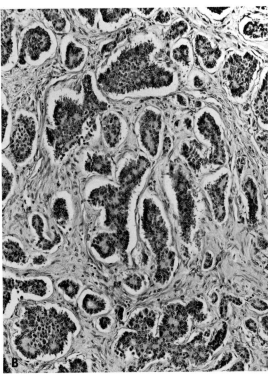

**Figure 16–16.** Argentaffinoma (carcinoid) of the small intestine. *A,* Low-power view of the small lesion. It has expanded into the submucosa, and nests of cells are seen penetrating the muscularis. *B,* High-power detail reveals the uniformity in size of the cells. Some gland patterns are evident.

noma, small cell carcinoma of the stomach or pancreas, and other similar carcinomas, all of which presumably arise in precursors of endocrine APUD cells capable of elaborating bioactive substances identical to those found with argentaffinomas. The main products thought to be responsible for the manifestations of the syndrome are 5-hydroxytryptamine (5-HT), histamine, bradykinin, and prostaglandins (in response to the tumor). It is generally believed that no single substance can induce all of the features of the syndrome. For example, 5-HT, elaborated by all functional carcinoids, is a likely candidate to induce the intestinal hypermotility and could possibly be responsible for the fibrosing, usually right-sided, cardiac lesions (since it is inactivated in a single pass through the lungs). The vasomotor and bronchoconstrictive features of the syndrome are more reasonably attributed to the release of bradykinin or histamine. Other explanations might be mentioned, but all are speculative.

Although the diagnosis of the carcinoid syndrome may be obvious clinically, it usually requires documentation of increased levels of 5-hydroxy-indolacetic acid (5-HIAA) or other metabolites of 5-HT in the urine. The outlook for patients with intestinal carcinoids is materially brighter than would be the case with most carcinomas. In the absence of liver metastases, an 80 to 90% five-year survival can be antici-

pated after surgical excision of the primary lesion. Even with secondary tumors in the liver, the five-year survival was 43% in one analysis.[103] The prognosis is best with a carcinoid in the appendix, which only exceptionally spreads beyond its site of origin. For obscure reasons, individuals with an extraappendiceal argentaffinoma have a much greater risk of another cancer in the gut or elsewhere than controls and even a three to five times greater risk than patients having any other form of primary cancer.

**Table 16–16. CLINICAL FEATURES OF THE CARCINOID SYNDROME**

**Vasomotor Disturbances**
Cutaneous flushes and apparent cyanosis (in almost all patients)
**Intestinal Hypermotility**
Diarrhea, cramps, nausea, vomiting (in almost all patients)
**Asthmatic Bronchoconstrictive Attacks**
Cough, wheezing, dyspnea (in about a third of cases)
**Cardiac Involvement**
Thickening and stenoses of the pulmonic valve leaflets and endocardial fibrosis, principally in right ventricle (in about one half of cases); bronchial carcinoids affect the left side of the heart
**Hepatomegaly**
Sometimes nodular; related to hepatic metastases (clinically apparent only in some cases)

# Colon

Colonic disorders are everyday problems in clinical practice. Carcinoma of the large bowel is second only to bronchogenic carcinoma as a cause of cancer death. Diarrheal diseases often related to ulceroinflammatory lesions are common causes of morbidity and, sometimes, mortality. Diverticula have notably increased in frequency in many industrialized nations. Thus the colon and the stomach are the levels of the gastrointestinal tract most frequently the seat of clinically significant lesions.

## HIRSCHSPRUNG'S DISEASE

Hirschsprung's disease is a form of *megacolon* caused by a failure in development of Meissner's submucosal and Auerbach's myenteric plexuses in the colon. Normally, the intramural innervation develops in a cephalocaudal direction and reaches the rectum at about 12 weeks of development. *Arrest of this process leaves various lengths of the terminal colon aganglionic.* In all cases, ganglion cells are lacking at the anorectal junction; in most cases the rectum and sometimes portions of the sigmoid also remain noninnervated. In perhaps 10 to 20% of patients a longer length of colon is affected or, rarely, even the entire colon—*aganglionosis coli.* Characteristic of all is distention of the intestine *proximal* to the noninnervated aperistaltic segment.

The mode of transmission of this congenital defect is unknown, but about 4% of siblings of index cases are affected. It is associated with various congenital anomalies, particularly Down's syndrome, but also with megaureter, megacystis, cryptorchidism, and defects in the heart, kidney, and other organs.

Congenital megacolon must be differentiated from *acquired megacolon* secondary usually to some obstructive process (Fig. 16–17). The many conditions leading to acquired megacolon include obstruction caused by a meconium plug in the neonate, neoplastic obstruction of the colon, infective destruction of the intestinal ganglia by *Trypanosoma cruzi* (Chagas' disease), and functional disorders causing constipation. Only rarely is the bowel distention in acquired megacolon as massive as that in the congenital disorder. *Critical to the diagnosis of the congenital form is rectal mucosal biopsy to document the absence of ganglion cells in Meissner's submucosal plexus.*

With Hirschsprung's disease, there is hyperplasia and an abnormal distribution of the cholinergic nerve fibers in the aganglionic segment.[104] Immunohistochemical staining for cholinesterase and neuron-specific enolase facilitates the visualization of the ganglia and nerve fibers, if they are present.[105] The innervated portion of the colon undergoes progressive dilation. Thus, **in the most common pattern in which the rectum and a portion of the sigmoid are affected, the dilatation is first evident in the descending colon, but over the span of months,**

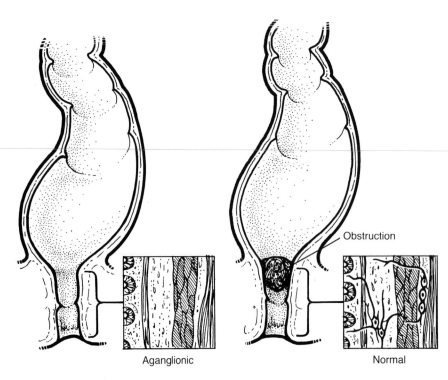

Aganglionic

Obstruction

Normal

Congenital (Hirschsprung's) megacolon

Acquired megacolon

Figure 16–17. Megacolon. To the left is seen the congenital form (Hirschsprung's), with its distal aganglionic functional obstruction. On the right the acquired form is depicted with normal innervation; there are various causes for obstruction, most often an intraluminal mass.

**it may extend back to the cecum.** In the infant, the enlargement may be quite massive and achieve a diameter of 15 to 20 cm. Rarely, the dilatation involves the appendix and even the terminal small intestine. Although there is hypertrophy of the muscularis in the distended colon, it is usually more than neutralized by the dilatation. In most cases, the mucosal lining is intact except when stercoral ulcers have developed.

Clinically, there is delay in the initial passage of meconium, which is followed by vomiting in 48 to 72 hours. Results from a barium enema may not be diagnostic at the outset because insufficient time may have elapsed for the characteristic dilatation to develop. When megacolon is not corrected surgically, there may be continued failure of passage of stools, but in some instances, there are alternating periods of obstruction and sudden passage of diarrheal stools. The principal threats to life in this disorder are superimposed enterocolitis, with fluid and electrolyte disturbances, and perforation of the distended colon or appendix with peritonitis.

## DIVERTICULAR DISEASE

The frequency of this condition, marked by saccular outpouchings of the colon, is increasing in individuals in the economically privileged populations of the western world. Near the turn of the century, its prevalence in autopsies in the United States, United Kingdom, and Australia was 5%. Currently, in these countries colonic diverticula are found in 30 to 50% of human autopsy subjects of either sex and over 60 years of age. In contrast, diverticular disease is rare in the economically deprived rural populations of Africa and Asia. These epidemiologic data have given rise to the theory that this condition is a "western disease" related to the growing consumption of fiber-poor diets in developed countries.[106]

In the past, much was made of the separation of *diverticulosis* from *diverticulitis*. The former term was applied to the presence of diverticula free of inflammatory changes that were assumed to be asymptomatic. Clinical manifestations such as lower abdominal pain were thought to arise only when inflammation in and about the diverticula—namely, diverticulitis—developed. Although diverticulitis is more likely to be symptomatic, it may also be silent. Conversely, those with diverticulosis may have abdominal complaints, for reasons soon to be explained. Altogether, only about 10 to 15% of individuals having diverticula, whether inflamed or not, are likely to be symptomatic. For these reasons it is current practice to use the noncommital term *"diverticular disease."* The pathogenesis of these lesions is best considered after the morphology.

**MORPHOLOGY.** In approximately 95% of patients, involvement is limited to the sigmoid colon. Infrequently, more proximal levels are affected as well.

**Three distinctive anatomic patterns are recognized: (1) prediverticular disease; (2) diverticulosis; and (3) diverticulitis. Prediverticular disease** refers to hypertrophy of both the circular and longitudinal musculature (teniae) of the colon ("myochosis coli") in the absence of demonstrable saccular outpouchings. The thickening of the teniae often induces shortening and puckering of the intervening colonic wall.

**Diverticulosis** implies the presence of outpouchings, from 1 mm up to several centimeters in diameter, that protrude into the pericolic fat or the appendices epiploicae. Typically, they are found between the mesenteric and antimesenteric teniae; rarely between the antimesenteric teniae (Fig. 16–18).[107] Histologically, **the wall of the saccule is composed of only the mucosa and submucosa and is usually devoid of any muscular layer** (Fig. 16–19). The saccules thus appear to represent hernations through the muscular coat. Often a saccule is filled with feces, which may not be readily extruded because the neck of the diverticulum is narrower than the sac. In most cases, but not all, there is the hypertrophy of the musculature and puckering of the colonic wall, as in the prediverticular stage. By definition, inflammatory changes are not present.

**Diverticulitis,** or secondary inflammation of one or more diverticula, develops when feces become impacted within the saccules and there is a subsequent secondary infection with *E. coli* and other enteric organisms. Frequently small perforations of the saccule develop. A nonspecific acute or chronic peridiverticulitis ensues and may eventually spread to the adjacent colonic wall. When multiple, closely adjacent diverticula are inflamed, the chronic inflammatory reaction may cause an irregular colonic stenosis that is sometimes difficult to differentiate

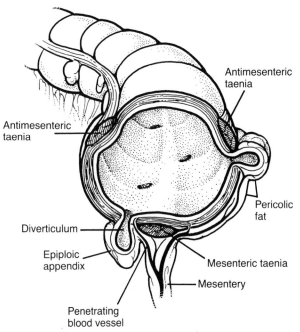

Figure 16–18. Diverticulosis of the colon. The favored locations for the diverticula (alongside the taeniae) and the penetrating mesenteric vessels are shown.

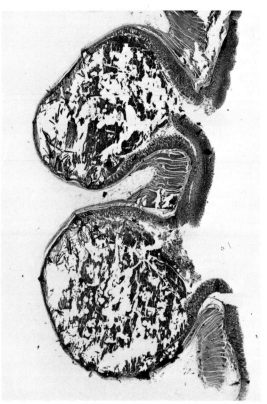

**Figure 16–19.** Diverticulosis of the colon. A low-power microscopic view of two diverticula, showing their thin walls and absence of muscular coats. There is no evidence of inflammation, but they are stuffed with fecal matter.

on radiographs or gross examination from an infiltrative carcinoma. Perforations may also lead to pericolic abscesses or, less frequently, to generalized peritonitis. Rarely, sinus tracts or fistulous communications with neighboring viscera develop.

**PATHOGENESIS.** Two influences are thought to be important in the genesis of diverticula: (1) *loci of weakness in the colonic wall* and (2) *a gradient of pressure between the colonic lumen and the peritoneal cavity.* There is a well-defined predilection of diverticula to form alongside penetrating vessels where the investing connective tissue provides avenues of lowered resistance through the colonic musculature. Supporting this notion is the early development of diverticula in individuals with such connective tissue disorders as Marfan's and Ehlers-Danlos syndromes. Furthermore, diverticular disease is uncommon under the age of 30; with aging, there is presumably loss of tensile strength of collagen and therefore favorable conditions for the development of diverticula.

With respect to especially high intraluminal pressure, the evidence is controversial.[108] One strongly held view proposes that low-fiber diets resulting from increased use of refined foods underly this condition.[108a] It is contended that these diets, by reducing the bulk and plasticity of the stool, demand increased peristaltic activity, which in turn raises intraluminal pressure. The augmented peristaltic waves may transiently sequester short segments of the colon from the adjacent colonic lumen—*segmentation.* In such sequestered segments the increased intraluminal pressure, instead of propelling the feces forward, is exerted laterally on the colonic wall and favors herniation. The sigmoid colon, as the narrowest portion, would be most vulnerable to segmentation. Although this concept appears convincing, it has come under challenge. It has been shown that asymptomatic patients with diverticula do not necessarily have increased intraluminal pressure or decreased stool weight. As noted earlier, not all patients with diverticula have hypertrophy of the colonic musculature. Nonetheless, increased peristaltic activity and increased bowel motility were associated with lower abdominal pain. Moreover, fiber supplementation of the diet often relieves these symptoms. However, there is no documentation in humans that the development of diverticula can be prevented by a high-fiber diet from early life. We must leave it that on balance, *the evidence supports the belief that a low-fiber diet is important in the induction of symptoms, but whether it is solely responsible for the development of diverticula remains uncertain.*

**CLINICAL COURSE.** Usually, most patients with diverticula are asymptomatic, but close questioning will often disclose a history of vague manifestations of disturbed bowel function, such as lower abdominal discomfort, transitory attacks of cramping pain relieved by a bowel movement, and episodes of constipation. Symptomatic patients have more of the same and sometimes bleeding. The pain, as noted above, results from excessive segmental contraction of the colon and so may be encountered with prediverticular disease as well as with radiologically demonstrable diverticula. When inflammation—diverticulitis—complicates the picture, well-defined left lower quadrant, persistent pain accompanied by fever and leukocytosis is likely to appear. Palpation may reveal tenderness in the left lower quadrant and sometimes a tender, sausage-shaped mass representing an involved sigmoid loop. However, the fever may be mild to absent, the elevated white count not impressive, and the tenderness minimal to absent, particularly when the inflammatory disease is re-

**Table 16–17.** MAJOR COMPLICATIONS OF DIVERTICULAR DISEASE

**Rectal Bleeding**
   Seen in 10 to 30% of patients with diverticular disease
   Massive in 3 to 5%; requiring transfusions and sometimes
     emergency surgery
**Infections Caused by Extension of Diverticulitis**
   Pericolic abscess
   Sinus or fistulous tract
   Generalized peritonitis—may be fatal
**Bowel Narrowing**
   Induced by long-standing chronic diverticulitis
   May be mistaken for an infiltrative bowel carcinoma on
     colonoscopy or barium enema

stricted. In such instances, it may be impossible to differentiate diverticulitis from diverticulosis.

The three principal complications are shown in Table 16–17. Currently there is near agreement that high-fiber foods (such as coarse wheat bran) in many instances will provide relief from symptoms, in some part because patients are known to have said, "The cure is worse than the disease."[106] Surgical intervention is only necessary for control of severe hemorrhage or relief of obstruction.

## VASCULAR LESIONS

Ischemic lesions including, of course, infarction of the colon were already considered together with those of the small intestine on page 526. Only two other disorders, angiodysplasia and hemorrhoids, need comment here.

### ANGIODYSPLASIA (VASCULAR ECTASIA)

This vascular anomaly and diverticular disease collectively are the cause of about 75% of all massive rectal bleeding. *Angiodysplasia is a focus of abnormal dilatation of the submucosal veins, usually in the cecum but sometimes in the right colon.*[109] Although the mucosal and submucosal telangiectatic anomalies may represent congenital malformations, more likely they are acquired over the span of decades and thus become manifest relatively late in life.[110] According to physical laws, tension in the wall of a cylinder is a function of intraluminal pressure and radius. Because the cecum has the greatest radius in the colon, it develops the greatest wall tension; peristaltic contractions thereby predispose the thin-walled veins, where they pass through the muscularis to intermittent occlusion in one localized area. The thicker-walled arterial supply remains patent, and thus progressive dilatation of the submucosal and mucosal veins ensues, leading eventually to possible rupture. Only awareness of the importance of this condition as a possible cause of bleeding and use of special diagnostic procedures (optimally selective angiography) will disclose its presence.

### HEMORRHOIDS

Hemorrhoids, also known as "piles," are variceal dilatations of the hemorrhoidal venous plexuses. It is estimated that 50% of the population over the age of 50 years have minimal or significant hemorrhoids. In the great majority of these individuals, they are asymptomatic. *Internal hemorrhoids* are varicosities of the superior and middle hemorrhoidal veins; they appear above the anorectal line and are covered by rectal mucosa. *External hemorrhoids* are dilatations of the inferior hemorrhoidal plexus, which appear below the anorectal line and are covered by anal

mucosa. Both forms result from elevated venous pressure within the hemorrhoidal plexuses. Most commonly they are the consequence of chronic constipation over the span of years and straining at stool. Repeated pregnancies with pelvic venous stasis is another important predisposition. *More rarely but of much greater clinical significance, hemorrhoids may arise in individuals having portal hypertension, usually related to cirrhosis of the liver.*

Histologically, hemorrhoids consist of thin-walled dilated typical varices that protrude beneath the anal or rectal mucosa. In their exposed situation, they are subject to trauma and may become thrombosed. This is particularly true of internal hemorrhoids, which may prolapse during defecation and become transiently trapped in the compressive circle of the anal sphincter (strangulation). In addition to the considerable discomfort (pain and itching) they may produce, they are a common cause of rectal bleeding. Too often, however, rectal bleeding is ascribed to hemorrhoids without meticulous exclusion of far more serious origins, such as rectal carcinoma.

## ENTEROCOLITIS

As used here, this heading is intended to refer to a group of diseases marked by clinically significant diarrhea and ulceroinflammatory, or sometimes only mild inflammatory, changes that usually occur in the colon (but sometimes are seen in the small intestine); hence the term "enterocolitis." Many of these diarrheal diseases have specific microbial causes, but the two most important in the Western world—Crohn's disease and ulcerative colitis—are of unknown origin. Furthermore, diarrhea and inflammatory intestinal changes may have other causes (e.g., radiation, uremia, cytotoxic drugs, heavy metal poisoning, and laxative abuse). Indeed, diarrhea, when defined as an increase in stool water leading to an increase in volume of each bowel movement or an increase in the number of bowel movements, is as basic to a diversity of intestinal disorders as fever is to infections.[111] Here our consideration is limited to the more common and significant infective causes of diarrhea and to idiopathic ulcerative colitis. Crohn's disease has already been considered on page 528. It should be particularly noted that in any large series of patients with diarrhea, after all known causes, ulcerative colitis, and Crohn's disease have been excluded, as many as one third of the cases remain of mysterious origin.

In considering the known infective causes of diarrheal enterocolitis, we must first *differentiate those conditions related to ingestion of preformed enterotoxins from those resulting from colonization of the intestines by pathogenic microorganisms.* The former category is conventionally referred to as "food poisoning," and the main offenders are *Clostridium perfringens, Clostridium botulinum, Staphylococcus aureus,* and *Bacillus cereus.* Any one of these organ-

**Table 16–18.** CAUSES OF INFECTIVE
ENTEROCOLITIS

**Viruses**
  Rotaviruses
  Norwalk virus
**Bacteria**
  *Vibrio cholerae*
  *Salmonella* species
  *Shigella* strains
  *Campylobacter jejuni*
  *Yersinia enterocolitica*
  *Escherichia coli* strains
  *Clostridium difficile*
**Protozoa**
  *Entamoeba histolytica*
  *Giardia lamblia*

isms may find appropriate conditions for growth in certain foods inadequately cooked and inadequately cooled, refrigerated, and stored. Each to an extent has its own preferred foods; for example, *C. perfringens* "delights" in preserved meats, whereas *S. aureus* "loves" custards. But it would be foolhardy to believe that only these dietary items pose risks. Characteristic of all food poisonings are the short interval (hours) between the ingestion of the contaminated food and the abrupt, sometimes violent onset of vomiting, which is followed soon by diarrhea in some cases. Furthermore, the attack is self-limited and usually brief. Thus little is known about the intestinal morphologic changes in these conditions.

In contrast to these intoxications, *the remaining microbial causes of enterocolitis result from replication of the organism within the intestinal lumen.* The most common and significant offenders are listed in Table 16–18. Some of these agents "set up shop" mainly in the small bowel—the vibrios, salmonellae (principally *S. typhi*), enterotoxigenic serotypes of *E. coli*, rotaviruses, Norwalk virus, *Giardia*—but others localize mainly in the large bowel—shigellae, *E. coli* serotypes, *Campylobacter*, and *Entamoeba histolytica*. However, often these preferences are not followed rigidly, and so lesions may be found in both large and small bowel (as is the case with *Campylobacter*) or unpredictably in one or another site (as with *Yersinia enterocolitica*).[112]

*Enteric pathogens cause diarrheal disease in one of two ways: (1) by production of an enterotoxin without invasion of the bowel wall or (2) by invasion of the bowel mucosa, usually resulting in ulcerations.* Occasionally strains can do both. Some basic generalizations relative to these two mechanisms follow.

*Enterotoxigenic organisms,* of which the two major prototypes are *Vibrio cholerae* and enterotoxigenic *E. coli,* are mainly characterized by the following features:

1. The organism preferentially colonizes the small intestine, does not invade the mucosa, but adheres to the epithelial surface.

2. There are no mucosal ulcerations.

3. Bacterial invasion of the blood stream does not occur.

4. In the absence of mucosal destruction, leukocytes are not present or are scant in number in the diarrheal discharge.

5. The diarrhea results from excessive intestinal mucosal secretion, which overwhelms the absorptive capacity of the colon (further described in the consideration of cholera).

In contrast, *diseases caused by invasive organisms—Shigella, Salmonella, Campylobacter,* enteroinvasive *E. coli, Yersinia,* and *Clostridium difficile*—have the following characteristics:

1. The principal sites of injury are the colon and the ileum.

2. There is morphologic evidence of epithelial and mucosal destruction, usually with the formation of ulcerations.

3. The diarrheal effluent almost always contains a varying number of leukocytes and sometimes has a mucopurulent exudate.

4. Bacteremia may be induced.

5. The pathophysiology of the diarrhea is poorly understood but could involve (a) damage to the absorptive surface, such that absorption cannot keep pace with even normal levels of secretion; (b) elaboration of an enterotoxin, at least in the initial phases, that increases fluid secretion; and (c) augmented local synthesis of prostaglandins increasing fluid secretion.

These generalizations about the toxigenic and invasive organisms permit a simple, almost bedside clinical approach to the differential diagnosis of intestinal infections on the basis of the presence or absence of leukocytes in the diarrheal effluent, as indicated in Table 16–19.

Against this background, we can turn to a consideration of some of these entities.

## CHOLERA

This drastic diarrheal disease, endemic in the watershed of the Ganges, has in the past caused pandemics that have spread widely into areas of Asia, Africa, and Europe. The awesome toll it has exacted and still exacts among children, particularly in the rural areas of India, Bangladesh, and Indonesia, is almost entirely related to the massive fluid and electrolyte losses caused by the purging diarrhea.

**Table 16–19.** ORGANISMS RELATED
TO PRESENCE OF FECAL LEUKOCYTES
IN ENTEROCOLITIS

| Abundant to Many Leukocytes | Scant to Absent Leukocytes |
|---|---|
| *Shigella* strains | *V. cholerae* |
| *Salmonella* species | Toxigenic *E. coli* |
| Invasive *E. coli* | Enteroadhesive *E. coli* |
| *Campylobacter* species | Rotavirus |
| *Yersinia* species | Norwalk virus |
| *Clostridium difficile* | *Giardia lamblia* |
|  | *Entamoeba histolytica* |

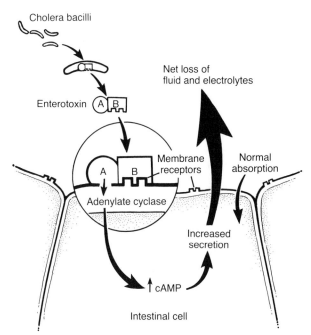

Figure 16–20. A schema of the mechanisms of action of the cholera enterotoxin in its induction of excessive mucosal secretory activity.

The pathogenicity of the gram-negative, comma-shaped major strain—*V. cholerae*—derives from its capacity to elaborate an enterotoxin that induces extreme secretory activity in the mucosal epithelial cells of the small intestine.[113] The classic "rice-water" stools are essentially an isotonic fluid that is rich in chloride ions and contains flecks of mucus but almost no leukocytes. *The organism does not invade the bowel mucosa, which remains essentially intact, except possibly for minimal desquamation of scattered epithelial cells. The only changes to be seen are congestion and a modest infiltration of mononuclear inflammatory cells in the lamina propria of the mucosa.*[114] Alterations in the normal villus-to-crypt ratio, accompanied sometimes by hyperplasia of Peyer's patches, mesenteric lymph nodes, and spleen, are likely to be secondary to concurrent malnutrition and other enteric pathogens.

Study of the enterotoxin of *V. cholerae* has unraveled the mode of action of all enterotoxigenic agents. Pathogenic biotypes of the cholera bacillus elaborate a protein molecule (the enterotoxin) containing, in simplified version, an enzymatically active "A" subunit linked to a peptide "B" subunit. (In reality, there is more than one "A" subunit and "B" subunit.) The latter binds to receptors on the intestinal cell surface, and the "A" subunit then activates membrane adenylate cyclase, which increases intracellular levels of cAMP and initiates cell secretion of chloride ions and water (Fig. 16–20).[115] *The fluid and electrolyte losses are the result of secretion in excess of reabsorption.* This understanding has made it possible to reduce the mortality rate of cholera to less than 1% by fluid and electrolyte replacement; anti-biotics serve to shorten the duration of the diarrhea. However, because death can occur within hours, prompt diagnosis and therapy are critical.

## ENTEROPATHOGENIC *E. coli*

It was recently said that "travel expands the mind and loosens the bowels."[116] There are potentially many causes for such "traveler's diarrhea," but studies suggest that in tropical and subtropical countries over half of the cases are caused by enteropathogenic strains of *E. coli. Four and possibly more mechanisms underlie the pathophysiology of the diarrhea, which is induced by specific serotypes:*[117] (1) the elaboration of a heat-labile (LT) enterotoxin; (2) the elaboration of a separate heat-stable (ST) toxin; (3) the ability of enteroinvasive strains to penetrate and multiply within colonic epithelial cells; and (4) an ability to adhere to the microvilli of epithelial cells. Each of these mechanisms is transmitted to specific strains through plasmids and so some serotypes acquire more than one (e.g., the ability to produce both ST and LT).

The *enterotoxigenic E. coli* strains belong mainly to the O-group. The LT enterotoxin produces diarrhea in exactly the same manner as the cholera toxin. It stimulates membrane-bound adenylate cyclase and the secretion of fluid and electrolytes into the intestinal lumen, principally in the small intestine. Colonization of this level of gut is favored by specific adhesion factors that provide the opportunity for the proliferation of the offenders to disease-producing levels. This mechanism appears to be the main cause of "Montezuma's revenge" in adult travelers. The ST enterotoxin is also produced by serotypes within the O-group and, although the mechanism of action closely parallels that of the LT enterotoxin, it differs inasmuch as guanylate cyclase is activated. As pointed out, some strains produce both ST and LT. Lack of sufficient prior exposure renders the nonimmune traveler at risk to these enterotoxigenic strains.

*Enteroinvasive E. coli* does not produce ST or LT. Instead, it directly invades and proliferates within intestinal epithelial cells, principally in the colon. It is suspected that the induction of diarrhea is related to impaired absorption of fluids owing to cell damage, but local synthesis of prostaglandins or the elaboration of some toxin has not been ruled out.

The fourth mechanism of diarrhea induction is associated with so-called *enteroadhesive serotypes* of *E. coli*, which also belong to the O-group. It is the least understood of the mechanisms but is involved in most cases of *E. coli*–related infantile summer diarrhea.[118] Studies to date suggest that neither ST or LT enterotoxins nor enteroinvasiveness are involved in this disease, and some isolates have demonstrated an apparent cytotoxin distinct from the better characterized enterotoxins. Other isolates have demonstrated a particular ability to adhere to the epithelial mucosa in the small intestine by mechanisms distinct from those seen with the enterotoxigenic strains. We do not yet know whether the ability to adhere and the cytotoxicity may occur together. It is clear that plasmid-transmitted properties have greatly increased the versatility of the once-thought-to-be-banal *E. coli* of the gut.

## SHIGELLOSIS (BACILLARY DYSENTERY)

*The term "dysentery" is applied to diarrheal disorders characterized by lower abdominal pain and the passage of watery stools containing pus.* The presence of pus denotes mucosal damage, usually with ulceration. Unless otherwise qualified, the designation "bacillary dysentery" is restricted to *Shigella*-induced disease.[119] There are four species of *Shigella: S. dysenteriae, S. flexneri, S. boydii,* and *S. sonnei.* The first three can be further subdivided into many serotypes. *S. dysenteriae* and *S. flexneri* produce the severest form of bacillary dysentery and are found mainly in Central and South America. In the United States and Europe, *S. sonnei* is now the principal offender.

Pathogenic shigellae (1) possess in their cell walls a lipopolysaccharide antigen, an endotoxin; (2) have genes encoding for the ability to invade and proliferate within mucosal epithelial cells; and (3) elaborate an exotoxin after cell invasion.[119] The precise mechanism of induction of the diarrhea is, however, still uncertain. This much is now known: lysates of pathogenic organisms will cause hindquarter paralysis in animals, and so the causative factor is called a neurotoxin or, alternatively, the Shiga toxin. Paralysis is not a feature of bacillary dysentery in humans, but severe infections in children are sometimes accompanied by convulsions that could be secondary to the action of neurotoxin. It is now clear that the Shiga exotoxin is also cytotoxic and so is presumably responsible for the mucosal damage.[120] Whether this Shiga toxin also stimulates small intestinal secretion is still unclear, but it does not activate adenyl cyclase in the manner of the cholera toxin.

Only humans and the higher apes are natural hosts of shigellae. The organisms are usually transmitted from infected humans by contaminated food or water or by person-to-person contact. As few as ten bacilli can induce disease in a healthy adult. They appear to be able to traverse the stomach and colonize the ileum and colon. They may induce hypersecretion in the small intestine, but the main site of attack is the colon.

Morphologically, the mucosa of the colon becomes hyperemic and edematous, and enlargement of the lymphoid follicles creates small projecting nodules. Within a day or so, a fibrinosuppurative, pseudomembranous, yellow-gray exudate covers the mucosa. **Superficial irregular ulcerations appear, and in severe infections, large tracts may be denuded.** Despite their extent, these ulcerations tend to remain superficial, but may perforate, and spread of the organisms into the blood rarely occurs. Histologically, there is a dominantly mononuclear leukocytic infiltrate within the lamina propria away from the denuded areas. The shallow ulcers are rimmed by and covered with an acute suppurative neutrophilic exudate. Congestion, edema, and thromboses of the small underlying vessels are also present.

Classically, within one to two days of ingestion of organisms, crampy abdominal pain and watery diarrhea appear. Soon thereafter, the diarrhea becomes more profuse, mucopurulent, and bloody. Fever is variable but may be hectic in children and accompanied by convulsions. In severe attacks, intestinal perforation and severe protein loss can be life-threatening. Extraintestinal complications such as arthritis, purulent keratitis, and the hemolytic-uremic syndrome may appear, but these are not related to dissemination of the organism; they are the result of an endotoxemia and circulating immune complexes. Confirmation of the diagnosis requires that the shigellae be isolated from the stools during the early stages of the disease or that antibodies be demonstrated during the second week.

## SALMONELLOSIS (INCLUDING TYPHOID FEVER)

The gram-negative salmonellae include three species, *S. typhi, S. cholerae-suis,* and *S. enteritidis,* the last separable into 1700 antigenically distinct serotypes. *There are six more or less distinctive clinical syndromes caused by the salmonellae, but the most important is typhoid fever, which is caused solely by S. typhi.* The remaining five syndromes caused by any of the other salmonellae comprise (1) gastroenteritis (the most common pattern); (2) bacteremia, with or without gastrointestinal involvement; (3) enteric fevers, which are essentially milder forms of typhoid fever; (4) localized infections in, for example, bones, joints, and meninges; and (5) a carrier state in asymptomatic individuals who harbor the organisms in their gallbladders. Only typhoid fever will be further described.

*Typhoid fever* is best characterized as a prolonged, systemic illness that is marked by an initiating bacteremia and hectic fever and is followed by spread of organisms to the mononuclear-phagocyte reticuloendothelial (RE) system throughout the body.[121] The main reservoir of *S. typhi* is humans, and infection is spread through the fecal-oral route from infected individuals, who may be convalescents or chronic carriers. Contaminated food, water, and insects may serve as intermediate vectors.

The pathophysiology of the disease is still uncertain, but it is known that *S. typhi,* like all salmonellae, possesses flagellar, somatic, and outer-coat antigens named H, O, and Vi antigens. In experimental animals the organism is cytotoxic to the intestinal epithelium and causes sloughing of villus cells, thereby providing an entry into the mucosa.[122] Also, a cholera-like enterotoxin has been identified that stimulates adenylate cyclase (p. 545).[123] Presumably, this enterotoxin contributes to the induction of diarrhea. After oral ingestion by humans and an incubation period of 1 to 2 weeks, the organism penetrates the small bowel mucosa and rapidly enters the lymphatics and thence the blood stream. The blood-borne organisms are picked up by macrophages and monocytic cells throughout the RE system. Replication within and destruction of macrophages leads to reemergence of organisms and the induction of recurrent waves of bacteremia. It is the seeding of the Peyer's patches in the terminal ileum that induces the intestinal changes. A similar sequence accounts for the reticuloendothelial hyperplasia throughout the body, producing both splenic enlargement and so-called typhoid nodules in the liver, bone marrow, and lymph nodes.

In the terminal ileum, the Peyer's patches are enlarged and appear as sharply delineated plateau-like elevations. The luminal surface overlying the patches is shed, resulting in oval ulcers with their long axes in the axis of the bowel. The ulcers are usually superficial, but rarely they may perforate. However, they are not infrequently the source of bleeding. Histologically, **the Peyer's patches are converted into masses or nodular aggregates of large, rounded, epithelioid macrophages, which often contain bacilli (during the height of the disease) and red cells (erythrophagocytosis).** Scattered lymphocytes and plasma cells are distributed among these macrophages, but neutrophils are surprisingly scarce.

The spleen is markedly enlarged, soft, and bulging as a result of striking proliferation of mononuclear phagocytes in the red pulp. Phagocytized bacilli and erythrophagocytosis may be evident. Similar changes are found in the lymph nodes throughout the body. The liver classically contains focal aggregates of phagocytic mononuclear cells originating from both Kupffer's cells and monocytes and creating **"typhoid nodules."** As with other salmonellae, S. typhi can localize in many sites, including the bones, joints, meninges, and gallbladder (where it may persist to create a chronic carrier state).

The clinical features of typhoid fever can largely be deduced from the pathogenetic sequence of events. The infection begins with malaise and a fever with afternoon spikes that progressively mount each day. Recurrent bacteremic chills may accompany the fever spikes. Abdominal pain, colic, and constipation alternating with diarrhea appear with the intestinal involvement. Despite the high fever, the pulse is remarkably slow and the peripheral white count low because of a neutropenia. *The combination of fever, bradycardia, and neutropenia is usually sufficiently distinctive to suggest the diagnosis.*

During the second week, the spleen enlarges, and a transient classic rash, referred to as *rose-spots*, appears. At this time, the fever becomes continuous.

When untreated, the fever persists into the third week and is often accompanied by confusion and sometimes delirium. Pneumonia, kidney, bone, or joint infections and, rarely, infective endocarditis may now appear. Feared complications are intestinal hemorrhage and perforation, the latter being more likely in those with significant intestinal bleeding. Even when untreated, the disease begins to defervesce in the fourth week, followed by recovery, but with appropriate antibiotic therapy much sooner. Plasmid-borne resistance factors have begun to appear in some strains, and so drug-susceptibility tests are indicated.

The diagnosis can be confirmed by isolation of the organisms from the blood during the first week (in 90% of cases), from the stools during the third to fifth weeks, and the demonstration of antibodies responsible for the Widal reaction after the third week of illness. (There are, however, false-positives and occassional false-negatives.)

Any hemoglobinopathy, such as sickle cell disease (presumably because it induces RE blockade) and *Schistosoma* infections, renders individuals vulnerable to typhoid fever and to prolonged bacteremia. Moreover, they are prone to develop localized infections, especially osteomyelitis, and the chronic carrier state.

## PSEUDOMEMBRANOUS COLITIS (PMC)

*When conditions permit the proliferation of Clostridium difficile in the colon, its cytopathic toxin will cause severe inflammation and focal necroses of the surface epithelium, which becomes covered with an inflammatory coagulum creating a pseudomembrane.* Pseudomembranous inflammation in the gut caused by C. *difficile* can be mimicked by other enteroinvasive infections (e.g., shigellosis) and ischemic injuries with secondary infection. C. *difficile* is normally a minor commensal in the gut; when patients are administered antibacterial agents that reduce the normal microflora, it is provided the opportunity to proliferate. Nearly all antimicrobial agents have at one time or another been implicated in this effect, but the most common offenders are clindamycin, lincomycin, ampicillin, and cephalosporin.[124] A notable exception is vancomycin, which is effective against C. *difficile* and so is used in the treatment of PMC. However, PMC sometimes occurs in the absence of prior antibiotic treatment, such as after surgery (particularly colonic, gastric, or pelvic), severe burns, shock, Crohn's disease, and other serious illnesses; indeed, it has occasionally developed in otherwise healthy young individuals. There has been a recent suggestion that C. *difficile* also elaborates a noncytopathic enterotoxin that could contribute to the diarrhea.[125]

The lesions are patchy and mainly confined to the colon. They are usually found in the rectosigmoid region

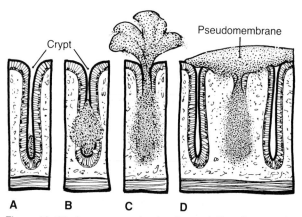

Figure 16–21. A sequence showing the evolution of a pseudomembrane. *A*, The crypt abscess; *B*, its expansion; *C*, extrusion of the exudate onto the surface of the bowel; and *D*, formation of a pseudomembrane by coalescence of multiple extrusions.

or in the hepatic flexure, but occasionally they also involve the distal small intestine or, rarely, the small intestine only. The intestinal mucosa is edematous, sometimes friable, with distinct adherent, yellow-white to dirty gray, raised, plaque-like pseudomembranes that range from a few millimeters to many centimeters in longest dimension. When the pseudomembranes are wiped off, superficial necrosis is evident but distinct ulcerations are uncommon. Microscopically, **the earliest change is suppurative inflammation beginning within a crypt that eventually breaks through the crypt wall and erupts through the surface in volcano-like fashion, extruding an inflammatory coagulum containing mucus, fibrin, neutrophils, and leukocytic and epithelial cell debris.** Coalescence of such exudative lesions yields the larger pseudomembranes (Fig. 16–21). Usually the inflammatory changes do not destroy the entire thickness of the mucosa. Typically, the immediately adjacent mucosa is edematous and hyperemic and contains a mixed inflammatory infiltrate in which plasma cells are numerous. In more remote intervening areas, the mucosa is normal.

Patients with PMC can be divided into two subsets. The first comprises patients who develop diarrhea while receiving antibiotic therapy. This pattern is self-limited within one to two weeks when the antibiotic is discontinued. A more serious subset consists of those who develop diarrhea days to weeks after the antibiotic course has been completed. The diarrhea is typically profuse, laden with leukocytes, and sometimes grossly bloody; it rapidly leads to fluid and electrolyte imbalances. Prior to vancomycin therapy, some of these patients died.

PMC must be differentiated from colitis caused by other invasive organisms. Required is the identification of the toxin of *C. difficile* in the gut, which until now largely depended on the cytopathic effect of the organism in tissue culture or on the detection of antibodies that were cross-reactive against a similar toxin of *C. sordellii*. More rapid diagnostic tests that use counter-immunoelectrophoresis and ELISA assays are now under study.

## AMEBIC COLITIS

It has been said that about 5 to 10% of the population of Europe and North America are asymptomatic carriers of *Entamoeba histolytica*. This prevalence is spuriously high because of confusion of pathogenic strains of *E. histolytica* with nonpathogenic strains and other nonpathogenic species that inhabit the human intestinal tract (e.g., *Entamoeba coli, Entamoeba nana*). Whatever the precise frequency, it is clear that amebic dysentery, although uncommon, is still encountered sporadically in the Western world, particularly among homosexual men and travelers from endemic foci in the tropics, where over half of the population may be infected.

The infection is transmitted by fecal contamination of water or food by the encysted organisms. The cysts are resistant to drying and gastric digestion, whereas the vegetative trophozoites are vulnerable to both. The encysted form is up to 20 μm in diameter and contains four nuclei. Only within the small bowel are the invasive trophozoites released. These are ameboid forms, up to 40 μm in diameter, that have a single small nucleus. Within the colon (most often the cecum and ascending colon, where the fecal stream is most fluid), the trophozoites enter the crypts of the colonic glands and release cytopathic lysosomal enzymes, which destroy epithelial cells.[126] In this manner the amebae prepare a pathway for invasion of the mucosa. For unknown reasons, concomitant bacterial growth is necessary for their survival.

The amebae burrow into the mucosa but are ultimately halted by the muscularis mucosa, which seems to constitute a barrier to their further progress. At this level, they fan out to create a characteristic undermined ulceration that has a flask shape (i.e., a narrow neck and a broad base). As the undermining progresses, the surface mucosa is deprived of its blood supply and tends to slough. **Histologically, the most important features of these lesions are the ameboid trophozoites (that often have phagocytized red cells) in the margins of ulcers, which are rendered distinctive by the relative absence of inflammatory infiltration.** Only when there is secondary bacterial infection is there a significant local leukocytic response.

Clinically, these patients have mild to severe abdominal cramps, diarrhea, and, occasionally, melena. Constitutional symptoms may be minimal or absent, unless there is secondary bacterial invasion. In about 40% of patients, trophozoites are drained to the liver, to produce solitary or multiple abscesses. These have a shaggy fibrinous lining and contain a chocolate-colored paste that consists of partially digested debris and blood. Similar abscesses may develop in the lung, either by drainage of parasites through the blood or by direct penetration through the diaphragm. Blood-borne spread may also lead to brain abscesses. Stool examination reveals the amebae proved to be pathogenic by enzyme analysis.

## IDIOPATHIC ULCERATIVE COLITIS

This serious common, chronic, recurrent diarrheal disease of unknown cause is characterized by severe ulcerations that occur principally in the rectum and rectosigmoid but sometimes extend throughout the colon. Although the clinical course and anatomic features are somewhat distinctive, the primary diagnosis of ulcerative colitis as a cause of diarrhea should not be made before other disorders of known etiology, such as amebiasis, shigellosis, *E. coli*–induced disease, have been ruled out. There are, as was pointed out earlier (p. 529), many similarities between ulcerative colitis and Crohn's disease, and indeed both are referred to as "inflammatory bowel disease." Suffice it here to recall the familial parallels; the association of both conditions with systemic complications such as migratory polyarthritis, sacroiliitis, ankylosing spondylitis, and erythema nodosum; and the increased frequency of HLA-B27 in those with either intestinal disorder who also have ankylosing spondylitis. But there are also many differences.

○ Ulcerative colitis is restricted to the large bowel except possibly in the case of "backwash ileitis," when there is total colonic involvement.[127]

○ The ulceroinflammatory process in ulcerative colitis is nonspecific, whereas in many cases of Crohn's disease it is marked by a granulomatous reaction.

○ Crohn's disease is characterized by transmural inflammation, but in ulcerative colitis it tends to be limited to the mucosa and submucosa.

○ Patients with ulcerative colitis are at far greater risk of developing colorectal cancer than are those with Crohn's granulomatous colitis.

The annual incidence of ulcerative colitis in the United States and other Western countries is about five to seven cases per 100,000 population. Unlike Crohn's disease, there is no evidence that the incidence is rising. Ulcerative colitis begins most often in the second to fourth decades of life, but occasionally it occurs in older individuals. Females are affected slightly more often than males, and whites more often than blacks.

**ETIOLOGY AND PATHOGENESIS.** The current state of uncertainty about the cause or causes of ulcerative colitis and Crohn's disease was detailed earlier. The many parallels between the two conditions raises the suspicion that both have similar origins but differ in the tissue response in particular individuals. It would be unproductive to repeat all of the still-indeterminate studies cited on page 529. It will suffice, therefore, to recall that the lines of investigation have focused on the search for (1) an etiologic bacterial agent, (2) an etiologic virus, and (3) immunopathogenetic mechanisms.[127, 128] We must leave it that there is much yet to be learned about the causation of ulcerative colitis. Indeed, many pathways may lead to the morphologic changes to be described.

**MORPHOLOGY. Ulcerative colitis begins in the rectum and spreads proximally in continuity. "Skip"** lesions, such as are seen in regional enteritis, **do not occur.** In most cases the disease remains confined to the rectosigmoid, but it sometimes extends to more proximal levels and, in about 10% of cases, affects the entire colon.

In the acute stage of the disease, the mucosa is hyperemic, edematous, and friable, and in most instances discloses small mucosal hemorrhages and apthoid ulcers consisting of minute foci of suppurative ulceration. **In time, and with progression, coalescence of these ulcers leads to irregular large ulcers ranging up to many centimeters in longest dimension. They are broadly based and typically extend through the mucosa and submucosa down to the muscularis. Coalescence of adjacent ulcerations may literally denude large tracts of the colon, but in the process, undermining may leave tenuous mucosal bridges between adjacent ulcers.** Residual edematous reactive islands of mucosa may create what are referred to as **"pseudopolyps,"** giving a cobblestone appearance (Fig. 16–22). With chronicity, there is some fibrous induration of the bowel wall, possibly with stricture formation; it is rarely as marked as that found in regional enteritis. In perhaps

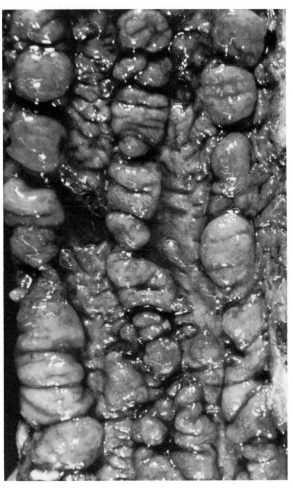

Figure 16–22. Ulcerative colitis. The many interconnecting ulcerations have created innumerable "pseudopolyps," which impart a "cobblestone" appearance to the surface.

5 to 10% of cases of chronic disease, the mucosal ulcerations penetrate more deeply to produce anal fissures or fistulas, perianal or ischiorectal abscesses, and recto-vaginal fistulas. Two very infrequent grave complications are "toxic" dilatation of the colorectum (seen in severe, acute expressions of extensive disease) and free perforation of the bowel.

The histologic features can be deduced largely from the gross changes. The acute stage of the disease is marked by hyperemia, edema, and microhemorrhages within the mucosa. Scattered neutrophils and mononuclear inflammatory cells are present in the lamina propria. More definitive is the appearance of minute abscesses beginning within the colorectal crypts—**crypt abscesses**—which induce suppurative necrosis of the overlying mucosa. Extension of this process leads to lateral spread of the suppurative necrosis, producing ulcerations with overhanging margins (Fig. 16–23). The walls and bases of these ulcers are heavily infiltrated with neutrophils, surrounded in turn by lymphocytes, plasma cells, and occasional mast cells. Sometimes the subjacent vessels disclose acute vasculitis and thromboses. Histologically, the pseudopolyps represent islands of mucosa

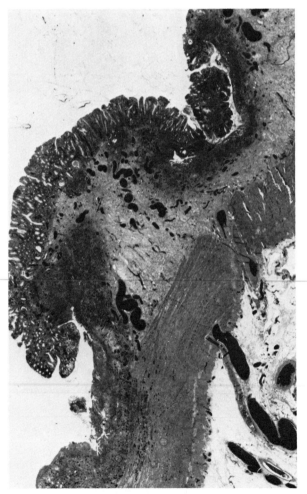

Figure 16–23. Ulcerative colitis. A low-power transection reveals two ulcerations extending into the submucosa and an intervening polypoid mucosal island.

containing edematous granulation tissue and having a rich inflammatory cell infiltration. In chronic disease with persistent or recurrent ulcerations, a fibrosing reaction may supervene. The mucosa and submucosa bear the brunt of the changes but, as indicated, they sometimes extend into the muscularis or even through the wall. **The subserosal and fibrosing reaction in chronic disease is not as pronounced as that seen in regional enteritis, nor are there granulomas.**

Particularly important in active colitis are the epithelial changes that appear in the margins of ulcers and often in the intervening mucosa. They consist of mucous depletion and inflammatory metaplasia, but far more important are varying degrees of atypical dysplasia, which have been classified as low to high grade.[129] The regrettable next step is the development of carcinoma. **The severity of the dysplasia and risk of carcinoma are most strongly correlated with the extent of the colorectal involvement and its duration. With "universal colitis" (entire colorectum), the incidence of carcinoma is about 1% for less than 10 years of disease, 3.5% at 15 years, 10 to 15% at 20 years, and in some studies over 30% at 30 years.** However, some reports suggest a substantially lower risk (12% after 26 years). The risk with long-standing disease confined to the rectosigmoid is about 3 to 5%. The cancers tend to be infiltrative and rapidly invasive lesions that spread to regional nodes and metastasize early. Because they often do not produce intraluminal masses, they are easily overlooked on endoscopy and barium enema studies against the background of the ulceroinflammatory disease.

Although the progression of changes encountered in active colitis have been emphasized to this point, it is necessary to note that **between bouts of activity, mucosal regeneration occurs,** depending on the chronicity of the disease, its severity, and duration of the remission. In the fortunate patient who has a single attack and no recurrences, restoration of an intact mucosa is possible, but in those with recurrent bouts and some fibrosis, the most that can be achieved is a simplified mucosa with shallow crypts and nondifferentiated surface epithelium.

**CLINICAL COURSE.** Most commonly, ulcerative colitis develops insidiously over the course of several months, manifesting itself by diarrhea that often consists of a mixture of blood, mucus, and flecks of feces; tenesmus and colicky lower abdominal pain, relieved by defecation; and variable constitutional signs, including fever and weight loss. Grossly bloody stools are far more common than with Crohn's disease, and the blood loss may be considerable. The extragastrointestinal complications mentioned are also more common with ulcerative colitis than with Crohn's disease. About 15% of patients develop, for obscure reasons, hepatic lesions (e.g., fatty change, pericholangitis, and sclerosing cholangitis).

The course of ulcerative colitis is variable. Most patients follow a chronic relapsing, remitting course, with exacerbations often triggered by emotional or physical stress. During severe exacerbations and also when the onset is acute with explosive diarrhea, the colon becomes markedly distended; this condition is known as *toxic dilatation* or *toxic megacolon* and requires emergency colectomy. Other life-threatening complications include massive hemorrhage and perforation with peritonitis. Strictures of the colorectum are easily confused with carcinoma.

Because involvement of the rectosigmoid colon is common, the diagnosis can usually be made on endoscopy and biopsy. Specific infectious causes must always be ruled out. The prognosis with ulcerative colitis varies with the clinical activity of the disease. The mortality is highest in the first months and improves with chronicity. About 8% of patients whose onset of disease is severe and unremitting die within one year of peritonitis, sepsis, hemorrhage, or fluid and electrolyte disturbances. The darkest cloud on the horizon is the development of colonic cancer, as was pointed out. It is therefore standard practice to closely monitor patients by repeated endoscopies and multiple mucosal biopsies, at least yearly or more often, depending on the severity of the epithelial changes in the prior biopsies.[132]

# TUMORS

Tumors of the colorectum are among the most common forms of neoplasia in humans. Colorectal carcinoma is the second commonest cause of cancer death in the United States and in other industrialized nations. When discovered at an early stage, it is resectable and curable. Polyps of the colorectum are found in 25 to 50% of older adults.[133] Certain forms of polyps, as will be seen, are now considered to be precursors of carcinomas of the colorectum; their early discovery and removal has been shown to reduce markedly the incidence of colorectal carcinoma. Diagnostic modalities (colonoscopy and barium radiographic studies) are widely available for the detection of these benign or malignant neoplasms before incurable disease has developed. Thus, the approximately 50,000 deaths caused by colorectal cancer annually can each be considered a preventable tragedy.

Although a wide range of benign or malignant mesenchymal neoplasms may arise in the colorectum, they are all extremely rare. Colorectal lymphomas and carcinoids, too, are uncommon. Only polyps and carcinoma occur with sufficient frequency to merit further consideration.

## POLYPS

"Polyp" is the macroscopic term for any lesion that protrudes above a mucosal surface. Although an expanding submucosal lipoma or intramural leiomyoma may create a polyp, unless qualified, the term "polyp" as used here implies an epithelial lesion. Colorectal polyps can be divided into the following categories: (1) hyperplastic; (2) adenomatous, of which

there are three variants: tubular, tubulovillous, and villous; and (3) polyposis syndromes, which are usually hereditary. *Hyperplastic polyps are best viewed as benign controlled proliferations.* In contrast, *adenomatous polyps are neoplasms that range from benign to those that may have begun as benign lesions but later acquired areas of carcinomatous transformation, giving rise to the concept of an "adenoma-carcinoma sequence."*[134] The polyposis syndromes are relatively uncommon, albeit clinically important, and will be considered after the far more common hyperplastic and adenomatous lesions.

Reports do not agree on the frequency of the different types of epithelial polyps. Nevertheless, hyperplastic polyps are the most common form in adults and are the preponderant very small polyp (less than 5 mm in diameter). Among the adenomatous lesions, tubular adenomas represent about 90%, tubulovillous about 5 to 10%, and villous about 1 to 2%. The frequency of epithelial polyps increases with age, thus they are found in 20 to 30% of individuals under the age of 50 and rise in frequency to about 50% in those aged 60 to 70.[135] Males and females are affected equally. Polyps may occur singly, but when one is found, there is a 20 to 50% likelihood of others, perhaps five or more. There are hints of genetic predisposition to the common types of adenomatous polyps and to common colorectal cancers, so that certain pedigrees have an increased frequency of these lesions.[136] Data vary on the distribution of polyps within the colorectum. In years past it was said that 50 to 60% occurred in the rectosigmoid, within reach of the sigmoidoscope, and only about 15% were found in the right colon. Current studies indicate that the distal part of the large intestine is still the favored site in younger individuals. However, as polyps progressively appear during life they tend to involve the right colon, so that in older individuals only about 40 to 45% are found in the rectosigmoid and relatively more occur in the right colon (25%).[137] The remainder are distributed throughout the rest of the colon. With this overview of the spectrum of epithelial polyps, we can turn to specific categories.

### Hyperplastic Polyps

This type of polyp is formed by an exaggerated but controlled proliferation of crypt epithelium. Normally, in the crypts of the large intestine cell division is restricted to the lowest third. The cells then migrate toward the mucosal surface while differentiating into mature goblet and absorptive cells, and they are then desquamated at the surface. If the proliferative zone is expanded, the excess of cells creates a polyp.

Grossly, hyperplastic polyps are small, tan-pink, hemispheric protrusions that usually sit on top of a mucosal fold. Over 90% are less than 5 mm in diameter. Rarely they are slightly larger and may become pedunculated. Their gross appearance is usually quite distinctive from that of tubular and villous adenomas (Fig. 16–24). Histologically, they have slightly expanded crypts lined by somewhat immature cells that, as they ascend the crypt wall, mature into goblet cells admixed with some absorptive cells. The epithelial overgrowth may cause some buckling of the normal single-layered palisade to create a serrated lining. The nuclei appear essentially normal and remain basally oriented. The crypts are separated by a scanty stroma, which may possibly contain a few mononuclear inflammatory cells.[138]

On the basis of their orderly cytologic characteristics and apparent genesis, *hyperplastic polyps are not believed to have cancerous potential*. However, a hyperplastic polyp occasionally contains an adenomatous focus. The interpretation of such lesions is uncertain, but there is little likelihood of their becoming cancerous. The only significance of hyperplastic polyps is their differentiation from the more ominous adenomatous lesions.

### Tubular Adenoma (Pedunculated Polyp)

The great preponderance of all adenomatous polyps are tubular adenomas, and so, unless qualified, the term "adenomatous polyp" refers to them. Because most have a well-developed stalk and since the tu-

bulovillous and villous lesions tend to be sessile, the term *"pedunculated polyp"* is also equated with tubular adenoma.

Reference has already been made in the introductory section to their usual distribution in the colon and to the fact that although they may be solitary, often they are not, and sometimes two to ten (and even more) are present concurrently. Furthermore, the individual having one or more polyps has an increased risk of developing subsequent lesions attributed to the abnormal growth kinetics of the surface epithelium over wide areas of the large bowel. **The typical individual lesion has a raspberry-like head, usually less than 1 cm in diameter that sits on top of a slender stalk ranging up to many centimeters in length** (Fig. 16–24). Uncommonly, the head of a pedunculated lesion exceeds 1 cm in diameter, and rarely is it greater than 3 to 4 cm; it is usually tan-red, firm, and slightly nobby, but the stalk is covered with yielding, normal colorectal mucosa, apparently superficially attached to the underlying submucosa. They are uncommonly found to be semisessile and are infrequently sessile.

Histologically, these polyps range from the entirely benign to those having areas of carcinomatous transformation. **In all there is loss of normal differentiation of the colonic epithelium into specialized cell types**

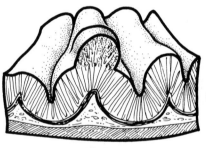

Hyperplastic polyp

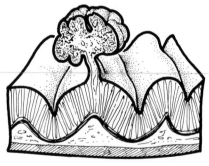

Tubular adenoma

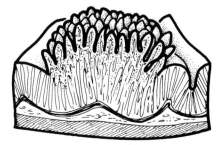

Villous adenoma

Figure 16–24. A diagrammatic representation of the three principal forms of colonic polyps. The hyperplastic polyp (*above*) sits as a hemispheric dome on top of the mucosal fold. The tubular (pedunculated) adenoma (*middle*) has a slender stalk and a knobby, "raspberry-like" head. The sessile villous adenoma (*below*) has a broad base and myriad delicate papillae protruding into the lumen.

**distinguishing adenomatous polyps from hyperplastic polyps.** The clearly benign lesions have a thickened mucosal layer (polypoid hyperplasia) composed of closely aggregated elongated tubules and glands that are well demarcated from the intervening scant connective tissue stroma (Fig. 16–25). The lining cells are abnormally tall, columnar, and well oriented albeit somewhat crowded. They have slightly enlarged hyperchromatic nuclei that are no longer basally oriented and therefore are pseudostratified. These epithelial elements are separated from the underlying submucosa by the muscularis mucosae, which is more or less continuous through the stalk and head of the lesion. Mitoses are scant to numerous but are not atypical. At the other end of the spectrum, the tubules and glands are more closely packed. Sometimes they lack intervening stroma and are thus "back-to-back," producing on occasion a cribriform pattern. The orderly orientation is replaced by a disarray of larger cells, and the nuclei are more hyperchromatic, vary in size and shape, and have numerous mitotic figures that are sometimes abnormal.

Tubular adenomas often contain foci of villous growth (p. 554)—areas where the adenomatous epithelium takes a papillary configuration. By general agreement, if the villous pattern composes less than 20 to 25% of the total adenoma, the lesion is still referred to as a tubular adenoma. **The greatest atypism, and indeed carcinomatous transformation, is likely to be found in these villous areas. Pure tubular adenomas only rarely have cancerous change, and so the risk is related to the proportion of the villous pattern, which in turn is correlated with the size of the pedunculated lesion.**

Although tubular adenomas may attract attention by bleeding, more often they are discovered incidentally. Critical to the clinical management of the patient is the determination of whether the cancerous alterations are confined to the epithelial lining of the tubules, glands, and papillae (*intraepithelial*); whether the atypical growth is restricted to the lamina propria (*intramucosal*); or whether it has extended below the muscularis mucosae within the head of the lesion and into the submucosa (*invasive cancer*). *Intraepithelial and intramucosal foci of cancer are not thought to have ominous biologic significance because removal of the polyp by transection of the base of the stalk will be curative. In contrast, invasion below the muscularis mucosae brings the neoplastic cells into potential contact with the lymphatics, creating a clinically significant lesion capable of metastasis.* Obviously, deep penetration of the stalk of the adenoma bodes even more poorly. Thus, the longer the stalk, the better the outlook even with invasion, and, conversely, the more sessile the lesion, the more significant invasion is likely to be. *The likelihood of carcinoma being present increases with (1) size of the adenoma, (2) the amount of villous growth in turn related to the size of the lesion, and (3) the tendency of larger lesions to be sessile.*[134] In general, when less than 1 cm in diameter, tubular adenomas have a 1% chance of containing a focus of carcinoma that, in many instances, has not penetrated the muscularis mucosae and so is not biologically significant. The risk of invasive cancer rises to 5 to 10% in those polyps 1 to 2 cm in diameter and is

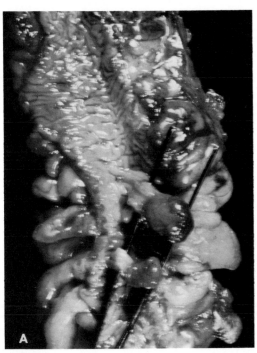
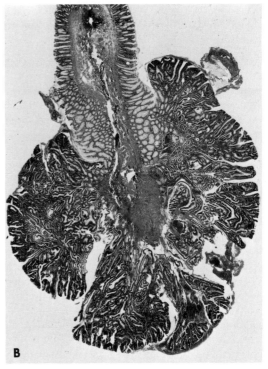

Figure 16–25. *A,* Two pedunculated adenomas of the colon, displayed on top of the forceps. The berry-like heads are attached on elongated, slender stalks. *B,* Low-power view of one of these lesions, showing the normal mucosa covering the stalk and the polypoid hyperplasia of the epithelium in the head of the polyp.

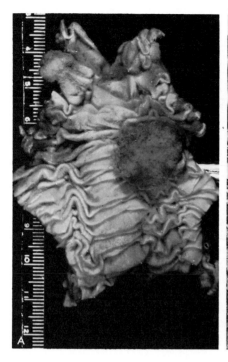 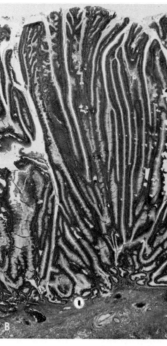

Figure 16–26. *A*, Villous adenoma of the colon, seen grossly. *B*, High-power detail of the long, villous glandular fronds. There is no evidence of cellular atypicality or of carcinoma in the view given.

significantly higher when they are of larger size. Overall, most tubular adenomas are small, so the incidence of invasive carcinoma is about 3 to 5%.[139]

## Villous Adenoma

Any colorectal adenoma more than 50% (some say 75%) papillary in architecture is referred to as a villous adenoma. These lesions are the least common epithelial polyps but are most likely to harbor carcinomatous areas.

**These polyps tend to be larger than tubular adenomas. Over half exceed 2 cm in diameter and only infrequently are less than 1 cm; most are sessile, but rarely they have a stalk.** Found anywhere in the large bowel, they tend to be distributed mostly in the rectosigmoid and slightly less frequently in the right colon. Typically, they are firm gray-tan, and lobular; they have a cauliflower appearance and protrude 1 to 3 cm above the surrounding mucosa (Fig. 16–24, p. 552). Focal hemorrhages or surface ulcerations may be present.

Histologically, at least half of the lesion is composed of papillary, sometimes branching fronds, but the residual portion may have tubular features. There is a direct correlation between the proportion of villous component and size of the polyp.[140] The papillae have fibrovascular, finger-like cores covered by epithelium. In a series of these lesions, the epithelium ranges from fairly orderly, tall, columnar cells that have little dysplasia but no differentiation into mature colonic types, to disorderly, multilayered arrangements with overt anaplasia (Fig. 16–26). Sometimes the anaplastic cells form "back-to-back" glands, cribriform patterns, or aggregations into compact nests abutting similar nests. These anaplastic cells often invade the lamina propria, and **in 25 to 45% of instances they penetrate the muscularis mucosae to constitute invasive carcinoma.**[139] Metastases to regional nodes are present in many of the invasive lesions by the time they are discovered.[141]

Villous adenomas are much more frequently symptomatic than other forms of epithelial polyps. Most commonly they cause rectal bleeding, and sometimes they elaborate sufficient quantities of potassium- and protein-rich secretions to produce diarrhea, hypoalbuminemia, and hypokalemia. Overshadowing these consequences is the fact that *approximately one third of them harbor invasive cancer.* Thus all villous adenomas require as early diagnosis as possible and adequate resection. However, what constitutes "adequate resection" is controversial but, fortunately, beyond our scope.

## Tubulovillous Adenoma

This designation is applied to any colorectal epithelial polyp that has, by definition, a 25 to 50% villous component; the remainder of the polyp conforms to the tubular pattern. Thus, the risk of cancer is intermediate between the tubular and villous adenomas.

The distribution of these adenomas is essentially the same as that of the tubular lesions. Moreover, they are intermediate in size; about half are 1 to 2 cm in diameter, and the rest are distributed equally above and below this range. They may have a stalk, be semisessile, or be sessile. The histologic features can be deduced from the bridging position they occupy between tubular and villous adenomas.

Most tubulovillous polyps are asymptomatic. A few cause occult bleeding; discovery is by chance during barium enema or colonoscopy. *About 10 to 15% of these lesions harbor cancer, and the risk is directly related to their size, which is, in turn, related to the proportion of villous growth.*

### Adenoma-Carcinoma Sequence

There is now fairly wide agreement from clinical and experimental studies that all three types of adenomatous polyps may give rise to colorectal carcinoma and, in many instances, invasive lesions that have already spread to regional nodes.[142, 143] Still controversial, however, is the issue of whether most (perhaps all) colorectal carcinomas arise in preexisting polyps. There are those who contend from experimental studies that adenomas and the usual colorectal carcinomas are separate and unrelated lesions.[144, 145] On the other hand, there is the extremely high frequency of carcinoma in individuals who have a profusion of adenomas in the familial multiple polyposis syndromes (to be described) and the general parallel between the frequency of epithelial polyps and colorectal carcinomas in various populations. The issue is more than academic. In a 25-year study of a large number of individuals receiving periodic sigmoidoscopic examinations and removal of all identified mucosal protrusions, the incidence of rectosigmoid carcinoma was reduced by 85%.[146] Preponderant opinion therefore favors the view that most or at least a substantial fraction of colorectal carcinomas arise in preexisting adenomas. On these grounds, no polyp can be considered to be benign when it exceeds 1 cm in diameter until it has been completely excised and submitted to adequate histologic examination. The colonic polyp often demands anatomic and clinical judgments that would tax even Solomon.

## POLYPOSIS SYNDROMES

There are several syndromes marked by numerous, sometimes hundreds of polyps within the gastrointestinal tract. These disorders can be divided into familial and nonfamilial groups. The best characterized are the familial polyposis syndromes: (1) familial polyposis coli; (2) Gardner's syndrome; (3) Turcot's syndrome; and (4) Peutz-Jeghers syndrome. All are inherited as autosomal dominant diseases. In the first three, the polyps are adenomatous neoplasms, but in the Peutz-Jeghers syndrome, the polyps are probably hamartomous in nature and so rarely undergo carcinomatous transformation. Brief descriptions will be limited to the four familial syndromes.

### Familial Polyposis Coli

In about 80% of these cases, there is clear evidence of autosomal dominant inheritance; in the remainder it is less well established. Usually beginning after puberty, typical adenomatous polyps begin to appear in the colon. Rarely, lesions are found in the small intestine and stomach. At first sparse, small, and stalked, they progressively become more numerous and may literally carpet the colon. Some enlarge and become sessile, and unless the entire colon is removed surgically, one or more *carcinomas almost always appear within one to two decades.*[146a]

A member of a family who has not developed intestinal polyps by the age of 30 has probably not inherited the mutant gene. Overt carcinomas usually appear by age 40, sometimes much earlier. Thus efforts have been made to identify at an early age those who have inherited the mutant gene so that total removal of the colon might be performed even before it becomes significantly involved. Holding great promise as a marker of this condition is increased activity of the enzyme ornithine decarboxylase in biopsies of apparently normal-appearing colonic mucosa.[147] This is a rate-limiting enzyme in the polyamine synthesis required for cellular proliferation. This finding suggests some defect in regulation or control of mucosal cell turnover in those affected; the result is myriads of neoplasms that at first are benign and then progressively turn into carcinomas. In passing, it should be noted that the near inevitability of carcinoma in multiple polyposis is taken as strong evidence in the support of the adenoma-carcinoma sequence in the general population.

### Gardner's Syndrome

*Gardner's syndrome may well be a variant of familial polyposis coli because the mode of inheritance is the same; also similar are the presence of numerous adenomatous polyps of the colon that are followed by carcinoma.* However, in Gardner's syndrome, adenomatous polyps are also commonly seen in the small intestine and stomach. In addition, the disorder exhibits one or more of the following features: osteomas (especially of the mandible and cranium), soft tissue tumors (fibromas, lipomas, sebaceous cysts, epidermoid cysts), desmoid tumors (p. 721), small intestinal carcinoma (especially periampullary), and, rarely, malignant transformation of osteomas or soft tissue tumors. Most patients do not have the full spectrum of lesions; the three most common are colonic polyposis in about 70%, multiple soft tissue tumors in about 60%, and osteomas in about 30%. In one analysis this triad was present only in 20% of patients.[148] The expression of the pleiotropic gene among family members is highly variable and may be manifest only as colonic polyposis or as the concurrence of two or more of the other features in an individual who lacks colonic polyps at least at the time of examination.

### Turcot's Syndrome

Better identified as the *polyposis-glioma syndrome*, this entity may merely be a variant of the two preceding familial polyposis syndromes. In its classic expression, Turcot's syndrome manifests adenomatous polyps in the colon that are followed by carcinoma of the colon if the patient survives long enough, because intercurrent glioma in the brain may bring about an early death. In some instances, the glioma appears first in patients not having polyposis.

### Peutz-Jeghers Syndrome

This curious disorder is better called "mucocutaneous pigmentations associated with gastrointestinal hamartomatous polyps." It, too, is thought to be transmitted by a single pleiotropic autosomal dominant gene with incomplete penetrance, but this is less certainly established than with the other familial syndromes. The two main features of the Peutz-Jeghers syndromes are (1) multiple, usually pedunculated, polyps of the colon and (2) irregular melanin pigmentations, found most often around the mouth, lips, buccal mucosa, and tips of the fingers. Less frequently, the pigmentations occur on the feet and perianal and genital regions. The polyps in this condition have a different distribution and nature from those in the preceding polyposis syndromes. *They are distributed less abundantly in the colon and rectum and are more common in the small intestine and the stomach.* The individual lesions are hamartomas in which the head of the polyp is composed of epithelial glands, tubules, and microcysts separated by a prominent arborizing network of smooth muscle that is sometimes continuous with the underlying muscularis mucosae. Carcinomatous transformation of the polyps is very uncommon. The rare reports of gastrointestinal malignancy in this syndrome refer to carcinomas most often in the duodenum, jejunum, and stomach. The question is, Do the malignancies indeed arise in the typical hamartomatous polyps or from concurrent adenomatous polyps?[149] In addition, ovarian neoplasms, particularly sex cord tumors, coexist in about 12% of cases. These sometimes appear in the second decade of life. There is also an increased frequency of cervical cancers, benign and malignant breast neoplasms, and many other different neoplasms in various organs, leading to the conclusion that although the hamartomas themselves do not usually become malignant, there is a genetic generalized predisposition to the development of neoplasms that are often malignant.[150]

## CARCINOMA OF THE COLORECTUM

At least 95% of all malignant tumors of the colorectum are carcinomas; the remainder include lymphomas (p. 369), carcinoids (p. 536), and diverse sarcomas. Colorectal cancer is currently number two on the roster of cancer-killers in the United States and causes approximately 60,000 deaths. Only lung cancer kills more men, and lung and breast cancer kill more women.

**EPIDEMIOLOGY.** In general, *carcinomas of the large bowel are uncommon before age 40, except when they represent a complication of ulcerative colitis, granulomatous colitis, familial multiple polyposis, Gardner's and Turcot's syndromes, and the rare family cancer syndromes unassociated with polyps.* In the general population, the risk of colorectal cancer significantly increases at age 50 and almost doubles with each successive decade. The incidence of colonic cancer, as distinct from rectal, has been slowly increasing over the past years in the United States but the incidence of rectal carcinoma has slightly decreased.[137] For unknown reasons the increase has been greater in blacks. Rectal carcinomas affect men slightly more often than women, but there is no sex preponderance for cancers in the remainder of the colon. These and other observations hint at the possibility that colonic and rectal carcinomas may be separate diseases having different causal influences. The following discussion therefore will, at times, differentiate colonic from rectal carcinoma.

Epidemiologic studies strongly suggest that environmental influences, notably the diet, play a significant role in the causation of colonic cancer, much more so than with rectal cancer.[151] Cancer of the colon is four to six times more common in most industrialized countries (Japan being a notable exception) where diets are higher in animal fat, protein, and refined carbohydrates but lower in fiber than the diets in Africa, Asia, many parts of South America, and Japan. Particularly high-risk areas include North America, Northern and Western Europe, and New Zealand. Significantly, the ratio of colonic cancer between the United States and Japan is 4–6:1, but for rectal cancer it is nearly 1:1. That dietary rather than racial factors may be involved is documented by the progressive rise over the span of years in the incidence of colonic cancer among the Japanese who migrate to Hawaii or mainland United States and adopt western dietary habits.[152]

Genetic influences may also contribute to the predisposition to this form of cancer. In addition to those for the well-defined mendelian polyposis-carcinoma syndromes, genetic predispositions to cancer may exist for the general population. First-degree relatives of a patient with colorectal carcinoma have a threefold greater risk than controls. An individual having this form of carcinoma has a 1.5 to 5% chance of developing a subsequent colorectal cancer. You should also recall the previously discussed (p. 555) important role of sporadic adenomatous polyps in the genesis of colorectal carcinoma.

**ETIOLOGY AND PATHOGENESIS.** *Experimental evidence and dietary surveys implicate the interaction of the following factors in colonic carcinogenesis: (1) high levels of consumption of beef and animal fat, (2) increase in the anaerobic microflora of the colon, (3) a tumor-producing effect of secondary bile acids, (4) a lack of dietary fiber, and (5) a possible deficiency of protective nutrients in the diet.* The following theory has been proposed—a diet high in beef and fat favors the development of an anaerobic fecal flora, notably clostridia and bacteroides. These organisms acting on the fat and bile increase the levels of fatty acids and secondary bile acids in the colon. Both the fatty and bile acids damage the colonic mucosa, initiating replicative activity, and simultaneously serve as promotors for other potentially carcinogenic compounds.[153] Contributing to the process may be the formation of a nitrosamide (a documented carcinogen in experimental animals) from the amines and amides released from meats in the diet (p. 251).[154] So it is speculated that meats and fats in the diet provide circumstances for the possible emergence of cancers. Simultaneously, it is proposed that a deficiency of dietary fiber reduces the stool bulk and slows the bowel transit time. At the same time, it reduces the dilution and binding of carcinogens.[155] Moreover, low-fiber diets are frequently a consequence of reduced consumption of fruit and vegetables containing the putative anti-cancer vitamins A, C, and E.

Dietary factors are thus thought to account for the lower incidence of colonic cancer among certain populations, such as rural Africans, who have diets rich in fiber. However, the dietary theory of colon carcinogenesis is not without challenge. A recent survey of two groups of nuns who ate little or no meat failed to identify any reduction in the incidence of colonic carcinoma.[156] Analogously, Mormons, whose intake of meat has steadily increased over the past years, have not experienced any change in their below-average incidence of colonic cancer. Other contrary evidence might be cited, so although dietary influences are suspected, they are far from established.

**MORPHOLOGY.** In the United States the distribution of carcinomas in the large intestine is: rectum, 25%; sigmoid, 30%; descending colon, 5 to 10%; transverse colon, 15 to 20%; and right colon, 20 to 25%. Infrequently, multiple carcinomas occur, most often in patients with familial polyposis syndromes, numerous sporadic adenomas, or ulcerative colitis.

It is extremely rare to find a small colorectal carcinoma arising de novo from normal mucosa, and so it is thought that most of these neoplasms arise in preexisting adenomas. At the time of discovery, carcinomas of the left side of the colon, including the rectum, generally have a different gross appearance from those of the right colon. **Most left-sided lesions have an annular configuration producing a so-called napkin-ring constriction of the bowel,** which accounts for early symptoms of obstruction (Fig. 16–27). It has been estimated that it takes approximately one to two years for a left-sided lesion to totally encircle the lumen, and therefore sometimes plaque-like lesions are encountered that do not involve the entire circumference. Often the mid-circumference of the ring or center of the plaque is ulcerated and the tumor penetrates the bowel wall, to appear as subserosal and serosal small white nodules. Advanced lesions may extend into the pericolic fat and metastasize to regional

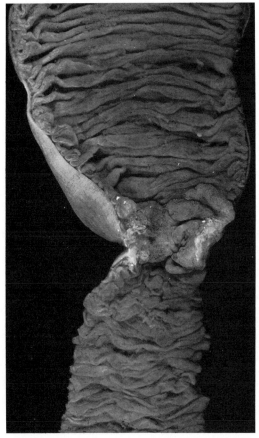

Figure 16–27. Carcinoma of the rectosigmoid. The narrow annular lesion has caused obstructive dilatation of the proximal bowel above.

lymph nodes and viscera, particularly the liver. On occasion, the penetration of the bowel wall produces pericolic abscesses or even peritonitis.

**Cancers in the right colon typically have a polypoid, fungating appearance and protrude into the lumen as cauliflower-like masses** (Fig. 16–28). Plaque-like or ulcerative lesions of the right side are much less common than polypoid forms. Whatever their gross morphology, the lesions eventually penetrate the wall and extend to the mesentery and regional lymph nodes. More distant dissemination to the liver and other sites may follow. Because they occur in the more capacious cecum and ascending colon, where the fecal stream is more fluid, these tumors rarely cause obstruction and so have a distressing tendency to remain silent clinically for long periods of time.

Uncommonly, but particularly in association with ulcerative colitis, colorectal cancers are insidiously infiltrative and do not produce readily recognized intraluminal lesions. Because of their invasiveness, they tend to spread at a relatively early stage into the regional nodes and to more distant sites.

Unlike their gross pathologic appearance, the histologic details of the right- and left-sided colorectal carcinomas are usually similar. Ninety-five percent are adenocarci-

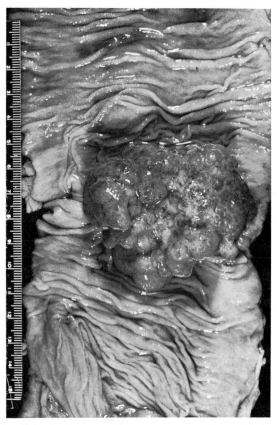

Figure 16–28. Carcinoma of the right colon. The polypoid cancer projects into the lumen but has not caused obstruction.

nomas; some secrete mucin and occasionally form signet-ring cells (p. 524). At the anorectal junction many different histologic types may be encountered, including squamous cell carcinomas, adenocanthomas (having both squamous cell and adenocarcinomatous differentiation, p. 645), and, rarely, melanocarcinomas.

A system for staging carcinomas of the rectum was originally devised by Dukes; it utilized three stages—A, B, and C. This system has since been extensively modified and applied to all colorectal carcinomas. The following stages (in simplified terms) are currently in use:[157]

Stage A:  Tumor confined to the bowel, not penetrating beyond muscularis propria
Stage B:  Tumor beyond muscularis propria, possibly with involvement of serosa
Stage C:  Lymph node metastases
Stage D:  Incomplete resection or distant metastases

Under this system of staging, at the time of resection, 25 to 40% of colorectal cancers have spread to regional nodes (Stage C), and 15% of rectal, 25% of left colonic, and 35% of right colonic neoplasms are Stage D, emphasizing the insidious nature of those in the right colon.

**CLINICAL COURSE.** Colorectal cancer is unfortunately too often silent during its developmental stages. When left-sided lesions induce manifestations, they usually take the form of a change in bowel habit, decrease in caliber of the stool, crampy left lower quadrant discomfort, or sometimes only occult or gross blood in the stools. In contrast, right-sided lesions are often entirely silent. There may be some vague discomfort in the right lower quadrant, but more often they are found because they produce bleeding, usually occult. Indeed, these tumors are sometimes discovered in the course of investigation of the cause of an iron-deficiency anemia. *It is a clinical maxim that this type of anemia in a male means GI cancer, usually in the right colon, unless other obvious causes such as malnutrition or chronic inflammatory bowel disease are present.* In the female, menstrual losses, multiple pregnancies, abnormal uterine bleeding, or dietary inadequacies are more likely to explain such an anemia. Only infrequently do large-bowel cancers cause massive rectal bleeding. Systemic manifestations such as weakness, malaise, and weight loss only appear when the neoplasm has disseminated, and at this time hepatomegaly may point to metastases to the liver. Local spread of rectal neoplasms may result in rectovaginal or rectovesical fistulas or back pain, and sometimes dissemination of colorectal lesions into the peritoneal cavity induces intestinal obstruction.

The diagnosis of most developed colorectal carcinomas is usually readily made by barium enema sigmoidoscopy or colonoscopy with biopsy. Attempts to find serum markers that would permit detection of neoplasms early in their development have been largely unsuccessful to date. Elevated blood levels of carcinoembryonic antigen (CEA) (p. 226) are unreliable for early detection because these lesions produce diagnostic levels only when there is a significant burden of neoplasm and only rarely in stages A and B. Moreover, as pointed out on page 226, a variety of cancers and benign disorders may also cause elevation of the CEA level. However, CEA assays are of great use in postoperative surveillance. Removal of the tumor is followed by a fall in the CEA level; reversal of the falling titer or reappearance of significantly elevated blood levels indicates recurrent, usually metastatic, disease.[158] Similarly, the CEA blood levels provide a rough quantitation of the effectiveness of chemotherapy. Among the many other potential markers of colorectal carcinoma of great current interest is the ornithine decarboxylase assay of mucosal biopsies. Further studies are needed to determine whether an elevated level of this mucosal enzyme is as useful a marker of colorectal cancers as it appears to be of familial multiple polyposis.[147] At the present time, fecal occult blood testing and endoscopy are still the most reliable methods for the screening of populations at risk and for early detection of tumors.

The prognosis for patients with colorectal carcinoma is primarily dependent on the stage of the neoplasm at time of diagnosis (and, therefore, its resectability) and secondarily on its level of differentiation and responsiveness to radiation and chemotherapy. The five-year survival rate for patients with tumors in Stages A and B, after therapy, is approximately 75 to 80%; this rate falls to about 45% with Stage C and 10% with Stage D. Regrettably, the best hope for cure is surgical resection; radiation and chemotherapy prolong survival in Stages C and D, but whether they can achieve a cure remains uncertain.

# Appendix

Only appendicitis and tumors, including mucocele, will be described here.

## APPENDICITIS

Acute appendicitis is one of the most common gastrointestinal diseases and the most frequent cause of an "acute abdomen." Surveys several decades ago indicated that as many as 10% of individuals developed appendicitis during their lifetimes, most often in the second and third decades of life. However, for unexplained reasons the overall incidence appears to be declining while the proportion of patients in the later decades of life is rising.[159] Males are affected slightly more often than females.

ETIOLOGY AND PATHOGENESIS. Despite its frequency, acute appendicitis has an etiology that is only incompletely understood. Most probably, the usual inciting event is obstruction of the appendiceal lumen by a fecalith, although there are other uncommon causes (e.g., tumors, pinworms). With obstruction, the outflow of mucus secretion is blocked and the appendix becomes distended. Possibly this distention compromises the blood flow within the wall of the appendix, thereby rendering it vulnerable to invasion by ordinarily harmless native bacteria. In cases in which no obvious luminal obstruction can be found, such vagaries as kinking, viral-induced lymphoid hyperplasia, and fibrosing strictures with aging are raised as possible causes.

MORPHOLOGY. In early acute appendicitis, there is a scant neutrophilic exudation throughout the mucosa, submucosa, and muscularis. The subserosal vessels are congested and are often surrounded by a neutrophilic emigration. The congestion transforms the normally glistening serosal covering into a reddened, dull, granular membrane. As the process develops, the neutrophilic exudate becomes more marked, and the serosa is covered by a fibrinopurulent material (Fig. 16–29). Foci of suppurative necrosis develop within the wall of the appendix, and at this stage the process may be termed acute suppurative appendicitis. Eventually, the inflammatory edema compromises the blood supply, and gangrenous necrosis is superimposed on it, resulting in large areas of greenish hemorrhagic ulceration of the mucosa and green-black foci of necrosis extending throughout the wall to the serosa. This stage, acute gangrenous appendicitis, immediately precedes rupture of the appendix. At surgery, a fecalith is commonly but not invariably found within the lumen.

The histologic picture during these stages of acute appendicitis is entirely nonspecific and follows the typical patterns of acute inflammation, suppuration, and gangrenous necrosis in any tissue. Because some degree of superficial inflammation may follow drainage of exudate into the appendix from a more proximal lesion, such as ileitis, the histologic diagnosis of acute appendicitis requires some involvement of the muscularis.

The entity of **chronic** appendicitis is a subject of some controversy. Involved is the issue of whether recurrent acute attacks that spontaneously subside should be termed chronic disease. Truly persistent, smoldering chronic inflammation of the appendix does occur, but it is rare. It is characterized grossly by a thickened fibrotic appendix. Histologically, there is a mononuclear leukocytic infiltrate throughout the wall, principally in the subserosa but sometimes aggregated into large lymphoid follicles.

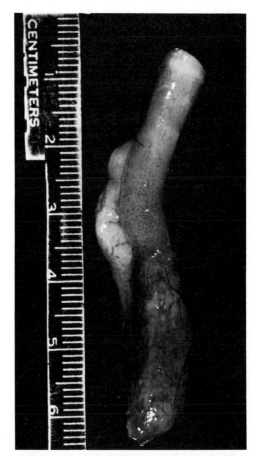

Figure 16–29. The distal half of the appendix (below) is swollen and darker in color because of inflammatory congestion, and the serosa is layered by a fibrinopurulent exudate.

**CLINICAL COURSE.** The classic case of acute appendicitis, which develops over the course of a day or two, begins with a mild periumbilical discomfort, followed by anorexia, nausea, and vomiting. As the appendix becomes distended, the discomfort begins to localize in the right lower quadrant of the abdomen and becomes a deep, constant ache, accompanied by tenderness to palpation. Later, when the inflammation becomes well advanced, bacteria are able to permeate the damaged wall, even before actual perforation has occurred. Involvement of the overlying parietal peritoneum results, causing severe pain and rebound tenderness. Fever and leukocytosis are present at this stage.

When surgical removal of the appendix is delayed beyond this point, the following complications may ensue: (1) generalized peritonitis; (2) periappendiceal abscess formation; (3) pylephlebitis, with thrombosis of the portal venous drainage; (4) hepatic abscess formation; or (5) septicemia. Generalized peritonitis may or may not imply actual rupture of the appendix. Ironically, rupture is sometimes accompanied by a temporary dramatic relief of pain.

The diagnosis of even the classic case just described presents many problems. The following disorders may have a similar or even identical clinical presentation: (1) mesenteric lymphadenitis, occurring in children in response to a viral systemic infection that produces enlargement and tenderness of all nodes, particularly the mesenteric; (2) gastroenteritis with mesenteric adenitis; (3) pelvic inflammatory disease (PID, p. 625); (4) intraperitoneal hemorrhage from any cause, such as a ruptured ectopic pregnancy or a ruptured ovarian follicle (mittelschmerz); (5) Crohn's disease (p. 528); and (6) Meckel's diverticulitis (p. 525). *To further complicate matters, deviations from the classic clinical pattern abound, particularly in infants and very aged individuals.* In the latter the pain is often minimal and there may be no fever. Thus the diagnosis of acute appendicitis can at times be difficult, and it has been said that it should never be excluded in the differential diagnosis of any acute abdominal problem. "The mortality of appendicitis is the mortality of delay."[160] The operative mortality rate before perforation has occurred is 0 to 0.3%, but it is at least 1% after perforation, rising to 15% in elderly individuals.[161]

# TUMORS, INCLUDING MUCOCELE AND PSEUDOMYXOMA PERITONEI

**CARCINOID (ARGENTAFFINOMA, ENDOCRINE CELL TUMOR).** This is the most common neoplasm in the appendix, as was detailed on page 536. It is usually an incidental finding and rarely spreads beyond the appendix.

**MUCOCELE OF THE APPENDIX AND PSEUDOMYXOMA PERITONEI.** *Mucocele of the appendix refers to progressive cystic dilatation of the lumen by accumulated mucinous material.* The cause of the dilatation is still controversial. There is, however, agreement that several categories can be recognized: (1) an entirely innocuous form related to retention of mucus (perhaps secondary to an obstructive process) or to hyperplastic secretory activity of the mucosa, (2) a benign neoplastic reaction (i.e., a mucinous cystadenoma of the appendix), and (3) a form produced by a cystadenocarcinoma of the appendiceal mucosa.[162, 163] *Only the last category, mucinous cystadenocarcinoma, leads to pseudomyxoma peritonei, the filling of the peritoneal cavity by glairy, mucinous secretions containing free-floating and implanted mucinous carcinomatous cells.* To be noted, *mucinous cystadenocarcinomas of the ovary with spread to the peritoneal cavity may induce an identical pseudomyxoma peritonei.*

**Non-neoplastic mucocele** is not associated with epithelial atypia. In some cases there is diffuse mucosal hyperplasia producing changes analogous to those found in the colonic hyperplastic polyp (p. 551). These changes are not associated with extension beyond the appendix. In other instances there is no mucosal hyperplasia; instead, there is dilatation of the lumen (sometimes up to 7 cm) and pressure atrophy of the mucosa. It is assumed without proof that some luminal obstruction induces the retention mucocele. In both of the previous circumstances, **the excessive mucinous dilatation does not lead to pseudomyxoma peritonei** and the changes are usually asymptomatic and only discovered as incidental findings.

A second category of mucocele is best referred to as **mucinous cystadenoma of the appendix**. It is the counterpart of the analogous ovarian neoplasm (p. 650). This is the most common cause of appendiceal mucocele and sometimes creates a globular cystic dilatation up to 10 to 12 cm in diameter. It is marked by benign neoplastic papillary proliferation of the mucin-secreting mucosal epithelium. **Most often these lesions are unruptured. Occasionally, however, the thinned appendiceal wall ruptures; this event is accompanied by spilling of mucus into the peritoneal cavity or, sometimes, only around the site of rupture.** The intraperitoneal mucus is usually devoid of neoplastic cells, but when they are present, they are not anaplastic and usually not implanted on peritoneal surfaces (i.e., they represent spillage rather than cancerous infiltration). The secretions in such cases do not fill the peritoneal cavity, as opposed to cancerous pseudomyxoma peritonei. The condition is most often an unsuspected surgical finding during abdominal exploration for other reasons. Occasionally, there is a palpable mass or manifestations reminiscent of acute appendicitis. **Appendectomy is curative even when the contents of the mucocele have spilled into the peritoneal cavity.**

**Mucinous cystadenocarcinoma** is the counterpart of the same type of tumor in the ovary (p. 650). This is the least common form of mucocele. It is most often symptomatic, with right lower quadrant pain, and it is the only appendiceal cause of bona fide pseudomyxoma peritonei (accounting for over half of all cases of pseudomyxoma).

**The lesion is clearly a malignant neoplasm, and the spread into the peritoneal cavity is a manifestation of cancerous extension beyond the primary site.** Thus the peritoneal cavity becomes filled with mucinous secretion that microscopically contains clearly identifiable cancer cells that sometimes float free, at other times grow on remote peritoneal surfaces, but rarely penetrate into the substance of the viscera. As with the pseudomyxoma peritonei caused by ovarian cancers, there is only rarely extraabdominal spread or distant metastases. Nonetheless, the intraperitoneal dissemination of the cancer slowly exacts its toll, causing death over the span of five to ten years.

## References

1. Miskovitz, P. F., and Steinberg, H.: Diverticula of the gastrointestinal tract. DM 29:1, 1982.
2. Cohen, S.: Motor disorders of the esophagus. N. Engl. J. Med. 301:184, 1979.
3. Smith, B.: The neurological lesion in achalasia of the cardia. Gut 11:388, 1970.
4. Cohen, S., et al.: Role of gastrin supersensitivity in the pathogenesis of lower esophageal sphincter hypertension in achalasia. J. Clin. Invest. 50:1241, 1971.
5. Russel, C. O., and Hill, L. D.: Gastroesophageal reflux. Curr. Prob. Surg. 20:205, 1983.
6. Muñoz, N., et al.: Precursor lesions of oesophageal cancer in high-risk populations in Iran and China. Lancet 1:876, 1982.
7. Crespi, M., et al.: Oesophageal lesions in Northern Iran. A premalignant lesion. Lancet 2:217, 1979.
8. Mason, S. J., and O'Meara, T. F.: Drug-induced esophagitis. J. Clin. Gastroenterol. 3:115, 1981.
9. Sjögren, R. W., Jr., and Johnson, L. F.: Barrett's esophagus: A review. Am. J. Med. 74;313, 1983.
10. Cameron, A. J., et al.: The incidence of adenocarcinoma in columnar-lined (Barrett's) esophagus. N. Engl. J. Med. 313:857, 1985.
11. Larson, D. E., and Farnell, M. D.: Upper gastrointestinal hemorrhage. Mayo Clin. Proc. 58:371, 1983.
12. Soderlund, C.: Variceal haemorrhage. A study of unselected patients with massive bleeding from oesophageal varices. Acta Chir. Scand. 148:275, 1982.
13. Sugawa, C., et al.: Mallory-Weiss syndrome. A study of 224 patients. Am. J. Surg. 145:30, 1983.
14. Stern, A. I., et al.: The Mallory-Weiss lesion as a cause of upper gastrointestinal bleeding. Aust.-N.Z. J. Surg. 49:13, 1979.
15. Mannell, A.: Carcinoma of the esophagus. Curr. Probl. Surg. 19:553, 1982.
16. Yang, C. S.: Research on esophageal cancer in China: A review. Cancer Res. 40:26, 1980.
17. Mandard, A. M., et al.: Cancer of the esophagus and associated lesions: Detailed pathologic study of 100 esophagectomy specimens. Hum. Pathol. 15:660, 1984.
18. Takita, H., et al.: Squamous cell carcinoma of the esophagus: A study of 153 cases. J. Surg. Oncol. 9:547, 1977.
19. Morton, J.: Alimentary tract cancer. In Rubin, P. (ed.): Clinical Oncology for Medical Students and Physicians. 3rd ed. Rochester, N.Y., American Cancer Society, 1970–1971, p. 115.
20. Akiyama, H.: Surgery for carcinoma of the esophagus. Curr. Probl. Surg. 17:53, 1980.
21. Gryboski, J., and Hillemeir, C.: Pyloric stenosis—Acquired or congenital. J. Clin. Gastroenterol. 4:72, 1982.
22. Croft, D.: Gastritis. Br. Med. J. 4:164, 1967.
23. Editorial: Susceptibility to aspirin bleeding. Br. Med. J. 2:436, 1970.
24. Dajani, E. Z.: Is peptic ulcer a prostaglandin deficiency disease. Hum. Pathol. 17:106, 1986.
25. Editorial: Pyloric campylobacter finds a volunteer. Lancet 1:1021, 1985.
26. Marshall, B. J., et al.: Attempt to fulfill Koch's postulates for pyloric campylobacter. Med. J. Austr. 142:436, 1985.
27. Lev, R., et al.: Effects of salicylates on the canine stomach: A morphological and histochemical study. Gastroenterology 62:970, 1972.
28. Valman, H. B., et al.: Lesions associated with gastroduodenal haemorrhage in relation to aspirin intakes. Br. Med. J. 4:661, 1968.
29. Ihamäki, T., et al.: Long-term observation of subjects with normal mucosa and with superficial gastritis: Results of 23–27 years follow-up examination. Scand. J. Gastroenterol. 13:771, 1978.
30. de Aizpurua, H. J., et al.: Autoantibodies cytotoxic to gastric parietal cells in serum of patients with pernicious anemia. N. Engl. J. Med. 309:625, 1983.
31. Sipponen, P., et al.: Atrophic chronic gastritis and intestinal metaplasia in gastric carcinoma. Cancer 52:1062, 1983.
32. Skillman, J. J., and Silen, W.: Acute gastroduodenal "stress" ulceration: Barrier disruption of varied pathogenesis? Gastroenterology 59:478, 1970.
33. Menguy, R.: The prophylaxis of stress ulceration (Editorial). N. Engl. J. Med. 302:461, 1980.
34. Chapman, M. L.: Peptic ulcer: A medical perspective. Med. Clin. North Am. 62:39, 1978.
35. Kurata, J. H., et al.: Sex differences in peptic ulcer disease (Abs.). Gastroenterology 86:1147, 1984.
36. Sontag, S., et al.: Cimetidine, cigarette smoking, and recurrence of duodenal ulcer. N. Engl. J. Med. 311:689, 1984.
37. Wormsley, K. G.: Duodenal ulcer: Does pathophysiology equal aetiology? Gut 24:775, 1983.
38. Grossman, M. I., et al.: Peptic diseases. Gastroenterology 69:1071, 1975.
39. Stabile, B. E., and Passaro, E., Jr.: Duodenal ulcer: A disease in evolution. Curr. Probl. Surg. 21:1, 1984.
40. Szabo, S., et al.: Role of local secretory and motility changes in the pathogenesis of experimental duodenal ulcer. Scand. J. Gastroenterol. 92 (Suppl.):106, 1984.
41. Baron, J. H.: Current views on the pathogenesis of peptic ulcer. Scand. J. Gastroenterol. 80 (Suppl.):1, 1982.
42. Ippoliti, A., and Walsh, J.: Newer concepts in the pathogenesis of peptic ulcer disease. Surg. Clin. North Am. 56:1479, 1976.
43. Editorial: Acid reduction or mucosal protection for peptic ulcer? Lancet 2:473, 1982.
44. Messer, J., et al.: Association of adrenocorticosteroid therapy and peptic-ulcer disease. N. Engl. J. Med. 309:21, 1983.
45. Editorial: Gastric ulcer or cancer? Lancet 1:202, 1985.
46. Ming, S.-C.: The adenoma-carcinoma sequence in the stomach and colon. II. Malignant potential of gastric polyps. Gastrointest. Radiol. 1:121, 1976.
47. Haenszel, W., and Correa, P.: Developments in the epidemiology of stomach cancer over the past decade. Cancer Res. 35:3452, 1975.
48. Ruddell, W. S., et al.: Gastric juice nitrate. A risk factor for cancer in the hypochlorhydric stomach? Lancet 2:1037, 1976.
49. Schlag, P., et al.: Are nitrite and N-nitroso compounds in gastric juice risk factors for carcinoma in the operated stomach? Lancet 1:727, 1980.
50. Joossens, J. V., and Geboers, J.: Nutrition and gastric cancer. Proc. Nutr. Soc. 40:37, 1981.
51. Sipponen, P., et al.: Atrophic chronic gastritis and intestinal metaplasia in gastric carcinoma. Comparison with a representative population sample. Cancer 52:1062, 1983.
52. Schrumpf, E., et al.: Mucosal changes in the gastric stump 20–25 years after partial gastrectomy. Lancet 2:467, 1977.
53. Grundmann, E.: Early gastric cancer—Today. Pathol. Res. Pract. 162:347, 1978.
54. Green, P. H. R., et al.: Early gastric cancer. Gastroenterology 81:247, 1981.

55. Dupont, J. B., et al.: Adenocarcinoma of the stomach. Review of 1,497 cases. Cancer 41:941, 1978.

56. Ming, S.-C.: Gastric carcinoma, a pathobiological classification. Cancer 39:2475, 1977.

57. Laurén, P.: The two histological main types of gastric carcinoma: Diffuse and so-called intestinal-type carcinoma. An attempt at a histoclinical classification. Acta Pathol. Microbiol. Scand. 64:31, 1965.

58. Antonioli, D. A., and Goldman, H.: Changes in the location and type of gastric adenocarcinoma. Cancer 50:775, 1982.

59. Pagnini, C. A., and Rugge, M.: Gastric cancer: Problems in histogenesis. Histopathology 7:699, 1983.

59a. Chejfec, G., and Gould, V. E.: Malignant gastric neuroendocrinomas. Ultrastructural and biochemical characterization of their secretory activity. Hum. Pathol. 8:433, 1977.

60. Moss, A. A., et al.: Gastric adenocarcinoma: A comparison of the accuracy and economics of staging by computed tomography and surgery. Gastroenterology 80:45, 1981.

61. Hirota, T., et al.: Clinicopathologic study of minute and small early gastric cancers. Pathol. Annu. 15 (Part 2):1, 1980.

62. Gray, G. M., et al.: Lymphomas involving the gastrointestinal tract. Gastroenterology 82:143, 1982.

63. Weingrad, D. N., et al.: Primary gastrointestinal lymphoma. A thirty-year review. Cancer 49:1258, 1982.

64. Isaacson, P., and Wright, D. H.: Malignant lymphoma of mucosa-associated lymphoid tissue. A distinctive type of B-cell lymphoma. Cancer 52:1410, 1983.

65. Ottinger, L. W.: Acute mesenteric ischemia. N. Engl. J. Med. 307:535, 1982.

66. Swerdlow, S. H., et al.: Intestinal infarction: A new classification. Arch. Pathol. Lab. Med. 105:218, 1981.

67. VerSteeg, K. R., and Broders, C. W.: Gangrene of the bowels. Surg. Clin. North Am. 59:869, 1979.

68. Marshak, R. H., et al.: Ischemia of the colon. Mt. Sinai J. Med. 48:180, 1981.

69. Pillai, D. K., and Matts, S. G. F.: Chronic inflammatory bowel disease. Br. J. Clin. Pract. 37:165, 1983.

70. Kirsner, J. B., and Shorter, R. G.: Recent developments in "nonspecific" inflammatory bowel disease. N. Engl. J. Med. 306:775, 837, 1982.

71. Gilat, T.: Incidence of inflammatory bowel diseases—Going up or down? Gastroenterology 85:196, 1983.

72. Achord, J. L., et al.: Regional enteritis and HLA concordance in multiple siblings. Dig. Dis. Sci. 27:330, 1982.

73. Sachar, D. B.: Aetiologic theories of inflammatory bowel disease. Clin. Gastroenterol. 9:231, 1980.

74. Dvorak, A. M., et al.: Crohn's disease: A scanning electron microscopic study. Hum. Pathol. 10:165, 1979.

75. Cave, D. R., Mitchell, D. N., and Brooke, B. N.: Crohn's disease and ulcerative colitis: A review of the evidence for transmissibility. In Jerzy-Glass, G. B. (ed.): Progress in Gastroenterology. Vol. 3. New York, Grune & Stratton, 1977, p. 839.

76. Morson, B. C.: Pathology of inflammatory bowel disease. Gastroenterol. Jpn. 15:184, 1980.

77. Simpson, S., et al.: The histologic appearance of dysplasia (precarcinomatous change) in Crohn's disease of the small and large intestine. Gastroenterology 81:492, 1981.

78. Greenstein, A. J., et al.: Patterns of neoplasia in Crohn's disease and ulcerative colitis. Cancer 46:403, 1980.

79. Isselbacher, K. J.: Malabsorption syndromes including disease of pancreatic and biliary origin. Curr. Concepts Nutr. 9:92, 1980.

80. Owen, R. L., and Brandborg, L. L.: Mucosal histopathology of malabsorption. Clin. Gastroenterol. 12:575, 1983.

81. Falchuk, Z. M.: Gluten-sensitive enteropathy. Clin. Gastroenterol. 12:475, 1983.

82. Congdon, P., et al.: Small bowel mucosa in asymptomatic children with celiac disease. Am. J. Dis. Child. 135:118, 1981.

83. Savilahti, E., et al.: IgA antigliadin antibodies: A marker of mucosal damage in childhood coeliac disease. Lancet 1:320, 1983.

84. Flores, A. F., et al.: In vitro model to assess immunoregulatory T-lymphocyte subpopulations in gluten-sensitive enteropathy (GSE) (Abs.). Gastroenterology 82:1058, 1982.

85. O'Farrelly, C., et al.: Suppressor-cell activity in coeliac disease induced by alpha-gliadin, a dietary antigen. Lancet 2:1305, 1984.

86. Swinson, C. M., et al.: Coeliac disease and malignancy. Lancet 1:111, 1983.

87. Cook, G. C.: Aetiology and pathogenesis of postinfective tropical malabsorption (tropical sprue). Lancet 1:721, 1984.

88. Comer, G. M., et al.: Whipple's disease: A review. Am. J. Gastroenterol. 78:107, 1983.

89. Feurle, G. E., et al.: Cerebral Whipple's disease with negative jejunal histology. N. Engl. J. Med. 300:907, 1979.

90. Keren, D. F.: Whipple's disease. A review emphasizing immunology and microbiology. CRC Crit. Rev. Clin. Lab. Sci. 14:75, 1981.

91. Dobbins, W. O., III: Current concepts of Whipple's disease (Editorial). J. Clin. Gastroenterol. 4:205, 1982.

92. McIver, M. A.: Acute intestinal obstruction. Am. J. Surg. 19:163, 1933.

93. Garvin, P. J., et al.: Benign and malignant tumors of the small intestine. Curr. Probl. Cancer 3:1, 1979.

94. Barclay, T. H. C., and Shapira, D. V.: Malignant tumors of the small intestine. Cancer 51:878, 1983.

95. Williamson, R. C. N., et al.: Adenocarcinoma and lymphoma of the small intestine. Ann. Surg. 197:172, 1983.

96. Van Bogaert, L.-J.: The diffuse endocrine system and derived tumours. Histological and histochemical characteristics. Acta Histochem. 70:122, 1982.

97. Pearse, A. G. E.: The cytochemistry and ultrastructure of polypeptide hormone-producing cells of the APUD series and the embryologic, physiologic, and pathologic implications of the concept. J. Histochem. Cytochem. 17:303, 1969.

98. Tapia, F. J., et al.: Neuron-specific enolase as produced by neuroendocrine tumours. Lancet 1:808, 1981.

99. Stevens, R. E., and Moore, G. E.: Inadequacy of APUD concept in explaining production of peptide hormones by tumours. Lancet 1:118, 1983.

100. Launay, J. M., et al.: The diffuse neuroendocrine system. Biomed. Pharmacother. 37:322, 1983.

101. Solcia, E., et al.: The contribution of immunohistochemistry to the diagnosis of neuroendocrine tumors. Semin. Diag. Pathol. 1:285, 1984.

102. DeLellis, R. A., et al: Carcinoid tumors (Editorial). Changing concepts and new perspectives. Am. J. Surg. Pathol. 8:295, 1984.

103. Mårtensson, H., et al.: Carcinoid tumors in the gastrointestinal tract—An analysis of 156 cases. Acta Chirurg. Scand. 149:607, 1983.

104. Ariel, I., et al.: Rectal mucosal biopsy in aganglionosis and allied conditions. Hum. Pathol. 14:991, 1983.

105. Hall, C. L., and Lampert, P. W.: Immunohistochemistry as an aid in the diagnosis of Hirschsprung's disease. Am. J. Clin. Pathol. 83:177, 1985.

106. Painter, N. S.: Lifestyle and disease. Diverticular disease of the colon. S. Afr. Med. J. 61:1016, 1982.

107. Parks, T. G.: The clinical significance of diverticular disease of the colon. Practitioner 226:643, 1982.

108. Weinreich, J., and Andersen, D.: Intraluminal pressure in the sigmoid colon. II. Patients with sigmoid diverticular and related conditions. Scand. J. Gastroenterol. 11:581, 1976.

108a. Berry, C. S., et al.: Dietary fiber and prevention of diverticular disease of the colon: Evidence from rats. Lancet 2:294, 1984.

109. Allison, D. J., et al.: Angiography in gastrointestinal bleeding. Lancet 2:30, 1982.

110. Editorial: Angiodysplasia. Lancet 2:1086, 1981.

111. Keusch, G. T., and Donowitz, M.: Pathophysiological mechanisms of diarrhoeal diseases: Diverse aetiologies and common mechanisms. Scand. J. Gastroenterol. 84:33, 1983.

112. Blaser, M. J., and Reller, L. B.: Campylobacter enteritis. N. Engl. J. Med. 305:1444, 1981.

113. Morris, J. G., Jr., and Black, R. E.: Cholera and other vibrioses in the U.S. N. Engl. J. Med. *312*:343, 1985.

114. Dammin, G. J.: Vibrio-caused diseases: Cholera. *In* Binford, C. H., and Connor, D. H. (eds.): Pathology of Tropical and Extraordinary Diseases. Washington, D.C., Armed Forces Institute and Pathology, 1976, p. 137.

115. Holmgren, J.: Actions of cholera toxin and the prevention and treatment of cholera. Nature *292*:413, 1981.

116. Gorbach, S. L.: Travellers' diarrhea. N. Engl. J. Med. *307*:881, 1982.

117. Editorial: Mechanisms in enteropathogenic *Escherichia coli* diarrhoae. Lancet *1*:1254, 1983

118. Rothbaum, R., et al.: A clinicopathologic study of enterocyte-adherent *Escherichia coli*: A cause of protracted diarrhea in infants. Gastroenterology *83*:441, 1982.

119. Levine, M. M.: Bacillary dysentery: Mechanisms and treatment. Med. Clin. North Am. *66*:623, 1982.

120. Olsnes, S., and Eiklid, K.: Isolation and characterization of *Shigella shigae* cytotoxins. J. Biol. Chem. *255*:284, 1980.

121. Blaser, M. J., and Newman, L. S.: A review of human salmonellosis. I. Infective dose. Rev. Infect. Dis. *4*:1096, 1982.

122. Koo, F. C. W., et al.: Pathogenesis of experimental salmonellosis: Inhibition of protein synthesis by cytotoxin. Infect. Immun. *43*:93, 1984.

123. Jiwa, S. F.: Probing for enterotoxigenicity among the salmonellae; An evaluation of biological assays. J. Clin. Microbiol. *14*:463, 1981.

124. Tedesco, F. J.: Pseudomembranous colitis. Pathogenesis and therapy. Med. Clin. North Am. *66*:655, 1982.

125. Taylor, N. S., et al.: Separation of an enterotoxin from the cytotoxin of *C. difficile*. Clin. Res. *28*:285A, 1980.

126. Harries, J.: Amoebiasis: A review. J. R. Soc. Med. *75*:190, 1982.

127. Kirsner, J. B., and Shorter, R. G.: Recent developments in "nonspecific" inflammatory bowel disease. N. Engl. J. Med. *306*:775, 837, 1982.

128. Johnson, W. R., et al.: Inflammatory bowel disease—Where are we? Med. J. Aust. *1*:226, 1982.

129. Riddel, R. H., et al.: Dysplasia in inflammatory bowel disease: Standardized classification with provisional clinical applications. Hum. Pathol. *14*:931, 1983.

130. Greenstein, A. J., et al.: Cancer in universal and left-sided ulcerative colitis: Factors determining risk. Gastroenterology *99*:290, 1979.

131. Dworken, H. J.: Ulcerative colitis: A clearer picture. Ann. Intern. Med. *99*:717, 1983.

132. Lennard-Jones, J. E., et al.: Cancer surveillance in ulcerative colitis. Experience over 15 years. Lancet *2*:149, 1983.

133. Chapman, I.: Adenomatous polyps of large intestine: Incidence and distribution. Ann. Surg. *157*:223, 1963.

134. Fenoglio-Preiser, C. M., and Hutter, R. V. P.: Colorectal polyps: Pathologic diagnosis and clinical significance. CA *35*:332, 1985.

135. Vatn, M. H., and Stalsberg, H.: The prevalence of polyps of the large intestine in Oslo: An autopsy study. Cancer *49*:819, 1982.

136. Burt, R. W., et al.: Dominant inheritance of adenomatous colonic polyps and colorectal cancer. N. Eng. J. Med. *312*:1540, 1985.

137. Greene, F. L.: Distribution of colorectal neoplasms. A left-to-right shift of polyps and cancer. Am. Surg. *49*:62, 1983.

138. Estrada, R. G., and Spjut, H. J.: Hyperplastic polyps of the large bowel. Am. J. Surg. Pathol. *4*:127, 1980.

139. Coutsoftides, T., et al.: Malignant polyps of the colon and rectum. A clinicopathologic study. Dis. Colon Rectum *22*:82, 1979.

140. Gillespie, P. E., et al.: Colonic adenomas—A colonoscopy survey. Gut *20*:240, 1979.

141. Grinnell, R. S., and Lane, N.: Benign and malignant adenomatous polyps and papillary adenomas of the colon and rectum. An analysis of 1,856 tumors in 1,335 patients. Intl. Abstr. Surg. (Surg. Gynecol. Obstet.) *106*:519, 1958.

142. DeCosse, J. J.: Malignant colorectal polyp. Gut *25*:433, 1984.

143. Friedman, E., et al.: A model for human colon carcinoma evolution based on the differential response of cultured preneoplastic, premalignant, and malignant cells to 12-0-tetradecanoylphorbol-13-acetate. Cancer Res. *44*:1568, 1984.

144. Day, D. W., and Morson, B. C.: The adenoma-carcinoma sequence. *In* Morson, B. C. (ed.): The Pathogenesis of Colorectal Cancer. Philadelphia, W. B. Saunders Co., 1978, p. 58.

145. Maskens, A. P., and Dujardin-Loits, R. M.: Experimental adenomas and carcinomas of the large intestine behave as distinct entities: Most carcinomas arise de novo in flat mucosa. Cancer *47*:81, 1981.

146. Gilbertsen, V. A.: Proctosigmoidoscopy and polypectomy in reducing the incidence of rectal cancer. Cancer *34* (Suppl.):836, 1974.

146a. Medical Staff Conference: Familial colonic cancer syndromes. West. J. Med. *139*:351, 1983.

147. Luk, G. D., and Baylin, S. B.: Ornithine decarboxylase as a biologic marker in familial colonic polyposis. N. Engl. J. Med. *311*:80, 1984.

148. Watne, A. L., et al.: The diagnosis and surgical treatment of patients with Gardner's syndrome. Surgery *82*:327, 1977.

149. Burdick, D., and Prior, J. T.: Peutz-Jeghers syndrome. A clinicopathologic study of a large family with a 27-year follow-up. Cancer *50*:2139, 1982.

150. Trau, H., et al.: Peutz-Jeghers syndrome and bilateral breast carcinoma. Cancer *50*:788, 1982.

151. Bresalier, R. S., and Kim, Y. S.: Diet and colon cancer. N. Engl. J. Med. *313*:1413, 1985.

152. Doll, R.: General epidemiologic considerations in etiology of colorectal cancer. *In* Winawar, S. J., Schottenfeld, D., and Sherlock P. (eds.): Progress in Cancer Research Therapy, Vol. 13. Colorectal Cancer: Prevention, Epidemiology, and Screening. New York, Raven Press, 1980, p. 3.

153. Weisberger, J. H., et al.: Nutritional factors and etiologic mechanisms in the causation of gastrointestinal cancers. Cancer *50*:2541, 1982.

154. Tannenbaum, S. R., et al.: Nitrite and nitrate are formed by endogenous synthesis in human intestine. Science *200*:1487, 1978.

155. Reddy, B. S.: Dietary fibre and colon cancer: Epidemiologic and experimental evidence. Can. Med. Assoc. J. *123*:850, 1980.

156. Kinlen, L. J.: Meat and fat consumption and cancer mortality: A study of strict religious orders in Britain. Lancet *1*:946, 1982.

157. Newland, R. C., et al.: The relationship of survival to staging and grading of colorectal carcinoma: A prospective study of 503 cases. Cancer *47*:1424, 1981.

158. McIntire, K.: Tumor markers. How useful are they? Hosp. Pract. *19*:55, 1984.

159. Peltokallio, P., and Tykkä, H.: Evolution of the age distribution and mortality of acute appendicitis. Arch. Surg. *116*:153, 1981.

160. Schrock, T. R.: Acute appendicitis. *In* Sleisenger, M. H., and Fordtran, J. S. (eds.): Gastrointestinal Disease. Pathophysiology, Diagnosis, Management. 3rd ed. Philadelphia, W. B. Saunders Co., 1983, p. 1274.

161. Lewis, F. R., et al.: Appendicitis. A critical review of diagnosis and treatment in 1,000 cases. Arch. Surg. *110*:667, 1975.

162. Higa, E., et al.: Mucosal hyperplasia, mucinous cystadenoma, and mucinous cystadenocarcinoma of the appendix. A reevaluation of appendiceal "mucocele." Cancer *32*:1525, 1973.

163. Wackym, P. A., and Gray, G. F., Jr.: Tumors of the appendix: I. Neoplastic and nonneoplastic mucoceles. South. Med. J. *77*:283, 1984.

# 17

# The Liver, the Biliary Tract, and the Pancreas

The liver, biliary tract, and pancreas, although treated separately, are all included in this chapter because of their anatomic proximity, closely interrelated functions, and the similarity of the symptom complexes induced by many of their disorders. The liver dominates this group because it is literally the crossroads of the body. The portal and systemic circulations join here to drain through a common venous outflow. The intermediary metabolism of all foodstuff occurs here. It is the major locus of synthetic, catabolic, and detoxifying activities in the body. Moreover, the liver is crucial in the excretion of heme pigments, and through its Kupffer cells it participates in the immune response.

## The Liver

It is fortunate that the liver has an enormous reserve capacity because it is one of the most frequently injured organs in the body. It has been shown in the experimental animal that removal of 80 to 90% of the hepatic parenchyma is still compatible with normal liver function. Thus, it requires diffuse disease to deplete the functional reserve. When such happens, it often causes jaundice and sometimes liver failure. Since these two syndromes are common to so many hepatic disorders, they will be considered first.

### JAUNDICE

*Jaundice*, or *icterus*, is a yellow discoloration of the skin and sclerae that is produced by accumulations of bilirubin in the tissues and interstitial fluids. Under optimal conditions (daylight), it usually becomes visible when the bilirubin levels exceed 2 to 3 mg/dl of serum. The intensity of the jaundice depends on many factors, including the level of hyperbilirubinemia, the rate of diffusion of bilirubin from the plasma into the interstitial fluid, and the binding of this pigment in the tissues.

A consideration of the mechanisms of jaundice involves an understanding of the formation, transportation, metabolism, and excretion of bilirubin (Fig. 17–1).[1] Our review can only be brief.

Approximately 75% of the bilirubin is derived from the breakdown of red cells with the conversion of the heme pigment by heme oxygenase to biliverdin, which is then reduced to bilirubin by a reductase.

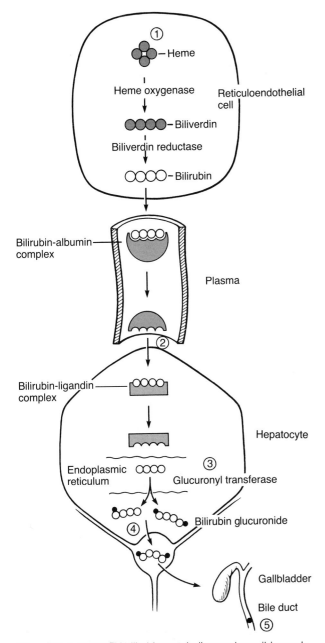

**Figure 17–1.** Outline of bilirubin metabolism and possible mechanisms of jaundice: (1) excessive production of bilirubin, (2) reduced hepatic uptake, (3) impaired conjugation of bilirubin, (4) impaired intrahepatic excretion of bilirubin, and (5) extrahepatic biliary obstruction.

This conversion occurs within the cells of the mononuclear phagocyte (RE) system, principally in the spleen. Most of the remaining bilirubin (25%) is derived from breakdown of nonhemoglobin heme proteins in the liver (e.g., cytochrome P-450), but a small fraction is produced by the lysis of immature red cells in the bone marrow. This latter pathway becomes particularly important in hematologic disorders associated with excessive intramedullary hemolysis of abnormal red cells ("ineffective erythropoiesis," p. 358).

*Whatever its origin, bilirubin formed outside the liver is bound principally to albumin and transported via the blood to the liver. Its further metabolism can be divided into four steps: (1) transfer into the liver cell from the hepatic sinusoidal blood, (2) intracellular binding to specific cytosolic proteins, (3) conjugation to one or two molecules of glucuronic acid, and (4) transport of conjugated bilirubin into the bile canaliculi.* The mechanisms involved in the uptake of bilirubin from the blood to its eventual excretion into the bile canaliculi are complex and poorly understood. Some aspects as they relate to specific diseases will be pointed out later.

Once in the canaliculus, the bilirubin enters the bile flow and eventually reaches the intestines, where the glucuronides are split and the bilirubin converted by bacterial action into urobilinogens, most of which are excreted in the feces. Approximately 20% of the urobilinogens formed are reabsorbed in the ileum and colon, to be returned to the liver, from which they are promptly excreted into the bile. A very small amount that escapes reexcretion by the liver reaches the kidneys and is excreted with urine.

There are important pathophysiologic differences between unconjugated bilirubin and the conjugated form. *Unconjugated bilirubin is soluble in lipids and is tightly complexed to albumin, in which form it cannot be excreted in the urine even when the blood levels are high.* Normally, a very small amount of unconjugated bilirubin is present as an albumin-free diffusible anion in normal plasma. High blood levels of diffusible unconjugated bilirubin may enter the tissues, particularly the brain, and produce toxic injury. This occurs especially in the newborn with erythroblastosis fetalis because of the immature blood-brain barrier, producing serious brain damage known as kernicterus. In contrast, *conjugated bilirubin is water soluble, nontoxic, and only loosely bound to albumin. Because of its solubility and weak association with albumin, conjugated bilirubin, when present in excess (as in obstructive jaundice), is excreted in the urine.*

Having reviewed bilirubin metabolism, we can turn now to the pathophysiologic mechanisms that cause jaundice. Hyperbilirubinemia is the hallmark of jaundice. Normal serum bilirubin levels vary between 0.3 and 1.0 mg/dl and are maintained within this range because bilirubin production is fairly evenly matched by its hepatic uptake, conjugation, and biliary excretion. Jaundice occurs when the equilibrium between the production and disposal of bilirubin is disturbed by one or more of the following three mechanisms: *(1) excessive production of bilirubin; (2) impaired liver cell uptake and conjugation, or secretion; and (3) inhibition of the outflow of bile (cholestasis).* As is evident from the following discussion and Table 17–1, each of these three pathogenetic mechanisms is responsible for jaundice in fairly well-defined clinical settings. It should be noted, however, that more than one mechanism may be operative in some disorders. This is particularly true in hepatocellular diseases such as hepatitis and cirrhosis, in which there may be simultaneous disruption of bilirubin uptake, conjugation, and outflow into bile canaliculi.

When a patient presents with jaundice, a knowledge of the predominant form of plasma bilirubin (i.e., conjugated or unconjugated) is of great clinical value in arriving at the possible cause of hyperbilirubinemia. For example, unconjugated hyperbilirubinemia indicates excessive production of bilirubin, as occurs in hemolytic anemias, whereas the presence of conjugated bilirubin points to a disorder "distal" to the hepatic conjugating enzyme systems. The latter is exemplified by biliary tract obstruction, which leads to regurgitation of conjugated bilirubin into the blood. As was alluded to earlier, conjugated hyperbilirubinemias are associated with the presence of bilirubin in the urine, whereas unconjugated hyperbilirubinemias do not cause bilirubinuria. With this general discussion, we can now illustrate some specific examples of jaundice with respect to the type of accumulated bilirubin and the mechanism of hyperbilirubinemia (Table 17–1).

**UNCONJUGATED HYPERBILIRUBINEMIA.** Predominantly unconjugated hyperbilirubinemia is said to exist when 80% or more of the serum bilirubin is unconjugated. It is caused by three major mechanisms:

1. *Excessive production of bilirubin.* Hemolytic disease (an increased rate of red cell destruction) is the most common cause of excessive bilirubin production and is called *hemolytic jaundice.* However active the hemolysis may be, the hyperbilirubinemia rarely exceeds 5 mg/dl, because the normal liver is capable of handling most of the overload. On occasion, patients who have had a pulmonary hemorrhage or infarction, or massive hemorrhage in any site in the body, may become icteric, presumably as a result of resorption of the heme pigment of the destroyed cells.

2. *Reduced hepatic uptake of bilirubin.* This is a much less common mechanism of unconjugated hyperbilirubinemia. It is encountered in some cases of the genetic disorder called Gilbert's syndrome (to be discussed later) and after administration of drugs such as rifampin.

3. *Impaired conjugation of bilirubin.* Bilirubin is conjugated in the smooth endoplasmic reticulum of the hepatocytes, through the action of glucuronyl transferase. The activity of glucuronyl transferase is low at birth and does not reach normal levels until about two weeks after birth. Thus almost every newborn develops transient and mild unconjugated hyperbilirubinemia (often called *neonatal jaundice* or *physiologic jaundice of the newborn).* More important are several conditions caused by a genetic or acquired lack of the conjugating enzyme. Gilbert's syndrome and Crigler-Najjar syndrome are characterized by hereditary glucuronyl transferase deficiency and are described later. Acquired deficiency may result from any cause of diffuse hepatocellular damage. However, since hepatic parenchymal diseases are often associated with impaired secretion of bile into the canaliculi as well, conjugated bilirubin also accumulates. Indeed, since transport of bile into the canaliculi is the rate-limiting step in bilirubin excretion, the hyperbilirubinemia of hepatocellular diseases is predominantly of the conjugated type.

**CONJUGATED HYPERBILIRUBINEMIA.** Conjugated hyperbilirubinemia is said to exist when more than half of the serum bilirubin is conjugated. This occurs when the secretion or excretion of conjugated bilirubin is impaired at the level of the liver cell membrane, within the bile canaliculi, or at any level within the excretory duct system (cholestasis). *Depending on the level of the derangement, disorders of bilirubin secretion or excretion are usually divided into intrahepatic and extrahepatic causes of cholestasis.* The *Dubin-Johnson* and *Rotor's syndromes* are hereditary disorders in which the defect appears to reside in the transfer of bilirubin and other organic anions across the hepatocyte membrane. Various *drugs* (to be discussed later) may cause intrahepatic cholestasis. Acute viral infection of the liver *(viral hepatitis)* and the various cirrhoses may act at several

**Table 17–1.** PATHOPHYSIOLOGIC
CLASSIFICATION OF JAUNDICE

**I. Predominantly Unconjugated Hyperbilirubinemia**
  A. Excess production of bilirubin
    a. Hemolytic anemias
    b. Resorption of blood from large areas of hemorrhage (e.g., pulmonary infarcts)
  B. Reduced hepatic uptake
    a. Drugs
    b. Some cases of Gilbert's syndrome
  C. Impaired bilirubin conjugation
    a. Gilbert's syndrome
    b. Crigler-Najjar syndrome
    c. Neonatal jaundice
    d. Diffuse hepatocellular disease

**II. Predominantly Conjugated Hyperbilirubinemia**
  A. Impaired intrahepatic excretion of bilirubin
    a. Dubin-Johnson syndrome
    b. Rotor's syndrome
    c. Drug-induced (e.g., oral contraceptives)
    d. Hepatocellular disease (e.g., viral hepatitis)
  B. Extrahepatic biliary obstruction (e.g., gallstones, carcinoma of pancreas, biliary atresia)

levels. Damage to the liver cells may impair the conjugating or secretory mechanisms, or the swelling and disorganization of liver cells can compress and block the canaliculi or cholangioles. All of these disorders are intrahepatic causes of cholestasis (discussed on p. 581).

Extrahepatic cholestasis results from obstruction of the extrahepatic bile ducts. Frequent causes include *gallstones* impacted in the common or main hepatic ducts and *carcinoma* of the extrahepatic bile ducts, ampulla of Vater, or head of the pancreas (which may then impinge on the common bile duct). Less common causes for such obstruction exist. Acute infections within the biliary tract (*cholangitis*) may fill the lumens with pus. In the newborn or infant, atresia or agenesis of the extrahepatic bile ducts will lead to extrahepatic obstruction. Obviously, strategically localized inflammatory or neoplastic lesions near the porta hepatis may block the major hepatic ducts by enlargement of impinging lymph nodes. Tumors or inflammatory lesions strategically located at the outflow of the hepatic ducts behave as extrahepatic obstructions.

When the blockage of the bile ducts is complete, bile disappears from the stools altogether (acholic stools). The characteristic brown color of the stools is lost, and they are instead gray and putty-like. Obviously, urinary urobilinogen also disappears. However, the urine contains bilirubin, since conjugated bilirubin is water soluble and can be filtered by the kidney. Since bile is necessary for the absorption of fats from the small intestine, there is malabsorption of fats and fat-soluble vitamins as well. Impaired absorption of vitamin K induces hypoprothrombinemia and thus predisposes to hemorrhage—a particular threat in those who may require surgery—for example, on the biliary tract. In all forms of obstructive jaundice, whether intrahepatic or extrahepatic, bile salts as well as bilirubin may be regurgitated into the blood. Bile salts produce intense itching, a particularly agonizing symptom to patients with obstructive lesions. Cholestasis is also associated with significant elevations of plasma cholesterol levels and, indeed, these patients may develop localized accumulations of macrophages laden with cholesterol in the skin (xanthomas). Another feature quite characteristic of cholestatic jaundice is the elevation of serum alkaline phosphatase. The increased enzyme levels result from increased synthesis rather than decreased excretion. It should be remembered, however, that since alkaline phosphatase is a widely distributed enzyme (in bones, kidneys, white cells, intestines), elevated levels may also be encountered in nonhepatic disorders. If diseases affecting other tissues rich in alkaline phosphatase can be excluded, an increase in the level of this enzyme provides a very sensitive marker of impaired biliary excretion.

A recapitulation of some of these patterns of jaundice is provided in Table 17–1 and Fig. 17–1. Overall, the most frequent causes of jaundice in adults are viral hepatitis, cirrhosis, extrahepatic biliary obstruction, and drug reactions.

# HEPATIC FAILURE

The ultimate consequence of many liver diseases is hepatic failure. This may come about by slow, cell-by-cell insidious erosion of the enormous functional reserve of the liver, by repetitive discrete waves of parenchymal damage, or in some cases by sudden or relatively sudden massive hepatic destruction. Whatever the sequence, the hepatic damage must ultimately be widespread because focal lesions, such as primary or metastatic tumors, focal infections, or traumas, rarely deplete the functional reserve. In some instances, diffuse liver injury is compatible with marginal compensation, but intercurrent disease (as, for example, a severe infection or a massive hemorrhage) tips the balance and leads to hepatic failure.

The morphologic disorders causing liver failure can be divided into three categories: (1) *ultrastructural lesions that do not necessarily produce obvious liver cell necrosis*, (2) *chronic liver disease*, and (3) *massive hepatic necrosis*.[2] The major conditions, many of which will be cited in greater detail later, falling within these categories are as follows:

1. *Without apparent significant liver cell necrosis.* These disorders are Reye's syndrome in children, tetracycline toxicity, and the acute fatty liver of pregnancy.

2. *Chronic liver disease.* The commonest disorders in this category are chronic active hepatitis and the many types of cirrhosis, all to be described later.

3. *Widespread massive necrosis.* Destruction of virtually the entire liver is most often caused by fulminant viral hepatitis. In addition, massive necrosis may follow exposure to drugs and chemicals such as acetaminophen, the anesthetic halothane, monoamine oxidase inhibitors used as antidepressants, agents employed in the treatment of tuberculosis, and industrial chemicals such as phosphorus and carbon tetrachloride.

Whatever the basis, liver failure manifests itself in a host of clinical dysfunctions. Disturbance of any one of the hundreds of liver functions may dominate the symptom complex. Certain features are, however, usual.

*Jaundice* is an almost invariable finding. With hepatocellular failure, all steps of bilirubin metabolism are affected to a variable degree. However, since the rate-limiting step is excretion of conjugated bilirubin, most often conjugated hyperbilirubinemia predominates.

*Fetor hepaticus*, a characteristic odor variously described as "musty" or "sweet and sour," occurs in some but not all instances. It is related to the formation of mercaptans by the action of gastrointestinal bacteria on the sulfur-containing amino acid methionine.

*Neuropsychiatric abnormalities*, also called *hepatic encephalopathy*, may also appear. They are characterized by variable disturbances in consciousness ranging from confusion to stupor to deep coma and fluctuating neurologic signs such as rigidity, hyperreflexia, and, rarely, seizures. Particularly characteristic is a peculiar "flapping tremor" of the outstretched hands (asterixis). The genesis of this encephalopathy is uncertain. It has been attributed variously to elevated blood levels of ammonia, short-chain fatty acids, false neurotransmitters such as octopamine, and other substances. With each of them the evidence is largely inferential, based on correlations between blood levels and manifestations of the encephalopathy.[3] Whatever the precise agent inducing the encephalopathy, two factors appear to be important: (1) shunting of blood around the liver, as may occur from spontaneous connections developed in the course of intrahepatic disease or as a consequence of surgical portosystemic shunts; and (2) severe loss of hepatocellular function, as may occur in fulminant hepatic necrosis. In either case, potentially neurotoxic substances present in the portal blood reach the systemic circulation. The implicated agent appears to be of nitrogenous origin derived from the action of gastrointestinal bacteria on the contents of the gut. Thus coma can be worsened by increased dietary protein or gastrointestinal bleeding and ameliorated by antibiotics that destroy the flora of the gut.

The brains of patients who have died in hepatic coma show a striking absence of significant morphologic findings. Most common is hyperplasia of protoplasmic-type astrocytes, principally in the cortex but also in other parts of the brain. In some individuals, there is cerebral edema, and it is proposed that the edema fluid may interfere with synaptic junctions. In a few instances, there are band-like cerebral cortical necroses.

*Renal failure* may occur in patients with extensive liver disease. It may, of course, be caused by some toxic agent, such as carbon tetrachloride or mycotoxins, which simultaneously damages kidney and renal parenchyma. Analogously, hepatic and renal disease is seen in Wilson's disease due to copper toxicity. Mysteriously, however, hepatic failure alone may cause renal failure referred to as the *hepatorenal syndrome*, or *hepatic nephropathy*. This syndrome may also follow surgical procedures for obstructive jaundice. Few terms in medicine have caused more confusion than "hepatorenal syndrome." The present consensus would restrict the term to patients with combined hepatic (or biliary obstructive) disease in whom the *renal failure is not associated with visible morphologic changes in the kidneys*. Indeed, kidneys from such patients have been successfully used for transplantation and have functioned normally in their new "homes."[4] The cause of renal failure is still uncertain, but increasingly the evidence points to reduction of renal blood flow due to generalized renal vasoconstriction induced by gut-derived bacterial endotoxins that escape normal clearance by the liver.[5] The effects of the endotoxins may be amplified by activation of the kallikrein-bradykinin system, catecholamines, and platelet activation with the release of their vasoactive substances, further deranging renal flow.

A host of *other abnormalities* may be encountered in hepatic failure secondary to altered hepatic metabolism. Useful diagnostically is evidence of *hypogonadism and gynecomastia* secondary to impaired degradation of estrogens. *Palmar erythema* (a reflection of local vasodilatation) and *"spider angiomas"* of the skin have also been attributed to hyperestrinism but with little proof. Each angioma is a central, pulsating, dilated arteriole from which small vessels radiate. Nonspecific changes include weight loss; muscle wasting; hypoglycemia; prolongation of the prothrombin time because of impaired synthesis of blood clotting factors II, VII, IX, and X, which may lead to a bleeding tendency; and respiratory and circulatory abnormalities.

As might be expected, liver function tests such as total serum protein concentration, albumin-globulin ratio, prothrombin level, hepatic enzyme assays, and Bromsulphalein excretion are useful in confirming the presence of serious injury to the liver. The outlook is grave, so grave that liver transplantation has been resorted to in a few clinics. Despite such "heroics," a rapid downhill course is usual, with death occurring within weeks to a few months. A fortunate few can be tided over an episode of acute necrosis until regeneration restores adequate hepatic function.

## HEREDITARY DISORDERS OF BILIRUBIN METABOLISM

There are a number of conditions, all quite rare, characterized by hyperbilirubinemia related to an inherited defect in the metabolism of bilirubin.[6] Most are quite innocuous and make the patient "more yellow than sick," but one disorder, the Crigler-Najjar syndrome, may be lethal. The importance of these disorders lies in the insight they provide into the dynamics of bilirubin metabolism, and because they may biochemically mimic some of the more ominous acquired hepatobiliary disorders. Hence, they should be kept in mind when dealing with the differential diagnosis of jaundice.

As with all other causes of jaundice, the genetic disorders of bilirubin metabolism can be classified into those associated with unconjugated hyperbilirubinemia and those in which the predominant form of bilirubin is conjugated. Gilbert's syndrome and the Crigler-Najjar syndromes (type I and type II) are characterized by unconjugated hyperbilirubinemia due to variable degrees of glucuronyl tranferase deficiency. *Gilbert's syndrome* is the most common and, happily, the most innocuous of all. It affects up to 7% of the population and is transmitted as an autosomal dominant with incomplete penetrance. In addition to a mild deficiency of glucuronyl transferase, which is present in most cases, some patients also exhibit reduced uptake of bilirubin and a mild decrease in red-cell survival (hemolysis). Thus Gilbert's syndrome may represent a constellation of disorders rather than a discrete entity. Except for the presence of hyperbilirubinemia, the liver functions are normal and there are no anatomic changes of note. The prognosis is excellent.

*Crigler-Najjar syndrome type I* is an extremely rare autosomal recessive disorder characterized by a virtual absence of hepatic glucuronyl transferase activity. Plasma bilirubin concentrations often exceed 20 mg/dl and death occurs in infancy, owing to the neurotoxic effects of unconjugated bilirubin (kernicterus, p. 362). *Crigler-Najjar syndrome type II* lies between the type I variant and Gilbert's disease, with respect to both the degree of enzyme deficiency and clinical features. The serum bilirubin is usually less than 20 mg/dl and can be further reduced by treatment with phenobarbital. This drug induces glucuronyl transferase activity in the liver and thus promotes conjugation of bile. The mode of inheritance appears to be autosomal dominant with variable penetrance.

In contrast to the syndromes described above, the *Dubin-Johnson* and *Rotor's syndromes* are characterized by predominantly conjugated hyperbilirubinemia. They are both autosomal recessive disorders and share an inability to secrete conjugated bilirubin into the bile canaliculi. The defect, which is believed to reside in the liver cell membrane, extends to other organic anions such as Bromsulphalein (BSP) and certain radio-opaque dyes excreted by the liver into bile. Thus the gallbladder cannot be visualized by oral cholecystography. The liver is histologically normal in Rotor's syndrome, but in the case of Dubin-Johnson syndrome, although the liver cells are otherwise normal, there is an accumulation of a dark pigment in the hepatic lysosomes. This imparts a black-brown color to the liver that is visible macroscopically. The pigment has been variously claimed to resemble melanin or lipofuscin.[7] In any event, it is totally innocuous and the patients have no symptoms referable to hepatocellular dysfunction.

## CIRCULATORY DISORDERS

*Hepatic chronic passive congestion (CPC) and central hemorrhagic necrosis (CHN)* are two circulatory changes representing essentially a continuum encountered in right-sided heart failure. They were discussed on page 315, and it suffices to state here that CPC of the liver is an extremely common postmortem finding, since some degree of circulatory failure is almost inevitable in the agonal stage of life. CHN, in contrast, is less common, and although it is encountered in severe right-sided heart failure it may also be caused by disorders that cause arterial hypoperfusion of the liver, such as left-sided heart failure or shock due to other causes. Since the central zone of the liver lobule is most susceptible to hypoxic injury, it succumbs to ischemia more readily than the peripheral portions. *Cardiac sclerosis* sometimes follows CHN and, more rarely, long-standing CPC. It is characterized by a delicate fibrosis about the central veins of the liver lobules. The older designation "cardiac cirrhosis" is inappropriate, since the pattern of liver damage does not fulfill all of the criteria required for the diagnosis of cirrhosis detailed on page 582. Nonetheless, the fibrotic process and destruction of central hepatocytes may slightly reduce the size of the liver and create a fine pigskin-like granularity to the serosal covering. Cardiac sclerosis almost never leads to any of the sequelae encountered with cirrhosis of the liver or to liver failure, but it may reduce the hepatic reserve to marginal levels, potentiating functional insufficiency during periods of stress.

*Infarctions* within the liver, with its double blood supply (hepatic artery and portal vein), are understandably quite rare. Nonetheless, they are encountered when an intrahepatic branch of the hepatic artery is occluded, such as may occur in polyarteritis nodosa. More rare origins are embolism, neoplastic or inflammation-induced thromboses, and, even more rarely, accidental surgical ligation of an arterial branch. The typical pale or anemic infarcts are similar to those encountered in other solid parenchymal organs and require no further description.

*Hepatic vein thrombosis* is also known as the *Budd-Chiari syndrome*. Although highly signficant clinically, it is sufficiently rare to warrant only brief consideration.[8] Known causes of the Budd-Chiari syndrome include (1) hematologic disorders with thrombotic tendencies, especially polycythemia vera, and paroxysmal nocturnal hemoglobinuria; (2) use of oral contraceptives; (3) tumors, particularly hepatocellular carcinoma and renal cell carcinoma, both of which tend to invade the hepatic vein; (4) intrahepatic infections, such as amebic abscesses; and (5) mysterious membranous webs, which develop in the venous outflow of the liver or within venae cavae and are found mostly in Japan and other parts of the Orient. They may represent congenital anomalies. In addition, several cases of hepatic vein thrombosis have been reported during pregnancy or shortly after delivery. These may relate to the increased risk of thrombosis in pregnancy. In approximately 30% of the cases, hepatic vein thrombosis appears without apparent cause. Whatever its origins, it is inevitably followed by painful, tender liver enlargement, ascites, portal hypertension (p. 583), and esophageal varices. Unless the obstruction can be surgically bypassed, death follows, usually within months. The anatomic changes are those of severe central passive congestion rapidly progressing to central hemorrhagic necrosis.

*Portal vein thrombosis* may be initiated by encroaching intrahepatic or intraabdominal sepsis or by invading cancers. It also occurs in association with cirrhosis. However, in the great majority of instances it appears de novo. When it is related to sepsis, inflammatory involvement of the wall of the portal vein or its major radicals creates what is known as *pylephlebitis*. Very infrequently, a thrombus initiated in a small radical of the portal vein by upper abdominal surgery propagates to obstruct the portal vein. Unlike the case with hepatic vein thrombosis, the liver is not enlarged or tender, and there is little or no ascites. Nonetheless, esophageal varices frequently develop as a manifestation of the portal hypertension (p. 583). Rupture of a varix may cause death, but in some cases the variceal bleeding can be controlled. In all instances, procedures such as a splenorenal shunt are required to bypass the obstruction.

## REYE'S SYNDROME

This disorder, characterized by fatty change in the liver and sometimes fatal encephalopathy, afflicts young people between six months and 17 years of age[9] and is fatal in 10 to 40% of the cases. Milder forms are entirely reversible and are believed to outnumber the more severe and dramatic expressions of this disease. Typically, Reye's syndrome follows an otherwise innocuous childhood viral illness, most commonly influenza A or B, or varicella. During recovery from the viral infection there is a sudden reversal of the course, heralded by recurrent vomiting and in some instances followed by lethargy, delirium, convulsions, and coma. In severe cases, death may occur within 24 to 48 hours after the onset of vomiting and results from increasing cerebral edema, with brain herniations.

Laboratory investigations reveal elevated serum transaminases, hyperammonemia, fatty acidemia, lactic acidemia, and prolonged prothrombin time, all pointing to hepatocellular dysfunction. Jaundice, however, is absent.

Morphologic changes are seen primarily in the liver and central nervous system. **There is panlobular fatty change seen as multiple small cytoplasmic vacuoles, without significant liver cell necrosis or inflammation.** Fatty change is also seen in the kidneys, heart, and skeletal muscles. The brain reveals marked cerebral edema, without any evidence of inflammation or viral infection. Ultrastructural changes affecting the mitochondria, such as swelling, irregularity of mitochondrial membranes, and reduction in number, have been noted in both the liver cells and the neurons.

Two decades of research have failed to reveal the cause of Reye's syndrome. About the only statement that can be made with assurance is that despite the universal association with viral illnesses, direct virus-induced injury is not the cause of this disorder. As usual, many hypotheses have sprouted, all of which will not be detailed here. We will consider only the role of aspirin, which according to epidemiologic data is somehow implicated in the pathogenesis of Reye's syndrome. Briefly, there seems to be a correlation between the administration of aspirin for the control of fever during the initial viral illness and the subsequent development of Reye's syndrome.[10] However, the amount of aspirin ingested is not large enough to be toxic by itself. Therefore, the emerging consensus seems to be that Reye's syndrome evolves from a complex interaction between the combined effects of certain viruses and salicylates. Since the disease does not affect everyone who is treated with salicylates during a viral infection, some genetic predisposition is invoked. Conceivably, in the genetically susceptible host mitochondrial damage occurs. A decrease in the activity of mitochondrial enzymes can explain most of the biochemical abnormalities such as hyperammonemia and lactic acidemia. Elevations in the levels of these and other toxic metabolites are believed to be responsible for the neurologic changes, which ultimately prove fatal. As an extension of this hypothesis, it has been suggested that other drugs or chemicals, rather than aspirin, may in some cases act as cofactors with viral infections. Thus Reye's syndrome appears to be a multifactorial disorder whose origins may be related to a combination of microbiologic, genetic, and one or more environmental factors.

## CHOLANGITIS AND LIVER ABSCESS

The designation *cholangitis* refers to inflammation of the bile ducts and should be distinguished from *cholangiolitis*, which implies involvement of smaller bile ductules, such as occurs in viral hepatitis. Cholangitis is almost always caused by bacteria. In the usual case, biliary tract disease and partial or complete obstruction to the outflow of bile underlie the development of the infection. As might be anticipated, the common organisms are *Escherichia coli*, enterococci, other gram-negative rods, and the salmonellae. The flora then is the same as that associated with acute cholecystitis (p. 601). In the great majority of cases, the cholangitis is associated with cholecystitis and is to be considered an extension of the same inflammatory process. The morphologic changes are typical of acute suppurative inflammation, which may extend upward and produce liver abscess.

*Liver abscesses* arise most commonly as complications of acute ascending cholangitis, and as such they are frequently associated with some obstructive disease of the biliary tract such as gallstones or malignancy. The next most common cause is blood-borne infection in a patient with bacteremia, as may occur in association with bacterial endocarditis. Since the advent of antibiotics, extension of infection along the portal vein secondary to intraabdominal sepsis is a much less frequent cause. As might be expected from their frequent association with ascending cholangitis, gram-negative rods such as *E. coli* and *Klebsiella* are commonly isolated from liver abscesses. However, with improvements in culture techniques, it is becoming obvious that liver abscesses are often polymicrobial in origin.[11] Pathogens other than gram-negative rods include anaerobes such as *Bacteroides fragilis* and *Fusobacterium* species as well as microaerophilic streptococci. Staphylococci are also encountered, although less frequently than the other pathogens listed.

The lesions vary from microscopic foci to massive areas of suppurative necrosis. In general, they are from 1 to 3 cm in diameter and are usually multiple. Rupture through the capsule may lead to subhepatic or subdiaphragmatic abscesses and peritonitis. On rare occasion, the infection may trek from the subdiaphragmatic location into the thoracic cavity. Liver abscesses may be totally silent if they are small and few in number. When they evoke symptoms, the clinical disease is usually indistinguishable from acute cholangitis, which, of course, is a frequent accompaniment.

There remains only one other form of liver abscess, to be briefly described.

*Amebic abscesses* of the liver are one of the serious complications of amebic dysentery (p. 548). The parasites reach the liver through the portal vein. *The abscess is most commonly located in the upper part of the right lobe and is solitary in 70% of the cases.* It characteristically contains a brown paste-like exudate rather than pus. The diagnosis depends on the demonstration of the parasites or their antigens in the aspirate material. Serologic tests are also of value.[12] From the liver, these abscesses may burrow through the subdiaphragmatic space to enter the lungs and occasionally embolize from there to the brain.

# VIRAL HEPATITIS

A number of viral agents, such as the Epstein-Barr virus of infectious mononucleosis, cytomegalovirus, yellow fever virus, and the herpes virus, may all cause systemic infections that sometimes involve the liver. However, the term "viral hepatitis" is generally reserved for primary hepatic infections caused by one of a group of specifically hepatotropic viruses. Two of these agents, hepatitis A virus (HAV) and hepatitis B virus (HBV), have been well characterized. But in addition, at least one, or possibly two or more, agents have now been implicated, known by the guarded term "non-A, non-B viruses (NANBV)." Yet another virus, the so-called delta agent that is replication defective and hence must rely on hepatitis B virus

for its multiplication, has also been found to cause hepatitis.

Invasion of the liver by these agents leads to a range of syndromes varying from asymptomatic occult infection to acute debilitating disease (acute icteric hepatitis), to several forms of chronic hepatitis, and in rare instances to fulminating submassive to massive hepatic necrosis. Moreover, there is a carrier state that may appear following certain of these syndromes, but is sometimes discovered in individuals who do not have a history of an overt preceding viral infection of the liver. The several causative agents vary in their propensity to cause all of the clinical patterns of infection cited, as will be detailed later. Presumably host-invader factors are involved in these variable outcomes, but in truth they are not well understood.

In the following discussion each of the causative agents will be characterized first, followed by a consideration of the pathogenesis of the disease and then of the range of clinical expressions.[13–15]

## CAUSATIVE AGENTS

**HEPATITIS B VIRUS (HBV).** More is known about the HBV than about the other hepatotropic viruses and so it is considered first. Logically, the disease it evokes is now referred to as hepatitis B but was formerly known as "serum hepatitis" or "long-incubation hepatitis." *This virus may cause acute hepatitis or may be involved in any of the patterns of viral infection mentioned earlier, ranging from the carrier state to fulminant hepatitis.* The complete virus particle is a sphere about 42 nm in diameter composed of a central 27 nm partially double-stranded DNA core (associated with its own DNA polymerase) enclosed within a lipoprotein coat (Fig. 17–2). These virions are sometimes called *Dane particles* (Fig. 17–3) in recognition of the investigator who first described them.[16] During active infection they can be readily visualized in infected hepatocytes but less commonly in serum. Dane particles transmit the infection to volunteers and chimpanzees but have not yet been grown in vitro.

There are three well-defined antigens associated

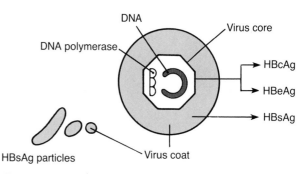

Figure 17–2. Schematic diagram of the structure of hepatitis B virus.

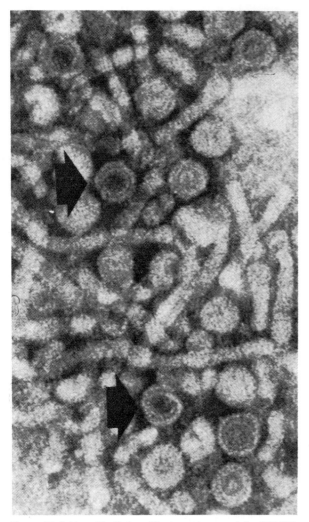

Figure 17–3. Hepatitis B virus. Electron micrograph (× 220,000 of negatively stained pellet prepared from the serum of a patient with chronic hepatitis. Numerous Dane particles (*arrows*) and 22-nm tubules are present. (Courtesy of Dr. Michael Gerber, Associate Professor of Pathology, Mount Sinai School of Medicine, New York.)

circulation is highly correlated with the presence of HBV-specific DNA polymerase, HBV-DNA and hence with the infectivity of the blood. HBeAg is never present in the blood in the absence of HBsAg. The antigens associated with HBV evoke specific antibodies: anti-HBs, anti-HBc, and anti-HBe.

Both the antigens and their antibodies constitute important immunologic markers of the infection and its course. The incubation period of hepatitis B ranges from 45 days to six months (average, two to three months). The following comments relative to the rise and fall of antigens and their antibodies are best understood by repeated reference to Figure 17–4, where they are depicted. HBsAg is first detected in blood during the incubation period, in some cases as early as one week after infection. Following on the heels of the surface antigen, virus particles and HBeAg appear in the blood; HBeAg disappears early, during the course of acute illness, usually two to three weeks before the clearance of HBsAg. In a typical case of acute hepatitis B, the HBsAg level begins to decline after the onset of illness and usually is undetectable three months after exposure. Persistence beyond six months usually indicates chronic disease (p. 578). Although the free core antigen HBcAg is never found in the serum, antibodies against it, anti-HBc, are the first antiviral antibodies to become detectable after exposure to HBV. Anti-HBc appears toward the end of the incubation period and persists during the acute illness (providing a valuable diagnostic marker) and for several months to years thereafter. The initial anti-HBc response is IgM, followed six to 18 months later by IgG antibodies. These antibodies are not protective and are detectable in the face of chronic disease. Anti-HBe appears in the serum as the HBeAg begins to disappear, early during the course of acute illness. Its presence indicates the onset of resolution of acute hepatitis. Anti-HBs is detected during convalescence

with HBV, two of which (HBcAg and HBeAg) are associated with the virus core, whereas the third, hepatitis B surface antigen (HBsAg), is the major antigenic determinant of the outer surface coat. HBsAg, of which there are several subtypes, is produced in abundance by the infected liver cells. Excess outer coat can be visualized within the involved liver cells and in the serum as spherical particles 22 nm in diameter and also as long, tubular, filamentous forms 22 nm thick (Figs. 17–2 and 17–3). HBsAg is sometimes called "*Australia antigen*" because it was first identified by Blumberg in the serum of an Australian aborigine. Unlike HBsAg, the hepatitis B core antigen (HBcAg) is never found free in the circulation, since naked core particles do not circulate. The other core-associated antigen, HBeAg, on the other hand, may be found in the serum as a soluble (nonparticulate) protein. Its presence in the

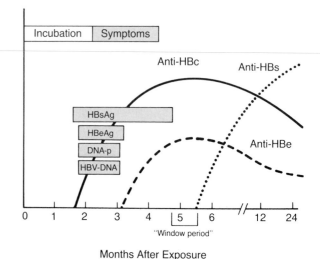

Figure 17–4. Correlation of the clinical course and serologic findings in acute type B hepatitis. DNA-p = DNA polymerase.

(several weeks to months after the disappearance of HBsAg), and it usually persists for life. The interval between the disappearance of HBsAg and the appearance of anti-HBs is called the "window period," during which the presence of anti-HBc may be the only serum marker of hepatitis B infection. A high titer of anti-HBs confers immunity to HBV. The persistence of HBsAg and its relationship to chronic hepatitis B infection is discussed later.

*In summary, during the presymptomatic stage of acute hepatitis B, the principal serum markers of the infection are first HBsAg and then HBeAg. As the patient becomes symptomatic, antibody to core antigen becomes detectable, followed after a variable period of weeks to months by anti-HBe and anti-HBs, in that order.*

*Blood and body fluids of infected individuals are the most important reservoirs of infection.* The HBV is most often transmitted by the parenteral (percutaneous) route—blood transfusions; infusions of plasma, fibrinogen, or other blood fractions; hypodermic needles; dental and surgical instruments; and razors. There is therefore a high risk of transmission with hemodialysis and transplantation. Not unexpectedly, HBsAg can be found in over half of all heroin addicts. Transmission may also occur accidentally to health care personnel (physicians, dentists, nurses, and laboratory workers). In recent years the nearly universal screening of blood donors for HBsAg has significantly reduced the incidence of HBV-induced post-transfusion hepatitis. Currently HBV is believed to be responsible for approximately 10% of all cases of post-transfusion hepatitis; most of the others are caused by non-A, non-B viruses, as discussed later.

The infection may also be contracted through other routes. The virus has been shown to be present in oropharyngeal secretions, in seminal fluid, in menstrual blood, in urine, and in the stool. Thus the infected individual sheds virus through literally every orifice, and it is no surprise that intimate personal contact is an important mode of spread. Consequently, high attack rates occur in spouses or sexual contacts of affected patients, in family members of chronic carriers, among male homosexuals, and among institutionalized patients (particularly children with Down's syndrome). Spread by close personal contact may also account for the so-called vertical transmission from mothers who have hepatitis B infection to their infants during the perinatal period. This method of spread is believed to account for the high carrier rate of HBV in some African and Asian populations.

**HEPATITIS A VIRUS (HAV).** This virus, like HBV, is hepatotropic and causes acute hepatitis that resembles acute hepatitis B. However, the similarities between the two viruses end here. Unlike HBV (a DNA virus), the causative agent of hepatitis A is a genetically distinct nonenveloped RNA virus. The disease that it evokes is called hepatitis A, which is

a benign, acute, self-limited disorder and which, unlike hepatitis B, does not lead to chronicity nor to a carrier state. Only rarely does hepatitis A cause massive liver necrosis. Hepatitis A was formerly referred to as *"infectious hepatitis"* or *"short-incubation hepatitis,"* since the incubation period (relative to hepatitis B) is short and varies from 15 to 45 days (average two to four weeks). The first evidence of HAV infection is the presence of the virus in the stools. Fecal shedding (which corresponds to the period of peak infectivity) begins before the symptoms appear, during the final week of the incubation period, and continues into the initial (prodromal) phase of illness. There is a transient viremia that begins during the prodrome and rapidly clears with the onset of clinical illness. Unlike the case of HBV, the virus is not shed in any significant quantities from the saliva, urine, or semen.

HAV evokes the formation of antibodies (anti-HAV) initially of the IgM type, followed rapidly by the IgG isotype. As seen in Figure 17–5, the appearance of IgM anti-HAV antibodies coincides roughly with the decline in fecal shedding of the virus. After several weeks to months, the titer of IgM antibodies falls, whereas the IgG antibodies persist for several years and confer long-term immunity.

Transmission of HAV occurs almost exclusively by the fecal-oral route. Since there is no carrier state nor chronicity to the infection, spread occurs only from acutely infected individuals, often before they reveal symptoms, or from clinically inapparent (mild) cases. As might be expected from the mode of transmission, spread of HAV is favored by poor personal hygiene, close contact, and overcrowding. *Hepatitis A may appear as a sporadic or epidemic infection.* Nonimmune adults are at particular risk when traveling in high-endemic areas. The prevalence of this infection can be judged by the fact that over 80% of blood donors in such countries as Taiwan, Israel, Yugoslavia, and Belgium have anti-HAV antibodies. In the United States the comparable rate is

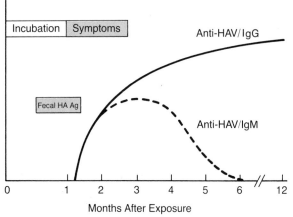

**Figure 17–5.** Correlation of the clinical course and serologic findings in acute type A hepatitis.

about 40%. Most of these individuals were never even aware that they had become infected. Clearly a large majority of those who are exposed to HAV develop a trivial or asymptomatic infection (p. 576). Sporadic infections may also be contracted by the consumption of raw or steamed shellfish (oysters, mussels, clams), which concentrate the virus from contaminated seawater. As with hepatitis B, there seems to be an increased incidence among promiscuous male homosexuals. Infections may occur in epidemics, particularly in institutions for small children, as well as among people of developing countries who live under overcrowded, unsanitary conditions. Such epidemics are often water-borne or related to food handlers. The virus can be transmitted to chimpanzees and marmosets, and infection has occurred in handlers of these primates. Since the viremia is transient, blood-borne transmission of HAV is rare.

**NON-A, NON-B VIRUSES (NANBV).** The development of sensitive assays for virologic and serologic markers of HBV and HAV has led to the awareness that almost 90% of cases of transfusion-associated hepatitis are due to one or possibly several non-A, non-B viruses. There are several hints (such as wide variations in incubation period) that more than one agent, very likely two, exist, but to date no clearly distinctive immunologic markers of one or more viruses have been established.

Electron microscopy has revealed an array of virus-like particles in the serum and liver of patients with NANB hepatitis.[17] Viral particles have also been observed in chimpanzees who develop the disease by transfer of patient sera.[18] However, the morphologic diversity of the virus-like particles described and the absence of well-defined immunologic reagents that react with the implicated agents have so far frustrated all efforts to identify definitively the NANB viruses.

Transmission of NANBV is usually by the parenteral route by infusion of blood or blood products. As such, the high-risk groups include not only patients who receive therapeutic blood transfusions but also patients undergoing hemodialysis, renal transplant recipients, drug addicts, and medical personnel exposed to blood or its derivatives. Like HBV, however, nonpercutaneous transmission involving spread resulting from close personal contact must also be involved. Such transmission is most likely responsible for the spread of NANB hepatitis in male homosexuals as well as that within institutions. Although fecal-oral transmission has not been documented in the Western world, several water-borne epidemics of NANB hepatitis have been described in Southeast Asia, North Africa, and Japan.[19] In the absence of serologic markers for NANB hepatitis, it is not possible to state whether the agent or agents involved in these epidemics are similar to those responsible for the sporadic form of the disease.

The clinical spectrum of NANB hepatitis spans the entire gamut from asymptomatic carrier state to acute hepatitis, chronic hepatitis, and sometimes fulminant disease. Its potential therefore parallels HBV. As compared with HBV, however, the acute hepatitis caused by NANB viruses is mild, but it has a higher propensity for transition to chronicity.

**DELTA HEPATITIS.** This most recent addition to the group of human hepatotropic viruses is a unique RNA virus that is replication defective.[20] The virus core, which contains the delta antigen, is surrounded by HBsAg necessary for its replication. Thus the delta virus (HDV), although taxonomically distinct from HBV, is absolutely dependent upon the genetic information provided by HBV for multiplication. Not surprisingly, therefore, HDV can cause hepatitis only in the presence of HBV, under the following three situations: (1) as an acute hepatitis with concurrent acute hepatitis B, (2) as an acute hepatitis in a chronic HBV carrier, and (3) as a chronic hepatitis in a chronic HBV carrier. Delta hepatitis is endemic in the Mediterranean area, the Middle East, and parts of Africa but occurs sporadically all over the world. In the United States delta hepatitis is uncommon and occurs mainly in those who have had repeated parenteral exposures (e.g., drug addicts and multiply transfused patients).[21] The delta antigen evokes the formation of both IgM and IgG antibodies.[22]

## PATHOGENESIS

The mechanism or mechanisms by which the hepatotropic viruses injure liver cells are uncertain, as indeed is the issue of whether all act alike. Bits of evidence raise the possibility that the pathogenetic pathways differ. *Two possibilities exist: (1) a direct cytopathic effect and (2) the induction of immune responses against viral antigens or virus-modified hepatocyte antigens that damage virally infected hepatocytes.*

Although not definitely ruled out, a direct cytopathic effect, particularly for the HBV and NANBV, is argued against by most of the available evidence.[23] The long incubation period and the fact that viral replication is maximal during the incubation period when the hepatocytic injury is not maximal are both inconsistent with the usual behavior of cytopathic viruses.

The short incubation period of HAV does raise the possibility of direct cytopathic effect, but the replication of the virus in subhuman primate cells is not associated with cell injury.

*The most popular current theory about the mechanism of action of these viral agents proposes that the immune response to the viral antigens is the ultimate mediator of liver cell injury.* Most of the available evidence relates to the HBV, but a number of observations suggest that the diseases caused by the NANBV and the HAV have similar origins. It is clear from the earlier discussion that the hepatotropic viruses induce a humoral immune response to viral antigens, but in addition, as with all viral infections, the main reaction is cell mediated. Thus it is proposed that cytotoxic T-cell reactions against virus-specific antigens or virus-modified cell membrane antigens injure the liver cells (Fig. 17–6).[24, 25] It is also conceivable that antibody-coated hepatocytes might be destroyed by antibody-dependent cellular cytotoxicity. There is evidence, albeit fragmentary, to support each of these mechanisms.[26]

It is further proposed that the variable clinical expressions of infection with the HBV and possibly with the other viruses are determined by the strength of the immune response. An adequate host immune reaction in acute viral hepatitis might cause cellular injury but at the same time eliminate the virus, thus resulting in a self-limited disease. The strength of this immune response would determine whether the virus was promptly eliminated, leading to destruction of many cells and a fairly severe but short-lived infection, or more slowly eliminated, with less damage to hepatocytes, inducing thereby a milder, longer, but nonetheless self-limited acute hepatitis or an asymptomatic infection. Within this framework, an overwhelming immune response would induce fulminant, massive liver necrosis, but the virus would be totally eliminated.[27] It is relevant to this conception that patients who survive such massive liver damage seldom become chronic carriers. At the opposite end of the spectrum of immune responses are those individuals who mount a marginal immune response and so cannot eliminate the virus. In such cases hepatocytes expressing viral antigens such as HBcAg, or virus-modified self-antigens would persist, leading to continued low-level destruction (i.e., development of chronic hepatitis).[25] Finally, the carrier state could be explained as a total failure of the immune response, with perpetuation of the viremia but little or no liver damage. This interesting view of the pathogenesis of liver injury is supported by the observation that viral antigens are abundant in the hepatocytes of carriers but are rare to absent in the liver cells in fulminant hepatitis. Seductive as this schema may be, it has not been possible to document a generalized suppression of immune responsiveness in patients with chronic hepatitis or the carrier state.

Although cell-mediated immune responses have been invoked as the major mechanism of liver cell injury in viral hepatitis, antiviral antibodies are undoubtedly involved in the pathogenesis of several extrahepatic manifestations. Circulating immune complexes containing viral antigens and antibodies are responsible for such manifestations as vasculitis, polyarthritis, and immune complex–mediated glomerulonephritis, seen in some patients with acute hepatitis B.

## CLINICAL SYNDROMES

As has been alluded to earlier, viral infection of the liver may be expressed (or unexpressed) in a range of clinical syndromes. The spectrum can be outlined as follows:
1. Carrier state
   a. Following subclinical illness
   b. Following chronic hepatitis
2. Acute hepatitis
   a. Anicteric
   b. Icteric
3. Chronic hepatitis
   a. Chronic persistent hepatitis
   b. Chronic active hepatitis
4. Subacute to massive hepatic necrosis (fulminant hepatitis)

As has been emphasized, not all of the viruses previously described evoke each of these clinical syndromes.

### The Carrier State

The use of the term "carrier" in the context of hepatitis virus differs somewhat from the conventional definition, which usually implies an asymptomatic, "healthy" carrier who can transmit the disease. In the case of viral hepatitis, one type of "carrier" is an individual who has virologic or serologic markers of infection but who is entirely asymptomatic and, indeed, has no evidence of liver damage. Such indi-

**HBV INFECTION**

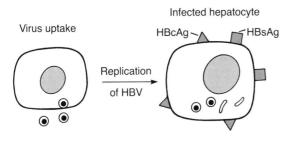

**IMMUNE RESPONSE AGAINST INFECTED HEPATOCYTE**

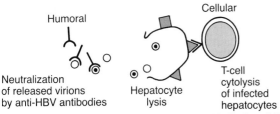

Figure 17–6. Immune response against hepatitis B virus (HBV) and its possible role in liver cell injury. Anti-HBV antibodies may not only neutralize hepatitis B virions (as shown) but may also coat hepatocytes, rendering them susceptible to antibody-dependent cell-mediated lysis.

viduals are identified as carriers in the course of screening programs for blood donation. The other category of carrier comprises patients with symptomatic or asymptomatic chronic liver disease who have definite evidence of liver cell injury and who have persistent infections.[28]

Since carriers may or may not have had a recognized prior infection but nonetheless can transmit the infection (sometimes for the remainder of their lives), the absence of a history of viral hepatitis in a blood donor does not exclude possible infectivity. *The carrier state is well recognized for HBV, HDV with HBV, and NANBV but is not associated with HAV.* Since HBV carriers can be detected by the presence of HBsAg but there are no markers for NANBV, adequate data are available only on the prevalence of carriers of hepatitis B. It ranges from 0.1 to 0.5% in the United States, but it is much higher in certain Asian and African populations (5 to 15%).[29] Perinatal transmission from an HBsAg carrier mother seems to be an important mode of maintenance of the high carrier rate in developing countries. Transmission from mother to offspring is correlated with the serum titer of HBeAg and inversely related to serum level of anti-HBeAg. In general, individuals at particular risk of developing the carrier state are those with impaired immune responses, whether constitutional or related to immunosuppressive therapy; patients who have received multiple transfusions or hemodialysis; drug addicts; and mentally retarded persons in institutions. In such high-risk populations the carrier rate may be as high as 15%, even in the Western countries.

**MORPHOLOGY.** In the "healthy" carrier the liver morphology is basically normal. However, striking changes can be seen within the hepatocytes containing HBV.[30] The cytoplasm of hepatocytes has a "ground-glass" appearance. Ultrastructurally, this can be resolved as marked proliferation of the endoplasmic reticulum, which is diffusely filled with tubular and spherical particles proved by immunofluorescent and immunoperoxidase techniques to be HBsAg. These particles can be readily demonstrated in formalin-fixed tissues by the orcein and aldehyde fuchsin stains. Immunofluorescent techniques may also disclose HBcAg within some nuclei. Carriers with chronic liver disease have histologic evidence of liver cell injury (chronic hepatitis, to be described later), as well as the cytoplasmic and nuclear changes described above. It is interesting to note that although healthy carriers have numerous clusters of antigen-bearing cells, those with chronic hepatitis have only scattered cells containing HBsAg. This observation supports the hypothesis discussed earlier that the healthy carrier state is associated with an inefficient immune response against virus-infected cells.

Despite the fact that healthy carriers have little or no evidence of liver damage, they have an increased risk of developing hepatocellular carcinoma, as do chronic carriers (p. 598).

## Acute Viral Hepatitis

The *sporadic attacks* of acute hepatitis caused by all of the hepatotropic viruses are essentially identical and are caused most commonly by HAV. When caused by HAV or HBV it can be related to these agents only by virologic or serologic criteria. NANBV hepatitis can currently be diagnosed only by exclusion of HAV and HBV. However, when the infection occurs within an *epidemic outbreak*, it is highly likely that it is due to HAV, save for the uncommon NANBV, water-borne epidemics described earlier. After contraction of infection there is an incubation period, which, as has been explained, is shortest in hepatitis A, longest in hepatitis B, and intermediate and quite variable in non-A, non-B hepatitis. During the incubation period, the individual is asymptomatic, but some weeks before symptoms appear, evidence of liver injury can be detected in the form of elevated levels of serum glutamate oxaloacetate transaminase (SGOT, also called aspartate aminotransferase, or AST), serum glutamate pyruvate transaminase (SGPT, also called alanine aminotransferase, or ALT), and lactic dehydrogenase (LDH). In some instances, particularly with hepatitis A, no symptoms or an extremely mild illness similar to that of many other viral infections may follow. Indeed, probably no more than 5% of cases of hepatitis A become more pronounced. In other instances, whatever the agent, there is a preicteric phase for a few days, with fever, malaise, nausea, vomiting, and weakness, often accompanied by a distaste for cigarettes. The physical examination at this stage may reveal a mildly enlarged and tender liver. The onset of these symptoms tends to be more abrupt in patients with hepatitis A than in those with hepatitis B. From this point, one of two clinical patterns may follow. In one, no elevation of the serum bilirubin levels ever appears, and after a period of weeks the patient recovers; this variant is referred to as *anicteric hepatitis*. In the other, the nonspecific symptoms are more marked, with higher fever, shaking chills, and headache, sometimes accompanied by right upper quadrant pain and tender liver enlargement. With this pattern, jaundice usually develops *(icteric hepatitis)* and, surprisingly, with the appearance of the jaundice, the other symptoms begin to abate. The jaundice is usually due to elevated levels of both conjugated and unconjugated bilirubin and is accompanied by dark-colored urine related to the presence of the conjugated bilirubin. The stools often become light-colored when the swollen liver cells obstruct the flow of bile through the biliary canaliculi (cholestasis, p. 581). In such patients the retention of bile salts may cause distressing skin itching (pruritus). When the manifestations of bile retention are particularly prominent, the disease may be referred to as *cholestatic viral hepatitis*. A variety of extrahepatic manifestations may confuse the clinical picture. Early in the preicteric stage, urticaria, skin rashes, and arthralgia are sometimes seen. These serum sickness–like changes are ascribed to circulating antigen-antibody complexes, although such immune complexes have been detected only in hepatitis B. Late in the disease, particularly in hepatitis B, glomerulonephritis, arthritis, or a variety of forms of systemic vasculitis such as polyarteritis nodosa may develop, owing to prolonged antigenemia and circulating immune complexes.

The clinical course of acute icteric hepatitis is extremely variable and is significantly affected by the specific causative viral agent. Typically, with hepatitis A the jaundice and elevated serum enzyme levels begin to subside within two weeks, and recovery is complete in four to six weeks. With hepatitis B, the illness is somewhat more protracted, but clinical and biochemical recovery is usually complete within 12 to 16 weeks. Most cases of acute non-A, non-B hepatitis are mild with minimal biochemical changes and clinical findings. In 1% or fewer of the patients, particularly those with hepatitis B and those with non-A, non-B hepatitis, the acute infection flares and leads to subacute or massive hepatic necrosis. Only about 10 to 30% of these unfortunate individuals survive the acute liver failure. Another possible outcome that occurs in about 5 to 10% of patients with hepatitis B, and much more frequently in those with posttransfusion NANB hepatitis but virtually never in those with hepatitis A, is the development of a carrier state. In a variable number of patients, persistence of the virus leads to progressive liver injury, to be discussed later (p. 578).

**MORPHOLOGY.** The anatomic changes are the same with all viruses. Although quite characteristic, they are not pathognomonic and can be mimicked, for example, by other viral infections and by adverse reactions to drugs. As seen by laparoscopy, the liver is slightly enlarged, reddened, and, depending on the amount of bile stasis, discolored green.

Histologically, **the dominant features are (1) relatively diffuse liver cell injury, (2) spotty or isolated liver cell necrosis, (3) Kupffer cell reactive changes and inflammatory changes, and (4) liver cell regeneration during the recovery phase.**[31] The liver cell injury takes the form of diffuse swelling of hepatocytes, referred to as "ballooning degeneration," so that the cytoplasm looks empty and contains only scattered wisps of cytoplasmic remnants. This change is most prominent in the centrilobular areas and is due to marked swelling of the endoplasmic reticulum and detachment of ribosomes and polyribosomes. Mitochondrial swelling may also be present. Autophagic bodies containing lipofuscin or ceroid may appear at this stage. Fatty change is rarely seen and indeed, if present, challenges the diagnosis of viral hepatitis. This stage may be followed by death of isolated hepatocytes or small nests of cells. Two patterns of cell necrosis are seen. In the first, there appears to be rupture of cell membranes followed by cytolysis. The necrotic cells appear to have "dropped out," followed by collapse of the reticulin framework where the cells have disappeared. The second pattern of cell death is more conspicuous and takes the form of condensation of entire

cells accompanied by loss of the nuclei, yielding acidophilic (Councilman) bodies, which are eventually phagocytosed by macrophages.[32] Two other patterns, called "piecemeal necrosis" and "bridging necrosis," are seen less frequently. Since they are more consistently observed in chronic active hepatitis or submassive necrosis, they are described later (p. 579). Although uncommon (contrary to previous opinions), "bridging" or "piecemeal" patterns of necrosis are not considered to be definite indicators of progression to chronic hepatitis. These lesions assume prognostic significance only if they are detected three to six months after the onset of illness.

During the height of the disease reactive and inflammatory changes appear. Particularly prominent is marked hypertrophy (and probably hyperplasia) of Kupffer cells and portal macrophages, whose cytoplasm is often packed with lipofuscin pigment as well as other cell debris. Concomitantly, a portal inflammatory infiltrate appears, composed principally of lymphocytes admixed with macrophages, and sometimes eosinophils and neutrophils (Fig. 17–7). Occasionally, similar inflammatory cells appear in foci of cell necrosis within the hepatic lobule. Plasma cells are distinctly uncommon in the typical case. Bile stasis may not be present in anicteric hepatitis but may be prominent in icteric patients, in which case droplets of bile pigment are found in ballooned hepatocytes and Kupffer cells and in the form of bile plugs in canaliculi compressed between swollen liver cells. During the recovery phase, cell regeneration becomes evident

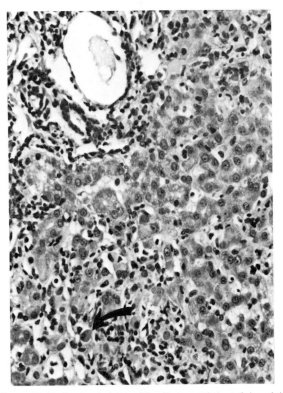

Figure 17–7. Acute viral hepatitis. The portal tract (*above*) is rimmed with a mononuclear infiltrate. The hepatocytes show focal necrosis and an inflammatory infiltrate. The arrow points to an acidophilic body. (Courtesy of Dr. Edwin Eigenbrodt, Southwestern Medical School, Dallas, Texas.)

with enlargement of nuclei in surviving liver cells and the appearance of mitotic figures and occasional binucleate cells.

Several additional features are worthy of note. The inflammatory reaction does not commonly extend to any significant degree from the portal areas into the hepatic substance. Neither special stains nor immunocytochemical methods reveal either intranuclear HBcAg or intracytoplasmic HBsAg save in widely scattered cells in the typical case of acute hepatitis caused by the HBV.[30]

In the classic case, with complete recovery the liver architecture is completely restored over the span of weeks to a few months, the inflammatory infiltrate disappears, and at some later date it would be impossible to ascertain that the patient had ever had viral hepatitis. However, as discussed below, acute hepatitis B or NANB hepatitis may lead to chronic hepatitis. Extensive liver necrosis is another potential complication of HBV or NANBV but rarely of HAV infections.

### Chronic Hepatitis

When there is biochemical or symptomatic evidence of persisting liver disease for more than six months following an attack of acute viral hepatitis, the condition is arbitrarily considered to have become chronic.[33] Of the several variants of chronic hepatitis, only two are well characterized by histopathologic criteria: (1) chronic persistent hepatitis and (2) chronic active hepatitis, sometimes called chronic aggressive hepatitis. Differentiation of these two patterns is of considerable clinical importance. Chronic active hepatitis implies continuing destruction of the liver, which may lead to cirrhosis and hepatic failure. Chronic persistent hepatitis, on the other hand, is a benign disorder that is ultimately self-limited. *It is estimated that 10 to 30% of HBsAg-positive carriers following acute hepatitis B and up to 60% of those with persisting elevations of ALT 6 months after acute NANB hepatitis develop chronic active hepatitis. In contrast, acute hepatitis A is not followed by chronicity.*[18, 28, 35]

Unfortunately, there are no reliable criteria during the stage of acute viral hepatitis to identify those persons at risk of developing chronic hepatitis. In particular, the severity of the acute attack bears no correlation with the persistence of viral infection. Serologic findings suggestive of chronicity in hepatitis B are the continued presence in the serum of HBsAg, HBeAg, high titers of anti-HBc, serum HBV-DNA, and DNA polymerase. In some patients, after a variable period of 1 to 20 years, the spontaneous appearance of anti-HBe antibodies heralds the control of viremia and cessation of further liver damage (Fig. 17–8).[35] *Chronicity is most likely to develop in males; in the very young and very elderly; in those having some immunologic deficiency or receiving immuno-*

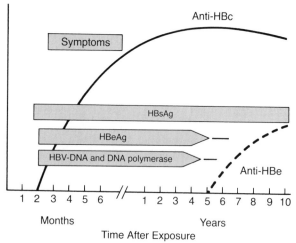

**Figure 17–8.** Clinical and serologic course of chronic hepatitis B infection.

*suppressant therapy; in individuals with Down's syndrome; and in patients on renal dialysis.*

Although there are two distinctive patterns of chronic hepatitis, occasional cases fall in the intermediate zone and others (fortunately uncommon) appear to progress from chronic persistent hepatitis to chronic active hepatitis.

***Chronic Persistent Hepatitis.*** *Chronic persistent hepatitis is a relapsing, remitting, benign, self-limited condition that is not associated with progressive liver damage and does not lead to liver failure or cirrhosis.* In some instances it may take as long as several years to clear.[36] This pattern of disease may follow an overt icteric or occult anicteric infection with either the HBV or the NANBV. During this extended recovery period, the patient may be symptomatic (with fatigue, malaise, loss of appetite, and possibly mild jaundice) or may be entirely asymptomatic. Characteristically, the serum transaminase levels are elevated, and sometimes this is the only clinical evidence of chronic persistent hepatitis. HBsAg can be identified in the serum in from 20 to 30% of these patients, and the remaining cases must be assumed to be due to non-A, non-B hepatitis.

The morphologic changes are mild and not pathognomonic. The liver architecture is basically preserved, and the dominant features comprise a portal inflammatory infiltrate of lymphocytes admixed with plasma cells and macrophages. This reaction does not spill over significantly into the adjacent liver cords. "Piecemeal" necrosis of liver hepatocytes, which is characteristic of chronic active hepatitis, is unusual but may be present during a relapse. Even when the ultimate recovery takes years, the hepatic structure is generally well preserved, and only in the very rare case does this form of benign chronic hepatitis become transformed into the more ominous chronic active hepatitis. In those cases caused by HBV, "ground-glass" hepatocytes, seen best in orcein or aldehyde fuchsin stains, are sometimes present.

*Chronic Active Hepatitis. In contrast to the previous condition, chronic active hepatitis is a "bad" disease characterized by progressive destruction of hepatocytes over the span of years, continued erosion of the hepatic functional reserve, and the eventual development of cirrhosis in most cases.* It is a disorder that can be caused by a variety of etiologic agents, including HBV and NANB viruses. Approximately 20 to 30% of the patients have serologic evidence of HBV infection, with or without concomitant infection with the delta agent. Of the remaining 70 to 80% of the cases, an undetermined number are caused by non-A, non-B viruses. No well-documented cases have been attributed to HAV. An essentially similar clinical and morphologic disorder may also result from toxic reactions to a variety of drugs, such as oxyphenisatin, methyldopa, isoniazid, and acetaminophen; from alpha-1-antitrypsin deficiency; or from Wilson's disease. In addition it may be closely mimicked by primary biliary cirrhosis. In many cases the etiology is unknown and an apparent autoimmune reaction *(lupoid hepatitis)* has been suspected. Identification of the specific origin depends heavily on historic data and on immunocytochemical or serologic evidence of viral infection. The viral forms of the disease are more common in men.

The so-called *autoimmune form of chronic active hepatitis* is somewhat distinctive clinically. It occurs predominantly in women, usually before or at the menopause, and is associated with a variety of immunologic findings—hypergammaglobulinemia, antibodies against DNA (hence the term *"lupoid" hepatitis*), a positive LE cell phenomenon in some patients, as well as antibodies against smooth muscle cells (more specifically, against actin).[37] In addition, an autoantibody directed against lipoproteins within the plasma membrane of hepatocytes has also been demonstrated in some cases. The origin of these apparent autoimmune reactions is unclear, but an increased frequency of HLA-B1, HLA-B8, DRw3, and DRw4 antigens in these patients suggests a genetic susceptibility. It must be confessed, however, that the existence of a truly autoimmune form of chronic active hepatitis is not proven, since similar immunologic findings are sometimes encountered in patients with other forms of chronic hepatitis. Thus the autoimmune reactions may result from liver injury, rather than be the cause of liver damage.

**MORPHOLOGY.** The major histologic hallmarks of chronic active hepatitis, whether of viral or other origin, are (1) a portal and periportal infiltrate of lymphocytes, plasma cells, macrophages and occasional scattered eosinophils and neutrophils, (2) active destruction of hepatocytes, particularly at the interface between the periportal inflammatory infiltrate and adjacent hepatic cords ("piecemeal necrosis"), (3) collapse of the reticulin framework of the lobule where hepatocytes are destroyed, which often creates bridges between portal tracts and central veins ("bridging necrosis"), and (4) progressive replacement of these bridges and periportal necrotic cells by fibrosis with the possible eventual development of cirrhosis.[37a] The inflammatory infiltrate in chronic active hepatitis spills out of the portal tracts into the surrounding parenchyma. Sensitized T lymphocytes surround and isolate single or small groups of hepatocytes, which undergo progressive fragmentation and eventual engulfment by macrophages, a process that is referred to as **"piecemeal necrosis"** and has also been called **"apoptosis."**[38] Such piecemeal necrosis may destroy sleeves of periportal parenchyma and be followed by collapse of the reticulin framework, leading to interconnections between adjacent portal tracts. At the same time, isolated cells and nests of cells within the lobule may undergo ballooning degeneration and acidophilic transformation similar to that described in acute viral hepatitis (p. 577). The confluence of such foci of necrosis may bring about **"bridging necrosis"** between portal tracts, and between portal tracts and central veins (Fig. 17–9). Eventually, the cell necrosis about the portal areas initiates a fibrogenic response, as also occurs in the areas of bridging necrosis, and in this manner cirrhosis may evolve. In addition to all these changes, there may be bile stasis in hepatocytes and canaliculi and evidence of hepatocytic regeneration as well as Kupffer cell hypertrophy and hyperplasia, particularly in proximity to areas of cell death. Sometimes these phagocytic cells are laden with lipofuscin (ceroid) and bile pigment. The only histologic feature that differentiates chronic active hepatitis of hepatitis B origin from that of other causes mentioned earlier is the "ground-glass" hepatocyte.

**CLINICAL CORRELATION.** About 30% of individuals who develop chronic active viral hepatitis have had an obvious preceding acute attack of icteric hepatitis. In such patients, the signs and symptoms of liver disease persist, such as fatigue, anorexia, low-grade fever, and sometimes persistent or recurrent jaundice. In others the chronic disease becomes evident without an apparent history of acute hepatitis and often is discovered by the chance finding of abnormal results of liver function tests. In yet other instances, the chronic hepatitis only attracts attention when the late manifestations of cirrhosis appear, such as ascites, bleeding varices, and liver failure. Uncommonly vasculitis, glomerulonephritis, or arthritis constitutes the presenting feature, each of which is related to prolonged antigenemia and circulating immune complexes. The clinical course is extremely variable. Some patients have progressive active liver destruction with the development of cirrhosis in a few years. *Patients who are positive for HBsAg as well as the delta agent are particularly prone to develop severe liver injury with a high mortality.*[39] Conversely, most cases that follow NANB posttransfusion hepatitis tend to remit spontaneously. Overall, with cases of HBV origin, there is a 25 to 50% mortality within five years if bridging necrosis is present.[40] An additional hazard in HBV-related chronic active hepatitis is the development of hepatocellular carcinoma.

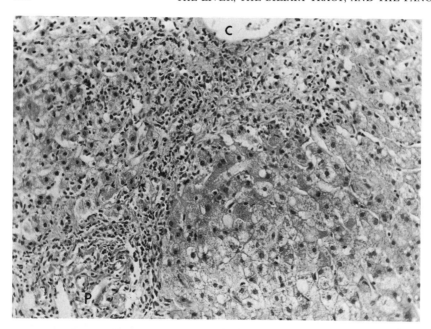

Figure 17–9. Bridging necrosis. A zone of intralobular necrosis extends from the central vein (C) to the portal tract (P). (From Robbins, S. L., and Cotran, R. S.: Pathologic Basis of Disease. 2nd ed. Philadelphia, W. B. Saunders Co., 1979, p. 1040.)

### Submassive and Massive Hepatic Necrosis (Fulminant Viral Hepatitis)

Fulminant hepatitis with submassive to massive necrosis of the liver is fortunately one of the rare expressions of viral hepatitis. It occurs in about 1 to 3% of cases of acute viral hepatitis caused by HBV (especially if associated with the delta agent) or NANBV. It is even more rare with HAV. Nonetheless, fulminant viral infection is the commonest cause of extensive liver necrosis.[41] A variety of chemicals and drugs may also cause massive destruction of the liver, principal among which are the anesthetics halothane (p. 582) and chloroform, carbon tetrachloride, the mycotoxins of the mushroom *Amanita phalloides*, monoamine oxidase inhibitors, methyldopa, and isoniazid.

In the usual case, soon after the onset of the viral infection or toxic exposure, the hepatic dysfunction rapidly worsens with deepening jaundice and other manifestations of liver failure, including metabolic encephalopathy. Sometimes this untoward turn of events appears later (one to four weeks) in the course of what would seem to be a typical attack of acute viral hepatitis. Regrettably, there are no reliable premonitory signs or symptoms.

MORPHOLOGY. The anatomic changes in the liver depend on the severity of the necrotizing process and duration of survival of the patient. The extent of destruction is extremely variable, as the term "submassive to massive" implies. The process may be limited to patchy foci dispersed throughout the liver, may involve large (2 to 5 cm) nonconfluent areas, an entire lobe, or even the whole liver.

Early in the course of massive necrosis, the liver is normal in size, but later, as the necrotic areas are resorbed, it is transformed into a shrunken, limp organ weighing as little as 500 gm (Fig. 17–10). With submassive necrosis and survival, regeneration may produce irregular, yellow-brown to green, firm nodules that bulge above the surrounding surface.

Microscopically, in submassive necrosis the involvement may be confined to the centers of the lobules, with many areas of bridging necrosis (p. 579). With more extensive destruction, innumerable contiguous, entire lobules are destroyed and there is collapse of the reticulin framework, sometimes capriciously leaving islands of preserved parenchyma. The cells appear to have undergone total coagulation, followed by liquefactive necrosis. There is surprisingly little inflammatory infiltrate accompanying this extensive destruction. The loss of hepatocytes produces an apparent convergence of portal tracts. With survival of the patient, irregular nodules of regeneration appear. Some time later there may be surprisingly little residual scarring with submassive necrosis. In larger areas of necrosis, pseudolobules of functional hepatocytes separated by bands or masses of fibrous tissue may be formed. Obviously, more massive necrosis and early death preclude scarring.

Submassive necrosis of the liver carries a poor prognosis. Overall, mortality rates range from 70 to 90%; otherwise healthy young adults fare better than older individuals. The only happy note that can be recorded for these seriously ill patients is that they almost never become carriers and almost always develop lifelong immunity to the particular causative viral agent.

## DRUG-INDUCED DISEASE

It is most gratifying to both patient and physician when jaundice and other manifestations of liver disease can be alleviated by simple withdrawal of a

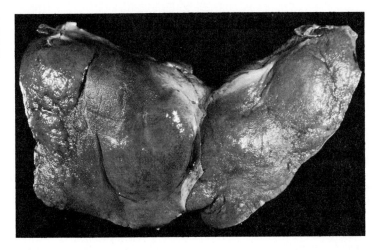

Figure 17–10. Massive hepatic necrosis. The destruction of liver substance has caused irregular collapse and irregular wrinkling of the capsule. The gross lobularity is due to the random areas of preserved hepatic substance.

drug. This possibility must always be borne in mind because adverse drug reactions may faithfully mimic more serious conditions, as, for example, viral hepatitis. The hepatic drug reactions range from ultrastructural or biochemical "lesions" unassociated with overt cell necrosis or inflammation (so-called intrahepatic cholestasis) to a spectrum of patterns of hepatitis extending from mild inflammation to massive necrosis of the liver. These diverse reactions can be conveniently divided into two major categories—cholestasis and hepatocellar damage—but, as might be guessed, in some instances there is overlap.

The term *cholestasis* can be applied to either impaired formation of canalicular bile, representing *intrahepatic (medical) cholestasis*, or blockade of its exit from the liver, constituting *extrahepatic (surgical) cholestasis* (p. 566). The differentiation of these two forms of jaundice is obviously a clinical problem of great importance and often of urgency, since extrahepatic cholestasis caused by such conditions as a gallstone or carcinoma blocking the common bile duct requires prompt surgical relief. *In the context of drug injury, we are concerned with intrahepatic cholestasis—namely, the secretion of bile into the canaliculus and its flow into the biliary ductules, which drain into the interlobular ducts. Morphologically it is associated with bile plugs in distended canaliculi and droplets of bile in liver cells and Kupffer cells.* Often these changes are accompanied by mild degenerative changes in the hepatocytes, referred to as "feathery degeneration," and attributed to retained bile acids. In "pure" intrahepatic cholestasis, the parenchymal architecture is undisturbed and there is no portal or sinusoidal inflammation.

*Clinically, intrahepatic cholestasis is marked principally by elevated levels of bile acids and alkaline phosphatase in the serum and usually, but not invariably, by elevated levels of conjugated bilirubin.* These biochemical abnormalities induce pruritus, jaundice, and, in some cases, steatorrhea because of malabsorption of fats. With the major role that bile plays in the excretion of cholesterol from the body,

intrahepatic cholestasis may also cause hyperlipidemia related principally to hypercholesterolemia, which may lead to the formation of skin xanthomas.

It is beyond the scope of this book to delve deeply into the pathophysiology of intrahepatic cholestasis. It suffices to state that it must arise from defects distal to the site of conjugation of bilirubin involving either the transmembrane passage of bilirubin from the hepatocyte into the canaliculus or the flow of bile through the canaliculus.[42]

*Hepatocellular damage is the other pattern of liver change encountered in adverse drug reactions.* It ranges from mild liver cell injury in the form of fatty change through lesions that resemble viral hepatitis to massive hepatic necrosis. In some instances hepatocellular and portal inflammation may coexist with cholestasis. The severity of the reaction to a single medicinal agent modifies the pathophysiologic consequences. An agent may begin with a cholestatic reaction, which progresses in time to parenchymal damage. By the same token, individual susceptibility, called idiosyncrasy, may lead to cholestasis in one individual but parenchymal damage in another, and indeed on occasion may cause massive necrosis. Against this background we can turn to a consideration of the major drugs involved in cholestasis or hepatocellular damage, or both.

A virtually limitless roster of drugs have at one time or another caused liver injury. Some are called *predictable hepatotoxins* and have been responsible repeatedly for hepatic reactions. Characteristic of predictable hepatotoxins are dose dependence, a relatively short interval between drug ingestion and the adverse reaction, and the ability to induce similar changes when administered to laboratory animals. Other medicinal agents are classified as *nonpredictable hepatotoxins*. With these there is no dose dependence, weeks to months passing between the drug ingestion and the adverse reaction, and, frequently, accompanying manifestations such as fever, arthralgia, and eosinophilia, all pointing to a hypersensitivity reaction. Presumably, the agent or its

**Table 17–2.** SOME COMMON DRUGS
INVOLVED IN HEPATIC REACTIONS

| Principally Cholestasis | Principally Hepatocellular Damage |
|---|---|
| *Predictable reactions* | *Predictable reactions* |
| Methyltestosterone | Isoniazid |
| Estrogens | Acetaminophen |
| Oral contraceptives | Aspirin |
| | Methotrexate |
| | Daunorubicin |
| | Tetracycline |
| | Chloramphenicol |
| | Methyldopa |
| *Nonpredictable reactions* | *Nonpredictable reactions* |
| Chlorpromazine | Chlorpromazine |
| | Halothane |
| | Rifampicin |
| | Phenylbutazone |
| | p-Aminosalicylic acid |
| | Oxyphenisatin |
| | Methyldopa |

metabolites serve as haptens to form sensitizing antigens.[43] Some of the more common drugs and the basic pattern of hepatic reaction are presented in Table 17–2. This categorization is admittedly arbitrary, and moreover some of these agents may in one instance cause cholestasis but in another hepatocellular damage (e.g., chlorpromazine).

*The two agents most commonly responsible for adverse reactions are chlorpromazine and halothane.* Chlorpromazine typically produces intrahepatic cholestasis, usually with variable amounts of spotty hepatocyte necrosis and portal inflammation. The prognosis of chlorpromazine-induced liver disease is quite favorable. Rarely, patients progress to a condition resembling primary biliary cirrhosis.

The anesthetic halothane, despite its much less frequent use relative to chlorpromazine, has been responsible for more than twice as many deaths. Indeed, *viral hepatitis and halothane reactions are the two most frequent causes of massive liver failure.* Two distinct forms of halothane-induced liver injury have been identified. Mild focal hepatocellular necrosis accompanied by an elevation in serum aminotransferase occurs in up to 20% of the patients following a single exposure to halothane. This reaction, which presumably reflects direct toxicity mediated by some metabolite of halothane, is usually noted in the second postoperative week. It is usually mild and completely reversible.[44] The other more serious and potentially fatal reaction is characterized by massive liver cell necrosis. Virtually all patients who experience the severe reaction have been exposed to halothane on one or more previous occasions. This suggests development of hypersensitivity, but firm evidence is lacking. Recent studies seem to implicate reactive metabolites of halothane as mediators of hepatic injury.[45] Risk factors for halothane hepatitis include female sex, obesity, and a history of

allergy. From a practical point of view, it is important to assess these factors carefully if the patient requires more than one exposure to halothane.

## CIRRHOSIS

In the United States and Great Britain, and probably globally, cirrhosis of the liver has shown an appalling increase in frequency, related in large part to the growing problem of alcoholism. In 1985, it was expected to be the eighth most common cause of death in the United States. It is reported to be the third leading cause of death among those 25 to 65 years of age.[46] Despite its frequency, there is no universally accepted definition of cirrhosis. Widely accepted and having the virtue of simplicity is the following: *Cirrhosis is a diffuse process characterized by fibrosis and a conversion of normal architecture into structurally abnormal nodules.*[47] Several aspects of this definition, shown schematically in Figure 17–11, merit emphasis. (1) The process must be diffuse and involve the whole liver; focal areas of fibrosis or scarring do not constitute cirrhosis. (2) The fibrosis may range from delicate interlacing bands to large, sometimes massive scars. The fibrosis is often progressive and is generally considered to be irreversible, although there are hints to the contrary. Collagen, even in scars, is in a constant state of turnover. When the underlying cause of the cirrhosis can be controlled, regression of fibrous septa has been observed in experimental animals and in the cirrhosis of humans associated with iron overload.[48] (3) Nodularity is a sine qua non of cirrhosis. The fibrous scarring may enclose a single lobule by bridging portal tract to portal tract; may traverse the lobule, joining central vein to portal tract to create very small nodules; or may encircle many contiguous lobules to create large nodules. Regeneration of he-

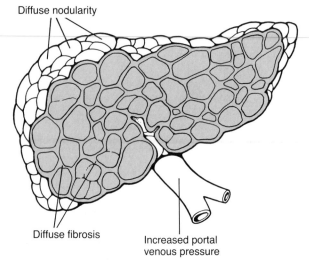

Figure 17–11. Schematic drawing of the hallmarks of cirrhosis.

patocytes surrounded by fibrous scars may contribute to the nodularity, but often the morphologic evidence of this process may have disappeared by the time the patient comes to study. (4) In most instances (largely because its causation cannot be controlled), cirrhosis is a progressive disorder that has the potential of leading to portal hypertension and liver failure.

The classification of the cirrhoses has been a topic of debate, it would seem for millennia, largely because there is no satisfactory method to categorize most of the cases. The etiology of many forms is poorly understood. The morphology is not always distinctive. The same morphologic pattern can result from a variety of causations and, conversely, a single cause can produce a variety of morphologic appearances. Retreat has been made by some experts to two large categories: *micronodular and macronodular cirrhosis, based on measurement of the nodules at autopsy. The dividing line is usually set at 3 mm for the majority of nodules.* Unfortunately, it may be extremely difficult in many cases to determine the precise dimensions of most nodules. Moreover, it is well recognized that with progression of the disease, micronodular cirrhosis may be converted into macronodular cirrhosis, thus producing intergrades. We therefore deal with uncertain origins and inconstant morphologic patterns. For this reason, we revert here to a historically sanctified, although admittedly imperfect, classification, as follows. An approximate relative frequency is given as a percentage after each type.

|  | Per cent |
|---|---|
| ○ Cirrhosis associated with alcohol abuse | 60–70 |
| ○ Postnecrotic cirrhosis | 10–15 |
| ○ Biliary cirrhosis (primary and secondary) | 10 |
| ○ Pigment cirrhosis (in hemochromatosis) | 5 |
| ○ Cirrhosis associated with Wilson's disease | rare |
| ○ Cirrhosis associated with alpha-1-<br>    anti-trypsin deficiency | rare |
| ○ Cryptogenic cirrhosis | 10–15 |

The relative frequencies given apply largely to North America and Europe. In South America, Asia, and Africa, the relative contribution of alcoholism is substantially lower.

These disorders are the most important causes of portal hypertension, which often dominates their clinical courses. It is appropriate, therefore, to discuss this pathophysiologic syndrome next.

## PORTAL HYPERTENSION

Elevation of the pressure within the portal circulation is a serious complication of a variety of disorders that affect the liver and its blood flow. These conditions have been variously classified but can be most simply divided into (1) posthepatic, (2) intrahepatic, and (3) prehepatic categories.

The major *posthepatic* disorders leading to portal hypertension are the Budd-Chiari syndrome (p. 569),

severe right-sided heart failure, and constrictive pericarditis.

The dominant *intrahepatic causes of portal hypertension* are the cirrhoses, which will be discussed below. All are characterized by widespread injury to the liver resulting in diffuse fibrous scarring, which causes diffuse nodularity, distorting the connective tissue and vascular framework of the liver. The various cirrhoses together account for over 90% of all cases of portal hypertension. Less common causes of intrahepatic portal hypertension include chronic active hepatitis, granulomatous disease (tuberculosis and sarcoidosis) involving the portal triads, and schistosomiasis. The pathophysiology of the elevation in portal blood pressure in the cirrhoses is complex and not entirely understood. The major factor is an increased resistance to portal blood flow at the level of the sinusoids, owing to perisinusoidal deposition of collagen in the spaces of Disse and the consequent narrowing of the sinusoids. Compression of central veins by the regenerative nodules may also contribute to the outflow resistance, but contrary to previous beliefs, this is not a major mechanism.[49] Arteriovenous anastomoses develop in the fibrous septa, bringing to bear hepatic arterial pressure on the portal circulation. Thus the elevation in portal pressure is a consequence of many hemodynamic alterations.

*Prehepatic portal hypertension* is related to obstruction of the main portal vein, previously discussed (p. 570).

*Whatever the cause of the portal hypertension, the clinical consequences are the same. The four most important features are (1) ascites; (2) the formation of systemic anastomotic channels, particularly in the submucosa of the esophagus (esophageal varices), which may rupture; (3) splenomegaly; and (4) occasionally, hepatic (metabolic) encephalopathy secondary to the entrance of portal blood into the systemic circulation prior to detoxification in the liver.*

Ascites is an intraperitoneal accumulation of watery fluid containing small amounts of protein, in the range of 1 to 2 gm/dl. Many liters may collect, causing abdominal distention. Although the fluid may contain a scant number of mesothelial cells and lymphocytes, it does not, in the uncomplicated case, contain polymorphonuclear leukocytes or red cells. Solutes such as glucose, sodium, and potassium have essentially the same concentrations in the ascitic fluid as in the blood. A considerable amount of sodium and albumin may be lost when large volumes of ascitic fluid are tapped to relieve the abdominal distention.

*The genesis of ascitic fluid is complex* (Fig. 17–12). *Scarring within the liver increases hydrostatic pressure within the portal system, not only through obstruction but also through the creation of arteriovenous communications within the scars. Transudation of plasma into the peritoneum results from the portal hypertension. Cirrhosis also impairs synthesis of albumin and lowers the colloid osmotic pressure of the plasma. Another key factor is retention of*

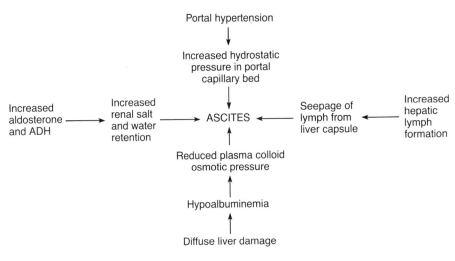

Figure 17–12. Pathogenic factors in the formation of ascites.

*sodium and water.*[50] With portal hypertension and the resultant sequestration of a large volume of blood within the splanchnic bed, renal blood flow and glomerular filtration rate fall. This in itself leads to sodium retention. In addition, aldosterone and ADH are elaborated, further augmenting salt and water retention. Since these hormones are metabolized in the liver, severe hepatic dysfunction may result in even higher levels. *Thus although the effective circulating blood volume may be lower than normal, a constellation of influences tends to increase fluid retention within the splanchnic bed and the accumulation of even larger volumes of ascitic fluid.* The fluid is not only a plasma transudate; an additional factor is increased formation of lymph within the liver and the abdominal viscera. This lymph fluid may leak through the liver capsule, but in addition, it probably weeps from all peritoneal surfaces within the abdomen. In about 20% of patients, the ascitic fluid passes through transdiaphragmatic lymphatics into the pleural cavities, particularly on the right, to cause *hydrothorax.*

*Collateral systemic anastomotic venous channels* might also be referred to as *portal vein bypasses.* When the pressure rises in the portal vein, collateral vessels are enlarged wherever the systemic and portal circulations share common capillary beds. The most important collateral channels are found in the lower esophageal plexus, where the portal and azygous systems intermingle. When portal flow is obstructed, the esophageal plexus becomes engorged, and dilatation of these veins results. Some appear beneath the esophageal mucosa in the form of varices (p. 510). Once such varices rupture, bleeding is difficult to control, and the hematemesis frequently is fatal.

*These varices occur in about 67% of patients with advanced cirrhosis, cause hematemesis in about 40% of patients, and indeed are the principal cause of death in almost this same number.* Varices may also develop in the anorectal region, where the superior mesenteric vein of the portal system communicates via the inferior mesenteric system with the hemor-

rhoidal plexus of the caval system. Thus a third to half of all patients with cirrhosis develop hemorrhoids. Perhaps because the hemorrhoidal communications are remote from the liver, the pressures in these anorectal varices are not as high as those in the esophagus. Serious hemorrhage does not often arise from rupture of hemorrhoids. If the fetal umbilical vein fails to become obliterated, it may communicate with veins about the umbilicus to produce an externally visible vascular pattern called *caput medusae.*

*Splenomegaly* is readily attributed to the prolonged congestion of the spleen. Such spleens may achieve weights of up to 1000 gm. A variety of hematologic abnormalities may appear secondary to the splenic enlargement, including anemia, leukopenia, and thrombocytopenia. All these hematologic alterations are attributed to *hypersplenism* and may be encountered in any form of splenic enlargement (p. 403). It is important to remember, however, that liver failure itself may lead to anemia and a bleeding diathesis, quite apart from any associated hypersplenism. The salient clinical manifestations of portal hypertension are summarized in Figure 17–13.

Hepatic (metabolic) encephalopathy, another major consequence of portosystemic shunts, has already been presented on page 568.

Against this background, we can turn to the major causes of portal hypertension—i.e., the various forms of cirrhosis.

## ALCOHOLIC LIVER DISEASE AND CIRRHOSIS

Long-term excessive consumption of alcohol is the single most important cause of liver disease in the United States and much of the Western world. Chronic abuse of alcohol can produce three patterns of change in the liver—fatty liver, alcoholic hepatitis, and cirrhosis. Each one of these may be the sole manifestation of alcoholic liver disease or may coexist with one or both of the other two. *Fatty liver,* the

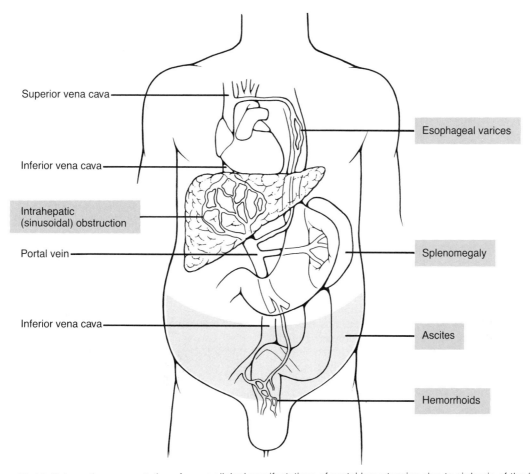

Figure 17–13. Schematic representation of some clinical manifestations of portal hypertension due to cirrhosis of the liver.

most innocuous of all, appears early and may be completely asymptomatic as well as fully reversible. *Alcoholic hepatitis, on the other hand, is associated with liver cell necrosis and inflammation* and produces clinical manifestations reminiscent of viral or toxic hepatitis. Alcoholic hepatitis may be reversible, especially if the initial injury is mild and further exposure to alcohol is prevented. However, repeated bouts of liver cell necrosis and the subsequent fibrosis associated with recurrent alcoholic hepatitis may lead to the final and irreversible stage of alcohol-induced liver disease—*alcoholic cirrhosis.* As will be discussed in greater detail later, alcoholic cirrhosis may also develop without preceding alcoholic hepatitis.

Alcoholic cirrhosis is the most common form of cirrhosis in North America and Europe, and it is also increasing in frequency at an incredible rate.[51] In the United States, in the interval from 1950 to 1974, the number of deaths from cirrhosis climbed more than 70%, whereas mortality from many other causes, especially cardiovascular disease, declined. Although at one time this was almost exclusively a male disorder, changing conventions have made it clear that women are just as susceptible. The mortality rate among both male and female nonwhites in urban areas in the United States doubles that of whites.

The morphology will be presented first because it facilitates the consideration of the pathogenesis.

**MORPHOLOGY.** Since the three patterns of hepatocellular changes associated with alcoholic liver disease may exist independent of each other and do not necessarily represent a continuum of changes, each will be described separately.[52]

The **fatty liver** in the chronic alcoholic does not differ at the outset from that related to other causations, as described on page 17. However, in the alcoholic the liver may be massive, up to 4 to 6 kg, and a soft, yellow, greasy, readily fractured organ. The fatty change is initially centrilobular, but later on it involves the entire lobule (diffuse). The hepatocytes are virtually transformed into lipocytes with peripherally compressed nuclei. Occasionally the fat accumulates in small droplets without nuclear displacement, as seen in Reye's syndrome. With excessive fat accumulation the plasma membranes of adjacent hepatocytes rupture to create so-called fatty cysts.[53] There is little or no obvious increase in fibrous tissue at the outset, but subtle sclerotic changes, described later, develop insidiously. **Up to the time of appearance of these fibrosing reactions, the fatty change is reversible if there is abstention from further alcohol intake.** In some cases the very delicate fibrosis mentioned above may be observed early, while the liver is fatty and has not yet developed grossly evident scarring. Such deposition of collagen may occur around central veins, (pericentral), around sinusoids (perisinusoidal), or as fine strands around individual hepatocytes (pericellular). Lieber has attributed considerable significance to **perivenular central fibrosis**, implying that when present, it is a warning sign that permits identification of patients likely to develop cirrhosis.[54] At present the accuracy of this contention is still being assessed.

**Alcoholic hepatitis** refers to a morphologic pattern of alcoholic liver disease characterized by (1) **swelling and necrosis of scattered hepatocytes,** (2) **neutrophilic reaction in and about the foci of necrosis,** and (3) **in many patients the presence of alcoholic hyalin or Mallory bodies within the affected liver cells** (Fig. 17–14).[55] These changes begin around the central veins, and hence the centrilobular areas are the most severely affected. The swelling of the liver cells results from accumulation of fat and water (hydropic change) as well as proteins. A characteristic but not diagnostic feature of alcoholic hepatitis is the presence of **alcoholic hyalin or Mallory bodies** appearing as irregular or discrete clumps of prominent eosinophilic material, often located around the nucleus of swollen or dead hepatocytes. These structures are derived, in all likelihood, from intermediate

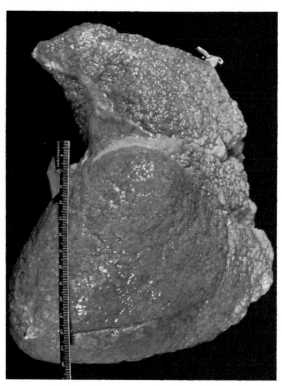

Figure 17–15. Cirrhosis of alcohol abuse, showing the characteristic diffuse micronodularity induced by the underlying fibrous scarring.

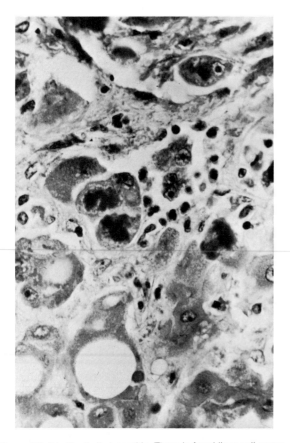

Figure 17–14. Alcoholic hepatitis. There is focal liver cell necrosis and a neutrophilic inflammatory reaction. The irregular, dark masses within the injured liver cells represent Mallory bodies (alcoholic hyalin). Many liver cells are swollen and vacuolated due to accumulation of fat and water.

filaments.[53] The term "Mallory" bodies is preferable, since similar material can also be seen within the hepatocytes in such diverse conditions as primary biliary cirrhosis, Wilson's disease, Indian childhood cirrhosis, and hepatocellular carcinoma. Necrosis of the liver cells induces an inflammatory reaction in which neutrophils predominate, with some admixture of lymphocytes as well as macrophages. Deviations from this typical picture may be seen. By far the most important is the presence of fibrosis in the centrilobular areas. Perivenular central sclerosis may obliterate the central veins and give rise to portal hypertension without any evidence of cirrhosis. In other cases continued alcohol abuse may lead to persistent or recurrent alcoholic hepatitis associated with widespread necrosis, inflammation, and fibrosis, which eventually evolve into alcoholic cirrhosis.

**Alcoholic cirrhosis,** the final and irreversible form of alcoholic liver disease, evolves slowly and usually insidiously. At first the liver is still enlarged but the smooth, tawny, fatty surface and transection become micronodular (1 to 3 mm in diameter) (Fig. 17–15). As the fibrosis increases with time, the fat content decreases and the liver becomes browner. In later stages, scattered larger nodules develop, presumably as a consequence of regeneration of liver cells; nodules range in size up to 1 cm in diameter to produce a so-called hobnail appearance. Ultimately, the scars become even larger and may in time produce a macronodular cirrhosis resembling the postnecrotic pattern (p. 590). Such livers are shrunken and reduced in weight. Histologically, the early nodular stage is characterized by slender, fibrous septa interconnecting portal areas and bridging portal areas to central veins. Thus, individual lobules may be encased or subdivided. The scarring and regeneration distort the normal lobular architecture. With progression, the fibrosis becomes more marked at the expense of the hepatic parenchyma (Fig. 17–16). Residual hepatocytes still contain some fat and, occasionally, changes of alcoholic hepatitis may be present. Portal tracts and central veins become buried within such scars and often become approximated as the intervening parenchyma disappears. A delicate lymphocytic infiltrate and reactive bile duct proliferation are sometimes found within the scarring. In this manner, the histology of advanced alcoholic cirrhosis approaches that of postnecrotic cirrhosis. The spectrum of morphologic changes associated with alcoholic liver disease are schematized in Figure 17–17.

**PATHOGENESIS.** There is now abundant evidence that alcohol or its metabolites are hepatotoxic and indeed toxic to other cells of the body as well.[54] The older view that the "empty calories" of alcohol and consequent malnutrition was the major cause of the alcohol-related liver disease is slowly fading. Instead it is now believed that secondary malnutrition, which is inevitably associated with chronic alcoholism, contributes to the organ damage initiated by the toxic effects of alcohol.[56] The pathogenesis of alcohol-induced liver injury can be conveniently considered within three contexts: (1) clinical and epidemiologic

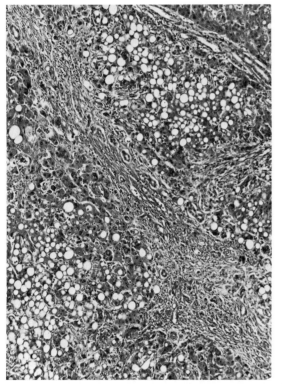

Figure 17–16. A low-power view of the cirrhosis associated with alcohol abuse. The fibrous scarring separates islands of hepatocytes, many of which contain fatty vacuoles of varying size.

evidence, (2) hepatic metabolism of ethanol, and (3) the mechanism of fibrogenesis.

*On clinical and epidemiologic grounds, there is an unmistakable association between the level and duration of alcohol consumption and the development of cirrhosis of the liver.* National surveys document a close correlation between per capita alcohol consumption and mortality from cirrhosis. Since susceptibility to alcohol-induced liver injury varies among individuals, it is difficult to define a "safe" upper limit of alcohol consumption. Nevertheless, it is generally accepted that a daily intake in excess of 60 to 80 gm for men and 20 gm for women over a period of 10 to 15 years incurs a high risk of developing cirrhosis. It should be pointed out, however, that only 17 to 30% of all alcoholics become cirrhotic. Individual, possibly genetic, susceptibility must exist, but as yet no definite genetic markers of susceptibility have been defined.

The *metabolic effects of alcohol* on the liver cell are complex and, to an extent, obscure. The liver contains three pathways for alcohol metabolism—the alcohol dehydrogenase pathway (ADH), the microsomal ethanol oxidizing system, and a catalase system.[54] Of these, the ADH-mediated conversion of ethanol to acetaldehyde seems to be the major pathway (Fig. 17–18). Acetaldehyde induces liver cell damage by covalent binding to proteins as well as by initiating lipid peroxidation of cell membranes. The conversion of alcohol to acetaldehyde and the subsequent oxidation of acetaldehyde require NAD, which in turn is reduced to NADH. These reactions alter the NADH/NAD ratio, leading to an increase in the reducing potential within the cell. This has ripple effects on the metabolism of pyruvates, urates, and fatty acids. In particular, fatty acid oxidation is impaired, contributing to the fatty liver associated with alcohol ingestion. Other factors important in the pathogenesis of alcohol-induced fatty liver include increased flux of free fatty acids into the liver, increased esterification to triglycerides, and reduced secretion of lipoproteins (p. 17).

Although acetaldehyde has received much attention as the mediator of alcohol toxicity, other mechanisms of liver injury, including immunologic factors, have also been implicated. Immunologic abnormalities, such as antibodies directed against liver cells, can be demonstrated in some alcoholics, but it is not yet proved whether the immune responses play any role in mediating liver cell necrosis. They are more likely to be involved in initiating or accentuating the fibrosis that characterizes the later stages of alcoholic liver disease.

The nature of the cells that lay down collagen and the stimuli that trigger *fibrogenesis* in the liver are not clear. As mentioned earlier, the centrilobular areas are the first to be involved by fibrosis. It has been suggested that collagen is secreted by myofibroblasts, which are normally present in the subendothelium of the central veins. In chronic alcoholics

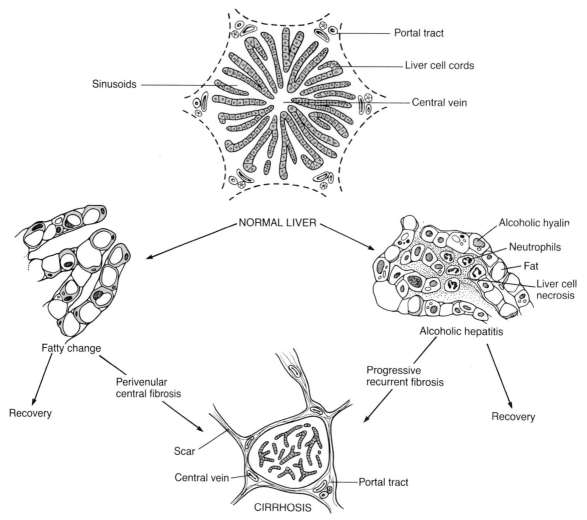

**Figure 17–17.** Schematic illustration of the morphologic changes associated with alcoholic liver disease, their possible interrelationships, and their consequences.

the number of myofibroblasts is increased even before fibrosis is obvious. Another cell believed to be involved is the Ito cell, present in the space of Disse. Early in the course of alcoholic liver disease the Ito cells accumulate fat, but in advanced stages fat tends to disappear and the cell assumes the morphology of a fibroblast. Signals that activate these mesenchymal cells to produce collagen remain elusive. Two pathways have been suggested. According to one theory, fibrosis is the consequence of alcoholic hepatitis, which according to some is the precursor of cirrhosis. Presumably, the inflammatory cells release soluble factors that induce myofibroblasts and Ito cells to synthesize collagen. Alcoholic hepatitis could also initiate autoimmune reactions against damaged liver cells, thus perpetuating both inflammation and fibrosis. An alternative pathway in the evolution of fibrosis is suggested by the baboon model of alcoholic liver disease.[57] Baboons fed an isocaloric diet containing excess alcohol develop fatty liver and eventually cirrhosis without an intervening stage of alcoholic hepatitis. To explain this sequence it has been postulated that ethanol itself or its metabolites may directly trigger cells with fibrogenic potential. Indeed, lactate and acetaldehyde can stimulate collagen synthesis in vitro,[58] but whether similar mechanisms operate in vivo is a matter of conjecture at the present time.

Although alcohol-induced fatty change may be followed by cirrhosis, it should be borne in mind that fatty change itself is not the cause of fibrosis. Fatty liver of kwashiorkor, marked obesity, and diabetes mellitus are not followed by cirrhosis, thus suggesting that factors other than accumulation of fat must come into play in the pathogenesis of alcoholic cirrhosis.

**CLINICAL COURSE.** There is a broad range of clinical presentations of alcohol-induced liver disease, some of which are depicted in Figure 17–19. At one end of the spectrum is the patient with the asymptomatic hepatomegaly of the fatty liver. Infrequently, there

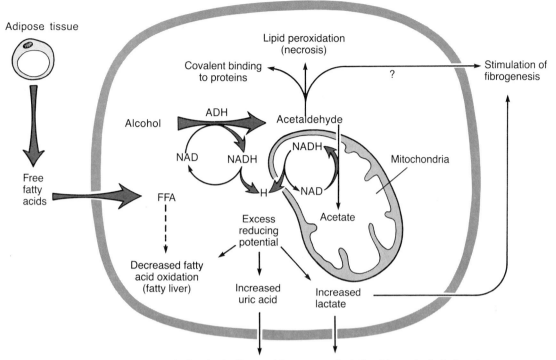

Figure 17–18. Alcohol metabolism in the liver and its proposed relationship to alcoholic liver injury.

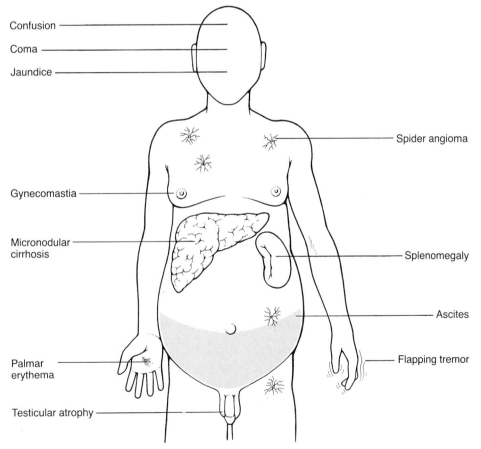

Figure 17–19. Clinical features associated with alcohol-induced cirrhosis of the liver.

is accompanying jaundice. At the other end is the wasted, jaundiced, cirrhotic patient with hepatic failure.

Usually the first signs of cirrhosis relate to portal hypertension, resulting in the classic picture of a grossly distended abdomen filled with ascitic fluid along with wasted extremities and a pathetically drawn face. In some cases, the first manifestation is jaundice. The hyperbilirubinemia is of both conjugated and unconjugated forms (p. 566). Not infrequently, despite the cirrhotic damage, the patient is asymptomatic until some stress upsets the balance. A massive hemorrhage from esophageal varices may be followed by hepatic insufficiency or even hepatic failure. Sometimes such bleeding is the first sign of the submerged cirrhosis. Intercurrent infections may also trigger hepatic decompensation. The host of abnormalities described as hepatic failure then becomes manifest.

*Alcoholic hepatitis* may be mild and virtually asymptomatic. More often it presents in the same manner as viral hepatitis, with nausea, vomiting, anorexia, jaundice, and tender hepatomegaly. Ascites, edema, and, in severe cases, hepatic encephalopathy may ensue. Alcoholic hepatitis may be superimposed on cirrhosis. Such acute exacerbations may occur at any stage in the development of cirrhosis and may be recurrent. Therefore, it must not be assumed that hepatic insufficiency or failure implies the advanced fibrotic stage of the disease. Each bout of alcoholic hepatitis carries with it a high mortality rate, ranging between 10 and 20%.[59]

The long-term outlook for patients with cirrhosis is very unpredictable. Numerous reports indicate that the disease can be arrested if the patient will abstain from alcohol. The five-year survival of abstainers approaches 90% in those without jaundice, ascites, or hematemesis, but drops to 50 to 60% in those who continue to imbibe. The causes of death are predominantly liver failure, intercurrent infections, gastrointestinal hemorrhage, and hepatocellular carcinoma, in that order. The source of the fatal hemorrhage is usually esophageal varices, but it may be peptic ulceration or esophageal laceration.

## POSTNECROTIC CIRRHOSIS

This term is a misnomer, since all forms of cirrhosis follow necrosis of liver cells, and hence the adjective "postnecrotic" is superfluous. Nevertheless, it persists in current vocabulary and is used to indicate a pattern of cirrhosis that is *characterized grossly by the presence of large irregular nodules separated by coarse irregular scars (macronodular cirrhosis)*. The pathogenesis of postnecrotic cirrhosis usually involves an extensive, sometimes confluent and often irregular loss of liver cells, followed by areas of stromal collapse and fibrosis (Fig. 17–20). Such injury to the liver may result from long-standing chronic active hepatitis

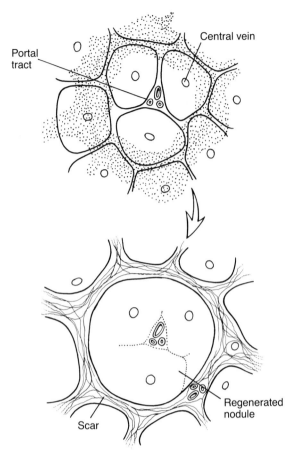

Figure 17–20. Schematic illustration of the pathogenesis of postnecrotic cirrhosis. Note that irregular and large areas of liver cell necrosis (*shaded areas in upper figure*) may leave a surviving island of liver cells, comprised of several intact and partially necrotic liver lobules. During regeneration, the remnants of the liver lobules merge to form a large nodule surrounded by a dense irregular scar, which replaces the necrotic liver cells.

B infection, which is responsible for about one fourth of the cases. Recall that in this form of chronic liver disease "piecemeal necrosis" and "bridging necrosis" progressively erode the liver parenchyma, leading to ever-enlarging scars and irregular regenerative nodules. Antecedent non-A, non-B chronic hepatitis may also result in postnecrotic cirrhosis, but owing to lack of serologic markers (for NANB viruses) it is difficult to estimate the contribution from this cause. Only infrequently is postnecrotic cirrhosis the result of submassive or fulminant liver necrosis. Either such patients succumb to massive liver destruction, or, if it is sufficiently limited to permit survival, regeneration of the destroyed hepatocytes ensues, leaving surprisingly little scarring. Nonetheless, massive necrosis, whether it be due to a fulminant viral infection or a hepatotoxic agent (discussed earlier, p. 580), may destroy portions of the liver, sparing large tracts. Such instances may be followed by massive scarring. Some would refer to this sequence of events as postnecrotic *scarring* rather than postnecrotic *cirrho-*

Figure 17–21. Postnecrotic cirrhosis, characterized by irregular, random areas of massive fibrosis alternating with other areas of more delicate scarring, producing the finer nodularity. The lobe on the left has been almost totally destroyed.

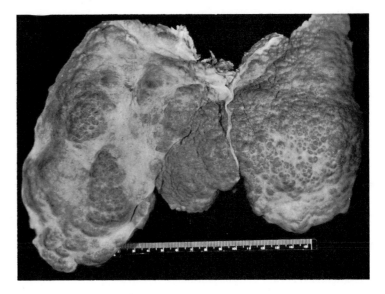

*sis*, but this is an issue for the purists. As discussed earlier, some cases of alcoholic micronodular cirrhosis develop coarse scars and large, irregular nodules so as to merit the morphologic designation of postnecrotic cirrhosis. It must be admitted, however, that in the *vast majority of cases no antecedent cause for postnecrotic cirrhosis can be identified.* Such cases, highlighting our ignorance, are dignified by the term "cryptogenic cirrhosis."

The gross appearance of postnecrotic cirrhosis depends on the distribution of the parenchymal destruction and the duration of survival following the necrotizing process. At the outset, the liver may be almost normal in size but more often is slightly shrunken. In time, the scarred areas become progressively larger and eventually contract, leading to liver shrinkage accompanied by accentuation of the nodules. The nodules are of all sizes, but typically some are very large (5 to 8 cm in diameter). Usually, they are the color of normal liver substance, save when retention of bile leads to greenish discoloration. The diagnostic features of postnecrotic scarring are the large size of the scars and the large nodules enclosed within the scars (macronodular cirrhosis) (Fig. 17–21). With extensive involvement, the liver may be dramatically reduced in size and weight.

Histologically, the classic features are the very broad scars interposed between islands of disorderly regenerating hepatocytes or areas of relatively normal hepatic substance. Within these fibrous bands is an infiltrate of lymphocytes admixed with macrophages, accompanied by proliferating bile ducts and ductules (Fig. 17–22). Where extensive necrosis has occurred, two or more portal triads may be closely approximated within the scars. At the interface between the scars and hepatocytes, piecemeal necrosis is sometimes present in those cases related to chronic active hepatitis, indicating the continued activity of the viral infection (p. 579). Surviving hepatocytes may manifest fatty change in cases related

to hepatotoxic drugs or chemicals, but more often it is absent.

Clinically, a history of chronic active hepatitis or a well-defined episode of massive liver destruction may be obtained, but *in many cases postnecrotic cirrhosis appears mysteriously.* Signs of portal hypertension,

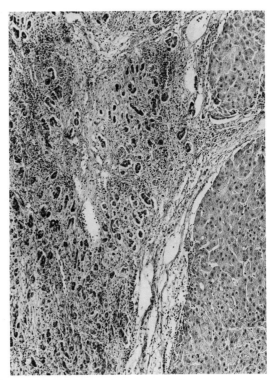

Figure 17–22. A view under low power of postnecrotic cirrhosis of the liver. The massive fibrous scar contains many closely crowded bile ducts, resulting from the total destruction of whole liver lobules. The islands of preserved liver cells on the right are free of fat.

such as ascites and splenomegaly, may be the first indication of underlying liver disease. Life-threatening complications such as massive bleeding from ruptured esophageal varices may occur, as in alcoholic cirrhosis. Liver failure manifested by jaundice, and in severe cases hepatic encephalopathy, are commonly seen, especially in patients with chronic active hepatitis. Most of these patients die within the first year; others follow a more indolent course, with slow erosion of hepatic function over the span of three to five years, eventuating in hepatic failure. There is also increased risk of developing hepatocellular carcinomas, especially in cases associated with hepatitis B virus infection.

## BILIARY CIRRHOSIS

This pattern of cirrhosis implies diffuse injury and scarring distributed throughout the liver in close relationship to the interlobular bile ducts. Whatever the nature of the injury, it appears to be localized at first to the biliary tract, and the scarring thus begins about these ducts and then involves the portal triads. Eventually, the fibrous tissue extends out to interconnect with adjacent portal areas and thus enclose individual lobules. *Several forms of injury have been identified, and biliary cirrhosis is divided into primary and secondary types* (Fig. 17–23). We can consider the *secondary type* first because its genesis is relatively simple. It is encountered in patients who have had extrahepatic obstructive jaundice or biliary tract infections. The major causes of extrahepatic biliary obstruction were discussed earlier (p. 566). Complete obstruction to the outflow of bile produces back pressure throughout the entire biliary system.

The interlobular bile ducts and cholangioles are damaged by the impacted, inspissated bile, and the injury leads to an inflammatory reaction and scarring. Obviously, such patients are jaundiced, sometimes intensely. Subtotal obstruction often leads to an ascending cholangitis and cholangiolitis as bacteria ascend within or about the ramifications of the biliary tract. The gram-negative bacilli and enterococci are the common culprits. Inflammation of the portal triads and periportal scarring ensue without striking evidence of inspissation of bile, and indeed jaundice may be absent.

*Primary biliary cirrhosis* is less clearly understood, but accumulating evidence suggests that it is an immunologic disorder.[60, 61] It is almost exclusively a disease of middle-aged women (although men are not exempt) that presents with manifestations of biliary tract obstruction—i.e., pruritus, elevated serum alkaline phosphatase levels, jaundice, and the eventual development of skin xanthomas secondary to hypercholesterolemia. As characterized by Sherlock, "*primary biliary cirrhosis or chronic destructive nonsuppurative cholangitis is a condition of chronic cholestasis in which small intrahepatic bile ducts in the portal zones of the liver become progressively destroyed and disappear.*[62] A variety of abnormalities of both cell-mediated and humoral immunity suggest an autoimmune causation. To begin with, there is an association between primary biliary cirrhosis and other autoimmune diseases, such as rheumatoid arthritis, Hashimoto's thyroiditis, and pernicious anemia. Immunologic derangements affecting both humoral and cellular immunity are present in almost every patient. Serum immunoglobulins, particularly IgM levels, are elevated and in addition, about 90% of patients have IgG antimitochondrial antibody of

SECONDARY                                                                 PRIMARY

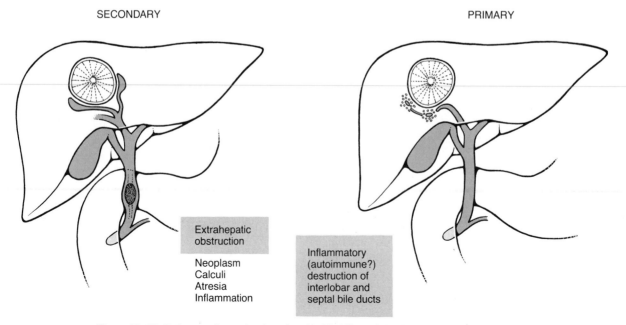

Extrahepatic
obstruction

Neoplasm
Calculi
Atresia
Inflammation

Inflammatory
(autoimmune?)
destruction of
interlobar and
septal bile ducts

**Figure 17–23.** Pathogenetic mechanisms involved in biliary cirrhosis, primary and secondary.

obscure significance. Smooth muscle antibody, anti-nuclear antibodies, and rheumatoid factor are also sometimes present. A variety of abnormalities affecting cellular immunity have been described. These include T- and B-cell lymphopenia, alterations in the ratios of helper and suppressor T cells, and evidence of T-cell sensitization to hepatobiliary antigens. As with other autoimmune disorders, reduced suppressor T-cell function, leading to unbridled activation of autoreactive T and B cells, has been proposed. Diminished natural killer-cell reactivity has also been observed. Despite all this evidence, the possibility cannot be excluded that the immunologic findings are secondary phenomena triggered by some primary cause of damage to interlobular bile ducts. In this connection, it is of interest that patients with primary biliary cirrhosis have very high copper concentrations in the liver. As will be seen, the accumulation of copper in the liver is thought to underlie the cirrhosis of Wilson's disease (p. 596) and by analogy may play a role in the causation of primary biliary cirrhosis. However, once again the question arises, is the elevated copper level primary or secondary, since this metal is largely excreted through the biliary tract? Impaired bile excretion from any cause would reasonably be expected to increase its concentration in the liver.

**MORPHOLOGY.** Common to all patterns of biliary cirrhosis is a diffuse, regular, and delicate scarring about each lobule, which gives a fine, sandpaper texture to the surface of the liver. The liver is usually dark green owing to cholestasis. Early in the evolution of biliary cirrhosis the liver may be normal in size or even slightly enlarged, particularly in the primary variant. Late in the course, the progressive scarring may cause a slight reduction in size in all variants.

Histologically, the principal characteristics of all forms of biliary cirrhosis are (1) regularity of fibrosis, extending out to interconnect portal triads (micronodular cirrhosis); (2) bile duct and ductular injury, proliferation, regeneration, and reduplication within the scars; and (3) a mononuclear infiltration, principally of lymphocytes admixed with macrophages, in the scars. Secondary features relate to the particular pathogenetic mechanism. **In the form induced by obstruction, bile stasis in the bile ducts, ductules, and canaliculi is prominent.** Accumulations of bile (referred to as **"bile lakes"**) may be present within the hepatic substance. When associated with ascending cholangitis, inflammatory cells, principally polymorphonuclear leukocytes, are scattered within the finer ramifications of the biliary tract.

In the **primary form of biliary cirrhosis**, the characteristic feature is a destructive inflammatory process of the cholangioles and interlobular bile ducts accompanied by a dense infiltrate of lymphocytes, macrophages, occasional plasma cells, and eosinophils. The lymphoid cells may aggregate in the form of follicles. Well-developed granulomas resembling those of sarcoidosis are seen in proximity to the damaged ducts and ductules in approximately 50% of the cases. The destruction of the

small ducts is accompanied by portal scarring and irregular ductal regeneration, producing abortive ductules and solid cords of cells. Later in the course of primary biliary cirrhosis, well-defined fibrous septa extend from the portal tracts to isolate individual lobules. At this stage of the disease, regeneration of hepatocytes may accentuate the nodularity. In about 25% of cases, hyaline inclusions similar to those seen in alcoholic hepatitis are present in the hepatocytes adjacent to portal tracts and connective tissue septa. The significance of these inclusions is obscure, and their number does not correlate with the severity of the disease. It should be noted that **in these patients there is no evidence of involvement of the larger intra- and extrahepatic biliary ducts.**

**CLINICAL COURSE.** The clinical findings are very variable and depend upon the genesis of the liver disease. Jaundice and itching are prominent particularly in those with the obstructive and primary forms of the disease. Fever, right upper quadrant pain, and marked leukocytosis are characteristic of the ascending infectious variety.

Primary biliary cirrhosis usually begins with the insidious onset of pruritus, with jaundice developing only later.[63] Hypercholesterolemia may be encountered. Indeed, these patients have skin xanthomas and often have florid atherosclerosis. The diagnosis of the primary form of biliary cirrhosis is supported by the demonstration of associated immunologic changes discussed earlier, particularly elevated serum levels of antimitochondrial antibody and of IgM, accompanied by other features pointing to obstructive biliary disease, such as elevated levels of serum bile acids and alkaline phosphatase (Table 17–3). Extrahepatic biliary tract obstruction must be ruled out by endoscopic retrograde cholangiopancreatography (ERCP), ultrasonography, and CT scan.

**Table 17–3. BILIARY CIRRHOSIS**

|  | Secondary | Primary |
|---|---|---|
| *Etiology* | Extrahepatic bile duct obstruction (e.g., congenital biliary atresia, gallstones, postoperative strictures, carcinoma of pancreatic head) | Possibly autoimmune; associated with Sjögren's syndrome, scleroderma, autoimmune thyroiditis |
| *Sex* | No special predilection | Females to males 9:1 |
| *Symptoms and Signs* | Pruritus, jaundice, bone pain, steatorrhea, hepatosplenomegaly | Same as secondary biliary cirrhosis |
| *Laboratory Findings* | Conjugated hyperbilirubinemia; increased serum alkaline phosphatase, bile acids, and cholesterol (all due to cholestasis) | Findings reflecting cholestatic jaundice and elevated serum IgM; presence of antimitochondrial antibody |

Because all forms of biliary cirrhosis yield deficient flow of bile into the duodenum, the malabsorption syndrome is more often encountered with this form of cirrhosis than with the others. Osteomalacia due to malabsorption of vitamin D and calcium is often clinically significant. A recent study suggests that women with primary biliary cirrhosis have an increased incidence of extrahepatic cancer, particularly breast cancer.[64] Whether this is related to a primary disorder in immunosurveillance or results from immunosuppressive therapy given to such patients is not entirely clear. In most cases of biliary cirrhosis, whatever the pathogenesis, hepatic failure ultimately ensues, but in contrast to the other cirrhoses *portal hypertension is uncommon*, as is hepatocarcinoma.

## PIGMENT CIRRHOSIS— HEMOCHROMATOSIS

Pigment cirrhosis, characterized by excessive deposition of ferritin and hemosiderin in hepatocytes and a micronodular cirrhosis is a cardinal feature of the iron storage disorder hemochromatosis. Excess iron is also deposited in parenchymal cells of other organs, particularly the pancreas, heart, endocrine glands, and joints, leading in time to functional impairment and possibly damage to all involved sites. In addition, *most patients have diabetes mellitus and skin pigmentation (hence the older designation "bronze diabetes"), which along with the pigment cirrhosis complete the classic triad of hemochromatosis.* The blood reflects the iron overload with abnormally high levels of plasma iron and ferritin, as well as excessive saturation of the total iron binding capacity, as will be discussed later. There are several causes of hemochromatosis (Table 17–4). Of these, the familial form called idiopathic hemochromatosis is clearly the most common. Next in frequency is hemochromatosis secondary to anemias associated with ineffective erythropoiesis.[65] The other causes of acquired or secondary hemochromatosis, listed in Table 17–4, are very rare.

*The key feature in all forms of hemochromatosis is the deposition of iron predominantly in parenchymal cells.* Some iron may be present in the cells of the mononuclear phagocyte system (e.g., Kupffer cells)

**Table 17–4.** CAUSES OF HEMOCHROMATOSIS*

1. Idiopathic (primary, genetic) hemochromatosis
2. Secondary hemochromatosis
   Secondary to anemia and ineffective erythropoiesis
      a. Thalassemia major
      b. Sideroblastic anemia
   Secondary to high iron intake
      a. Prolonged ingestion of medicinal iron
      b. Increased intake of iron with alcohol (South African blacks)

*From Halliday, J. W., and Powell, L. W.: Iron overload. Semin. Hematol. *19*:42, 1982.

but it is overshadowed by iron in the parenchymal cells. This is in contrast to *systemic hemosiderosis*, a form of iron overload characterized by storage of excess iron chiefly within the reticuloendothelial (RE, mononuclear phagocytic) cells. Little iron is present in the parenchymal tissues and hence, in contrast to hemochromatosis, organ injury or dysfunction is not a feature. Hemosiderosis is associated most commonly with excessive breakdown of red cells, as occurs in several hemolytic anemias and in patients receiving multiple blood transfusions. In some cases, systemic hemosiderosis, starting with a predominant increase in reticuloendothelial iron, seemingly evolves into secondary hemochromatosis. Whether the shift of iron into the parenchymal cells represents a "spillover" from the phagocytic cells (with increasing levels of body iron) or whether these individuals are carriers of the hemochromatosis gene is not entirely clear. Discussion of the pathogenesis of hemochromatosis requires brief comments on processes that affect iron absorption into the body.

**PATHOGENESIS.** The total content of body iron normally ranges from 2 to 5 gm. This amount is a closely guarded constant maintained by balancing gastrointestinal absorption of iron from the diet with the daily limited and relatively fixed losses. Without going into detail, we can say that the control point of intake appears to be at the level of intestinal mucosal cells, principally in the duodenum and jejunum. However, the mechanism is not perfect and is subject to a number of influences, some of which (mentioned below) have bearing on the possible development of iron overload.

○ Substances in the diet affect absorption; alcohol, for example, increases absorption, whereas phosphates and tannins (take note tea drinkers) have a contrary effect.
○ Anemia, even in the presence of excessive iron stores (such as occurs in ineffective erythropoiesis or hemolytic disorders), enhances absorption.
○ Increasing amounts of iron in the diet lead to higher levels of absorption, despite the fact that the proportion of absorbed to total dietary iron may be smaller.
○ Cirrhosis may predispose to enhanced absorption, but possibly only with an underlying genetic predisposition.

All of these influences may lead to a positive iron balance irrespective of the total body content. With this background we can turn to the spectrum of iron overload syndromes and their origins.

*Idiopathic hemochromatosis is a genetic disorder of iron metabolism characterized by excessive absorption of iron.* The total body iron may reach 40 gm (normal, 2 to 5 gm). The evidence that this disorder is genetic stems largely from the demonstration that these patients have an increased incidence of histocompatibility antigens HLA-A3 and HLA-B14. HLA-A3 occurs in approximately 70% of patients with hemochromatosis, a frequency that is approximately three times higher than in the general population. Apparently, tightly linked to the HLA-A region on chromosome 6 is a so-called susceptibility gene, which governs in some obscure manner absorption of dietary iron.[66] The gene behaves as a mendelian autosomal recessive; homozygotes develop full-blown idiopathic hemochromatosis, whereas heterozygotes may show some evidence of abnormal iron metabolism in the form of elevated plasma levels of iron and ferritin and increased saturation of the total iron-binding capacity. However, they do not develop the organ injury of hemochromatosis.

Although it is clear that the genetically predisposed individual progressively absorbs excessive iron over the span of years, the precise locus of the derangement is still obscure.[67] The primary defect may reside in the RE cell in the form of an inability to synthesize the regulatory signal for the intestinal mucosa, or it may be the inability of RE cells to store iron. Alternatively, the defect may lie at the level of the intestinal mucosa itself. Thus this genetic disease is generally called "idiopathic hemochromatosis."

Secondary hemochromatosis is encountered most commonly in *hemolytic anemias* associated with ineffective erythropoiesis (e.g., thalassemia major, p. 358). In these disorders, *the excess iron results not only from transfusions but also from increased absorption of iron, which accompanies ineffective erythropoiesis.* Transfusions alone—for example, in aplastic anemias—usually lead to systemic hemosiderosis.

*Alcoholic cirrhosis* is often associated with an increase in stainable iron within the liver cells. Whether this is due to an alcohol-induced increase in iron absorption or due to cell necrosis followed by uptake of released iron by surviving liver cells is not clear. In any event, most alcoholics with cirrhosis and increased liver iron do not have a significant increase in total body iron, and thus do not have hemochromatosis. The small number of alcoholics who do develop gross systemic iron overload and clinical features of hemochromatosis are suspected to be heterozygous for the hemochromatosis gene. Conceivably, in these patients the cumulative effects of alcohol and the hemochromatosis gene on iron absorption lead to significant iron overload and hemochromatosis. A similar speculation applies to those rare cases of hemochromatosis that seem to follow many years of oral (medicinal) iron ingestion. A rather unusual form of iron overload resembling idiopathic hemochromatosis develops in South African blacks, who ingest large quantities of alcoholic beverage fermented in iron utensils ("Bantu siderosis"). The increased absorption of iron is possibly due to the combined effect of excessive consumption of alcohol and iron (derived from the iron utensils).

Although it is clear that iron deposition in the parenchymal cells is fundamental to the pathogenesis of hemochromatosis, the mechanism of iron toxicity at the subcellular level is still not fully understood.

Currently favored is the view that with progressive iron loading, the capacity of cells to convert iron into ferritin is surpassed, leading thereby to an excess of "free iron." This in turn catalyzes the formation of oxygen-derived free radicals that interact with cellular membranes to cause lipid peroxidation and cell injury (p. 9).

The morphologic descriptions and clinical findings that follow present the full-blown classic idiopathic form of hemochromatosis.

**MORPHOLOGY. The morphologic changes in idiopathic hemochromatosis are characterized principally by (1) the deposition of hemosiderin in the following organs, in decreasing order of severity: liver, pancreas, myocardium, pituitary, adrenal, thyroid, and parathyroid glands, joints, and the skin; (2) cirrhosis of the liver; and (3) fibrosis of the pancreas. Fibrosis is relatively rare in the myocardium and the other organs.**

The evolution of cirrhosis occurs slowly. First, increased amounts of hemosiderin appear in Kupffer cells, parenchymal cells, and bile duct epithelium. In time, fibrous septa appear, extending out from portal triads to interconnect portal areas and sometimes also central veins to portal areas. Over the span of years, a diffuse, finely nodular pigment cirrhosis develops that is micronodular and, in terms of scarring, resembles that of alcoholic cirrhosis. However, the liver is usually enlarged, perhaps up to 3.0 kg, and is dense, radiopaque, and chocolate-brown. Hemosiderin can also be seen extracellularly, within the scars. As might be anticipated, iron stains such as the Prussian blue reaction are strikingly positive on transected surfaces of the liver as well as in tissue sections (Fig. 17–24). Ultrastructurally, the hemosiderin is located principally within lysosomes of surviving cells. In 8 to 22% of patients with advanced cirrhosis, a hepatocellular carcinoma develops.

**The pancreas is extensively pigmented and often has a diffuse interstitial fibrosis.** The hemosiderin is found in both the acinar cells of the exocrine glands and the islet cells. Pigment is also present in the interstitial stroma. There is some correlation between the levels of siderosis of the pancreas and the occurrence or severity of diabetes mellitus.

The **heart** often has hemosiderin granules within the myocardial fibers. Indeed, in some cases, the pigmentation is sufficiently extensive to cause a striking brown coloration.

Any or all of the **endocrine glands** may reveal brownish discoloration because of the accumulation of hemosiderin in parenchymal cells.

**Skin pigmentation** is one of the major presenting clinical features of hemochromatosis and, indeed, there is hemosiderin deposition in macrophages and fibroblasts about adnexal structures in the dermis. However, paradoxically, most of the skin pigmentation results from an increased production of melanin (for obscure reasons) within the basal layer of the epidermis.

The **joints** may be the site of hemosiderin pigmentation

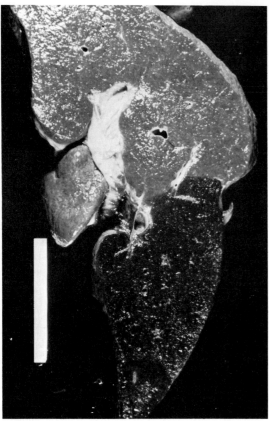

**Figure 17–24.** Transected surface of a finely nodular liver with pigment cirrhosis. A Prussian blue iron stain has been applied to the lower half, and the contained hemosiderin has produced the black discoloration.

of the synovium in 25 to 50% of cases. It is frequently accompanied by excessive deposition of calcium pyrophosphate, leading to severe damage to the articular cartilage and sometimes disabling arthritis (pseudogout).

The **testes** are usually little affected by hemosiderin, despite the fact that hypogonadism is sometimes a prominent clinical feature.

**CLINICAL COURSE.** The clinical manifestations of the idiopathic hemochromatosis will be described here. The findings in the secondary variants are more or less the same, depending on the severity of the iron overload and the resultant parenchymal and organ injury. Idiopathic hemochromatosis is preponderantly a male disease, in a ratio of 9:1. It rarely becomes manifest before the age of 40 years, requiring this time for the accumulation of the excess iron. Females are thought to be protected because of losses of iron incurred by menstruation and pregnancy. It should be noted, however, that the accumulation of iron probably begins at birth, and so strenuous efforts are now being made to identify young individuals at risk by HLA typing and other studies to detect excessive iron absorption in the precirrhotic stage of the disease, thus permitting interventions aimed at controlling the iron overload. The signs and symptoms of idiopathic hemochromatosis relate to tissue

changes in a variety of organs. Prominent, however, are skin pigmentation (80% of patients), hepatomegaly (75%), mild diabetes mellitus (45%), and gonadal insufficiency (40 to 50%). Splenomegaly and ascites may or may not be present. Cardiac involvement may present as heart failure or as life-threatening arrhythmias.[68] The arthropathy found in up to 50% of cases sometimes dominates the clinical course.

*Although the diagnosis can generally be established by the triad of skin pigmentation, diabetes, and hepatomegaly, these are late manifestations.* Evidence of iron overload can be detected much earlier by laboratory studies. The plasma iron level is elevated, sometimes up to 300 μg/dl (normal 50 to 150 μg/dl). The per cent transferrin saturation increases from a normal range of 25 to 50%, to 50 to 100%. The serum ferritin level is markedly increased, up to 6000 ng/ml (normal, 10 to 200 ng/ml). There is an increased urinary excretion of iron, and the amount of iron that can be mobilized by the administration of a chelating agent such as desferrioxamine may rise to 10 mg in the urine in 24 hours (normal, less than 2 mg). Ultimately, in patients with an excessive load of parenchymal iron, biochemical analysis of hepatic tissue obtained at biopsy may reveal 600 to 1800 μg of iron per 100 mg dry weight (normal 30 to 140 μg).

The natural long, protracted downhill course of this disease has been materially altered by a variety of interventions, such as administration of chelating agents, repeated phlebotomies, dietary regimens, and controlled use of transfusions, all aimed at creating a negative iron balance. The major causes of death in untreated patients are cardiac failure, hepatocellular failure, portal hypertension, and liver cancer. The risk of developing hepatocellular carcinoma is particularly high with this form of cirrhosis (p. 598). Most of these complications can be prevented by early institution of therapy. Since hepatocellular carcinoma develops only in patients who have developed cirrhosis, prevention of this fatal sequela can be achieved only by detection and treatment in the precirrhotic phase. Family studies must be initiated when a case is diagnosed to prevent iron overloading in those at increased risk. The five-year mortality rate is 11% for those receiving intensive iron-draining therapy, in contrast to 67% in the untreated group.

## OTHER FORMS OF CIRRHOSIS

*Wilson's disease,* a familial autosomal recessive disorder of copper metabolism, was discussed on p. 110. As pointed out, this condition is often called "hepatolenticular degeneration" because the major sites of copper toxicity are the brain and the liver, although the eye and the kidney are also affected. The basic changes were described in this earlier presentation and here it need only be emphasized that a form of cirrhosis may develop as a consequence of the toxicity of the copper accumulation in the liver. In some instances, the cirrhosis is micronodular, caused by the development of fine, fibrous trabeculae radiating out from the portal triads, quite similar to the pattern encountered in chronic active hepatitis. In other instances, or perhaps at a later stage, the scarring becomes more coarse, producing a macronodular cirrhosis reminiscent of the postnecrotic pattern. It should be noted that in the evolution of this late stage of hepatic injury, the hepatocytes often are laden with fat vacuoles and sometimes contain hyaline inclusions similar to those seen in alcoholic hepatitis (p. 586), creating the potential for confusion of these two conditions on liver biopsy.

*Alpha-1-antitrypsin (A1AT) deficiency*, discussed in an earlier chapter (p. 419), is a genetic disorder that may lead to pulmonary emphysema and hepatic injury.[69] The mechanism by which a deficiency of this protease inhibitor causes liver disease is unknown, and, significantly, only a minority of individuals with the most marked deficiency state develop liver disease. A variety of hepatic syndromes associated with A1AT deficiency have been recognized. The most common form is *neonatal hepatitis*, presenting within days to weeks after birth. It is characterized by the following:

○ Marked cholestasis
○ Liver cell necrosis
○ Mononuclear inflammatory reaction
○ Presence of globular PAS-positive inclusions that represent A1AT

The hepatitis may subside or in some cases progress to cirrhosis. Sometimes the initial presentation is cirrhosis in childhood without preceding hepatitis. Although a marked deficiency of A1AT is uncommon, it is a frequent cause of cirrhosis in children. The exact frequency of liver disease in adults with A1AT deficiency is not known. It may manifest as chronic non-B hepatitis or cryptogenic cirrhosis and affect both homozygotes and heterozygotes. Rarely, hepatocellular carcinoma complicates the liver disease in adults.

*Syphilitic cirrhosis* in the adult is known as *hepar lobatum*. It is now a very rare condition caused by the scarring associated with multiple hepatic gummas in tertiary syphilis. A different pattern of syphilitic cirrhosis may be seen in congenital syphilis, in which the liver is diffusely scarred by an interstitial fibrosis that may separate one liver plate from another. This form of the disease is related to widespread invasion of the liver by the treponemes, which invoke the inflammatory reaction.

# TUMORS

Metastatic implants from primary cancers arising in the portal area of drainage are the commonest form of neoplastic involvement of the liver. Bizarre distortions and enormous hepatomegaly may appear in such cases, but surprisingly, functional insufficiency is rare because sufficient intervening parenchyma is spared. Primary tumors of the liver are uncommon relative to such neoplasms as bronchogenic carcinoma in the male and breast carcinoma in the female. However, the most frequent primary neoplasm, the hepatocellular carcinoma (loosely termed hepatoma), is no rarity. Before discussing the more important primary hepatic neoplasms, a few comments will be made about two oddities: (1) liver cell adenoma and (2) hepatic angiosarcoma. *Liver cell adenomas* are, as the name implies, encapsulated masses of well-differentiated hepatocytes that may indeed form pseudocanaliculi and bile as well. Their importance derives from the facts that the use of oral contraceptives favors their development and so they most often arise in young women, and, on occasion, despite their innocent morphologic appearance, they have ruptured to cause life-threatening hemorrhages.[70] The second "oddity" is the *hepatic angiosarcoma*, which merits passing mention because of the substantial evidence that it may be induced by exposure to vinyl chloride,[71] Thorotrast (once used in cholangiography), and arsenic.

## PRIMARY CARCINOMA

There are three types of primary carcinoma of the liver: (1) hepatocellular carcinoma (80%), (2) intrahepatic bile duct carcinoma or cholangiocarcinoma (20%), and (3) mixed hepatocholangiocarcinoma (uncommon). In 60 to 80% of the instances, hepatocellular carcinoma arises in cirrhotic livers; the cholangiocarcinoma, by contrast, has no association with cirrhosis.

There are striking differences in the frequency of hepatocellular carcinoma among the nations of the world. In the United States, Canada, and Great Britain, the incidence rates are low, ranging about 1 to 1.5 per 100,000 population in males and about 0.5 in females. The rates are strikingly higher in some African countries, such as Mozambique, with 104 per 100,000 population for males, 31 for females, and South Africa, with 20 to 28 for males, 7 to 10 for females. It is evident that there is a pronounced male preponderance throughout the world, of the order of about 3:1, believed to be related to the greater prevalence of alcoholism, chronic liver disease, and, in particular, hepatitis B infection among males. In the high-incidence areas, the tumor generally arises in young adult life, whereas in the low-incidence areas, such as the United States, it is most often encountered in the sixth and seventh decades.

PATHOGENESIS. Three influences are thought to make major contributions to the causation of hepatocellular carcinoma: (1) chronic hepatitis B virus infection, (2) cirrhosis of liver, and (3) possible hepatocarcinogens in food. They apparently play no role in cholangiocarcinoma.

The evidence linking HBV and liver cancer is voluminous and is derived from epidemiologic, serologic, and molecular studies.[72, 73]

There is a direct correlation between the incidence of hepatocellular carcinoma and the frequency of chronic hepatitis B infection. Thus in parts of Africa and in Southeast Asia where the incidence of HBV carriers is very high, liver cancer is extremely common. Prospective studies in Taiwan have demonstrated that HBsAg carriers have a 200 times greater risk of developing hepatocellular cancer, as compared with those with no serologic evidence of HBV infection.[73] Conversely, patients who develop hepatocellular carcinoma are much more likely to have evidence of HBV infection as compared with controls. Molecular probing of tumor cells in HBsAg-positive patients has demonstrated that HBV-DNA is integrated into the tumor cell's genome. Despite all this evidence linking HBV with hepatocellular cancer, it is still not clear whether HBV itself causes transformation or renders liver cells susceptible to malignant change by other agents. This dilemma arises because studies of the HBV have failed to demonstrate any transforming sequences in the viral genome. This is in contrast to other known oncogenic DNA viruses. A recent analysis of liver cancer cells suggests that integration of HBV-DNA into the genome brings about structural rearrangements of flanking cellular DNA. Conceivably such a change may result in activation of some cellular oncogene (p. 209), which in turn causes neoplastic transformation.[74] This interesting possibility, which is reminiscent of the transforming activity of certain retroviruses, is currently under investigation.

As stated earlier, *60 to 80% of hepatocellular carcinomas arise in cirrhotic livers*. The risk of developing cancer is particularly high with macronodular (postnecrotic) cirrhosis associated with chronic hepatitis B infection, somewhat lower with pigment cirrhosis, and lowest with alcoholic cirrhosis. It has been traditional to ascribe the development of hepatocellular carcinoma in cirrhosis to long-standing regenerative hyperplastic reactions, which become transformed in time into neoplasia. There are, however, other possible explanations. Both the cirrhosis and tumor may be caused by the same agent, or alternatively, the cirrhosis may render the liver susceptible to the carcinogenic effects of environmental agents.[75] Clearly, cirrhosis is not a necessary precursor, since it is not present in 20 to 40% of cases.

Among the potential *food carcinogens* that may play a role in the causation of this form of cancer, greatest interest attaches to aflatoxin, as was discussed earlier (p. 203). This product of *Aspergillus flavus* in microgram amounts is an unmistakable carcinogen in experimental animals. Moreover, in Africa and Southeast Asia, where the fungus flourishes on improperly stored grains and ground nuts (peanuts), there is a well-defined correlation between the dietary content of aflatoxin and the incidence of hepatic carcinoma.[76] An interesting question has been raised—does the aflatoxin act indirectly by suppressing the immune system and thereby favor the development of hepatitis B infection? Other, more exotic food products have also been implicated, but they are of little general consequence in the origin of these neoplasms.

In closing, attention should be drawn to the causative role of liver flukes in the increased incidence of cholangiocarcinoma in the Orient.

**MORPHOLOGY.** Both the hepatocellular carcinoma and the cholangiocarcinoma as well as the rare mixed pattern may occur as (1) a solitary massive tumor, which sometimes produces marked hepatomegaly; (2) multiple nodules scattered throughout the liver, inducing less striking hepatomegaly; or (3) a diffuse infiltration of the entire hepatic substance, difficult to discern against the background of an underlying cirrhosis. In all three patterns the tumors are usually yellow-white, but well-differentiated hepatocellular carcinomas may elaborate sufficient bile to produce a green coloration. Foci of hemorrhage and necrosis are frequently present in the larger masses. Sometimes the margins of cholangiocarcinomas are also bile-stained, presumably by obstruction of bile ducts. In all variants, it may be difficult to differentiate large regenerative nodules of hepatic parenchyma in the cirrhotic liver from small nodules of neoplasm. These cancers (particularly the hepatocarcinoma) have a propensity for invading blood vessels and may obstruct the hepatic vein, producing the Budd-Chiari syndrome (p. 569), or they may block the portal vein, producing portal hypertension.

Histologically, the hepatocellular carcinoma ranges from well-differentiated lesions that virtually reproduce hepatocytes, arranged in cords or small nests, to poorly differentiated lesions often made up of large multinucleate anaplastic tumor giant cells. **In the better differentiated variants, globules of bile may be found within the cytoplasm of cells as well as in the pseudocanaliculi between cells.** In addition, acidophilic hyaline inclusions within the cytoplasm may be present, resembling alcoholic hyalin. There is surprisingly scant stroma in most hepatocellular carcinomas and it is the poor vascularization that leads to the necrosis of central regions of the tumor. The cholangiocarcinoma appears as a more or less well differentiated adenocarcinoma, typically with an abundant fibrous stroma (desmoplastic). **No bile pigment or hyaline inclusions are found within cells.** The histologic differentiation of a multicentric cholangiocarcinoma from metastatic adenocarcinoma may at times be treacherous.

Typically all primary carcinomas of the liver tend to remain localized to the organ for some long time, but eventually, by the time of death, about half have spread to such extrahepatic sites as regional lymph nodes, lungs, bones, adrenal glands, and other sites.

**CLINICAL COURSE.** Although primary carcinomas in the liver may present as silent hepatomegaly, they are often encountered in patients with cirrhosis of the liver who already have symptoms of the underlying disorder. In these circumstances, rapid increase in liver size, sudden worsening of ascites, or the appearance of bloody ascites, fever, and pain calls attention to the development of a tumor. The fever is attributed to resorption of necrotic tumor products. Jaundice may be absent; if present, it is typically mild.

Ninety per cent of patients with hepatocellular carcinoma have elevated serum levels of alpha-fetoprotein.[77] This is not true of those with cholangiocarcinoma.[77] This serum globulin is normally present in the fetus, but it disappears after birth. Its appearance in patients with hepatocarcinoma suggests that in the neoplastic liver cells the coding for this protein is derepressed. Unfortunately, this tumor marker lacks specificity, since elevated levels are also encountered in a variety of other conditions such as cirrhosis, chronic hepatitis, pregnancy, and germ cell tumors of the gonads. It is said that very high levels of AFP (>1000 ng/ml) are unusual in other conditions, and hence strongly suggestive of liver cell cancer. A variety of procedures, including radionuclide scans, CT scans, and angiography, are helpful in the diagnosis. The prognosis with either hepatocellular carcinoma or cholangiocarcinoma is poor. Although cures have been accomplished by radical partial hepatectomy, they are rare. Most deaths occur within a year of diagnosis, from liver failure or metastatic disease. Because of the association of liver cancer with HBV, it is hoped that immunization against the hepatitis virus may be preventive, especially in high-risk populations.[78]

# The Biliary Tract

Complaints referable to disease of the biliary tract are extremely common in clinical practice. Cholelithiasis and the closely associated cholecystitis account for the great preponderance of these complaints. Next in order of frequency, but much less common, are tumors involving the biliary tract. Together these conditions account for over 95% of clinical problems related to the biliary tract, permitting limitation of the following discussion to cholelithiasis, cholecystitis, and tumors.

## CHOLELITHIASIS

Gallstones and inflammatory disease of the gallbladder are intimately interrelated but may occur separately. When they coexist, it is still uncertain as to which precedes. Autopsy studies reveal that in the United States gallstones occur in 8% of men and 20% of women over 40 years of age. They are rare in the first two decades of life. The four "F's"—fat, female, fertile (multiparous), and forty—characterize the population with the highest incidence. Several other risk factors, to be described later, have also been identified.

Although gallstones may form anywhere in the biliary tract, the great preponderance arise in the gallbladder. In about 80% of cases, cholesterol is the chief component of gallstones (**cholesterol stones**). Usually they also contain calcium carbonate, phosphate, or bilirubinate, but infrequently they are pure. Cholesterol stones are classically 1 to 3 cm in diameter, pale yellow to tan, often multiple, round, or faceted owing to tight apposition. **Pigment stones**, composed of calcium bilirubinate, are next in importance to cholesterol stones. Unlike cholesterol stones, they are often fairly pure, in which case they are jet-black "jack-stones" or, when mixed, spheroids usually under 1 cm in diameter. They almost never occur singly and may be present in great numbers. Enough calcium carbonate is found in 10 to 20% of all gallstones to render them radiopaque, but pure calcium carbonate stones are rare.

Gallstone formation can be divided into three stages: (1) formation of supersaturated bile, (2) nucleation or initiation of stone formation, and (3) growth by accretion. Cholesterol solubility is the crux of the problem in the genesis of all stones save the pigment stones. *Supersaturation of bile with cholesterol results when the ratio of bile acids and phospholipids (principally lecithin) to cholesterol falls below a certain level.*[79] Normally, cholesterol is insoluble in an aqueous medium. In bile it is maintained in solution by the formation of micelles having a central core of cholesterol surrounded by a hydrophilic shell of bile salts and phospholipids (lecithin) (Fig. 17–25). *Thus excessive secretion of cholesterol (since bile is a major path of exit of this substance from the body) or low bile acid or lecithin secretion is lithogenic* (Table 17–5). Obesity, as we shall discuss, predisposes to excessive biliary cholesterol secretion. A deficiency of bile acids may result from accelerated loss or impaired synthesis, perhaps secondary to disturbances in the feedback regulation of bile acid synthesis. Bile acids that enter the gut are reabsorbed and returned to the liver through the enterohepatic circulation. Although theoretically, diminished hepatic phospholipid synthesis could play a role in producing lithogenic bile, no such condition has been identified.

We come next to the issue of what initiates stone formation. Supersaturation of bile is necessary but not enough for cholesterol stone formation.[80] Stone formation is initiated only when a nidus or nucleus for cholesterol precipitation is available. It seems reasonable to propose that at high levels of supersaturation cholesterol crystallizes out of solution to form

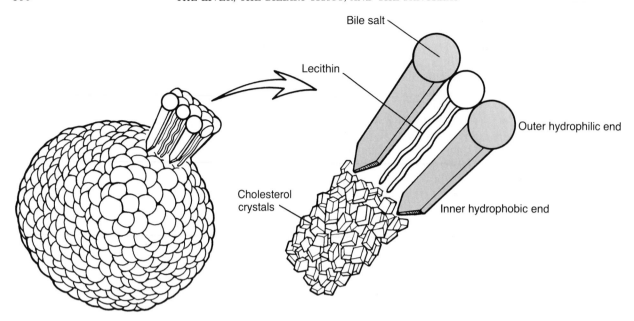

**Figure 17–25.** Cholesterol transport in bile. Cholesterol is contained within the hydrophobic core of a complex lipid micelle, which is maintained in aqueous solution by an outer hydrophilic shell of bile acids and lecithin.

a nidus on which further accretion may occur. At lower levels of saturation, the bile is said to be in a "metastable" state, and in this case perhaps bacteria, parasite fragments, desquamated epithelial cells, or other particulate debris are required to serve as seed crystals.

Growth of a gallstone obviously requires that it remain within its gallbladder nest and not be rudely cast off downstream before "it was growed." Once again we come to mystery, but this issue is raised because it may be relevant to conditions that predispose to gallstone formation, to be discussed next.

In addition to the four "F's" already mentioned, several other risk factors have been identified.[81] There are many instances of *ethnic* and possibly *genetic* predisposition to gallstones. A rather striking example is the extremely high incidence of cholelithiasis in certain American Indian tribes. Decreased

### Table 17–5. BILIARY COMPOSITION AND RISK FACTORS FOR CHOLESTEROL GALLSTONES

**Decreased Bile Acids**
Hereditary defect in synthesis: Cerebrotendinous xanthomatosis

Acquired inhibition of synthesis: induced by estrogens due to "hyperactive" feedback inhibition

Excessive loss: ileal resection, ileal diseases (e.g., Crohn's disease), malabsorption (e.g., cystic fibrosis)

**Increased Cholesterol**
Estrogen induced
Associated with obesity
Associated with high-calorie diet
Induced by clofibrate therapy

hepatic bile acid synthesis owing to "hyperactive" feedback inhibition by the bile acids absorbed in the ileum has been invoked to explain this predisposition. Malabsorption of bile acids from the ileum seems to be the basis of increased risk associated with ileal resection, Crohn's disease, and cystic fibrosis with pancreatic insufficiency. The use of *estrogens*, including those contained within *oral contraceptives*, roughly doubles the risk of gallstone formation, possibly contributing to the female preponderance of this condition. The mechanism of action is thought to be excessive cholesterol secretion coupled with defective bile acid synthesis. Clofibrate, used in an attempt to lower serum lipids and to inhibit atherogenesis, significantly increases the incidence of gallstones by increasing biliary cholesterol secretion. Obesity, as mentioned, also increases the cholesterol content of bile. Perhaps related to obesity is the increased risk of gallstones encountered with high intake of calories and simple sugars. Impaired gallbladder emptying as may occur with pregnancy or diabetes mellitus favors lithogenesis presumably by allowing gallstone growth. In contrast to the plethora of risk factors, the "social set" will be happy to know that moderate intake of alcohol appears to be protective.[82]

Little as we know about cholesterol stones, less is known about the formation of pigment stones. Most critical appears to be an increased concentration of unconjugated bilirubin in the bile.[83] How unconjugated bilirubin gets into the bile is a mystery. It could be formed directly within the biliary tract by the action of glucuronidase, which might split off glucuronide from the conjugated bilirubin. However, what is the source of the glucuronidase? A theoretical possibility is bacteria, but bile is usually sterile. Thus an origin from biliary epithelium or hepatocytes is currently favored. A better-defined cause of excess unconjugated bilirubin is increased secretion by the liver in patients having excessive hemoglobin breakdown, such as occurs in hemolytic anemia. For completely obscure reasons cirrhosis also predisposes to pigment stones.

Whatever the clinical setting, gallstones may have little or great clinical significance. Approximately 50% of cases have no symptoms ("silent stones") when the stones are discovered. The majority of individuals with silent gallstones tend to remain asymptomatic for extended periods of time. In others gallstones are not so innocuous. They may (1) play a role in the induction of cholecystitis and its complications (as is discussed next), (2) give rise to calculous obstruction of the common bile duct manifested by excruciating pain (biliary colic, p. 602), (3) predispose to suppurative cholangitis (p. 570), (4) lead to obstructive jaundice, and, most controversial of all, (5) favor the formation of carcinoma of the gallbladder.

## CHOLECYSTITIS

Inflammation of the gallbladder may be acute, chronic, or acute superimposed on chronic. In the United States, cholecystitis is one of the most common indications for abdominal surgery. Its distribution in the population closely parallels that of gallstones, and indeed stones are present in 80 to 90% of all patients with cholecystitis.

The roles of chemical injury, bacterial infection, and gallstones in the initiation of cholecystitis are subjects of contention. The central issues are the following: Can cholecystitis be initiated by chemical injury that predisposes to infection, or is bacterial invasion required? Could stone formation in the noninflamed gallbladder be the initial event, which is followed by mechanical injury and bacterial invasion?

Bacteria can be cultured from about 80% of all acutely inflamed gallbladders. When only chronic inflammation is present, the incidence falls to about 30%. The most common offenders are *Escherichia coli* and enterococci. On occasion, *Salmonella typhi* localize in the gallbladder after a systemic infection. Bacteria are indisputably absent in some cases. Therefore, it has been proposed that supersaturation or imbalances in the constituents of the bile, such as high levels of bile salts or acids, may induce chemical inflammation. Secondary invasion by bacteria may then ensue. On the other hand, the development of cholecystitis during a systemic bacterial infection suggests an initial bacterial invasion.

Stones could contribute to both mechanisms. If they arise first, they might cause trauma to the wall of the gallbladder and predispose to bacterial invasion. They might also cause obstruction and stasis and thus favor supersaturation, with resultant chemical injury. Obstruction of the cystic or common duct would distend the gallbladder and impair the blood supply and lymphatic drainage. Indeed, stones are frequently found in the cystic duct and neck of the gallbladder in acute cholecystitis and are believed to be the major factors in the initiation of acute inflammation. Although chronic cholecystitis is also frequently associated with gallstones, it is doubtful that stones play a direct role in the initiation of chronic inflammation. More likely supersaturation of bile predisposes to stone formation as well as chemical injury to the gallbladder wall. In any event, cholelithiasis and cholecystitis are virtual Siamese twins.

In **acute cholecystitis**, the gallbladder is usually enlarged, tense, edematous, fiery red, and often covered with a fibrinosuppurative exudate. Areas of black, gangrenous necrosis may be evident. The wall is characteristically thickened and edematous, and there is generally extensive inflammatory ulceration of the mucosa (Fig. 17–26). As was mentioned, stones are almost invariably present, and not infrequently one is impacted within the neck of the gallbladder, strongly suggesting that it triggered the flareup. The histologic changes are characteristic of any acute inflammatory response. Sometimes the lumen is filled with frank pus, creating **empyema of the gallbladder**.

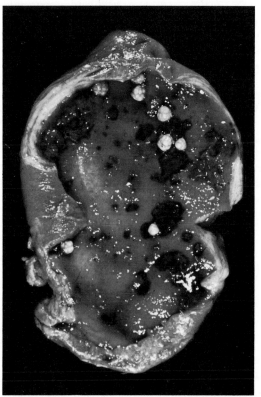

Figure 17–26. Acute cholecystitis. The gallbladder has been opened to show the edematous, thickened wall and the glazed, congested mucosa on which rest some small multifaceted gallstones. The dark, irregular patches are areas of mucosal ulceration.

In **chronic cholecystitis**, the gallbladder may be large, but more often it is contracted. The serosa may be smooth or dulled by subserosal fibrosis. The wall is variably thickened, gray-white, and tough. Stones are usually present, as was already mentioned. Mucosal ulcerations are not frequent. The inflammatory reaction is that of a mononuclear infiltrate, and the submucosal and subserosal levels are often fibrosed. Not infrequently the changes of chronic cholecystitis are found with a superimposed acute inflammatory reaction.

On occasion, when a stone has been impacted in the neck of the gallbladder or cystic duct for long periods of time, resorption of the bile solids (excluding the stones) occurs, leaving only a clear, mucinous secretion. This pattern is designated **hydrops or mucocele of the gallbladder**.

Cholecystitis has many potential consequences. The acute form announces itself loudly with severe, steady, upper abdominal pain, often radiating to the right shoulder. Sometimes, when stones are present in the neck of the gallbladder or in ducts, the pain is colicky. Fever, nausea, leukocytosis, and prostration are classic. The right subcostal region is markedly tender and may feel rigid owing to spasm of the abdominal muscles. In approximately one third of the cases, however, a tender, distended gallbladder can be palpated, confirming the diagnosis. Slow penetration of the bacteria yields pericholecystic abscesses, or the gangrenous gallbladder may suddenly rupture, producing a violent, acute peritonitis. The bacterial infection may ascend the bile ducts, resulting in intrahepatic ascending cholangitis. Liver abscesses may follow.

The chronic form of the disease does not have the striking manifestations of the acute form but is characterized instead by recurrent attacks of either steady or colicky epigastric or right upper quadrant pain. Nausea, vomiting, and intolerance of fatty foods are frequent accompaniments. The diagnosis of both the acute and chronic disease often rests on ultrasonography revealing the presence of gallstones, dilatation of the bile ducts, or both conditions. It hardly needs to be stated that in the absence of obstructing stones or infection within the common duct, jaundice will not be present.

## CARCINOMA OF THE GALLBLADDER

Among the cancers of the biliary tract, carcinoma of the gallbladder is most common. In 60 to 90% of cases, gallstones are also present and, indeed, the incidence of this form of neoplasia follows the pattern of cholelithiasis, affecting females about three times as often as males, most often in the 70- to 75-year age group. Most surgeons believe that gallstones play a causal role in the genesis of cancer by producing chronic irritation of the gallbladder mucosa, but this

relationship is still a matter of controversy. In this connection, the close similarity between bile acids and the carcinogen methylcholanthrene raises yet another possibility.

**Most cancers of the gallbladder are adenocarcinomas**, some secreting mucin. These grow either in an infiltrative pattern, thickening the gallbladder wall, or as exophytic lesions fungating into the lumen. About 5 to 10% are squamous cell carcinomas or adenoacanthomas. Presumably these arise from metaplastic squamous epithelium. All generally spread by local extension. Direct permeation of the liver is characteristic of those arising in the liver bed of the gallbladder. Many situated near the neck of the gallbladder evoke symptoms highly reminiscent of gallstones or cholecystitis. Some grow along the cystic duct, eventually obstructing the common bile duct. Those arising in the fundus of the gallbladder remain silent until their advance impinges upon some structure or function that evokes clinical manifestations. The gallbladder is palpable in about two thirds of patients. Although jaundice eventually develops in most patients, it is relatively mild. Spread to the porta hepatis nodes and liver is frequent. Although widespread metastatic dissemination may occur, it is uncommon.

About half of the patients come to clinical attention because of complaints referable to the biliary tract.[84] Indeed, the symptoms may be indistinguishable from those of cholecystitis or cholelithiasis—symptoms that may be all too familiar to these patients, hence not particularly alarming. In the remaining cases, the disease is entirely occult until anorexia and weight loss make their ominous appearance. The five-year survival rate is a tragic 3%.

## CARCINOMA OF EXTRAHEPATIC BILE DUCTS, INCLUDING AMPULLA OF VATER

Cancers arising in the extrahepatic ducts and ampulla of Vater are extremely insidious and generally produce silent jaundice. In contrast to the situation with gallbladder cancers, males are more often affected.[85] The locations of these tumors, in descending order of frequency, are (1) the common bile duct, especially its lower end; (2) the junction of the cystic, hepatic, and common duct; (3) the hepatic ducts; (4) the cystic duct; and (5) the duodenal portion of the common bile duct, including the periampullary region. Collectively, these neoplasms are less common than those arising in the gallbladder. Attempts to relate gallstones to the genesis of these tumors have been unconvincing and, moreover, they are only present in about one third of cases.[86] However, liver flukes are thought to be predisposing influences in the Orient, but the frequency of these infections may make the association fortuitous.

Almost all are extremely small, presumably because, in their strategic locations, they produce extrahepatic obstructive jaundice and hepatic decompensation very early. Accordingly, they rarely metastasize widely but infiltrate locally and sometimes spread to the lymph nodes of the porta hepatis or to the liver. Some infiltrate the wall of the duct, causing thickening and narrowing of the lumen, whereas others fungate directly into the lumen. Almost all are adenocarcinomas, more or less well differentiated, and some have papillary patterns. Mucin secretion is sometimes present. Rarely they appear as adenoacanthomas.

Gallstones are found less frequently in these cancers than in carcinomas of the gallbladder. One would expect the gallbladder to be enlarged with these tumors, according to **Courvoisier's law**. This law states that neoplasms that obstruct the common bile duct result in enlargement of the gallbladder, whereas obstructing calculi do not, since the gallbladder is too scarred from chronic disease to permit enlargement. However, in practice, Courvoisier's law is not very reliable. Indeed, only about a third of cancers of the bile ducts and ampulla of Vater are associated with a palpably enlarged gallbladder.

The clinical diagnosis is initiated by painless obstructive jaundice and pruritus. Many of the clinical features are shared by non-neoplastic obstructive lesions of the bile ducts such as calculous disease. In general, obstructive jaundice due to cancer is painless and associated with weight loss, but these features are not absolute. Radiographic techniques such as transhepatic or retrograde cholangiography usually demonstrate ductal dilatation and can localize the site of obstruction. Ultimately, surgical exploration may be necessary. *Intermittent biliary tract obstruction* was once thought to point to calculous obstruction, but it should be noted that necrosis and ulceration of these neoplasms may also produce waxing and waning of obstruction. The periampullary lesions offer the best hope for cure. If discovered early, they permit a 33% five-year survival. For most other cancer locations, death usually occurs within one year of diagnosis.

# The Pancreas

With the exception of diabetes mellitus, already discussed, the remaining disorders of the pancreas are relatively uncommon in clinical practice as compared with those of the liver. The four most frequent, to be discussed in the following sections, are acute pancreatitis, chronic pancreatitis, carcinoma of the pancreas, and tumors of the islets. All of these have clinical importance out of proportion to their prevalence. Acute pancreatitis produces a calamitous acute abdomen, which may lead to death within a few days. Chronic pancreatitis is a cause of less severe abdominal pain, which is nonetheless disabling and at the same time difficult to diagnose. Carcinoma of the pancreas is a silent disease that only comes to attention when far advanced and almost always beyond cure. Tumors of the islets, on the other hand, may produce dramatic endocrinopathies such as potentially lethal hypoglycemia, which can be gratifyingly cured by resection of a benign, sometimes minute, neoplasm. Thus, pancreatic diseases represent diagnostic clinical challenges requiring a constant awareness of their possible occurrence.

## ACUTE PANCREATITIS (ACUTE HEMORRHAGIC PANCREATITIS, ACUTE PANCREATIC NECROSIS)

Acute pancreatitis is better thought of as *acute hemorrhagic pancreatic necrosis*, since it constitutes sudden enzymic destruction of pancreatic substance and fat by activated pancreatic enzymes, accompanied by rupture of local vessels. Thus, *the diagnostic features of this condition are areas of necrosis of pancreatic parenchyma and focal enzymic necrosis of fat in and about the pancreas, accompanied by hemorrhage into and about the pancreatic substance.* This suddenly developing necrotizing condition is frequently associated with alcoholism and biliary tract disease.

It is advantageous to consider the morphology of acute pancreatic necrosis before exploring its etiology and pathogenesis.

**MORPHOLOGY.** The morphology of acute pancreatic necrosis stems directly from the action of activated enzymes.

The basic histologic changes are four in number: (1) proteolytic destruction of pancreatic substance, (2) necrosis of blood vessels with subsequent hemorrhage, (3) necrosis of fat by lipolytic enzymes, and (4) an accompanying inflammatory reaction. The extent and contribution of each of these alterations depend upon the duration and severity of the process and vary from one case to the other. In the very early stages, the changes consist only of edema, vascular congestion, and a neutrophilic infiltration of the pancreatic interstitium. With progression, there is focal enzymic necrosis of the exocrine and endocrine cells, with relative preservation of the stroma. This represents the **proteolytic destruction** of the parenchyma. **Hemorrhagic extravasation** may be minimal to extreme. In the milder cases, the interstitium is suffused with red blood cells and fibrin clots; in severe cases, large areas of the pancreatic substance are virtually converted to a mass of blood clot. Perhaps the hallmark of acute pancreatic necrosis is **enzymic fat necrosis**. This process was described briefly on page 16 and will be recapitulated here. Enzymic fat necrosis occurs in the peripancreatic fat and in fat depots throughout the abdominal cavity, as well as in the pancreas itself. Liberated lipase enzymically cleaves the triglycerides stored in the fat cells. Histologically, these cells appear as shadowy outlines of cell membranes filled with pink, granular, opaque precipitate. Presumably, this granular material is derived from the hydrolysis of fat. The liberated glycerol is reabsorbed, and the released fatty acids combine with calcium to form insoluble salts that precipitate in situ. Depending on the amount of calcium deposition, amorphous basophilic precipitates may be visible within the necrotic focus. The **leukocytic reaction** appears between the areas of hemorrhage and necrosis, and in particular rims the foci of fat necrosis (Fig. 17–27). If the patient survives, milder lesions may resolve completely. Occasionally, liquefied areas are walled off by fibrous tissue to form cystic spaces, known as **pancreatic pseudocysts**.

Grossly, acute pancreatic necrosis is easily recognized. It is characterized by areas of blue-black hemorrhage interspersed with other areas of gray-white necrotic softening, sprinkled with foci of yellow-white, chalky fat necrosis (Fig. 17–28). In individual cases, any one of these three components may dominate. Typically, there are accompanying changes in the remainder of the abdominal cavity. In the majority of instances, the peritoneal cavity contains a serous, slightly turbid, brown-tinged fluid in

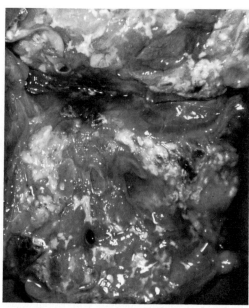

Figure 17–28. Acute pancreatic necrosis. The pancreas has been sectioned across to reveal focal areas of pale fat necrosis and darker areas of hemorrhage. Often there is more extensive hemorrhage.

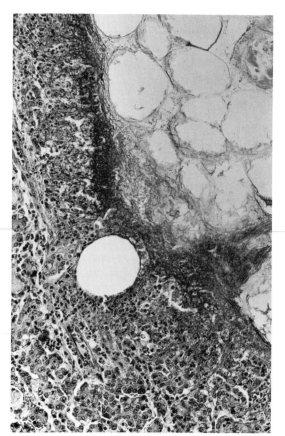

Figure 17–27. Acute pancreatic necrosis. The microscopic field shows a focus of necrosis of the fat cells at upper right, rimmed by an inflammatory hemorrhagic reaction. Preserved pancreatic parenchyma is seen at the bottom left.

which globules of oil can be identified (so-called chicken broth fluid). The liquid fat globules result from the lipolytic actions of enzymes on adult fat cells. In late cases, this fluid may become secondarily infected, to produce suppurative peritonitis. Additionally, foci of fat necrosis may be found in any of the fat depots, such as the omentum, mesentery of the bowel, and periperitoneal deposits. Occasionally, fat necrosis has been described in fat depots outside the abdominal cavity.

It should be emphasized that the characteristic chalky, white foci of fat necrosis and the presence of peritoneal fluid are important findings in establishing the diagnosis of pancreatic necrosis on laparotomy.

**ETIOLOGY AND PATHOGENESIS.** The pathogenesis of acute hemorrhagic pancreatic necrosis is still a mystery. A variety of etiologic factors have been identified which can be grouped under four major categories (Table 17–6).[87] Most commonly associated with acute pancreatitis are gallstones and alcoholism, together accounting for approximately 80% of the cases. Hypercalcemia and hyperlipoproteinemia (especially types I and IV) are less frequent, but important, predisposing conditions. Even when all associated and possible contributing influences are taken into account, a significant fraction of cases (20 to 25%) arise de novo without apparent predisposing influences.

*The anatomic changes, as pointed out, strongly suggest autodigestion of the pancreatic substance by inappropriately activated pancreatic enzymes.* The tissue lesions appear to be the consequence of proteolysis, lipolysis, and weakening of vessels. Thus two questions arise—which of the many pancreatic enzymes initiate the process, and how are they

**Table 17–6.** ETIOLOGIC FACTORS IN
ACUTE PANCREATITIS*

**Metabolic**
Alcohol
Hyperlipoproteinemia
Hypercalcemia
Drugs
Genetic

**Mechanical**
Gallstones
Postoperative (gastric, biliary)
Posttraumatic

**Vascular**
Polyarteritis nodosa
Atheroembolism

**Infectious**
Mumps
Coxsackievirus

*Modified from Ranson, J. H. C.: Acute pancreatitis: Pathogenesis, outcome and treatment. Clin. Gastroenterol. *13*:843, 1984.

activated? Among the many possible candidates, current thinking attributes a major role to trypsin, which in turn activates chymotrypsin, phospholipase A, and elastase. The action of trypsin could well explain the proteolytic destruction of pancreatic substance and the activation of other enzymes. Trypsin also converts prekallikrein to its activated form, thus bringing into play the kinin system and, by activation of Hageman factor, the clotting and complement systems as well. In this way, the inflammation and small-vessel thromboses (which may lead to congestion and rupture of already weakened vessels) are amplified. Thus it is widely believed that activation of trypsinogen is a probable trigger event in the initiation of acute pancreatic necrosis.

Activation of phospholipase A may well contribute to the necrotizing process by destroying cell membranes. At the same time, activated phospholipase A converts lecithin in bile to the highly toxic lysolecithin. Once the fat cells are disrupted, lipase would be free to split the triglycerides to release fatty acids.

Conversion of proelastase to elastase by trypsin provides a mechanism for damage of elastic fibers of blood vessels and ducts, rendering them vulnerable to rupture. In this manner, hemorrhages can be explained. The ductal damage in turn probably contributes to release and activation of enzymes, creating an autocatalytic reaction extending the amount of tissue destruction.

As mentioned earlier, even if activated pancreatic enzymes cause the tissue damage, how are they activated and liberated into the pancreatic substance? Endless theories have been proposed, but all are speculative and can be briefly considered under two categories: (1) duct obstruction and (2) acinar cell injury (Fig. 17–29).

*Obstruction to the outflow of bile or pancreatic juices, or both,* along with possible reflux into the pancreas is considered central to the pathogenesis of acute pancreatitis associated with gallstones and alcoholism. It may be recalled that the common bile duct is joined by the main pancreatic duct in 70% of normal individuals. It is proposed that obstruction of the common outflow channel, say by a stone impacted in the ampulla of Vater, raises the intrapancreatic pressure and, more importantly, causes a *reflux of bile into the pancreas.* The mixture of bile with pancreatic juice may well lead to the activation of proenzymes as well as the formation of highly toxic lysolecithin, as described earlier. This view is supported by the fact that in 75 to 80% of patients with cholelithiasis and pancreatitis, gallstones can be found in the ampulla or in the stools. In most patients pancreatic reflux can also be demonstrated by operative cholangiography.[88] When obstructive stones are not found, it is proposed that impaction of gallstones in the ampulla with subsequent passage into the duodenum damages the sphincter of Oddi and allows reflux of the duodenal juices into the pancreas. The enterokinase present within the duodenal juice may then activate the pancreatic enzymes within the substance of the pancreas.

Obstruction at various levels of the biliary-pancreatic duct system has also been invoked in the pathogenesis of pancreatitis associated with alcoholism.[89] It should be noted that alcohol causes both acute and chronic pancreatitis. Acute pancreatitis is often superimposed on chronic pancreatitis and usually follows 10 to 15 years of heavy drinking. Alcohol affects the pancreas in many ways. It increases the tone of the sphincter of Oddi, thus favoring reflux of bile into the pancreatic ducts. Spasm of the sphincter acting in concert with alcohol-induced stimulation of pancreatic secretion could conceivably build sufficient pressure to rupture small pancreatic ductules and initiate autodigestion. Sustained action of alcohol on the sphincter of Oddi may render it incompetent, thus allowing duodenopancreatic reflux. *Small duct obstruction, as opposed to large duct obstruction, is*

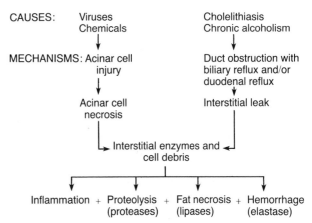

**Figure 17–29.** Etiology and pathogenesis of pancreatitis. (Modified from Longnecker, D. S.: Pathology and pathogenesis of disease of the pancreas. Am. J. Pathol. *107*:103, 1982.)

*believed to underlie alcohol-induced chronic pancreatitis.* According to Sarles and colleagues, chronic alcohol ingestion causes secretion of protein-rich pancreatic juice, leading to deposition of protein plugs in small pancreatic ducts. The acini drained by the obstructed ducts then undergo degeneration and are replaced by fibrous tissue.[90]

*Direct injury to the acini* may lead to intrapancreatic release and activation of enzymes. This mechanism is most clearly involved in the pathogenesis of acute pancreatitis caused by certain viruses and drugs and following trauma,[91] and it is suspected to be involved in the genesis of pancreatitis not associated with alcoholism or biliary disease ("idiopathic pancreatitis"). Although both hypertriglyceridema and hypercalcemia increase the risk of developing acute pancreatitis, the mechanism for such association is unknown.

*In summary, acute pancreatitis results from autodigestion of the pancreas caused by intrapancreatic activation of pancreatic enzymes. Most commonly this process is initiated by reflux of bile or duodenal contents into the pancreas after mechanical or functional obstruction of the ducts. Direct chemical, viral, or vascular injury to the pancreatic acini may be involved in some cases.*

**CLINICAL COURSE.** As might be anticipated, the onset of acute pancreatic necrosis is usually calamitous, manifested by severe abdominal pain often followed by shock. It is closely mimicked by other causes of "acute abdomen" such as perforated peptic ulcer and infarction of the bowel, from which it must be differentiated. Elevated serum levels of amylase are very important diagnostic findings. The amylase level rises within the first 12 hours and then often falls to normal within 40 to 72 hours. It should be cautioned that a variety of other diseases may secondarily affect the pancreas and produce elevation of these serum enzymes. These include perforated peptic ulcer, carcinoma of the pancreas, intestinal obstruction, peritonitis, and indeed any disease that secondarily impinges upon the pancreas; however, most of these conditions are associated with lesser degrees of elevations. Serum lipase is also increased and this is more specific for pancreatitis. Until recently, however, serum lipase measurements have not been widely used, but this test may become more popular owing to the recent development of a simple and sensitive assay. Direct visualization of the enlarged inflamed pancreas by high resolution CT scanning is useful in the diagnosis of pancreatitis and its complications such as pseudocysts and suppuration.[92] Hypocalcemia often develops, presumably because calcium is depleted as it binds with fatty acids in the abdomen. Jaundice, hyperglycemia, and glycosuria appear in fewer than half of the patients. The mortality rate with acute pancreatic necrosis is high, about 10 to 15%. Death is usually caused by shock, secondary abdominal sepsis, or the adult respiratory distress syndrome. After recovery, the patient must

be investigated for the presence of gallstones; if present, cholecystectomy is indicated to prevent future acute attacks.

# CHRONIC PANCREATITIS

This entity might better be referred to as *chronic relapsing pancreatitis,* since it is characterized by repeated mild bouts of inflammation eventuating in months to years by replacement of much of the pancreatic acinar tissue by fibrous tissue. The disease is protean in its manifestations, as will be discussed later. Middle-aged males, particularly alcoholics, are most frequently affected. Biliary tract disease plays a less important role in chronic pancreatitis than in the acute form of the disease. Hypercalcemia and hyperlipoproteinemia also predispose to chronic pancreatitis. Almost half of the patients have no apparent predisposing influences.[93]

The pathogenesis of chronic relapsing pancreatitis is even more obscure than that of acute pancreatic necrosis. One speculative proposal suggests that chronic ethanol ingestion, by increasing cholinergic tone, stimulates protein secretion by the pancreas and that inspissation of the protein-rich secretion causes ductal obstructions. Protein-calorie malnutrition has also been suggested as a potential causative mechanism and may indeed play a role in so-called tropical pancreatitis encountered in Asia and parts of Africa.

**MORPHOLOGY.** Basically, the changes constitute a fibrosing atrophy of the exocrine glands, sometimes with remarkable sparing of the islets. In other instances, the islets are overrun by the fibrous tissues. The distribution of these changes permits differentiation of two morphologic variants. In one pattern, the involvement tends to have a lobular distribution and is associated with proteinaceous and calcifying plugs in the ducts within the affected lobules, hence the sometimes-used designation **calcifying pancreatitis.** Sometimes the ducts are extremely dilated and contain grossly visible calcified concretions. The lining epithelium may be atrophic or hyperplastic or may have undergone squamous metaplasia. Pseudocysts similar to those described in acute pancreatic necrosis may appear in this variant of chronic pancreatitis. This is the pattern most often associated with alcoholism.

The other variant of chronic pancreatitis shows more widespread atrophic changes, such as would follow obstruction to the main excretory ducts. Although there may be ductal dilatation, it is not usually marked, and calculi and calcifications are infrequent. This pattern of so-called **chronic obstructive pancreatitis** may indeed be associated with a gallstone impacted in the sphincter of Oddi or stenosis of the sphincter secondary to cholelithiasis.

**CLINICAL COURSE.** A presentation of the many clinical faces of chronic pancreatitis would far exceed the spatial limitations of this book. It may present as repeated attacks of moderately severe abdominal pain, recurrent attacks of mild pain, or persistent abdominal and back pain. Yet again, the local disease may be entirely silent until pancreatic insufficiency and, more rarely, diabetes develops. In still other instances, the condition may present as recurrent episodes of mild jaundice or vague attacks of indigestion. The diagnosis of chronic pancreatitis requires a high index of suspicion. During an attack of pain, there may be mild elevations of serum amylase and serum lipase levels, but when the disease has been present for a long time, the destruction of acinar cells precludes such diagnostic clues. A very helpful finding, when present, is the visualization of calcifications within the pancreas by radiography. CT scan and ultrasonography may reveal calcifications missed by routine radiographs. These newer techniques also help to localize pseudocysts and rule out carcinoma of the pancreas, which may also present with vague abdominal complaints. Other, more sophisticated techniques attempt to demonstrate inadequate pancreatic enzyme responses to such stimulants as secretin and cholecystokinin. The condition is more disabling than life-threatening but can, as mentioned, lead to severe pancreatic exocrine insufficiency and the wasting of chronic malabsorption.

## CARCINOMA OF THE PANCREAS

The term "carcinoma of the pancreas" is meant to imply carcinoma arising in the *exocrine* portion of the gland. (The much less frequent islet tumors will be discussed in the next section.) Carcinoma of the pancreas is now the fifth most frequent cause of death from cancer in the United States, preceded only by lung, colorectal, prostate, and breast cancers. Moreover, its incidence has been steadily and rather rapidly increasing over the years. Currently 25,000 new cases are identified every year, of which more than 24,000 are expected to result in the death of the patient within five years. These figures are even more distressing when one considers that there are virtually no clues as to the etiology of pancreatic cancer.[94] Two possibly significant associations have been noted. This form of cancer appears to be about two to three times more common in smokers than in nonsmokers. For reasons unexplained, pancreatic cancer is more common in diabetics than in nondiabetics. One study has linked coffee drinking (but not caffeine) to pancreatic cancer, but this finding has not been widely corroborated.[95] The peak incidence occurs between 60 and 80 years of age.

**MORPHOLOGY.** Approximately 60% of the cancers of this organ arise in the head of the organ, 15% in the body, and 5% in the tail; in 20% the tumor diffusely involves the entire gland. Virtually all of these lesions are adenocarcinomas arising in the ductal epithelium. Some may secrete mucin, and many have an abundant fibrous stroma.[96] These desmoplastic lesions therefore present

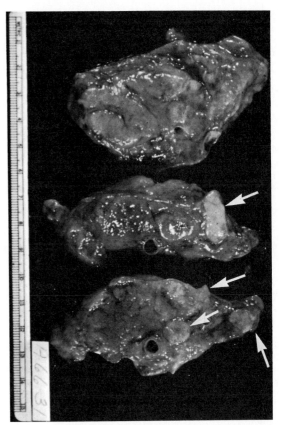

Figure 17–30. Carcinoma of the pancreas. The cross sections of the gland show the nodules of pale tumor that virtually replace the entire gland in the top slice and are evident as nodules (*arrows*) in the lower slices.

as gritty, gray-white, hard masses. The consistency of these cancers is not too dissimilar from that of a pancreas with chronic inflammatory changes or even of the normal pancreas, a point of importance to the surgeon attempting to identify such lesions by palpation of the organ. The tumor, in its early stages, infiltrates locally and eventually extends into adjacent structures (Fig. 17–30).

With carcinoma of the head of the pancreas, the ampullary region is invaded, obstructing the outflow of bile. In this infiltrative growth, it frequently surrounds and compresses, and less commonly directly invades, the common bile duct or ampulla of Vater. Ulceration of the tumor into the duodenal mucosa may occur. As a consequence of the involvement of the common bile duct, there is marked distention of the gallbladder in about half of the patients with carcinoma of the head of the pancreas. Because of the strategic location of carcinomas of the head of the pancreas, patients usually die of obstructive jaundice and hepatobiliary dysfunction while the tumor is still relatively small and not widely disseminated.

In marked contrast, carcinomas of the body and tail of the pancreas remain silent for some time and may be quite large and widely disseminated by the time they are discovered. They impinge upon the adjacent vertebral column, extend through the retroperitoneal spaces, and occasionally invade the adjacent spleen and adrenals. They may extend into the transverse colon or stomach.

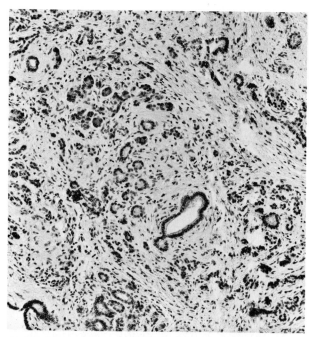

Figure 17–31. Carcinoma of the pancreas. The desmoplastic adenocarcinoma has almost totally replaced the native architecture. Only one normal duct (*below center*) remains. The cancer grows in small nests and strands of cells scattered in an abundant stroma. Occasionally it reproduces gland-like patterns.

Peripancreatic, gastric, mesenteric, omental, and portahepatic nodes are frequently involved, and the liver is often strikingly seeded with tumor nodules, producing hepatic enlargement of up to two to three times the normal size. Such massive hepatic metastases are quite characteristic of carcinoma of the tail and body of the pancreas and are attributed to invasion of the splenic vein that courses directly along the margins of the pancreas. Distant metastases occur, principally to the lungs and bones.

Microscopically, there is no difference between carcinomas of the head of the pancreas and those of the body and tail of the pancreas. Most grow in more or less well differentiated glandular patterns (Fig. 17–31). As mentioned, they may be either mucinous or nonmucin-secreting. In some cases, the gland patterns are atypical, irregular, and small, and the glands lined by anaplastic cuboidal to columnar epithelial cells. Other variants grow in a totally undifferentiated pattern. Rarely, there are adenosquamous patterns, or extremely anaplastic tumors with giant cell formation, numerous mitoses, and bizarre pleomorphism.

**CLINICAL COURSE.** From the preceding discussion, it should be evident that carcinomas in the pancreas remain silent until their extension impinges upon some other structure. It is when they erode to the posterior wall of the abdomen and affect nerve fibers that pain appears. There has long been a prevalent misconception that carcinoma of the pancreas is a painless disease. Many large series have clearly documented that pain is usually the first symptom,

although unfortunately, by the time pain appears, these cancers have already encroached on adjacent structures. *Those arising in the head of the pancreas eventually cause jaundice, whereas those of the body and tail remain difficult to diagnose until weight loss and pressure on adjacent organs make evident the cause of the pain.* Unfortunately, there are no early signs and symptoms specific enough to offer a clue to the diagnosis. Obstructive jaundice, which is usually severe and progressive, is associated with most cases of carcinoma of the head of the pancreas. Spontaneously appearing *phlebothrombosis*, also called *migratory thrombophlebitis*, is sometimes seen with carcinoma of the pancreas, particularly those of the body and tail (*Trousseau's sign*). But, as was mentioned, this syndrome is not pathognomonic of cancer in this organ (p. 307).

Because of the insidiousness of these lesions, there has long been a search for biochemical tests indicative of their presence. Levels of many enzymes and antigens (e.g., carcinoembryonic antigen) have been found to be elevated, but no single marker has proved to be specific for pancreatic cancer. Several new imaging techniques such as ultrasonography and CT scanning have proved of great value in the diagnosis of carcinomas localized to the head. With these imaging modalities it is possible in some cases to perform percutaneous needle biopsies, obviating the need for exploratory laparotomy. Five-year survival is only 2%, and most patients survive less than a year after diagnosis.

## ISLET CELL TUMORS

There are several cell types in the islets of Langerhans that can be differentiated by their staining properties, by the ultrastructural morphology of their granules, and by their hormonal content.[97] Of these, the four most important cell types are: B (beta), A (alpha), D (delta), and PP (pancreatic polypeptide) cells. The *B (beta) cells* contain insulin and compose 70% of the islet cell population. Beta cell tumors, also called insulinomas, are the most common form of islet cell neoplasia, producing the important clinical syndrome of hyperinsulinism. *A (alpha) cells* elaborate glucagon, and they compose 20% of the islet. Tumors of alpha cells, called glucagonomas, are very rare. *D (delta) cells* contain somatostatin, which suppresses the release of glucagon and insulin. D cells make up 5 to 10% of the islet cell population and their tumors (somatostatinomas) are extremely rare. *PP cells* are found not only within the islets but also scattered within the exocrine part of the pancreas. Within the islets they constitute 1 to 2% of all cells, and they contain a unique pancreatic polypeptide. The physiologic function of pancreatic polypeptide is unknown. When injected into animals it produces diarrhea and hypermotility. Tumors of PP cells are also very rare.

In addition to all of these secretory products, ACTH or ACTH-like peptides, MSH, vasopressin, gastrin, norepinephrine, serotonin, and chorionic gonadotropin or its subunits have also been associated with tumors of islet cells.

Among the many distinctive clinical syndromes associated with products of the islet cells,[98] only three are sufficiently common to merit description: (1) beta-cell lesions and hyperinsulinism, (2) hypergastrinemia and the Zollinger-Ellison syndrome, and (3) multiple endocrine neoplasia. The last-mentioned is characterized by the occurrence of tumors (generally adenomas) in several endocrine glands and so is described in the chapter on endocrine disease (p. 701).

## BETA-CELL LESIONS (HYPERINSULINISM)

Hyperinsulinism, as you would know, causes hypoglycemia and frequently neuropsychiatric disturbances. The hypoglycemic attacks are precipitated by fasting and promptly relieved by glucose administration or by food. The critical laboratory findings are high circulating levels of insulin relative to the glucose levels and often increased proportions of circulating proinsulin-like products.[99]

**MORPHOLOGY.** The morphologic lesions of the beta cells encountered with hyperinsulinism are as follows: solitary adenomas—70%; multiple adenomas—10%; diffuse hyperplasia of the islets, usually in newborns or children of diabetic mothers, or adenomas in ectopic pancreatic tissue—10%; carcinomas—10%. The adenomas are usually small (rarely over 5 cm in diameter), encapsulated, pale to red-brown nodules located anywhere in the pancreas (Fig. 17–32). Rarely, they are extremely large and exceed 1000 gm. Histologically, these benign tumors look remarkably like giant islets and there is preservation of the regular cords of cells and their orientation to the vasculature. Not even the malignant lesions present much evidence of anaplasia and may also appear deceptively encapsulated. Thus, the diagnosis of cancer rests largely on unmistakable evidence of destructive invasion beyond the pancreas, or, more securely, on metastatic spread to such sites as the regional lymph nodes or the liver. Under the electron microscope neoplastic beta cells, like their normal counterparts, display distinctive granules. They are round and contain polygonal or rectangular dense crystals that are separated from the enclosing membrane by a clear halo. By immunocytochemistry insulin can be localized in tumor cells. Without the identification of the typical granules and their content it is impossible to differentiate beta-cell tumors from other forms of islet cell neoplasia or indeed to establish the fact that the neoplasms are hormonally active. However, it should be cautioned that granules may be present in the absence of clinically significant hormonal activity.

Diffuse hyperplasia of the islets causing hyperinsulinism, as mentioned, is mostly encountered in newborn infants and young children of diabetic mothers. Prolonged exposure to maternal hyperglycemia seems to underlie the development of this lesion.

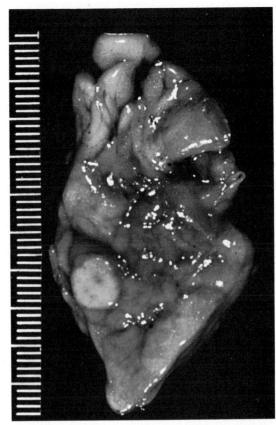

Figure 17–32. A pale beta-cell adenoma of the pancreas (*lower left*). Despite its small size, the tumor produced hyperinsulinism.

In closing, it is important to note that there are many other causes of hypoglycemia besides beta-cell lesions. The differential diagnosis of this frequently obscure metabolic abnormality is beyond our scope, but it might include such conditions as insulin sensitivity, diffuse liver disease, the glycogenoses, and ectopic formation of insulin by retroperitoneal or mediastinal fibromas and fibrosarcomas. Indeed, most patients with hypoglycemia have no overt morphologic cause for their disease.

## HYPERGASTRINEMIA—ZOLLINGER-ELLISON SYNDROME

Marked hypersecretion of gastrin usually has its origin in gastrin-producing tumors (gastrinomas), most often arising in the pancreas but sometimes in the gastrin-producing cells found in the duodenum and stomach.[100] Zollinger and Ellison first called attention to the association of pancreatic islet cell lesions with hypersecretion of gastric acidity and peptic ulceration. At that time attention was focused on the aberrant location of the peptic ulcers, as, for example, in the jejunum; but since then it has become evident that most often the ulcers occur in the usual sites within the stomach and duodenum. Ulcers are present in 90 to 95% of these individuals; the ratio of duodenal to gastric is 6:1 (p. 518).

The cell of origin of the gastrinomas of the pancreas is uncertain. Gastrin cannot be found in any cell of the normal adult islets. By electron microscopy, the tumor cells resemble normal gastrin-producing (G) cells found in the stomach and intestines.

**MORPHOLOGY.** In a review of a large series of cases of the Zollinger-Ellison syndrome, 60% of the gastrin-producing lesions were malignant, two thirds had metastasized by the time of discovery, 30% were adenomas, and 10% revealed only hyperplasia of the islets. In some instances, multiple adenomas are encountered in patients having other endocrine tumors, thus conforming to multiple endocrine neoplasia I (p. 701). As with the insulin-secreting lesions of the pancreas, there is rarely marked anaplasia, and the establishment of malignancy requires unmistakable evidence of invasion or spread to lymph nodes and extrapancreatic sites. The peptic ulcers, sometimes multiple, are identical to those found in the general population. They differ only in their intractability to usual modalities of therapy. However, when present in the jejunum, suspicion of the Zollinger-Ellison syndrome should be raised.

In the classic case of the Zollinger-Ellison syndrome, the gastric hyperacidity is associated with peptic ulcers, which in only 25% of the cases occur within the jejunum. Multiple ulcerations are found in about 10% of patients. However, it should be noted that the gastric hypersecretion does not always produce ulcerations but sometimes only abdominal pain, diarrhea, and gastrointestinal bleeding associated with hypertrophic gastric mucosa. The hypergastrinemia can be alleviated by excision of the neoplasms, but often they are malignant and invasive or extremely difficult to find because of their small size or aberrant extrapancreatic location. Too often metastases are present at the time of exploration. Further surgical difficulty may be occasioned when the lesions, even though benign, are multiple. However, total resection of the neoplasm, when possible, is curative of the syndrome.

## References

1. Whitmer, D. I., et al.: Mechanisms of formation, hepatic transport, and metabolism of bile pigments. Prog. Clin. Biol. Res. 152:29, 1984.
2. Popper, H.: Pathogenesis of hepatic failure. Kidney Int. 10:S-225, 1976.
3. Fraser, C. L., and Arieff, A. J.: Hepatic encephalopathy. N. Engl. J. Med. 313:865, 1985.
4. Koppel, M. H., et al.: Transplantation of cadaveric kidneys from patients with hepatorenal syndrome. Evidence for the functional nature of renal failure in advanced liver disease. N. Engl. J. Med. 280:1367, 1969.
5. Editorial: Hepatorenal syndrome of hepatic nephropathy? Lancet 1:801, 1980.
6. Gollan, J. L., and Knapp, A. B.: Bilirubin metabolism and congenital jaundice. Hosp. Pract. 20:83, 1985.
7. Swartz, H. M.: On the nature and excretion of the hepatic pigment in the Dubin-Johnson syndrome. Gastroenterology 76:958, 1979.
8. Mitchell, M. C., et al.: Budd-Chiari syndrome: etiology, diagnosis and management. Medicine 61:199, 1982.
9. Trauner, D. A.: Reye's syndrome. West. J. Med. 141:206, 1984.
10. Waldman, R. J., et al.: Aspirin as a risk factor in Reye's syndrome. J.A.M.A. 247:3089, 1984.
11. McDonald, M. I., et al.: Single and multiple pyogenic liver abscesses. Natural history, diagnosis and treatment, with emphasis on percutaneous drainage. Medicine 63:291, 1984.
12. Knight, R.: Hepatic amebiasis. Semin. Liv. Dis. 4:277, 1984.
13. Dienhardt, F.: The agents of human viral hepatitis, and control of the disease. Prog. Med. Virol. 30:14, 1984.
14. Minkoff, H.: Hepatitis. Clin. Obstet. Gynecol. 26:178, 1983.
15. Zhkarinsky, E., et al.: The biology of viral hepatitis. Monogr. Pathol. 23:156, 1982.
16. Dane, D. S., et al.: Virus-like particles in serum of patients with Australia antigen-associated hepatitis. Lancet 1:695, 1970.
17. Fagan, E. A., and Williams, R.: Non-A, non-B hepatitis. Semin. Liv. Dis. 4:314, 1984.
18. Bradley, D. W., and Maynard, J. E.: Etiology and natural history of post-transfusion and enterically transmitted non-A, non-B hepatitis. Semin. Liv. Dis. 6:56, 1986.
19. Maynard, J.: Epidemic non-A, non-B hepatitis. Semin. Liv. Dis. 4:336, 1984.
20. Bonino, F., and Smedile, A.: Delta agent (Type D) hepatitis. Semin. Liv. Dis. 6:28, 1986.
21. Jacobson, I. M., et al.: Epidemiology and clinical impact of hepatitis D virus (Delta) infection. Hepatology 5:188, 1985.
22. Purcell, R. H.: Hepatitis delta virus infection of the liver. Semin. Liv. Dis. 4:340, 1984.
23. Gerber, M. A., and Thung, S. N.: Molecular and cellular pathology of hepatitis B. Lab. Invest. 52:572, 1985.
24. Vento, S., et al.: T-lymphocyte sensitization to HBc Ag and T cell mediated unresponsiveness to Hbs Ag in hepatitis B virus related chronic liver disease. Hepatology 5:192, 1985.
25. Mondelli, M., and Eddleston, A. L. W. F.: Mechanism of liver cell injury in acute and chronic hepatitis B. Semin. Liv. Dis. 4:47, 1984.
26. Edgington, T. S.: Antihepatocyte antibodies and hepatitis. Hepatology 4:346, 1984.
27. Zuckerman, A. J.: The enigma of fulminant viral hepatitis. Hepatology 3:568, 1984.
28. Sampliner, R. E.: Follow-up and management of hepatitis B carriers. In Gerety, R. J. (ed.): Hepatitis B. New York, Academic Press, 1985, p. 155.
29. Szmuness, W.: Recent advances in the study of the epidemiology of hepatitis B. Am. J. Pathol. 81:629, 1975.
30. Huang, S.-N., and Neurath, A. R.: Immunohistologic demonstration of hepatitis B viral antigens in liver with reference to the significance in liver injury. Lab. Invest. 40:1, 1979.
31. Phillips, M. J., and Roucell, S.: Modern aspects of the morphology of viral hepatitis. Hum. Pathol. 12:1060, 1981.
32. Ishak, K. G.: Light microscopic morphology of viral hepatitis. Am. J. Clin. Pathol. 65:787, 1976.
33. Sherlock, S.: Chronic hepatitis and cirrhosis. Hepatology 4(Suppl. 1): 25, 1984.
34. Vyas, G. N., and Blum, H. E.: Hepatitis B virus infection current concepts of chronicity and immunity. West. J. Med. 140:754, 1984.
35. Seeff, L. B., and Koff, R. S.: Evolving concepts of the clinical and serologic consequences of hepatitis B virus infection. Semin. Liv. Dis. 6:11, 1986.
36. Dietrichson, O.: Chronic persistent hepatitis. A clinical serological and prognostic study. Scand. J. Gastroenterol. 10:249, 1975.
37. Lidman, K., et al.: Anti-actin specificity of human smooth muscle antibodies in chronic active hepatitis. Clin. Exp. Immunol. 24:266, 1977.
37a. Popper, H.: Pathology of viral hepatitis. Isr. J. Med. Sci. 15:240, 1979.
38. Kerr, J. F. R.: The nature of piecemeal necrosis in chronic active hepatitis. Lancet 2:827, 1979.
39. Nishioka, N., and Dienstag, J. L.: Delta hepatitis. A new scourge? N. Engl. J. Med. 312:1515, 1985.
40. Weissberg, J. I., et al.: Survival in chronic hepatitis B. Ann. Int. Med. 101:613, 1984.
41. Rakela, J., et al.: Fulminant hepatitis. Mayo Clinic Experience with 34 cases. Mayo Clin. Proc. 60:289, 1985.

42. Ockner, R. K., Drug-induced liver disease. *In* Zakim, D., and Boyer, T. (eds.): Hepatology. Philadelphia, W. B. Saunders Co., 1982, pp. 691–772.

43. Mitchell, J. R., and Lauterberg, B. H.: Drug-induced liver injury. Hosp. Pract. *13*:95, 1978.

44. Neuberger, J., and Williams, R.: Halothane anesthesia and liver damage. Br. Med. J. *289*:1136, 1984.

45. Brown, B. R.: Halothane hepatitis revisited. N. Engl. J. Med. *313*:1347, 1985.

46. Lieber, C. S.: Pathogenesis and early diagnosis of alcoholic liver injury. N. Engl. J. Med. *298*:888, 1978.

47. Anthony, P. P., et al.: The morphology of cirrhosis: definition, nomenclature and classification. Bull. WHO 55:521, 1977.

48. Powell, L. W., and Kerr, J. F. R.: Reversal of "cirrhosis" in idiopathic haemochromatosis following long-term intensive venous section therapy. Australas. Ann. Med. *19*:54, 1970.

49. Groszman, R. J., and Atterbury, C. E.: The pathophysiology of portal hypertension: A basis for classification. Semin. Liv. Dis. 2:177, 1982.

50. Rocco, V. K., and Ware, A. J.: Cirrhotic ascites. Pathophysiology, diagnosis and management. Ann. Intern. Med. *105*:573, 1986.

51. Schenker, S.: Alcoholic liver disease: Evaluation of natural history and prognostic factors. Hepatology 4(Suppl. 1): 36S, 1984.

52. Zakim, D., et al.: Alcoholic liver disease. *In* Zakim, D., and Boyer, T. (eds.): Hepatology. Philadelphia, W. B. Saunders Co., 1982, p. 739.

53. Fleming, K. A., and McGee, J. O. D.: Alcohol-induced liver disease. J. Clin. Pathol. 37:721, 1984.

54. Leiber, C. S.: Alcohol and liver: 1984 update. Hepatology 4:1243, 1984.

55. Maddrey, W. C.: Alcoholic hepatitis. *In* Williams, R., and Maddrey, W. C. (eds.) Gastroenterology 4. Liver. London, Butterworths, 1984, p. 226.

56. Mendenhall, C. L., et al.: Protein-caloric malnutrition associated with alcoholic hepatitis. Am. J. Med. 76:211, 1984.

57. Popper, H., and Lieber, C. S.: The histogenesis of alcoholic fibrosis and cirrhosis in the baboon. Am. J. Pathol. *98*:695, 1980.

58. Savolainen, E. R., et al.: Acetaldehyde and lactate stimulate collagen synthesis of cultured baboon liver myofibroblasts. Gastroenterology *87*:777, 1984.

59. Rubin, E., et al.: Fatty liver, alcoholic hepatitis and cirrhosis produced by alcohol in primates. N. Engl. J. Med. *290*:128, 1974.

60. James, S. P., et al.: Primary biliary cirrhosis. A model autoimmune disease. Ann. Int. Med. *99*:500, 1983.

61. James, S. P.: Primary biliary cirrhosis. N. Engl. J. Med. *312*:1055, 1985.

62. Sherlock, S.: Primary biliary cirrhosis. Am. J. Med. *65*:217, 1978.

63. Beswick, D. R., and Boyer, J. L.: Primary biliary cirrhosis. Hepatology 4(Suppl. 1):29S, 1984.

64. Wolke, A. M.: Malignancy in primary biliary cirrhosis. High incidence of breast cancer in affected women. Am. J. Med. 76:1075, 1984.

65. Halliday, J. W., and Powell, L. W.: Iron overload. Semin. Hematol. *19*:42, 1982.

66. Bothwell, T. H., et al.: Idiopathic hemochromatosis. *In* Stanbudy, J. B., et al.: The Metabolic Basis of Inherited Disease, 5th ed. New York, McGraw-Hill Book Co., 1983, pp. 1269–1298.

67. Bassett, M. L., et al.: Genetic hemochromatosis. Semin. Liv. Dis. 4:217, 1984.

68. Milder, M. S., et al.: Idiopathic hemochromatosis, an interim report. Medicine 59:34, 1980.

69. Gadek, J. E., and Crystal, R. G.: α1-Antitrypsin deficiency. *In* Stanbury, J. B., et al.: The Metabolic Basis of Inherited Disease, 5th ed. New York, McGraw-Hill Book Co., 1983, p. 1450.

70. Mays, E. T., and Christopherson, W.: Hepatic tumors induced by sex steroids. Semin. Liv. Dis. 4:147, 1984.

71. Tamburro, C. H.: Relationship of vinyl monomers and liver cancers: angiosarcoma and hepatocellular carcinoma. Semin. Liv. Dis. 4:170, 1984.

72. Sherman, M., and Shafritz, D. A.: Hepatitis B virus and hepatocellular carcinoma: Molecular biology and mechanistic considerations. Semin. Liv. Dis. 4:98, 1984.

73. Beasley, R. P., and Hwang, L.: Hepatocellular carcinoma and hepatitis B virus. Semin. Liv. Dis. 4:113, 1984.

74. Mizusawa, H., et al.: Inversely repeating integrated hepatitis B virus DNA and cellular flanking sequences in the human hepatoma-derived cell line huSP. Proc. Natl. Acad. Sci. U.S.A. 82:208, 1985.

75. Ken, M. D., and Popper, H.: Relationship between hepatocellular carcinoma and cirrhosis. Semin. Liv. Dis. 4:136, 1984.

76. Newberne, P. M.: Chemical carcinogenesis. Mycotoxins and other chemicals to which humans are exposed. Semin. Liv. Dis. 4:122, 1984.

77. Chen, D. S., and Sung, J. L.: Serum alphafetoprotein in hepatocellular carcinoma. Cancer 40:779, 1977.

78. WHO Scientific group: Prevention of primary liver cancer. Lancet *1*:463, 1983.

79. Weisberg, H. F.: Pathogenesis of gallstones. Ann. Clin. Lab. Sci. *14*:243, 1984.

80. Whiting, M. J., and Watts, J. M.: Supersaturated bile from obese patients without gallstones supports cholesterol crystal growth but not nucleation. Gastroenterology 86:243, 1984.

81. Boucher, I. A. D.: Debits and credits: A current account of cholesterol gallstone disease. Gut 25:1021, 1984.

82. Scragg, R. K. R., et al.: Diet alcohol, and relative weight in gallstone disease: A case control study. Br. Med. J. 288:1113, 1984.

83. Ostrow, J. D.: Bilirubin solubility and etiology of pigment gallstones. Prog. Clin. Biol. Res. 152:53, 1984.

84. Donaldson, L. A., and Busutil, A.: A clinico-pathologic review of 68 carcinomas of the gallbladder. Br. J. Surg. 62:27, 1975.

85. Bismuch, H., and Malt, R. A.: Carcinoma of the biliary tract. N. Engl. J. Med. *301*:704, 1979.

86. Sako, K., et al.: Carcinoma of extrahepatic bile ducts. A review of the literature and report of six cases. Surgery *41*:416, 1957.

87. Ranson, J. H. C.: Acute pancreatitis: Pathogenesis, outcome and treatment. Clin. Gastroenterol. *13*:843, 1984.

88. Kelley, T. R.: Gallstone pancreatitis. Ann. Surg. *200*:479, 1984.

89. Wilson, J. S., and Pirola, R. C.: Pathogenesis of alcoholic pancreatitis. Aust. N.Z. J. Med. *13*:307, 1983.

90. Sarles, H.: Epidemiology and pathophysiology of chronic pancreatitis and the role of pancreatic stone protein. Clin. Gastroenterol. *13*:895, 1984.

91. Longnecker, D. S.: Pathology and pathogenesis of disease of the pancreas. Am. J. Pathol. *107*:103, 1982.

92. Moosa, A. R.: Current concepts: Diagnostic tests and procedures in acute pancreatitis. N. Engl. J. Med. *311*:639, 1984.

93. Worning, H.: Chronic pancreatitis: Pathogenesis, natural history and conservative treatments. Clin. Gastroenterol. *13*:871, 1984.

94. Gold, E. B., et al.: Diet and other risk factors for cancer of the pancreas. Cancer 55:460, 1985.

95. Bentley, F. R., and Cohn, I., Jr.: Pancreatic cancer. Int. Adv. Surg. Oncol. 7:47, 1984.

96. Morohoshi, T., et al.: Exocrine pancreatic tumors and their histologic classification. A study based on 167 autopsy and 97 surgical cases. Histopathology 7:645, 1983.

97. Mukai, K.: Functional pathology of pancreatic islets: Immunocytochemical exploration. Pathol. Ann. *18*(pt. 2):87, 1983.

98. Freisen, S. R.: Tumors of the endocrine pancreas. N. Engl. J. Med. *306*:580, 1982.

99. Sherman, B. M., et al.: Plasma proinsulin in patients with functioning pancreatic islet cell tumors. J. Clin. Endocrinol. 35:271, 1972.

100. Hansky, J.: Gastrin and Gastrinomas. Postgrad. Med. J. 60:767, 1984.

# 18

# The Male Genital System

In this chapter the major anatomic subdivisions of the male genital system—the penis, the scrotum and its contents, and the prostate—will be considered individually. Although there is some overlap, diseases tend initially or predominantly to affect only one of these structures. An exception to this anatomic consideration is the grouping of the venereal diseases together at the end of the chapter. Because the pathologic processes are quite similar in both sexes, and to facilitate comparison, the effects of venereal disease in the female are also discussed in this section. No derogation of either sex is intended by this arrangement.

# Penis

The principal lesions of the penis are infectious, congenital, or neoplastic. In most cases they affect the surface of the penis, and hence are readily visible to the patient. The more important infectious processes are venereally transmitted and are discussed at the end of the chapter. Remaining to be described here are the congenital anomalies *hypospadias, epispadias,* and *phimosis,* and two neoplastic lesions, *Bowen's disease* (representing carcinoma in situ) and invasive *carcinoma of the penis.*

## HYPOSPADIAS AND EPISPADIAS

Among the more frequent congenital anomalies of the penis is termination of the urethra at the ventral surface of the penis *(hypospadias)* or at its dorsal surface *(epispadias).* Because the abnormal opening is often constricted, partial outflow obstruction, with its attendant risk of urinary infection and hydronephrosis, may result. In addition, these anomalies may be causes of sterility when the abnormal orifice is situated near the base of the penis. Frequently, hypospadias and epispadias are associated with failure of normal descent of the testes and with malformations of the bladder; sometimes they are associated with more serious congenital deformities.

## PHIMOSIS

When the orifice of the prepuce is too small to permit its retraction over the glans penis, the condition is designated *phimosis.* This may be a congenital anomaly, or it may be acquired by inflammatory scarring. In either case, phimosis permits the accumulation of secretions and smegma under the prepuce, favoring the development of secondary infection and further scarring. The nonspecific infection of the glans and prepuce that often accompanies phimosis is termed *balanoposthitis.* Forcible retraction of the prepuce may cause constriction, with pain and swelling of the glans penis, a condition known as *paraphimosis.* Urinary retention may develop in severe cases.

## BOWEN'S DISEASE

Bowen's disease refers to carcinoma in situ. It is not specific to the penis but may occur on the skin or on mucosal surfaces, including the vulva and the oral cavity. Its importance lies in the potential for its transformation into invasive squamous cell carcinoma. The frequency of conversion from the premalignant (in situ) stage to frank malignancy is not well established but is considered to be no more than 11%. According to some authors, Bowen's disease is associated with a high incidence of visceral cancer, but others have failed to find such an association.[1, 2]

## CARCINOMA OF THE PENIS

In the United States, squamous cell carcinoma of the penis accounts for no more than 0.5% of cancer in the male. Other forms of cancer of the penis are even more rare. This lesion is extremely rare among men who were circumcised early in life. The protection conferred by circumcision has been traditionally ascribed to its effectiveness in preventing accumulation of unidentified carcinogens, contained in smegma. However, recent evidence suggests that, as with certain cancers of the female genital tract (p. 638), human papilloma virus (subtypes 16 and 18) may be involved in the causation of penile cancer.[2a] It is conceivable, therefore, that the prophylactic effect of circumcision may relate to the associated improvement of general hygiene, thereby lessening exposure to potentially oncogenic viruses. The incidence of this cancer is highest in those over 40 years of age.[3] As mentioned, this form of cancer may be preceded by Bowen's disease.

Morphologically, squamous cell carcinoma of the penis usually initially appears as a small, grayish, crusted papule on the glans or prepuce, near the coronal sulcus. When the plaque reaches about 1 cm in diameter, the center usually ulcerates and develops a necrotic, secondarily infected base with ragged, heaped-up margins. Less frequently, the tumor takes a papillary form, resembling the benign papilloma. This form enlarges to produce a cauliflower-like fungating mass. Both patterns are locally destructive and may cause large necrotizing erosions. Histologically, the appearance is that of squamous cell carcinomas occurring anywhere on the skin or mucosa (see p. 228).

Carcinoma of the penis tends to follow a slow, indolent course. Metastases to the inguinal nodes are present in only 25% of patients at the time of diagnosis although many more have reactive lymphadenopathy. Widespread dissemination is uncommon until late in the course. For all stages, five-year survival is about 70%.[4]

# Scrotum, Testis, and Epididymis

The more important disorders of the scrotum and its contents involve the testes. *Some of these disorders produce testes that are smaller than normal, and others cause enlargement.* In the first category are congenital abnormalities that result in failure of the testes to develop normally at puberty. These include *cryptorchidism*, to be described later, and *Klinefelter's syndrome*. In addition, a variety of disorders result in atrophy of previously normal-sized testes.

A number of diseases cause enlargement of the testes. By far the most important are *testicular tumors*, which are usually associated with insidious painless enlargement. Second in importance are *infections (orchitis)*. These usually produce more rapid, painful swelling. A third, relatively infrequent cause of testicular enlargement is *torsion of the testis*. In this case, violent movement or physical trauma causes twisting of the spermatic cord, with consequent impairment of blood flow to and from the testis. Usually there is some underlying structural abnormality—such as incomplete descent of the testis, absence of the gubernaculum testis, or testicular atrophy—that permits excessive mobility of the testis within the tunica vaginalis. Because the thick-walled arteries are less vulnerable to compression than are the veins, there is intense vascular engorgement and, in severe cases, extravasation of blood into the interstitial tissue of the testis and epididymis, with consequent hemorrhagic infarction. There is usually little doubt about the diagnosis because of the intense pain and rapid swelling, often with bloody discoloration of the scrotum.

It is important to remember that the clinical distinction between enlargement of testicular origin and that due to disorders within the epididymis or scrotum itself is not always easily made. Indeed, swelling due to infection more often originates in the epididymis than in the testis. In addition, abnormal collections of fluid or herniated intestinal loops in the scrotal sac may initially be confused with a testicular mass. Although they are of relatively trivial consequence compared with, say, carcinoma of the testis, these disorders of the scrotum are extremely common. They will be described briefly before discussing testicular tumors and infections in more detail.

A clear serous accumulation within the tunica vaginalis—the serosa-lined sac enclosing the testis and epididymis—is termed a *hydrocele*. It may be a response to neighboring infections or tumors, or it may be a manifestation of generalized edema from any cause. Often, however, it develops slowly and painlessly, without apparent cause. *Hydroceles are frequent and are the most common cause of scrotal enlargement.* They may be differentiated from true testicular masses by transillumination.

Much less frequent are *hematoceles*, that is, blood in the tunica vaginalis as a result of tissue trauma or bleeding diatheses, and *chyloceles*, an accumulation of lymphatic fluid resulting from lymphatic obstruction.

With an *inguinal hernia*, loops of intestine may

descend into the tunica vaginalis, causing marked scrotal enlargement. This is easily differentiated from testicular disease by the presence of bowel sounds in the scrotum and by the reduction of the hernia through the widened inguinal ring. This is also a common cause of scrotal enlargement in children, since inguinal hernias are seen in 1% of the pediatric population.

## CRYPTORCHIDISM

Normally the testes descend from their initial embryonic position in the coelomic cavity to the pelvic brim in the third month of fetal life, a process termed *internal descent*. During the last two months of intrauterine life, *external descent,* or passage of the testes through the inguinal canals to the scrotal sac, takes place. When either process is incomplete, resulting in the *malpositioning of the testis anywhere along this pathway, the condition is termed cryptorchidism.* It is a common condition, seen in about 0.7% of the adult male population.[5]

Cryptorchidism is best considered a syndrome with various causes. Primary anatomic abnormalities (hereditary or developmental) such as a short spermatic cord or a narrow inguinal canal are observed in some, but in the vast majority of the cases no obvious mechanical factor can be recognized. Since a normally functioning hypothalamic-pituitary-testicular axis is considered essential for testicular development and descent, it is suspected that hormonal factors are primary in most cases. A transient deficiency of testosterone resulting from primary luteinizing hormone deficiency has been noted in some patients.[6]

Cryptorchidism is unilateral in the vast majority of the cases, affecting the right testis somewhat more frequently than the left. Progressive atrophy of the malpositioned testis begins early. Developmental arrest of the germ cells may be noted as early as two years of age and is evident in most by five to six years. Grossly visible atrophy, characterized by diminution in size and an increase in consistency as a result of progressive fibrosis, is obvious by 13 years of age. Microscopically, the tubules become atrophic, outlined by prominent, thickened basement membranes, and eventually they become virtually totally replaced by fibrous tissue. There may be an accompanying hyperplasia of the interstitial cells of Leydig as well as of the stroma. **Such testicular atrophy is nonspecific and may be seen in many other conditions, including progressive arteriosclerotic encroachment on testicular blood supply, end-stage orchitis, hypopituitarism, prolonged administration of female sex hormones, cirrhosis of the liver, some forms of malnutrition, and obstruction to the outflow of semen, as well as following irradiation.**

It should be apparent that bilateral cryptorchidism, present in 25% of the cases, results in sterility. However, infertility is also noted in a significant number of cases with unilateral cryptorchidism. In addition, the undescended testis is at a greatly increased risk of developing testicular cancer. Hence the undescended testis demands surgical correction. There is no unanimity, however, regarding the ideal age at which the placement of the testis in the scrotum (orchiopexy) should be performed. Histopathologic studies suggest that orchiopexy should be performed early, preferably before two years of age, to prevent progressive atrophy. However, orchiopexy does not preclude the possibility of a cancer developing at a later stage, nor can fertility be taken for granted. These results suggest that in some cases there is an intrinsic defect in the testis, unrelated to its position, which cannot be corrected by anatomic repositioning.

## KLINEFELTER'S SYNDROME

This syndrome is characterized by primary failure of the testes to develop at puberty, with resultant eunuchoidism (Fig. 18–1). It is responsible for about 3% of cases of infertility in males. This disorder is described on page 123.

## TESTICULAR TUMORS

*Testicular tumors are the most important cause of firm, painless enlargement of the testis.* About 95%

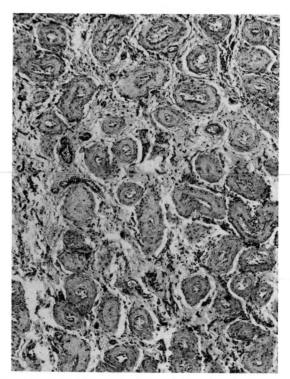

Figure 18–1. Klinefelter's syndrome. The spermatic tubules are totally atrophic and hyalinized and appear as doughnut-shaped masses of collagenous tissue.

of testicular tumors arise from germ cells. Almost all of these are malignant. Most of the remaining 5% originate from the interstitial cells of Leydig or the Sertoli cells, and these are usually benign, although they may elaborate steroids and thus cause endocrinopathies. Here we will consider only the germ cell tumors.

The average incidence of testicular germ cell tumors in the United States is approximately two per 100,000 males. Their peak incidence is in the 15- to 34-year-old age group. Moreover, in this age group there has been a steady increase in the frequency of these tumors over the past several years.

The etiology of testicular cancer is unknown. However, some predisposing factors have been identified. Reference has already been made to the increased incidence of tumors (10- to 40-fold) in undescended testes. Epidemiologic studies suggest that genetic influences also play a role in the etiology. Blacks in Africa as well as in the United States have an extremely low incidence of germ cell tumors. Among whites in the United States, Jews are affected twice as frequently as non-Jews.

**CLASSIFICATION AND HISTOGENESIS.** The classification of testicular germ cell tumors has been somewhat controversial. This stems in part from differing views on their histogenesis. Here we will present the WHO classification (Table 18–1), most widely used in the United States, followed by the proposed histogenesis of these neoplasms. Details of alternative classifications have been reviewed by Mostofi.[7]

Testicular germ cell tumors may be divided into two categories, based on whether they are composed of a single histologic pattern or more than one histologic pattern.[8] Tumors with a *single* histologic pattern constitute about 60% of all testicular neoplasms and are listed in Table 18–1. In approximately *40%* of the tumors, there is a *mixture of two or more of the histologic patterns.* The most common of these mixtures is that of teratoma and embryonal carcinoma *(teratocarcinoma),* which constitutes 25% of all testicular neoplasms. This classification is based on the view that all of the previously mentioned tumors

**Table 18–1. CLASSIFICATION OF TESTICULAR GERM CELL TUMORS**

**I. Tumors of One Histologic Pattern (60%)**
Seminoma
Spermatocytic seminoma
Embryonal carcinoma
Yolk sac tumor
Polyembryoma
Choriocarcinoma
Teratoma
  Mature
  Immature
  With malignant transformation

**II. Tumors of More Than One Histologic Pattern (Mixed Tumors) (40%)**
Specify the type and estimate amount of each component

arise in totipotential cells ("germ cells") (Fig. 18–2). *The totipotential cells may give rise to a seminoma, representing gonadal differentiation, or they may transform into totipotential tumor cells, represented by embryonal carcinoma.* According to this concept, embryonal carcinoma is the stem cell for all nonseminomatous germ cell tumors. Depending on the degree and the line of differentiation of embryonal carcinoma cells, tumors with different histologic patterns result. The most undifferentiated state is represented by pure embryonal cell carcinoma, whereas choriocarcinoma and yolk sac tumor represent commitment of the tumor stem cells to differentiate into specific extraembryonic cell types. Teratoma, on the other hand, results from differentiation of the embryonic carcinoma cells along all three of the germ cell layers, and therefore teratomas contain the greatest variety of neoplastic cells and tissues. With this background of histogenesis, we will present the morphology of the more common individual tumors, to be followed by comments on their clinical course.

**SEMINOMA.** This is the most common germ cell tumor, which accounts for approximately 40% of testicular neoplasms. In the great majority of cases it is characterized by sheets or cords of fairly well differentiated uniform polygonal cells, with distinct cell membranes, central

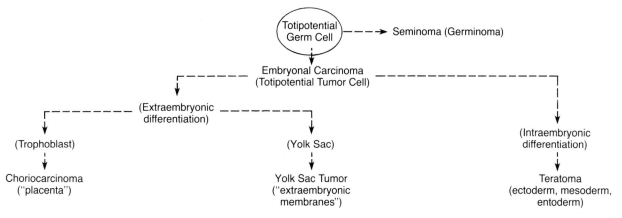

**Figure 18–2.** Histogenesis of testicular tumors. (After Morse, M. J., and Willet, W. F.: Neoplasms of the testis. *In* Walsh, P. C., et al. (eds.): Campbell's Urology. 5th ed. Philadelphia, W. B. Saunders Co., 1986, p. 1537.)

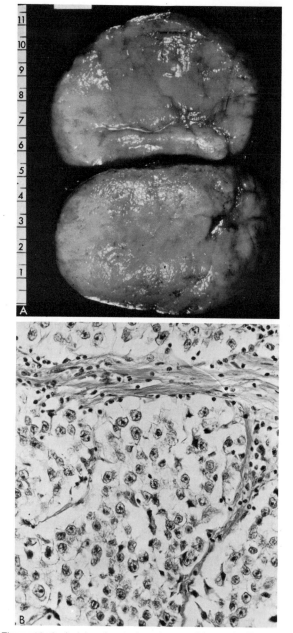

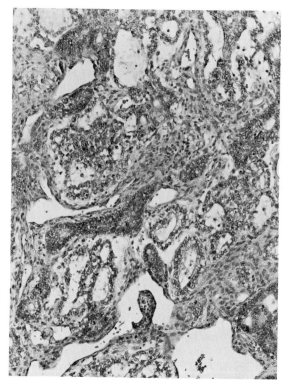

Figure 18–4. Embryonal carcinoma of the testis. An acinar, tubular, and papillary pattern is seen in this neoplasm.

Figure 18–3. *A*, A hemisected seminoma of the testis. The gray-white, fleshy mass totally replaces the testis. Note that its size is approximately 5 × 7 cm and it has therefore caused testicular enlargement. *B*, A high-power detail of a seminoma of the testis, showing sheets of neoplastic cells with clear cytoplasm and regular nuclei. The cell membranes are best seen in the lower left field. The fibrous stroma contains a relatively scant lymphoid infiltrate.

round nuclei, and clear cytoplasm. Approximately 10% of the cases show syncytial giant cells, which contain human chorionic gonadotropin (HCG). These probably represent mixed tumors with a minor element of choriocarcinoma. Typically, there is a variable fibrous stroma with a prominent lymphocytic infiltrate and occasional granulomatous formations. These tumors tend to grow rapidly as large, gray-white, fleshy masses (Fig. 18–3) but remain confined within the tunica albuginea until late in their course.

**EMBRYONAL CARCINOMA.** In contrast to the seminoma, embryonal carcinomas are poorly differentiated. They constitute 10 to 20% of all testicular neoplasms and are generally smaller than seminomas, appearing grossly as discrete, gray-white nodules, often with areas of hemorrhage and necrosis. Microscopically, the cells may be completely undifferentiated and arranged in sheets or, alternatively, they may assume an acinar, tubular, or papillary pattern (Fig. 18–4). The neoplastic cells are large and pleomorphic and, unlike seminoma cells, have indistinct cell borders. The stroma is scanty and devoid of lymphocytes.

**YOLK SAC TUMOR.** This tumor is variously known as infantile embryonal carcinoma, endodermal sinus tumor, and orchioblastoma. Although in its pure form the yolk sac tumor is rare, constituting less than 1% of all testicular tumors, it is the commonest tumor affecting the testes of children under three years of age. Yolk sac elements are frequently found admixed with embryonal carcinoma in adults. The tumor cells are undifferentiated and vary from endothelium-like to cuboidal or columnar cells. These cells occur in glandular, papillary, or solid formation. With immunoperoxidase techniques it is possible to demonstrate alpha-fetoprotein (AFP) within the tumor cells, a finding highly characteristic of yolk sac tumor.

**CHORIOCARCINOMA.** Choriocarcinoma, a highly malignant neoplasm, accounts for only 1% of testicular cancers in its pure form. The lesion may cause testicular enlargement, but more often the primary tumor is very small and cannot be palpated. Nonetheless, it is highly malignant, metastasizing via the bloodstream early and widely. His-

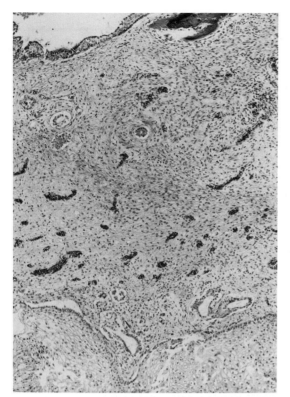

Figure 18–5. Histologic detail of a testicular teratoma. A spicule of bone (*top center*) is immediately to the right of a cystic space lined by columnar, respiratory-appearing epithelium. The center of the field shows areas, resembling white matter of the brain, in which small glands are scattered. At the bottom is a large nest of stratified squamous epithelium.

tologically, these tumors reproduce the two components of placental tissue—cytotrophoblast, composed of masses of cuboidal cells with central round nuclei, and syncytiotrophoblast, appearing as sheets of syncytial epithelium with an abundant pink, vacuolated cytoplasm and large, pleomorphic nuclei. HCG has been identified within the syncytiotrophoblast. These two cellular elements, both of which are requisite for diagnosis, are not arranged as in placental villi but instead grow in disorderly array.

**TERATOMA.** Teratoma of the testis is characterized by a histologic pattern in which tissues from all three germ cell layers may be present. Three variants based on the degree of differentiation are recognized.[7] The fully differentiated variant, called the **mature teratoma,** is found most often in children. Microscopically, these tumors are composed of well-differentiated elements such as neural tissue, muscle, cartilage, fat, squamous epithelium, bronchial epithelium, and bits of intestinal wall (Fig. 18–5) These elements lie helter-skelter with no definite pattern or orientation. The **immature teratoma** contains similar elements, which are incompletely differentiated but can be easily identified as embryonic tissues. Although this variant displays malignant behavior, the tissues may not show cytologic features of malignancy. On the other hand, in **teratoma with malignant transformation,** derivatives of one or more of the germ cell layers are frankly malignant. Thus there may be a focus of squamous cell

carcinoma, mucin-secreting adenocarcinoma, or sarcoma. Immature and frankly malignant teratomas occur more commonly in adults. Since benign mature teratomas are rare in adults, every teratoma in the adult must be regarded as malignant. Owing to the great variety of tissues present in teratomas, the gross appearance of these tumors is understandably variable. In general, the cut surface reveals cystic areas and a variegated appearance with foci of cartilage, bone, or soft myxomatous tissue. Together the three variants of teratoma constitute approximately 10% of all testicular tumors.

**MIXED TUMORS.** Mixed tumors constitute 40% of all testicular tumors and contain combinations of the various histologic patterns already described. However, recent studies that utilize the tumor markers AFP and HCG suggest that approximately 60% of the testicular germ cell tumors possess more than one element.[9] Most common is the mixture of teratoma and embryonal carcinoma (teratocarcinoma), but all conceivable patterns of mixtures have been described. It is important to note that in general the prognosis of a mixed tumor is determined by the more malignant element.

**CLINICAL COURSE.** Testicular tumors present most often as a painless enlargement of the testis.[10] Indeed, the overwhelming majority of intratesticular masses are malignant germ cell tumors. As already pointed out, in some instances the more aggressive variants, such as choriocarcinoma, may present initially with disseminated metastases and a small intratesticular primary lesion. Tumors of the testis have a characteristic mode of spread, the knowledge of which is essential in clinical staging as well as in treatment. In general, testicular tumors spread first to the common iliac and para-aortic lymph nodes and later to the mediastinal and supraclavicular nodes. Seminomas typically spread by lymphatics after having remained localized for a long time. Hematogenous spread to the lungs, brain, bones, and other organs is usually a late event. Some variants, however, especially embryonal carcinoma, choriocarcinoma, and mixed tumors with an element of choriocarcinoma, tend to metastasize early via the blood. Choriocarcinomas are the most aggressive, and in most cases lungs and liver are already involved at the time of diagnosis.

Staging of testicular tumors is being progressively refined with the addition of newer diagnostic techniques, including computed tomography, inferior venacavography, lymphangiography, and studies of tumor markers. Three stages are defined:

○ Tumor confined to the testis (Stage I).
○ Distant spread limited to the retroperitoneal nodes below the diaphragm (Stage II).
○ Metastases outside the retroperitoneal nodes or above the diaphragm (Stage III).

Major advances in the diagnosis and management of testicular cancer have been made possible by the development of sensitive and specific radioimmunoassays for the detection of tumor-associated polypep-

**Table 18–2.** SUMMARY OF TESTICULAR TUMORS

| Tumor | Frequency | Peak Age | Morphology | Tumor Markers | Prognosis |
|---|---|---|---|---|---|
| *Seminoma* | 40% | 40–50 yrs | Sheets of uniform polygonal cells with lymphocytes in the stroma | 10 to 15% have elevated HCG | Excellent |
| *Embryonal Carcinoma* | 10–20% | 20–30 yrs | Poorly differentiated, pleomorphic cells in cords, sheets, or papillary formation | 90% have elevated HCG or AFP | Good in Stages I and II |
| *Yolk Sac Tumor* | 1% | 3 yrs | Poorly differentiated endothelium-like, cuboidal, or columnar cells | 100% have elevated AFP | Same as embryonal carcinoma |
| *Choriocarcinoma (Pure)* | 1% | 20–30 yrs | Cytotrophoblast and syncytiotrophoblast without villus formation | 100% have elevated HCG | Poor |
| *Teratoma* | 7–10% | All ages | Tissues from all three germ cell layers with varying degrees of differentiation | 50% have elevated HCG or AFP | Better in children; in adults, like other nonseminomatous tumors |
| *Mixed Tumors* | 40% | 15–30 yrs | Variable, depending on mixture; commonly teratoma and embryonal carcinoma | 90% have elevated HCG or AFP | Like other nonseminomatous tumors |

tides. Two such markers, AFP and HCG, have proved to be of considerable value. AFP is normally synthesized by fetal tissues (liver, yolk sac, and intestines), whereas HCG is a product of the placental syncytiotrophoblast. As might be expected from the histogenesis and morphology, elevations in the levels of these markers are seen most often in patients with nonseminomatous tumors. All patients with choriocarcinoma have increased levels of HCG, whereas almost 90% of those with embryonal carcinoma or teratocarcinoma have elevated levels of HCG or AFP, or both. In approximately half of the patients with teratoma, one or both of these markers is elevated. Seminoma is associated with increased HCG in less than 10% of cases. Many investigators believe that such an association is an ominous indicator of coexisting choriocarcinomatous elements. In addition to their value in diagnosis, tumor markers are also helpful in studies of staging and follow-up. For example, an elevated serum level following orchiectomy is a clear indication of Stage II disease; similarly, a rise in marker levels following therapy can predict recurrences, often well in advance of clinical expression of relapse.

The prognosis of testicular cancer varies with the histologic type and the clinical stage. Seminoma, which is extremely radiosensitive and tends to metastasize late, has the best prognosis. Close to 95% of patients in Stages I and II survive five years and may be considered cured. Recent improvements in the treatment of nonseminomatous tumors allow for 80 to 90% survival for those in Stages I and II.[11] Among the nonseminomatous tumors, histologic type has little impact on the survival and therefore they are treated as a group. Table 18–2 summarizes the salient features of testicular tumors.

# INFLAMMATIONS

## EPIDIDYMITIS AND ORCHITIS

In general, infections are more common in the epididymis than in the testis but may ultimately reach the testis by direct or lymphatic spread. Most cases of epididymitis are secondary to urinary tract infection or to prostatitis. In sexually active men under the age of 35 years, two sexually transmitted pathogens, *Neisseria gonorrhoeae* and *Chlamydia trachomatis*, are the most frequent causes of epididymitis. On the other hand, in men over 35 years, *Escherichia coli* and *Pseudomonas* are responsible for most of the infections.[12] In addition to these organisms, which cause nonspecific epididymitis, genitourinary tuberculosis may also involve the epididymis and produce typical lesions of tuberculosis. The testis may be infected by an extension of the infection from the epididymis. Thus orchitis may develop in association with gonococcal or tubercular epididymitis. On the other hand, organisms such as *Treponema pallidum* and the mumps virus tend to infect the testis without prior epididymitis. Gonorrhea and syphilis, which are sexually transmitted, will be discussed later in this chapter.

With nonspecific infections, the early changes are limited to the epididymis and consist of edema and a nonspecific leukocytic infiltration of the interstitial tissue. Later, the tubules are filled with exudate and there may be abscess formation or a generalized suppurative necrosis. Retrograde spread involves the testis. Any such nonspecific inflammation may become chronic. Pressure within the edematous testis or fibrous scarring of the tubules often leads to sterility. The hardier cells of Leydig usually are spared, so that endocrine function and libido remain intact.

In about 25 to 33% of cases of *mumps* in adult males, an acute interstitial orchitis, usually unilateral but occasionally bilateral, develops about one week after the swelling of the salivary glands. Rarely, cases of mumps orchitis have been described without significant involvement of the salivary glands.

The affected testis swells and, histologically, shows interstitial edema and a patchy mononuclear leukocytic infiltration. Although there is often some degree of atrophy on healing, the patchy nature of the process tends to permit preservation of fertility, even when the process is bilateral. However, when there has been especially intense generalized edema, compression of the blood supply may induce generalized atrophy and lead to sterility.

# Prostate

There are three important lesions of the prostate: *inflammation*, usually as a result of nonspecific infection; *nodular hyperplasia*, commonly known as benign prostatic hypertrophy (BPH); and *carcinoma*. All three cause some degree of enlargement of the prostate. Because the prostate encircles the urethra, any lesion that causes significant prostatic enlargement may easily encroach on the lumen of the urethra. Thus, diseases of the prostate commonly manifest themselves by urinary symptoms. These symptoms are variable but usually include such indications of partial obstruction as frequency of urination, nocturia, and difficulty in initiating or maintaining the stream of urine.

## PROSTATITIS

Inflammations of the prostate may be acute or chronic and are further classified on the basis of bacteriologic findings and examination of prostatic secretions obtained by transrectal prostatic massage.[13] *Bacterial prostatitis*, both acute and chronic, is caused by the same microorganisms that are commonly associated with urinary tract infections (UTI). As might be expected, bacterial infections of the prostate are associated with the presence of inflammatory cells in the prostatic secretions. However, in many patients with symptoms of chronic prostatitis, bacteriologic findings are negative but the presence of prostatic inflammation can be documented by the presence of increased numbers of leukocytes in prostatic secretions. Such *chronic abacterial prostatitis* is perhaps the most common form of prostatitis seen today.[12]

Bacterial prostatitis is caused most commonly by *E. coli*, but other gram-negative pathogens of the urinary tract may also be involved. In acute prostatitis the organisms usually reach the prostate by direct extension from the posterior urethra or the bladder. Chronic bacterial prostatitis may be a sequel to acute prostatitis, but more often it appears insidiously. The etiology of *chronic abacterial prostatitis* is unclear. Since the affected patients are usually 30- to 45-year-old sexually active males, several sexually transmitted pathogens have been implicated. The prime suspects in this group include *Chlamydia trachomatis* and *Ureaplasma urealyticum*, which have also been implicated in the causation of nongonococcal urethritis (p. 625).

Acute prostatitis is characterized by suppuration, either in the form of minute, discrete abscesses or as large, coalescent areas of involvement. Diffuse involvement often leads to soft, boggy enlargement of the entire prostate. Histologically, the gland lumens may become virtually packed with a neutrophilic exudate, and the stroma characteristically contains a nonspecific leukocytic infiltrate.

Because some degree of lymphocytic infiltration of the prostate is a normal accompaniment of aging, the diagnosis of chronic prostatitis should not be made unless other mononuclear leukocytes and neutrophils are also present, along with some evidence of tissue destruction and fibroblastic proliferation.

The development of granulomas without caseous centers may occur as a nonspecific inflammatory response to inspissated prostatic secretions.

Clinically, both acute and chronic prostatitis may be associated with low back pain, dysuria, frequency, and urgency. Sometimes the prostate is enlarged and tender. With acute disease, systemic signs of acute inflammation, including fever and malaise, may be present. In contrast, many cases of chronic bacterial prostatitis are asymptomatic. Since most antibiotics penetrate the prostate poorly, bacteria find safe haven in the parenchyma and constantly seed the urinary tract. Thus *in men chronic bacterial prostatitis is the most common cause of recurrent UTI caused by the same pathogen.*

## NODULAR HYPERPLASIA OF THE PROSTATE (BENIGN PROSTATIC HYPERTROPHY)

This is an extremely common disorder charcterized by the development of large, fairly discrete nodules within the prostate. By long-standing tradition, this entity is known as "benign prostatic hypertrophy" or BPH. This, however, is a misnomer, since the basic process is hyperplasia rather than hypertrophy and, in either case, the qualification "benign" is redundant.

Beginning in the fifth decade of life, there is a progressive increase in incidence of nodular hyperplasia with age, until about 95% of men beyond the age of 75 years are affected. Fortunately, most of those affected are not seriously inconvenienced.

The cause of this lesion is unknown, but current opinion favors an endocrine basis.[14] Both androgens and estrogens are involved. Dihydrotestosterone, which is the biologically active metabolite of testosterone, is believed to be the ultimate mediator of hyperplasia. It has been suggested that estrogens "sensitize" the prostatic tissues to the growth-promoting effects of dihydrotestosterone. This would explain the synergism between estrogens and androgens observed in experimentally induced prostatic hyperplasia in the canine model. In humans, it is postulated that the increase in the level of estrogens that occurs with aging may facilitate the action of androgens within the prostate, even in the face of declining testicular output of testosterone.

**MORPHOLOGY.** In the typical case, the prostatic nodules weigh between 60 and 100 gm; aggregate weights of up to 200 gm are seen. The nodules characteristically originate around the urethra in the median lobe and more central portions of the lateral lobes. The ducts of the affected glands almost always drain proximal to the verumontanum. **This distribution is in striking contrast to that of prostatic carcinoma, which usually involves the posterior lobe.** Although the nodules do not have a true capsule, they are well demarcated on cross section because of the compression of the surrounding parenchyma. The urethra may be compressed to a slitlike orifice by nodules on its lateral aspects. The hyperplastic median lobe projects up into the floor of the urethra in a hemispheric mass, sometimes having the effect of a ball valve (Fig. 18–6).

In most cases, the hyperplasia is seen microscopically to result primarily from glandular proliferation, although smooth muscles and fibroblasts are also frequently involved.[15] The new glands are variable in size, often lined by hypertrophic tall columnar epithelium that is characteristically thrown into numerous papillary buds and infoldings. The gland formations are well developed and are separated from each other by stroma, however scant. Numerous small foci of hyaline concretions, termed corpora amylacea, are nested within these glands. Aggregates of lymphocytes are commonly found within the stroma. Sometimes the hyperplasia is predominantly fibromuscular, and in these cases the nodules may appear microscopically as almost solid masses of spindle cells. Whether glandular or fibromuscular, small areas of ischemic necrosis surrounded by margins of squamous metaplasia may be seen within the nodules or in the surrounding prostatic tissue. In addition, squamous metaplasia of the periurethral glands, which may be mistaken for carcinoma, is a common accompaniment of nodular hyperplasia.

**CLINICAL COURSE.** The clinical significance of nodular hyperplasia lies entirely in its tendency to produce urinary tract obstruction by impinging upon the urethra. Despite the prevalence of this disorder, however, not more than 10% of men with this condition require surgical relief of the obstruction. Early symptoms include difficulty in starting, maintaining, and stopping the stream of urine. There may also be frequency and nocturia, presumably because the raised level of the urethral floor leads to retention in the bladder of a large volume of residual urine after micturition. Hydronephrosis may ensue (see p. 486), as may infection, the all-too-frequent companion of obstruction. It had been suggested that patients with nodular hyperplasia of the prostate have a higher risk of developing cancer. However, current opinion does not favor nodular hyperplasia as a premalignant lesion.

## CARCINOMA OF PROSTATE

Carcinoma of the prostate is an extremely common cancer. Approximately 75,000 new patients are diagnosed every year in the United States, of whom 25,000 succumb to their disease. Its incidence, estimated to be 19% of all cancers in men, is second

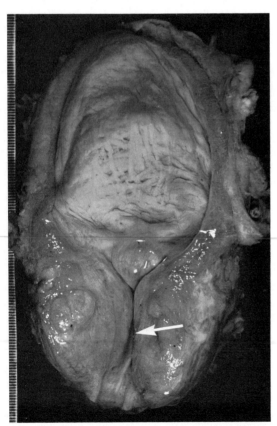

Figure 18–6. Nodular hyperplasia of the prostate. The urinary bladder and prostatic urethra have been opened. The enlargement of the prostate is seen as the two masses flanking the urethra (*arrow*). A median lobe projects under the floor of the bladder as a hemispheric mass.

only to lung cancer (22%). Prostatic cancer is a disease of men over the age of 50, reaching a peak incidence around 75 years, when it is the second leading cause of cancer death in males. In addition to these clinically evident tumors, there are many more latent, small foci of cancer found incidentally at autopsy or on histologic examination of glands removed for nodular hyperplasia. As will be discussed later, most of these localized lesions, classified as Stage $A_1$ cancers, progress so slowly that those who harbor them die of unrelated causes.

**ETIOLOGY AND PATHOGENESIS.** The etiologic influences responsible for carcinoma of the prostate are not definitely known. As with nodular hyperplasia, its incidence increases with age, and it is speculated that the endocrine changes of old age are related to its origin. Support for this general thesis lies in the inhibition of these tumors that can be achieved with orchiectomy or estrogen therapy. Neoplastic epithelial cells, like their normal counterparts, possess steroid (androgen and estrogen) receptors, which would suggest responsiveness to hormones. However, no significant or consistent alterations in the metabolism of the steroid hormones have been disclosed in any studies. It seems more likely, therefore, that the role of hormones in this malignancy is essentially permissive. Androgens are required for the maintenance of the prostatic epithelium, which is then transformed by agents not yet characterized.

Epidemiologic studies are of interest in seeking the causation of carcinoma of the prostate. The Scandinavian countries show a very high death rate from this form of cancer, whereas at the other extreme, the Japanese are relatively free of the disease. The United States occupies an intermediate position. Immigrants from low-risk to high-risk geographic areas acquire an intermediate risk of developing this tumor, suggesting a role for environmental factors.

Genetic influences also seem to be involved, since there is a tendency toward familial aggregation and in the United States blacks are affected much more frequently than whites.

**MORPHOLOGY.** Prostatic carcinoma usually begins in the peripheral zones of the prostate but can arise anywhere in the gland, usually in multiple foci, which fuse to form a single mass. Grossly, the tumor often blends imperceptibly into the background of the gland, although it may be apparent by its firm, gritty texture or by a color somewhat yellower than the surrounding tissue. Histologically, most of these lesions are adenocarcinomas of varying degrees of differentiation (Fig. 18–7). In well-differentiated tumors the acini are smaller than normal, closely spaced (back to back), and lined by a single layer of cuboidal epithelium. The neoplastic epithelium may be thrown into folds, which may fuse and give rise to a cribriform pattern. When gland formation is orderly, it may be difficult histologically to distinguish carcinoma of the prostate from nodular hyperplasia. In these cases, the distinction may rest on the presence of invasion of blood vessels, perineurial and perivascular spaces, or the pros-

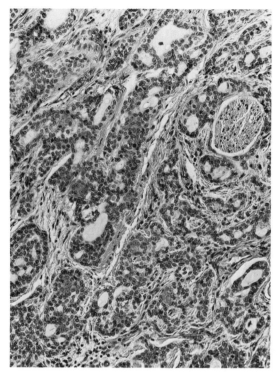

Figure 18–7. Carcinoma of the prostate. The neoplastic gland patterns are small and disorderly and, at the upper right, have encircled and permeated a perineurial space.

tatic capsule. In the undifferentiated tumors the malignant epithelial cells may diffusely infiltrate the stroma without any gland formation. Concomitantly, the cells display obvious cytologic features of malignancy. Several grading systems based on the degree of differentiation, glandular architecture, and extent of cellular atypicality have been described.[16] In general there is an excellent correlation between the degree of differentiation, anatomic extent (stage), and prognosis. Hence grading is of considerable value in the treatment of prostate cancer.

Stroma in between the glands is sometimes abundant and fibrous. This may be responsible for the hard (scirrhous) consistency. Distant spread of prostatic cancer occurs via both lymphatics and the bloodstream. Metastases to the regional lymph nodes occur early and may often precede vascular spread. Osseous metastases constitute the most common form of hematogenous spread. Metastatic lesions in the bones, involving mainly the axial skeleton (pelvis, ribs, spine), may be osteoclastic (destructive) or more commonly osteoblastic (bone-forming).

**CLINICAL COURSE.** The symptoms as well as prognosis depend upon the anatomic extent and spread of the tumor. Four clinical stages (Fig. 18–8) are defined. As might be expected, Stage A tumors are asymptomatic and discovered on histologic examination of prostatectomy specimens. The incidence of Stage A cancers increases with age and approaches 60% or more in men past the age of 80 years. Due to their slow rate of progression, Stage $A_1$ lesions are lethal only in a small percentage of patients. Stage

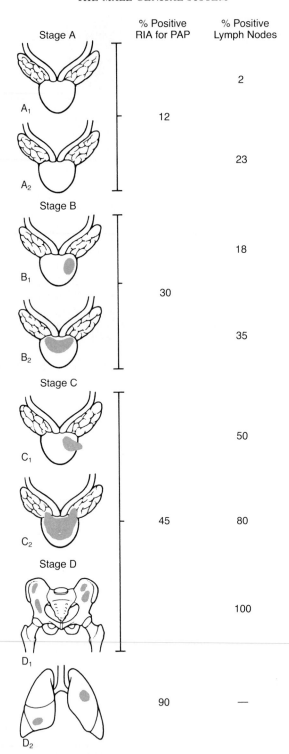

|  | % Positive RIA for PAP | % Positive Lymph Nodes |
|---|---|---|
| Stage A | | |
| $A_1$ | 12 | 2 |
| $A_2$ | | 23 |
| Stage B | | |
| $B_1$ | 30 | 18 |
| $B_2$ | | 35 |
| Stage C | | |
| $C_1$ | 45 | 50 |
| $C_2$ | | 80 |
| Stage D | | |
| $D_1$ | 90 | 100 |
| $D_2$ | | — |

**Figure 18–8.** Schematic illustration of a staging system for cancer of the prostate. For each stage, the percentage of cases with elevated prostatic acid phosphatase (PAP), detected by radioimmunoassay (RIA), and the frequency of lymph node involvement are also indicated. In Stage A, the tumor is microscopic. It is either unifocal and well differentiated (Stage $A_1$), or it is multifocal or poorly differentiated, or both (Stage $A_2$). Stage B cancers are palpable by digital rectal examination but confined to the prostate. Stage $B_1$ cancers involve only one lobe, whereas lesions in Stage $B_2$ extend into more than one lobe. Stage C includes tumors that have involved the periprostatic tissue but have not produced distant metastases. Cancers in Stage $C_1$ do not involve seminal vesicles and are less than 70 gm in weight, whereas those in Stage $C_2$ are larger than 70 gm and extend into the seminal vesicles. Stage D defines tumors with distant metastases. In Stage $D_1$ the metastases are confined to regional (pelvic) nodes, but the presence of extrapelvic metastases indicates Stage $D_2$. (Data from Catalona, W. J.: Prostate Cancer. New York, Grune & Stratton, Inc., 1984, p. 60.)

$A_2$ lesions, however, are more ominous, leading to death with distant metastases in 20% of untreated cases. Stage B prostate cancers are palpable by rectal digital examination. However, because of their peripheral location and small size, they do not encroach upon the urethra, and hence urinary symptoms are absent. Up to 35% of Stage B cancers have lymph node metastases. Patients with lesions in Stage C or D usually present with urinary symptoms such as dysuria, slow urinary stream, or urinary retention. Local pain in the perineum and rectum are late symptoms. Some patients in Stage D may present initially with bone pain produced by osseous metastases.

Careful digital rectal examination is a very useful and direct method for detection of early prostatic carcinoma, since the posterior location of most tumors renders them easily palpable. A transperineal or transrectal needle biopsy can confirm the diagnosis. Lymphangiography and CT scans provide tools for detection of lymph node metastases. Osseous metastases may be detected by x-rays or the much more sensitive radionuclide bone scanning. Immunohistochemical stains for prostatic acid phosphatase and prostate-specific tissue antigen are helpful in deciding whether a metastatic tumor originated in the prostate.

Acid phosphatase is normally released into the blood in small quantities by the prostate. Elevated levels detected by enzymatic assays are found mainly in patients with advanced prostatic cancer (Stages C and D). Radioimmunoassays for prostatic acid phosphatase are more sensitive than the enzymatic assays, but their value as screening tests for early (Stage A) prostatic cancer has not been proved.

Cancer of the prostate is treated by surgery, radiotherapy, and hormonal manipulations. As might be expected, surgery and radiotherapy are most suited for treatment of patients with localized (Stage A or B) disease. Fifty to 80% of patients in this group can expect to live for 10 years. Endocrine therapy is the mainstay for treatment of advanced, metastatic carcinoma. Since prostatic cancer cells are dependent on androgens for their sustenance, the aim of endocrine manipulations is to deprive the tumor cells of testosterone. This is readily achieved by orchiectomy or administration of estrogens or synthetic agonists of luteinizing hormone–releasing hormone (LHRH). Although estrogens can inhibit testicular androgen synthesis directly, their principal effect appears to be suppression of pituitary luteinizing hormone (LH) secretion, which in turn leads to reduced testicular output of testosterone. Synthetic analogs of LHRH act similarly. Long-term administration of LHRH agonists (after an initial transient increase in LH secretion) suppress LH release, achieving in effect a pharmacologic orchiectomy. Despite all the treatments, patients with disseminated cancers have a 10 to 40% ten-year survival rate.

# Venereal Disease

The term "venereal disease" refers to disorders that are sexually transmitted. Historically, five "classic" venereal diseases have been recognized—syphilis, gonorrhea, chancroid, granuloma inguinale, and lymphogranuloma venereum. In the past decade, however, the spectrum of sexually transmitted disease (STD) has widened considerably (Table 18–3). A new group of syndromes primarily affecting homosexual men has emerged. These include infections by enteric pathogens such as *Entamoeba histolytica, Giardia lamblia,* and *Shigella* sp., acquired probably by oral-anal contact. In addition, venereal transmission of viral infections such as hepatitis B and possibly cytomegalovirus (agents that are predominantly spread by other routes) is also becoming increasingly recognized.

In epidemiologic studies, sexual preference has clearly emerged as an important factor in the incidence of most STD. Homosexual males appear to be at increased risk for the enteric pathogens mentioned above; in addition, the infection rates of virtually all the major STDs, including syphilis and gonorrhea, are significantly higher in homosexual men.[17] HTLV-III, the virus believed to be responsible for the acquired immunodeficiency syndrome (AIDS) is also transmitted by the venereal route in homosexual males (p. 176). Discussion of the entire range of venereal disease listed in Table 18–3 is beyond our scope. Some, such as hepatitis B, are discussed elsewhere (p. 571); others, such as *Trichomonas vaginitis,* do not cause serious morbidity and will not be presented.

## GONORRHEA

With the possible exception of nongonococcal urethritis, gonorrhea is the most frequent of the venereal diseases. If affects approximately 2,000,000 Americans per year, with about 60% of reported cases occurring in males. Most infections occur in the 15- to 30-year age group; the peak is between 20 and 24 years of age.

The organism that causes gonorrhea is *Neisseria gonorrhoeae,* a gram-negative diplococcus identical in appearance to the meningococcus. Much has been learned about the basis for the virulence of the gonococcus.[18] Several components of its cell wall are associated with virulence:

○ *Pili,* which are seen as filamentous protrusions under the electron microscope, are believed to

### Table 18–3. CLASSIFICATION OF IMPORTANT SEXUALLY TRANSMITTED DISEASES*

| Pathogens | Disease or Syndrome and Primary Population Affected | | |
| --- | --- | --- | --- |
| | *Male* | *Both* | *Female* |
| *Viruses:* | | | |
| Herpes simplex virus | | Primary and recurrent herpes Neonatal herpes | Carcinoma of cervix (?) |
| Hepatitis B virus | †Hepatitis | | |
| Human papilloma virus (genital wart virus) | Cancer of penis(?) | Condyloma acuminatum | Cervical dysplasia and cancer, vulvar cancer (?) |
| Cytomegalovirus (?) | | Congenital infection, infant mortality, birth defects | Cervicitis (?) |
| HTLV-III/HIV | †AIDS | | |
| *Chlamydia:* | | | |
| *Chlamydia trachomatis* | Urethritis Epididymitis Proctitis | Lymphogranuloma venereum | Urethral syndrome Cervicitis Salpingitis Bartholinitis |
| *Mycoplasmata:* | | | |
| *Ureaplasma urealyticum* | Urethritis | | Salpingitis |
| *Bacteria:* | | | |
| *Neisseria gonorrhoeae* | Epididymitis Prostatitis Urethral stricture | Urethritis Proctitis Pharyngitis Disseminated gonococcal infection | Cervicitis Endometritis Bartholinitis Salpingitis and sequelae (infertility, ectopic pregnancy, recurrent salpingitis) |
| *Treponema pallidum* | | Syphilis | |
| *Haemophilus ducreyi* | | Chancroid | |
| *Calymmatobacterium granulomatis* | | Granuloma inguinale (donovanosis) | |
| *Shigella* | †Enterocolitis | | |
| *Campylobacter* | †Enterocolitis | | |
| *Protozoa:* | | | |
| *Trichomonas vaginalis* | Urethritis Balanitis | | Vaginitis |
| *Entamoeba histolytica* | †Amebiasis | | |
| *Giardia lamblia* | †Giardiasis | | |

*Modified from Krieger, J. N.: Biology of sexual transmitted diseases. Urol. Clin. North Am. *11*:15, 1984.
†Most important in homosexual populations.

favor adherence to mucosal cells, inhibit phagocytosis, and attach to sperm.

○ Components of the *outer membrane protein* induce adherence to epithelial cells and also promote intergonococcal association. Clumps of organisms are less readily phagocytosed.

○ *Lipopolysaccharide*, found in the cell wall, is toxic to ciliated fallopian tube cells and may also confer resistance to complement-mediated lysis.

Infection with the gonococcus does not confer immunity, and reinfection may occur virtually as often as the individual is exposed. The record that nobody seems interested in "besting" is said to be 45 acute attacks. Although urethral and vaginal secretions from infected patients contain secretory IgA and IgG directed against pili, many pathogenic strains contain specific proteases that neutralize the effects of these antibodies. Like the other pyogenic cocci, this organism evokes a nonspecific, neutrophilic inflammatory reaction manifested by the production of copious amounts of yellow pus.

**MORPHOLOGY.** Two to seven days after exposure, the anterior urethra and meatus of the male become hyperemic and edematous and exude a mucopurulent material. At this stage the major symptoms are dysuria and increased frequency. Symptomatic men who seek treatment are easily cured and the disease does not progress any further. **However, males with mild symptoms who fail to obtain treatment become the major reservoir of infection.**

Unless there is prompt and adequate therapy, gonorrhea tends to spread upward in the genital tract. In the male, the prostate, seminal vesicles, and epididymides may become involved, producing marked perineal or scrotal pain and fever. With chronicity, abscess formation and tissue destruction occur in these organs. The testes are relatively resistant to gonococcal infection. Urethral strictures may develop, sometimes leading to hydronephrosis and serious secondary pyelonephritis. Most of these complications are fairly uncommon in countries with adequate health care delivery systems.

In the female, the initial involvement is in the urethra and the endocervical canal. Reddening and edema of the urethral meatus, however, is less conspicuous than in males. Bartholin's and Skene's glands are also involved early in the course of infection. The stratified squamous epithelium of the vagina is resistant to infections, hence vaginitis does not occur. The symptoms of gonococcal infection in the female reflect the involvement of the lower urogenital tract and include dysuria, excessive vaginal discharge, and intermenstrual bleeding. As in the male, untreated gonorrhea tends to spread upward and in the female involves one or both fallopian tubes. In sexually active females the upward spread of gonococci is believed to occur by their ability to adhere to human sperm. The gonococci thus "hitch-hike" on the sperm on their upward journey.[18] Approximately 30% of women with gonorrhea develop salpingitis. The lumens of the affected oviducts become filled with purulent exudate, creating a **pyosalpinx** (pus tube). At first, the exudate may leak out of the tubal fimbriae, but often the fimbriae eventually become sealed, sometimes against the ovary, producing a **salpingo-oophoritis.** As pus collects in these sealed tubes, they become distended, occasionally attaining a diameter of 10 cm or more. A localized pelvic peritonitis commonly is present, with a tendency toward formation of extensive adhesions. This pattern of inflammatory involvement in the female is known as **pelvic inflammatory disease (PID).** Since gonococcal salpingitis is just one of a number of causes of PID, this entity is also described in Chapter 19. Permanent sterility almost always results when cases of gonorrhea are neglected in either sex.

In homosexual males, and less frequently in heterosexual males or females, anorectal and pharyngeal infections may be the initial sites of infection. **Disseminated gonococcal infection (DGI)** occurs in 1 to 3% of recently infected patients and can occur in two settings.[19] Most commonly it occurs in asymptomatic carrier males and is caused by strains of gonococci that are uniquely resistant to complement-mediated lysis by antibodies present in normal serum (called AHU auxotype). The other setting is composed of individuals genetically deficient in late-acting complement components C6, C7, and C8. A strong association has also been noted between disseminated meningococcal infection and complement deficiency. The dissemination of gonococci occurs via the bloodstream, and the most common manifestation is the **arthritis-dermatitis syndrome.** The joint involvement takes the form of suppurative arthritis or tenosynovitis, and the skin lesions take the form of petechiae, pustules, or hemorrhages. Other manifestations of DGI include endocarditis and meningitis. A tragic complication of gonorrhea that has become rare due to the use of prophylactic antibiotics is gonococcal **ophthalmia neonatorum,** caused by contamination of an infant's eyes as it passes through the birth canal of its infected mother.

In summary, gonorrhea may be an asymptomatic infection or may produce local symptoms in the lower urogenital tract, which can be readily treated without any long-term sequelae. Approximately 80 to 90% of the cases remain uncomplicated in the United States. Local complication in the urogenital tract is uncommon but leads to serious morbidity. The spectrum of

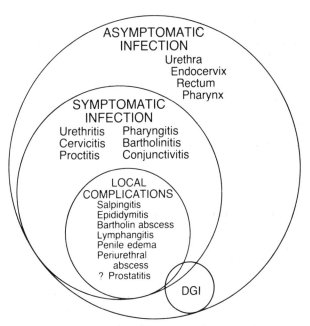

Figure 18–9. Clinical spectrum of gonococcal infection. DGI = disseminated gonococcal infection. (From Holmes, K. K., et al. (eds.): Sexually Transmitted Diseases. New York, McGraw-Hill Book Co., 1984, p. 207. Reproduced by permission.)

gonococcal infections is depicted in Figure 18–9. The diagnosis of gonorrhea rests on identification of typical gram-negative diplococci within the leukocytes in Gram-stained smears obtained from discharge or by culture. By these techniques almost 100% of the cases can be diagnosed.

Penicillin has been the mainstay of treatment for several decades. However, recently penicillinase-producing gonococci have been identified in several parts of the world. The incidence of infections with such penicillin-resistant organisms in the United States has been steadily increasing for the last several years.

## NONGONOCOCCAL URETHRITIS

Nongonococcal urethritis (NGU) is a venereal disease that mimics gonococcal urethritis in males. It is not a reportable disease in the United States and hence accurate estimates of its incidence are not available. However, recent data suggest that NGU is much more prevalent than gonorrhea.[20]

Various organisms have been implicated in the etiology of NGU. These include *Chlamydia trachomatis*, which is responsible for 40 to 50% of cases, and *Ureaplasma urealyticum*, suspected to be the causative agent in 30% of the cases. In the remaining cases (approximately 20%), no etiologic agent can be identified. The chlamydiae, like viruses, are obligate intracellular organisms but they contain both RNA and DNA and possess ribosomes and cell walls,

**Table 18–4.** HUMAN DISEASES CAUSED
BY CHLAMYDIA*

| Species | Serotype† | Disease |
| --- | --- | --- |
| C. psittaci | Many unidenti- fied serotypes | Psittacosis |
| C. trachomatis | L-1, L-2, L-3 | Lymphogranuloma venereum |
| C. trachomatis | A, B, Ba, C | Hyperendemic blinding trachoma |
| C. trachomatis | D, E, F, G, H, I, J, K | Inclusion conjunctivitis (adult and newborn), nongonococcal urethritis, cervicitis, salpingitis, proctitis, epididymitis, and pneumonia of newborns |

*From Schachter, J.: Chylamydial infection. N. Engl. J. Med. 298:428, 1978. Reprinted by permission of the New England Journal of Medicine.

†Predominant, but not exclusive, association of serotype with disease.

thereby resembling gram-negative bacteria. They require tissue culture techniques for isolation and are classified as a group distinct from bacteria and viruses.[21] The diseases caused by chlamydiae are listed in Table 18–4. Although the evidence supporting a pathogenic role for *C. trachomatis* is fairly strong, the same cannot be said for *U. urealyticum.*[22] Definitive evidence implicating *U. urealyticum* in the causation of NGU is complicated by the fact that approximately 50 to 70% of sexually experienced men and women are asymptomatic carriers of this mycoplasma. Nevertheless, most authorities accept that in some individuals *U. urealyticum* is indeed pathogenic and gives rise to urethritis in men and possibly pelvic inflammatory disease in women.

The clinical features of NGU resemble those of gonococcal urethritis, already discussed. However, the symptoms are usually milder, and serious complications are much less common. NGU, unlike gonorrhea, responds to tetracyclines but not to penicillin; this is an important reason to distinguish between the two conditions. *The diagnosis is established by exclusion of gonococcal urethritis by smear and culture.*

Positive identification of *C. trachomatis* by culture is not available routinely. Detection of chlamydial antigens in secretions is possible by reaction with monoclonal antibodies, and this method is becoming increasingly useful in the diagnosis.[23] Whether there is a female counterpart of NGU is uncertain. By convention, the term NGU is not used in women, although it is very likely that *C. trachomatis* is responsible for some cases of urethritis in women.

## SYPHILIS (LUES)

Syphilis is far less frequent than gonorrhea, and efforts to control it have been more successful. Its incidence increased dramatically during World War II; then, with the advent of penicillin and the return to peacetime conditions, it declined to a low point in 1977. Since then, there has been some resurgence

in the incidence of syphilis, but, fortunately, its occurrence is still well below World War II levels. Syphilis is now increasingly a disease of younger males, approximately 50% of whom are homosexual or bisexual.[24]

The causative organism of syphilis is the spirochete *Treponema pallidum,* which is transmitted either by venereal contact or by an infected mother to the fetus in utero. The extreme vulnerability of *Treponema* to drying probably precludes any other mode of transmission. These organisms can rapidly traverse intact mucous membranes and abraded skin, but little is known about their precise mechanism of toxicity. Isolation of toxins and characterization of treponemal antigens have been greatly hampered by the inability to culture these bacteria in vitro. The immune responses and immunologically mediated protection against syphilis have remained enigmatic. Those who develop an initial infection (primary syphilis) usually heal spontaneously and develop resistance to reinfections. Yet most of these apparently "resistant" individuals go on to develop disseminated (secondary) syphilis. The presence of a humoral immune response can be inferred from the appearance of two distinct antibodies in the serum: (1) a *nontreponemal antibody,* which by long tradition is called reagin although it is not an IgE, and which reacts with a lipid antigen derived from beef heart (cardiolipin), and (2) *specific antibodies to treponemal antigens.* These antibodies are not protective, but their detection is an important step in the diagnosis of syphilis. The reaginic antibody is commonly detected by a flocculation test, called the VDRL (Venereal Disease Research Laboratory) test, and the rapid plasma reagin test. These tests are not specific, and there are a number of biologic false-positive (BFP) results with other disorders such as infectious mononucleosis, mycoplasmal pneumonia, autoimmune diseases (e.g., systemic lupus erythematosus), and nearly any acute febrile illness. One commonly used method for detection of specific treponemal antibody is the fluorescent treponemal antibody (FTA) test. The FTA is based on indirect immunofluorescence. False-positive test results are relatively infrequent. The detailed application of these tests has been recently reviewed.[25]

**MORPHOLOGY.** Syphilis may affect nearly any organ or tissue in the body. **In all sites, it evokes one of two morphologic patterns of tissue injury.** One of these is a type of vasculitis, termed obliterative endarteritis, which is characterized by a concentric endothelial and fibroblastic proliferative thickening of the small vessels in an involved area and a surrounding mononuclear (principally plasma cell) inflammatory infiltrate, known as **perivascular cuffing.**

The second pattern of tissue injury seen years after the initial infection is a lesion known as a **gumma,** which, on occasion, may be difficult to distinguish from the lesions of tuberculosis. Gummas consist of a center of coagulative necrosis in which the native cells are barely discernible as shadowy outlines. This focus is surrounded by macrophages (some resembling epithelioid cells) admixed with mononuclear leukocytes (principally plasma cells) and enclosed by a fibroblastic wall. The small vessels in the enclosing inflammatory wall may show obliterative endarteritis and perivascular cuffing. With difficulty, treponemes may be demonstrated in the reactive inflammatory zone. Gummas are infrequent late lesions and may occur in any site of the body, most often in the liver, bones, and testes. They vary in size from microscopic defects to grossly visible tumorous masses of necrotic material. Erosion of a cutaneous or mucosal gumma may yield a persistent, shaggy ulcer that shows a surprising resistance to local therapeutic measures.

**CLINICAL COURSE.** *Clinically, acquired (untreated) syphilitic infection is characterized by three fairly distinct stages,* which will be discussed separately. The disease is infectious only in the first two stages. In addition, congenital syphilis may be looked upon as a fourth distinctive entity.

*Primary Syphilis.* This stage is marked by the development of a *chancre* at the site of inoculation, usually on the penis or on the vulva or cervix, within one week to three months after exposure. Usually there is an accompanying, painless, nonspecific regional lymphadenopathy. The primary chancre begins as a single indurated, button-like papule, up to several centimeters in diameter, which erodes to create a clean-based, shallow ulceration on an elevated base. The most distinctive histologic feature, deep within the base, is the obliterative endarteritis with perivascular plasma cell cuffing, so characteristic of lues. The more superficial reaction consists of a nonspecific diffuse mononuclear leukocytic infiltrate. Although a systemic spirochetemia occurs within a day of infection and persists for weeks to years, the patient feels well at this state. The results of nontreponemal antibody tests are positive in approximately 25%, 50%, and 75% of the patients within the first, second, and third weeks, respectively. *Since the serologic test results may be negative in early cases, direct demonstration of the treponemes by dark-field examination of the exudate is extremely important in the diagnosis of primary syphilis.* The chancre slowly heals spontaneously. Approximately 50% of female patients and 30% of males do not notice the primary lesion.

*Secondary Syphilis.* From one to three months after the development of the primary chancre, a *widespread patchy or diffuse mucocutaneous rash* ensues, accompanied by a generalized, nonspecific lymphadenopathy. This marks the second systemic stage of syphilis. The lesions that constitute the rash are extremely variable. Most commonly, they are bilaterally symmetrical and maculopapular; each red-brown lesion is 5 to 10 mm in diameter. In other cases, however, follicular, pustular, annular, or scaling lesions may be seen. Histologically, the lesions show typical vasculitis, perhaps with a less marked

mononuclear infiltrate, and spirochetes are present. In the external genital and anogenital regions the lesions may take the form of large, elevated plaques, designated *condylomata lata.* Constitutional symptoms such as fever, malaise, and weight loss may also be experienced. Hepatitis, arthritis, and meningeal involvement are seen only in a small minority of cases. By this stage serologic test results are positive in almost all patients.

*Latent Syphilis.* Virtually all the untreated patients with secondary syphilis remit spontaneously within four to 12 weeks and enter a phase called *latent syphilis.* During this period, they are asymptomatic, but serologic markers of previous syphilitic infection remain positive. The outcome of latent syphilis is extremely variable. Some patients develop relapses of secondary syphilis; others remain asymptomatic for several years before they develop lesions characteristic of tertiary or late syphilis. Pregnant females may transmit the infection to their offspring, who are born with congenital syphilis. The vast majority, however, remain asymptomatic and never develop progressive disease.

*Tertiary Syphilis.* In only about one third of patients with untreated syphilis does the disease ever progress to this stage, and, of these, about half remain asymptomatic. When tertiary syphilis develops after a period of latency lasting from one to 30 years it may affect any part of the body, but it shows a predilection for the cardiovascular system (80 to 85%) and the central nervous system (5 to 10%). Cardiovascular syphilis and its complications are discussed on page 301. Other organs may be involved, singly or concurrently, giving rise to truly protean and often confusing clinical findings. In the liver, gummas may produce the coarsely nodular pattern of cirrhosis, termed *hepar lobatum* because of the simulation of multiple irregular lobes by the deep scars. Bone and joint gummas lead to areas of cortical and articular destruction. Pathologic fractures and joint immobilization may result. Testicular gummas often cause painless enlargement of the affected testis, thus simulating a tumor. In general, tertiary syphilis is becoming increasingly rare.

*Congenital Syphilis.* Syphilis may be transmitted to the fetus by an infected mother for a variable period of months to years after she contracts the disease, presumably until the spirochetemia has abated. Transmission may occur at any time during gestation, but the stigmata of congenital syphilis develop only in fetuses affected after the fourth month. Depending upon the magnitude of the infection, the fetus may die in utero or soon after birth, or it may survive. Surviving infants usually show a widespread, rather fulminant infection with spirochetemia that differs from any of the classic stages of acquired syphilis. The most striking lesions affect the mucocutaneous surfaces and the bones. A diffuse maculopapular rash develops, which differs from that of acquired syphilis by its tendency to cause extensive desquamation of the skin. A generalized osteochondritis and perichondritis are present. Destruction of the vomer of the nose produces the characteristic *saddle deformity*, inflammatory proliferation of the anterior surface of the tibiae causes the typical anterior bowing of *saber shins*, and dental malformations create wedge-shaped notched incisors (hutchinsonian incisors) and "mulberry molars." A diffuse interstitial inflammatory reaction with prominent fibrosis may affect any organ of the body. In particular, the liver and lungs are frequently involved and can exhibit severe functional impairment. The eyes commonly show an interstitial keratitis or a choroiditis, and sometimes there are areas of abnormal pigmentation of the retinae.

Occasionally, congenital syphilis remains latent until early adulthood and then simulates tertiary syphilis in its manifestations, with the formation of gummas and the frequent development of neurosyphilis.

## PAPILLOMA (CONDYLOMA ACUMINATUM)

This sexually transmitted disease takes the form of a benign tumor and is caused by human papilloma virus (subtypes 6 and 11). It is related to the common wart (verruca vulgaris) and may occur on any moist mucocutaneous surface of the external genitals in both males and females. It should not be confused with the condyloma lata of secondary syphilis.

In males most often, the tumors are seen about the coronal sulcus and inner surface of the prepuce and range from minute sessile or pedunculated excrescences of 1 mm in diameter to large, raspberry-like masses several centimeters in diameter. Histologically, there is a villous connective tissue stroma covered by hyperplastic epithelium that shows perinuclear vacuolization (koilocytosis, p. 633). Such cells are characteristic of human papilloma virus infection. The basement membrane is intact, and there is no evidence of invasion of the underlying stroma. Malignant transformation to carcinoma of the penis, although reported in some cases, is uncommon.

## CHANCROID, GRANULOMA INGUINALE, AND LYMPHOGRANULOMA VENEREUM

These are three distinct venereal diseases caused by three different infectious organisms. The diseases, however, are often confused because of their *common tendency to produce ulcerative lesions of the external genitalia and sometimes tender inflammatory swelling* (buboes) *of the inguinal lymph nodes.*

**CHANCROID (SOFT CHANCRE).** This is an acute process caused by the gram-negative coccobacillus *Haemophilus ducreyi.* It is characterized by the development of a necrotic ulcer at the site of inoculation on the genitals and by suppurative inflammation in the regional lymph nodes.

Within three to five days after exposure, a small maculopapular lesion appears on the penis or vulva, followed over the next few days by rapid pustule formation and sloughing of the overlying skin, producing an ulcer between 1 and 3 cm in diameter. This bears a superficial resemblance to the chancre of syphilis, but unlike the syphilitic "hard chancre" it is painful and lacks induration. Histologically, the superficial necrotic debris covers a zone of granulation tissue and vasculitis, and this in turn overlies a zone of chronic inflammatory changes, with fibroblastic proliferation and mononuclear leukocytic infiltration. Often, autoinoculation produces multiple lesions. In about 50% of cases, within two weeks after the appearance of the ulcer, the inguinal lymph nodes become enlarged and exquisitely tender. The histologic changes in the lymph nodes are essentially similar to those of the skin ulcer. There may be central abscess formation. Sometimes these abscesses drain to the surface.

Diagnosis is by tissue biopsy and identification of the organisms in smears or by culture. The course is usually self-limited, leaving only fibrous induration of the affected nodes and a scar at the site of the skin lesion.

**DONOVANOSIS.** This disorder is also known as *granuloma inguinale,* and in contrast to chancroid, it is a chronic rather than an acute process caused by the gram-negative coccobacillus *Calymmatobacterium granulomatis.* It is distinctive in its tendency to produce large, irregular ulcers that form keloid-like scars upon healing. Lymph nodes are generally spared. However, the extensive scarring may eventually produce lymphatic obstruction, which results in elephantiasis of the external genitalia. Although the sexual partners of patients are not always affected, it is thought to be a venereal disease, possibly of relatively low infectivity.

The initial lesion is a papule at the site of inoculation, usually on the external genitalia, which develops into a spreading, necrotic ulcer with a raised inflammatory border. Microabscesses form in the advancing margin of the lesion, and satellite papules and ulcers may appear along the course of lymphatic drainage. The lesion is characterized histologically by nonspecific acute and chronic inflammation, accompanied by an exuberant granulation tissue. The most distinctive finding is of large, vacuolated macrophages containing many faintly blue, dot-like phagocytized organisms, termed Donovan bodies.

Diagnosis is by the demonstration of Donovan bodies either in smears or in tissue biopsies. Rarely, the organism becomes widely disseminated, and may even cause death.

**LYMPHOGRANULOMA VENEREUM (LYMPHOGRANULOMA INGUINALE).** This disorder is caused by *Chlamydia trachomatis.* As seen in Table 18–4 (p. 626), lymphogranuloma venereum and NGU are caused by distinct serotypes of the same organism.

The disease is characterized by ulceration of the external genitalia, but unlike the case in donovanosis, there is prominent involvement of the lymph nodes. In most cases the genital ulcers are small and inconspicuous, and the patients present initially with lymphadenopathy. Histologically, the lesions show a granulomatous reaction with central suppuration. In late stages the lymph nodes become matted, and lymphatic obstruction leads to elephantiasis of the genitalia. The late sequelae tend to be much more serious in the female. Whereas in males the nodal involvement remains limited to the inguinal region, in females vaginal or posterior perineal lesions lead to involvement of the perirectal and deep pelvic nodes. Such involvement produces chronic fibrosis about the rectum, with resultant rectal strictures.

Lymphogranuloma venereum, then, should be considered when rectal obstruction in the female is evaluated. The laboratory diagnosis depends upon a complement fixation test. The Frei skin test is less sensitive and no longer widely used.

## HERPES GENITALIS

Herpes genitalis is caused by the herpes simplex virus (HSV). Although most (75 to 80%) of the cases are infected by HSV type II, some are caused by the closely related HSV I, which is commonly associated with oral infections.[26] As such, genital herpes is the venereal counterpart of oral "fever blisters" or gingivostomatitis. Along with NGU, herpes genitalis is now an extremely common sexually transmitted disease. Its prevalence correlates fairly closely with the sexual activity of the population under study. As with other venereal diseases, increasing numbers of homosexual males are developing genital herpes. Two clinical forms are recognized: primary and recurrent, both associated with vesicular and ulcerative lesions. However, due to the absence of any immunity, the lesions in the first episode of genital herpes are numerous, bilateral, and more painful; they are associated with tender inguinal lymphadenopathy and systemic signs such as fever, headache, and malaise. In contrast, recurrent lesions are less extensive and milder, and systemic illness is not usually noted.[27]

In both sexes herpetic lesions are found on the external genitalia. In women, the cervix is involved in over 90% of the primary infections. Involvement of the urethra may also occur. Extragenital lesions, resulting from autoinoculation of the virus, may be found on the thighs, buttocks, or fingers. Proctitis may be the presenting feature in male homosexuals. Grossly, the lesions appear as small vesicles, 1 mm or more in diameter, surrounded by marked erythema and edema. These rapidly rupture to form shallow ulcerations. *Histologically, the hallmark of herpetic infection is the presence of multinuclear giant cells of epithelial origin that contain intranuclear inclusions.* Such cells are found in Papanicolaou smears, indicating herpetic cervicitis. The clinical manifestations of primary herpes genitalis last three to four weeks. *Recurrent* herpes genitalis is characterized by the periodic development of vesiculoulcerative lesions on an erythematous base. There is less edema and inflammatory response than with the primary disease, and the lesions disappear within a week to 10 days. More than 80% of the patients with HSV II genital herpes have one or more recurrences yearly for several years.

A grave complication of herpes genitalis in pregnant women is the risk of transmission to neonates. Among pregnant women infected near the time of delivery, about 50% of newborns delivered vaginally develop *neonatal herpes.* This is a severe, generalized disease that is often fatal. Another potentially serious effect of herpes genitalis is its possible contribution toward the development of *carcinoma of the vulva and cervix.* This subject is fully explored in Chapter 19. It suffices to say that prospective studies suggest that women with herpes genitalis have a higher risk of developing vulval and cervical cancer than women not infected by HSV II.[28]

## References

1. Graham, J. H., and Helwig, E. G.: Bowen's disease and its relationship to systemic cancer. Arch. Dermatol. 83:738, 1961.
2. Andersen, S. L. C., et al.: Relationship between Bowen disease and internal malignant tumors. Arch. Dermatol. 108:367, 1973.
2a. McCance, D. J., et al.: Human papillomavirus types 16 and 18 in carcinomas of the penis from Brazil. Int. J. Cancer 37:55, 1986.
3. Harty, J. I., and Catalona, W. J.: Carcinoma of the penis. In Javadpour, N. (ed.): Principles and Management of Urologic Cancer. 2nd ed. Baltimore, Williams & Wilkins, 1983, p. 581.
4. Nelson, R. P., et al.: Epidermoid carcinoma of the penis. Br. J. Urol. 54:172, 1982.
5. Colodny, A. J.: Undescended testes—Is surgery necessary? N. Engl. J. Med. 314:510, 1986.
6. Job, J. C., and Gendrel, D.: Endocrine aspects of cryptorchidism. Urol. Clin. North Am. 9:353, 1982.
7. Mostofi, F. K.: Pathology of germ cell tumors of testis. A progress report. Cancer 45:1735, 1980.
8. Mostofi, F. K., and Davis, C. J.: Pathology of tumors of testis. In Javadpour, N. (ed.): Principles and Management of Urologic Cancer. 2nd ed. Baltimore, Williams & Wilkins, 1983, p. 102.
9. Mostofi, F. K.: Tumor markers and pathology of testicular tumors. In Kurth, K. H., et al (eds.): Progress and Controversies in Oncologic Urology. New York, Alan R. Liss, 1984, p. 69.
10. Hainsworth, J. D., and Greco, F. A.: Testicular germ cell neoplasms. Am. J. Med. 75:817, 1983.
11. Silverberg, E.: Cancer statistics, 1985. CA 35:32, 1985.
12. Ireton, R. C., and Berger, R. E.: Prostatitis and epididymitis. Urol. Clin. North Am. 11:83, 1984.
13. Meares, E. J.: Prostatitis and related disorders. In Walsh, P. C., et al. (eds.): Campbell's Urology. 5th ed. Philadelphia, W. B. Saunders Co., 1986, p. 868.
14. Walsh, P. C.: Human benign prostatic hyperplasia: Etiological considerations. Prog. Clin. Biol. Res. 145:1, 1984.
15. McNeal, J. E.: Anatomy of the prostate and morphogenesis of BPH. Prog. Clin. Biol. Res. 145:27, 1984.
16. Catalona, W. J., and Scott, W. W.: Carcinoma of the Prostate. In Walsh, P. C., et al. (eds.): Campbell's Urology. 5th ed. Philadelphia, W. B. Saunders Co., 1986, p. 1463.

17. Ostro, D. G.: Homosexuality and sexually transmitted diseases. *In* Holmes, K. K., et al. (eds.): Sexually Transmitted Diseases. New York, McGraw-Hill Book Co., 1984, p. 99.

18. Britigan, B. E., et al.: Gonococcal infection: A model of molecular pathogenesis. N. Engl. J. Med. *312*:1683, 1985.

19. Mills, J., and Brooks, G. F.: Disseminated gonococcal infection. *In* Holmes, K. K., et al. (eds.): Sexually Transmitted Diseases. New York, McGraw-Hill Book Co. 1984, p. 229.

20. Bowie, W. R.: Nongonococcal urethritis. Urol. Clin. North Am. *11*:55, 1984.

21. Schacter, J.: Chlamydia trachomatis. *In* Holmes, K. K., and Mardh, P. (eds.): International Perspectives on Neglected Sexually Transmitted Diseases. New York, McGraw-Hill Book Co., 1983, p. 7.

22. Berger, R. E.: Sexually transmitted disease. *In* Walsh, P. C., et al. (eds.): Campbell's Urology, 5th ed. Philadelphia, W. B. Saunders Co., 1986, p. 900.

23. Smith, T. F.: Sexually transmitted infections due to *Chlamydia trachomatis:* Rapid detection by immunofluorescence microscopy. Mayo Clin. Proc. *60*:204, 1985.

24. Drusin, L. M.: Syphilis: Clinical manifestations, diagnosis, and treatment. Urol. Clin. North Am. *11*:121, 1984.

25. Hart, G.: Syphilis tests in diagnostic and therapeutic decision making. Ann. Intern. Med. *104*:368, 1986.

26. Corey, L., and Spear, P. G.: Infections with herpes simplex viruses. N. Engl. J. Med. *314*:748, 1986.

27. Mertz, G., and Corey, L.: Genital herpes simplex virus infections in adults. Urol. Clin. North Am. *11*:103, 1984.

28. Nelson, J. H., Jr., et al.: Dysplasia, carcinoma in situ, and early invasive cervical carcinoma. CA *34*:306, 1984.

# 19

# The Female Genital System and Breast

# Vulva

The vulva is a less frequent site of disease than is the cervix, uterus, or ovary. The major pathologic changes of the vulva can be conveniently divided into the following categories: (1) inflammatory disorders (vulvitis), (2) epidermal hyperplasias or atrophies (dystrophies), (3) cysts, and (4) tumors (benign and malignant). The first three categories can be distressing to the patient because frequently they are asso-ciated with either intense itching or painful inter-course, but fortunately they are not life-threatening. Malignant neoplasms, on the other hand, are uncom-mon but too often lethal. The only congenital anomaly worthy of mention is the imperforate hymen; it may be unnoted until menstrual flow is impounded and collected within the vagina (*hematocolpos*) and the uterus (*hematometria*).

## VULVITIS

The moist hair-bearing skin and delicate membrane of the vulva are vulnerable to many nonspecific microbial-induced inflammations and dermatologic disorders. Intense itching (pruritus) and subsequent scratching often worsens the primary condition. There are also many specific forms of microbial vulvitis related to the sexually transmitted diseases. These often evoke distinctive findings such as the suppurative infections of the vulvo-vaginal glands, caused by gonococci and other agents; the chancre of syphilis; the ulcerative infections of donovanosis, lymphogranuloma venereum (with its prominent lymphadenopathy), and chancroid; the characteristic gray-white curdy exudate of monilial infection; and the vesicular eruption of herpes virus. Details on these venereal diseases are given on page 623

## VULVAR DYSTROPHIES

*The epithelium of the vulval mucosa may undergo atrophic thinning or hyperplastic thickening.* For want of a better term, these alterations are collectively referred to as *dystrophies*.[1] All variants may appear macroscopically as depigmented white lesions, referred to in the past as *"leukoplakia."* However, similar white patches or plaques are seen with (1) vitiligo (loss of pigment) of the skin, (2) a variety of benign dermatoses such as psoriasis and lichen planus, (3) carcinoma in situ, (4) Paget's disease (described later), and (5) invasive carcinoma. Thus *"leukoplakia" is merely a descriptive term that gives no indication of its underlying nature* (Fig. 19–1). Only biopsy and microscopic examination can differentiate among these widely differing but similar-appearing lesions. Here hyperplastic and atrophic dystrophy are discussed separately, but in a significant number of instances both patterns occur concurrently, referred to as *"mixed dystrophy."*

*Hyperplastic dystrophy (with and without atypia)* presents clinically as ill-defined or discrete areas of leukoplakia anywhere on the vulvar epithelium. Similar lesions may appear on the penis, in the oral cavity (particularly in habitual smokers), or in relation to a locus of chronic irritation. Sometimes the lesions are scaly or significantly thickened. The underlying changes range from orderly epidermal hyperplasia to all degrees of epithelial atypicality bordering on carcinoma in situ. Clinical studies indicate that *carcinoma develops in 5 to 10% of hyperplastic lesions* and so not surprisingly more than half of the patients who have cancer of the vulva have hyperplastic dystrophy elsewhere on the vulva. Such evidence underscores the importance of biopsy of leukoplakic lesions, a problem that is compounded by the fact that multiple discrete areas of leukoplakia may appear in the individual patient.

*Atrophic dystrophy (lichen sclerosus)* occurs most often in postmenopausal or prepubertal white females. Blacks are rarely affected. These epithelial alterations may also be encountered elsewhere on the skin. They have been attributed without substantial proof to estrogen deficiency, but uncommonly they develop during the reproductive years. In essence, the changes comprise atrophy and thinning of the epidermis accompanied by a dermal fibrosis with a scant perivascular, mononuclear inflammatory cell infiltrate. Atypical changes may be present but rarely are as marked as those found in the hyperplastic variant. Macroscopically, the lesions appear as smooth, white plaques or papules that in time may extend and coalesce. The surface of the lesions appears smoothed out and sometimes parchment-like. When the entire vulva is affected, the labia become somewhat atrophic and stiffened and the vaginal orifice constricted (hence, the older designation *"kraurosis vulvae"*). In the postmenopausal woman, these changes may be progressive and extend beyond the labia majora onto the thighs, groin, and perianal region. In the prepubertal girl, similar progression may occur, but usually the changes regress spontaneously at puberty. Most authorities do not consider this variant of vulvar dystrophy to be precancerous,[2] but this unfortunate complication has occurred rarely.

It should be noted that in about one third of cases, areas of hyperplastic dystrophy and atrophic dystrophy develop concurrently—*mixed* dystrophy—and, furthermore, hyperplastic lesions may convert to atrophic and vice versa.

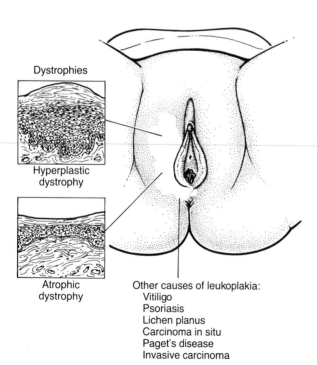

Dystrophies

Hyperplastic
dystrophy

Atrophic
dystrophy

Other causes of leukoplakia:
Vitiligo
Psoriasis
Lichen planus
Carcinoma in situ
Paget's disease
Invasive carcinoma

**Figure 19–1.** A representation of an area of leukoplakia on the labia majora and its possible causes.

## CYSTS OF THE VULVA

Cysts, sometimes multiple, may arise in the sub-clitoral or periurethral areas or in the regions of Bartholin's glands on the vulva in women of any age. More often they occur as single lesions usually in relation to Bartholin's glands. Those arising in the Bartholin's glands or their excretory ducts may reach a diameter of 5 cm and are most often the result of obstruction of one of the major excretory ducts and subsequent progressive accumulation of mucinous secretion. Such cysts are lined by either the transitional or cuboidal epithelium of the ducts, but it may become markedly flattened or almost disappear owing to the intracystic pressure. Besides causing local pain and discomfort, these cysts are vulnerable to secondary infection, producing a *Bartholin's abscess*. Cysts in other locations are thought to arise from embryonic rests; they are generally small (1 to 2 cm in diameter) and are lined by columnar to cuboidal mucinous or ciliated epithelium that occasionally undergoes metaplastic change into squamous epithelium.[3] Not having connections with the vulval vestibule, these cysts uncommonly become infected.

## TUMORS

### CONDYLOMAS

Condylomas are essentially anogenital warts, but in the moist environment of the vulva, they tend to be large. Most fall into two distinctive biologic forms, but more rare types also exist. (1) *Condylomata lata*, rarely seen today, are flat, moist, minimally elevated lesions occurring in secondary syphilis (p. 627) (2) The more common—*condylomata acuminata*—may be papillary and distinctly elevated or somewhat flat and rugose. They occur anywhere on the anogenital surface, sometimes singly but more often in multiple sites. On the vulva, they range from a few millimeters to many centimeters in diameter and are red-pink to pink-brown. The histologic appearance of these lesions was described earlier (p. 628), but *particularly significant is a characteristic cellular morphology, namely perinuclear cytoplasmic vacuolization with nuclear angular pleomorphism—koilocytosis* (Fig. 19–2). *Such cells are considered to be hallmarks of human papillomavirus (HPV) infection.* Although condylomata acuminata are frequently accompanied by herpes genitalis, there is a stronger association with at least two genotypes (6 and 11) of the human papillomavirus identical to or closely related to the viruses causing common warts.[4] The HPV can be transmitted venereally; identical lesions occur on the penis and around the anus in men. Vulvar condylomas are associated with intraepithelial neoplasia, as is discussed later,[5] but usually the genotypes of HPV isolated from the cancers differ from those most often found in condylomas.

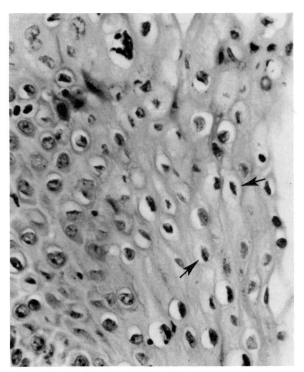

Figure 19–2. A high-power detail of koilocytes with cytoplasmic clearing and striking angulated nuclear pleomorphism (*arrows*).

## PAGET'S DISEASE OF THE VULVA

Vulvar Paget's disease is a rare form of intraepithelial carcinoma that is analogous to the more common Paget's disease of the breast (p. 666) and so is often referred to as "extramammary Paget's disease."[6] It sometimes extends into the perianal region. Clinically, it presents as an indurated or nodular, fairly well defined area of varying shades of red, usually on the labia majora. Sometimes the lesions have a scaling or even eroded surface. This appearance invites the misdiagnosis of dermatitis. Only infrequently can a small underlying tumor be palpated. *The histologic hallmarks of Paget's disease in all locations are large anaplastic cancer cells lying singly or in small clusters within the epidermis (Paget's cells). These anaplastic cells have perinuclear cleared cytoplasm (produced by vacuoles of PAS-positive polysaccharides), creating the appearance of a halo around the nucleus* (Fig. 19–3). Sometimes these cells extend down into the intraepithelial segments of the secretory ducts of the adnexal appendages, but in most cases the tumor cells are restricted to the epidermis and indeed may persist in this location for decades without invading the dermis. Such lesions are amenable to curative resection, but because of lateral intraepithelial spread, recurrence may follow incomplete removal. Infrequently they become invasive. In a few cases there is a well-defined small cancer of apparently apocrine or sweat-gland origin that underlies the epidermis. *When there is well-defined invasion or a subepithelial tumor, the prognosis is poor.*

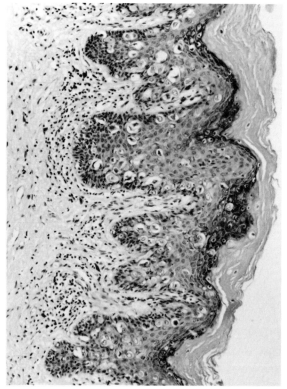

Figure 19–3. Paget's disease of the vulva, showing the intra-epithelial cancer cells accentuated by their cleared "halos."

The origin of the Paget's cells in the vulva remains controversial. Immunochemical studies favor an origin from the adnexal ductal cells traversing the epidermis because Paget's cells often contain either carcinoembyronic antigen (CEA), present in normal sweat gland and apocrine epithelium, or a protein characteristic of apocrine cells, or both.[7, 8] Neither CEA nor the protein is found in normal epidermal cells.

## CARCINOMA OF THE VULVA (NONINVASIVE AND INVASIVE)

Because in situ carcinomas of the vulva do not inevitably become invasive cancers, it is best to consider them separately.

*Carcinoma in situ of the vulva (vulvar intraepithelial neoplasia, VIN) is also called Bowen's disease of the vulva.* Identical lesions may develop on the penis (p. 612).

Macroscopically, it appears as a discrete (sometimes multiple) leukoplakia-like epidermal thickening or as red-brown papules (hence the designation "papulosis") arising on the labia minora or majora, about the clitoris, or in the perianal region. The wide variation in the clinical appearance may reflect differing causal influences. There is equal variability in the histologic appearance. Some

lesions have moderate degrees of intraepithelial cellular atypia and an increased number of normal mitoses in the stratum basalis, often associated with koilocytotic changes (p. 633) in the superficial and sometimes deep layers. Other lesions have more marked atypia or overt anaplasia and abnormal mitoses, some of which are well above the basalis, but no well-defined koilocytosis. By definition, whatever the pattern, there is no evidence of penetration into the underlying dermis.

The wide range of morphologic changes, both gross and microscopic, is accompanied by an equally wide range of clinical behavior. Only about 5 to 10% of in situ vulvar carcinomas progress to invasive carcinoma, and this occurs principally in elderly or immunosuppressed patients. In the remainder, the changes appear to be indolent over the span of many years, or, in women in the early decades of life, they may regress.[9] The interpretation of these morphologic and clinical findings is still uncertain, but a few speculations will be offered.

There is a growing body of evidence that herpes simplex virus II (HSV II)[10] and types 16 and 18 mainly of papillomavirus (HPV) are involved in the genesis of instances of vulvar and cervical neoplasia (p. 638).[11] Indeed, VIN and cervical cancer frequently coexist, suggesting a "field effect." Both HPV and HSV are sexually transmitted. Condylomata acuminata (p. 633) associated with particular genotypes of HPV are present in about 25% of cases of VIN, particularly those instances occurring in younger women. However, the usual genotypes of HPV found in carcinomas and condylomas differ as has been noted, but there are overlaps. Viral-associated lesions often have a nonprogressive course or may spontaneously regress, but a few progress into invasive lesions.[12] In elderly women, even though the condition may be virally related (more likely to HSV II), the most important antecedent is hyperplastic dystrophy. Moreover, in such settings the lesion is characterized by more marked cellular atypism but not koilocytosis and is more likely to progress to invasive cancer. Thus there may be more than one biologic form of VIN, accounting for the variable behavior. *Attractive as such an interpretation of the findings may be, it is at present speculative.* All that can be said with certainty is that not all instances of VIN are destined to become progressively invasive carcinoma, and so cautious long-term observation is necessary.

*Invasive carcinoma of the vulva* is an uncommon malignancy encountered most often in those over the age of 50. The most frequent antecedent is hyperplastic dystrophy; rarely, it is atrophic dystrophy. Condylomas are associated with about 10% of invasive carcinomas. Although invasive carcinoma must be preceded by an in situ stage, only about 5 to 10% of in situ cancers progress to the invasive stage for reasons noted above. Conceivably, the virally induced in situ changes require some additional promoting or potentiating influence to produce an invasive lesion.

Most invasive cancers of the vulva are squamous cell carcinomas. The remaining few are either melanocarcinomas, basal cell carcinomas, or adenocarcinomas arising in adnexal appendages. Squamous cell neoplasms begin as small grayish areas of firm, elevated thickening that eventually become fissured and ulcerated. Microscopically, they are usually well differentiated and have keratohyaline pearls and prickle cells. Occasionally, they are relatively undifferentiated. These neoplasms have a distressing potential for early spread; involvement of regional lymph nodes may occur when the lesions are small and have only a 5-mm depth of microinvasion.[13] In time, more widespread dissemination to internal viscera follows. Thus, patients with tumors less than 2 cm in diameter have a 60 to 80% five-year survival rate following vulvectomy and lymphadenectomy, but larger lesions with significant invasion and overt lymph node metastasis yield less than a 10% five-year survival.

Circumstantial evidence implicates HSV and more direct evidence, HPV in the genesis of at least some invasive cancers. For example, about 10% of invasive cancers arise in individuals who have or have had HPV-induced condylomas. Both viruses are related to intraepithelial neoplasia, and clinical studies document the development of invasive cancers from some in situ lesions. However, to date more direct documentation of viral footprints within the frankly anaplastic cancer cells of invasive neoplasms is fragmentary—one report has identified HSV-specific polymerase in the cells of invasive vulvar cancers and their metastases.[14] We must leave it then that viruses may be involved in some instances, but whether they play roles in most is unknown.

# Vagina

The vagina of the adult is seldom the site of primary disease. More often, it is secondarily involved in the spread of cancer or infections arising in close proximity (e.g., cervix, vulva, bladder, rectum). The only primary disorders meriting brief comment are (1) a few congenital anomalies, (2) vaginitis, and (3) primary tumors.

*Congenital anomalies* of the vagina are fortunately uncommon, comprising such entities as total absence of the vagina, a septate or double vagina (usually associated with a septate cervix and, sometimes, uterus), and congenital small lateral *Gartner's duct cysts* arising from persistent embryonic remnants.

*Vaginitis*—inflammation of the vaginal mucous membrane that often involves the cervix and vulva—is by far the most common primary disorder of the vagina. It occurs mainly in infants or in young women during active reproductive life. These infections account for about 5 to 10% of patient visits to gynecologists. The most common causes are cited in Table 19–1. Any of these agents, most notably HSV, HPV, and chlamydia (a frequent cause of urethritis in males), can be sexually transmitted.[15] But many of the agents, such as the candidal species and *Trichomonas gardnerella*, are normal inhabitants of the vagina; *Candida*, for example, can be found in about one third of apparently healthy women. Thus it is uncertain whether an attack of monilial vaginitis implies sexual transmission of new strains to which prior immunity is lacking or instead reflects accentuation of some predisposing influence (e.g., diabetes mellitus, marked sexual activity, pregnancy, or exposure to broad-spectrum antibiotics or oral contraceptives).

Although most attacks of vaginitis are more uncomfortable than serious, some have particular importance. Herpetic infections of the genital tract may lead to serious infections in the newborn. The toxic shock syndrome (rash, fever, hypotension, multisystem involvement) has been traced (most often) to the growth of exotoxin-producing strains of staphylococci that flourish in certain types of vaginal tampons saturated with menstrual flow.[16] It should be noted that *Neisseria gonorrhoeae* is not responsible for primary vaginitis in the adult because the mature vaginal mucosa is resistant to this pathogen. None-

## Table 19–1. CAUSES OF VAGINITIS

| Causes | Comments |
|---|---|
| *In the Newborn* | |
| Neisseria gonorrhoeae | Now uncommon because of postdelivery prophylaxis |
| *In the Infant and Young Child* | |
| N. gonorrhoeae | May be epidemic in nurseries, schools—indirect spread by contaminated articles |
| *In Young Adults* | |
| Common Agents | |
| Gardnerella vaginalis | Normal commensal—may require mixed flora |
| Trichomonas vaginalis | Normal commensal—may require predisposing influence |
| Candida spp. | Normal commensal—may require predisposing influence |
| *Less Common Agents* | |
| Chlamydia trachomatis | |
| Mycoplasma hominis | |
| Herpes virus type II | Associated vesicular genital herpes |
| Human papillomavirus | Associated condylomata |
| Staphylococci (exotoxic strains) | Toxic shock syndrome—(rash, fever, hypotension, multisystem involvement) |

theless (as has been detailed on p. 625), it often induces suppurative inflammation involving vulvar and endocervical glands and so may produce a vaginal discharge that must be differentiated from primary vaginitis. However, in the newborn and infant it can cause suppurative vulvovaginitis.

Whatever the causative agent, the local changes comprise erythema and sometimes superficial erosions of the vaginal mucosa. The clinical symptoms are nonspecific and include excessive vaginal discharge (sometimes purulent—leukorrhea), itching, and localized discomfort. Although certain features of the infection may be clinically distinctive, such as the vesicular eruption of herpes in the vagina and on the vulva, the curdy white exudate of candidiasis, and the sometimes frothy yellow-green exudation of trichomoniasis, the differential diagnosis ultimately depends upon identification of the causative agent.

Specific infections may also occur in postmenopausal women, but nonspecific vaginitis is more common because atrophy of the vaginal mucosa, secondary to diminished estrogenic function, induces increased vulnerability.

*Neoplasms* are fortunately rare. Among these rarities, *squamous cell carcinoma* is most common. Of particular interest is the vaginal *clear cell adenocarcinoma*, encountered usually in girls in their late teens whose mothers had taken diethylstilbestrol during pregnancy (p. 208).[17] Sometimes these cancers have not appeared until the third or fourth decades of life. The overall risk is small, approximately one or less per thousand.[18] In about one third of the instances, these cancers arise in the cervix. Much more frequently, perhaps in over half of the population at risk, small glandular or microcystic inclusions appear in the glandular mucosa—*vaginal adenosis*. These benign lesions appear as red granular foci and are lined by mucus-secreting or ciliated columnar cells. It is from such inclusions that the more rare clear cell adenocarcinoma arises. *Sarcoma botryoides*, producing soft polypoid masses, is another fortunately rare form of primary vaginal cancer that is encountered usually in infants and children under the age of five. It is basically a subtype of rhabdomyosarcoma, which may occur in other sites, such as the urinary bladder and bile ducts, and so is described on page 722.

# Cervix Uteri

The cervix lives a troubled life: it must serve as a barrier to the ingress of air and the microflora of the vagina, yet must permit the escape of menstrual flow and sustain the mild (albeit possibly pleasurable) buffeting of intercourse and, worst of all, the trauma of childbirth. No small wonder it is often the seat of disease. Fortunately, most of its lesions are relatively banal inflammations—cervicitis—but it also is the site of one of the most common cancers in women—squamous cell carcinoma, responsible for about 5% of all cancer deaths. These common disorders are discussed below, but first a few comments on some developmental anomalies are presented.

*Congenital anomalies* of the cervix are uncommon and take the forms of hypoplasia, causing stenosis of the cervical os (to be differentiated from inflammatory stenosis), and of septate cervix with a septate or double uterus. Atresias and stenoses are generally probe-patent, but with sufficient narrowing of the os, they may impound menstrual flow and induce *hematometria* or cause sterility.

## CERVICITIS

Inflammations of the cervix are so common they have been called "the birthright of all women." Traditionally, they have been divided into specific infections (those caused by the agents responsible for the sexually transmitted diseases, discussed on p. 623), and nonspecific infections (those caused by all

other organisms, many of which are normal inhabitants of the vagina). It is only necessary here to point out that among the specific pathogens, *Chlamydia trachomatis* has replaced gonococci as the leading cause of specific cervicovaginal infections.[19]

Much more common is the relatively banal *nonspecific cervicitis*, present to some degree in almost every multiparous woman. Although this baffling entity is known to be associated with a variety of organisms, including coliforms, bacteroides, streptococci, and staphylococci, the pathogenesis of the infection is poorly understood. Trauma of childbirth and from instruments used during gynecologic procedures, hyperestrinism, hypoestrinism, excessive secretion of the endocervical glands, alkalinity of the cervical mucus, and congenital eversion (described later) of the endocervical mucosa have all been cited as predisposing influences.

Nonspecific cervicitis may be either *acute* or *chronic*. Excluding gonococcal infection, which causes a specific form of acute disease, the relatively uncommon *acute nonspecific* form is virtually limited to postpartum women and is usually caused by staphylococci or streptococci. The acute inflammatory infiltrate tends to remain largely limited to the superficial endocervical mucosa and endocervical glands (*endocervicitis*) and is accompanied by swelling of the cervix and reddening of the exocervical mucosa.

The *chronic* form is the nearly ubiquitous entity usually referred to by the unqualified term "nonspecific cervicitis."

It begins as a slight reddening, swelling, and granularity near the squamocolumnar junction. With persistence of the inflammation, it encroaches on the exocervical mucosa, and superficial irregular erosions or ulcerations develop. **Eventually, in severe cases, the continual inflammatory-reparative process results in distortion of the exocervix by irregular, friable nodules and ulcerations which may, on inspection, be confused with carcinoma of the cervix.** Histologically, a predominantly mononuclear inflammatory infiltrate admixed with some polymorphonuclear leukocytes is found subjacent to the endocervical mucosa, close to the squamocolumnar junction. This infiltrate typically extends beneath the adjacent exocervical epithelium (which becomes depleted of glycogen), surrounds the endocervical mucous glands, and fills their lumens. Usually the overlying endocervical epithelium undergoes some degree of inflammatory metaplastic change and, in severe cases, may show considerable dysplasia, with downward growth into the mouths of the endocervical glands, referred to as **epidermidalization.** Such changes can be mistaken for invasion by a squamous cell carcinoma. Other morphologic features include cystic dilatation of the endocervical glands caused by inflammatory stenosis of their outlets **(nabothian cysts),** protrusion of the endocervical mucosa onto the external aspect of the cervix **(eversion),** and the development of lymphoid follicles **(follicular cervicitis).**

Nonspecific chronic cervicitis commonly comes to attention on routine examination or because of marked leukorrhea. When the lesion is severe, differentiation from carcinoma may be difficult even with colposcopy and may require a biopsy. The depletion of glycogen in the mucosal cells further complicates the differentiation because it is also a characteristic of preneoplastic and neoplastic cells, as is discussed on page 639. Cervicitis per se is not a precancerous lesion, but the secondary epithelial dysplastic changes may constitute a favorable subsoil for carcinogenic influences such as viruses (p. 638). Severe cervicitis may lead also to sterility through deformation and exudative blocking of the cervical os while simultaneously producing an unfavorable environment for sperm.

# TUMORS OF THE CERVIX

Although a wide variety of tumors may develop in the cervix uteri, all are rare except the relatively unimportant polyp and squamous cell neoplasia and its sometimes accompanying condylomata (p. 633).

## POLYP

Although *polyps* are common, occurring in 2 to 5% of adult females, they are innocuous, occasionally being important as a cause of abnormal bleeding that must be differentiated from that due to more ominous causes.

These lesions typically arise within the endocervical canal. They may be sessile, hemispheric masses or pedunculated, spherical lesions up to 3 cm in diameter. Those with long stalks may be seen on clinical examination, hanging down through the exocervical os and causing dilatation of the cervix. Characteristically, cervical polyps are soft, almost mucoid. Their histologic nature is that of a loose fibromyxomatous stroma containing cystically dilated endocervical glands. Although the covering epithelium is usually columnar and secretes mucus, superimposed chronic inflammation may lead to squamous metaplasia and ulcerations. Malignant transformation rarely, if ever, occurs.

## CARCINOMA OF THE CERVIX

The decline in the number of deaths caused by cancer of the cervix in the United States and in other developed nations is a dramatic and gratifying testament to the benefits of early diagnosis. Once one of the leading causes of cancer death, cervical cancer now ranks seventh or eighth among the cancer-killers of females in the United States, causing about 6,500 deaths, according to a 1985 estimate.[20] In sharp contrast, there are about two to three times as many newly diagnosed cases of invasive carcinoma of the cervix yearly and seven to eight times as many new patients discovered with in situ carcinoma. It is evident that *well over half of invasive cancers are cured by effective therapy and, even more important, most lesions are discovered while still in situ and amenable to eradication by timely and appropriate treatment.* Thanks for these dramatic gains are owed largely to the effectiveness of the Papanicolaou cytologic test (p. 224) in detecting cervical carcinoma during its incipiency and by the fortuitous accessibility of the cervix to colposcopy and biopsy. The widespread application of the "Pap smear" in mass screening programs and in routine physical examinations followed by biopsy to evaluate and confirm abnormal cytologic findings has documented that carcinoma of the cervix arises in a series of stepwise epithelial changes ranging from progressively more severe dysplasia to invasive carcinoma.[21] More is known about the life history of this form of cancer than of any other.

**INCIDENCE AND EPIDEMIOLOGY.** Both in situ and invasive carcinomas are diagnosed now at an earlier age than in past decades. Indeed, cervical intraepithelial neoplasia (CIN) is now being discovered in teenagers and young adults![22] The peak incidence is at about 30 years of age. Similarly, invasive carcinoma is now appearing as early as the third decade of life with a peak incidence at about age 40 (i.e., about 10 to 15 years later). Deaths begin in the fourth decade, and the mortality rate rises throughout life.[23] Only a few decades ago, all of these unfortunate events were delayed at least 10 years, strongly suggesting that oncogenic influences, possibly viruses (as will be noted later), are now at work earlier in life.

### Table 19–2. CORRELATIONS BETWEEN HSV AND CERVICAL CARCINOMA*

| | |
|---|---|
| Serum antibodies to a viral antigen | Present in 50 to 90% of patients with invasive carcinoma vs. 5–10% of controls |
| | Present in 30 to 70% of patients with in situ cancer vs. 5% of controls |
| Herpes genitalis infection of the genital tract | Higher incidence of cervical cancer than in noninfected controls |
| HSV-2 antigen | Present in 50 to 90% of cervical carcinoma biopsies vs. 10% of matched-control biopsies |
| HSV-2 viral DNA, mRNA, viral proteins | Identified in cells in some cases of cervical carcinoma |
| HSV-2 DNA sequences | Identified in malignant cells by recombinant DNA techniques in some cases |

*From Nelson, J. H., Jr., et al.: Dysplasia, carcinoma in situ, and early invasive cervical carcinoma. CA *34*:306, 1984.

Many risk factors for cervical carcinoma have been identified. Among them, the following are most important:

○ Early age at first intercourse
○ Multiple sexual partners
○ "High risk" male sexual partners—i.e., those who are promiscuous, who have a former wife with cervical cancer, or who have a history of penile condylomas[24]

All other risk factors can be related to these three influences, such as the higher incidence of cervical carcinoma in lower socioeconomic groups, the higher incidence in married women (increasing with the number of marriages and children), the rarity of cervical carcinoma in virgins, and the high incidence in prostitutes. No longer considered significant risk factors are cigarette smoking, birth control pills, vague agents in semen, and a lack of circumcision in the male sexual partner (implicating some putative carcinogen within smegma).

**ETIOLOGY AND PATHOGENESIS.** The epidemiology of cervical cancer strongly suggests sexual transmission of an oncogen, and particularly incriminated are the herpes simplex virus (HSV) type II and human papillomavirus (HPV), particularly types 16 and 18.[25] Despite the many observations associating one or both of these viruses with cervical carcinoma, it must not be overlooked that the evidence is still incomplete.[26] Conceivably, either or both viruses may have an affinity for abnormal and neoplastic cells, or viral infection and development of neoplasia could be coincidental events that are both related to sexual practices. Table 19–2 summarizes the major observations relating to HSV. The evidence implicating HPV is more persuasive.[11] Condylomas, particularly flat condylomas, are considered to be precursors to cervical neoplasia; they are of established HPV origin. Moreover, the "telltales" of viral infection (i.e., viral DNA sequences) are frequently present in the cells. When dysplasia (often accompanied by koilocytosis) supervenes to produce what have been called precancerous changes, HPV types 16 and 18 are usually present. A summary of some of the more important observations relating to HPV is presented in Table 19–3.

Regarding the etiology of cervical cancer, two points need emphasis; (1) even if HSV and HPV play causal roles, it is highly likely that other influences are also necessary to carry the changes to the stage of invasive cancer (i.e., multifactorial causation) and (2) viruses may not be involved in all cases, and other quite separate pathways may exist.

### Table 19–3. CORRELATIONS BETWEEN HPV AND CERVICAL CARCINOMA*

| | |
|---|---|
| Penile condylomas | Often present in consorts who develop cervical neoplasia |
| Cervical condylomas | Coexist with marked dysplasia or carcinoma in situ in 5 to 55% of cases; sometimes have cellular atypia |
| Koilocytotic cells | Hallmark of HPV; is frequent in dysplasia and carcinoma in situ but is uncommon with invasive cancer |
| HPV-viral proteins, viral antigens, DNA sequences | Identified in cells of 80 to 90% of cases of invasive neoplasia |

*From Meisels, A., et al.: Human papillomavirus (HPV). Venereal infections and gynecologic cancer. Pathol. Annu. *18*(Part 2):277, 1983.

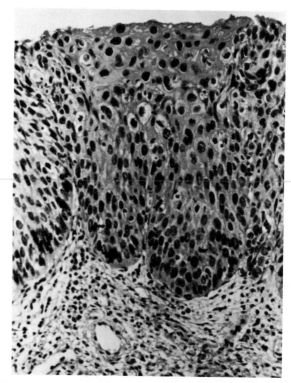

**Figure 19–4.** Focus of carcinoma in situ of the cervix (CIN Grade III), showing markedly atypical cells that occupy the full thickness of the epithelium. (Courtesy of Dr. D. Antonioli, Beth Israel Hospital, Boston.)

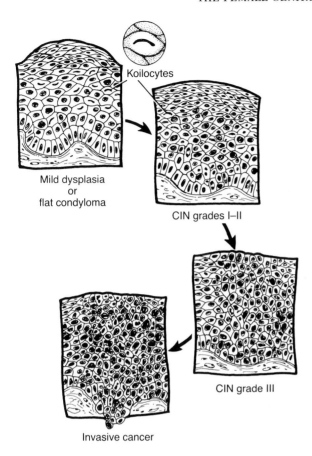

Koilocytes

Mild dysplasia
or
flat condyloma

CIN grades I–II

CIN grade III

Invasive cancer

CIN = Cervical intraepithelial neoplasia

Figure 19–5. Representation of the progressive evolution of invasive carcinoma of the cervix.

earlier document that the progression from mild dysplasia to carcinoma in situ to invasive cancer evolves slowly over the span of many years (10 to 15). It is difficult to interpret the repeated claims that some in situ lesions may spontaneously regress. Conceivably, in situ changes of viral origin may indeed regress. Alternatively, pregnancy or HPV infection with or without the formation of condylomas may introduce epithelial changes readily overdiagnosed as in situ carcinoma, or in situ lesions may be small and be eradicated by the biopsy or such influences as trauma, delivery, douches, or even secondary infections (cervicitis). In any event, it is impossible to predict "regression" and dangerous to depend on it.

Epithelial atypicalities and carcinoma of the cervix almost always begin at or close to the squamocolumnar junction of the external os. **In the CIN stages there are no changes visible to the naked eye,** but atypical cells can be detected by cytologic examination in most cases. In addition, colposcopy provides a magnified look at the cervix and often reveals abnormal areas not visible to the naked eye. Foci of epithelial changes can also be rendered more apparent by either painting the cervix with iodine solution—the Schiller test (the normal mucosa stains red-brown owing to the glycogen content of the cells but the atypical cells are glycogen depleted and appear pale)—or with dilute acetic acid, which for unknown reasons renders abnormal foci pale white. Ultimately, biopsy and histologic examination is requisite and reveals changes that range from mild dysplasia to carcinoma in situ, as has been amply detailed.

Although the etiology of cervical carcinoma is still uncertain, there is general agreement that this form of cancer begins with *mild dysplasia,* either in the usual cervical epithelium or in a *flat condyloma* marked by koilocytotic changes. The dysplasia becomes more disorderly and may be associated with some variation in cell and nuclear size and with normal-appearing mitoses above the basal layer of either the usual cervical mucosa or flat condyloma; this stage is designated *moderate dysplasia.* Although *these changes are reversible,* they are often called *CIN (cervical intraepithelial neoplasia) Grades I–II.* The superficial layer of cells is still well differentiated but in some cases shows koilocytotic changes. The next step in the sequence is *severe dysplasia (CIN Grade III),* marked by greater variation in cell and nuclear size, disorderly orientation, hyperchromasia, and mitoses, normal or abnormal, sometimes near the surface layer (Fig. 19–4). Differentiation of surface cells and koilocytotic changes have usually disappeared or are found very uncommonly. In CIN Grade III the epithelial changes have not invaded the underlying stroma but may extend into endocervical glands; this stage represents *carcinoma-in-situ. The next stage is invasive cancer* (Fig. 19–5). Sequential biopsies and the epidemiologic data cited

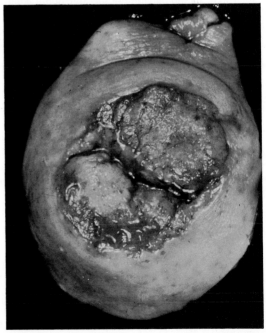

Figure 19–6. Carcinoma of the cervix, well advanced. (From Robbins, S. L., Cotran, R. S., and Kumar, V.: Pathologic Basis of Disease. 3rd ed. Philadelphia, W. B. Saunders Co., 1984, p. 1127.)

Invasive carcinoma takes one of three distinct macroscopic forms. The most frequent is a **fungating** tumor, which begins as a nodular thickening of the epithelium and eventually appears as a cauliflower-like mass projecting above the surrounding mucosa, sometimes completely encircling the external os (Fig. 19–6). The second is an **ulcerative** form, characterized by necrotic sloughing of the central surface of the tumor. The least frequent variety is the **infiltrative,** which tends to grow downward into the underlying stroma, rather than outward. With time these forms tend to merge as they infiltrate the underlying tissue, obliterate the external os, grow upward into the endocervical canal and lower uterine segment, and eventually extend into and through the wall of the fundus into the broad ligaments. Advanced lesions may extend into the rectum or base of the urinary bladder, sometimes to obstruct one or both of the ureters. Only relatively late is there involvement of lymph nodes or distant metastases. The lymph nodes first affected are the internal iliac and hypogastric chains, followed later by periaortic nodal involvement. Distant metastases, when present, usually affect the lungs, bones, and liver.

The histologic character of 95% of carcinomas of the cervix is that of a typical **squamous cell carcinoma** of varying differentiation. The remaining 5% are **adenocarcinomas,** presumably arising in the endocervical glands or mixed squamous and adeno- forms, termed **adenosquamous carcinomas.**

Both a grading system, based on the degree of cellular differentiation, and a staging system, based on tumor spread, have been devised. Grades I through III refer to progressively undifferentiated lesions. The details of the currently used staging system are beyond our needs. In brief, it recognizes Stage 0—carcinoma in situ—and then Stages 1 to 4, based on whether the carcinoma is strictly confined to the cervix (Stage I) or has extended beyond the cervix ultimately to reach Stage 4, marked by extension beyond the uterus into the pelvis and by involvement of adjacent organs or metastatic dissemination.

**CLINICAL COURSE.** Results of a Pap smear may first become abnormal with mild dysplasia in asymptomatic teenagers or young adults. Even frank carcinoma in situ is usually asymptomatic except possibly for the presence of some leukorrhea, which is more often related to concomitant cervicitis or vaginitis. The cervix may still appear normal to the naked eye, but colposcopy and the Schiller or acetic acid tests may disclose an abnormal area. When invasive carcinoma appears, usually in the fourth or fifth decade of life or sometimes later, it is often associated with irregular vaginal bleeding, leukorrhea, painful coitus, and dysuria. All invasive lesions except possibly for those with an infiltrative pattern are usually readily evident on palpation and inspection. Biopsy is always necessary to confirm the cytologic findings and to evaluate the depth of penetration of the lesion.

*The mortality from this form of cancer is more often related to its local effects (i.e., obstruction of the ureters or penetration into the bladder or rectum) than to distant metastases.* Death from this disease is a particularly lamentable tragedy because at least a decade lapses between the in situ and invasive stages, providing ample opportunity for early diagnosis. Neither is there any need for hasty ill-considered treatment. If the interpretation of a biopsy is in doubt, there is time to permit the lesion to declare itself.

Survival with this disease, assuming appropriate management (usually surgery or radiotherapy, or both), depends largely on the stage when first discovered, as the following data on five-year survival indicate:

Stage 0—100%
Stage 1—85–95%
Stage 2—70–75%
Stage 3—35%
Stage 4—10%

# Corpus Uteri and Endometrium

The corpus with its endometrium is the principal seat of gynecological pathology. Many disorders of this organ are common, often chronic and recurrent, and sometimes disastrous. Only the more frequent and significant are considered.

## ENDOMETRITIS

The endometrium is relatively resistant to infection. However, uncommonly *acute endometritis* develops, usually after abortion or full-term delivery and retention of placental fragments. Implicated organisms are principally streptococci or staphylococci.

*Chronic endometritis*, although not frequent, is more common than the acute form. Its origins are poorly understood, and microbiologic investigations to date have not been satisfactory. Most instances are believed to be caused by infectious agents—chlamydia, mycoplasma, toxoplasma, bacteroides, cytomegalovirus, and others. Although the endometrium is relatively resistant to the gonococcus, chronic endometrial infection rarely appears as a component of gonococcal pelvic inflammatory disease (p. 625). An intrauterine device (IUD) itself induces inflammatory changes and is an important predisposing cause of secondary infection. Because of uncertainties about the origins of chronic endometritis, a possible autoimmune etiology has been raised.

Except for tuberculous endometritis, the histologic findings are quite nonspecific. The endometrial glands become irregular and there is variable stromal edema accompanied by an inflammatory infiltrate of lymphocytes (sometimes in focal aggregates), occasional neutrophils, and, notably, plasma cells. Although much emphasis has been placed on the identification of plasma cells, in some instances they are remarkably sparse.

Despite the vagueness of the etiologic and morphologic findings, chronic endometritis is a valid entity and is associated with abnormal bleeding, discharge, and, most important, infertility in some cases.[27]

## ENDOMETRIOSIS AND ADENOMYOSIS

Although adenomyosis is sometimes referred to as "internal endometriosis," it is completely distinct pathogenetically and clinically from endometriosis and so will be considered separately.

*Adenomyosis* refers to the growth of the basal layer of the endometrium down into the myometrium. Thus nests of endometrial stroma or glands, or both, are found well down in the myometrium between the muscle bundles. In the fortuitous microscopic section, continuity between these nests and the overlying endometrium can be established. As a consequence, the uterine wall often becomes thickened. Cyclic bleeding into the penetrating nests, producing hemosiderin pigmentation, is extremely unusual because the stratum basalis of the endometrium, from which the penetrations arise, is nonfunctional. Marked involvement may produce menorrhagia, dysmenorrhea, and pelvic pain prior to the onset of menstruation.

*Endometriosis* is a far more important clinical condition than adenomyosis; it often causes infertility, dysmenorrhea, pelvic pain, and other problems. *The condition is marked by the appearance of foci of more or less recognizable endometrium in the pelvis (ovaries, pouch of Douglas, uterine ligaments, tubes, and rectovaginal septum), less frequently in more remote sites of the peritoneal cavity, and about the umbilicus.* Uncommonly, the lymph nodes, lungs, and even heart or bone are involved. Three possibilities (not mutually exclusive) have been invoked to explain the origin of these dispersed lesions.[28] (1) The *regurgitation theory* proposes menstrual backflow through the fallopian tubes and subsequent implantation. Indeed, menstrual endometrium is viable and survives when injected into the anterior abdominal wall. However, this theory cannot explain lesions in the lymph nodes or lungs, for example. (2) The *metaplastic theory* proposes endometrial differentiation of coelomic epithelium, which in the last analysis is the origin of the endometrium itself. This theory, too, cannot explain endometriotic lesions in the lungs or lymph nodes. (3) The *vascular or lymphatic dissemination theory* has been invoked to explain extrapelvic or intranodal implants. Conceivably, all pathways are valid in individual instances (Fig. 19–7).

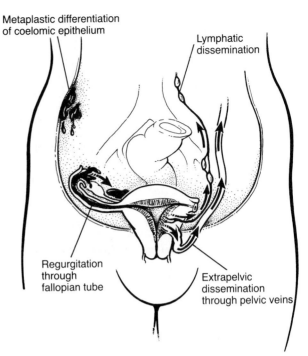

Figure 19–7. Depiction of the three potential origins of endometrial implants.

In contrast to adenomyosis, **endometriosis almost always contains functioning endometrium, which undergoes cyclic bleeding.** Because blood collects in these aberrant foci, they usually appear grossly as red-blue to yellow-brown nodules or implants. They vary in size from microscopic to 1 to 2 cm in diameter and lie on or just under the affected serosal surface. Often, individual lesions coalesce to form larger masses. When the ovaries are involved, small lesions appear as red-blue subcortical foci, but in time they form large blood-filled cysts that are transformed into so-called **chocolate cysts** as the blood ages (Fig. 19–8). These cysts may become as large as 8 to 10 cm in diameter. With long-standing extensive disease, seepage and organization of the blood leads to widespread fibrosis, adherence of pelvic structures (a "frozen" pelvis), obliteration of the pouch of Douglas, sealing of the tubal fimbriated ends, and distortion of the oviducts and ovaries. The histologic diagnosis at all sites depends on the finding within the lesions of two of the following three features: endometrial glands, stroma, or hemosiderin pigment. When the disease is far advanced, with extensive scarring, both the gross and histologic diagnosis may be difficult because the characteristic features may largely be replaced by nonspecific fibrosis.

The clinical manifestations of endometriosis depend upon the distribution of the lesions. Extensive scarring of the oviducts and ovaries often produces discomfort in the lower quadrant and eventually causes sterility. Pain on defecation reflects rectal wall involvement, and dyspareunia (painful intercourse) and dysuria reflect involvement of the uterine and

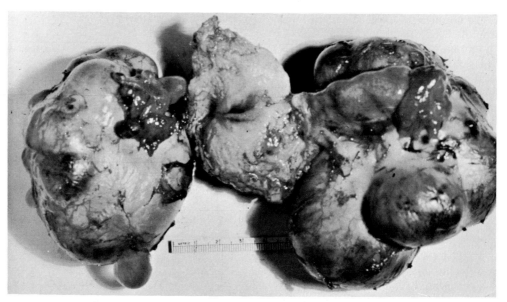

**Figure 19–8.** Endometriosis. The ovaries are converted into enlarged, irregular masses by large "chocolate cysts." (Courtesy of Dr. Arthur Hertig.)

bladder serosa, respectively. *In almost all cases, there is severe dysmenorrhea and pelvic pain as a result of intrapelvic bleeding and periuterine adhesions.* For unclear reasons, menstrual irregularities are common.

## DYSFUNCTIONAL UTERINE BLEEDING AND ENDOMETRIAL HYPERPLASIA

By far, the most common problem for which women seek medical attention is some disturbance in menstrual function—*menorrhagia* (profuse or prolonged bleeding at the time of the period), *metrorrhagia* (irregular bleeding between the periods), or *ovulatory (intermenstrual) bleeding.* Common causes include polyps, leiomyomas, endometrial carcinoma, endometritis, endometriosis, and, of interest here, dysfunctional uterine bleeding and endometrial hyperplasias.

### DYSFUNCTIONAL UTERINE BLEEDING

Abnormal bleeding in the absence of a well-defined organic lesion in the endometrium or uterus is called dysfunctional uterine bleeding. In many cases, it arises from a normal secretory endometrium and then is attributed to excessive fibrinolytic activity or changes in prostaglandin production within the uterus.[29] The commonest cause, however, is failure of ovulation and anovulatory bleeding.[30] As a consequence, there is no luteal or secretory phase of the endometrium, and under the influence of prolonged estrogenic activity, the proliferative endometrium

develops mild hyperplasia characterized by persistent mitotic activity and an increase in gland size. The diagnostic feature is a proliferative endometrium in the last half of the menstrual cycle when secretory changes would be expected.

Anovulatory cycles are most common at menarche and premenopausally, but they can occur throughout life. Oral contraceptives also block ovulation, but the combination of contained estrogens and progestogens is intended to prevent the development of the endometrial changes seen in dysfunctional uterine bleeding. In most instances anovulatory cycles (in the absence of oral contraceptives) are of obscure origin, but a number of endocrine-metabolic derangements alter ovulation; these include pituitary, adrenal, and thyroid disease; functioning ovarian tumors (p. 652); marked obesity; chronic inanition; and emotional stress or excessive physical activity as occurs in marathon runners and ballet dancers. Whatever the cause, long-standing anovulatory endometrial changes are associated with an increased incidence of endometrial carcinoma, presumably because of the unbalanced estrogenic stimulation.

### ENDOMETRIAL HYPERPLASIA

Endometrial hyperplasia is not only a cause of abnormal bleeding but also, in its more severe expressions, a forerunner of endometrial carcinoma. Hyperplasia has classically been divided into subtypes. The mildest form is called *cystic hyperplasia.* More advanced changes are termed *adenomatous hyperplasia,* and the most severe form is variously called *atypical hyperplasia* or *atypical adenomatous hyperplasia.* Because these patterns represent a continuum and sometimes blend with one another, it is recommended that they be simply classified as *mild, moderate,* and *atypical hyperplasia.*[31] Considerable importance attaches to the severity of the hyperplastic changes, since the "bad" end of the spectrum often progresses to carcinoma.[32]

Encountered most often in perimenopausal women, hyperplasias are caused by a relative or absolute hyperestrinism, such as is seen with polycystic ovaries, chronic failure of ovulation, functioning estrogenic ovarian tumors, adrenocortical hyperfunction, and prolonged use of exogenous estrogens.[33] Oral contraceptives are not implicated, presumably because of their progestogen content.

**Mild hyperplasia,** because of the pathologist's penchant for comparing distasteful lesions to tasteful foods, is often called **"Swiss cheese" hyperplasia** because the dilated glands produce a grossly visible lacunar appearance. In addition, the endometrium is thickened and velvety. Microscopic examination reveals hyperplasia of the more or less normal-appearing, regularly arrayed columnar or cuboidal epithelium lining the dilated glands or cysts (rarely there is multiple layering) and hyperplasia of the stroma. Frequently, normal mitoses are present in the epithelium and stroma. Note should be made that **cystic dilatation of the glands without the hyperplasia is frequently encountered in postmenopausal women, but it is accompanied by stromal atrophy and hence called senile cystic atrophy.**

**Moderate (adenomatous) hyperplasia** is marked by a lush, velvety, thickened endometrium that does not contain cystic spaces visible to the naked eye. In more advanced expressions, polypoid projections may appear. Histologically, there is an increase in the number and marked variability in the size and shape of the endometrial glands. The lining epithelium is cuboidal to columnar, often multilayered, has increased mitotic activity, and may buckle into the gland lumens in papillary buddings. Although the stroma is also hyperplastic, the overall appearance is of **"too many glands and too little stroma."** With this form of hyperplasia, there is a well-defined but not markedly increased incidence of transition to endometrial carcinoma.

**Atypical hyperplasia** is the most severe form of the condition. Although indistinguishable grossly from adenomatous hyperplasia, microscopic examination discloses a range of changes. There is crowding of glands of variable size, so that some lie "back to back" and sometimes glands are apparently within glands. The epithelium is no longer regularly arrayed; sometimes it is multilayered or forms bridges that traverse the lumen. The epithelial cells have prominent nuclei of variable size and shape and show numerous mitoses. With increasing severity, occasional glands are lined by large, pale-pink, anaplastic cells, justifying the diagnosis of **carcinoma in situ.** The spectrum of abnormalities shown in Figure 19–9 represents a biologic sequence that can sometimes be followed to carcinoma, which appears in the course of two or more years in approximately 25 to 35% of untreated cases of atypical hyperplasia.

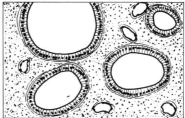
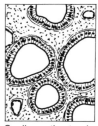

Cystic "Swiss cheese" hyperplasia    Senile cystic atrophy

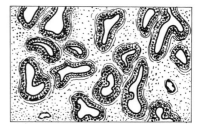

Moderate (adenomatous) hyperplasia

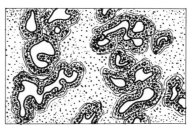

Atypical hyperplasia

**Figure 19–9.** Several patterns of endometrial hyperplasia that document progressive cellularity. A comparison between cystic hyperplasia and senile cystic atrophy is also shown.

Not only is curettage necessary to control the abnormal bleeding caused by endometrial hyperplasia, it is also requisite to establish the nature and severity of the glandular changes, which in some cases must be monitored over time by repeated endometrial biopsy or curettage to ascertain possible recurrence or progression.

## TUMORS OF THE ENDOMETRIUM AND MYOMETRIUM

The most common neoplasms are *endometrial polyps, leiomyomas,* and *endometrial carcinomas.* In addition, exotic mesodermal tumors are encountered, such as the stromal sarcoma botryoides (also encountered in the vagina), described on page 722. *All tend to produce bleeding from the uterus as the earliest manifestation.*

### ENDOMETRIAL POLYP

These are sessile, usually hemispheric (rarely pedunculated) lesions, from 0.5 to 3 cm in diameter. Larger polyps may project from the endometrial mucosa into the uterine cavity. On histologic examination, they are covered with columnar cells; some have an edematous stroma with essentially normal endometrial architecture, but more often they have cystically dilated glands similar to those seen with cystic hyperplasia.

Although endometrial polyps may occur at any age, they develop more commonly at the time of menopause. Probably their only clinical significance lies in the production of abnormal uterine bleeding.

## LEIOMYOMA AND LEIOMYOSARCOMA

Benign tumors arising in the myometrium are properly termed "leiomyomas," although often they are referred to as "fibroids." *These are the most common benign tumors in females, developing in about one in four women during active reproductive life.* Although the etiology and pathogenesis are unknown, leiomyomas, once developed, seem to be estrogen dependent, as evidenced by their rapid growth during pregnancy and their tendency to regress following menopause. Whether or not hyperestrinism alone can actually initiate the formation of these tumors is, however, unclear.

Leiomyomas usually occur as multiple, sharply circumscribed but unencapsulated, firm, gray-white masses, with a characteristically **whorled cut surface.** They vary in size from barely visible seedings to massive tumors that may simulate a pregnant uterus. They may be embedded within the myometrium **(intramural)** or be **subserosal** or lie directly beneath the endometrium **(submucosal)** (Fig. 19–10). Subserosal lesions may become pedunculated and, rarely, become attached to a loop of bowel, develop

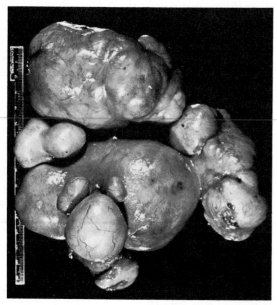

**Figure 19–10.** Leiomyomas of the uterus. The multiple subserosal, pedunculated, irregular tumors are viewed in the removed uterus. The uterine corpus is distorted beyond recognition. Only the cervix is identifiable as the lowermost projection.

a blood supply from it, and then, by attenuation of the original stalk, free themselves from the uterus to become a "parasitic leiomyoma." The submucosal tumors may project as polyps into the uterine cavity. Larger leiomyomas contain areas of yellow-brown to red softening, known as **necrobiosis** or **red carnaceous degeneration.** Proteolysis of these necrotic areas yields foci of cystic degeneration. After menopause they tend to shrink, become firmer and more collagenous, and sometimes undergo partial or even complete calcification. Histologically, the tumors are characterized by whorling bundles of smooth muscle cells, duplicating the normal muscle bundles of the myometrium. Foci of fibrosis, calcification, ischemic necrosis with hemorrhage, and more or less complete proteolytic digestion of dead cells may be present. After menopause, the smooth muscle cells tend to atrophy, eventually being replaced by fibrous tissue.

Leiomyomas of the uterus are often entirely asymptomatic and are discovered on routine pelvic examination as a mass or asymmetry of the uterine fundus. The most frequent manifestation is menorrhagia, with or without metrorrhagia. The exact basis for bleeding is unknown. Concomitant hyperestrinism has been suggested, but the endometrium is usually not hyperplastic. Large masses may produce a dragging sensation in the pelvic region. When situated in the lower uterine segment, they may create problems during childbirth.

*Leiomyosarcomas arise from the myometrium directly. Whether or not uterine leiomyomas ever undergo malignant transformation to become leiomyosarcomas is a controversial point.* If they do, such transformation is indeed rare, because the benign tumors are commonplace, but their malignant counterparts are rare.

Grossly, **leiomyosarcomas** develop in several distinct patterns: as bulky masses infiltrating the uterine wall; as polypoid lesions projecting into the uterine cavity; or as structures with deceptively discrete margins that masquerade as large benign leiomyomas. Histologically, they show a wide range of differentiation, from well-differentiated growths similar to the leiomyomas to wildly anaplastic lesions approximating undifferentiated sarcomas. The well-differentiated tumors may be difficult to differentiate from "cellular leiomyomas." The number of mitoses per high power field (hpf) has been used as the differential feature. When there are fewer than 4 mitoses per hpf the tumor is considered benign.

The five-year survival rate with overt malignancy is about 20 to 40%. After surgical removal, leiomyosarcomas show a striking tendency toward local recurrence, and some metastasize widely.

## CARCINOMA OF THE ENDOMETRIUM

The incidence of this disease has remained at about the same level for many years. Although invasive carcinoma of the cervix was once much more common than cancer of the endometrium, the dramatic control that has been seen with the former (p. 637) has not been achieved with endometrial carcinoma and so it is now more common than invasive cervical carcinoma. Cytologic diagnosis with endometrial carcinoma is far less effective than with cervical cancers. However, endometrial lesions tend to arise postmenopausally and cause irregular bleeding, permitting their diagnosis while still confined to the uterus and therefore curable by surgery or radiotherapy. Thus, endometrial carcinoma accounts for about 3000 deaths annually in the United States, less than half as many as caused by invasive cervical carcinoma.[20]

**INCIDENCE.** Carcinoma of the endometrium is uncommon in women under age 40. The peak incidence is in the 55- to 65-year age range. *An increased frequency of this form of neoplasia is seen with: (1) obesity; (2) diabetes or, merely, glucose intolerance; and (3) infertility.* An increased frequency of hypertension has also been noted in some studies but denied in others.[34] There are plausible explanations for the roles of obesity and infertility, as will become evident, but the concurrence of diabetes with this form of neoplasia remains largely unexplained, except for the well-known association of the metabolic disease with obesity. Infrequently, both endometrial and breast carcinomas arise in the same patient.

**PATHOGENESIS.** The evidence is quite convincing that endometrial carcinoma arises as a progression from ever more florid endometrial hyperplasia under the influence of prolonged estrogen stimulation.[35] The supporting observations can be summarized as follows:

○ Adenomatous hyperplasia progressing to atypical hyperplasia (clearly related to hyperestrinism) frequently antedates the appearance of endometrial carcinoma. Indeed, it is difficult to segregate morphologically atypical hyperplasia from carcinoma.[31]

○ Exogenous estrogens, particularly when used to control menopausal symptoms, are associated with an increased risk.[36]

○ Estrogen-secreting ovarian neoplasms (e.g., granulosa cell tumors) induce an increased incidence of endometrial carcinoma.

○ Obesity predisposes because of increased synthesis of estrogens in fat depots from adrenal and ovarian precursors.

○ The cancer is more common in infertile women, related to ovulatory failure and prolonged estrogen stimulation unopposed by postovulatory progestins.

○ The development of tumors at the time of or after the menopause reflects the continued influence of estrogens of adrenal origin unopposed by progestins.

○ The role of oral contraceptives (OCs) remains contentious. OCs currently available that have both estrogens and progestin are generally thought not to increase the risk or even to protect, but a few reports suggest a slightly increased risk.[37, 38]

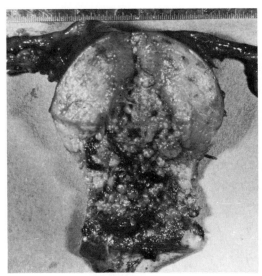

Figure 19–11. Endometrial carcinoma, presenting as a fungating mass in the fundus of the uterus. (From Robbins, S. L., Cotran, R. S., and Kumar, V.: Pathologic Basis of Disease. 3rd ed. Philadelphia, W. B. Saunders Co., 1984, p. 1138.)

**MORPHOLOGY.** Endometrial carcinomas are believed to arise as in situ lesions, which, after a period of years, assume one of two macroscopic appearances.[39] Either they infiltrate, causing diffuse thickening of the affected uterine wall, or they assume an exophytic form (Fig. 19–11). In both cases, they eventually fill the endometrial cavity with firm to soft, partially necrotic tumor tissue, and in time they extend through the myometrial wall to the serosa and thence by direct contiguity to periuterine structures. Late in the course, metastases to regional lymph nodes and later to distant organs occur. In about 85% of these tumors, the histologic form is that of an **adenocarcinoma,** with well-defined gland patterns lined with anaplastic cuboidal to columnar epithelial cells. They range from well differentiated to poorly differentiated. Rarely, these cells have mucinous secretory activity, but most are nonsecretory and recapitulate the proliferative phase of the endometrial cycle. The remaining 15% of endometrial carcinomas are **adenoacanthomas** and **adenosquamous** carcinomas. These two should be clearly distinguished. Adenoacanthoma is characterized by metaplastic transformation of neoplastic columnar cells into squamous cells along part of the circumference of the glands. The squamous element is mature and well differentiated. Despite such curious and aberrant differentiation, these tumors behave like adenocarcinomas. Adenosquamous carcinomas, on the other hand, consist of clearly malignant squamous elements mixed with adenocarcinoma, both usually poorly differentiated (Fig. 19–12). Because the "adeno-" component is poorly differentiated, these neoplasms have a worse prognosis than adenoacanthomas.[35]

Like most cancers, endometrial carcinoma is graded according to cellular differentiation and staged according to the extent of the disease at diagnosis. The grades are

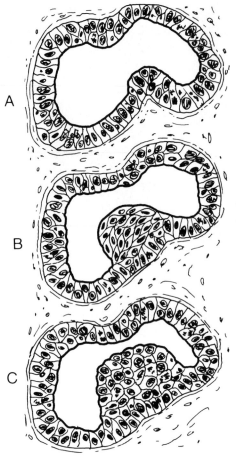

**Figure 19–12.** A comparison of (*A*) adenocarcinoma, (*B*) adenoacanthoma with a focus of well-differentiated squamous metaplasia, and (*C*) adenosquamous carcinoma with poor differentiation of both patterns of epithelium.

I to III, from well differentiated to undifferentiated. The staging system most widely used recognizes:

Stage I—confined to uterine corpus
Stage II—involvement of corpus and cervix
Stage III—extension outside of uterus but not outside true pelvis
Stage IV—extension beyond Stage III

**CLINICAL COURSE.** The first clinical indications of endometrial carcinoma are usually marked leukorrhea and irregular bleeding. This reflects erosion and ulceration of the endometrial surface. Even at this stage, the cervix may appear completely normal. With progression, the uterus may be palpably enlarged, and in time it becomes fixed to surrounding structures by extension of the cancer beyond the uterus. Fortunately, these are usually late-metastasizing neoplasms, but dissemination eventually occurs with involvement of regional nodes and more distant sites (e.g., liver, lungs). Radiotherapy and surgery have long been the standard modes of therapy, but many adenocarcinomas possess estrogen and progesterone receptors and respond favorably to antiestrogens.[40] Various chemotherapy protocols are also under study, but surgical excision and radiotherapy are still the most effective forms of treatment because other modalities may retard progression but rarely achieve cures. Curiously, receptor-positive neoplasms also yield better results following surgery, perhaps because they tend to be better differentiated. When all therapeutic modalities are utilized, Stage I carcinoma is associated with a 90% five-year survival rate. This rate drops to 30 to 50% in Stage II and to less than 20% in Stages III and IV.

# Fallopian Tubes

These should be the most beloved organs in the body to the pathology student because they are so seldom the site of primary disease. Their most common afflictions are inflammations, almost always as part of pelvic inflammatory disease, or PID (p. 625). Much less often they are affected by ectopic (tubal) pregnancy (p. 655), followed in order of frequency by endometriosis (p. 641) and the rare primary tumors. Only a few comments on salpingitis and tumors are necessary.

*Inflammations of the tube* are almost always bacterial in origin. With the declining incidence of gonorrhea, nongonococcal organisms such as chlamydia, *Mycoplasma hominis*, coliforms, and, in the postpartum setting, streptococci and staphylococci are now the major offenders. The morphologic changes produced by gonococci conform to those already described in PID. Nongonococcal infections differ somewhat inasmuch as they are more invasive, penetrating the wall of the tubes and thus tending

more often to give rise to blood-borne infections and seeding of the meninges, joint spaces, and sometimes the heart valves. Rarely, tuberculous salpingitis is encountered, almost always in combination with involvement of the endometrium as a part of miliary tuberculosis. All forms of salpingitis, whatever the cause, are of importance. They may produce fever, lower abdominal or pelvic pain, sometimes right upper quadrant pain when the organisms trek up to the liver and cause perihepatitis, and pelvic masses when the tubes become distended with either exudate or later burned-out inflammatory debris and secretions (*hydrosalpinx*) (Fig. 19–13). Even more serious is the potential for obstruction of the tubal lumens, which sometimes produces permanent sterility.

*Primary adenocarcinomas may arise in the tubes.* They are curiosities that are usually undiscovered until they spread. In time they may cause death.

Figure 19–13. Pelvic inflammatory disease. The uterus is flanked by large bilateral tubo-ovarian masses resulting from the accumulation of exudate within the sealed-off tubes and ovaries. Note the shaggy hemorrhagic surface responsible for pelvic adhesions.

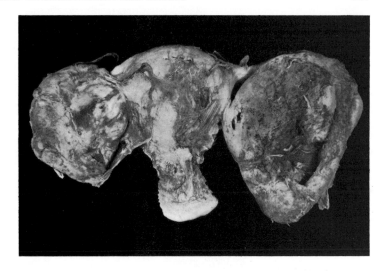

# Ovaries

The ovaries are infrequently the primary site of any disease except, notably, neoplasms. Indeed, carcinomas of the ovaries account for more deaths (about 12,000) than cancers of the cervix and uterine corpus together. It is less their frequency than their lethality that makes them so evil. Non-neoplastic cysts are commonplace but generally are not serious problems. Primary inflammations of the ovary are rarities, but salpingitis of the tubes frequently causes a periovarian reaction called salpingo-oophoritis. As discussed earlier, the ovary is frequently secondarily affected in endometriosis. Only the non-neoplastic cysts and neoplasms merit further consideration.

## FOLLICLE AND LUTEAL CYSTS

*Follicle and luteal cysts* in the ovaries are so commonplace as to be almost physiologic variants.

These innocuous lesions originate in unruptured graafian follicles or in follicles that have ruptured and have immediately been sealed. Such cysts are often multiple and develop immediately subjacent to the serosal covering of the ovary. Usually they are small—1 to 1.5 cm in diameter—and are filled with clear serous fluid, but occasionally they accumulate enough fluid to achieve diameters of 4 to 5 cm and may thus become palpable masses and indeed produce pelvic pain. They are lined by granulosal lining cells or luteal cells when small, but as the fluid accumulates under pressure, it may cause atrophy of these cells. Thus, the larger cysts often have only a compressed stromal enclosing wall. On occasion, these usually innocuous lesions rupture, producing intraperitoneal bleeding and acute abdominal symptoms.

## POLYCYSTIC OVARIES

Oligoamenorrhea, hirsutism, infertility, and sometimes obesity may appear in young women, usually in the postmenarchal girl, secondary to excessive production of estrogens and androgens (mostly the latter) by multiple cystic follicles in the ovaries. This condition is also called *polycystic ovaries* or *Stein-Leventhal syndrome*.[41]

The ovaries are usually twice normal in size, are gray-white with a smooth outer cortex, and are studded with subcortical cysts 0.5 to 1.5 cm in diameter. Histologically, there is a thickened fibrosed outer tunica, sometimes referred to as "cortical stromal fibrosis," beneath which are innumerable cysts lined by granulosal cells with a hypertrophic and hyperplastic luteinized theca interna. There is a conspicuous absence of corpora lutea.

The principal biochemical abnormalities that can be identified in most patients are excessive production of androgens, high levels of luteinizing hormone, and low levels of follicle-stimulating hormone. For years, these endocrine abnormalities were attributed to some primary ovarian dysfunction because large wedge resections of the ovaries reversed the clinical and endocrinologic abnormalities and restored fertility in most patients. However, it is now believed that the ovarian and hormonal changes are probably the result of unbalanced or asynchronous release of FSH and LH by the pituitary, which is in turn related to some disruption of hypothalamic control of pituitary secretion.[42] Presumably, reduction in size of the ovarian mass by wedge resections corrects the condition because it reduces the volume of ovarian tissue that can respond to pituitary hormones.

## TUMORS OF THE OVARY

Ovarian neoplasms come in an amazing variety of histogenetic types and shapes. This diversity is attributable to the three cell types making up the normal ovary—the multipotential surface (coelomic) covering epithelium, the totipotential germ cells, and the multipotential sex cord–stromal cells (Fig. 19–

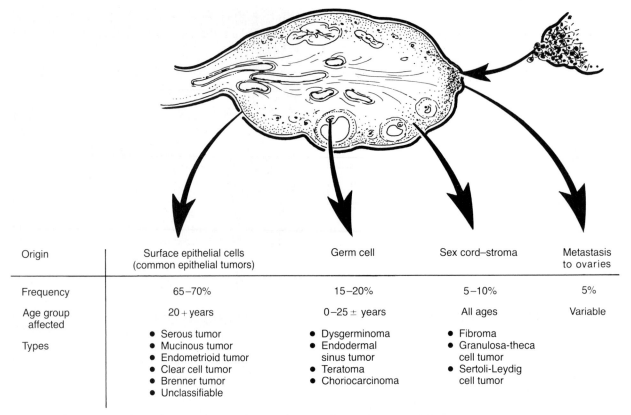

| Origin | Surface epithelial cells (common epithelial tumors) | Germ cell | Sex cord–stroma | Metastasis to ovaries |
|---|---|---|---|---|
| Frequency | 65–70% | 15–20% | 5–10% | 5% |
| Age group affected | 20 + years | 0–25 ± years | All ages | Variable |
| Types | • Serous tumor<br>• Mucinous tumor<br>• Endometrioid tumor<br>• Clear cell tumor<br>• Brenner tumor<br>• Unclassifiable | • Dysgerminoma<br>• Endodermal sinus tumor<br>• Teratoma<br>• Choriocarcinoma | • Fibroma<br>• Granulosa-theca cell tumor<br>• Sertoli-Leydig cell tumor | |

Figure 19–14. Derivation of various ovarian neoplasms and some data on their frequency and age distribution.

14). You recall that coelomic epithelium lines the embryonic furrows that form the Müllerian ducts and covers the ovaries. Thus tumors of the coelomic epithelium may be composed of epithelium recapitulating the lining of the fallopian tubes (ciliated and serous columnar cells), the endometrial lining (nonciliated columnar cells), or the endocervical glands (columnar mucus-secreting nonciliated cells). These neoplasms of surface epithelial origin account for about 65 to 70% of all primary ovarian tumors and, in their malignant forms, for almost 90% of all ovarian cancers, justifying their being called *"common epithelial tumors."*[43] In addition to the clearly benign and malignant neoplasms, some common epithelial tumors occupy an intermediate zone and are called "borderline malignant." They are characterized by epithelial anaplasia without stromal invasion.[44] The totipotential germ cells give rise to a variety of neoplasms, ranging from teratomas (mature and immature) to other forms of neoplasia, which represent unidirectional differentiation of the germ cells and account collectively for about 15 to 20% of all ovarian tumors but only 2 to 4% of ovarian cancers. The sex cord–stromal cells may differentiate along granulosal, thecal, fibromatous, and Sertoli-Leydig cell lines, as well as others representing 5 to 10% of all ovarian tumors and 2% of ovarian cancers.[45] Were this complexity not sufficient, there remain unclassified tumors and cancers metastatic to the ovaries. Only the more common among this large array of neoplasms will be considered, but a more complete presentation has been provided by Scully.[46]

All ovarian neoplasms pose formidable clinical challenges because they produce no symptoms or signs until well advanced in their development. Indeed, many are discovered on routine gynecologic examination. Thus the cancers are often not discovered until they have extended beyond the ovaries. Unlike the case with cancers of the cervix, deaths from malignant neoplasms of the ovary have not declined in frequency over the years and now rank fourth among the cancer-killers of women (behind those of the lung, breast, and large intestine).[20] The contributions of the various types of ovarian cancer to these deaths is presented in Table 19–4.

Little is known about the origins of these neoplasms, but a few risk factors have been identified. Blacks have a lower incidence of epithelial neoplasms than whites and about a third less ovarian cancer. Rare families are predisposed to the malignant neoplasms, which sometimes occur in association with breast carcinoma. The frequency of cancer is high in unmarried women and is inversely related to parity. Controversy persists, but several studies suggest that exogenous estrogens increase the risk. On the other hand, oral contraceptives containing both estrogens and progestins exert a modest protective effect. First we will turn to the morphology of the more common

**Table 19–4.** FREQUENCIES OF MALIGNANT TUMORS

| Type of Tumor | Approximate Proportion of Ovarian Cancers (%) |
|---|---|
| Serous tumors | 40 |
| Endometrioid tumors | 20 |
| Mucinous tumors | 10 |
| Undifferentiated carcinoma | 10 |
| Granulosa cell tumors | 5 |
| Metastatic | 6 |
| Clear cell carcinoma | 5 |
| Teratoma | 1 |
| Dysgerminoma | 1 |
| Others | 2 |

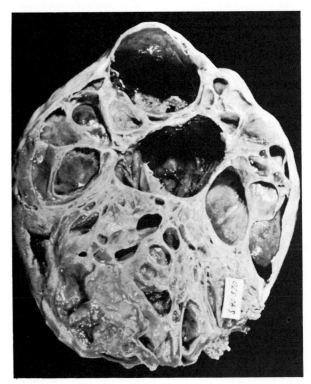

Figure 19–15. Multilocular serous cystadenoma of the ovary, on cross section. (From Robbins, S. L., Cotran, R. S., and Kumar, V.: Pathologic Basis of Disease. 3rd ed. Philadelphia, W. B. Saunders Co., 1984, p. 1145.)

ovarian neoplasms, after which some general comments will be made about the clinical features common to all.

## COMMON EPITHELIAL TUMORS

Although it is traditional to divide neoplasms into benign and malignant categories, with the common epithelial tumors an intermediate—borderline—category has been established. These neoplasms appear to be low-grade cancers with low invasive potential. Thus they have a much better prognosis than their uglier cousins, as will be evident.[43]

### Serous Tumors

These are the most frequent of the ovarian tumors, encountered usually between the ages of 30 and 40. Although they may be solid, they are usually cystic, hence they are commonly known as *cystadenomas* or *cystadenocarcinomas. About 25% are benign, 10% borderline, and 65% malignant, yielding a 3:1 malignant to benign ratio.* Combined borderline and malignant lesions account for about 40% of all ovarian cancers.

Grossly, serous tumors may be small (5 to 10 cm in diameter) but most are large, spherical to ovoid, cystic structures, up to approximately 30 to 40 cm in diameter. **About 33% of the benign forms are bilateral, whereas 66% of the more aggressive lesions are bilateral.** In the benign form, the serosal covering is smooth and glistening. In contrast, the covering of the cystadenocarcinoma shows nodular irregularities, which represent penetration of the tumor to or through the serosa. On transection, the small cystic tumor may reveal a single cavity, but larger ones are usually divided by multiple septa into a multiloculated mass (Fig. 19–15). The cystic spaces are usually filled with a clear serous fluid, although a considerable amount of mucus may also be present. Jutting into the cystic cavities are polypoid or papillary projections, which become more marked in malignant tumors, accompanied by neoplastic infiltration through the walls of the cystic cavities. **In general, the more exuberant the papillations, the more abundant the solid areas, and the more prominent the subserosal or serosal nodularity or papillation, the more likely the lesion is malignant** (Fig. 19–16).

Histologically, the benign tumors are characterized by a single layer of tall columnar epithelium which lines the cyst or cysts. The cells are in part ciliated and in part dome-shaped secretory cells. Microscopic papillae, consisting of a delicate fibrous core covered by a single layer of epithelium, may be present. Psammoma bodies (concentrically laminated concretions) are common in the tips of papillae. When the stromal component is abundant, these lesions are often termed **cystadenofibromas.** With the development of frank carcinoma, microscopic examination discloses most importantly anaplasia of the lining cells. Invasion of the stroma is usually readily evident, and papillary formations are complex and multilayered with invasion of the axial fibrous tissue by nests or totally undifferentiated sheets of malignant cells. Between these clearly benign and obviously malignant forms are the so-called "borderline tumors" with obvious epithelial anaplasia in the absence of stromal invasion. These may implant locally on the peritoneum, after which a rare "less borderline" lesion spreads through vascular or lymphatic channels. The overt carcinomas tend to spread contiguously within the pelvis and, by seeding the frequently associated ascitic fluid, implant throughout the peritoneal cavity. Often the implants glaze all peritoneal surfaces, but uncommonly they penetrate the underlying viscera.

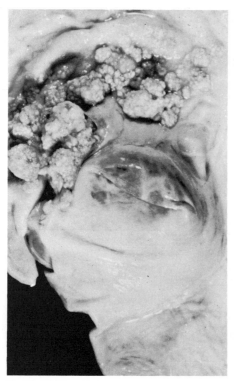

Figure 19–16. Multilocular serous cystadenocarcinoma of the ovary—close-up of the papillary excrescences that have penetrated the covering serosa. (From Robbins, S. L., Cotran, R. S., and Kumar, V.: Pathologic Basis of Disease. 3rd ed. Philadelphia, W. B. Saunders Co., 1984, p. 1145.)

Spread to regional lymph nodes is frequent, but distant lymphatic and hematogenous metastases are infrequent.

The prognosis for the patient with clearly invasive serous cystadenocarcinoma after surgery, which is sometimes followed by radiation and chemotherapy, is poor and depends heavily on the stage of the disease at the time of diagnosis; an overall 10-year survival rate is only 13%. In contrast, the borderline cancers yield an overall 10-year survival of about 80 to 85%.

### Mucinous Tumors

They are in most respects entirely analogous to the serous tumors, differing essentially in that the epithelium consists of mucin-secreting cells similar to those of the endocervical mucosa. These tumors occur in patients in the same age range as those with serous tumors, but mucinous lesions *are considerably less likely to be malignant, having a malignant to benign ratio of 1:5 and accounting for about 10% of all ovarian cancers.* Benign lesions (*cystadenoma*) predominate—75%; borderline represent 10%, and malignant (*cystadenocarcinoma*), 15%. When stromal proliferation is marked, the benign lesion may be termed a *cystadenofibroma.*

Only about 5% of benign and 20% of malignant tumors are bilateral, much less often than the case with their serous counterparts. On gross examination, they may be indistinguishable from serous tumors except by the mucinous nature of the cystic contents. However, **they are more likely to be larger and multilocular, and papillary formations are less common. Prominent papillation, serosal penetration, and solidified areas point to malignancy.**

Histologically, these mucinous tumors are identified by the apical vacuolation of the tall columnar epithelial cells and by the absence of cilia. Occasionally, mixtures of ciliated and mucinous epithelium are encountered. Metastases or rupture of mucinous cystadenocarcinomas may give rise to the clinical condition designated **pseudomyxoma peritonei.** The peritoneal cavity becomes filled with a glairy mucinous material resembling the cystic contents of the tumor. Multiple tumor implants are found on all the serosal surfaces, and the abdominal viscera become matted together. This form of pseudomyxoma peritonei is analogous to that encountered with rupture of a carcinomatous mucocele of the appendix (p. 560). Local extension and visceral metastasis may also occur.

The prognosis of mucinous cystadenocarcinoma is better than that with the serous counterpart. The overall 10-year survival rate is about 35%. Borderline mucinous tumors are associated with an 85% 10-year survival rate.

### Endometrioid Tumors

*These tumors are characterized by the formation of tubular glands, similar to those of the endometrium, within the linings of cystic spaces. Although benign and borderline forms exist, endometrioid tumors are usually malignant.* They are bilateral in about 30% of cases, and *15 to 30% of patients with these ovarian tumors have a concomitant endometrial carcinoma.* The relationship between the ovarian and the endometrial lesions is unclear, but it is likely that they represent separate primary tumors.

Grossly, the ovarian lesion may be solid or cystic. The cystic forms are usually indistinguishable on gross inspection from the serous and mucinous lesions just described. Sometimes these tumors develop as a mass projecting from the wall of an endometriotic cyst filled with chocolate-colored fluid. Microscopically, the cells lining the glandular formations are usually columnar, producing an **adenocarcinoma.** Sometimes, foci of metaplastic squamous cells are found, thus recapitulating the **adenoacanthoma** of the endometrium of the uterus. Varying degrees of anaplasia are present.

When these tumors are relatively well differentiated, there is a 62% five-year survival rate. However, the more aggressive carcinomas permit only a 23% five-year survival.

### Clear Cell Carcinomas

These rare neoplasms are marked by large glycogen-filled clear cells bearing a strong resemblance to those of renal cell carcinomas. There is little doubt but that they arise from Müllerian epithelium; analogous tumors arise in the endometrium, and in some instances they are associated with pelvic and ovarian endometriosis, supporting their Müllerian origin.

Grossly, they tend to be smaller than serous and mucinous tumors, are unilateral in 90% of cases, may be solid or cystic, and often have foci of necrosis and hemorrhage.[47] Histologically, the clear cells may form tubules or papillary projections into cystic spaces. The more anaplastic lesions may penetrate the capsule and spread locally or to distant organs. The overall five-year survival rate is about 50%, but with tumor limited to the ovary, the outlook is excellent.

Of particular interest, these tumors sometimes produce hypercalcemia as a paraneoplastic syndrome.

### Brenner Tumor

*The Brenner tumor* is an uncommon ovarian solid, usually benign tumor consisting of an abundant stroma **containing nests of transitional epithelium resembling that of the urinary tract.** Occasionally, the nests are cystic and lined by columnar mucus-secreting cells. Brenner tumors generally are smoothly encapsulated and gray-white on transection and range from a few centimeters to 20 cm in diameter.

Possibly these tumors arise from the surface epithelium, but it is also hypothesized that they spring from rests of urogenital epithelium trapped within the germinal ridge. They are generally incidental findings and *sometimes appear as a focal area within a mucinous cystadenoma.*

## GERM CELL TUMORS

Tumors of germ cell origin comprise about 15 to 20% of ovarian neoplasms.[48] Over half arise in the first two decades of life and, unfortunately, the younger the patient, the greater the likelihood of malignancy. About 90 to 95% are benign cystic mature teratomas readily identified morphologically. Most of the residual represent immature and often malignant teratomas, dysgerminomas, choriocarcinomas, or other lines of development of germ cells. Only the better defined lesions will be discussed.

### Teratoma

Teratomas, you recall, contain elements representative of more than one germ layer. Similar tumors may also arise in the testis and, rarely, in extragonadal sites (p. 617). In the ovary 99% differentiate mainly along ectodermal lines and, fortunately, are benign cystic teratomas. The small remainder of immature teratomas are much more likely to be malignant. Rarely, unusual patterns of specialized differentiation are encountered; two are briefly characterized later—struma ovarii and carcinoid.

***Benign (Mature) Cystic Teratoma.*** These interesting neoplasms are marked by ectodermal differentiation with the formation of cysts, which are, to all appearances, lined by normal-appearing skin that is often replete with adnexal appendages; hence the common designation "dermoid cysts." About 80% occur in patients between 20 and 30 years of age.

Most are unilateral, most often on the right, but in 10% of cases they are bilateral. Typically, they are less than 10 cm in diameter and are covered by a glistening serosa. On sectioning there is a thin cystic wall lined by well-differentiated skin having adnexal glands, including hair. The cystic space is filled with a thick, sebaceous secretion containing matted hair (Fig. 19–17). Sometimes teeth protrude from a nodular projection and (children take note) they are unbrushed and may be carious! Occasionally, foci of bone, cartilage, nests of bronchial or gastrointestinal epithelium, and other recognizable structures are present in the nodular projection.

Excision of these tumors is almost always curative. In about 1% of dermoid cysts there is malignant transformation of one of the tissue elements, usually taking the form of a squamous cell carcinoma. Of interest, *torsion of the tumor occurs in about 10 to 15% of cases, producing an acute surgical emergency.*

***Immature Teratoma.*** As the name indicates, this often malignant neoplasm is composed of random mixtures of immature tissue derived from any or all of the three germ layers. Sometimes immature teratomas also have components representing other types of germ cell neoplasia, such as foci of choriocarcinoma

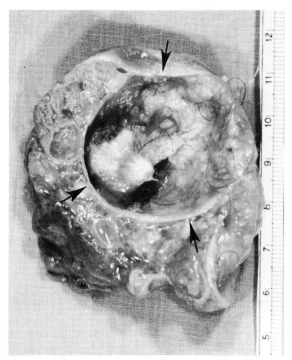

Figure 19–17. A small, opened, benign cystic teratoma (dermoid cyst) of the ovary.

or dysgerminoma, to which the terms "teratocarcinoma" or "malignant teratoma" are sometimes applied. It is recommended that with ovarian lesions these mixed patterns be excluded from the category of immature teratoma. So defined, immature teratomas occur in patients under 40 years of age, and a significant number occur before puberty.

They are generally unilateral, often cystic masses up to 25 cm in diameter. The external surface is smooth and the cut surface is of varying consistence (reflecting the contained tissue elements) and red to pink with areas of hemorrhage and necrosis. Microscopically, there is a wide range of cellular differentiation, with variable maturation toward mature tissues.[49] Most have immature but recognizable cartilage, bone, and, particularly, neuroepithelial and glial elements. But many other tissues, such as gastrointestinal, bronchial, and squamous epithelia, may be identified. Tumors having more or less well-differentiated components may remain confined to the ovary, but with progressive immaturity (most often within the neuroepithelial elements) penetration through the capsule and metastases may appear.

The prognosis is dependent on the most immature component having the greatest degree of anaplasia, the presence of metastases, and the level of anaplasia in the metastases. Unfortunately, most of these neoplasms grow rapidly and extend beyond the ovary, yielding about a 25 to 30% five-year survival. The better differentiated lesions confined to the ovary can be cured by excision.

*Monodermal (Specialized) Teratomas.* These merit brief comment only because they are medical curiosities. Very rarely teratogenous, unidirectional differentiation produces an ovarian mass composed of red-brown thyroid tissue *(struma ovarii)*. These lesions are of interest because the ectopic tissue has in some cases participated along with the thyroid gland in causing hyperthyroidism. Equally exotic is the *carcinoid*, which occasionally induces the carcinoid syndrome (p. 538).

### Dysgerminoma

This uncommon, usually malignant ovarian tumor is composed of primordial germ cells and so is the counterpart of the seminoma of the testis (p. 615).[50]

It occurs in children and young adults, generally as a solid unilateral (90%) mass ranging up to 25 cm in diameter. Most are quite distinctive histologically, having nests and aggregates of large vesicular cells with cleared cytoplasm and centrally placed nuclei separated by trabeculae that have a lymphocytic infiltrate and, occasionally, syncytial-type giant cells and granuloma formations.

Although the tumors are invasive and have a propensity for early spread to regional and then para-aortic nodes before metastasizing elsewhere, they are responsive to radiotherapy (and some to chemotherapy), yielding a 65 to 95% five-year survival. A well-defined association with congenital malformations of the genitals and with Turner's syndrome (p. 124) has been noted.

### Endodermal Sinus (Yolk Sac) Tumor

This rapidly growing, highly malignant tumor is analogous to the yolk sac tumor of the testis (p. 616). The age range is one to 45 years, with a median of 19 years.

The tumors seem to appear abruptly and enlarge under observation, sometimes producing masses extending into the abdomen. Although they have a smooth external surface, there is frequently rupture through it. Although the tumor is usually unilateral in origin, spread to the opposite ovary sometimes occurs. Microscopically, the pattern recapitulates the yolk sac, comprising a loose meshwork of cysts and channels lined by flattened or vacuolated cells. The cells may contain intracellular droplets, which can be shown to be rich in alpha-1-antitrypsin, alpha-fetoprotein (AFP), or both. Sometimes epithelial-covered projections into the cystic spaces have a central glomerulus-like tuft with a vascular core (the Schiller-Duval body). Metastases are usually widespread.

At one time, these tumors were almost universally fatal within a year, but chemotherapeutic regimens now achieve a few cases of long-term survivals. Helpful in the diagnosis of these neoplasms and in monitoring possible recurrences are the elevated serum AFP levels.

### Choriocarcinoma

This rare tumor is analogous anatomically to its counterparts in the testis (p. 616) and in the placenta (p. 657). When primary in the ovary, they are usually part of a mixed germ cell tumor; "pure" choriocarcinoma is most often a metastasis from a tumor arising in the placenta, where the neoplasm is described.

## SEX CORD–STROMAL TUMORS

These neoplasms are composed of varying combinations of sex cord and stromal derivatives capable of differentiating in an ovarian direction (granulosa cells, theca cells), in a testicular direction (Sertoli cells, Leydig cells), or in the stromal direction to remain fibromatous.[51] Neoplasms in this category comprise about 5 to 10% of all ovarian tumors but only about 2% of cancers. Nonetheless, they are of clinical importance because many elaborate steroid hormones, which are usually estrogenic but sometimes androgenic.

### Granulosa Cell Tumor

Although uncommon, these neoplasms account for most sex cord–stromal cancers. Most arise in postmenopausal women, but younger women and occasionally prepubertal girls may be affected. *About 75% of these tumors in adults induce hyperestrinism, resulting in endometrial hyperplasia and a variety of menstrual disorders, notably postmenopausal uterine bleeding and, occasionally, adenocarcinoma of the endometrium.* In the young child, they induce precocious puberty.

Rarely bilateral, these neoplasms are typically well encapsulated, but rupture is common. They range in size up to 30 cm in diameter. Transection reveals either a solid gray-yellow mass, punctuated by areas of hemorrhagic necrosis and cysts, or a unilocular or multilocular tumor. There is great diversity in the microscopic appearance. In the most recognizable pattern, the granulosa cells form large islands or broad anastomosing cords in which there are microfollicular spaces, which sometimes harbor an aggregate of debris or degenerated tumor cells that create a resemblance to an ovum **(Call-Exner body).** Less easily recognized patterns have trabeculae of granulosal cells that occasionally form gland patterns, whereas others are solid masses of granulosa cells, and in others the cells occasionally become spindled and sarcomatoid. The stromal component may be minimal or abundant, but the neoplasm is called a granulosa cell tumor as long as even a minor feature comprises well-differentiated granulosa cells. Local invasion is moderately common but metastasis rare.

Although complete surgical removal of these neoplasms is usually possible, the prognosis is affected by (1) rupture of the tumor and (2) size of the mass. With lesions less than 5 cm in diameter there is almost 100% 10-year survival, but with larger masses, the survival is 25 to 50%.[52] As noted above, high levels of circulating estrogens are usually present, leading in rare cases to endometrial carcinoma.

### Fibroma-Thecoma-Luteoma Tumors

Individual tumors within this category range from typical fibroblastic lesions (*fibroma*) to neoplasms in which the plump fibroblasts contain abundant intracytoplasmic lipid (*thecoma*) to those containing areas largely composed of typical epithelium-like lutein cells (*luteoma*). Paralleling these histologic characteristics are the functional activities of the neoplasms; the fibroma is nonfunctional but the thecomas are estrogenic and the luteomas androgenic.

The **fibroma** is composed of spindled fibroblasts arrayed in interweaving bands (storiform pattern) with a variable amount of intercellular collagen. Generally small, these tumors are hard, solid gray-white encapsulated masses rarely exceeding 10 cm in diameter. About half of the larger lesions are associated with ascites and, sometimes, hydrothorax (usually right-sided) in a condition called the **"Meigs' syndrome."** Most patients are over 40 years of age. It should be noted, then, that **an ovarian neoplasm with effusions into the peritoneal and pleural cavities does not necessarily spell dissemination of an ovarian cancer.** The ascitic fluid is thought to represent transudate or lymphatic weepage from the tumor. Occasional fibromas have increased mitotic activity and cellular atypicality and are referred to as "cellular fibromas" or even "fibrosarcomas."

**Thecomas** look like yellowed fibromas, although they may be more rubbery. Microscopic examination reveals spindle-shaped or oval cells that have granular or frankly vacuolated cytoplasm containing abundant lipid, which biochemical analysis proves to be at least in part composed of estrogens. Most patients are postmenopausal and have uterine bleeding, and almost a quarter develop endometrial carcinoma.

Blending imperceptibly, on histologic grounds, with thecomas are tumors that contain collections of luteinized cells. These neoplasms may be called **"luteinized thecomas"** or, when the luteal component is dominant, **"luteomas."** In contrast to thecomas, luteinized tumors induce masculinization, most often in postmenopausal women but occasionally in much younger individuals.

These tumors are principally of importance because of their hormonal effects. The effects of thecomas are analogous to those of granulosa cell tumors, whereas the luteomas induce masculinization. The diagnosis of these tumors is facilitated by the identification of either estrogens or androgens in the blood. Resection of the ovarian neoplasm corrects the endocrinopathy, but somatic features of marked virilization (e.g., enlargement of the clitoris) may persist.

### Sertoli-Leydig Cell Tumors (Androblastoma, Arrhenoblastoma)

In the embryo, the primitive gonads, composed largely of undifferentiated mesenchyme, may differentiate along male or female lines; the result is presumably dictated by the sex chromosomes. Sertoli-Leydig cell neoplasms are thought to represent masculine differentiation of primitive mesenchymal elements within the ovary. Most of these tumors synthesize a variety of androgens and cause masculinization. A few are estrogenic, but some are apparently nonfunctional.

Resembling small granulosa cell tumors macroscopically, these tumors assume one of many histologic patterns. On the one extreme, they may be composed of cords or trabeculae of cuboidal Sertoli cells, with pale, granular lipid-laden cytoplasm and rounded nuclei, recapitulating early testicular development. Other tumors have an admixture of Sertoli cells and Leydig cells, the latter appearing as large polygonal cells with granular eosinophilic cytoplasm that sometimes contain rounded or pointed crystals of Reinke and central, small, round hyperchromatic nuclei. Most Leydig cells contain lipid that can be proved to be steroids. At the other extreme are tumors composed largely of Leydig cells. Heterologous elements such as bone, cartilage, and epithelial glands are sometimes found in the stroma. In addition to this range of cytologic composition, individual neoplasms may be well to poorly differentiated.[53]

The prognosis is largely dependent on the degree of differentiation of the neoplastic cells and so the five-year survival rate ranges from 100% to 50 or 60%. Recurrences and metastases account for the deaths.

## CLINICAL CORRELATIONS FOR ALL OVARIAN TUMORS

The clinical presentation of all ovarian tumors is remarkably similar despite their great morphologic diversity, except for the functioning neoplasms that have hormonal affects. Ovarian tumors are usually asymptomatic until they become large enough to cause local pressure symptoms, (e.g., pain, gastrointestinal complaints, urinary frequency). Indeed, about 30% of all ovarian neoplasms are discovered incidentally on routine gynecologic examination. Larger masses, notably the "common epithelial tumors," may cause an increase in abdominal girth. In addition to this common background, there are a number of clinical features related to specific neoplasms. Smaller masses, particularly dermoid cysts, may become twisted on their pedicles (torsion), producing severe abdominal pain and an acute abdomen. Fibromas and malignant serous tumors often cause ascites, the latter owing to metastatic seeding of the peritoneal cavity, so that tumor cells can be identified in the ascitic fluid. Mucinous cancers may literally fill the abdominal cavity with a gelatinous neoplastic mass (pseudomyxoma peritonei). Functioning ovarian tumors often come to attention because of the endocrinopathies they induce, as has already been noted.

The major challenge is the early detection of ovarian cancers. To this end an intense search has been made for circulating markers.[54, 55] Regrettably, only a few have proved to have limited value because of difficulties with sensitivity and specificity. The better established markers and their applications are presented in Table 19–5. However, their diagnostic usefulness is limited because significantly elevated blood levels may not appear until the neoplasms are quite large; their principal utility is in the monitoring of possible recurrences in patients with elevated levels prior to therapy.

Elaborate treatment protocols involving surgery, radiation, and chemotherapy (intraperitoneal and systemic) have been established for ovarian cancers. To

**Table 19–5. TUMOR MARKERS FOR OVARIAN CANCER**

| Marker | Tumor | % Positivity |
|---|---|---|
| Carcinoembryonic antigen | Serous carcinoma | 50–70 |
| | Mucinous carcinoma | 25–50 |
| Alpha-fetoprotein | Endodermal sinus | 80–90 |
| | Immature teratoma | 20–25 |
| Human chorionic gonadotropin | Choriocarcinoma | Most |
| | Dysgerminoma | 5–35 |
| Common epithelial antigen (CA-125) | Common epithelial tumors | 80 |

evaluate the efficacy of the many different protocols, a detailed and complex staging system has been devised. A simplified version is as follows:

Stages of Primary Carcinoma of the Ovary (International Federation of Gynecology and Obstetrics)
Stage I— Growth limited to ovaries with possibly ascites
Stage II— Growth involving one or both ovaries with pelvic extension
Stage III— Growth involving one or both ovaries with intraperitoneal metastases outside of pelvis and/or positive retroperitoneal nodes
Stage IV— Growth involving one or both ovaries with distant metastases or positive pleural effusion or metastases to liver

Further details have been reported by Richardson and colleagues.[43] Despite all efforts to achieve early diagnosis and effective methods of treatment, the overall five-year survival for the common epithelial cancers is a disappointing 30 to 35%. These poor results are in large part attributable to the fact that (as in years past) over half of these cancers are in Stages III and IV at the time of discovery.

## TUMORS METASTATIC TO THE OVARY

Metastases to the ovary most often arise from the gastrointestinal tract or nearby pelvic organs. The term *Krukenberg tumor* refers to bilateral ovarian metastases characterized by mucin-secreting "signet ring" cells. Commonly, such lesions are primary in the stomach, but they may also be metastatic from the colon, breast, or, indeed, any other organ having mucin-producing cells.

# Diseases of Pregnancy

This discussion will concern itself only with those disorders having prominent morphologic lesions— i.e., ectopic pregnancy and proliferative lesions of trophoblastic tissue. The toxemias of pregnancy often are associated with disseminated intravascular coagulation and are mentioned on page 395.

# ECTOPIC PREGNANCY

*Ectopic pregnancy* refers to implantation of the fertilized ovum in any site other than the normal uterine location. The condition occurs in up to 1% of pregnancies. *In over 90% of these cases, implantation is in the oviducts (tubal pregnancy); other sites include the ovaries, the abdominal cavity, and the intrauterine portion of the oviducts (interstitial pregnancy).* Any factor that retards passage of the ovum along its course through the oviducts to the uterus predisposes to an ectopic pregnancy. In about half of the cases such hindrance is based on chronic inflammatory changes within the oviduct, although intrauterine tumors and endometriosis may also hamper passage of the ovum. Occasionally, ectopic pregnancies are associated with the use of intrauterine contraceptive devices. In approximately 50% of tubal pregnancies, no anatomic cause can be demonstrated; these have been ascribed to functional disorders such as delayed ovulation. Ovarian pregnancies probably result from those rare instances of fertilization with trapping of the ovum within its follicle just at the time of rupture. Gestation within the abdominal cavity occurs when the fertilized egg drops out of the fimbriated end of the oviduct and implants on the peritoneum.

In all sites, ectopic pregnancies are characterized by fairly normal **early** development of the embryo, with the formation of placental tissue and amniotic sac and decidual changes. An abdominal pregnancy is occasionally carried to full term. With tubal pregnancies, however, the invading placenta eventually burrows through the wall of the oviduct or so weakens it that tubal rupture, with intraperitoneal hemorrhage, usually ensues, typically about two to six weeks after the onset of pregnancy. In addition, the tube is usually locally distended up to 3 to 4 cm by a contained mass of freshly clotted blood in which may be seen bits of gray placental tissue. The histologic diagnosis depends on the visualization of placental villi or, rarely, of the embryo. Less commonly, poor attachment of the placenta results in death of the embryo, with spontaneous proteolysis and absorption of the products of conception. Sometimes, in these cases, the embryo is not digested but rather becomes calcified, forming a **lithopedion.**

Until rupture occurs, an ectopic pregnancy may be indistinguishable from a normal one, with cessation of menstruation and elevation of serum and urinary placental hormones. Under the influence of these hormones, the endometrium (in about 50% of cases) undergoes the characteristic hypersecretory and decidual changes. *However, absence of elevated gonadotropin levels does not exclude this diagnosis, because poor attachment with necrosis of the placenta is common.* Rupture of an ectopic pregnancy is catastrophic, with the sudden onset of intense abdominal pain and signs of an acute abdomen, often followed by profound shock. Prompt surgical intervention is life-saving.

# GESTATIONAL TROPHOBLASTIC DISEASE

Traditionally, *the gestational trophoblastic tumors have been divided mainly into three overlapping morphologic categories—hydatidiform mole, invasive mole (chorioadenoma destruens), and choriocarcinoma.* They range in level of aggressiveness from the hydatidiform moles, most of which are benign, to the highly malignant choriocarcinomas. All elaborate human chorionic gonadotropin (HCG) that can be detected in the circulating blood and urine at titers considerably higher than those found during normal pregnancy. In addition to aiding in diagnosis, the fall or, alternatively, rise in the level of the hormone in the blood or urine can be used to monitor the effectiveness of treatment. Clinicians therefore prefer the term "gestational trophoblastic diseases" because the response to therapy as judged by the hormone titers is significantly more important than any arbitrary anatomic segregation of one lesion from another. Nonetheless, it is necessary to understand their individual characteristics to appreciate the spectrum of lesions.[56]

## HYDATIDIFORM MOLE

The typical hydatidiform mole comprises a voluminous mass of swollen, sometimes cystically dilated, chorionic villi covered by variable amounts of banal to highly atypical chorionic epithelium. More recently, two distinctive subtypes have been segregated—*"complete" and "partial" moles.*[57] *The complete hydatidiform mole never contains an embryo, umbilical cord, or amniotic membranes. All the chorionic villi are abnormal, and the chorionic epithelial cells usually have a 46 XX karyotype. The partial hydatidiform mole contains an embryo, umbilical cord, and amniotic membranes, has some normal chorionic villi, and is almost always triploid* (Fig. 19–18). The latter is much less common, so the following remarks will relate largely to the former.

The incidence of complete hydatidiform mole is about 1 to 1.5 per 2,000 pregnancies in the United States and other Western countries. For unknown reasons, there is a much higher incidence in Asian countries. They are much more common in women under 20 and over 40 years of age. Paternal age does not contribute to the frequency of occurrence. Current studies indicate that moles begin at conception as a form of neoplasia and so probably never represented potentially viable embryos. They usually present clinically with painless vaginal bleeding on average 16 to 17 weeks after conception. The uterus is

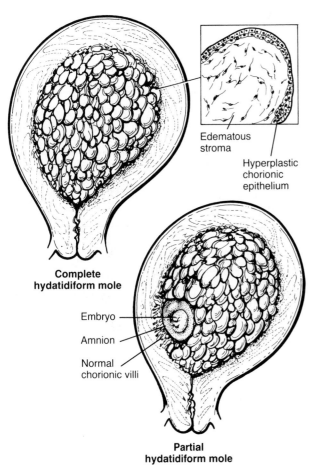

**Complete hydatidiform mole**

Edematous stroma

Hyperplastic chorionic epithelium

Embryo

Amnion

Normal chorionic villi

**Partial hydatidiform mole**

Figure 19–18. Comparison between the complete and partial hydatidiform moles. Note the presence of an embryo in the partial mole.

become invasive moles, and not more than 2 to 3% give rise to choriocarcinoma. Monitoring the postcurettage blood and urine levels of HCG, particularly the more definitive beta subunit of the hormone, permits detection of incomplete removal or a more ominous complication and the institution of appropriate therapy, including in some cases chemotherapy, which is almost always curative.

## INVASIVE MOLE (CHORIOADENOMA DESTRUENS)

Biologically, *an invasive mole is intermediate between a benign mole and choriocarcinoma.* It is more invasive locally, but it does not have the aggressive metastatic potential of a choriocarcinoma.

An **invasive mole retains hydropic villi,** which penetrate the uterine wall deeply, possibly causing rupture and sometimes life-threatening hemorrhage. Local spread to the broad ligament and vagina may also occur. Microscopically, the epithelium of the villi is markedly hyperplastic and atypical, with proliferation of both cuboidal and syncytial components.

Although the marked invasiveness of this lesion makes removal technically difficult, metastases do not occur. Hydropic villi may embolize to distant organs, such as the lungs or the brain, but these emboli do not constitute true metastases and may actually regress spontaneously. Owing to the greater depth of invasion of the myometrium, invasive mole is usually not removed completely by curettage, and therefore HCG levels continue to be elevated. This alerts the

"too large for dates," and no fetal parts or heart sounds are present. Elevated levels of HCG are present in maternal blood and urine, and ultrasonography provides a positive diagnosis.

**The mole appears as a delicate mass of translucent cystic structures, not unlike a large bunch of grapes** (Fig. 19–19). The individual locules vary in size from tiny swollen villi to cysts ranging up to 3 cm in diameter. The enclosed stroma is edematous and usually devoid of blood vessels. **The chorionic epithelial covering ranges among moles from those having a nearly normal-appearing double layer of cells (cytotrophoblast and syncytiotrophoblast) to those having piled-up chorionic (usually syncytial) epithelium with variable levels of atypia, sometimes bordering on choriocarcinoma.** By contrast, **partial moles are rarely followed by choriocarcinoma.** Recognition of the atypia is difficult because even normal syncytial epithelium is marked by variability in cell morphology. Nonetheless, experts such as Driscoll are capable of distinguishing three grades of increasing atypia, associated with worsening prognosis.[58]

Overall, at least 80% of complete moles are benign and cured by thorough curettage. Approximately 15%

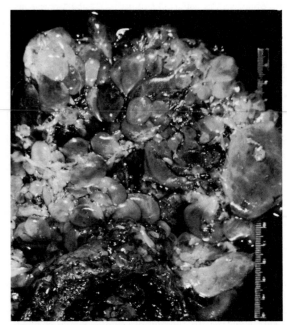

Figure 19–19. Hydatidiform mole evacuated from the uterus. The "bunch-of-grapes" appearance of the lesion is readily evident.

clinician to the need for further treatment. Fortunately, in most cases cure is possible by chemotherapy.

## CHORIOCARCINOMA

This highly aggressive malignant tumor arises either from gestational chorionic epithelium or, less frequently, from totipotential cells within the gonads or elsewhere. Choriocarcinomas are rare in most Western cultures and in the United States occur in about one in 40,000 to 70,000 pregnancies. They are much more common in Asian and African countries, reaching a frequency of one in 1000 pregnancies. The risk is somewhat elevated in those under the age of 20 and is significantly elevated in those 40 or older.[57] *In about 50% of cases, it follows a complete hydatidiform mole but only rarely a partial mole. About 25% arise after an abortion, and most of the remainder occur in a previously normal pregnancy.* Stated in another way, the more abnormal the conception, the greater the hazard of developing gestational choriocarcinoma. Most cases are discovered by the appearance of a bloody brownish discharge accompanied by a rising titer of HCG, particularly the beta subunit, in blood and urine and by the absence of marked uterine enlargement such as would be anticipated with a mole. In general, the titers are much higher than those associated with a mole. In those instances that follow abortion or pregnancy, the fact that maternal age influences the frequency of this neoplasm suggests origin from an abnormal ovum rather than retained chorionic epithelium.

Choriocarcinomas appear usually as very hemorrhagic, necrotic masses within the uterus. Sometimes the necrosis is so complete as to make anatomic diagnosis difficult because there is deceptively little recognizable viable neoplasm. Indeed, the primary lesion may self-destruct and only the metastases tell the story. Very early, the tumor insinuates itself into the myometrium and into vessels. **In contrast to the case with hydatidiform moles and invasive moles, chorionic villi are not formed; instead, the tumor is purely epithelial, composed of anaplastic cuboidal cytotrophoblast and syncytiotrophoblast** (Fig. 19–20). However, identification of such atypicality can be difficult because normal chorionic epithelium is so variable in cytomorphology.[59]

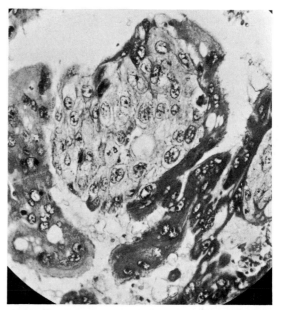

Figure 19–20. High-power detail of choriocarcinoma, illustrating the two types of epithelial cells—cytotrophoblast and syncytiotrophoblast. (From Robbins, S. L., Cotran, R. S., and Kumar, V.: Pathologic Basis of Disease. 3rd ed. Philadelphia, W. B. Saunders Co., 1984, p. 1161.)

By the time most neoplasms are discovered, widespread dissemination via the blood is usually present, most often to the lungs (50%), vagina (30 to 40%), brain, liver, and kidneys. Lymphatic invasion is uncommon.

Despite the extreme aggressiveness of these neoplasms, which made them nearly uniformly fatal in the past, present-day chemotherapy has achieved remarkable results. Nearly 100% cures have been obtained with neoplasms that have not spread beyond the pelvis, vagina, and lungs.[60] Almost a 75% remission rate has been achieved with even widely disseminated neoplasms. Equally remarkable are the many reports of healthy infants borne by these survivors.

Of interest is the possible synergistic role of a host immune response against these tumors. The tumor tissue is derived from the fertilized ovum and has antigens of paternal origin; it is therefore composed of cells "foreign" to the patient. Thus an immune response against paternal antigens is possible. This is supported by the relatively poor response to chemotherapy of choriocarcinomas that arise in the gonads (ovary or testis) and are "native" to the patient.

# Breast

At least in one respect, there can be no argument that being female can be a great disadvantage; lesions of the female breast are much more common than lesions of the male breast, which is remarkably seldom affected. They usually take the form of palpable, sometimes painful, nodules or masses. Fortunately, most are innocent, but as is well known, up to 1985 in the United States breast cancer was the foremost

cause of cancer deaths in women. In 1986 it was supplanted by carcinoma of the lung. By contrast, carcinoma of the male breast is about 100 times *less* common. The following discussion therefore deals largely with lesions of the female breast and concludes with several lesions of the male breast. The conditions to be described should all be considered in terms of their possible confusion clinically with a

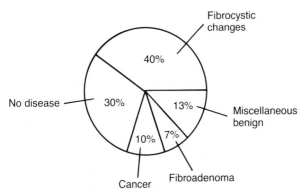

Figure 19–21. Representation of the findings in a series of women seeking evaluation of apparent breast "lumps."

malignancy. This problem is most acute with fibrocystic change because it is the commonest cause of breast "lumps" and because of the continuing controversy about the association of particular variants with breast carcinoma.

An overall perspective of the frequency of various breast problems can be gained from a recent analysis of a large series of patients with breast complaints who were seen in a surgical outpatient department of a London general hospital.[61] About 30% of the women were considered, after careful evaluation, to have no breast disease. Almost 40% were diagnosed by their criteria as having fibrocystic changes. Slightly over 10% had biopsy-proven cancer, and about 7% had a benign tumor (fibroadenoma). The remainder were suffering from a miscellany of benign lesions (Fig. 19–21). Three features of this study deserve particular note: (1) *a significant proportion of women having no recognizable breast disease have sufficient irregularity of the "normal" breast tissue to cause concern and to necessitate clinical evaluation,* (2) *fibrocystic changes are the dominant breast problem,* and (3) *cancer is all too frequent.*

## FIBROCYSTIC CHANGES

This designation is something of a wastebasket, since it is applied to a miscellany of changes in the female breast that range from those that are entirely innocuous to the relatively infrequent patterns associated with an increased risk of breast carcinoma. The only unifying feature is that all these alterations produce palpable "lumps." Included are stromal fibrosis, concurrent stromal and epithelial hyperplasia (often inducing micro- or macrocysts), various patterns of banal epithelial hyperplasia, and the more serious atypical hyperplasias. It is widely accepted that *this range of changes is the consequence of an exaggeration and distortion of the cyclic breast changes that occur normally in the menstrual cycle.*[62] Estrogenic therapy and oral contraceptives do not appear to increase the incidence of these alterations.[63]

In years past, these breast alterations have been called fibrocystic *disease.* However, great dissatisfaction has been expressed with this term on two levels. First, it is extremely difficult to draw a line between "physiologic nodularity," most prominent during the menstrual cycle, and changes meriting the appellation "disease." Various reports in the past have cited histologic evidence of "fibrocystic disease" in 60 to 90% of autopsies on women.[64, 65] Love and coworkers (as well as others) have therefore asked—"Is it reasonable to define as a disease any process that occurs clinically in 50% and histologically in 90% of women?"[66] Second, most of the changes encompassed within the diagnosis "fibrocystic disease" have little clinical significance except for their causing nodularity; only a small minority represent forms of epithelial hyperplasia having clinical importance. Thus the term "fibrocystic changes" is preferred, since it does not stigmatize the subject with "a disease."[67] Despite this semantic and conceptual controversy, it should not be overlooked that there are valid lesions encompassed under the term "fibrocystic changes"; they sometimes produce masses requiring differentiation from cancer, and the distinction between the trivial variants and the not so trivial can only be made by biopsy and histologic evaluation. *In a somewhat arbitrary manner, these alterations have been subdivided into categories discussed below, but there is considerable overlap among them, and in a single patient or even within a single lesion, all patterns may be present.* All tend to arise during reproductive life but may persist after the menopause.

## FIBROSIS OF THE BREAST

Some degree of fibrosis is present in most forms of fibrocystic change. Occasionally, however, usually in women 30 to 40 years of age, a clinically manifest breast lump is removed and is found to be composed almost entirely of fibrous tissue unaccompanied by macrocysts or epithelial hyperplasia. As noted, there is considerable disagreement in the literature as to whether such "masses" are true pathologic lesions or merely physiologic aberrations.

The usually solitary mass is poorly defined, from 2 to 10 cm in diameter, and of a rubbery consistency. On cut section, the appearance is of a tough, rubbery, gray-white, homogeneous connective tissue that is devoid of fat and within which tiny yellow-pink areas of glandular parenchyma may be barely visible. On histologic examination, the mass can be seen to consist of fibrous tissue that sometimes encloses involuted ducts, lobules, and microcysts.

Fibrosis of the breast typically presents as a painful, tender (particularly prior to the menstrual period), usually poorly delimited area of increased consistence. Often the induration and tenderness regress after the period. There is no evidence that it predisposes to carcinoma.

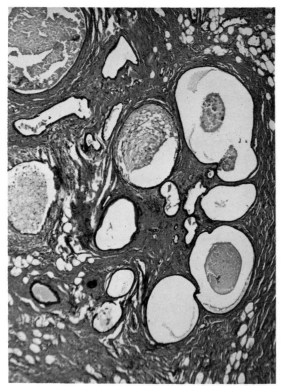

**Figure 19–22.** Cystic change of the breast. The microscopic view shows numerous small cysts, some containing inspissated secretions. The epithelium is flattened and inactive.

## CYSTIC CHANGES

This pattern is in the center of the "fibrocystic controversy" mentioned above. Microcysts are extremely common in breasts of women in the last half of reproductive life. Thus it is suggested that the term "cystic changes" and the less satisfactory term "cystic disease" should be applied only to macrocysts over 3 mm in diameter, which occur in less than 10% of women in this age group. They represent cystic dilatation of the ducts resulting from epithelial hyperplasia and are usually accompanied by stromal hyperplasia.

Macrocysts, as defined above, may occur as solitary lesions that are sometimes up to 2 to 3 cm in diameter. More often they are multifocal and often bilateral. When multiple they may impart a diffuse nodularity. Aggregations of multiple cysts may produce a large, irregular, multilobular mass. Typically, they are filled with a thin, turbid fluid that imparts a blue cast to the unopened cyst, hence the older term **"blue dome cyst."** Escape of the fluid usually reveals a smooth, glistening lining. Intracystic hemorrhage or inspissation of secretions may modify the cystic contents. Sometimes organization of the hemorrhage leads to thickening or calcification of the walls. The lobular stroma surrounding the cysts is often densely fibrotic.

Histologically, the smaller lesions are lined by cuboidal to columnar epithelium that is sometimes multilayered in areas. Proliferation of the epithelium may lead to small papillary projections, but the enclosing ductal membrane remains intact. Rarely there are outbuddings of epithelium into the surrounding stroma, interpreted as pressure extensions rather than invasion. As the cysts enlarge, the epithelium becomes progressively atrophic and may sometimes apparently disappear (Fig. 19–22). Foci of calcification may be present. Occasionally, individual cysts within a multicystic breast are lined by large cells having abundant acidophilic cytoplasm with regular central nuclei, resulting from what is called **apocrine metaplasia.** Papillary projections and epithelial multilayering are frequent in such cysts, but the changes are almost never malignant. In somewhat less than half of the cases, other patterns of fibrocystic changes are present along with the cysts.

Multiple cysts, particularly when bilateral, are usually readily distinguished from a carcinoma because cancers are almost always solitary masses. The large solitary cyst causes greater alarm, but ultrasonography and needle aspiration can usually confirm its benign nature. However, the microcalcifications, when seen on mammography, raise the suspicion of breast cancer. *Cysts per se incur no increased risk of carcinoma unless there is a family history of breast carcinoma, as is discussed on page 661 in greater detail.* However, concurrent epithelial hyperplasias add a new dimension.

## SCLEROSING ADENOSIS

This variant has significance because its clinical and morphologic features may be deceptively similar to carcinoma. There is, in this lesion, marked intralobular fibrosis and proliferation of small ductules and acini. This disorder affects an age range intermediate between that of fibrosis and cystic disease, roughly between ages 35 and 45 years.

Sclerosing adenosis is usually, but not invariably, unilateral and tends to affect the upper outer quadrant of the breast. Grossly, the circumscribed lesion has a hard, rubbery consistency, similar to that of breast cancer (a point worthy of note by surgeons). Histologically, sclerosing adenosis is characterized by reduplication of glands or terminal ducts, often revealing the biphasic layering of epithelial and myoepithelial cells. In some cases, the proliferative element is largely myoepithelial. Aggregated glands or proliferating ductules may be virtually back to back, with single or multiple layers of epithelial cells in contact with one another **(adenosis).** Always accompanying the adenosis is marked stromal fibrosis, which may compress and distort the proliferating epithelium, hence the designation "sclerosing adenosis." In some cases, **this overgrowth of fibrous tissue completely compresses the lumens of the acini and ducts so that they appear as solid cords of cells.** This pattern then may be difficult to distinguish histologically from an inva-

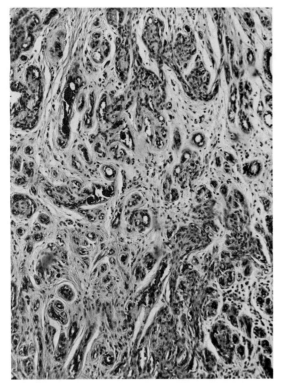

Figure 19–23. Sclerosing adenosis of the breast. The epithelial hyperplasia has produced the nests of cells, which appear quite disorderly. The overgrowth of fibrous tissue enmeshes and partially obliterates many of the epithelial nests, creating a pattern closely similar to the infiltrative growth of a cancer. Compare with Figure 19–28.

sive scirrhous carcinoma (Fig. 19–23). Helpful when there appear to be solid cords of cells is the recognition that many are double layered (approximation of walls) and the identification of myoepithelial elements.

*Sclerosing adenosis is not thought to predispose to carcinoma.* Nonetheless, it can be difficult to distinguish clinically from cancer because it usually produces a firm, well-delineated mass on palpation. Often the "lump" is painful or tender, particularly premenstrually, helping to differentiate it from the nontender carcinoma. When the cystic pattern is concurrently present, particularly when multifocal, it adds comfort to the judgment—"not carcinoma." Furthermore, mammography uncommonly discloses microcalcifications, a prevalent finding in breast carcinoma. Despite all the hints militating against cancer, the ultimate differentiation usually requires biopsy.

## EPITHELIAL HYPERPLASIA

The term "epithelial hyperplasia" encompasses a range of proliferative lesions within the ductules, terminal ducts, and, sometimes, lobules of the breast. Some of the epithelial hyperplasias are mild and

orderly and incur little risk of carcinoma, but at the other end of the spectrum are the more florid atypical hyperplasias that impose a significantly increased risk commensurate with the severity and atypicality of the changes as is discussed later.[68] The epithelial hyperplasias often are accompanied by other histologic variants of fibrocystic change, but they nonetheless may be the dominant pattern morphologically. As in the case of sclerosing adenosis, women between the ages of 35 and 45 years are most commonly affected.

The gross appearance of epithelial hyperplasia is not distinctive and is often dominated by coexistent fibrous or cystic changes. Rarely, ropey thickening of the small ducts is palpable. Histologically, there is an almost infinite spectrum of proliferative alterations. The ducts, ductules, or lobules may be filled with orderly cuboidal cells, within which small gland patterns can be discerned **(cribriform pattern)**. Sometimes the proliferating epithelium projects in multiple small papillary excrescences into the ductal lumen **(ductal papillomatosis)**. Occasionally, the proliferative changes extend into lobules or sometimes are dominant within the lobules. The latter pattern is, however, uncommon. Most often the hyperplastic cells are not more than four layers deep and are quite normal

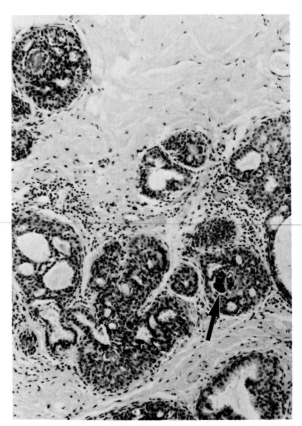

Figure 19–24. Florid intraduct hyperplasia, producing in places a cribriform pattern. The changes border on atypical hyperplasia. Note the microcalcification (*arrow*).

cytologically with intact ductal and lobular basement membranes. Such changes are called **"mild hyperplasia."** Moreover, myoepithelial cells underlying the lining epithelial cells are preserved. When the epithelial hyperplasia is more than four cells deep, it is called **"moderate to florid"** (Fig. 19–24). In some instances the hyperplastic cells are more multilayered and disorderly, with variation in nuclear and cell size and slight hyperchromasia; in short, they have changes approaching those of "in situ carcinoma" (p. 639). Such irregular hyperplasia is called **atypical.** The line separating the epithelial hyperplasias without atypia from atypical hyperplasia is poorly defined, just as is the line demarcating atypical hyperplasia from in situ carcinoma, but these distinctions have importance, as will soon become clear.

Epithelial hyperplasia *per se* does not often produce a clinically discrete breast mass. Occasionally, it produces microcalcifications on mammography, raising grave doubts about cancer. Such nodularity as may be present usually relates to other concurrent variants of fibrocystic disease. However, florid papillomatosis may be associated with a serous or serosanguineous nipple discharge. The significance of this condition lies principally in its relationship to cancer, discussed next.

## RELATIONSHIP OF FIBROCYSTIC CHANGES TO BREAST CARCINOMA

Here we enter a stormy arena filled with claims and counterclaims. Only some reasonably supportable summary statements are possible. As previously mentioned, the diagnosis of "fibrocystic disease" lends itself to abuse because it is difficult to draw the line between physiologic aberrations and pathologic alterations. Because it encompasses a constellation of lesions of widely varying potential, the term has lost much of its clinical utility with respect to its role in the induction of carcinoma.[69] The term "fibrocystic changes" is equally unsatisfactory but at least less chilling. With respect to the relationship of the various patterns of fibrocystic change to cancer, the following statements represent the current most informed opinion.[67, 70]

○ *No increased risk of breast carcinoma:*
Fibrosis, cystic changes (micro or macro), apocrine metaplasia, sclerosing adenosis, mild hyperplasia
○ *Slightly increased risk—1.5 to 2 times:*
Hyperplasia moderate to florid, ductal papillomatosis (marked)
○ *Significantly increased risk—5 times:*
atypical hyperplasia
○ *A family history of breast cancer increases the risk in all categories*—e.g., to about 10-fold with atypical hyperplasia.

*Moderate to florid hyperplasia and ductal papillomatosis account for about 26% of all biopsies that show fibrocystic change. In contrast, only about 4% of biopsies reveal atypical epithelial hyperplasia. Thus the great majority of women having "lumps" related to fibrocystic change can be reassured that there is little or no increased predisposition to cancer.* The need to differentiate among the many variants and the grounds for dissatisfaction with the unqualified terms—"fibrocystic changes" or, even worse, "fibrocystic disease"—are apparent. The risks inherent in the various patterns are shown in Figure 19–25.

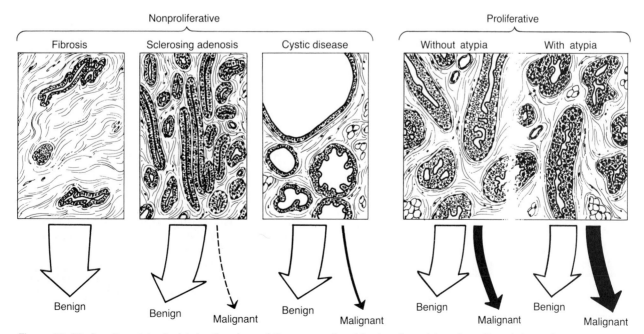

**Figure 19–25.** An attempt to depict, by the sizes of the arrows, the risk of malignant transformation of the various patterns of fibrocystic change.

# INFLAMMATIONS

Inflammations of the breast are uncommon and usually cause pain and tenderness in the areas of involvement during the acute stages. However, in the later healing or healed stage they become non-painful and sometimes leave residual scarring that is palpable as a breast "lump." Included in this category are several forms of mastitis and traumatic fat necrosis, none of which incurs an increased risk of cancer.

## MASTITIS (INCLUDING BREAST ABSCESS)

*Acute mastitis* develops when bacteria gain access to the breast tissue either through the ducts when there is inspissation of secretions or through fissures in the nipples, which usually develop during the early weeks of nursing. Nonspecific dermatologic conditions involving the nipple may also provide avenues of ingress. The invading organisms are usually staphylococci or streptococci.

**Staphylococcal infections induce single or multiple abscesses** accompanied by the typical clinical acute inflammatory changes when they are near the surface. They are usually small, but when sufficiently large in the course of healing may leave residual foci of scarring that are palpable as localized areas of induration. **Streptococcal infections generally spread throughout the entire breast, causing pain, marked swelling with enlargement, and tenderness** of the breast. Resolution of these infections rarely leaves residual areas of induration.

*Periductal or plasma cell mastitis* is a nonbacterial inflammation of the breast secondary to inspissation of breast secretions in the main excretory ducts. Ductal dilatation with ductal rupture leads to reactive changes in the surrounding breast substance. It is an uncommon condition encountered usually in women who have borne children and most often in those late in reproductive life. The genesis of these changes is poorly understood but is vaguely attributed to prior injuries to the excretory ducts during nursing. Presumably, secretions build up behind narrowed ducts, possibly leading to ductal rupture. Microbial invasion is not involved.

Usually the inflammatory changes are confined to an area drained by one or several major excretory ducts opening into the nipple. There is increased firmness of the tissue and, on cross section, dilated ropey ducts are apparent from which thick, cheesy secretions can be extruded. Histologically, the ducts are filled by granular debris, sometimes containing leukocytes, principally lipid-laden macrophages. The lining epithelium is generally destroyed. **Most distinguishing is the prominence of the lymphocytic and plasma cell infiltration in the periductal stroma.**

Mammary duct ectasia is of principal importance because it leads to induration of the breast substance and, more significantly, to retraction of the skin or nipple, mimicking the changes caused by some carcinomas.

## TRAUMATIC FAT NECROSIS

This is an uncommon and innocuous lesion that is significant only because it produces a mass. Most, but not all, patients give a history of some preceding trauma to the breast.

During the early stage, the lesion is small, often tender, rarely over 2 cm in diameter, and sharply localized. It consists of a central focus of necrotic fat cells surrounded by neutrophils and lipid-filled macrophages, and, later, by an enclosing wall of fibrous tissue and mononuclear leukocytes. Eventually, the central debris is either removed by the macrophages and giant cells and is replaced by scar tissue or the debris becomes encysted within the scar. Calcifications may develop in either the scar or cyst wall. A tendency for the fibrous tissue to adhere to the overlying skin sometimes results in dimpling or retraction, a finding that may also be caused by cancer.

# TUMORS OF THE BREAST

These constitute the most important lesions of the female breast. Although tumors within the breast may arise from any one of its component tissues (i.e., connective tissue and epithelial structures), it is the latter that give rise to the common breast neoplasms. Here we will describe fibroadenoma, papilloma and papillary carcinoma, and carcinomas of the breast.

## FIBROADENOMA

The encapsulated fibroadenoma is by far the most common benign tumor of the female breast. An absolute or relative increased estrogen activity is thought to play a role in its development and indeed, similar lesions, perhaps less discretely encapsulated, may appear with fibrocystic changes (*fibroadenosis*). Fibroadenomas usually appear in prepubertal girls and in young women; the peak incidence is in the third decade of life.

The fibroadenoma, in contrast to fibroadenosis, occurs as a discrete, encapsulated, usually solitary, freely movable nodule. Rarely, multiple tumors are encountered. Differentiation clinically from a solitary cyst is most difficult but is readily accomplished by sonography. Typically, they are about 3 cm in diameter, but they may be considerably larger. **As the name implies, these tumors are composed of both fibrous and glandular tissue.** Grossly, they are firm, with a uniform gray-white color on cut section, punctuated by softer yellow-pink specks representing the glandular areas. Histologically, there is a loose fibroblastic stroma containing duct-like, epithe-

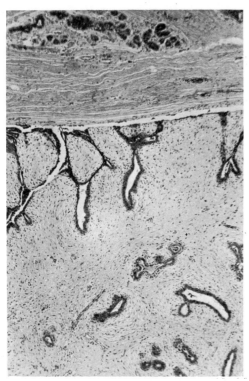

Figure 19–26. Fibroadenoma of the breast. The margin of the nodule shows clear demarcation from the compressed breast substance above. The tumor is in part intracanalicular, particularly near the capsule. Toward the bottom of this view, the pattern is pericanalicular.

lium-lined spaces of various forms and sizes. Although in some lesions the ductal spaces are round to oval and fairly regular **(the pericanalicular fibroadenoma),** others are compressed by extensive proliferation of the stroma so that on cross section they appear as slits or irregular, star-shaped structures **(the intracanalicular fibroadenoma).** These duct-like or glandular spaces are lined with single or multiple layers of cells that are regular and have a well-defined, intact basement membrane (Fig. 19–26).

Fibroadenomas that reach dimensions of 10 to 15 cm in diameter are commonly termed **giant fibroadenomas.** These may markedly distort the breast and even cause pressure necrosis of the overlying skin, sometimes with rupture of the tumor through its capsule to the surface. Although such alarming behavior does not of itself imply malignancy, the epithelium or stroma in a few of these larger lesions undergoes malignant transformation. Even then, however, their behavior is relatively innocent, and although a few do metastasize to regional nodes, surgical excision effects a cure. To these giant fibroadenomas the unfortunate designation **cystosarcoma phyllodes** has been given.

## PAPILLOMA AND PAPILLARY CARCINOMA

Papillary formations within ducts or cysts may occur as a single isolated neoplasm or as a diffuse process—*ductal papillomatosis,* a component of fibrocystic disease (see p. 660). *In either case, these lesions are rarely large enough to be palpable and usually manifest themselves by a serous, turbid, or bloody discharge from the nipple.*

The benign isolated neoplastic papilloma usually occurs in the fourth or fifth decade of life. It is a small lesion, usually less than 1 cm in diameter, growing within a cyst or dilated duct, usually close to the nipple. It may be sessile or pedunculated. On microscopic examination, it can be seen to have a delicate central connective tissue framework covered by one or two layers of regular cuboidal epithelial cells. Apocrine metaplasia and foci of hyalinization are frequently found. Although most of the solitary papillary lesions are benign, some malignant and intermediate forms (papillary carcinoma) are characterized by progressive epithelial atypicality, anaplasia, and invasion of the stroma of the stalk or even the periductal tissue. Histologic differentiation of benign, borderline, and malignant papillomas may be difficult, unless several tissue sections are examined to assess the severity of atypia, mitotic rate, and stromal infiltration.

It is relatively easy to differentiate histologically the benign end of the spectrum of epithelial changes from the clearly malignant end, but in the middle are many difficult diagnostic problems. An old aphorism states "If in doubt, the lesion will behave as a benign process." The basis for this belief is the growing evidence that benign papillomas are *not* precursors of papillary carcinomas, which begin de novo as malignant lesions. However, ductal *papillomatosis* as a component of fibrocystic changes may have atypical epithelial hyperplasia and, as such, incurs the increased risk of breast carcinoma seen with all forms of atypical hyperplastic fibrocystic change.

## CARCINOMA

As noted earlier, carcinoma of the breast has just been supplanted as the number one cause of cancer deaths in females in the United States; this is also likely to occur in other Western countries. Unhappily, this fall from predominance reflects an alarming increase in the frequency of lung cancer in women rather than a decline in the death rate from carcinoma of the breast, which has held steady for many years. However, it should not be overlooked that women are now living longer, and thus the aggregate number of risk-years has substantially increased. Whatever the variables, carcinoma of the breast continues to account for almost 20% of cancer deaths in women in the United States. The only happy note is that there are many more new cases of invasive carcinoma discovered each year than there are deaths, indicating that many women are cured of their disease. In contrast, breast carcinoma is extremely rare in men.

**EPIDEMIOLOGY.** The following risk factors for carcinoma of the breast have been identified.[71, 72, 73]

○ *Geographic influences*: Five times more common in the United States than in Japan and Taiwan.

○ *Genetic predisposition*: Well-defined. The magnitude of risk is in proportion to number of close relatives with breast cancer and age when cancer occurred in relatives. The younger the relatives at time of developing cancer and bilateral cancers, the greater the genetic predisposition. There are uncommon high-risk families with apparent autosomal dominant transmission and familial association of breast and ovarian carcinomas.

○ *Increasing age*: Uncommon before age 20, but then a steady rise to the time of menopause, followed by a slower rise throughout life.

○ *Length of reproductive life*: Risk increases with early menarche and late menopause.

○ *Parity*: More frequent in nulliparous than in multiparous women.

○ *Age at first child*: Increased risk when over 30 at time of first child.

○ *Obesity*: Increased risk attributed to synthesis of estrogens in fat depots.

○ *Exogenous estrogens*: Still controversial, but some data show moderately increased risk with high-dosage therapy of menopausal symptoms.

○ *Oral contraceptives*: No clear-cut increased risk; attributed to balanced content of estrogens and progestins in currently used OCs.

○ *Fibrocystic changes with atypical epithelial hyperplasia*: Increased risk, as noted in earlier discussion of this condition.

○ *Carcinoma of the contralateral breast or endometrium*: Increased risk.

**ETIOLOGY AND PATHOGENESIS.** Despite extensive studies the ultimate origin or origins of breast carcinoma remain an enigma enshrouded in mystery. The only clues point to genetic influences and hormonal imbalances. The former enthusiasm for an oncogenic virus has largely waned, but there are still champions of dietary influences.

*Genetic predisposition* undoubtedly exists, as the above-mentioned data indicate. However, there is no understanding of how genetic factors operate in the induction of the neoplasm. Conceivably, they may influence the availability of hormone receptors in breast epithelial cells (as will be discussed), but this is speculative.

*Endogenous hyperestrinism* is thought to play a significant role. Many of the risk factors mentioned—long duration of reproductive life, nulliparity, and late age at first child—all imply increased exposure to the estrogen peaks during the menstrual cycle. There are the additional findings of the association with fibrocystic epithelial hyperplasia (presumed to reflect estrogenic influences), the modestly increased (albeit disputed) risk imposed by exogenous estrogens, and the rarity of breast carcinoma in prepubertally castrated girls. There are hints of how the estrogens might act. It is well known that normal breast epithelium possesses estrogen and progester-

one receptors (the latter controlled by the level of estrogen-binding receptors). The estrogen receptor-hormone complex is translated into the nucleus, where the hormones turn on genes leading to cell division and synthesis of progesterone receptors. Steroid receptors have been identified in some (but not all) breast cancers, providing a plausible mechanism by which unbalanced estrogenic effects may serve as promoters in the carcinogenic process.[74] Receptor assays of tissue biopsies are now being used in an attempt to predict the responsiveness of particular neoplasms to hormonal therapy, as will be discussed later.

A *mammary tumor virus (MTV)* capable of causing breast cancer in mice was brilliantly documented by Bittner in 1936.[75] Subsequently, there were many hints of the existence of an analogous virus in breast cancers of humans; the findings have not been very conclusive at present, but there are tantalizing leads (e.g., the similarity of a protein in cancer cells to one induced by MTV).

*Dietary influences* have been talked about for years but remain controversial. Nonetheless, there are staunch advocates of the thesis that high dietary fat constitutes a significant predisposition.[76] Most of the evidence is derived from epidemiologic surveys, as was noted in an earlier discussion (p. 251), and in brief consists of a correlation between the dietary intake of animal fat in various countries and the incidence of breast cancer. However, without doubt there is a long lag time between initiation of a neoplasm and its development, calling into question the significance of current analysis of diet and the reliability of historical data on diet. Coffee addicts will be pleased to know, there is no substantial evidence that caffeine consumption increases the risk.

**MORPHOLOGY.** Cancer of the breast affects the left breast slightly more often than the right. In 4 to 10% of patients there are bilateral primary tumors or a second primary tumor develops subsequently. The locations of the tumors within the breast are as follows:

|  | *Per Cent* |
|---|---|
| Upper outer quadrant | 50 |
| Central portion | 20 |
| Lower outer quadrant | 10 |
| Upper inner quadrant | 10 |
| Lower inner quadrant | 10 |

Tumors may arise in the ductal epithelium (90%) or within the lobular epithelium (10%). Unless otherwise specified, the term "breast carcinoma" implies ductal origin. Both ductal and lobular cancers are further divided into those that have not penetrated the limiting basement membranes (**noninfiltrating**) and those that have done so (**infiltrating**). Thus, the chief forms of carcinoma of the breast can be classified as follows:

A. Arising in ducts
  1. Noninfiltrating—
    a. **Intraductal carcinoma (comedocarcinoma)**
    b. **Intraductal papillary carcinoma** (p. 663)

2. Infiltrating
   a. **Simple or usual type (includes scirrhous carcinoma)**
   b. **Medullary carcinoma**
   c. **Colloid (mucinous) carcinoma**
   d. **Paget's disease**
   e. **Tubular carcinoma**
B. Arising in lobules
   1. Noninfiltrating—**in situ lobular carcinoma**
   2. Infiltrating—**lobular carcinoma**

Of these, the infiltrating ductal (scirrhous) carcinoma is by far the most common. The morphology of each type will be discussed separately.

***Intraductal Carcinoma (Comedocarcinoma).*** This type represents about 5% of carcinomas of the breast. The tumor may present as a clinically palpable mass (up to 5 cm in diameter)[68] or as ropy cords within the breast, created by proliferation of the ductal epithelium, which tends to grow within the ducts without invading the ductal basement membrane and underlying breast tissue. Eventually, the ducts become filled with cheesy necrotic tumor tissue, which can be extruded with slight pressure when the ducts are transected (hence the name **comedocarcinoma**). Histologically, the neoplastic cells may initially assume a glandular pattern or pile up within the ducts to create irregular excrescences. Often the proliferating cells form bridges that traverse the duct or, alternatively, create large arches about the circumference. Continued replication fills the ducts with compressed tumor cells until all architectural detail is lost. At this point they appear as solid cords of anaplastic cells. Whether all intraductal cancers are fated in time to become invasive is at present not clear. Reports suggest that about 70% become invasive.[77] Whether the remainder would in time become invasive is moot. Significantly, **about 5 to 15% of patients acquire an invasive cancer in the other breast.**[78]

***Infiltrating Duct Carcinoma (Usual Type).*** This is the most common form of breast cancer, accounting for roughly 75% of carcinomas of the breast. Clinically, it is a deceptively delimited mass, rarely over 3 to 4 cm in diameter, of stony hard consistency, hence the commonly used designation **scirrhous carcinoma** (Fig. 19–27). On cut section, the tumor is obviously infiltrative and retracted below the surrounding fibrofatty tissue, and it has a gritty texture that produces a grating sound when the tumor is scraped with a knife. Foci of chalky white necrosis and sometimes calcification are often evident on the cut surface. Extension of the growth may cause dimpling of the skin, retraction of the nipple, or fixation to the chest wall. Histologically, the lesion is composed principally of dense fibrous stroma in which are found widely scattered nests or cords of tumor cells (Fig. 19–28). These are round to polygonal, or compressed, and contain fairly uniform, small, dark nuclei with remarkably few mitotic figures. At the margins of the tumor, the neoplastic cells can be seen infiltrating the surrounding tissue and frequently invading perivascular and perineurial spaces as well as blood vessels.

***Medullary Carcinoma.*** Medullary carcinoma represents about 5% of breast carcinoma. The morphology of

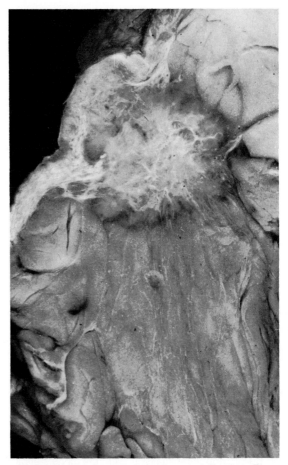

Figure 19–27. Carcinoma of the breast, infiltrating. The cut surface illustrates the lack of demarcation, the fixation to the skin, and the chalky foci of necrosis within the mass. (From Robbins, S. L., Cotran, R. S., and Kumar, V.: Pathologic Basis of Disease. 3rd ed. Philadelphia, W. B. Saunders Co., 1984, p. 1182.)

these tumors is in sharp contrast to that of the usual breast carcinoma. They tend to be soft and fleshy, rather than stony hard, and often become large (up to 10 cm in diameter). On cut section, the tumor bulges above the surrounding tissue, rather than retracting below it. The reason for these differences is apparent on histologic examination. Unlike the scirrhous carcinoma, the medullary carcinoma has a scant stroma. The tumor cells grow in large, irregular sheets of undifferentiated polygonal to spindled cells, although occasionally well-differentiated gland formations are present, meriting the designation medullary adenocarcinoma. There is usually a moderate to marked lymphocytic infiltration between the tumor cells and particularly in the margins of the tumor mass. This feature is presumed to represent a host response to the tumor, and, correspondingly, these tumors have a distinctly better prognosis than the usual infiltrating breast carcinoma.

***Colloid (Mucinous) Carcinoma.*** This form is even more uncommon than the medullary carcinoma. It is characterized by the production of mucin, intracellularly and extracellularly. Grossly, these lesions are extremely

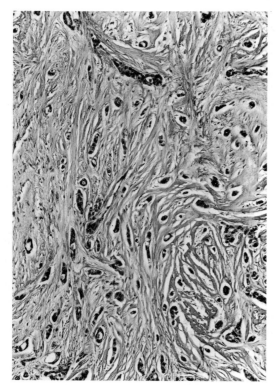

Figure 19–28. A high-power detail of a scirrhous adenocarcinoma of the breast. The scattered islands of cancer cells are trapped in the striking desmoplastic stromal overgrowth.

soft, bulky, gray-blue masses with the consistency of gelatin. There may be central cystic softening and hemorrhage. Histologically, one or more of three patterns are present. In the first pattern, the tumor cells are seen as small islands, or even isolated cells, floating in a large lake of basophilic mucin that flows into contiguous tissue spaces and planes of cleavage. At least some of the tumor cells have a vacuolated appearance because of the presence of intracellular mucin. In the second pattern, the neoplastic cells grow in well-defined glandular arrangements, the lumens of which contain mucinous secretions. Again, the neoplastic cells may be vacuolated. The third pattern consists of a disorganized mass of undifferentiated tumor cells, most of which are of the signet-ring type; that is, they are distended with large vacuoles of mucin. The prognosis of these variants is better than that of the usual infiltrative neoplasm.

***Paget's Disease of the Breast.*** This is an unusual form of ductal breast cancer that affects women in a slightly older age group than the other forms. It begins as a typical intraductal carcinoma but involves the main excretory ducts, from which it extends to infiltrate the skin of the nipple and areola. As a consequence, eczematoid changes in the nipple and areola antedate the formation of any palpable mass in the breast. The involved areolar and periareolar skin is frequently fissured, ulcerated, and oozing. There are surrounding inflammatory hyperemia and edema, and superimposed bacterial infections are common. The histologic hallmark of this tumor is the invasion of the epidermis by pathognomonic neoplastic cells termed **Paget cells**. These are large, hyperchromatic cells surrounded by a clear halo, which represents intracellular accumulation of mucopolysaccharides. In other respects the morphology of Paget's disease is similar to that of an intraductal carcinoma, and despite extension to the skin, has a favorable prognosis. Similar lesions may appear in the anogenital region, particularly in women; this condition is often called "extramammary Paget's disease" (p. 633).

***Lobular Carcinoma.*** Lobular carcinoma arises from the acini or terminal ductules of the lobule. Not only does it differ from the ductal carcinomas in its origin, but it is characterized by a peculiar tendency to multicentricity within the same breast and to have a high incidence (20%) of bilaterality.[79] Two forms are described, lobular carcinoma in situ and infiltrating lobular carcinoma. **Lobular carcinoma in situ** is nonpalpable and can be defined only histologically. With the microscope, an entire lobule reveals acini (terminal ductules), which are distended with neoplastic cells (Fig. 19–29). The cells are somewhat larger than normal and loosely cohesive, and they have oval or round nuclei and small nucleoli. In general, mitotic figures and pleomorphism are lacking. The distention of the acini (terminal ductules) is a particularly characteristic feature. The significance of lobular carcinoma in situ lies in the possibility of its transition into infiltrating carcinoma.

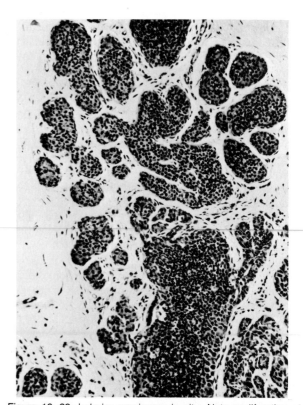

Figure 19–29. Lobular carcinoma in situ. Note proliferation of well-differentiated tumor cells in terminal ducts and acini. (From Robbins, S. L., Cotran, R. S., and Kumar, V.: Pathologic Basis of Disease. 3rd ed. Philadelphia, W. B. Saunders Co., 1984, p. 1186.)

Somewhere between 4 and 25%, depending on morphologic criteria and tissue sampling, become invasive in time, but when carcinoma in the contralateral breast is also included, the frequency climbs to about 35%.[80]

**Infiltrating lobular carcinoma** is poorly circumscribed and usually rubbery in consistency. Sometimes the lesion may be hard and scirrhous. Histologically, in the classic form, strands of tumor cells often one cell in width (Indian file pattern) are loosely dispersed in a fibrous stroma. In most cases, the tumor cells are small and uniform, with little pleomorphism. Occasionally, they surround normal-appearing acini or ducts, the so-called "bull's eye pattern," which is considered characteristic. Not uncommonly, the tumors have histologic features of both ductal and lobular patterns. It is therefore difficult to obtain a precise incidence of infiltrating lobular carcinoma. Most studies report that they constitute 5 to 10% of breast carcinoma. Despite their infrequent occurrence, these tumors are considered important owing to the high incidence of bilaterality, which mandates a careful clinical and histologic evaluation (by biopsy) of the contralateral breast.

**FEATURES COMMON TO ALL CANCERS.** In all of the forms of breast cancer discussed previously, progression of the disease leads to certain local morphologic features. These include a tendency to become adherent to the pectoral muscles or deep fascia of the chest wall, with consequent **fixation** of the lesion, as well as adherence to the overlying skin, with **retraction** or **dimpling** of the skin or nipple. The latter is an important sign, because it may be the first indication of a lesion, observed by the patient herself during self examination. Involvement of the lymphatic pathways may cause localized **lymphedema**. In these cases the skin becomes thickened around exaggerated hair follicles, a change known as "orange peel." Sometimes, particularly in pregnancy, the tumor spreads so rapidly that it excites an acute inflammatory reaction, with swelling, redness, and tenderness. This picture has been referred to as **"inflammatory carcinoma."** However, it is not a distinct morphologic pattern but simply reflects rapid growth of any pattern. The advent of mammography as a diagnostic tool has called attention to the frequency of microcalcifications in breast carcinoma. Although certain variants (e.g., intraductal carcinoma) only infrequently have such calcifications, they are common in the usual infiltrative scirrhous lesion, so that overall, they are found in 60 to 80% of breast cancers. However, they may also be present in the epithelial proliferation of fibrocystic changes.[81]

Spread through lymphatic and hematogenous channels eventually occurs. Nodal metastases are present in about two thirds of cases at the time of diagnosis. Outer-quadrant and centrally located lesions typically spread first to the axillary nodes. Those in the inner quadrants often involve the lymph nodes along the internal mammary arteries. The supraclavicular nodes are sometimes the primary site of spread but may only become involved after the axillary and internal mammary nodes are affected. More distant dissemination eventually ensues,

with metastatic involvement of almost any organ or tissue in the body. Favored locations are the lungs, skeleton, liver, and adrenals and, less commonly, the brain, spleen, and pituitary. But no site is exempt. **Metastases may appear many years after apparent therapeutic control of the primary lesion, sometimes 15 years later.** However, with each passing year the scene brightens. Breast cancer is an ugly lesion for many reasons, not the least being its potential to reappear so many years later.

**GRADING AND STAGING.** These neoplasms have been graded on the basis of their level of anaplasia (Grades I to III) and have been divided into three categories, based on their biologic aggressiveness:

*Nonmetastasizing:* Intraductal carcinoma without stromal invasion; in situ lobular carcinoma

*Uncommonly metastasizing:* Colloid carcinoma; medullary carcinoma with lymphocytic infiltration; infiltrating papillary

*Moderately-to-highly metastasizing:* All other types

In addition, there are staging systems—regrettably, too many in current use. All attempt to create stages based on the size of the primary lesion, the possible presence of nodal metastases, and the possible presence of distant dissemination. A simplified version of the presently recommended system is provided in Table 19–6.

**CLINICAL COURSE.** Breast cancer is usually discovered by the patient or her physician as a deceptively discrete, solitary, painless, and movable mass. At this time the lesion is typically less than 4 cm in diameter, although, as mentioned, involvement of the regional lymph nodes (most often axillary) is already present in about two thirds of patients. Much less often (in about 15% of instances) an occult lesion is detected by a routine mammogram. Admittedly, "mammos" incur radiation risks and increased costs and worry produced by questionable findings (calcifications are

**Table 19–6. AMERICAN JOINT COMMITTEE ON CANCER STAGING OF BREAST CARCINOMA***

| | |
|---|---|
| Stage Tis | In situ cancer (in situ lobular, pure intraductal, and Paget's Disease of the nipple without palpable tumor) |
| Stage I | Tumor 2 cm or less in greatest diameter and without evidence of regional or distant spread |
| Stage II | Tumor more than 2 cm but not more than 5 cm in greatest dimension, but without distant spread |
| Stage III (A) | Tumor of up to and more than 5 cm in diameter with or without homolateral regional (local) spread that may or may not be fixed, but without distant spread |
| Stage III (B) | Tumor of up to and more than 5 cm in diameter with homolateral metastatic supraclavicular and intraclavicular nodes |
| Stage IV | Tumor of any size with or without regional spread but with evidence of distant metastases |

*From Beahrs, O. H.: Staging of cancer of the breast as a guide to therapy. Cancer 53:592, 1984.

also seen with fibrocystic changes). Nonetheless, currently there is an apparent consensus for mammography every one to two years beginning at about age 40 unless there is a family history of cancer or a history of atypical hyperplastic fibrocystic change, in which case screening should begin earlier. This technique is well established as a valuable diagnostic modality in the differentiation of cancerous from benign breast masses. However, controversy continues about its reliability as a screening tool for the discovery of small, perhaps nonpalpable masses. The false-negative rate as reported in the literature ranges from about 10% to over 50%.[81, 82] But in experienced hands, mass screening of women over the age of 40 has achieved a significant reduction in mortality from this disease.[83]

A prognosis for this disease is difficult to express because so many variables influence the outlook, but of principal significance are stage at diagnosis and the method of therapy (currently an area of stormy debate). Traditional approaches have relied heavily on radical mastectomy—removal of the entire breast along with the axillary nodes and the pectoral muscles in continuity—or less radical surgery preserving the pectoral muscles (simple mastectomy). Currently, there is a growing conviction that less mutilating procedures such as segmental mastectomy followed in some cases by local irradiation to the breast and axilla may yield as good or even better results than the traditional approaches. The recent report of a large-scale multicenter study indicates that with tumors less than 4 cm in diameter, whether or not axillary nodes are affected, segmental resection with tumor-free margins coupled with radiation and sometimes chemotherapy yielded about a 90% tumor-free five-year survival—results that were at least as good as those obtained in a comparable group having only total mastectomy.[84] The 10-year results of this therapeutic approach are not yet available.

For many years it has been known that a variety of hormonal manipulations aimed at lowering or counteracting estrogenic stimulation may affect the course of breast cancers. In earlier years, ovariectomy was performed in premenopausal women and, sometimes, also adrenalectomy and hypophysectomy in patients with metastatic disease, particularly those having pain arising in bone metastases, in the hope of palliating the disease and possibly prolonging life. Currently favored are antiestrogenic agents (e.g., tamoxifen). Overall, about one third of human breast carcinomas are responsive to such hormonal manipulation. Now assays of the neoplasm for estrogen and progesterone receptors permit identification of those patients most likely to be benefited. Recent studies suggest that the level of progesterone receptors is a better predictor of a favorable response than the level of estrogen receptors, presumably because the presence of progesterone receptors implies better differentiation of the cancer cells.[85] Tumors possessing both receptors have an almost 80% likelihood of

responding to hormonal therapy. Moreover, the presence of these receptors appears to correlate with longer survival after mastectomy, perhaps again reflecting the level of differentiation of the neoplasm.[86]

There can be no question but that breast cancers progressively enlarge with time, and therefore early diagnosis is more likely to yield small primary masses. However, there is a strong suspicion that some tumors are biologically more aggressive than others and so may spread to nodes or more widely even when small. Nonetheless, in the past somewhere between 10 and 25% of cancers were inoperable at the time of discovery, but today mammography and public education have resulted in fewer inoperable cases. Overall, the current 10-year survival rate for patients with any tumor amenable to resection and adjunctive therapy is about 60%. Regrettably, even 10-year survival does not preclude the possibility of a recurrence at a later date; carcinoma of the breast is notorious for unpredictability. Whether earlier diagnosis and the newer modes of therapy will achieve the long-hoped-for brighter outlook, only time will tell. But not to be forgotten is the increased incidence of cancer (perhaps years later) in the contralateral breast.

# MALE BREAST

The rudimentary male breast is relatively free from pathologic involvement. Only two disorders occur with sufficient frequency to merit consideration—*gynecomastia* and *carcinoma*.

## GYNECOMASTIA

As in the female, the male breast is subject to hormonal influences, but it is considerably less sensitive than the female breast. Nonetheless, enlargement of the male breast, or *gynecomastia*, may occur in response to absolute or relative estrogen excesses. *Gynecomastia, then, is the male analogue of fibrocystic change in the female.* The most important cause of such hyperestrinism in the male is cirrhosis of the liver, with consequent inability of the liver to metabolize estrogens. Other causes include Klinefelter's syndrome, estrogen-secreting tumors, estrogen therapy, and occasionally, digitalis therapy. Physiologic gynecomastia often occurs in puberty and in extreme old age.

The morphologic features of gynecomastia are similar to those of intraductal hyperplasia. Grossly, a button-like, subareolar swelling develops, usually in both breasts but occasionally in only one.

## CARCINOMA OF THE MALE BREAST

This is a rare occurrence, with a frequency ratio to breast cancer in the female of 1:125. It occurs in advanced age. Because of the scant amount of breast substance in the male, the tumor rapidly infiltrates the overlying skin and underlying thoracic wall. These tumors resemble the invasive scirrhous carcinomas in the female both morphologically and biologically. Surprisingly, considering the size of the male breast, almost half spread to regional nodes and more distant sites by the time of discovery.[87]

## References

1. Lavery, H. A.: Vulval dystrophies: New approaches. Clin. Obstet. Gynaecol. 11:155, 1984.
2. Sanchez, N. P., and Mihm, M. C., Jr.: Reactive and neoplastic epithelial alterations of the vulva. J. Am. Acad. Dermatol. 6:378, 1982.
3. Robboy, S. J., et al.: Urogenital sinus origin of mucinous and ciliated cysts of the vulva. Obstet. Gynecol. 51:347, 1978.
4. Kryzek, R. A., et al.: Anogenital warts contain several distinct pieces of human papillomavirus. J. Virol. 36:236, 1980.
5. Editorial: Genital warts, human papilloma viruses, and cervical cancer. Lancet 2:1045, 1985.
6. Jones, R. E., Jr., et al.: Extramammary Paget's disease. A critical reexamination. Am. J. Dermatopathol. 1:101, 1979.
7. Nadji, M., et al.: Paget's disease of the skin. A unifying concept of histogenesis. Cancer 50:2203, 1983.
8. Mazoujian, G., et al.: Extramammary Paget's disease—Evidence for an apocrine origin: An immunoperoxidase study of gross cystic disease fluid protein-15, carcinoembryonic antigen and keratin proteins. Am. J. Surg. Pathol. 8:43, 1984.
9. Friedrich, E. G., Jr., et al.: Carcinoma in situ of the vulva: A continuing challenge. Am. J. Obstet. Gynecol. 136:830, 1980.
10. Kaufman, R. H., et al.: Herpesvirus-induced antigens in squamous-cell carcinoma in situ of the vulva. N. Engl. J. Med. 305:483, 1981.
11. Howley, P. M.: On human papillomaviruses. N. Engl. J. Med. 315:1089, 1986.
12. Crum, C. P., et al.: Vulvar intraepithelial neoplasia (severe atypia and carcinoma in situ). Cancer 54:1429, 1984.
13. Magrina, J. F., et al.: Stage I squamous cell cancer of the vulva. Am. J. Obstet. Gynecol. 134:453, 1979.
14. Schwartz, P. E., and Naftolin, F.: Type 2 herpes simplex virus and vulvar carcinoma in situ (Editorial). N. Engl. J. Med. 305:517, 1981.
15. Lossick, J. G.: Sexually transmitted vaginitis. Urol. Clin. North Am. 11:141, 1984.
16. Schneider, G. T.: Vaginal infections: How to identify and treat them. Postgrad. Med. 73:255, 1983.
17. Herbst, A. L.: Clear cell adenocarcinoma and the current status of DES exposed females. Cancer 48:484, 1981.
18. Herbst, A. L.: Diethylstilbesterol exposure—1984. N. Engl. J. Med. 311:1433, 1984.
19. Brunham, R. C., et al.: Mucopurulent cervicitis—The ignored counterpart in women of urethritis in men. N. Engl. J. Med. 311:1, 1984.
20. Silverberg, E.: Cancer statistics 1985. CA 35:19, 1985.
21. Nelson, J. H., Jr., et al.: Dysplasia, carcinoma in situ, and early invasive cervical carcinoma. CA 34:306, 1984.
22. Sadeghi, S. B., et al.: Prevalence of cervical intraepithelial neoplasia in sexually active teenagers and young adults. Results of data analysis of mass Papanicolaou screening of 796,337 women in the United States in 1981. Am. J. Obstet. Gynecol. 148:726, 1984.
23. Devesa, S. S.: Descriptive epidemiology of cancer of the uterine cervix. Obstet. Gynecol. 63:605, 1984.
24. Campion, M. J., et al.: Increased risk of cervical neoplasia in consorts of men with penile condylomata acuminata. Lancet 1:943, 1985.
25. Kadish, A. S., et al.: Human papillomaviruses of different types in precancerous lesions of the uterine cervix. Histologic, immunocytochemical and ultrastructural studies. Hum. Pathol. 17:384, 1986.
26. Kaufman, R., et al.: Statement of caution in the interpretation of papillomavirus-associated lesions of the epithelium of the uterine cervix (Editorial). Acta Cytol. 27:107, 1983.
27. Greenwood, S. M., and Moran, J. J.: Chronic endometritis: Morphologic and clinical observations. Obstet. Gynecol. 58:176, 1981.
28. Fox, H., and Buckley, C. H.: Current concepts of endometriosis. Clin. Obstet. Gynaecol. 11:279, 1984.
29. Sheppard, B. L.: The pathology of dysfunctional uterine bleeding. Clin. Obstet. Gynaecol. 11:227, 1984.
30. Poindexter, A. N., and Ritter, M. B.: Anovulatory uterine bleeding. Compr. Ther. 9:65, 1983.
31. Norris, H. J., et al.: Endometrial hyperplasia and carcinoma. Diagnostic considerations. Am. J. Surg. Pathol. 7:839, 1983.
32. Sherman, A. I., and Brown, S.: The precursors of endometrial carcinoma. Am. J. Obstet. Gynecol. 135:947, 1979.
33. Morrow, C. P.: The benefits of estrogen to the menopausal woman outweigh the risks of developing endometrial cancer. Opinion: Con. CA 34:220, 1984.
34. Davies, J. L., et al.: A review of the risk factors for endometrial carcinoma. Obstet. Gynecol. Surv. 36:107, 1981.
35. Silverberg, S. G.: New aspects of endometrial carcinoma. Clin. Obstet. Gynaecol. 11:189, 1984.
36. Vessey, M. P.: Exogenous hormones in the aetiology of cancer in women. J. R. Soc. Med. 77:542, 1984.
37. Center for Disease Control: Oral contraceptive use and the risk of endometrial cancer. J.A.M.A., 249:1600, 1983.
38. Trapido, E. J.: A prospective cohort study of oral contraceptives and cancer of the endometrium. Int. J. Epidemiol. 12:297, 1983.
39. Gusberg, S. B., et al.: Precursors of corpus cancer. II. A clinical and pathological study of adenomatous hyperplasia. Am. J. Obstet. Gynecol. 68:1472, 1954.
40. Martin, J. D., et al.: The effect of estrogen receptor status on survival in patients with endometrial cancer. Am. J. Obstet. Gynecol. 147:322, 1983.
41. Stein, I. F., and Leventhal, M. L.: Amenorrhea associated with bilateral polycystic ovaries. Am. J. Obstet. Gynecol. 29:181, 1935.
42. Vaitukaitis, J. L.: Polycystic-ovary syndrome—What is it? N. Engl. J. Med. 309:1245, 1983.
43. Richardson, G. S., et al.: Common epithelial cancer of the ovary. N. Engl. J. Med. 312:415, 474, 1985.
44. Russell, P.: Borderline epithelial tumours of the ovary: A conceptual dilemma. Clin. Obstet. Gynaecol. 11:259, 1984.
45. Zaloudek, C., and Kurman, R. J.: Recent advances in the pathology of ovarian cancer. Clin. Obstet. Gynaecol. 10:155, 1983.
46. Scully, R. E.: Ovarian tumors. A review. Am. J. Pathol. 87:686, 1977.
47. Eastwood, J.: Mesonephroid (clear cell) carcinoma of the ovary and endometrium. A comparative prospective clinico-pathological study and review of literature. Cancer 41:1911, 1978.
48. Kurman, R. J., and Norris, H. J.: Germ cell tumors of the ovary. Pathol. Annu. 13(Part 1):291, 1978.
49. Steeper, T. A., and Mukai, K.: Solid ovarian teratomas: An immunocytochemical study of thirteen cases with clinicopathologic correlation. Pathol. Annu. 19(Part 1):81, 1984.
50. Resta, L., et al.: Ovarian dysgerminoma. A clinico-pathologic study. Neoplasma 31:459, 1984.
51. Young, R. H., and Scully, R. E.: Ovarian sex cord–stromal tumours: Recent advances and current status. Clin. Obstet. Gynaecol. 11:93, 1984.
52. Björkholm, E., and Silfverswärd, C.: Prognostic factors in granulosa-cell tumors. Gynecol. Oncol. 11:261, 1981.
53. Zaloudek, C., and Norris, H. J.: Sertoli-Leydig tumors of the ovary. A clinicopathologic study of 64 intermediate and poorly differentiated neoplasms. Am. J. Surg. Pathol. 8:405, 1984.

54. Umbach, G.: Review of tumor markers for ovarian cancer. Med. Hypoth. *13*:329, 1984.

55. van Nagell, J. R., Jr.: Tumour markers in ovarian cancer. Clin. Obstet. Gynaecol. *10*:197, 1983.

56. Elston, C. W.: The pathology of trophoblastic disease: Current status. Clin. Obstet. Gynaecol. *11*:135, 1984.

57. Bracken, M.B., et al.: Epidemiology of hydatidiform mole and choriocarcinoma. Epidemiol. Rev. *6*:52, 1984.

58. Driscoll, S. G.: Gestational trophoblastic neoplasms: Morphologic considerations. Hum. Pathol. *8*:529, 1977.

59. Driscoll, S. G.: Trophoblastic growths: Morphologic aspects and taxonomy. J. Reprod. Med. *26*:181, 1981.

60. Goldstein, D. P., and Berkowitz, R. S.: The role of regional centers for gestational trophoblastic disease. *In* Pattillo, R. A., and Hussa, R. O. (eds.): Human Trophoblast Neoplasms. New York, Plenum Press, 1984, p. 383.

61. Ellis, H., and Cox, P. J.: Breast problems in 1,000 consecutive referrals to surgical out-patients. Postgrad. Med. J. *60*:653, 1984.

62. Golinger, R. C.: Hormones and the pathophysiology of fibrocystic mastopathy. Surg. Gynecol. Obstet. *146*:273, 1978.

63. Parazzini F., et al.: Risk factors for pathologically confirmed benign breast disease. Am. J. Epidemiol. *120*:115, 1984.

64. Davis, H. H., et al.: Cystic disease of the breast: Relationship to carcinoma. Cancer *17*:957, 1964.

65. Kramer, W. M., and Rush, B. F.: Mammary duct proliferation in the elderly. A histopathologic study. Cancer *31*:130, 1973.

66. Love, S. M., et al.: Fibrocystic "disease" of the breast—A non disease? N. Engl. J. Med. *307*:1010, 1982.

67. Consensus Statement by the Cancer Committee of the College of American Pathologists: Is "fibrocystic disease" of the breast precancerous? Arch. Pathol. Lab. Med. *110*:171, 1986.

68. McDivitt, R. W.: Breast carcinoma. Hum. Pathol. *9*:3, 1978.

69. Hutter, R. V. P.: Goodbye to "fibrocystic disease." N. Engl. J. Med. *312*:179, 1985.

70. Dupont, W. D., and Page, D. L.: Risk factors for breast cancer in women with proliferative breast disease. N. Engl. J. Med. *312*:146, 1985.

71. Kalache, A., and Vessey, M.: Risk factors for breast cancer. Clin. Oncol. *1*:661, 1982.

72. Rico, M.: Breast cancer: Risk factors and etiology. Mt. Sinai J. Med. *51*:300, 1984.

73. The Cancer and Steroid Hormone Study of the Centers for Disease Control and the National Institute of Child Health and Human Development: Oral-contraceptive use and the risk of breast cancer. N. Engl. J. Med. *315*:405, 1986.

74. Wittliff, J. L.: Steroid hormone receptors in breast cancer. Cancer *53*:630, 1984.

75. Bittner, J. J.: Some possible effects of nursing on mammary gland tumor incidence in mice. Science *84*:162, 1936.

76. Wynder, E. L., and Rose, D. P.: Diet and breast cancer. Hosp. Pract. *19*:73, 1984.

77. Editorial: Intraduct carcinoma of the breast. Lancet *2*:24, 1984.

78. von Rueden, D. G., and Wilson, R. E.: Intraductal carcinoma of the breast. Surg. Gynecol. Obstet. *158*:105, 1984.

79. Wheeler, J. E., and Enterline, H. T.: Lobular carcinoma of the breast: In situ and infiltrating. Pathol. Annu. *11*:161, 1976.

80. Rosen, P. P.: Lobular carcinoma in situ of the breast. Am. J. Surg. Pathol. *2*:225, 1978.

81. Kopans, D. B., et al.: Breast imaging. N. Engl. J. Med. *310*:960, 1984.

82. Skrabanek, P.: False premises and false promises of breast cancer screening. Lancet *2*:316, 1985.

83. Tabár, L., et al.: Reduction in mortality from breast cancer after mass screening with mammography. Lancet *1*:829, 1985.

84. Fisher, B., et al.: Five-year results of a randomized clinical trial comparing total mastectomy and segmental mastectomy with or without radiation in the treatment of breast cancer. N. Engl. J. Med. *312*:665, 1985.

85. Mirecki, D. M., and Jordan, V. C.: Steroid hormone receptors and human breast cancer. Lab. Med. *16*:287, 1985.

86. Editorial: Steroid receptors and prognosis of breast cancer. Lancet *1*:887, 1984.

87. Vercoutere, A. L., and O'Connell, T. X.: Carcinoma of the male breast. Arch. Surg. *119*:1301, 1984.

# 20

# The Endocrine System

**PITUITARY GLAND**

HYPERPITUITARISM—ADENOMAS

HYPOPITUITARISM
  Nonfunctional Adenomas
  Sheehan's Syndrome
  Empty Sella Syndrome
POSTERIOR PITUITARY SYNDROMES

**THYROID GLAND**

THYROTOXICOSIS—HYPERTHYROIDISM

HYPOTHYROIDISM
  Cretinism
  Myxedema
THYROIDITIS
  Hashimoto's Thyroiditis (Struma Lymphomatosa)
  Subacute (de Quervain's, Granulomatous) Thyroiditis
  Chronic Painless Thyroiditis
GRAVES' DISEASE (BASEDOW'S DISEASE)
DIFFUSE (SIMPLE) AND MULTINODULAR GOITER
THYROID NEOPLASMS
  Adenomas
  Carcinomas
      Papillary carcinoma
      Follicular carcinoma
      Anaplastic carcinoma
      Medullary amyloidotic carcinoma

**PARATHYROID GLANDS**

HYPERPARATHYROIDISM
  Primary Hyperparathyroidism
      Adenoma
      Primary hyperplasia
      Carcinoma of the parathyroids
      Clinical features of primary hyperparathyroidism
  Secondary Hyperparathyroidism
HYPOPARATHYROIDISM

**ADRENAL CORTEX**

ADRENAL CORTICAL HYPERFUNCTION
(HYPERADRENALISM)
  Cushing's Syndrome
  Hyperaldosteronism
  Adrenal Virilism—Congenital Adrenal Hyperplasia
HYPOFUNCTION OF THE ADRENAL CORTEX
  Addison's Disease
  Acute Adrenocortical Insufficiency
CORTICAL NEOPLASMS

**ADRENAL MEDULLA**

PHEOCHROMOCYTOMA

NEUROBLASTOMA

**THYMUS**

HYPERPLASIA

THYMOMA

**MULTIPLE ENDOCRINE NEOPLASIA (MEN) SYNDROMES**

Endocrine disorders are among the most rewarding in medicine. They frequently present a jigsaw puzzle of signs and symptoms that, when correctly perceived, can be fit together into a satisfying diagnosis. Even more important, whereas many are potentially lethal, they can often be corrected and even cured. Although single gland involvement is the rule, polyglandular endocrinopathies are sometimes encountered in the multiple endocrine neoplasia (MEN) syndromes (p. 701). In addition, nonendocrine cancers sometimes are responsible for endocrinopathies referred to as paraneoplastic syndromes (p. 215). Nonetheless, most endocrinopathies arise out of lesions in a single gland, as the following discussions indicate.

## Pituitary Gland

The normal pituitary is a minute gland (about 0.5 gm) with anterior and posterior lobes nestled within the sella turcica of the sphenoid bone in the base of the skull. The sella is roofed over by an extension of the dura, the diaphragma sellae. The anterior lobe is derived from an outpouching of the primitive oral canal (Rathke's pouch). While the cephalad tip persists, the pedicle regresses, separating the anterior lobe from its embryonic origins. The posterior lobe (neurohypophysis) is formed by a downward exten-sion of the floor of the third ventricle. Persistence of the connection creates the pituitary stalk, which passes through a small aperture in the diaphragma sellae. There is no well-defined intermediate lobe in humans. The capillary network of the anterior and posterior lobes has two vascular supplies—one from branches of the internal carotids that brings arterial blood and the other from a so-called portal system that takes origin in capillaries in the floor of the third ventricle—these anastomose to form vessels that course along the pituitary stalk to reach the gland and its capillary bed. Thus, factors elaborated in the hypothalamus can be delivered directly to the pituitary.

The neurogenous posterior lobe is composed of tangled nerve fibers and scattered glia-like pituicytes. The posterior pituitary hormones (oxytocin and antidiuretic hormone—ADH) are synthesized in the hypothalamus and conveyed to the posterior lobe within nerve fibers, in which they can be visualized by electron microscopy (EM) as secretory granules awaiting discharge. The anterior lobe is composed of small polygonal secretory cells that traditionally have been divided into acidophils, basophils, and chromophobes, based on the abundance of cytoplasmic granules and their reactions to usual tissue stains. However, this approach has not yielded satisfactory correlations between specific cell types and secretory activity. Greater precision is now possible with EM, which reveals quite distinctive cytoplasmic granules constituting the storage forms of each anterior lobe hormone coupled with immunocytochemical methods using monoclonal antibodies for each hormone.[1] Such techniques permit identification of the five cell types secreting hormones that are (a) adrenocorticotropic (ACTH), (b) thyrotropic (thyroid-stimulating hormone, TSH), (c) gonadotropic (follicle-stimulating hormone, FSH; luteinizing hormone, LH), (d) lactotropic (prolactin, PRL), and (e) somatotropic (somatotropin, or growth hormone, GH). In addition, there are cells that have the conformation of secretory cells under the light microscope but have cytoplasm that is more or less cleared. They are neither basophilic nor acidophilic and so are called chromophobes. It was always assumed that they were nonfunctional, but electron microscopy reveals that some are indeed sparsely granulated and react weakly (if at all) with any of the hormonal immunocytochemical stains (hereafter referred to as "immunostains"). It is now clear that marked secretory activity of any anterior lobe cell leads to progressive degranulation (Table 20–1).

The release of pituitary tropic hormones, as you know, is under hypothalamic control. Hypothalamic releasing factors have been well characterized for TSH, LH, FSH, ACTH, and, probably, GH. Control of GH is also exerted by somatostatin, which functions as a release inhibitor. PRL secretion is similarly controlled by an inhibiting factor and by dopamine of neurogenic origin, which also inhibits its release. Another level of control is exerted by the hormones elaborated by target endocrine organs in negative feedback loops. For example, thyroid hormones inhibit thyrotroph activity and glucocorticoids inhibit the corticotrophs. With this cursory review of normal structure and function, we can turn to a consideration of the major disorders of the pituitary under the headings of hyperpituitarism, hypopituitarism, and posterior pituitary syndromes.

# HYPERPITUITARISM—ADENOMAS

Excess hormone production by the anterior pituitary is most often due to a pituitary adenoma. Carcinomas, particularly functioning ones, are exceedingly rare. Hyperplasia of a particular subtype of cells is equally rare; it may develop secondary to either some hypothalamic dysfunction or loss of feedback inhibition by the target organ hormone. In experimental animals, removal of the thyroid is followed by hyperplasia of the thyrotrophs and, eventually, in some animals a TSH-producing adenoma. *Despite the several possibilities, an excess of one of the anterior pituitary hormones implies the presence of an adenoma.*[2] Three types account for most of these adenomas—in order of frequency, those composed of prolactin cells (about 60% of all adenomas), growth hormone cells, and corticotroph cells. Strangely, adenomas producing the glycoprotein hormones (TSH, FSH, and LH) are uncommon.[3] Almost all adenomas are monoclonal and elaborate a single tropic hormone. Rarely, an adenoma is composed of two cell types or, rarely, only one cell type that produces both PRL and GH or other combinations; this is not unexpected, since all functional cell types stem from a common precursor. At the other extreme are the 10 to 30% of adenomas that are nonfunctional and are described on page 675.

Functional adenomas vary in size from large tumors (5 cm or greater in diameter) to microadenomas (less than 5 mm in diameter). Most are discretely encapsulated, but large lesions tend to expand the sella turcica, erode the anterior clinoid processes, and produce pressure defects in the optic chiasma or optic nerves. Some rupture through their capsules and diaphragma sellae to expand along broad fronts into the contiguous brain or cavernous and nasal sinuses to give the false impression of cancerous invasion. This phenomenon has given rise to the term "invasive adenoma." Microadenomas are, however, more common than grossly visible tumors and are found in about 25% of unselected autopsies.[4] They may or may not be encapsulated and so may be difficult to differentiate from a focus of hyperplasia. When the tumor can be visualized macroscopically it is soft, yielding, and usually red-brown on transection. Foci of ischemic necrosis are frequent in bulkier lesions, and indeed some appear to be largely necrotic, presumably because they compress their blood supply. Secondary hemorrhage may suddenly expand the neoplasm, producing what will be described as "pituitary apoplexy." The residual normal pituitary is more or less atrophic owing to the expansile pressure of the neoplasm, and sometimes it appears to be virtually obliterated.

Histologically, most adenomas are monomorphic and composed of sheets, cords, or nests of epithelial cells resembling one of the types of the normal pituitary. Sometimes, apparent glandular formations or papillary configurations are present. In the usual lesion, the cells

Table 20–1. THE NORMAL PITUITARY*

| Cell | Cell Size and Shape | Nucleus | Conventional Staining | Granularity | Granules | Immunoperoxidase Staining |
|---|---|---|---|---|---|---|
| **Somatotroph** Densely granulated (resting phase) | Medium; spherical to oval | Spherical and central, with prominent nucleoli | Acidophilic; PAS (−) | +++ to ++++ | Abundant; dense, spherical; 350–600 nm | GH (strong) |
| Sparsely granulated (secretory phase) | Medium; spherical to oval | Irregular | Weakly acidophilic to chromophobic; PAS (−) | + to ++ | Sparse; dense, spherical; 100–250 nm | GH (weak) |
| **Lactotroph** Densely granulated (resting phase) | Large; polyhedral to elongate | Oval to elongate | Acidophilic; PAS (−) | +++ to ++++ | Abundant; dense, spherical to oval, irregular; 500–800 nm | PRL (strong) |
| Sparsely granulated (secretory phase) | Medium; polyhedral to elongate | Oval | Weakly acidophilic to chromophobic; PAS (−) | + to ++ | Sparse; dense, irregular; 200–350 nm | PRL (weak) |
| **Corticotroph** | Medium; oval to polygonal | Spherical; eccentric | Basophilic; PAS (+) | ++ to +++ | Variable density, spherical to irregular; 300–350 nm (range 250–700) | ACTH |
| **Gonadotrophs** | Medium; oval | Spherical; eccentric | Basophilic; PAS (+) | ++ | Dense, spherical; 250–400 nm | FSH and LH |
| **Thyrotroph** | Medium; polygonal | Spherical; eccentric | Basophilic; PAS (+) | + to ++ | Dense, spherical; 150 nm | TSH |
| **Nonsecretory Cells** | Medium | Spherical | Chromophobic | ± | Sparse to none | None (weak) |

*Modified from Scheithauer, B. W.: Surgical pathology of the pituitary: The adenoma (Pt. II). Pathol. Annu. 19(Part 2):269, 1984.

are round, to oval, to polygonal and have abundant cytoplasm (often containing visible granules) and small central or eccentric regular nuclei. In occasional adenomas, the cells are more variable in size and shape and show some nuclear pleomorphism, raising the suspicion of malignancy, but to avoid overdiagnosis it is recommended that **evidence of metastatic dissemination must be present for a diagnosis of carcinoma**.

A few details about the more common specific types of adenoma follow.[1, 2]

○ **Prolactinomas** may be large, but most are microadenomas.[5] With conventional stains the cells may be acidophilic and on EM they may be densely granulated, but more often they look like chromophobes and are sparsely granulated, consistent with marked secretory activity and degranulation. Immunostains permit reliable identification of prolactinomas; the intensity of the reaction correlates with the degree of granularity. Some tumors associated with excess prolactin production are made up of sparsely granulated cells and yield weak to negative immunocytochemical reactions for prolactin.

○ **Growth hormone adenomas** range from small to large but are less commonly microadenomas than prolactinomas. The cells may be densely or sparsely granulated. Densely granulated cells are acidophilic by conventional stains and yield strong immunocytochemical rections for growth hormone. Sparsely granulated cells may appear chromophobic with conventional stains and yield weak reactions with immunostains.[2]

○ **Corticotroph adenomas** may be large, but in most series 75 to 80% are microadenomas.[6] They are made up of basophilic cells closely resembling their normal forebears. As might be anticipated, they yield strong reactions for ACTH with immunostains. Occasionally an apparent chromophobic lesion made up of sparsely granulated cells is found in these patients. Conversely, there are instances in which an adenoma yields a positive immunoreaction for ACTH but has no apparent functional effects, and it must be assumed that the tumor secretes nonfunctional products sharing antigenic specificities with ACTH.[7] The nontumor corticotrophs in the residual pituitary gland and, rarely, the cells of the adenoma exhibit cytoplasmic basophilic hyalinization, referred to as **"Crooke's hyalin change"** (p. 693).

○ There are other more rare types of adenoma that can be differentiated only by immunocytochemical methods. Some elaborate FSH-LH or, rarely, TSH, but a significant number (10 to 30%) are apparently nonsecretory and unassociated with clinical or biochemical evidence of hyperfunction and so are called "null" cell or chromophobe adenomas.

**CLINICAL COURSE.** Pituitary tumors may cause manifestations because of (1) the mass effect of the lesion, (2) the secretory function of the neoplasm, or both.[8]

*Mass effects* are seen only with large tumors (Fig. 20–1). They include disturbances in vision, head-

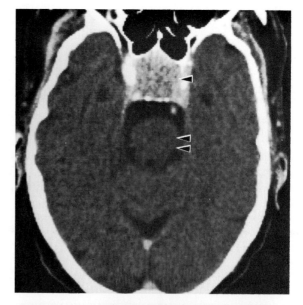

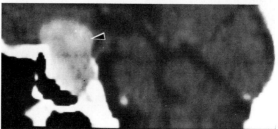

Figure 20–1. *Above*, CT scan of transverse plane of the skull at the level of the pituitary fossa, revealing enlargement of the sella caused by an expansile pituitary adenoma (*arrow*). Compare its size with the transverse dimension of the brain stem (*double arrow*). *Below*, Computer reconstruction of the same tumor in the sagittal plane (*arrow*). It has bulged out of the sella turcica, producing a moderately enlarged suprasellar mass. (Courtesy of Dr. Calvin Rumbaugh, Department of Radiology, Brigham and Women's Hospital, Harvard Medical School. Reprinted from Robbins, S. L., Cotran, R. S., and Kumar, V.: Pathologic Basis of Disease. 3rd ed. Philadelphia, W. B. Saunders Co., 1984, p. 1194.)

aches, cranial nerve palsies, and derangements in endocrine function of the nontumoral pituitary. In addition expansion of the sella turcica may be found by radiography, CT scans, or other scanning techniques; sometimes there is also erosion of the clinoid processes. Among these mass effects, the most characteristic are visual field defects, commonly taking the form of bitemporal hemianopsia related to pressure on the optic chiasm or nerves. The most frequent cranial nerve palsy involves the oculomotor nerves leading to diplopia or ptosis of the eyelids. Varying patterns of pituitary hypofunction may be manifest, stemming from tumorous compression and destruction of the uninvolved anterior lobe. However, well over half of all pituitary tumors are microadenomas and so more often than not the clinician is faced with the dilemma of evidence of pituitary hyperfunction in the absence of findings pointing to a mass effect.[9]

*Tropic hormone hypersecretion* is the most dramatic consequence of a functioning pituitary tumor. However, as indicated, perhaps one third of all pituitary adenomas are unassociated with hypersecretion of hormones. Such lesions can only be discovered by their mass effects or by their impingement on and destruction of the gland producing hypopituitarism. The major clinical syndromes produced by functional pituitary tumors are presented in capsule review in Table 20–2. Although the clinical features of the various hyperpituitary syndromes are for the most part quite distinctive, the diagnosis usually must be supported by radioimmunoassays documenting increased blood levels of specific pituitary tropic hormones as well as the biochemical markers of excessive function of the secondary endocrine target organs (e.g., adrenal steroids or their metabolites, thyroid hormones).

In conclusion, it is necessary to reemphasize that although increased levels of tropic hormones usually arise from hyperfunctioning pituitary tumors, rarely they have their origins in nonendocrine cancers and, even more rarely, in hypothalamic dysfunction such as may be caused by impinging meningiomas, metastases, gliomas, and craniopharyngiomas.

## HYPOPITUITARISM

A deficiency of anterior pituitary hormones may arise through three pathways: (1) lesions within the gland that destroy the secretory cells; (2) lesions within or adjacent to the pituitary stalk that block transmission of factors originating in the hypothalamus; and (3) lesions within the hypothalamus itself that impair the release of the anterior pituitary regulators. Note, the last two mechanisms would lead to *hyper*prolactinemia because of loss of the inhibitory factor. When the pituitary itself is the site of injury, a deficiency of two or three of the anterior lobe hormones usually results; GH, ACTH, and gonadotropins are frequently involved.[10] Multihormonal deficiencies become clinically evident in the following temporal sequences; FSH-LH, GH, ACTH, TSH, and, lastly, PRL. On the other hand, the hypopituitarism may be expressed as a single hormone deficiency—usually, a lack of growth hormone. Single or bihormonal deficiencies are more likely to arise from extrasellar lesions such as craniopharyngiomas resembling ameloblastomas (p. 503), meningiomas (p. 744), gliomas (p. 741), and germ cell tumors (p. 614). *Multihormonal deficiencies are usually related to destructive disorders of the pituitary gland itself. They are diverse and include sarcoidosis, tuberculosis, suppurative infections such as an extension of meningitis, surgical or radiation ablation of the pituitary, and histiocytosis X, but the three most common are nonsecretory adenomas, Sheehan's pituitary necrosis, and the empty sella syndrome,* to which the following comments are restricted (Fig. 20–2).

## NONFUNCTIONAL ADENOMAS

*Nonfunctional adenomas* account for about 10 to 30% of all pituitary tumors and represent the commonest cause of hypopituitarism.[11] When sufficiently large to cause pressure atrophy of the nontumorous anterior lobe, the adenomas are almost always accompanied by local mass effects (discussed earlier). The nonsecretory tumors are of two cytologic patterns. The more common is composed of chromophobic cells totally lacking granules and so failing to react with immunostains for all of the known tropic hormones. These are called "null cell" adenomas and

Table 20–2. SYNDROMES ASSOCIATED WITH HYPERSECRETING
PITUITARY ADENOMAS*

| Hormonal Excess | Syndrome | Clinical Features |
|---|---|---|
| GH | Gigantism (with onset before puberty) | Enlargement of head, body, extremities, and internal organs—the classic 8-foot "circus giant" prone to arthritis and neuromuscular dysfunction |
| | Acromegaly with postpubertal onset) | Acral "megaly" (i.e., enlargement of hands, feet, head); thickening of facial features, protuberant lower jaw; thick lips; large tongue; metabolic changes (e.g., osteoporosis, hypertension, glucose intolerance, diabetes mellitus) |
| Prolactin | Amenorrhea-galactorrhea syndrome | Amenorrhea or oligomenorrhea, variable galactorrhea; loss of libido, impotence in men |
| ACTH | Cushing's disease | Centripetal obesity, "moon facies," "buffalo hump," skin striae, ecchymoses, hirsutism, hypertension, glucose intolerance, psychiatric disturbances; must be differentiated from primary adrenal disease (p. 691) |
| TSH | Hyperthyroidism | Hypermetabolism with tachycardia, tremor, heat intolerance, sweating, weight loss, and other features discussed on page 677; must be differentiated from primary thyroid gland hyperfunction |
| LH, FSH | Hypergonadism | No specific features known |

*Modified from Tindal, G. T., and McLanahan, C. S.: Hyperfunctional pituitary tumors: Pre- and postoperative management considerations. Clin. Neurosurg. 27:48, 1980.

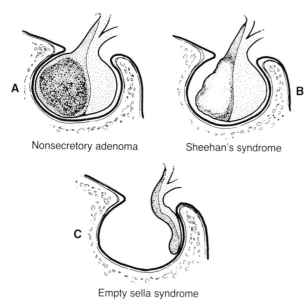

Nonsecretory adenoma

Sheehan's syndrome

Empty sella syndrome

FIGURE 20–2. Major causes of loss of anterior lobe and hypopituitarism. *A*, A nonfunctional adenoma; *B*, Sheehan's necrosis; and *C*, the mysterious "empty sella syndrome."

are thought to represent proliferation of undifferentiated precursor cells. The line of demarcation between a *"null cell"* adenoma and a secretory adenoma whose cells are extensively degranulated is exceedingly fine. Less commonly, the nonsecretory lesion is composed of epithelial cells having brightly eosinophilic granular cytoplasm (*oncocytomas*). Although both forms of neoplasia may cause global panhypopituitarism, more often they are manifested by deficiencies of gonadotropins and growth hormone.

## SHEEHAN'S SYNDROME

Also called *postpartum pituitary necrosis, Sheehan's syndrome* is another cause of hypopituitarism. During pregnancy, the anterior pituitary gland enlarges to about twice normal size, thereby compressing its vascularization. When there is a significant hemorrhage during or immediately following delivery, the hypotension or hemorrhagic shock further compromises the vascular supply of the anterior pituitary and thus may lead to infarction and necrosis. This complication may be immediately apparent when there is failure to lactate but may only be discovered much later when there is failure to resume menses. Sometimes the destruction of the gland does not become evident until a deficiency of tropic hormones appears years later. It is assumed, in these instances, that marginal cells had remained viable enough to maintain anterior pituitary function but they were trapped and progressively destroyed in the ensuing scarring. Rarely, infarction of the gland is seen in DIC, sickle cell anemia, and vasculitis syndromes, in either sex and at any age. Massive intrasellar necrosis, hemorrhage, and leakage into the

cerebrospinal fluid may produce sudden fever, stiff neck, and convulsions (pituitary apoplexy).

## EMPTY SELLA SYNDROME

This uncommon and curious cause of hypopituitarism is in essence the demonstration by special radiographic techniques (e.g., pneumoencephalography) of an empty sella in a patient with evidence of pituitary secretory hypofunction.[12] At autopsy, all that may remain is a small nubbin of fibrous tissue and, sometimes, the posterior pituitary lobe or a portion of it. In many instances, it is impossible to determine the basis for the mysterious disappearance. Occasionally, there is a reasonable explanation for the "missing" gland—e.g., pituitary necrosis, postsuppurative scarring, infarction and fibrosis of an adenoma, or radiation or surgical ablation. Often, however, there is no ready explanation, and herniation of the arachnoid through a diaphragmatic defect has been invoked. This might permit even minor or transient increases in CSF pressure to produce pressure atrophy of the pituitary over the course of years; sometimes in these cases the sella is not only empty but also enlarged and so is readily mistaken on radiographs or CT scan for an expansile nonsecretory pituitary neoplasm.

*The clinical manifestations* of hypopituitarism are extremely variable and depend largely on the age of onset and severity of the deficiency state. Children usually manifest growth retardation secondary to loss of GH when the hypopituitarism begins early in life. In the postpubertal or adult period, the panhypopituitarism tends to be expressed in the male as hypogonadism with loss of axillary and pubic hair, genital and breast atrophy, and failure to develop temporal recession of the hairline or baldness, but in the female it is manifest as amenorrhea. To be noted, cachexia (a false impression stemming from the older designation, "Simmond's cachexia") is lacking. Deficient function of other target organs may also be present; these include hypothyroidism, hypoadrenalism, and failure to lactate after childbirth. The critical evidence is the abnormally low serum levels of the various tropic hormones on radioimmunoassay.

## POSTERIOR PITUITARY SYNDROMES

Disordered posterior pituitary function is extremely rare. Its major expression is either a deficiency of antidiuretic hormone (ADH) or inappropriate release of it. *ADH deficiency induces diabetes insipidus*, characterized by polyuria and polydipsia. There are many possible causes of diabetes insipidus, including anterior lobe adenomas, metastatic cancer, and suppurative infections in association with meningitis, tuberculosis, sarcoidosis, surgical or radiation damage, or severe head injuries. When all these origins can be excluded, recourse is made to a wastebasket called "idiopathic." Rarely, the idiopathic form appears to be familial.

*Inappropriate ADH secretion* implies persistent release of ADH, unrelated to the osmolarity of the plasma. As a consequence, there is excessive reabsorption of water in the kidneys and expansion of the extracellular fluid volume, leading to hemodilution, hyponatremia, and the inability to excrete a dilute urine. Although injury to the posterior pituitary–hypothalamic axis may be responsible for this disorder, the great majority of cases arise from the paraneoplastic elaboration of ADH by nonendocrine tumors (bronchogenic carcinomas, thymomas, lymphomas, and others).

# Thyroid Gland

Disorders of the thyroid come to clinical attention because of (1) enlargement of the gland (goiter), which may be diffuse and symmetric, asymmetric, multinodular, or focal when it is caused by a neoplasm; (2) oversupply of thyroid hormone to the tissues of the body—thyrotoxicosis; or (3) inadequate hormone production—hypofunction. Often two or all of these derangements are present either concomitantly or in the course of the disease. Thus the patient with a goiter may also be thyrotoxic, and quite often a period of hyperfunction is followed by hypofunction. *Thyrotoxicosis* and *hypothyroidism* are threads that run throughout many of the diseases of the thyroid and so they will be discussed at the outset.

## THYROTOXICOSIS— HYPERTHYROIDISM

Thyrotoxicosis is the term applied to the hypermetabolic state induced by an oversupply of active thyroid hormone to the tissues of the body. *When the oversupply arises because of hyperfunction of the thyroid or of a tumor, it is referred to as hyperthyroidism.* However, in certain conditions (for example, some types of thyroiditis), the oversupply is related to excessive release of preformed thyroid hormone and not hyperfunction of the gland. Thus hyperthyroidism is only one cause of thyrotoxicosis. Despite these different implications, the two terms are nonetheless often loosely used interchangeably and we too must plead "mea culpa." *The principal causes of excess circulating thyroid hormone (i.e., thyrotoxicosis), accounting for 75 to 80% of all cases of thyrotoxicosis, are diffuse toxic hyperplasia (Graves' disease), toxic multinodular goiter, and toxic adenoma.* Rarely, thyroid hyperfunction is secondary to a TSH-producing pituitary adenoma or increased production of thyrotropin-releasing factor by the hypothalamus. Most of the remaining 20 to 25% of cases of thyrotoxicosis are referrable to certain forms of thyroiditis and are typically self-limited.

Whatever its origin, thyrotoxicosis causes the major clinical symptoms of nervousness, menstrual changes, emotional instability, fine tremors of the hands, warm skin with excessive sweating, heat intolerance, weight loss despite an increased appetite, and loss of strength. Cardiopulmonary symptoms are often prominent; they include dyspnea, rapid pulse, palpitations, and, in severe thyrotoxicosis, manifestations of cardiac failure. Despite the distinctive signs and symptoms of thyrotoxicosis, the diagnosis must always be confirmed by laboratory tests. Most commonly employed are measurements of the serum levels of thyroxin ($T_4$) and thyronine ($T_3$). The largest part of these hormones is bound to plasma proteins, principally a thyroid hormone–binding globulin (TBG). It is the small residual unbound fraction that has physiologic function, and so the levels of free $T_4$ and $T_3$ are particularly significant. To ascertain whether the increased level of hormone relates to thyroid hyperfunction rather than to abnormal release, a radioactive iodine uptake (RAIU) test can be performed. When there is increased RAIU, the thyrotoxicosis can be attributed to hyperfunction of the gland (i.e., hyperthyroidism); in thyrotoxicosis induced by abnormal release, RAIU is normal or even depressed. On occasion a radioimmunoassay for the serum TSH level is desirable to make certain that the primary dysfunction is not hypophyseothalamic.

The morphologic changes induced by excess thyroid hormone are surprisingly scanty and for the most part vague. They are more often seen with Graves' disease than in the other forms of thyrotoxicosis because this disease tends to produce the most severe and protracted elevations of thyroid hormone. Most prominent of the changes is cardiomegaly attributed to prolonged tachycardia and increased contractility.[13] Sometimes there are myocardial foci of lymphocytic and eosinophilic infiltration, mild interstitial fibrosis, and, occasionally, fatty change collectively designated **thyrotoxic cardiomyopathy**. Extracardiac alterations that are sometimes seen include variable atrophy and fatty infiltration of skeletal muscles, sometimes with focal interstitial lymphocytic infiltrates; generalized lymphoid hyperplasia with lymphadenopathy; occasionally, a mild nonspecific lymphocytic periportal infiltration and fatty change in the liver; and, even more rarely, osteoporosis.

Since any thyroid disorder responsible for an oversupply of active thyroid hormones to the body may induce the clinical syndrome of thyrotoxicosis, additional clinical findings are necessary to identify the specific underlying thyroid lesion, but sometimes fine-needle aspiration or open biopsy is required.

**Table 20–3.** CAUSES OF HYPOTHYROIDISM

**Deficiency Thyroid Parenchyma (Thyroprivic)**
Surgical or radiation ablation
Primary idiopathic myxedema (? autoimmune)
Agenesis, hypoplasia, or dysplasia of thyroid

*Goitrous Hypothyroidism*
Hashimoto's thyroiditis
Endemic iodine deficiency
Exogenous goitrogenic agents (para-aminosalicylic acid,
    cruciferous plants, phenylbutazone, lithium, cassava)
Congenital, often heritable, biosynthetic defects
Immune block of hormone synthesis

*Suprathyroidal Disorders (Trophoprivic)*
Hypopituitarism
Hypothalamic lesions

*Peripheral Resistance to Thyroid Hormone*

# HYPOTHYROIDISM

A deficiency of or peripheral resistance to thyroid hormone leads to the hypometabolic state of hypothyroidism. When the hormone lack appears in infancy it produces *cretinism*. In the older child or adult it results in *myxedema*, so called because of the edematous, doughy thickening of the skin that develops owing to the accumulation of hydrophilic mucopolysaccharides in connective tissues throughout the body. The disorders causing hypothyroidism are presented in Table 20–3. About 95% of cases of myxedema are caused by three conditions (in descending order of frequency); (1) surgical or radiation ablation of the gland incident to the therapy of Graves' disease or thyroid cancer, (2) Hashimoto's thyroiditis, and (3) the development of primary idiopathic myxedema of probable autoimmune origin (i.e., the formation of antibodies that block the TSH receptors).[14]

## CRETINISM

At one time hypothyroidism, particularly cretinism in the child, was endemic in the mountainous regions of the world and was mainly related to iodine deficiency, but the widespread iodination of salt has largely eradicated this global problem, which is now usually multifactorial in origin. Contributing mechanisms are mild iodine lack, hereditary biosynthetic defects, exogenous goitrogens, and antibody-mediated mechanisms such as the transplacental passage of autoantibodies from hypothyroid mothers to the embryo, which block TSH receptors and so impair thyroid hormone synthesis.[15] Hypophyseothalamic disorders impairing synthesis of TSH are rare causes.

Manifestations of thyroid hormone deficiency may be evident at birth but usually do not become apparent for several months. *Basically they comprise retardation in mental and physical development*, such as delay in the appearance of the normal milestones of infant development, short stature related to slowed epiphyseal bone growth, delayed dentition, coarse facial features with protruding tongue, dry skin, and protuberant abdomen. The mental retardation can become irreversible unless hormonal replacement therapy is instituted early. Fortunately, the diagnosis can be readily established by the depressed serum levels of total and free $T_4$ and $T_3$, accompanied by an increased level of TSH.

## MYXEDEMA

In the older child or adult, the manifestations of thyroid hormone deficiency appear insidiously and are often subtle. They usually begin with lethargy, cold intolerance, and, in the female, profuse menstrual flow. Over the span of months, slowing of mentation, speech, and movement become evident and are often accompanied by the distinctive myxedema, particularly noticeable about the eyes. The skin becomes cool, rough, and doughy. Other systems share in the hypodynamic state, and constipation sometimes progresses to adynamic ileus. The cardiac output is reduced and, typically, the heart becomes enlarged. The enlargement is caused mostly by chamber dilatation as the myocardium becomes flabby owing to an increase of interstitial mucopolysaccharide-rich edema (*myxedema heart*). Pericardial and pleural effusions may appear. Unless the condition is corrected, the patient with advanced hypothyroidism ultimately becomes stuporous and may even go into fatal coma. The diagnosis can be established at any point in the course by depressed RAIU and low levels of serum total and free $T_4$ and $T_3$. The TSH level is compensatorily elevated, unless the condition is primarily due to some hypophyseothalamic dysfunction.

With this overview of the systemic consequences of thyroid dysfunction, we can turn to the various lesions of the thyroid itself.

# THYROIDITIS

*This generic term is applied to thyroidal disorders marked by prominent infiltration of the gland by leukocytes, fibrosis, or both changes.* There are three distinctive forms of thyroiditis that merit description: Hashimoto's, subacute granulomatous, and chronic painless thyroiditis.[16] Before these are described, several uncommon variants should be mentioned. Seeding of the thyroid by bacteria, fungi, or, rarely, parasites is most uncommon and is usually caused by staphylococci and streptococci; less often it is caused by other bacteria. The resultant inflammatory changes are those encountered in any other localization of the particular offender, and in most instances the involvement is self-limited. Equally rare is *Riedel's fibrous thyroiditis*, in which the gland becomes virtually replaced by dense fibrosis that is idiopathic in origin. Some systemic dysfunction may be involved, because on occasion it is accompanied by mediastinal and retroperitoneal fibrosis.

## HASHIMOTO'S THYROIDITIS (STRUMA LYMPHOMATOSA)

There is abundant evidence that this most common form of thyroiditis is autoimmune in origin. It can arise at any age with a strong female preponderance (10 to 20 times more frequent than in males). Typically, the condition presents with variable goitrous enlargement and, in its fully developed stage, with hypothyroidism. However, the patient may have been euthyroid earlier, and in some instances during the course of the disease there may have been manifestations of thyrotoxicosis, giving rise to the term "hashitoxicosis." There is considerable clinical overlap between Graves' disease and Hashimoto's thyroiditis. Moreover, both conditions are thought to be autoimmune in origin and to have some similarities in the abnormal immune reactions. However, it should be noted that individuals with Hashimoto's thyroiditis have an increased frequency of HLA-DR5, whereas Graves' disease is associated with HLA-DR3.

**PATHOGENESIS.** Hashimoto's thyroiditis is the archetype of organ-specific autoimmune diseases; an experimental model of the disease can be produced in animals by sensitization to thyroidal antigens, and patients have a variety of autoantibodies to particular thyroidal antigens.[17] Among the autoantibodies most consistently present (about 95% of cases) are thyroidal antimicrosomal antibodies. Less frequent are antithyroglobulin antibodies. Some of these antibodies have been implicated in antibody-dependent, cell-mediated cytotoxicity against thyroid cells.[18] In addition, *a number of autoantibodies can be detected in many (but not all) patients against TSH receptors or closely related plasma membrane components.* One such antibody promotes thyroid growth and so is called "thyroid-growth immunoglobulin" (TGI). Another receptor-related antibody mimics pituitary thyrotropin and stimulates thyroid hormone synthesis—"thyroid-stimulating immunoglobulin" (TSI). This antibody is particularly associated with "hashitoxicosis" but disappears in those with advanced Hashimoto's when thyroid function is depressed.

What provokes the emergence of all of these autoimmune reactions? There are only speculations. An organ-specific defect in suppressor T-cell function is proposed. Presumably this defect is more likely in individuals of HLA-DR5 genotype. *It is then hypothesized that by chance an autoreactive clone of B cells is unrestrained by T-suppressor cells,* which presumably help to maintain self-tolerance. Thus, B cells are permitted to form the many antibodies (Fig. 20–3).[19] Conceivably, cytotoxic T cells for thyroid cells may participate along with antibody-mediated cellular cytotoxicity to cause the thyroid injury. Seductive as

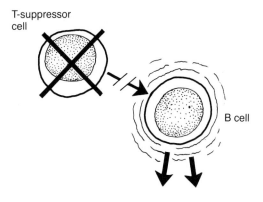

T-suppressor cell

B cell

Autoantibodies
Antimicrosomal antibody
Antithyroglobulin antibody
Thyroid-growth immunoglobulin
Thyroid-stimulating immunoglobulin

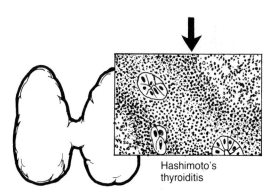

Hashimoto's thyroiditis

**Figure 20–3.** Diagrammatic representation of the possible pathogenesis of Hashimoto's thyroiditis.

these postulations may be, pieces of the puzzle are still missing—e.g., what is the nature of the genetic susceptibility? Clearly, some fundamental immunologic defect is present, since there is a greater than chance frequency in these individuals of other autoimmune diseases, including pernicious anemia, rheumatoid arthritis, systemic lupus erythematosus, insulin-dependent diabetes mellitus, and Addison's disease.

**MORPHOLOGY.** Typically, the gland is modestly enlarged, symmetric, firm, rubbery, and discrete. It may, however, be normal in size and even be contracted when there is significant fibrosis. Sometimes the enlargement is asymmetric and seemingly lobular to palpation. On transection, the normal red-brown, meaty, thyroidal substance is replaced by a pale, gray-white tissue that can even arouse concern at surgery about the possibility of a neoplasm, but the thyroid capsule remains intact. The classic features become evident microscopically. **There is extensive replacement of the thyroid architecture by lymphocytes (sometimes forming germinal centers), plasma cells, immunoblasts, and macro-**

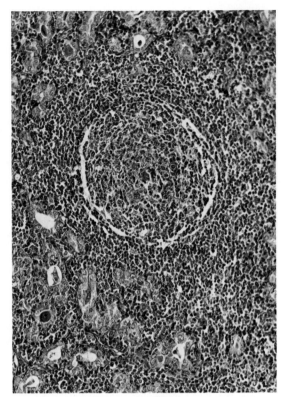

**Figure 20–4.** Hashimoto's thyroiditis. The microscopic field shows a prominent lymphoid follicle and a diffuse lymphocytic and plasma cell infiltrate interspersed among the atrophic thyroid follicles.

**phages.**[20] Indeed, entire microscopic fields may resemble a lymph node. However, here and there are isolated follicles or clusters of distorted follicles (Fig. 20–4). Frequently, the follicular epithelium is transformed into brightly acidophilic Hürthle cells (oncocytes) that have abundant granular cytoplasm. A delicate or fairly significant fibrosis is present, but the fibrosing reaction does not extend beyond the capsule.

Classically, this condition presents as a goiter in association with mild to significant hypothyroidism. In this circumstance the serum thyroxin levels are low and the TSH level elevated. However, early in the disease the patient may be euthyroid since the hypofunction develops slowly over the course of years. As noted earlier, occasionally patients develop thyrotoxicosis. In some instances, it is due to TSI and thus may be difficult to differentiate from the hyperthyroidism of Graves' disease. In other instances, the thyrotoxic state is transient and self-limited when it is incident to excessive release of thyroid hormones from injured follicular epithelium. Almost always present are high titers of antimicrosomal antibody and, less often, other types of autoantibodies. Infrequently, the clinical findings are not distinctive and needle biopsy is required. Lymphomatous transformation of the thyroidal infiltration is a rare complication.

## SUBACUTE (DE QUERVAIN'S, GRANULOMATOUS) THYROIDITIS

This acute to subacute inflammatory disorder is much less common than Hashimoto's thyroiditis. There is suggestive evidence that it is of viral origin since it is frequently preceded by an upper respiratory infection and is associated with prodromal symptoms typically associated with a systemic viral infection—malaise, fever, and muscle aching. A number of viruses have been implicated, particularly those causing mumps, measles, and influenza. There is no convincing evidence for an autoimmune origin.

The thyroid is usually somewhat enlarged (two to three times normal), often asymmetrically, with patchy foci of gray-white necrosis or fibrosis. Histologically, there are random foci of disruption and necrosis of the follicles, surrounded at first by a nonspecific acute to subacute inflammatory infiltrate, which later changes to a granulomatous pattern. The centers of the granulomas often contain irregular fragments of colloid surrounded by a foreign-body giant cell reaction, suggesting disruption of a follicle. Still later, the reactive foci undergo fibrosis with a residual lymphocytic infiltrate.

This condition is self-limited. At the outset, the thyroid is somewhat enlarged, perhaps irregularly tender and painful, and there may be signs and symptoms of thyrotoxicosis resulting from release of stored hormone. At this stage the serum concentrations of $T_4$ and $T_3$ are elevated. Within weeks, these manifestations abate as the patient becomes euthyroid; a few have a transient phase of hypothyroidism marked by elevated serum levels of TSH. In the great majority of individuals, there is complete resolution of the disease with no residual sequelae.

## CHRONIC PAINLESS THYROIDITIS

A better designation for this entity would be the cumbersome term "lymphocytic, painless thyroiditis with transient thyrotoxicosis" since it specifies the cardinal morphologic and clinical features. It accounts for 10 to 20% of cases of thyrotoxicosis.[21] Occurring at any age, it is somewhat more common in females, particularly postpartally.[22] The cause of this condition is unknown, and there is still debate about its being a variant of one or both of the two previously described forms of thyroiditis.

The gland is normal in size or sometimes modestly enlarged, usually symmetrically. The transection may reveal no changes or subtle foci of pallor. Histologically, the dominant findings are a diffuse or focal lymphocytic infiltration with injury to follicles in the areas of involvement but little fibrosis and no formation of germinal centers. The lymphoid infiltrate is less dense than that of Hashimoto's disease and lacks plasma cells. Granulomas such as are seen in subacute thyroiditis are not present. Ultimately, the changes resolve.[23]

Clinically, the disease appears silently, and manifestations of thyrotoxicosis or sometimes goitrous enlargement announce its presence. The gland is neither tender nor painful. The serum levels of $T_3$ and $T_4$ are elevated, and the major differential is the hyperthyroidism of Graves' disease. Critical in distinguishing these two conditions is measurement of RAIU, which is uniformly suppressed in painless thyroiditis but elevated in Graves' disease. Thus, the thyrotoxicosis arises from inappropriate release rather than production of hormones. In the usual case, the thyrotoxic phase passes in months (sometimes a year) and is followed by euthyroidism. However, a significant minority of cases have a subsequent transient phase of hypothyroidism. Ultimately, the condition resolves with no sequelae, albeit the goitrous enlargement, if present, may persist for a long time.

# GRAVES' DISEASE (BASEDOW'S DISEASE)

Graves' disease is the most common cause of thyrotoxicosis, in this condition related to hyperfunction and overproduction of thyroid hormone. *It is characterized by a triad of major manifestations: (1) hyperthyroidism, (2) infiltrative ophthalmopathy, and (3) infiltrative dermopathy.* One or two of these features may not be present. For example, in some patients, Graves' disease is marked by hyperthyroidism alone without eye or skin changes. Uncommonly, ophthalmopathy and dermopathy coexist in the absence of hyperthyroidism. Thus, it appears that *although the three features have closely related origins, they are independent variables.* Overall, hyperthyroidism is the most consistent feature and is accompanied by ophthalmopathy in about two thirds of cases and dermopathy in about a sixth.

Graves' disease may occur at any age but is most common in the third or fourth decades, particularly in women; females are affected five to seven times more frequently than males. The disease tends to be associated with HLA-DR3, suggesting a genetic predisposition, but many individuals have other HLA types and all with HLA-DR3 are not afflicted. Many findings point to an autoimmune pathogenesis and, as noted earlier, the same is true of Hashimoto's thyroiditis, but the latter is associated with HLA-DR5. In some patients, features of both disorders are present (i.e., "hashitoxicosis"). Not surprisingly, Graves' disease and Hashimoto's thyroiditis are associated with the same autoimmune disorders, such as pernicious anemia, systemic lupus erythematosus, rheumatoid arthritis, insulin-dependent diabetes mellitus, and Addison's disease.

**PATHOGENESIS.** Considerable evidence suggests an autoimmune pathogenesis for Graves' disease. Thyroid microsomal autoantibodies are present in about 85% of patients and thyroglobulin antibodies are found in about 30%.[24] More important from a pathogenetic viewpoint are a constellation of antibodies to the TSH receptor or membrane domains closely related to it. In most cases, there are thyroid-stimulating immunoglobulins (TSI), presumably responsible for hyperfunction of the follicular cells. The thyroid gland in this disorder usually has a diffuse lymphocytic infiltration, and some findings suggest that the TSI may at least in part be formed by these cells.[25] Sometimes thyroid-growth immunoglobulins (TGI) are also present; they are presumably involved in the hyperplasia responsible for the goitrous enlargement. Other receptor-related autoantibodies are sometimes present but, like sleeping dogs, will be let to lie.

Cell-mediated immunity also appears to be deranged. There is evidence for an organ-specific defect in T-suppressor cells.[26] It is proposed, therefore, that immune-response genes in the HLA-DR3 locus in some way increase the predisposition to the deranged suppressor cell function, permitting the unrestrained activity of autoreactive B cells. However, the trigger for the appearance of these abnormal immune reactions remains unknown.

The origins of the ophthalmopathy are uncertain, but a recent finding suggests that it is caused by a distinctive autoantibody that binds specifically to retroorbital antigens, principally within the extraocular muscles.[27] Nothing is known about the pathogenesis of the skin changes.

**MORPHOLOGY.** The thyroid gland is usually diffusely and symmetrically enlarged but, rarely, more than three times normal size. It has a red-brown, muscle-like appearance on transection. **The cardinal histologic features in the untreated case are "too many follicular cells and too little colloid."** The epithelial cells become columnar, crowded, and often buckle into the thyroid follicles to form small papillae. While there is some slight variation in size and shape of the cells, there is no significant atypicality. The colloid is more or less resorbed and has a thin, almost watery appearance when present, but many follicles are devoid of it (Fig. 20–5). There is a marked diffuse lymphocytic infiltrate in the interfollicular stroma along with lymphoid hypertrophy throughout the body, which causes enlargement of lymph nodes, thymus, and spleen. Increased vascularity of the gland is also present.

The classic histologic signs are significantly altered by preoperative medication. Iodides, which block lysis of the thyroglobulin-containing colloid, promote colloid storage, and the increased size of the follicles compresses the vascularization. Thioureas, on the other hand, suppress thyroid hormone synthesis, leading to a compensatory increase in TSH, which augments the hypercellularity.

When present, the exophthalmos is related to swelling of the extraocular muscles and retroorbital tissues, caused by a diffuse deposition of hydrophilic mucopolysaccharides associated with a lymphocytic infiltration (infiltrative ophthalmopathy).[28] The dermopathy is usually located over the dorsum of the legs or feet and so is

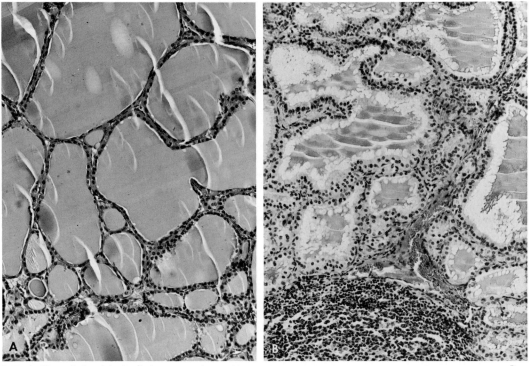

Figure 20–5. *A*, Normal thyroid gland, for comparison with the hyperplasia of the thyroid in *B*. Note the resorption of colloid, producing the peripheral scalloping, and the lymphoid aggregate below.

incongruously termed "pretibial myxedema." These changes are attributed to the accumulation of dermal and subcutaneous mucopolysaccharides accompanied by a lymphocytic infiltration.

The heart may be enlarged and have the changes previously described as **thyrotoxic cardiomyopathy** (p. 677).

**CLINICAL COURSE.** The major clinical features of Graves' disease were mentioned at the outset. The hyperthyroidism (p. 677) is caused by hyperfunctioning follicular cells and increased production of thyroid hormones. Thus, laboratory tests reveal increased RAIU and increased serum levels of total and free $T_4$ and $T_3$. Antimicrosomal or antithyroglobulin antibodies, or both, are present in most cases. Although appropriate assays will reveal other autoantibodies, these tests are rarely necessary for the clinical diagnosis. In the differential diagnosis it should be noted that hypersecretion of thyroid hormone is also encountered in other conditions such as toxic multinodular goiter, hyperfunctioning thyroid adenoma, and TSH-producing pituitary adenoma, and, as pointed out in previous discussions, thyrotoxicosis is seen with several forms of thyroiditis. However, none of these conditions causes the ophthalmopathy and dermopathy of Graves' disease. The eye changes, when present, are particularly striking. Related to the hyperthyroidism and therefore reversible with control of it are lid lag, lid retraction, and often a pronounced stare. Having their own autoimmune origins and seen in more advanced cases are perior-

bital swelling, conjunctivitis, and bulging of the eyes (proptosis). In many instances, incoordination of eye movement and ophthalmoplegia develop. Increases in intraocular pressure can become sufficiently extreme to produce blindness. The proptosis (sometimes called "malignant exophthalmos") is one of the most troubling aspects of Graves' disease, since it prevents closure of the lids and leads to corneal injury, infection, and, possibly, loss of the eyes. Moreover, it does not respond to control of the hyperthyroidism.

## DIFFUSE (SIMPLE) AND MULTINODULAR GOITER

*These two patterns of goiter are presented together because they have common origins; the multinodular variant arises as an extension of the diffuse lesion.* At the most elemental level, both types of goitrous enlargement are the consequence of "excessive replication of epithelial cells with subsequent generation of new follicles of widely differing structure and function."[29] Repeated cycles of hyperplasia and involution create nodules of varying size. The resultant physical stresses and encroachment on the vascularization lead to focal damage, with subsequent scarring and compensatory generation of new follicles, and enlargement of surviving follicles to thus produce multinodularity. *Both forms of goiter may occur endemically (in over 10% of the population) or sporadically.*[30] *Endemic goiter was formerly very common in iodine-deficient areas such as the mountainous regions of the Alps, Andes, and Himalayas,* but iodination of salt has to a considerable extent eradicated this problem. The iodine deficiency impairs the ability of the thyroid gland to elaborate hormone, and compensatory TSH secretion induces the growth of the gland. However, elevated TSH levels cannot always be identified, and so increased sensitivity to TSH has also been invoked.

*The sporadic patterns are in all likelihood multifactorial in origin. Possibly involved in one or another instance are mild lack of iodine, ingestion of goitrogenic substances, hereditary biosynthetic defects, and autoimmune reactions.* Goitrogens are present in foods (cabbage, cassava, cauliflower, turnip, Brussels sprouts) and infected water supplies, and certain drugs (lithium, phenylbutazone, para-amino salicylic acid) are goitrogenic. A variety of heritable metabolic errors in thyroid hormone synthesis have been identified as rare causes of goiter formation. Recently, the possibility of autoantibodies in the form of thyroid-growth immunoglobulins has been raised as another potential pathway.[31] Superimposed on all these influences are physiologic or pathologic stresses such as puberty, infection, and, notably, pregnancy that increase the demand for thyroid function and so contribute to the development of both diffuse and multinodular goiters. Consequently, women are affected more often than men.

**MORPHOLOGY.** With **diffuse colloid goiter**, the thyroid is firm and symmetrically enlarged, up to 200 to 300 gm, which is 10 times its normal size. The capsule is usually uninvolved. The transected surface is pale, brown-gray, glistening, brittle, and gelatinous. On histologic examination, large colloid-filled follicles are seen, lined by flattened epithelial cells and separated by a scant stroma. Sometimes there is evidence of preexisting hyperplasia in the form of occasional small acini lined by cuboidal to tall columnar cells.

**Multinodular colloid goiters** evolve over the course of years from diffuse goiters. They progressively enlarge without treatment, may be truly enormous, and, in general, are the largest type of goiter encountered, weighing up to 1000 gm. They may be markedly asymmetrical, consisting of masses of palpable nodules (Fig. 20–6). Expansion may occur downward behind the sternum to produce an **intrathoracic** or **plunging goiter**. Although the capsule is usually uninvolved, subcapsular hemorrhage sometimes causes adhesion to surrounding structures. Perhaps the most important histologic feature is the extreme variability of the tissue within these glands. Nodules of hyperplasia exist side by side with nodules composed of dilated, colloid-filled follicles. Grossly, this appears as meaty, red-brown parenchyma alternating with pale, gelatinous areas punctuated by small cysts, foci of red-brown hemorrhage, and pale fibrotic scars. Calcification is common in the scarred areas. **Although the nodules may give the false impression of encapsulation on gross examination, they are actually merely surrounded by compressed stromal tissue.**

**CLINICAL COURSE.** Both diffuse and multinodular colloid goiters usually come to attention because of progressive thyromegaly. *In general, the increase in size of these glands is sufficient to keep the patient euthyroid (nontoxic nodular goiter),* but sometimes hypothyroidism develops. With long-standing multinodular goiters, hyperthyroidism may appear. The

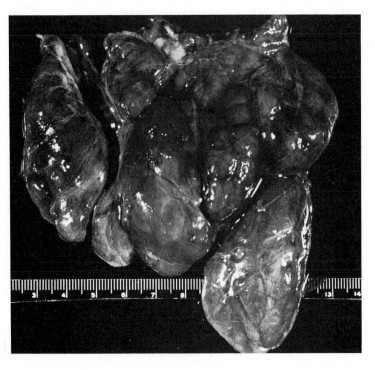

Figure 20–6. Multinodular colloid.

source of excess hormone can be localized on scinti-scans to hyperplastic hyperfunctioning nodules (*toxic nodular goiter*). The multinodular thyromegaly may become sufficient to compress the trachea or esophagus, particularly when the thyroid becomes trapped behind the sternum. The superior vena cava may also become compressed, producing congestion of the superficial veins in the neck and face. In such instances, surgical resection is necessary. A major clinical problem is the differentiation of multinodular goiter from a neoplasm, particularly when the goitrous enlargement seems to be restricted to a single focus. Ultrasonography and CT scans can be of great help by revealing the true diffuseness of the involvement in multinodular goiters, but frequently fine-needle aspiration or even open biopsy and histologic examination are necessary.

## THYROID NEOPLASMS

Neoplasms of the thyroid, whether benign or malignant, usually present as a solitary mass or nodule. The great majority of solitary nodules (about 80%) are adenomas. Uncommonly, they represent cancers. The remainder embrace a miscellany of lesions including a focus of a multinodular goiter, thyroid cysts, and focal thyroiditis. Few problems tax clinicians more than the noninvasive differentiation of adenomas from carcinomas. Involved in this clinical dilemma are the relative frequency of solitary nodules and how often they prove to be cancerous. Regrettably, the data are extremely variable, reflecting population differences, methods of analysis (e.g., palpation versus ultrasonography versus autopsy), and anatomic criteria for the diagnosis of benign and malignant neoplasms. Data derived from several older reports have made it gospel that approximately 4 to 7% of adults in the United States have clinically palpable thyroid nodules.[32, 33] Significantly higher prevalence rates are encountered in endemic goitrous and radiation-exposed populations. The frequency of malignancy in these nodules is a veritable quagmire of disagreement, with estimates ranging from 0.4% to 33%.[34] The grounds for this disagreement are too laborious to be detailed, but one variable merits mention—the rigor of the anatomic evaluation. Occult microscopic foci of carcinoma can be found, it is said, in 5 to 10% of the general population, when sought with sufficient vigor![35] Most of these microscopic cancers are not biologically threatening and probably are clinically irrelevant, but their inclusion in reported series significantly muddies the waters. Thus there are no universally accepted data for the prevalence of cancers in solitary thyroid nodules, but the following generalizations can be made.

○ Thyroid nodules, mostly adenomas, are common in the general population.
○ In contrast to the situation in females, a solitary nodule in a male is more likely to be tumorous, rather than a focus of multinodular goiter, because goiters are more common in females than in males.
○ Thyroid cancers are very uncommon, with an annual incidence of about 35 to 40 cases per million population.
○ In unselected, unbiased populations, only a tiny fraction of clinically palpable thyroid nodules are malignant.

Nonetheless, the patient is not a statistic!

## ADENOMAS

These benign tumors may arise at any age but become increasingly frequent with advancing years. They are the commonest cause of a solitary thyroid nodule in nonendemic areas. Rarely is there more than a single adenoma. Multiple nodules until proven otherwise imply a multinodular goiter.

Thyroid adenomas are usually spherical, completely encapsulated, and rarely exceed 4 cm in diameter. On transection, they vary from gray to brown, but a central focus of fibrosis and sometimes calcification may be present. Some lesions undergo cystic degeneration. These adenomas are derived from the epithelium of the follicle, and in the overwhelming majority there are readily recognized follicles on microscopy, so almost all could be designated **follicular adenomas**. Sometimes, however, they are divided into macrofollicular and microfollicular categories. They have been more elaborately subdivided according to the relative amounts of colloid and cellularity (Fig. 20–7). A **colloid adenoma** is composed

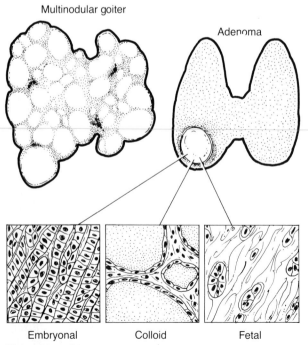

Multinodular goiter

Adenoma

Embryonal      Colloid      Fetal

**Figure 20–7.** Diagrammatic comparison of the morphology of multinodular goiter and a solitary thyroid adenoma with the three major histologic variants of adenoma.

of large follicles with abundant colloid and scant interfollicular stroma. The **simple adenoma** has colloid-bearing follicles of normal size with scant stroma. **Fetal adenomas** have microfollicles separated by an abundant interfollicular loose connective tissue. In **embryonal or trabecular adenomas**, the cells are disposed in cords or strands with scattered abortive follicles. In addition, there are encapsulated nodules having well-developed papillary formations covered by orderly epithelial cells; these may be called **papillary adenomas**. However, their segregation from well-differentiated papillary carcinomas is so difficult (as will be discussed later) that most experts prefer to consider all papillary lesions as cancerous or potentially cancerous.

Helpful in the differentiation of an adenoma from a nodule of a multinodular goiter are the following criteria. **(1) Adenomas are generally well encapsulated, whereas the apparent encapsulation of a nodule is imperfect. (2) The architecture within the adenoma is homogeneous, is distinctly different from that of the surrounding thyroid substance, and does not have the variability typical of a nodule within a multinodular goiter. (3) The adenoma produces compression of the more or less normal surrounding follicles.** An even more difficult problem is the histologic differentiation of a benign follicular adenoma from an encapsulated, well-differentiated follicular carcinoma, particularly when there is apparent, albeit minimal, capsular or vascular invasion. Such lesions, which straddle the line, have been termed "angioinvasive follicular adenomas" or "atypical adenomas" and have given rise to the controversial concept that follicular adenomas may become transformed into follicular carcinomas. It is believed that (1) **vascular invasion is an unreliable indicator of malignancy unless it is accompanied by unmistakable cytologic atypia,** and (2) **the notion of malignant transformation of an adenoma stems from failure of recognition of the cancerous nature of a very well differentiated follicular carcinoma.**[36] Thus adenomas are not construed as precursors of carcinoma, but a "baby carcinoma" may masquerade as an adenoma.

The interpretation clinically of an apparent solitary nodule within the thyroid is a common and vexing problem. In addition to adenomas and carcinomas, a solitary focus within a multinodular goiter, asymmetric Hashimoto's thyroiditis, and cysts may present as a solitary nodule. It is sometimes difficult but usually possible to segregate the non-neoplastic from the neoplastic lesion. The differentiation of an adenoma from a cancer is the heart of the problem. Many approaches are used; among them, ultrasonography and radionuclide imaging.[37] The former is capable of delineating the size, shape, homogeneity, and extent of encapsulation of the lesion. The latter evaluates its function (i.e., its ability to take up from the circulation $^{131}$I or sodium pertechnetate). *Functioning adenomas, which may indeed produce hyperthyroidism, avidly take these markers up and so appear on scintiscan as "hot" nodules.* Nonfunctional nodules are "cold," and there are, in addition, "warm" nodules. Most malignant lesions are "cold," and so the failure to take up the radiolabel points strongly toward malignancy but, alas, benign adenomas may also on occasion be "cold" and cancers "warm" to "hot." Ultimately, fine-needle aspiration, surgical biopsy, or excision is often required.

## CARCINOMAS

The frequency of thyroid cancers is obviously highly relevant to the likelihood of a lesion being malignant. Although they understandably cause great concern in all patients with a thyroid mass or nodule, they are, as previously noted, uncommon forms of cancers. About 7500 new cases are diagnosed each year in the United States. The incidence of these lesions has steadily risen, but it is unclear whether it is real or an artifact (of better case-finding); in Japan, however, there is no doubt about its validity, for reasons that will become clear.[38] The great preponderance of cancers are carcinomas; sarcomas and lymphomas are rarities. The carcinomas are divided into two categories: (1) *well-differentiated lesions,* further subclassified into papillary or follicular carcinomas, and (2) *poorly differentiated lesions,* embracing medullary carcinoma and undifferentiated carcinoma. As noted later, the various subtypes have widely differing prognoses. Females are affected two to three times more often than males. *Although cancers may arise at any age, the papillary and, to a lesser extent, follicular patterns often appear before age 30, particularly in individuals who have received radiation to the head and neck regions in the past.* Approximately 7% of the Japanese suvivors of the atomic bombs have developed thyroid carcinoma two or more decades later. Therapeutic doses of radiation to the neck and head for benign conditions such as skin disorders or tonsillar enlargement have yielded years later a similar frequency of thyroid carcinomas.[39] Indeed, when a young individual previously exposed to radiation develops a thyroid nodule, there is almost a 50% chance that it will prove to be malignant. Most are papillary carcinomas; the remainder are almost entirely follicular. Both patterns tend to be more aggressive than their analogs unrelated to radiation.

### *Papillary Carcinoma*

*The designation "papillary carcinoma" is applied to all thyroid malignancies having a "pure" papillary or a mixed papillary and follicular architecture or to all cancers composed of cells having "ground-glass," "optically clear" nuclei, whether papillary formations are present or not.* So defined, papillary carcinomas constitute about 60 to 70% of all thyroid cancers.[40] Some papillary neoplasms are extremely well differentiated, and a few have been called "papillary adenoma," but experience has taught that the line between these lesions and carcinomas is so fine that all are best considered cancerous.

They range from solitary, seemingly encapsulated lesions less than 1 cm in diameter to large or multifocal tumors possibly from intrathyroidal spread. Advanced tumors may penetrate the thyroid capsule into surrounding structures. The neoplastic foci are gray to brown and firm and sometimes have a furry appearance on transection. Some are almost entirely papillary. **True papillae, when present, have a central fibrovascular stalk covered by a single or multiple layers of cuboidal to low columnar epithelial cells**. Most are well differentiated; uncommonly, the cells are somewhat anaplastic, but mitoses are rare.[41] **Usually the cells have ground-glass nuclei**—the nuclear membranes are distinct, the nucleoli are small and marginated, and the nucleoplasm contains finely divided chromatin, imparting a cleared appearance to the nucleoplasm. Tumors having true papillae are regarded as papillary carcinomas even if they do not have ground-glass nuclei. In other neoplasms, there are mixtures of irregular follicles and papillary configurations, and occasionally there are variants in which the architecture is almost entirely follicular but the nuclei have a ground-glass appearance.[42] Other microscopic features that may be present include psammoma bodies within the tips of papillae, foci of squamous metaplasia, and lymphoid infiltration of the tumor stroma (Fig. 20–8).

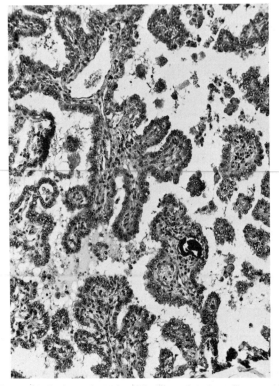

**Figure 20–8.** A moderately well differentiated papillary carcinoma of the thyroid. The epithelial cells display a slightly disordered array and show some variability in size.

Typically, these neoplasms spread through lymphatics to lymph nodes, usually within the neck, and sometimes even when the primary lesion is very small. Hematogenous spread is less common, but nonetheless 5 to 10% have metastasized to the lungs by the time of diagnosis. Spread to more distant sites (e.g., bones) is unusual unless the primary tumor has invaded beyond the thyroid.

As noted earlier, this form of carcinoma has the strongest association with prior irradiation.[43] It tends to occur in young individuals (under 30 years of age), particularly when there is a history of radiation exposure. Not infrequently, such a tumor will come to attention by discovery of a metastasis in an enlarged lymph node in the neck. *Occasional neoplasms hyperfunction and induce hyperthyroidism.* They are, on the whole, indolent lesions, yielding an overall 70 to 85% 10-year survival rate. Surprisingly, the initial presence or subsequent development of cervical lymph node metastases does not significantly influence the prognosis, because the nodal lesions too are indolent and readily excised. *Favorable prognostic features are young age, small tumor size, and encapsulation.* Conversely, unfavorable indicators are multicentricity, extrathyroid extension, and presence of distant metastases.

### Follicular Carcinoma

*The term "follicular carcinoma" is applied to cancers composed of cells arranged in follicles along with trabeculae, or sheets having no papillae or ground-glass nuclei.* As noted above, when ground-glass nuclei or even sparsely distributed papillae are present, the lesion is a papillary carcinoma, both anatomically and biologically.[44] Follicular carcinomas constitute about 20% of all thyroid cancers.

Macroscopically, **they may take the form of either an encapsulated gray-white nodule up to several centimeters in diameter or a massive, obviously invasive neoplasm that shows extension into perithyroidal structures**. The encapsulated pattern obviously mimics an adenoma and may also mimic it microscopically. There is great histologic variation among these cancers. The cells range from well differentiated to markedly anaplastic and can be arranged in small follicles containing remnants of collid or in trabecular cords, small nests, or solid sheets (Fig. 20–9).[45] The better levels of differentiation tend to be seen in lesions producing small follicles. The anaplastic lesions tend to have few follicles, many mitotic figures, and the pleomorphism typical of cancer. Vascular and capsular invasion is usually prominent in both the nodular and massive variants.

The differentiation of the small, encapsulated, well-differentiated follicular cancers from adenomas may be difficult. Although much stress has been laid on vascular invasion as a marker of malignancy, rarely adenomas may have occasional vessels seemingly penetrated by tumor cells, and therefore caution is required to avoid overdiagnosis of angioinvasive lesions.[46] Almost always

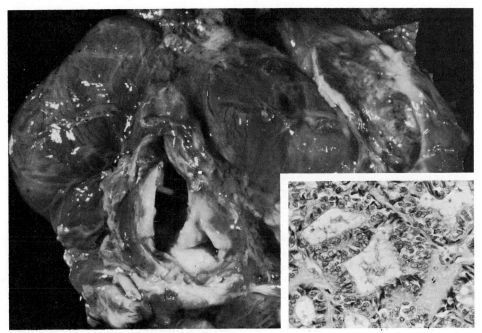

Figure 20–9. The gross appearance of a follicular carcinoma of the thyroid, viewed from above. The gray-white tumor tissue has penetrated the capsule to produce the extrathyroidal mass seen on the right. The trachea is compressed and is held open by a prop. The insert on the lower right shows the tumor to be a moderately well differentiated carcinoma.

when the vascular invasion has biologic significance, there is accompanying cytologic atypia, providing support for the diagnosis of malignancy. When follicular carcinomas disseminate, it is usually hematogenously, most often to the lungs, bone, liver, or brain and, strangely, sparing regional lymph nodes.

Large, invasive lesions with extrathyroidal extension usually can readily be recognized clinically as cancers, but the small encapsulated pattern may defy clinical differentiation from an adenoma until biopsy. Better differentiated lesions may elaborate thyroid hormone and induce hyperthyroidism. The outlook depends on the size and extent of the tumor. The prognosis of the small encapsulated lesion is almost as good as that of papillary carcinoma, but the large invasive, anaplastic cancers generally cause death within 10 years by widespread dissemination.

### Anaplastic Carcinoma

In contrast to the two types of thyroid cancer described previously, this is a highly malignant tumor that almost always causes death within two years. It affects older individuals, usually those between the ages of 60 and 80 years. Ten to 15% of thyroid carcinomas fall into this category.

By the time it is brought to medical attention, the tumor is usually a bulky mass that has obviously invaded beyond the thyroid capsule. The histologic pattern is totally undifferentiated. Sometimes the cells are spindled, reminiscent of an undifferentiated sarcoma, whereas in other instances they are large, highly variable in size and shape, and often multinucleated or squamoid.

Rapid advance in size, extension beyond the thyroid, and widespread metastases, all occurring within one year, are characteristic of this aggressive neoplasm.[47]

### Medullary Amyloidotic Carcinoma

These neoplasms may arise from the parafollicular C cells of the thyroid gland, which belong to the family of neurosecretory APUD cells (p. 537). Like other APUDomas producing bioactive products, thyroid medullary carcinomas elaborate calcitonin and, sometimes, other peptide hormones, including ACTH. Recently, however, mixtures and transitional forms of follicular and calcitonin-producing cells have been described in these cancers, suggesting common progenitors.[48] Moreover, it has been found that the cells in most medullary carcinomas elaborate carcinoembryonic antigen (CEA), which is also a feature of many non-APUD carcinomas. Thus the origin of all C cells and their carcinomas in neuroendocrine cells has been called into question. About 10% of these cancers occur in familial syndromes having autosomal dominant transmission; the remainder arise sporadically. The most frequent genetic settings constitute multiple endocrine neoplasia (MEN) syndromes II and III, discussed on page 701, in which the medullary carcinoma occurs along with pheochromocytomas, usually in the adrenals.

**The sporadic tumors** tend to be large, appear gray-white, and occupy or replace one lobe. They may have circumscribed or infiltrative margins, spread locally be-

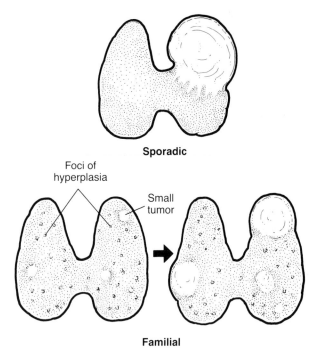

**Sporadic**

Foci of
hyperplasia

Small
tumor

**Familial**

Figure 20–10. Comparison between the solitary sporadic neoplasm (*above*) and the multicentric familial neoplasm (*below*) that probably arises in foci of C-cell hyperplasia.

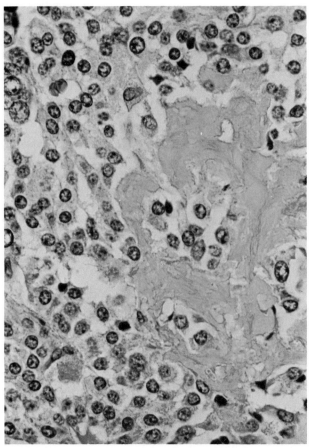

Figure 20–11. Medullary carcinoma with amyloid stroma. The high-power detail reveals the round to polygonal, neurosecretory-like tumor cells and an abundant intercellular amyloidic stroma. (Courtesy of Drs. M. Warhol and L. Weiss, Department of Pathology, Brigham and Women's Hospital, Harvard Medical School. Reprinted from Robbins, S. L., Cotran, R. S., and Kumar, V.: Pathologic Basis of Disease. 3rd ed. Philadelphia, W. B. Saunders Co., 1984, p. 1223.)

yond the thyroid, and contain foci of hemorrhage and necrosis. In the **familial settings the neoplasm tends to be multifocal**, with several nodules ranging up to many centimeters in diameter, sometimes involving both lobes of the gland; microscopically, focal hyperplasia of C cells is often present in the nontumorous gland. There is the suggestion then that this form of cancer arises from neoplastic transformation of foci of hyperplasia (Fig. 20–10). The two most common histologic patterns can be characterized as neurosecretory, small, round cells or sarcomatoid (spindled cells). **The cells are disposed in small nests separated by a fibrovascular stroma, which usually but not invariably has deposits of amyloid** (Fig. 20–11). The amyloid has the ultrastructure and staining reactions of all other forms of amyloid. Infrequently, there is follicular or trabecular disposition of cuboidal cells. Any of these histologic patterns may be observed in the sporadic or familial settings, and all have the same secretory capacity. Thus, ultrastructural studies reveal secretory granules that are bounded by distinct membrane and that can be shown with immunoperoxidase techniques to contain calcitonin and CEA. In time, the larger infiltrative neoplasms disseminate to regional nodes and then to distant sites.

Most sporadic tumors present as a painless thyroid mass. Familial lesions may be obviously multifocal

and bilateral. Strongly supporting the diagnosis is an elevated level of serum calcitonin. The serum CEA level is also frequently elevated, markedly, but this tumor product is a less specific marker than calcitonin. The overall survival of patients with sporadic disease is 40% at 10 years. Favorable indicators are young age, small tumor, and few mitoses.[49] The prognosis for familial medullary carcinoma is significantly better, with almost a 70% 10-year survival rate. In large part this improved outlook can be attributed to earlier diagnosis, owing to periodic screening of family members for elevated serum levels of calcitonin. Thus familial cancers are often diagnosed when small and confined to the thyroid and amenable to excision.

# Parathyroid Glands

All the disorders of these glands can be conveniently considered under the headings of hyper- and hypoparathyroidism.

## HYPERPARATHYROIDISM

*Hyperparathyroidism is classified as primary, when some parathyroid disorder underlies it, or secondary, when the hyperparathyroidism is the result of some disorder outside of the parathyroids,* most often chronic renal disease. In both forms there is a sustained elevation in the secretion of parathyroid hormone (parathormone or PTH). As will be apparent, *the primary form is characterized by hypercalcemia, but hypocalcemia is more typical of secondary hyperparathyroidism and serves as the stimulus to the parathyroid hyperplasia.* Some believe that prolonged secondary hyperfunction may in time lead to autonomous hyperparathyroidism.[50]

### PRIMARY HYPERPARATHYROIDISM

The "sine qua non" of primary hyperparathyroidism is hypercalcemia. Radioimmunoassays of circulating parathyroid hormone (parathormone) are less reliable, because parathormone circulates in the plasma as fragments of varying biologic activity and immunoreactivity and particular assays may not necessarily measure biologically active fragments. *Hypercalcemia has many origins other than primary hyperparathyroidism, including hypervitaminosis D; milk-alkali syndrome; granulomatous disease, principally sarcoidosis; use of thiazide drugs; long immobilization of the skeleton; and, sometimes, nonendocrine tumors.* The hypercalcemia associated with myeloma, bronchogenic and breast cancers, for example, is called "ectopic hyperparathyroidism" or, better, "pseudohyperparathyroidism." In these paraneoplastic syndromes, the basis for the hypercalcemia is uncertain (as is discussed on p. 216) but it is not necessarily related to elaboration of parathormone or its active fragments.[51]

Here we are concerned only with the hypercalcemia induced by primary parathyroid disease. *The parathyroid lesions underlying primary hyperfunction are adenomas (usually single, rarely double), primary hyperplasia, and carcinoma.* It has been traditional to attribute about 80% of all cases of primary hyperparathyroidism to a solitary adenoma. Recently, this view has been challenged by the contention that the great majority of putative "solitary adenomas" represent primary hyperplasia, which usually involves all glands but often asymmetrically so that only a single gland may be enlarged.[52] The issue is more than academic—removal may be expected to be curative if indeed the solitary gland

lesion is an adenoma, but if it is hyperplasia affecting largely a single gland, recurrence of the hyperparathyroidism is highly likely. Where pathologists disagree, mere mortals dare not tread, and so the relative frequency of the various lesions to be described is uncertain. However, it is clear that in about 5% of all cases, the parathyroid neoplasm or hyperplasia occurs in the setting of familial endocrine neoplasia (MEN) syndromes, usually types I and sometimes type II (p. 701) or other more rare familial syndromes.[53]

### Adenoma

These tumors appear at any age, more often in females than males. Almost always they occur singly, although rarely two may arise simultaneously in different glands, particularly in the familial syndromes.

About 75% occur in the lower glands. All are discrete, encapsulated, yellow-brown, soft nodules averaging 2 cm in diameter but ranging up to 5 cm (normal gland size is up to 1 cm), that replace most of a gland. Such residual gland as persists shows compression of the cells. Sometimes they are found in aberrant locations, such as within the thyroid, thymus, or adjacent neck tissues, much to the distress of the surgeon.[54] **They are generally monomorphic and most commonly composed of polygonal chief cells** having a pale acidophilic cytoplasm and central, somewhat variable nuclei. Others are made up predominantly of slightly larger cells having pale, somewhat cleared cytoplasm—"wasserhelle cells." Uncommonly, they are composed of cells having a granular, intensely eosinophilic cytoplasm—oxyphil cells. The wasserhelle and oxyphil cells are thought to be derived from chief cells, and so occasionally mixed cell patterns are observed. However, complete lobules made up of more than one cell type are rare in an adenoma but common in hyperplasia. Fat cells, which are normally present in the interstitium of the parathyroid gland, are notably absent from the adenoma, as is discrete lobulation. The cells in the adenoma are commonly arrayed in solid sheets but occasionally occur in cords or gland-like patterns. Usually they resemble those in the normal parathyroid, but sometimes there is considerable variation in cell size and morphology, raising the possibility of carcinoma (discussed below).

Virtually all adenomas are functional and produce primary hyperparathyroidism (to be described). It used to be thought that oxyphil adenomas in particular were nonfunctional, but recent studies dispel this concept.[55] Removal, which entails the sometimes formidable problem of finding the small offender, is curative.

### Primary Hyperplasia

Hyperplasia of the parathyroids, usually involving all glands albeit sometimes unequally, is character-

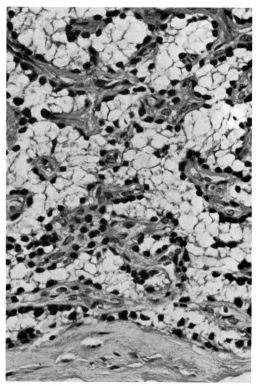

Figure 20–12. A detail of marked primary parathyroid hyperplasia showing the clear cell pattern. (From Robbins, S. L., Cotran, R. S., and Kumar, V.: Pathologic Basis of Disease. 3rd ed. Philadelphia, W. B. Saunders Co., 1984, p. 1229.)

istic of secondary hyperparathyroidism. *However, hyperplasia may appear in the absence of a recognized stimulus and therefore is called primary hyperplasia.* Little is known about the origins of this disorder, but elevation of the setpoint at which serum calcium suppresses parathyroid function has been proposed, which likens it to the persistent autonomous hyperfunction that sometimes follows secondary hyperparathyroidism.

In primary hyperplasia the glandular enlargement is often unequal and tends to be most marked in the superior glands; quite commonly, a single gland is significantly larger than the remainder. The problem of differentiating clinically such unequal enlargement from an adenoma has already been alluded to above. The hyperplastic gland sometimes exceeds in size the usual adenoma. Distinct lobulation is usually readily apparent. **In the great majority of cases, the lobules are composed of chief cells and the condition is referred to as "chief cell primary hyperplasia."** A less frequent variant is "clear cell primary hyperplasia" (Fig. 20–12). In both patterns there are usually discrete lobules of oxyphils. Regularity of cell morphology is the rule, but occasionally there is some pleomorphism. Strands of interlobular connective tissue containing fat persist as residuals of the normal parathyroid architecture. There is no discrete encapsulation, save for the expanded capsule of the normal gland. The features differentiating these changes from those of an adenoma (described above) should be evident.

## Carcinoma of the Parathyroids

Carcinoma of the parathyroids is an extremely rare cause of primary hyperparathyroidism, accounting for less than 1% of cases. Brevity is therefore indicated here. These malignant neoplasms grow and spread slowly and so rarely produce large masses. Like all malignancies, they eventually invade the surrounding tissues, metastasize first to regional nodes, and rarely spread to distant sites. *The differentiation of a small, localized carcinoma from an adenoma is difficult, and so three required criteria have been established: (1) evidence of local invasion; (2) metastasis to cervical lymph nodes or distant sites, such as lung, liver, and bone; and (3) well-defined cellular atypia, accompanied by capsular or vascular invasion.*[56] The last-mentioned criterion is a slender thread and so is discounted by many experts on the grounds that some cellular atypia is present in occasional adenomas and the interpretation of capsular and vascular invasion is difficult, so only metastasis is left. Some carcinomas are nonsecretory but, when functioning, induce clinical features of primary hyperparathyroidism with a few possible variations on the common theme (to be mentioned later).

## Clinical Features of Primary Hyperparathyroidism

The clinical presentation of hyperparathyroidism has undergone change over time. In almost half of the patients the condition is now being discovered at an early asymptomatic stage by the chance finding of hypercalcemia in a multiple-channel biochemical analysis of a patient's serum, performed for other reasons. As noted earlier, the hypercalcemia may have origins other than primary parathyroid disease. Signs and symptoms of hyperparathyroidism usually only become evident when the dysfunction has been present for years. *The two major systems affected are the kidneys and skeletal system.* Deposits of calcium in the tubules and peritubular tissue induce *nephrocalcinosis,* accompanied by decreased renal function and phosphate retention. *Renal stones,* composed of calcium salts, may develop, and these can cause hematuria, predisposition to urinary tract infection, and, when the stones pass into the ureter, induction of severe renal colic or urinary obstruction (p. 485). With protracted hyperparathyroidism, mobilization of calcium from the skeleton occurs. *The demineralization produces at first osteomalacia,* which, in time, becomes converted into the classic pattern of *osteitis fibrosa cystica.* Both of these skeletal osteopenic disorders are discussed elsewhere (p. 706), but full-blown osteitis fibrosa cystica is rarely seen today because of earlier diagnosis. Unexplained is the more frequent occurrence of renal and skeletal involvement with the hyperparathyroidism induced by carcinoma than that produced by benign parathyroid disease. The hypercalcemia may lead to *metastatic calcifications* in soft tissues, vessels, joints, and eyes (p. 26).

The deposits of calcium in the joints may induce a form of painful arthritis called "*chondrocalcinosis*." A so-called *band keratopathy*, when it appears, strongly suggests the diagnosis. It represents a white line on the lateral margin of the cornea that is caused by the deposition of calcium and phosphate.

In addition, hyperparathyroidism may be associated with signs and symptoms relating to the central nervous system, neuromuscular function, and the gastrointestinal tract. The CNS changes range from mild personality disturbances to psychoses. Muscle weakness, easy fatigability, and, occasionally, muscle atrophy may even mimic a primary neuromuscular disorder. Gastrointestinal manifestations may take the form of vague complaints of abdominal pain, but in about 25% of patients, peptic ulcers develop.[57]

The clinical impression is buttressed by the findings of hypercalcemia, hypercalciuria, and hypophosphatemia, but all of these values are equivocal at times. Elevated parathormone levels in the blood are often present but should be interpreted with caution because of the problems inherent in radioimmunoassay techniques mentioned at the outset. In sum, the diagnosis of hyperparathyroidism poses little difficulty when it has already reached the "stones and bones" stage, but it can be exceedingly challenging when the signs and symptoms are less well defined.

## SECONDARY HYPERPARATHYROIDISM

*Compensatory hyperfunction of the parathyroids occurs with several underlying disorders, all marked by hypocalcemia or peripheral resistance to parathormone.* The most common setting for secondary hyperparathyroidism is chronic renal insufficiency with its attendant hyperphosphatemia and hypocalcemia. Less common associations are osteomalacia (p. 706), calcium malabsorption, and deficient or deranged vitamin D metabolism. The low levels of serum calcium "turn on" parathyroid function, and hyperplasia results. The glandular enlargement may be symmetric or asymmetric, is usually not as striking as that in primary hyperplasia, and involves principally chief cells with scattered hyperplastic foci of oxyphils. The systemic consequences of the increased levels of parathormone are rarely as pronounced as in primary hyperplasia, so skeletal changes are uncommon, and, with the hypocalcemia, there is no predisposition to metastatic calcifications in the kidneys or elsewhere. Unlike primary hyperplasia, the secondary form is reversible if the underlying disorder can be corrected (e.g., renal transplant in those with chronic renal insufficiency). However, with long-standing secondary hyperplasia, complete reversion may not occur, raising the possibility of transformation into primary hyperplasia.

## HYPOPARATHYROIDISM

Hypoparathyroidism is basically a metabolic disorder characterized by hypocalcemia and consequent neuromuscular and mental changes. Anatomic consequences are exceedingly scant; they are intracranial calcifications, cataract formation, and disturbed dentition when the disorder affects the very young. The major causes of parathyroid insufficiency are unintentional removal of glands during thyroid surgery, radiation injury, developmental failure as in DiGeorge's syndrome (p. 174), and "idiopathic" hypoparathyroidism. The last mentioned, in some instances, is familial and accompanied by other endocrine deficiencies and autoimmune disorders. Often there is a concomitant predisposition to mucocutaneous candidiasis, strongly suggesting some defect in T-cell function. Thus, "idiopathic" hypoparathyroidism is attributed to deranged cell-mediated immunity and autoimmunity.[58]

# Adrenal Cortex

Disorders of the adrenal cortex will be considered under the headings of (1) adrenal cortical hyperfunction, (2) adrenal cortical hypofunction, and (3) neoplasms (since these may be functional or nonfunctional).

## ADRENAL CORTICAL HYPERFUNCTION (HYPERADRENALISM)

As you well know, the cortical steroids can be divided into glucocorticoids, mineralocorticoids, and adrenal androgens. Disorders related to hyperfunction of the cortex fall into three more or less distinctive syndromes based on which category of steroids is produced in excess. *Thus, overproduction of cortisol, the principal glucocorticoid, results in Cushing's syndrome; an excess of aldosterone, the principal mineralocorticoid, induces, not surprisingly, hyperaldosteronism; and excess adrenal androgens, usually arising in congenital adrenal hyperplasia, induce adrenal virilism.* Just as there are overlaps in the function of the three categories of steroids (e.g., glucocorticoids have weak effects on electrolyte metabolism), so are there sometimes overlaps in the three clinical syndromes they produce.

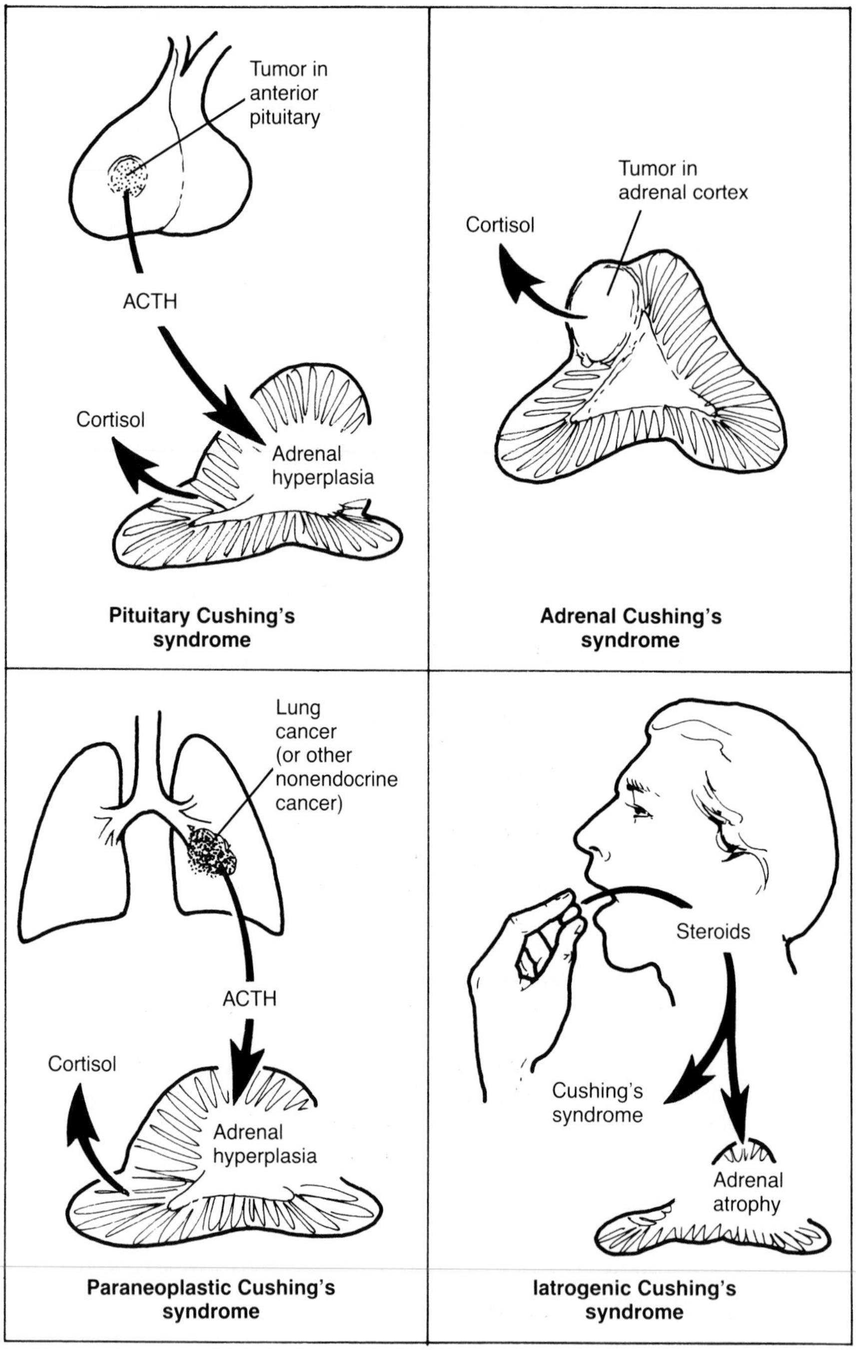

Figure 20–13. The four pathogenetic patterns of Cushing's syndrome.

## CUSHING'S SYNDROME

This clinical syndrome resulting from excess production of cortisol is characterized by a distinctive constellation of features—truncal obesity, plethoric "moon" facies, hypertension, abnormal glucose metabolism, muscle weakness, amenorrhea, hirsutism, acne, osteoporosis, and mental disturbances ranging from depression to euphoria to psychosis. These manifestations have four distinct pathogenetic origins (Fig. 20–13).

1. *About 60 to 70% of cases of Cushing's syndrome are related to excessive secretion of corticotropin and hence are most conveniently designated "pituitary Cushing's syndrome."* Because this pattern was first described by the neurosurgeon Harvey Cushing, it is sometimes called, confusingly, *"Cushing's disease"* to differentiate it from the other types of Cushing's syndrome. In many cases, there is a corticotropin-releasing pituitary adenoma, usually a microadenoma (p. 674). A small fraction have hypersecretion of ACTH by non-neoplastic corticotrophs, related to a

hypothalamic defect yielding excessive corticotropin-releasing factor.[59, 60] All are marked by an increased level of ACTH that in time produces bilateral adrenal hyperplasia (sometimes nodular hyperplasia), causing increased cortisol secretion.

2. *About 20% of cases have autonomous adrenal hyperfunction*, and these are most easily remembered as "adrenal Cushing's syndrome." In most, the adrenal cortical secretion emanates from a hyperfunctioning adenoma. Rarely, it is a carcinoma, and, even more rarely, it is nodular hyperplasia of obscure origin. The adrenal pattern of Cushing's syndrome is characterized by high serum levels of cortisol but low levels of ACTH, owing to cortisol suppression of the pituitary corticotrophs.

3. *About 10 to 15% of cases are called "paraneoplastic Cushing's syndrome" because they result from the ectopic production of ACTH, or some biologically active fragment, by a nonendocrine cancer.*[61] Bronchogenic carcinoma accounts for over half of these paraneoplastic syndromes; the remainder are related to thymomas, pancreatic islet cell tumors, and, more rarely, other neoplasms. As in the pituitary variant, the high levels of cortisol in the serum derive from elevated levels of ACTH, which in time induce bilateral adrenal hyperplasia.

4. *Iatrogenic Cushing's syndrome* is relatively common and arises from the long-term use of glucocorticoids (for example, as an immunosuppressant in transplant recipients). The exogenous steroids produce all of the clinical manifestations of Cushing's syndrome but at the same time result in bilateral adrenal cortical atrophy related to suppression of ACTH secretion.

**Morphology.** The fundamental anatomic changes are found in the pituitary and adrenal glands. In all variants of the syndrome, the increased serum levels of cortisol produce apparent feedback effects on the non-tumorous corticotrophs (and sometimes those within adenomas), referred to as **Crooke's hyaline degeneration of the basophils.** The usual cytoplasmic granularity imparted by the ACTH-containing granules is patchily or completely obscured by a basophilic hyalinization, which can be resolved as densely aggregated microfilaments. **In the pituitary variant a corticotroph (basophilic) adenoma, more usually a microadenoma** (p. 674), **is most often present,** but sometimes only hyperplasia of corticotrophs or even an anatomically unremarkable anterior lobe that is presumably hyperfunctioning is found.

The changes in the adrenals depend on the particular variant of Cushing's syndrome. **In the so-called pituitary and paraneoplastic patterns, the excess ACTH induces bilateral cortical hyperplasia, which is sometimes nodular** (Fig. 20–14). The adrenal enlargement may be subtle or may sometimes cause an increase many times greater than the normal weight of the adrenal. The hyperplasia is caused primarily by widening of the active non-lipid-laden cells of the zona reticularis so that they occupy the inner half of the cortex. These changes may be accompanied by some widening of the lipid-laden cells of the zona fasciculata. In some instances, particular foci of the cortex expand more rapidly than others, producing the nodular hyperplasia. **In "adrenal Cushing's syndrome" there is most often a discrete adenoma.** Uncommonly a large ominous-appearing carcinoma is found. Since these functioning neoplasms do not differ significantly from analogous nonfunctioning tumors, they will be described later (p. 696). With hyperfunctioning

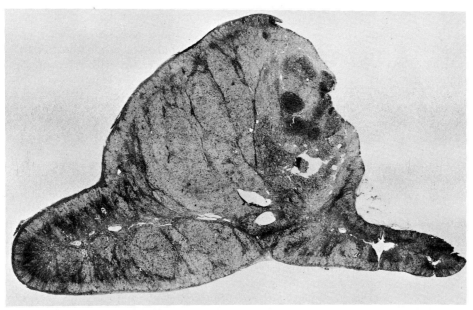

Figure 20–14. Irregular, nodular, adenomatous hyperplasia of an adrenal from a patient with Cushing's syndrome. (From Robbins, S. L., Cotran, R. S., and Kumar, V.: Pathologic Basis of Disease. 3rd ed. Philadelphia, W. B. Saunders, Co., 1984, p. 1239.)

neoplasms there is atrophy of the residual cortex about the tumor and atrophy of the contralateral uninvolved gland. Bilateral cortical atrophy appears in the "iatrogenic" form of Cushing's syndrome and, indeed, these individuals are vulnerable to acute adrenal hypofunctional crises if the exogenous administration of glucocorticoids is stopped too abruptly.

CLINICAL COURSE. Cushing's syndrome arises at all ages but mostly occurs in middle life. It is more frequent in women than in men. The clinical diagnosis of this condition usually poses no great problem because of the distinctive manifestations. It can be readily confirmed by the elevated cortisol levels in the plasma and urine. Much more difficult is the differential diagnosis of the various forms of Cushing's syndrome. Although the complete diagnostic algorithm is beyond our scope, several points are worthy of mention. Attempts to document a pituitary lesion by radiography or scanning techniques are of limited value because often the pituitary lesion, if present, is exceedingly small. A more reliable differentiation of Cushing's disease (i.e., "pituitary Cushing's syndrome") from the "ectopic" and "adrenal" syndromes is possible by the administration of a "high dose" of dexamethasone (a synthetic analog of cortisol) to the patient.[62] In those with the "pituitary" syndrome, ACTH release and adrenal steroid synthesis are partially suppressed, even though a pituitary adenoma is present. In contrast, in those with neoplastic ectopic ACTH production and with a primary adrenal disorder, the plasma cortisol levels are unaffected, but these two categories can be segregated by the serum levels of ACTH.

## HYPERALDOSTERONISM

As you recall, aldosterone promotes potassium excretion and sodium retention and so expands blood and extracellular fluid volumes. Thus *increased production of aldosterone is marked by hypokalemia, hypernatremia, and hypertension.* When the aldosterone excess appears without an apparent physiologic need it is called *"primary hyperaldosteronism."* In contrast, in *secondary hyperaldosteronism* it occurs as an appropriate compensatory reaction in disorders marked by edema and hypovolemia or decreased renal perfusion and blood flow (e.g., malignant hypertension with malignant nephrosclerosis, p. 482). Further comments about the *secondary pattern* are not required except to point out that the hyperaldosteronism is the consequence of increased elaboration of renin, which can be confirmed by an *elevated level of plasma renin activity.* In contrast to the case in *primary hyperaldosteronism*, the *plasma renin activity is depressed* because the sodium retention expands the blood volume, serving to downregulate renin release. Thus *primary hyperaldosteronism is marked by hypokalemia, hypernatremia, hypertension, and low plasma renin activity.*[63] The

low levels of potassium may induce muscular weakness, paralyses, and disturbances in cardiac function. Usually appearing in mid-adult life, this rare condition is twice as common in women as in men.

In about 90% of the cases of primary hyperaldosteronism, the excess steroid production derives from an adrenal adenoma. The remaining cases are attributable to primary bilateral adrenal hyperplasia (idiopathic hyperaldosteronism)[64] or, rarely, an adrenal carcinoma. In those cases with an adenoma, the condition is referred to sometimes as Conn's syndrome. The adenoma is located more often on the left, is usually less than 2 cm in diameter, is well encapsulated, and is composed of cells resembling those of the zona glomerulosa or zona fasciculata or sometimes hybrid forms. In idiopathic hyperaldosteronism, with its bilateral, diffuse, sometimes nodular hyperplasia, the adrenals are often enlarged several times normal by diffuse or focal hyperplasia of zona glomerulosa cells, which are sometimes admixed with fascicular cells. As is evident from the designation of the hyperplasia, its basis is uncertain, but recent studies have isolated a putative aldosterone-stimulating factor of pituitary origin.[65]

## ADRENAL VIRILISM—CONGENITAL ADRENAL HYPERPLASIA

Virilism may appear with any ovarian or adrenal cortical disorder responsible for excessive production of androgens. Excess adrenal androgens may be produced by hyperfunctioning adenomas, carcinomas, or cortical hyperplasia. The first two are encountered mainly in young adults. The hyperplasia usually develops in infancy but sometimes does not produce manifestations for many years. It is the consequence of a congenital deficiency of a particular enzyme involved in steroidogenesis that blocks cortisol synthesis. The unopposed ACTH then induces what is called "congenital adrenal hyperplasia." In some instances the enzyme block channels steroidogenesis into overproduction of only androgens, with resultant pure virilism; in other enzyme deficiencies not only are androgens elaborated in excess but there is also inadequate synthesis of aldosterone, yielding a "salt-wasting virilism."[66] Each of the various enzyme deficiencies and biosynthetic defects runs "true" within a family. All the defects have autosomal recessive patterns of inheritance.

About 95% of cases of congenital adrenal hyperplasia relate to a deficiency of the C21-hydroxylase that can be mild or severe. The gene encoding this enzyme has been localized to the short arm of chromosome 6, closely linked to the HLA-B locus. *A mild deficiency of C21 may induce "classic pure virilism,"* which usually becomes manifest by pure virilism of female infants and children. Recently it has been discovered that this same enzyme defect may produce "nonclassical virilism" inasmuch as it may not become

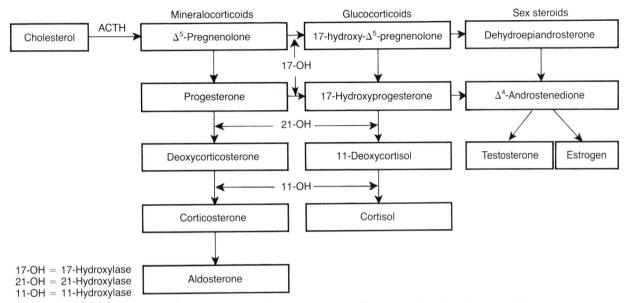

**Figure 20–15.** Diagrammatic representation of adrenal steroidogenesis. The sites of action of the crucial 17-, 21-, and 11-hydroxylases are indicated. A 21-hydroxylase deficiency, when mild, impairs synthesis of cortisol and possibly aldosterone but, when severe, totally interrupts the synthesis of both steroids.

evident until young adult life as infertility, premature sexual development, short stature, excessive facial hair in women, and acne.[67] In both variants males are unaffected at birth but have sexual precocity at an early age.

Another distinctive genetic defect is a severe 21-hydroxylase deficiency in which both cortisol and aldosterone production are decreased (Fig. 20–15). The result is the salt-losing form of adrenal virilism.[68] Other clinical patterns are rare and associated with other enzyme defects. In all, the adrenals are bilaterally hyperplastic and indistinguishable from those sometimes producing the other patterns of hyperadrenalism, already described. Analogously, the neoplasms producing virilism are morphologically indistinguishable from those involved in other hypersecretory states or, indeed, from nonfunctional neoplasms. It should be noted, however, that most virilizing tumors are carcinomas. Virilizing adenomas are rare.

# HYPOFUNCTION OF THE ADRENAL CORTEX

Insufficient output of adrenal steroids may arise because of extensive cortical destruction of both glands or because of ACTH insufficiency secondary to some hypophyseothalamic derangement such as a nonsecretory adenoma of the pituitary (p. 675). The disorders involving the adrenals produce so-called *primary adrenal cortical insufficiency, better known as Addison's disease,* whereas those relating to ACTH deficiency are sometimes referred to as *secondary adrenal cortical insufficiency.*

## ADDISON'S DISEASE

Clinically, overt, chronic adrenal insufficiency (i.e., Addison's disease) is uncommon, although it is likely that many undiagnosed borderline cases exist. Because of the large functional reserve of the adrenal cortex, about 90% of the parenchyma of both glands must be destroyed in order to produce symptoms of insufficiency. Most cases are seen in individuals between the ages of 20 and 50 years. Whereas in 1930 tuberculous destruction was the cause of 70% of Addison's disease, this lesion is now thought to cause less than 25% of cases. *Currently, most cases of Addison's disease are called idiopathic, but the condition may be autoimmune in origin.* Together tuberculosis and idiopathic atrophy account for over 80% of cases. Less frequent causes include the deep fungi, amyloidosis, and replacement of the adrenals by metastases. Atrophy of the adrenals secondary to the long-term administration of exogenous glucocorticoids, which suppress ACTH production, is an uncommon cause; the adrenal insufficiency only becomes evident when the exogenous steroids are suddenly stopped (rather than tapered).

Evidence for the autoimmune nature of *idiopathic Addison's disease* includes the following observations: (1) This disease is histologically similar to "autoimmune" Hashimoto's thyroiditis, characterized by parenchymal atrophy with a lymphocytic infiltrate. (2) From 50 to 67% of these patients have circulating autoantibodies to adrenal tissue. (3) Other autoantibodies, especially against the thyroid gland and the gastric mucosa, are often present in these patients. Indeed, concurrent Addison's disease and Hashimoto's thyroiditis (*Schmidt's syndrome*) develop with more than chance frequency. (4) Lesions similar to those of idiopathic Addison's disease can be produced experimentally by injecting autologous adrenal tissue and Freund's adjuvant.

**MORPHOLOGY.** Idiopathic Addison's disease reveals small, irregularly contracted adrenal glands, with a combined weight as low as 2.5 gm. On sectioning, it can be seen that the cortex has collapsed around an otherwise normal medulla. The histologic changes are atrophy and destruction of the adrenal cells, with replacement by fibrous scarring. The few remaining viable cortical cells may be enlarged with an eosinophilic, lipid-poor cytoplasm (compact cells). A variable lymphocytic infiltrate is present.

Tuberculous adrenal glands, on the other hand, are enlarged, firm, and nodular, with a thickened capsule. Histologically, they are characteristic of tuberculosis in any site, with confluent areas of caseation necrosis and tubercle formation. Focal calcification of the tuberculous lesions may provide useful radiologic clues to the etiology of the adrenal insufficiency.[69] Addison's disease caused by amyloidosis, usually seen with systemic so-called secondary amyloidosis, is also associated with enlargement of the adrenal glands, sometimes with a combined weight up to 40 gm. Grossly, these glands are firm and pale gray. On microscopic examination, most of the cortex is replaced by amyloid deposits. Metastatic involvement of the adrenals is common in all forms of disseminated cancer, particularly bronchogenic carcinomas. Surprisingly, even though the glands may appear to be almost totally obliterated by the cancerous implants, functional insufficiency is uncommon because sufficient islands of cortex usually persist between the implants to maintain adequate steroid output. Admittedly, the manifestations of adrenal insufficiency may be masked in some instances by the cachectic wasting of the patient.

**CLINICAL COURSE.** Addison's disease from any cause presents an insidious, rather ill-defined clinical picture. The first indications are often a vague weakness and fatigability *As the negative feedback on the hypothalamic-pituitary axis is abolished, ACTH (and perhaps MSH) levels rise, with a consequent increase in pigmentation of the skin, particularly of the mucous membranes, areolae, and any surgical scars.* The presence of pigmentation is helpful in differentiating primary adrenocortical hypofunction from the secondary pattern, which results from pituitary lesions. The latter is associated with low ACTH levels. Most patients develop gastrointestinal disturbances, including anorexia with weight loss, nausea, vomiting, and diarrhea. Blood sugar is low, and hypoglycemic symptoms may occasionally occur. Although some degree of hypotension is characteristic, actual syncope is uncommon. The heart becomes smaller, possibly because of its lightened work load as a result of chronic hypovolemia and hypotension.

When Addison's disease is full-blown, the diagnosis is generally apparent from the distinctive signs and symptoms. But the clinical manifestations may be extremely subtle in earlier phases when the diagnosis is most important because the adrenal dysfunction is correctable with exogenous steroids even though the underlying disease persists or progresses. Confirming the diagnosis are the lack of a normal steroid response to administered ACTH and hyponatremia with hyperkalemia owing to aldosterone deficiency.

Although patients with Addison's disease may continue indefinitely in their subactive precarious existence, any stress such as surgery, infection, or injury may precipitate an acute crisis, characterized by the sudden appearance, about 12 hours later, of profound weakness, hyperpyrexia progressing to hypothermia, coma, and vascular collapse. Without prompt steroid therapy, death may ensue.

## ACUTE ADRENOCORTICAL INSUFFICIENCY

Acute adrenocortical steroid insufficiency may be caused by (1) sudden withdrawal of long-term steroid therapy, (2) stress in patients with Addison's disease (see previous discussion), and (3) massive hemorrhagic destruction of the glands. Hemorrhage into the adrenals is seen in the newborn incident to the trauma of childbirth, in adrenal vein thrombosis, and, most importantly, with overwhelming septicemia, most often a meningococcemia (*Waterhouse-Friderichsen syndrome*) (Fig. 20–16). In the last instance, it is the overwhelming sepsis rather than acute steroid insufficiency that threatens life. It should be noted that small medullary hemorrhages may also occur in any of the bleeding diatheses but they must be massive to produce acute steroid insufficiency. Thus even with the Waterhouse-Friderichsen syndrome, in which the hemorrhage appears to have converted the adrenals into bags of blood, sufficient islands of cortical cells often survive to maintain adequate adrenal function.

## CORTICAL NEOPLASMS

As has been pointed out in previous discussions, a functional cortical adenoma, or carcinoma, or hyperplasia, may be the source of one or more excess steroids in all hyperadrenal syndromes. However, all adenomas and carcinomas do not elaborate steroids and, regrettably, it is not possible from morphologic examination alone to determine whether a tumor is functional, or which steroids it is elaborating. Biochemical analysis of the lesion, its venous efflux, or the plasma drawn from the patient are necessary to identify any or all specific products. Thus on morphologic grounds "a tumor is a tumor is a tumor," and so adenomas and carcinomas have not been well characterized to this point.

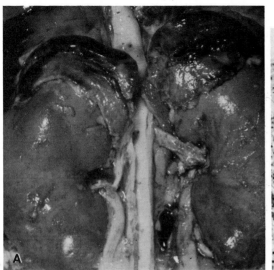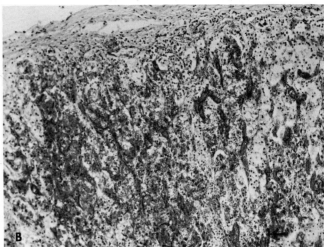

Figure 20–16. *A*, The kidneys and adrenals in situ in a child with the Waterhouse-Friderichsen syndrome. The dark adrenals are markedly hemorrhagic. *B*, Low-power section. The cortical cells between the extravasated blood have undergone ischemic necrosis.

**Adenomas** are common at autopsy and only rarely are associated with one of the hyperadrenal states. Nonetheless, they are the commonest cause of primary hyperaldosteronism and on rare occasion underlie Cushing's syndrome. They are discrete, encapsulated, yellow-brown nodules within the cortex that often project into the medullary cavity or subcapsularly and sometimes appear to be extracapsular. They range up to 5 cm in diameter (average 1 to 2 cm). The smaller lesions are usually composed of lipid-laden cells resembling those of the fasciculata, having cleared cytoplasm and regular small nuclei (Fig. 20–17). Occasionally, the cells have less lipid, a granular cytoplasm, and resemble those of the zona reticularis. Larger tumors may have areas of hemorrhage, cystic necrosis, and more variation in cell and nuclear size, with nuclear hyperchromasia and scattered mitoses. The line between such an "atypical" adenoma, particularly when poorly encapsulated, and a carcinoma is vague, but as a rule of thumb—**tumors less than 3 cm in diameter are benign unless they have marked cellular atypia and numerous mitoses** or are unmistakably aggressive (invasive or disseminated). Equally difficult is the differentiation of a focus of nodular hyperplasia from an adenoma, particularly when there are multiple small adenomas. Here the rule of thumb is—when well encapsulated or unilateral, the lesions are adenomas. As you well know, there are exceptions to all rules.[70]

**Cortical carcinomas**, in contrast to adenomas, are usually functional and therefore found in association with one of the hyperadrenal syndromes previously described. Whether functional or not, they are exceedingly uncommon and usually constitute bulky, obviously invasive masses that have obliterated the involved gland and have extended into the periadrenal fat and sometimes the adjacent kidney. The rare smaller lesion may appear deceptively encapsulated and be difficult to differentiate from an adenoma. On transection cortical carcinomas

present a variegated surface with areas of yellow, viable tumor surrounded by hemorrhage, necroses, and cystic foci. Histologically, they range from well-differentiated carcinomas having mild degrees of atypia, not dissimilar

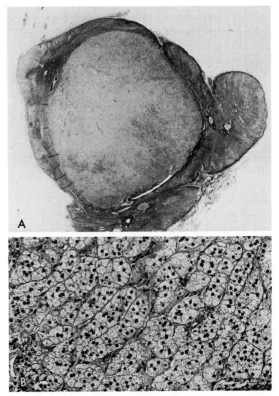

Figure 20–17. *A*, A slightly enlarged whole-organ mount of a section of an adrenal bearing an adenoma. The tumor has expanded into the medulla and is enclosed within a rim of adrenal cortex. The arrangement of the lipid-laden cortical cells in nests is seen in *B*.

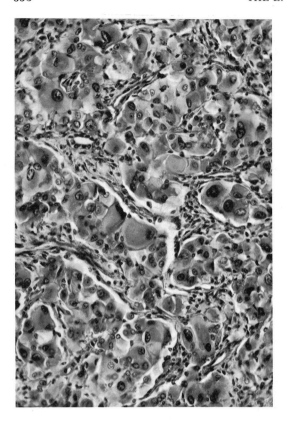

Figure 20–18. Adrenal carcinoma. There is marked anaplasia and pleomorphism of the neoplastic cells. (From Robbins, S. L., Cotran, R. S., and Kumar, V.: Pathologic Basis of Disease. 3rd ed. Philadelphia, W. B. Saunders Co., 1984, p. 1243.)

from that seen in some larger adenomas, to wildly anaplastic neoplasms composed of bizarre giant cells with extremely hyperchromatic pleomorphic nuclei that often bear mitoses (Fig. 20–18). Invasion of the veins, sometimes with extension into the vena cava, and permeation of lymphatics leads to widespread metastases to the lungs, bones, liver, and periaortic lymph nodes, accounting for a 10 to 25% five-year survival rate.[71]

# Adrenal Medulla

Disease primary in the medulla is a clinical rarity; the major rarities are pheochromocytomas and neuroblastomas.

## PHEOCHROMOCYTOMA

These uncommon neoplasms belonging to the family of APUDomas (p. 537) are of great clinical interest because they produce the catecholamines norepinephrine and epinephrine. Thus *they usually induce hypertension, most often sustained, but sometimes distinctively paroxysmal; removal of the offending tumor provides the gratifying opportunity to cure a form of hypertension.* However, they are found in only 0.1% of the hypertensive population. Derived from chromaffin cells, about 90% of these tumors are primary in the adrenal medullae, but the remainder arise from chromaffin cells in the paraaortic sympathetic ganglia (chiefly in the abdomen) and the organ of Zuckerkandl. The extraadrenal neoplasms are sometimes called *paragangliomas.* In all locations, they tend to occur in young to mid-adult life and slightly more often in females.

Although these lesions are most often sporadic, about 15 to 20% of pheochromocytomas are associated with a constellation of well-defined familial syndromes. The most frequent familial syndromes are MEN II (*Sipple's syndrome*) and MEN III (p. 701). Other associations are with neurofibromatosis, von Hippel-Lindau disease, and the poorly defined syndrome of familial pheochromocytoma unassociated with other endocrine lesions.

The pheochromocytoma is known as the "10% tumor"; in 10% of patients they occur bilaterally, 10% occur in extraadrenal locations, and 10% are malignant. **The sporadic tumors tend to occur singly and in the adrenals. In contrast, in the familial syndromes there is a greater frequency of extraadrenal and multiple tumors.** Moreover, in the MEN syndromes the pheochromocytoma is often accompanied by focal medullary hyperplasia bilaterally or, indeed, there may only be medullary hyperplasia. Thus there is a suggestion that in these genetic settings, hyperplasia antedates and in some instances leads to the neoplasm. These tumors vary markedly in size, ranging from a few grams to several kilos in weight, but they average about 200 gm. In general, the familial tumors tend to be smaller because periodic screening of affected family members for catechols or their metabolites leads to earlier discovery of any neoplasm(s). All tend to be well-demarcated, basically spherical masses bounded by the expanded adrenal capsule, the compressed stroma of the gland, or both. The cut surface is irregularly gray to brown to hemorrhagic. Areas of hemorrhage, necrosis, and cystic degeneration are common in the larger masses. When a sample of the tissue is placed in a dichromate fixative, it turns brownblack, owing to oxidation of the catecholamines stored within the granules of the chromaffin cells.

The histologic appearance is as variable as the size of these neoplasms. Most often and most distinctively, they are composed of small to large polygonal cells having abundant basophilic to eosinophilic granular cytoplasm and pleomorphic nuclei (Fig. 20–19). In tumors proved to be biologically benign, the nuclear size and shape are extremely variable, sometimes with bizarre lobulation, which creates the appearance of multiple nuclei. In other neoplasms the cells may be small and round or spindle-shaped with scant cytoplasm. Whatever the cytologic features, the cells are disposed usually in small nests or irregular trabeculae demarcated by a delicate fibrous stroma. Sometimes the cells form solid sheets.[72] Electron microscopy reveals the oval to round membrane-bounded cytoplasmic granules of stored catecholamines. Capsular and vascular invasion are not uncommon in clinically proven benign tumors. **Thus, the only reliable criteria of malignancy are metastases and extensive local invasion well beyond the confines of the capsule.**

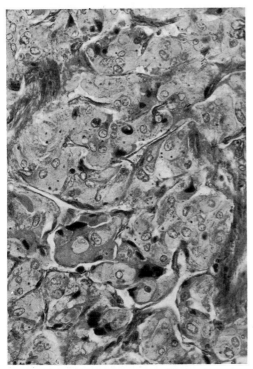

Figure 20–19. Pheochromocytoma. High-power cellular detail shows irregular nuclei and abundant granular cytoplasm. The chromatin pigment is not visible in the photograph.

Paroxysms of hypertension, accompanied by rapid pulse, profuse sweating, headache, and anxiety related to waves of catecholamine release are typical of this neoplasm. Unfortunately, more often there is sustained hypertension, but pressure over the neoplasm or vigorous palpation may be capable of precipitating an attack.[73] Other features may be present, including carbohydrate intolerance, the manifestations relating to polyendocrinopathies in the MEN syndromes, and cardiac irregularities ranging from arrhythmias to angina to myocardial infarction. The diagnosis of pheochromocytoma can be confirmed by the demonstration of elevated levels of catecholamines in the blood and their metabolites in the urine.

## NEUROBLASTOMA

This highly malignant tumor is a common cause of cancer death in children under 15 years of age. Most neuroblastomas arise in the adrenal medulla, but a significant number are found in the cervical, thoracic, and lower abdominal sympathetic chains. Retinoblastoma, a closely related tumor, arises in the retina. Like pheochromocytomas, most neuroblastomas elaborate catecholamines.[74] These cancers usually appear within the first five years of life; they appear infrequently up to age 15 but rarely in adults. In some instances there is well-defined familial clustering conforming to autosomal dominant transmission. Several additional observations underscore the role of one or more mutations, whether inherited or acquired, in the genesis of these tumors. Frequently, a deletion or rearrangement of the short arm of chromosome 1 can be identified in the genome of the tumor cells, and molecular probes of the genome have recently identified a DNA sequence called N-myc because of its homology to the well-known retroviral oncogene V-myc.[75]

These tumors commonly weigh between 80 and 150 gm and are lobular and soft, with a grayish cut surface. Often, areas of necrosis, hemorrhage, and calcification are present. Histologically, the tumor cells are small, dark, and either round or slightly elongated. They tend to grow in haphazard masses. The nuclei are hyperchromatic and regular, and the scant cytoplasm has granules of stored catecholamines. Careful searching near the periphery of the tumor usually reveals the cells arranged in characteristic rosettes, with young nerve fibrils growing into the center of each rosette. Varying degrees of differentiation are found in most neuroblastomas. The most differentiated form, called **ganglioneuroma**, contains ganglion cells scattered in a fibrous stromal background. Intermediate forms are referred to as **ganglioneuroblastomas**.

These are rapidly growing cancers, and when discovered in infants under one year of age are almost always localized masses. More often, in patients older than one year, these cancers are already disseminated when discovered. Over half of all patients have widespread metastases, particularly to bones or liver, or both. The combination of multiple bone metastases and elevated blood levels of catecholamines or urinary levels of their metabolites is virtually diagnostic. When the tumor is localized in infancy, the five-year survival rate following resection is approximately 75 to 80%. With disseminated tumor, it drops to 5 to 20%.[76] Rarely, and almost entirely in infants, a neuroblastoma undergoes spontaneous maturation to a ganglioneuroma that has a benign course. Immune mechanisms may be responsible for such differentiation.

# Thymus

Thymic hyperplasia and thymomas, the two most frequent (albeit uncommon) disorders of the thymus, are of particular interest because of their association with a variety of systemic disorders. Thymic lymphomas were discussed on page 369.

## HYPERPLASIA

The weight of the thymus is of little use in establishing the diagnosis of hyperplasia. There is wide variation in the weight of the normal thymus among individuals, and the progressive atrophy occurring during life pursues a variable course. Thus *hyperplasia of the thymus is best characterized by the appearance of lymphoid follicles within the medulla.* You may recall that the normal thymus is devoid of lymphoid follicles. Immunostaining techniques reveal that the follicles are rich in immunoglobulins, and, indeed, thymic hyperplasia is frequently present in patients with myasthenia gravis, considered to be an autoimmune disorder.[77] The relationship between the thymus and myasthenia gravis is discussed in detail on page 719, and so for now it suffices to state that B cells generated in the thymus and sensitized to its myoid cells are thought to underlie the autoimmune reaction to acetylcholine receptors at the neuromuscular junction, a characteristic of this grave neuromuscular disorder. Significantly, removal of a hyperplastic thymus is of benefit early in the disease.

## THYMOMA

Although the normal thymus is a lymphoepithelial organ, *the term "thymoma" is restricted to tumors in which epithelial cells constitute the neoplastic element.* Scant or abundant thymic lymphocytes may also be present in these tumors, but they are essentially normal thymocytes and not neoplastic. Lymphomas arising in the lymphoid elements of the thymus gland are therefore not classified as thymomas. Numerous subtypes of thymoma have been established, based on cytologic and biologic criteria.[78] For our purposes it suffices that they be divided into *benign and malignant thymomas*, omitting the other more rare, more aggressive malignancies called thymic carcinomas.

Both benign and malignant thymomas are gray-tan, lobulated neoplasms having great histologic diversity. As noted, all have neoplastic epithelial cells and a variable lymphocytic infiltrate. In most neoplasms, the epithelial cells resemble their normal counterparts by having poorly defined cytoplasmic outlines and large, pale nuclei. Less commonly, the epithelial cells are oval- to spindle-shaped and sometimes appear squamoid. Hassall's corpuscles are most frequently found in the squamoid neoplasms. Whatever their shape, the cells are disposed in sheets but sometimes arranged in isolated nests separated by sparse or abundant lymphocytes. **Based on the intensity of the lymphoid infiltrate, the tumors are sometimes further subdivided into (a) epithelial predominance; (b) lymphoid predominance; and (c) mixed lymphoepithelial composition.** Benign thymomas range up to 10 to 15 cm in diameter and are enclosed within a well-defined capsule. Their malignant counterparts extend beyond the capsule and are usually larger. They range up to 20 cm in diameter and sometimes metastasize. To be noted, **the diagnosis of malignant thymoma is not based on cytologic atypia but rather on the basis of capsular invasion or metastasis.**

All thymomas are rarities, the malignant more so than the benign. They may arise at any age but typically occur in mid-adult life. Frequently, they are silent and only discovered at autopsy or accidentally on chest radiographs, but sometimes they compress adjacent structures and produce cough, dyspnea, dysphagia, and vena caval compression. Most interestingly, they may be associated with a variety of systemic disorders, including myasthenia gravis, red-cell hypoplasia, hypogammaglobulinemia, systemic lupus erythematosus, and nonthymic cancers.[79] The most common association is with myasthenia gravis; about 10 to 15% of these patients, usually over 30, have a thymoma. Removal of the thymoma sometimes leads to improvement in the neuromuscular disorder, but this benefit is still in dispute. There is the suggestion, then, that the thymic neoplasm in some way contributes to the production of the autoantibody found in this condition (p. 719). Survival with a localized thymic neoplasm following resection is about 80% at 10 years, but the associated disease, when present, may exact its toll. Ten-year survival rates fall to about 20% with malignant thymomas.

# Multiple Endocrine Neoplasia (MEN) Syndromes

There are three genetically distinct MEN syndromes. Each is characterized by autosomal dominant transmission and by neoplastic or hyperplastic involvement of at least two (sometimes three or more) endocrine glands. Other associated nonendocrine lesions may also present.[80]

*The MEN I (Wermer) syndrome is chiefly characterized by hyperplasia, adenomas, or carcinomas of the pituitary, parathyroids, and pancreatic islets.* Less consistently there are similar changes in the adrenal cortices and thyroid, and there may be carcinoids in the lungs or foregut. All of these lesions are more or less functional, and those of the islets elaborate, among other products, gastrin. *Hypergastrinemia and consequent peptic ulceration (known as the Zollinger-Ellison syndrome, p. 609) are present in about 90% of patients with MEN I.* As might be anticipated, the clinical presentation is largely dependent on which lesion "acts out" the most, but in the great majority of patients hypercalcemia, peptic ulcer, hypoglycemia, and symptoms referable to a pituitary mass or hyperfunction constitute the major features.

*The MEN II or IIa (Sipple) syndrome is more easily remembered as the medullary thyroid carcinoma–pheochromocytoma syndrome. Sometimes there is also parathyroid hyperplasia,* but it is not clear whether it is a separate feature of the genetic syndrome or the consequence of the calcium-lowering effect of the calcitonin elaborated by the medullary thyroid carcinoma. As noted earlier, the pheochromocytomas are frequently bilateral and have a greater tendency to be extraadrenal. As you would expect, these patients present usually with hypertension or with a thyroid mass, but ectopic production of other products such as ACTH, gastrin, or prolactin by the thyroid tumor may induce confusing clinical complexes.

*MEN IIb or III is very similar to MEN II but has distinct differences. These patients typically have puffy lips and multiple mucocutaneous neuromas in the eyes, lips, mouth, skin, and other sites.* Other embryogenetic defects may also be present. Despite the overlaps between MEN II and III, the latter is not associated with parathyroid hyperplasia; it runs a more progressive course, terminating in death at a much earlier age from the ravages of the thyroid carcinoma; and, moreover, each pattern "breeds true" (i.e., no concurrence with a single family). An overview of the several MEN syndromes is provided in Table 20–4.

There is no satisfactory understanding of the origins of the multiple organ involvements in the MEN syndromes.[81] One theory proposes a central role for the pancreatic islets and their production of multiple bioactive products, which secondarily induce changes in other glands. However, this explanation could not account for MEN II and III. Accordingly, it is speculated that all of the syndromes arise because of some basic defect in control mechanisms in the cells of neural crest origin—the cells of the APUD system. But, clearly, the cells of the parathyroid cannot be construed as APUD cells. Better we admit ignorance.

## References

1. McCarthy, K. S., Jr., and Dobson, C. E., II: Pituitary pathology associated with abnormalities of prolactin secretion. Clin. Obstet. Gynecol. 23:367, 1980.
2. Asa, S. L., and Kovacs, K.: Histological classification of pituitary disease. Clin. Endocrinol. Metab. 12:567, 1983.
3. Saeger, W., and Ludecke, D. K.: Pituitary adenomas with hyperfunction of TSH. Virchows Archiv. (Pathol. Anat.) 394:255, 1982.
4. Burrow, G. N., et al.: Microadenomas of the pituitary and abnormal sellar tomograms in an unselected autopsy series. N. Engl. J. Med. 304:156, 1981.
5. Grossman, A., and Besser, G. M.: Prolactinomas. Br. Med. J. 290:182, 1985.
6. Robert, F., et al.: Pituitary adenomas in Cushing's disease: A histologic, ultrastructural, and immunocytochemical study. Arch. Pathol. Lab. Med. 102:448, 1978.
7. Scheithauer, B. W.: Surgical pathology of the pituitary: The adenomas. Pathol. Annu. 19(Part 2):269, 1984.
8. Howanitz, J. H., and Howanitz, P. J.: Pituitary tumors. Clin. Lab. Med. 4:643, 1984.
9. Editorial: Prolactinomas: Bromocriptine rules OK? Lancet 1:430, 1982.
10. Jialal, I., et al.: Hypopituitarism. A 3-year study. S. Afr. Med. J. 59:590, 1981.
11. Challa, V. R., et al.: Pathobiologic study of pituitary tumors: Report of 62 cases with a review of the recent literature. Hum. Pathol. 16:873, 1985.
12. Spaziante, R., et al.: The empty sella. Surg. Neurol. 16:418, 1981.
13. Skelton, C. L.: The heart and hyperthyroidism. N. Engl. J. Med. 307:1206, 1982.
14. Doniach, D.: Hashimoto's thyroiditis and primary myxoedema viewed as separate entities. Eur. J. Clin. Invest. 11:245, 1981.
15. van der Gaag, R. D., et al.: Role of maternal immunoglobulins

**Table 20–4.** MULTIPLE ENDOCRINE NEOPLASIA (MEN) SYNDROMES

| Lesions | MEN I | MEN II or MEN IIa | MEN IIb or III |
|---|---|---|---|
| Pituitary | + + + + | 0 | 0 |
| Medullary carcinoma of thyroid | + + | + + + + | + + + |
| Parathyroid | + + + + | + + | 0 |
| Adrenal cortex | + + | + | + |
| Pheochromocytoma | 0 | + + + + | + + + |
| Pancreatic islets | + + + + | 0 | 0 |
| Peptic ulcer | + + + + | 0 | 0 |
| Mucocutaneous neuromas | 0 | 0 | + + + + |
| Gastrointestinal carcinoids | + | 0 | 0 |

blocking TSH-induced thyroid growth in sporadic forms of congenital hypothyroidism. Lancet *1*:246, 1985.

16. Levine, S. N.: Current concepts of thyroiditis. Arch. Intern. Med. *143*:1952, 1983.

17. Selenkow, H. A., et al.: Autoimmune thyroid disease: An integrated concept of Graves' and Hashimoto's disease. Compr. Ther. *10*:48, 1984.

18. Bogner, U., et al.: Antibody-dependent cell mediated cytotoxicity against human thyroid cells in Hashimoto's thyroiditis but not Graves' disease. J. Clin. Endocrinol. Metab. *159*:734, 1984.

19. Strakosh, C. R., et al.: Immunology of autoimmune thyroid diseases. N. Engl. J. Med. *307*:1499, 1982.

20. Volpe, R.: The pathology of thyroiditis. Hum. Pathol. *9*:429, 1978.

21. Klein, I., and Levy, G. S.: Silent thyrotoxic thyroiditis. Ann. Intern. Med. *96*:242, 1982.

22. Amino, N., et al.: High prevalence of transient post-partum thyrotoxicosis and hypothyroidism. N. Engl. J. Med. *306*:849, 1982.

23. Inada, M., et al.: Reversible changes of the histological abnormalities of the thyroid in patients with painless thyroiditis. J. Clin. Endocrinol. Metab. *52*:431, 1981.

24. Baker, B. A., et al.: Correlation of thyroid antibodies and cytologic features in suspected autoimmune thyroid disease. Am. J. Med. *74*:941, 1983.

25. Kendall-Taylor, P., et al.: Evidence that thyroid-stimulating antibody is produced in the thyroid gland. Lancet *1*:645, 1984.

26. Okita, N., et al.: Suppressor T-lymphocyte deficiency in Graves' disease and Hashimoto's thyroiditis. J. Clin. Endocrinol. Metab. *52*:528, 1981.

27. Atkinson, S., et al.: Ophthalmopathic immunoglobulin in patients with Graves' ophthalmopathy. Lancet *2*:374, 1984.

28. Gorman, C.: Ophthalmopathy of Graves' disease (editorial). N. Engl. J. Med. *308*:453, 1983.

29. Studer, H., and Ramelli, F.: Simple goiter and its variants: Euthyroid and hyperthyroid multinodular goiters. Endocr. Rev. *3*:40, 1982.

30. Ramelli, F., et al.: Pathogenesis of thyroid nodules in multinodular goiter. Am. J. Pathol. *109*:215, 1982.

31. Doniach, D., et al.: The implications of "thyroid-growth-immunoglobulins" (TGI) for the understanding of sporadic nontoxic nodular goiter. Springer Semin. Immunopathol. *5*:433, 1982.

32. Vander, J. B., et al.: The significance of nontoxic thyroid nodules. Final report of a 15-year study of the incidence of thyroid malignancy. Ann. Intern. Med. *69*:537, 1968.

33. Stoffer, R. P., et al.: Nodular goiter. Incidence, morphology before and after iodine prophylaxis, and clinical diagnosis. Arch. Intern. Med. *106*:10, 1960.

34. Livolsi, V. A., and Merino, M. J.: Histopathologic differential diagnosis of the thyroid. Pathol. Annu. *16*(Part 2):357, 1981.

35. Sampson, R. J., et al.: Occult thyroid carcinoma in Olmsted County, Minnesota: Prevalence at autopsy compared with that in Hiroshima and Nagasaki, Japan. Cancer *34*:2072, 1974.

36. Lang, W., et al.: The differentiation of atypical adenomas and encapsulated follicular carcinomas in the thyroid gland. Virchows Arch. (Pathol. Anat.) *385*:125, 1980.

37. Rojeski, M. T., and Gharib, H.: Nodular thyroid disease. Evaluation and management. N. Engl. J. Med. *313*:428, 1985.

38. Weiss, W.: Changing incidence of thyroid cancer. J. Natl. Cancer Inst. *62*:1137, 1979.

39. DeGroot, L. J., et al.: Retrospective and prospective study of radiation-induced thyroid disease. Am. J. Med. *74*:852, 1983.

40. Carcangiu, M. L., et al.: Papillary carcinoma of the thyroid. A clinicopathologic study of 241 cases treated at the University of Florence, Italy. Cancer *55*:805, 1985.

41. Vickery, A. L., Jr.: Thyroid papillary carcinoma. Pathological and philosophical controversies. Am. J. Surg. Pathol. *7*:797, 1983.

42. Rosai, J., et al.: Papillary carcinoma of the thyroid. A discussion of its several morphologic expressions with particular emphasis on the follicular variant. Am. J. Surg. Pathol. *7*:809, 1983.

43. Editorial: Radiation-induced thyroid cancer. Lancet *2*:21, 1985.

44. Franssila, K. O.: Is the differentiation between papillary and follicular thyroid carcinoma valid? Cancer *32*:853, 1973.

45. Meissner, W. A.: Follicular carcinoma of the thyroid. Am. J. Surg. Pathol. *1*:171, 1977.

46. Rosai, J., and Carcangiu, M. L.: Pathology of thyroid tumors: Some recent and old questions. Hum. Pathol. *15*:1008, 1984.

47. Carcangiu, M. L., et al.: Anaplastic thyroid carcinoma. A study of 70 cases. Am. J. Clin. Pathol. *83*:135, 1985.

48. Harach, H. R., and Williams, E. D.: Glandular (tubular and follicular) variants of medullary carcinoma of the thyroid. Histopathology *7*:83, 1983.

49. Emmertsen, K.: Medullary thyroid carcinoma and calcitonin. Dan. Med. Bull. *32*:1, 1985.

50. Kraus, M. W., and Hedinger, C. E.: Pathologic study of parathyroid glands in tertiary hyperparathyroidism. Hum. Pathol. *16*:772, 1985.

51. Simpson, E. L., et al.: Absence of parathyroid hormone messenger RNA in nonparathyroid tumors associated with hypercalcemia. N. Engl. J. Med. *309*:325, 1983.

52. Ghandur-Mnaymneh, L., and Kimura, N.: The parathyroid adenoma. A histopathologic definition with a study of 172 cases of primary hyperparathyroidism. Am. J. Pathol. *115*:70, 1984.

53. Marx, S. J.: New insights into primary hyperparathyroidism. Hosp. Pract. *18*:55, 1984.

54. Thompson, N. W., et al.: The anatomy of primary hyperparathyroidism. Surgery *92*:814, 1982.

55. Bedetti, C. D., et al.: Functioning oxyphil cell adenoma of the parathyroid: A clinicopathologic study of 10 patients with hyperparathyroidism. Hum. Pathol. *15*:1121, 1984.

56. Shane, E., and Bilezikian, J. P.: Parathyroid carcinoma: A review of 62 patients. Endocr. Rev. *3*:218, 1982.

57. Lang, P. G., Jr.: The clinical spectrum of parathyroid disease. J. Am. Acad. Dermatol. *5*:733, 1981.

58. Arulanantham, K., et al.: Evidence for defective immunoregulation in the syndrome of familial candidiasis endocrinopathy. N. Engl. J. Med. *300*:164, 1979.

59. Krieger, D. T.: Physiopathology of Cushing's disease. Endocr. Rev. *4*:22, 1983.

60. Burch, W. M.: Cushing's disease. A review. Arch. Intern. Med. *145*:1106, 1985.

61. Imura, H., et al.: Studies on ectopic ACTH-producing tumors. II. Clinical and biochemical features of 30 cases. Cancer *35*:1430, 1975.

62. Orth, D. N.: The old and the new in Cushing's syndrome. N. Engl. J. Med. *310*:649, 1984.

63. Ganguly, A., and Donohue, J. P.: Primary aldosteronism: Pathophysiology, diagnosis, and treatment. J. Urol. *129*:24, 1983.

64. Melby, J. C.: Primary aldosteronism. Kidney Int. *26*:769, 1984.

65. Carey, R. M., et al.: Idiopathic hyperaldosteronism. A possible role for aldosterone-stimulating factor. N. Engl. J. Med. *311*:94, 1984.

66. Mininberg, D. T., et al.: Current concepts in congenital adrenal hyperplasia. Pathol. Annu. *17*(Part 2):179, 1982.

67. Speiser, P. W., et al.: High frequency of nonclassical steroid 21-hydroxylase deficiency. Am. J. Hum. Genet. *37*:650, 1985.

68. Holler, W., et al.: Genetic differences between the salt-wasting, simple virilizing, and nonclassical types of congenital adrenal hyperplasia. J. Clin. Endocrinol. Metab. *60*:757, 1985.

69. Vita, J. A., et al.: Clinical clues to the cause of Addison's disease. Am. J. Med. *78*:461, 1985.

70. van Slooten, H., et al.: Morphologic characteristics of benign and malignant adrenocortical tumors. Cancer *55*:766, 1985.

71. King, D. R., and Lack, E. E.: Adrenal cortical carcinoma: A

clinical and pathologic study of 49 cases. Cancer 44:239, 1979.

72. Madeiros, L. J., et al.: Adrenal pheochromocytoma: A clinicopathologic review of 60 cases. Hum. Pathol. 16:580, 1985.

73. Harris, R. B., and DelaRoca, R. R.: Pheochromocytoma: A medical review. Heart Lung 13:73, 1984.

74. Lopez-Ibor, B., and Schwartz, A. D.: Neuroblastoma. Ped. Clin. North Am. 32:755, 1985.

75. Seeger, R. C., et al.: Association of multiple copies of the N-myc oncogene with rapid progression of neuroblastomas. N. Engl. J. Med. 313:1111, 1985.

76. Berthold, F.: Current concepts on the biology of neuroblastoma. Blut 50:65, 1985.

77. Kornstein, M. J.: The immunohistology of the thymus in myasthenia gravis. Am. J. Pathol. 117:184, 1984.

78. Hofmann, W., et al.: Thymoma. A clinicopathologic study of 98 cases with special reference to three unusual cases. Pathol. Res. Pract. 179:337, 1985.

79. Verley, J. M., and Hollmann, K. H.: Thymoma. A comparative study of clinical stages, histologic features, and survival in 200 cases. Cancer 55:1074, 1985.

80. Schimke, R. N.: Genetic aspects of multiple endocrine neoplasia. Ann. Rev. Med. 35:25, 1984.

81. Schimke, R. N.: Multiple endocrine neoplasia. Search for the oncogenic trigger. N. Engl. J. Med. 314:1315, 1986.

# 21

# The Musculoskeletal System

Diseases of the musculoskeletal system are here divided into those of bones, joints, and muscles. The hypothesis that the head bone is connected to the neck bone seems reasonably well established (although the etiology remains disputed). Beyond this, matters become more complicated. Because of the many cell types constituting bone, lesions affecting it are many and varied. Some of these have been described elsewhere in this book. The myeloproliferative disorders are discussed in Chapter 12. The healing of bone fractures is described on page 54. In addition, bone is a favored site for metastatic disease. Indeed, about two thirds of malignant lesions in bone are secondary rather than primary. Since these metastatic neoplasms do not differ significantly from their primary tumors, their description will not be repeated. Plasma cell myeloma, the most common of the *primary* tumors, is discussed on page 392. There remains for consideration in this chapter the very common metabolic diseases of bone and a large group of infrequently occurring primary bone tumors. In addition, a brief review of infection as it affects bone will be given.

Discussion of joint diseases includes a presentation of the relatively common osteoarthritis and of the infrequently occuring synoviosarcoma. Septic arthritis is described briefly. Rheumatoid arthritis is discussed with other systemic disorders of immune pathogenesis in Chapter 5. Gout is considered with the genetic disorders in Chapter 4.

The muscles seem relatively resistant to disease. Only muscle atrophy, the progressive dystrophies, myasthenia gravis, and trichinosis occur frequently enough to warrant full description. Involvement of muscles by tumors, whether primary or secondary, is quite rare. The desmoid tumor and the rhabdomyosarcoma are briefly presented.

# Bones

## OSTEOPOROSIS (OSTEOPENIA)

*Osteoporosis refers to an absolute decrease in the amount of bone below the levels required for adequate mechanical support.* Some loss of skeletal mass and, indeed, the muscular mass is a universal attribute of aging. Only when the loss of bone becomes sufficiently advanced to induce symptoms does it merit the designation of osteoporosis. The bone structure, although reduced in amount, appears normal by histologic criteria, and the ratio of mineral to organic elements within the bone remains unchanged. Since the basic abnormality appears to be too little bone, this condition is also called *osteopenia*. Osteoporosis can be classified into two categories: *primary*, the more common form, and *secondary*, which refers to bone loss associated with a variety of well-defined pathologic syndromes. These include (1) malnutrition, the result of dietary protein deficiencies or of malabsorption syndromes; (2) various endocrinopathies, including Cushing's syndrome and thyrotoxicosis; and (3) prolonged immobilization. Of greater interest to us is the form of osteoporosis called primary—a polite term frequently used in medicine to express ignorance of etiology. This is the most common form of metabolic bone disease, and its incidence increases with age. Although males develop symptomatic osteoporosis between 50 and 70 years of age, it is predominantly a disease of postmenopausal women; for these reasons, primary osteoporosis is also called *senile* or *postmenopausal osteoporosis*. An estimated four million older Americans are affected by osteoporosis, leading annually to about one million fractures.

**PATHOGENESIS.** As you are well aware, the seemingly rigid and static skeletal mass is in a constant state of turnover. New bone formation and reabsorption occur throughout life. For bone mass to increase, osteogenesis has to exceed reabsorption; this occurs during the early growing years of life. Following the growth phase, an equilibrium is maintained well into the third decade of life. In about the fourth decade of life, the bony skeleton starts undergoing a progressive erosion of its mass, marking the beginning of osteoporosis. Whether this occurs because of excessive reabsorption, inadequate bone formation, or a combination of the two processes is still controversial.[1]

Osteogenesis and osteolysis are complex phenomena that are finely tuned by several metabolic, nutritional, and endocrine factors. Although a detailed review of the homeostasis of bone mass is beyond our scope, some salient features with relevance to the pathogenesis of osteoporosis are worthy of recall. Calcium, the major mineral component of bone, is clearly important for osteogenesis. Because of the obligatory fecal and urinary losses, adequate intake and absorption of calcium are crucial for positive calcium balance. The absorption of dietary calcium is favored by the active form of vitamin D (1,25-[OH]$_2$D$_3$), which in turn is synthesized in the proximal convoluted tubes of the kidneys. The enzyme 1-alpha-hydroxylase, responsible for the conversion of Vitamin D to its active form in the kidney, is activated by parathyroid hormone (PTH). Parathormone also has a powerful influence on osteoclasts, driving them to increase bone reabsorption, an effect that may be potentiated by a deficiency of estrogens. Derangement in any one or more of these regulatory mechanisms may tilt the balance in favor of bone loss over bone formation (Fig. 21–1). For example, dietary

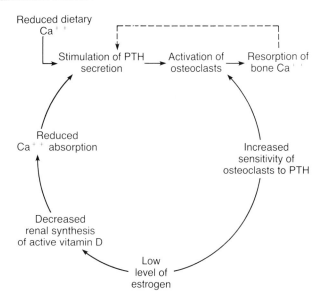

Figure 21–1. A possible schema for the pathogenesis of postmenopausal osteoporosis. Dotted line represents feedback inhibition.

deficiency of calcium may prevail in the elderly due to reduced intake of calcium-rich foods. Calcium absorption also seems to decrease in the aged, possibly due to decreased production of active vitamin D in the kidney. Together these two factors tend to lower serum calcium, but hypocalcemia does not occur, since calcium is mobilized from the bone under the influence of PTH. Thus, adequate serum calcium levels (important for neuromuscular transmission) are maintained at the expense of bone calcium. Approximately 15% of the patients with primary osteoporosis show increased levels of serum PTH, supporting the notion that the sequence outlined above may be relevant in the pathogenesis of osteoporosis in these patients.

Since there is a close association between bone loss and menopause, estrogen deficiency as a possible etiologic factor has received much attention. As mentioned earlier, low levels of estrogen increase the sensitivity of osteoclasts to PTH. In addition, relative estrogen deficiency may also impair the synthesis of active vitamin D by renal tubules and consequently reduce calcium absorption.[2]

The effects of bone loss are understandably more severe in individuals endowed with a delicate skeleton or low original density of bones. This may well underlie the differential occurrence of symptomatic osteoporosis in various racial and sex subgroups. In the United States, the maximal bone density achieved in young adults is greatest in black males and least in white females; white males and black females are at intermediate levels. Since the rate of age-related bone loss in these groups is similar, it would be expected that white females, who start with the lowest initial levels of bone density, would be at the greatest risk of developing osteoporosis. This prediction is borne out by the results of epidemiologic studies.

*In summary, primary osteoporosis is a multifactorial and possibly heterogeneous disorder. It has no single cause but rather is a common morphologic expression of a number of derangements associated most often with aging.*[3]

**MORPHOLOGY.** Except when it is secondary to prolonged immobilization of localized parts, osteoporosis is a systemic disorder affecting the entire skeleton. Nevertheless, bone loss is most severe in areas of skeleton that contain relatively large amounts of trabecular bone[4] and that are subject to prime weight-bearing stresses. Thus, the vertebrae and femoral neck are particular targets and are often the sites of fractures. Cortical bone is thinned, with resorption of cancellous bone spicules and enlargement of the medullary cavity. Nevertheless, osteoporotic bone, although reduced in mass, has the same composition as normal bone, with no evidence of inadequate mineralization because matrix formation and mineralization remain in balance.

**CLINICAL COURSE.** Bone pain, especially backache, is a common complaint of patients with osteoporosis. This results from collapse of fractured vertebral bodies. Other common sites of fracture are the femoral neck and lower end of the radius. Often these may follow trivial trauma. Radiographs sometimes show an increase in radiolucency of bone, frequently with compression fractures of vertebrae. Newer, more sensitive radiologic techniques such as dual-beam photon absorptiometry more accurately quantitate the mineral content of bone. Serum levels of alkaline phosphatase, calcium, and phosphorus are characteristically within normal limits, and this is an important point in distinguishing osteoporosis from osteomalacia, with which it may be identical on radiographs (see below). Several agents that retard bone reabsorption or favor osteogenesis are used in the treatment of primary osteoporosis. These include estrogens,[5] calcitonin, vitamin D, and calcium. Treatment to reverse changes is unsatisfactory and leads, at best, to prevention of further bone loss.

# RICKETS AND OSTEOMALACIA

These disorders are mainly caused by a lack of active vitamin D $(1,25\text{-}[OH]_2D_3)$. In children this deficiency produces rickets; osteomalacia is the adult counterpart. Both were described, along with vitamin D metabolism, in Chapter 8, and reference should be made to this earlier discussion. Suffice it to reiterate here that deficiency of the active form of vitamin D is a fairly common disorder, which may be seen in a number of clinical settings. The most important are (1) simple dietary inadequacy of vitamin D, often combined with a lack of exposure to sunshine; (2) intestinal malabsorption from any cause; and (3) chronic renal insufficiency, in which osteomalacia appears as a component of renal osteodystrophy (p. 459). It may also be recalled that osteomalacia, in contrast with osteoporosis, is characterized primarily by impaired mineralization of bone matrix. However, if calcification continues to be inadequate, the production of organic bone matrix also decreases. On the other hand, decrease in bone mass, which is characteristic of osteoporosis, must necessarily be associated with slowed mineralization. Thus the two disorders merge. Not surprisingly, therefore, the radiologic appearance of osteoporosis and osteomalacia may be very similar, and it may be difficult to distinguish them on the basis of x-ray findings alone.

# OSTEITIS FIBROSA CYSTICA GENERALISATA (VON RECKLINGHAUSEN'S DISEASE)

This is the pattern of bone disease associated with severe hyperparathyroidism, whether primary or secondary. The causes of hyperparathyroidism were discussed in Chapter 20; here we will only describe the associated skeletal changes. Because of its calcium-mobilizing effects, demineralization of bones is the hallmark of excessive secretion of parathormone. Subperiosteal resorption of bone in the phalanges and distal clavicles and loss of the lamina dura about the teeth are characteristic radiographic signs. In its advanced form primary hyperparathyroidism gives rise to the lesion known as *osteitis fibrosa cystica generalisata*, or *von Recklinghausen's disease of bone*. Its presence confirms the existence of hyperparathyroidism. More often, however, presumably because of early diagnosis, the nonspecific and less severe bony lesion osteomalacia is present.

The basic anatomic change with osteitis fibrosa cystica is osteoclastic resorption of bone, with fibrous replacement. Both microscopic and gross cysts form within the fibrous tissue. Frequently, the first manifestation of the well-developed lesion is a cystic lesion in the jaw. In many instances, the radiographic cysts are in reality soft tissue masses referred to as "brown tumors." Although these lesions resemble giant cell tumors of bone (presence of multinucleate osteoclasts in a fibrous stroma), they are non-neoplastic and better referred to as reparative giant cell granulomas. Removal of the cause of parathyroid hyperfunction may be followed by amazingly rapid reversion of the bone to normal, but cystic lesions may persist.

Secondary hyperparathyroidism resulting from chronic renal failure can also give rise to cystic changes in the bone, but rarely to the extent noted in primary hyperparathyroidism.

# OSTEITIS DEFORMANS
# (PAGET'S DISEASE)

Osteitis deformans is yet another skeletal disorder of unknown etiology characterized by continuous excessive destruction of bone and its simultaneous replacement by an abnormally soft, poorly mineralized matrix. This lesion is present in from 1 to 3% of elderly individuals and is almost never detected in patients below 40 years of age. In most cases Paget's disease is mild and asymptomatic, although more advanced cases are associated with intense pain in the involved bones.

The etiology of Paget's disease remains unknown. Genetically determined defects in connective tissue metabolism have been suspected on the basis of some reports of familial clustering of Paget's disease.[6] Based on the presence of tubular structures resembling paramyxoviruses in the nuclei of osteoclasts, a viral etiology has been suggested. Antigenically, these tubular structures seem to cross-react with the antigens of measles virus and respiratory syncytial virus. However, viruses have never been isolated from the lesions, and serum antibodies directed against the viral agents are not consistently seen. Hence, this currently favored hypothesis needs further substantiation. Since the etiology is unknown, therapy is directed toward reducing osteoclastic activity by administration of agents such as calcitonin and diphosphonates.[7]

**MORPHOLOGY.** Osteitis deformans may be polyostotic or monostotic. In the polyostotic form, the pelvis and sacrum are generally the first sites affected. The process may then extend to the skull, femur, spine, tibia, humerus, and scapula, in decreasing order of frequency. The monostotic form may affect only a portion of a single bone, most often the tibia. The lesions seem to evolve through three phases: (1) an initial osteolytic stage, followed by (2) a mixed osteolytic and osteoblastic phase, and (3) in many cases, a so-called burnt-out or osteoblastic, sclerotic phase of the disease. In the initial osteolytic phase, intense focal bone resorption by bizarre-looking osteoclasts with over 100 nuclei can be seen. Even at this stage, an osteoblastic response can occur that gets progressively more prominent in the mixed phase. The resorbed bone is replaced initially by highly vascular connective tissue and later by new lamellar bone. **Since mineralization of new osteoid lags, osteoid seams persist at the margin of the newly laid down bone to create a tile-like or mosaic pattern that is pathognomonic of Paget's disease** (Fig. 21–2). Concomitantly with these changes in the bone, the contiguous marrow cavity is replaced by loose, highly vascular connective tissue. Eventually, after many years, the third sclerotic phase may appear as osteoclastic activity wanes and there is predominantly osteoblastic activity. The neoosteogenesis may eventually increase bone thickness or

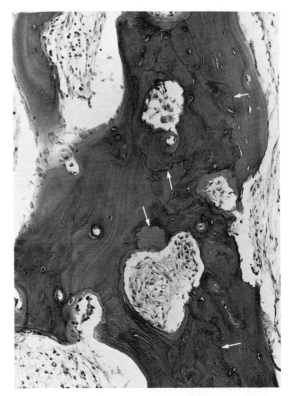

Figure 21–2. Paget's disease of bone. The thickened, irregular bony trabeculae show the classic mosaic pattern, outlined by the black lines traversing them (*arrows*). These lines are produced by bone resorption and irregular patterns of new bone formation.

size, but it is laid down in a haphazard manner, remains poorly mineralized, and is soft, porous, and lacking in structural strength. It can be easily deformed and can crumble under stress, as is discussed below.

**CLINICAL FEATURES.** Patients with Paget's disease may be entirely asymptomatic, in which case the disease may be detected only on radiographs taken for an unrelated disorder. The most common symptoms, when present, are pain or deformity related to the underlying skeletal change. Headache and pain in the face may result from impingement on cranial nerves by *enlarging skull bones*. There may be accompanying deafness or visual disturbances. Back pain may be caused by *pathologic fractures of the vertebrae* or compression of spinal roots. *Long bones are deformed by irregular swelling*, and gait may be affected. X-ray examination reflects the state of the disease; early in the course there are areas of radiolucency, but later the bones may be abnormally dense. In view of the excessive bone resorption, one might anticipate elevated levels of serum calcium. However, since new bone formation occurs almost simultaneously, serum calcium and inorganic phosphate levels are normal. On the other hand, *high* *rates of urinary hydroxyproline excretion and mark-edly elevated serum alkaline phosphatase levels result from excessive bone matrix degradation and new bone formation, respectively.*

Two additional complications of Paget's disease are worthy of note. The increased vascularization of the abnormal bone acts as multiple arteriovenous fistulae, which result in an increase work load for the heart and sometimes in high output heart failure. Most serious, however, is the development of osteogenic sarcoma in the bones affected by osteitis deformans. Such malignant transformation is reported in approximately 1% of cases and carries with it a particularly grave prognosis.

## FIBROUS DYSPLASIA OF BONE

This uncommon disorder is characterized by focal areas of fibrous replacement of bone. Although the etiology is unknown, it is believed to represent a disturbance of normal bone development, perhaps a malformation that results in progressive replacement of bone by fibrous tissue.[8]

Usually the lesion is monostotic, affects males slightly more often than females, and may appear at any time between infancy and middle age, with a median age in one series of 14 years. Occasionally, fibrous dysplasia is polyostotic, and in a very small percentage of cases, the polyostotic form is associated with scattered areas of melanotic pigmentation of the skin (*café au lait spots*) and with sexual precocity. The concurrence of these disparate features is known as *Albright's syndrome.* In contrast to the monostotic form of fibrous dysplasia, Albright's syndrome occurs primarily in females. Although the multisystem involvement suggests some congenital defect, no hereditary or familial pattern has been established.

**MORPHOLOGY.** The monostotic form shows a predilection for the long bones of the extremities, the ribs, and the bones of the skull and face. The lesion begins in the intramedullary cancellous bone and expands to involve the adjacent cortex. Although it is not encapsulated, it tends to remain enclosed within a shell of cortical bone. Histologically, there is a fibrous stroma containing variable amounts of bone spicules. The bone trabeculae are arranged haphazardly and comprise poorly formed woven bone having no internal lamellar structure. Bone appears to be formed by osseous metaplasia of the stroma.

The clinical course is more or less unpredictable. Sometimes the lesion grows slowly and may even, apparently spontaneously, become stationary. In other patients, unless it is cured by surgical excision, fibrous dysplasia progresses rapidly and inexorably, causing bone destruction and disfiguration. When the facial bones are involved, there may be severe distortions of the orbit, nose, and jaw. Malignant transformation occurs rarely.

## HYPERTROPHIC OSTEOARTHROPATHY

This mysterious entity has three separate components: (a) "clubbing" of the fingers, (b) periostitis with new bone formation at the distal ends of long bones as well as the metacarpals and proximal phalanges, and (c) swelling and tenderness of joints. These changes are seen in a multitude of clinical settings. The most common underlying causes of this triad are intrathoracic disease: lung cancer, chronic lung sepsis (for example, bronchiectasis), and chronic interstitial pneumonia. Clubbing alone may be seen in congenital cyanotic heart disease, bacterial endocarditis, biliary cirrhosis, ulcerative colitis, Crohn's disease, chronic myelogenous leukemia, and thyroid cancer.

The changes involved in clubbing of the fingers are edema, fibrous overgrowth at the tips of the fingers, and increased vascularization in the nail bed with rounding or "watchglass" deformity of the nail. The tips of the digits become enlarged and often are dusky or cyanotic. These changes are more or less readily discernible on inspection, and therefore clubbing is a valuable diagnostic sign.

Periosteal bone changes affect the distal radius, ulna, tibia, fibula, metacarpals, and proximal phalanges. The amount of new bone formation varies from radiographically barely visible tufting to the formation of a complete enclosing layer about the metacarpals and first and second phalanges. Although any of the disorders leading to clubbing may produce periosteal proliferation, the most important underlying condition is bronchogenic carcinoma. The recognition of hypertrophic osteoarthropathy may actually lead to the discovery of an unsuspected bronchogenic carcinoma.

Hypertrophic osteoarthropathy and clubbing are thought to involve increased blood flow to the bones, possibly as a result of some derangement in the autonomic nervous system or hormonal imbalances. Beyond this, the mechanism remains an enigma. With removal of the underlying disease, the bony changes promptly regress.

## BONE TUMORS

Bone is a complex structure that contains cartilage, hematopoietic elements, and fibrous tissue, in addition to bony (osseous) tissue itself. Hence, primary tumors in the bone may arise from any one of these elements. Tumors of hematopoietic cells and connective tissue have been described elsewhere; in this chapter, we will consider *osteoblastic* (bone-forming) and *chondromatous* (cartilaginous) tumors, along with two neoplasms of uncertain origin: Ewing's sarcoma and giant cell tumor. Before proceeding to the discussion of specific bone tumors, a few generalizations can be offered. First, primary bone tumors are usually malignant, in the ratio of approximately 3:1. The four most common malignant tumors of bone are osteogenic sarcoma, chondrosarcoma, Ewing's sarcoma, and malignant giant cell tumors. Osteogenic sarcoma is by far the most common. Most of the bone tumors have rather characteristic skeletal locations. For example, osteosarcomas almost always arise in the metaphyses, whereas giant cell tumors are epiphyseal in location. The age distribution of the more common bone tumors is also fairly characteristic. In general they tend to strike young people, often adolescents, which is ascribed to their propensity to arise in actively growing bone. Most important, however, is the radiologic appearance of bone tumors. Without the knowledge of the clinical and x-ray findings, the pathologist is severely handicapped in rendering an accurate diagnosis.

## BONE-FORMING (OSTEOBLASTIC) TUMORS

Tumors in this category are marked by the formation of osteoid matrix (that may become mineralized) and hence may be considered to have arisen from primitive mesenchymal cells that have differentiated along the osteoblastic pathway. These tumors have also been called osteogenic, a term we would like to avoid since it has also been applied to all the tumors arising in bone.

The three principal tumors in this category are the *osteoma*, the *osteoid osteoma*, and the *osteosarcoma*. By far the most important of these is the osteosarcoma.

### Osteoma

This is an infrequent and totally benign growth, found most often on the inner surface of the skull. It may project into the orbit or paranasal sinuses. Histologically, the growth is composed of dense normal bone. These tumors are of little clinical significance and are removed only for cosmetic reasons or if they cause local pressure effects.

### Osteoid Osteoma

This is a small benign neoplasm that involves the diaphyses of long bones. They are most likely to occur in persons under the age of 20 years and affect males twice as often as females. Although any bone may be involved, the femur and tibia are most commonly affected. The tumor typically arises within cortical bone, where it erodes the underlying normal bone, producing a discrete, red-brown nodule rarely over 1 cm in diameter. Immediately surrounding it is a zone of dense, sclerotic bone. The tumor itself is composed of an array of branching and anastomosing,

partially mineralized osteoid trabeculae with intervening vascular connective tissue. On radiographs, the osteoid osteoma appears as a distinctive lytic lesion surrounded by a rim of densely sclerotic bone. Despite its small size and benign nature, the lesion is extremely painful, and so it necessitates surgical removal.

### Osteosarcoma (Osteogenic Sarcoma)

This tumor, arising from mesenchymal cells, is characterized by osteoblastic differentiation of the neoplastic cells. As such, *formation of osteoid directly by the tumor cells is a hallmark of osteosarcoma.* The amount of osteoid and bone formation within a given tumor is variable. Furthermore, in view of the common origin of osteoblasts, chondroblasts, and fibroblasts, it is not surprising that some osteosarcomas also contain cartilage and collagen. Nevertheless, osteosarcomas must be clearly distinguished from chondrosarcomas and fibrosarcomas, which also arise in the bone. Osteosarcomas have a distinctive natural history characterized by an aggressive course and relatively poor prognosis.

Excluding multiple myeloma, osteosarcoma is the most common primary malignant tumor of the bone. A great majority of those afflicted by this neoplasm are young people between the ages of 10 and 25 years. Males are affected twice as frequently as females. A second, smaller peak is seen after 50 years of age. In this group there is a very high percentage of patients with preexisting Paget's disease.

ETIOLOGIC FACTORS. The etiology, like that of most other malignant neoplasms, is still an unsolved puzzle. Irradiation and oncogenic viruses, which have also been implicated in the genesis of other forms of cancer, have been suggested as causative agents. Genetic factors may also play a role. The risk of osteosarcoma in patients with hereditary retinoblastoma is increased 500 times over that of controls. As with retinoblastoma, deletions on the long arm of chromosome 13 have been reported.[9] Other hereditary conditions such as multiple enchondromatosis and multiple osteochondromatoses are also documented predispositions to this form of cancer.

MORPHOLOGY. The majority of the osteosarcomas in the younger age group (10 to 25 years) arise at the growing metaphyseal ends of long bones. The bones affected, in decreasing order of frequency, are the lower end of femur, upper end of tibia, upper end of humerus, and upper end of femur. About 50% of all osteosarcomas occur about the knee. Of the flat bones, the ilium is most often involved. However, virtually any bone in the body may be involved, and, in the older age group with Paget's disease, preferential involvement of ends of long bones is not seen. Since osteosarcomas grow rapidly, in most cases a visible mass is present when the patient is first seen. The tumor usually arises in and replaces the metaphyseal cancellous tissue and then erodes the cortex, finally invading the adjacent soft tissues. Spreading inwards, it replaces the medullary cavity (Fig. 21–3). Cartilage is less readily invaded by the tumor, and therefore invasion of the joint space through the articular cartilage or the epiphyseal plate is not common. As the advancing tumor extends beyond the outer surface of the bone, it lifts the periosteum from the cortex. At this point, there is delicate calcification between the elevated periosteum and the underlying cortex, creating the so-called Codman's triangle where the elevated periosteum meets the outer cortical contour. Codman's triangle is a useful radiographic feature of this form of tumor but it is not diagnostic of osteosarcoma. The cut surface of the tumor presents a gray-white appearance with areas of hemorrhage and cystic necrosis. The tumor consistency and appearance vary depending upon the proportion of various elements within it.[10] About 50% of the tumors are hard and gritty—the so-called **osteoblastic variety**—because they contain extensive mineralized osteoid. As mentioned earlier, osteosarcomas may also contain cartilage or collagen; in some cases these elements predominate and are sometimes called chondroblastic or fibroblastic variants, respectively. Histologically, all the tumors contain highly anaplastic mesenchymal cells, with **unmistakable evidence of osteoid formation by the**

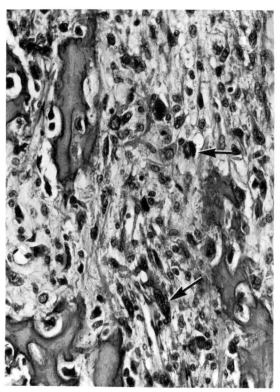

Figure 21–4. Osteogenic sarcoma. The high-power detail illustrates the anaplastic fibrous tissue with mitoses and tumor giant cell formation (*arrows*). Osteoid trabeculae have been produced by the neoplastic cells, and anaplastic tumor cells are found lying within apparent bone lacunae.

**tumor cells** (Fig. 21–4). The osteoid, which is pink and amorphous, may be abundant or localized to small areas. It is laid down in the form of islands surrounded by plump tumor cells or as intertwining strands enclosing nests of tumor cells. Calcification of the osteoid may impart to it a bluish appearance. Islands of cartilage formed by the tumor cells may also be present, and in some cases cartilaginous stroma may exceed the amount of osteoid. The tumor cells show all the classic cytologic features of malignancy—pleomorphism, hyperchromasia, abnormal mitoses and bizarre-appearing tumor giant cells.

The bloodstream is the major route of spread, and the lungs are the most frequent site of metastases. Other parenchymal organs may also be involved. It is unusual for osteosarcoma to spread to regional lymph nodes. In the great majority of cases, death is due to pulmonary metastases.

**CLINICAL FEATURES.** Unlike most other tumors, osteosarcoma manifests pain early. When pain is accompanied by local swelling and fever, the relatively innocuous diagnosis of osteomyelitis may be suggested. Growth of the tumor is very rapid, and visible changes in the tumor mass occur rapidly. The serum alkaline phosphatase level may be raised if there is enough osteoblastic activity in the tumor. X-ray films may show Codman's triangle and areas of bone destruction as well as soft tissue radiodensities

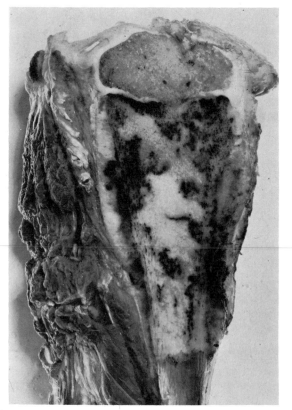

Figure 21–3. Osteogenic sarcoma, osteoblastic type, of the upper end of the tibia. The hard white tumor fills the marrow cavity but has not penetrated the epiphyseal plate. It has infiltrated through the cortex and lifted the periosteum on both lateral aspects. (From Robbins, S. L., Cotran, R. S., and Kumar, V.: Pathologic Basis of Disease. 3rd ed. Philadelphia, W. B. Saunders Co., 1984, p. 1339.)

representing new bone formation. Even the most suggestive clinical and roentgenographic findings are best confirmed by a biopsy, since the usual treatment includes amputation of the affected limb. In the past the prognosis of osteosarcoma has been uniformly poor, with a 10 to 20% five-year survival rate. The recent approach of amputation, chemotherapy, and aggressive surgery for pulmonary metastases appears to be more successful. Currently, the overall survival of patients without metastatic disease is 60 to 80%. Even with pulmonary metastases 40%, five-year survival has been reported.[9]

The above description applies to over 75% of osteosarcomas, which may be called primary or classic cases. Osteosarcoma may also arise secondarily in bones that are the sites of preexisting diseases.[10] The most important predisposing disease in this category is Paget's disease, already discussed. Osteosarcoma complicating Paget's disease often arises in flat bones having pagetic lesions; it occurs in individuals over 50 years of age and is extremely aggressive. Few patients survive more than two years.

## CHRONDROMA SERIES OF TUMORS

There are three important cartilaginous tumors: the *osteochondroma*, the *enchondroma*, and the *chondrosarcoma*.

### Osteochondroma (Exostosis Cartilaginea)

This knobby, benign, bony neoplasm protrudes from the metaphyseal surface of long bones, mostly the lower femur or upper tibia, and is capped by growing cartilage. The cartilage produces endochondral bone. As an isolated defect, it develops commonly in children and adolescents and follows a very indolent course, sometimes with apparent cessation of growth followed by complete ossification. Multiple exostoses occur as a hereditary disorder (*hereditary multiple cartilaginous exostoses*). These appear earlier than the isolated lesions, usually in infancy, and typically cease to enlarge before adolescence is reached. The major clinical significance of these lesions, particularly in the hereditary form, lies in their potential for malignant transformation to a chondrosarcoma or an osteogenic sarcoma.

### Enchondroma

This is also a benign cartilaginous tumor, but, unlike the exostoses, it occurs deep within the bone, in the spongiosa. Most frequently involved are the small bones of the hands and feet. Young adults are principally affected. Multiple enchondromas, or *enchondromatosis*, may occur in childhood, a condition known as *Ollier's disease*. When this pattern is accompanied by hemangiomas of the skin, the involvement is termed *Maffucci's syndrome*.

Grossly, the enchondroma appears as a firm, slightly lobulated, glassy, gray-blue, translucent lesion that abuts on and erodes the overlying cortical bone. Usually reactive bone formation maintains a thin outer bony shell. With the light microscope, the tumor is seen to be composed of small masses of mature hyaline cartilage merging gradually through transitional cell forms with a scant fibrous stroma. Foci of calcification and even ossification may be present within the cartilage.

The erosive nature of these lesions may cause pain, swelling, or pathologic fractures of the involved bone. On the other hand, the lesion may remain completely silent. As with the exostosis, malignant transformation is reported with the enchondroma, particularly the multiple patterns.

### Chondrosarcoma

Chondrosarcoma is a malignant tumor of chondroblasts; among bone cancers it is next to osteosarcoma in frequency. Chondrosarcomas differ from osteosarcomas in several respects. *They occur in an older age group (most tumors arising after the age of 35 years). Their growth is much slower and the prognosis is much better.* Unlike the case in osteosarcomas, pelvic bones are the most commonly affected, followed by the femur, ribs, and other bones. Some chondrosarcomas arise from malignant transformation of enchondromas and multiple exostoses; however, the great majority arise de novo.

MORPHOLOGY. Chondrosarcomas may originate in a central location within the bone or in a peripheral (cortical or periosteal) location. The gross appearance of most tumors betrays their cartilaginous nature; they are bulky and lobulated and have a bluish, glistening appearance. **Microscopically, some tumors may be very well-differentiated and difficult to distinguish from enchondromas on the histologic basis alone.** At the other end of the spectrum are tumors with obvious signs of malignancy. Features suggestive of a malignant cartilaginous tumor include cells with plump nuclei, multiple nuclei in a single cell, and the presence of several chondroblasts in a single lacuna (Fig. 21–5). In between the cells is a cartilaginous matrix that may be calcified or even ossified. As a matter of great practical significance, it is important to remember that **in chondrosarcomas bone formation occurs within the cartilage by a process similar to endochondral ossification, whereas in osteosarcomas, osteoid is formed directly by the malignant cells.**

Chondrosarcomas are slow-growing tumors, often present for years. Depending upon the degree of differentiation the five-year survival rates vary from 43 to 90%.

## OTHER BONE TUMORS

### Giant Cell Tumor (Osteoclastoma)

Giant cell tumors are set apart from other neoplasms of bone by having numerous multinucleated

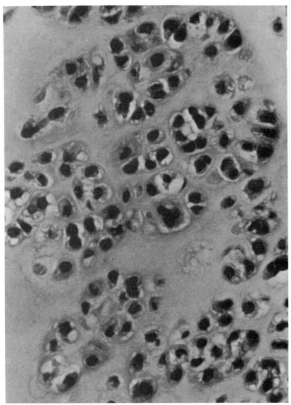

Figure 21–5. Chondrosarcoma. Anaplastic chondrocytes within lacunae are separated by cartilaginous matrix. (From Robbins, S. L., Cotran, R. S., and Kumar, V.: Pathologic Basis of Disease. 3rd ed. Philadelphia, W. B. Saunders Co., 1984, p. 1343.)

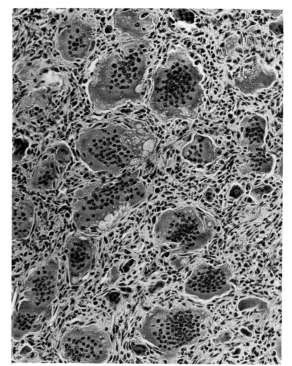

Figure 21–6. Giant cell tumor of bone. The large giant cells are separated by a scant benign-appearing spindle cell stroma.

giant cells in the spindle cell stroma that makes up these lesions. Most patients are over the age of 20 years, and slightly more females than males are affected.

**MORPHOLOGY.** In contrast to most bone cancers, giant cell tumors begin within the epiphyses and progressively expand outward, often reaching but not eroding the articular cartilage. They thus produce a club-like deformity of the end of the bone. The most frequently involved sites are the ends of long bones, particularly the lower femur, upper tibia, and lower radius. Reactive new bone formation about the cortex may maintain a thin enclosing outer shell. The tumor itself is gray-brown, firm, and friable, with scattered foci of hemorrhage and necrosis. Microscopically, the striking feature is the presence of numerous irregularly scattered giant cells resembling osteoclasts. **These are found within a background of plump or spindled fibroblast-like cells, which constitute the basic tumor element** (Fig. 21–6). **These stromal cells are the proliferating component and presumably give rise to the giant cells.** A recent study with monoclonal antibodies indicates that both the stromal and giant cell elements are related to cells of the monocyte-macrophage lineage.[11] Bone and cartilage formation typically do not occur in these tumors. On the basis of the degree of atypia of the stromal cells, giant cell tumors have been classified into grades 1 to 3. However, as discussed below, most workers feel that histologic grading is of little value in determining clinical behavior.

**CLINICAL COURSE.** The clinical presentation of giant cell tumors is nonspecific with pain, tenderness, and, occasionally, pathologic fractures. Sometimes there is an externally palpable mass. X-rays often reveal a distinctive but not pathognomonic soap bubble appearance—large cystic areas of bone rarefaction traversed by strands of calcification and surrounded by a thin shell of bone. The clinical course of these tumors is variable. Some tumors, even if histologically innocuous, metastasize early, but their incidence is believed to be fairly small.[12] Most others are not aggressive, at least initially, and are therefore treated by curettage. However, approximately 50% recur following such treatment. Sometimes the recurrent tumor is more ominous and may even metastasize.

Often inflammatory or reparative lesions of bone contain giant cells, but these are called "tumors" only as misnomers. These lesions include the "brown tumors" of hyperparathyroidism, the giant cell granuloma of the jaw bones in adolescents (also called *epulis*), and the giant cell tumor of synovial or tendon sheath origin. Histologically they may closely resemble giant cell tumors but should be referred to as "reparative giant cell granulomas."

## Ewing's Sarcoma

This rare and extremely malignant tumor arises within the marrow cavity of bone. There is much debate and uncertainty regarding the histogenesis of Ewing's tumor. Most of the currently available evidence suggests that it arises from primitive mesenchymal cells within the bone marrow.[13] Ewing's sarcoma affects adolescents, most frequently between the ages of 10 and 15 years. It is very rare in blacks.

The major sites of involvement are the long tubular bones of the lower extremity and the pelvis. Most tumors begin in the metaphyses, but origin in the diaphyses is also common. They grow rapidly, and by the time the patients seek medical attention, often the entire bone is involved, a fact which may not be evident on radiographs. Radiologically, bone destruction with fusiform expansion and extension into soft tissues may be evident. Periosteal reaction may produce a concentric "onion-skin" layering around the tumor in about 50% of the cases.

Grossly the tumor tissue is very soft, gray, or white with areas of necrosis and hemorrhage. Histologically, these tumors consist of diffuse sheets of cells with little stroma, or sometimes lobular aggregates separated by fine fibrovascular septae. The tumor cells are small, round, and undifferentiated. They have prominent nuclei and indistinct cytoplasm, which often contains PAS-positive glycogen granules. Mitotic figures are rarely numerous. Because of the undifferentiated "small round cell" morphology these tumors have to be carefully distinguished from metastatic neuroblastoma and from lymphoma of the bone.

Pain and tenderness are the dominant presenting clinical features of Ewing's sarcoma. Widespread dissemination, particularly to other bones and lungs, occurs early, and the prognosis is generally poor. In recent years combined treatment modalities (surgery, irradiation, and chemotherapy) have resulted in a 40 to 50%, five-year survival rate. Patients with pelvic lesions have the worst prognosis.

# OSTEOMYELITIS

The two most important infections of bone are (1) hematogenous pyogenic osteomyelitis and (2) tuberculosis. Fortunately, both forms are becoming progressively less frequent.

## Pyogenic Osteomyelitis

This usually develops in children. In most cases, the primary focus of bacterial infection cannot be demonstrated, and a transient bacteremia from trivial causes is presumed. Hematogenous pyogenic osteomyelitis is caused principally by *Staphylococcus aureus*, followed in importance by streptococci, pneumococci, gonococci, *Hemophilus influenzae*, and coliform bacilli. There are some important exceptions to this generalization. For example, salmonellae are the common causative organism in patients with sickle cell anemia. In the neonatal period, group B streptococci are emerging as frequent pathogens, and in drug addicts, *Pseudomonas* is most often the offending organism. In addition to the hematogenous route, direct contamination of bone exposed by trauma or spread of a neighboring soft tissue infection can cause osteomyelitis.

In children, the long bones are most commonly involved, and the infection begins in the metaphyseal marrow cavity. In adults, the spine is often the site of infection. In either location it develops as a characteristic suppurative reaction. As the inflammatory pressure increases within the rigidly confined focus of infection, the vascular supply is often compromised, adding an element of ischemic necrosis to the suppurative damage. Eventually, the inflammation may penetrate the cortex through the haversian system, often producing multiple sinus tracts opening on the overlying skin. The suppuration and ischemia may then cause necrosis of a fragment of bone known as a **sequestrum**. Extension into the joint is uncommon. In certain instances, the initial infection becomes walled off by inflammatory fibrous tissue, creating a localized abscess that may undergo spontaneous sterilization or become a chronic nidus of infection (**Brodie's abscess**). Reactive osteoblastic activity forms new bone (**involucrum**) that tends to enclose the inflammatory focus. The histologic changes depend upon the duration of osteomyelitis. In early stages, polymorphonuclear exudate predominates; as chronicity sets in, mononuclear and fibroblastic reaction can be seen. However, foci of neutrophils often persist even in chronic osteomyelitis. Areas of bone necrosis and reactive new bone formation are also seen.

Hematogenous osteomyelitis usually manifests itself as an acute systemic febrile illness, accompanied by local pain, tenderness, redness, and swelling. Results of blood cultures are usually positive during this stage. Necrosis of bone is typically not sufficiently advanced to be demonstrable on radiographs for the first seven to ten days. Although spontaneous healing may occur, the usual course in the absence of adequate therapy is toward chronicity, with destruction of bone and the risk of metastatic dissemination of infection.

## Tuberculous Osteomyelitis

Tuberculous osteomyelitis is no longer a significant clinical problem except in developing countries where the incidence of tuberculosis is high. Seeding of the bones usually occurs by the hematogenous route, but in many cases a primary focus in the lungs or elsewhere may not be identifiable. Unlike pyogenic osteomyelitis, tuberculous osteomyelitis tends to arise insidiously and to extend into joint spaces. Often it is not noted until destruction is widespread. The long bones of the extremities and the spine

(*Pott's disease*) are the favored sites of localization. In the spine tuberculous osteomyelitis can lead to serious deformities (kyphosis, scoliosis) due to the

destruction and malalignment of the vertebrae. The histologic reaction is typical of all tuberculous lesions and will not be repeated here.

# Joints

## ARTHRITIS

Arthritis is the most common form of joint disease, encompassing a variety of disorders of diverse causes. Some are truly inflammatory in origin, such as infective arthritis and rheumatoid arthritis. Osteoarthritis, on the other hand, is primarily a degenerative disorder with little inflammation. However, this designation, hallowed by years of use, persists despite efforts to rename the condition "degenerative joint disease." Here we will discuss infective arthritis and osteoarthritis. Since rheumatoid arthritis was discussed earlier, in Chapter 5, we will here offer only a comparison with osteoarthritis.

## INFECTIVE (BACTERIAL) ARTHRITIS

Joints may be involved by pyogenic bacteria or tubercle bacilli. *Pyogenic arthritis* usually represents hematogenous spread from a primary infection elsewhere.[14] The source may be readily identified (e.g., bacterial endocarditis, gonorrhea) or may not be obvious. The most frequent causative organisms are gonococci, staphylococci, streptococci, pneumococci, and gram-negative rods. In childhood, *H. influenza* is the common causative organism. Gonococcal arthritis is perhaps the most common form seen in sexually active young adults. This complication of gonorrhea is somewhat more frequent in women and homosexual males.

Characteristically, the infection is monoarticular and involves one of the large joints, such as the knee, hip, ankle, elbow, wrist, or shoulder. The anatomic changes are typical of a suppurative infection. The synovial membranes become edematous and congested, and the joint fills with purulent material. In severe cases, the inflammatory synovitis may ulcerate and involve the underlying articular cartilage, eventuating in destruction of the joint surfaces with scarring and, occasionally, calcification.

The clinical manifestations are those of an acute infection, with redness, swelling, tenderness, and pain, often with accompanying constitutional symptoms. Because of the destructive tendencies of chronic suppurative arthritis, the acute phase requires prompt recognition and therapy for the preservation of normal joint function.

*Tuberculous arthritis* most frequently occurs in the spine and represents simply an aspect of tuberculous osteomyelitis (*Pott's disease*), with extension into the

intervertebral discs. It may also occur as a monoarticular involvement in the large joints. Like tuberculous osteomyelitis, tuberculous arthritis is an extremely insidious destructive process that tends to erode into the underlying articular surface and destroy the bone. Early diagnosis is imperative to prevent permanent damage.

## LYME DISEASE (LYME ARTHRITIS)

This disorder was first described in 1976 as an epidemic of inflammatory arthritis clustered in Northeastern United States, near the town of Lyme, Connecticut.[15] It has now been reported from several locales within and outside the United States. With increasing experience, it has become apparent that this condition is a multisystem disease, and hence it was rechristened Lyme disease in 1979.

Lyme disease is caused by a newly identified spirochete, called *Borrelia burgdorferi*, that is transmitted by the tick *Ixodes dammini*. In a typical case the clinical manifestations begin days to weeks after a tick bite that may have gone unnoticed. The disease then evolves through three stages: Stage I is dominated by dermatologic and constitutional symptoms, Stage II is associated with cardiac and neurologic involvement, and Stage III is characterized by arthritis. Skin involvement begins with a rash, *erythema chronicum migrans*, that is characterized by a slowly enlarging annular lesion with red, hot margins and central pallor. The skin lesion may increase in size to several inches before it fades. Within several weeks to months, 10 to 15% of the patients develop cardiac abnormalities, (atrioventricular block or pericarditis) and neurologic abnormalities (meningitis, encephalitis, or cranial neuritis). Joint involvement occurs in over 50% of the cases and is manifested initially as a migratory polyarthritis. In some patients it evolves into a chronic arthritis affecting, most commonly, the knee joints. At this stage Lyme disease may resemble rheumatoid arthritis both clinically and histologically, but unlike the latter, small joints are rarely involved and rheumatoid factor is lacking.

Lyme disease is believed to result from the formation of immune complexes in response to the spirochete antigens. IgM antibodies directed against the spirochete and immune complexes can be detected in the serum after infection. When arthritis is present, immune complexes can be found in the joint fluid. Whether cell-mediated immunity also plays a role is not entirely clear.[16] The Lyme agent is sensitive to several antibiotics, including penicillin. Treatment early in the course of this disease is effective in preventing the major late sequelae such as arthritis.

## DEGENERATIVE JOINT DISEASE (OSTEOARTHRITIS)

Degenerative joint disease, more commonly known as osteoarthritis, is the commonest joint disease, affecting an estimated 40 million Americans, 85% of whom are above the age of 70 years. Since the major pathologic change appears to be degeneration of the articular cartilage and not inflammation, the term "degenerative joint disease" (DJD) is much preferred. DJD has been classified into two categories: primary, associated with aging, and secondary, which may occur in young persons when the articular cartilage has previously been damaged by injury, infection, or congenital deformities.

**MORPHOLOGY.** The spine and large joints of the body (i.e., those that are most subject to weight bearing) are principally affected, although small joints, including distal interphalangeal and the carpometacarpal joint of the thumb, may also be affected. The involvement may be either monoarticular or polyarticular. Unlike most arthritides, the major anatomic change is degeneration of the articular cartilage, rather than inflammation of the synovia. This degeneration manifests itself as fissuring and irregularity of the cartilaginous surfaces, followed by formation of vertical clefts in the cartilage, which may reach the subchondral bone (cartilage fibrillation). There is a decrease in the metachromatic staining capacity of the cartilage, which is thought to reflect depletion of proteoglycans. With moderately advanced disease, the chondrocytes show proliferative activity, presumably reparative. Ultimately, however, nearly all the chondrocytes undergo degeneration. The synovial membrane usually reveals some inflammatory changes by the time the disease is clinically apparent. In contrast to rheumatoid arthritis, however, the inflammation is not severe and there is no pannus formation (p. 160). With destruction of the articular cartilage, the underlying bone is exposed. This becomes thickened as a result of either compression or reactive new bone formation. Characteristic bony "spurs" project from the reactive bone at the margins of the joint space (Fig. 21–7). When large spurs project from opposing bones, they may come into contact with each other, causing pain and limiting motion. Either spurs or fragments of articular cartilage may break off, forming free intraarticular foreign bodies known as "joint mice."

**ETIOLOGY AND PATHOGENESIS.** The elasticity of the articular cartilage, and therefore its ability to withstand repeated load bearing, depends upon the pres-

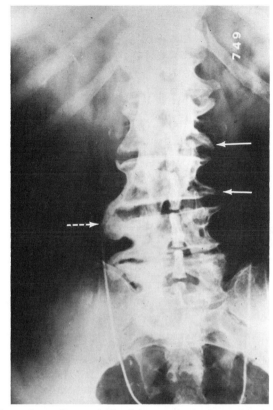

Figure 21–7. Osteoarthritis of the vertebral column. Prominent spur formation is seen along the intervertebral margins of the vertebral bodies (*solid arrows*). Fusion of the spurs has created a bony bridge (*dashed arrow*).

ence of water and several macromolecules in the cartilage matrix. The macromolecules include complexes containing proteins, glycosaminoglycan (proteoglycans), and type II collagen. Although it is clear that the degradation of the cartilage matrix is central to the pathogenesis of osteoarthritis, the etiologic factors that trigger this process have remained elusive. The common belief that changes in the cartilage result entirely from long-standing "wear and tear" has the merit of simplicity, but it is not entirely accurate.[17, 18] Current opinion favors DJD as a multifactorial process resulting from diverse influences, all of which affect the integrity of the joint. In addition to the degenerative changes that accompany aging, immunologically mediated tissue injury and ill-defined genetic factors are also presumed to contribute to the degradation of cartilage.

Regardless of the initiating factor, all lead to matrix depletion of the cartilage manifested as a decrease in proteoglycan content and an increase in water content. There are qualitative changes that affect chondroitin sulfate and other glycosaminoglycans as well. In response to these alterations, the normally quiescent chondrocytes are triggered into proliferation, and they attempt to replenish the matrix by increasing its synthesis. However, since the stimulated chondrocytes also secrete degradative enzymes, there is a continued net loss of proteoglycans. Recent evidence suggests that products of cartilage degradation such as collagen and cartilage fragments activate the synovial cells to liberate mediators such as IL-1 that in turn lead to further elaboration of hydrolytic enzymes by the chondrocytes.[19]

Coincident with changes in the cartilage is stiffening of the subchondral bone, which reduces its shock-absorbing capacity and predisposes the overlying cartilage to ever-increasing stress. Sclerotic changes in the subchondral bone are believed to result from attempted repair of microfractures, caused by years of repetitive trauma borne by the weight-bearing joints. Thus a vicious circle is set into motion and progressive joint damage ensues.

**CLINICAL COURSE.** In most cases, DJD appears insidiously as slowly progressive joint stiffness. Pain and crepitus on motion, as well as occasional swelling of affected joints, may be present. However, there are no constitutional signs of an inflammatory disease. Involvement of the spine may lead to compression of nerve roots and radicular pain. When spur formation affects the distal interphalangeal joints of the fingers, it appears clinically as firm, nodular enlargements of the joints, known as *Heberden's nodes*. These are more common in females than in males and constitute an important exception to the tendency of this form of arthritis to affect large, weight-bearing joints.

## RHEUMATOID ARTHRITIS

This very important type of arthritis is discussed in Chapter 5 because of its probable autoimmune pathogenesis and its systemic nature. Table 21–1 presents the major features that differentiate rheumatoid arthritis from osteoarthritis.

# TUMORS

## SYNOVIOSARCOMA

As its name implies, the synoviosarcoma is a malignant tumor arising in synovial membranes. These tumors are located, therefore, in the vicinity of joints and other synovium-lined structures such as tendon sheaths. Synoviosarcoma is the only tumor of joints that occurs with sufficient frequency to merit even a brief description. Often the misnomer "synovioma" is applied to it, despite its clearly malignant behavior. The tumor shows no sex preponderance and most often develops after middle age.

In 75% of cases, the lesion arises somewhere in the leg. It may grow rapidly, attaining a size of 15 cm or more in diameter. Histologically, the synoviosarcoma is quite pleomorphic, typically revealing a biphasic cell pattern tending to recapitulate the differentiation of cuboidal synovial cells from a more primitive spindle-shaped fibroblasts. Thus, there may be sheets of fusiform cells merging with cuboidal epithelium, which lines cleft-like spaces that may contain serous or mucinous secretion similar to the fluid found within joint spaces. Monophasic spindled or epithelium-like patterns are less common. The 10-year survival is about 50%.

## GANGLION

This is a small cystic swelling, up to 2 cm in diameter, that arises from a joint capsule or tendon sheath; it is usually found on the wrist but occasionally occurs on the foot or knee. Anatomically, it consists of a collagenous fibrous wall that is filled with mucoid fluid. They are thought to arise as a result of localized myxoid degeneration of connective tissue.

Table 21–1. MAJOR DIFFERENCES BETWEEN RHEUMATOID ARTHRITIS AND DEGENERATIVE JOINT DISEASE

| | Rheumatoid Arthritis | Degenerative Joint Disease |
|---|---|---|
| Age at onset | Third and fourth decades | Fifth and sixth decades |
| Weight | Normal or underweight | Usually overweight |
| Constitutional manifestations | Present | Absent |
| Joints involved | Any joint (classically bilateral symmetrical proximal interphalangeal and metacarpophalangeal joints) | Mainly knees, hips, spine, and distal interphalangeal joints |
| Appearance of joints | Soft tissue swelling | Bony swelling |
| Special deformities | Fusiform finger joints, ulnar deviation | Heberden's nodes |
| Subcutaneous nodules | Present in 20% | Never present |
| X-ray | Osteoporosis, erosions | Osteosclerosis and spurs |
| Joint fluid | Increased cells, poor mucin | Few cells; good mucin |
| Rheumatoid factors | Usually present | Usually absent |
| Blood count | Anemia and leukocytosis | Normal |
| Erythrocyte sedimentation rate | Markedly elevated | Normal |
| Course | Often progressive | Slow or stationary |
| Termination | Ankylosis and deformity; amyloidosis | No ankylosis and no amyloidosis |

# Muscles

## MUSCLE ATROPHY

At the outset we should distinguish between muscle atrophy and dystrophy, both of which may be associated with regressive changes in muscles. Muscle atrophy, as you would predict, is an acquired lesion secondary to some well-defined predisposing cause; muscular dystrophy, on the other hand, refers to a variety of genetically determined primary disorders of muscles, to be discussed later.

Atrophic shrinkage, death, and disappearance of muscle cells occur under a variety of circumstances, some generalized and some local. Among the systemic disorders are chronic malnutrition, panhypopituitarism, prolonged immobilization, SLE, dermatomyositis, and advanced age (which presumably leads to muscle atrophy on the basis of diffuse ischemia). In these disorders, entire muscles are affected more or less uniformly.

Localized muscle atrophy results from interference with the innervation and may be caused by traumatic denervation or by neuromuscular disorders such as polio, the peripheral neuritides, and a variety of fortunately rare degenerative neuropathies. Obviously, the distribution of the muscle atrophy depends upon the pattern of involvement of the nerves. Whole muscles, bundles of cells, or only a single neuromuscular unit may be affected.

When the process is generalized or when large bundles of myocytes are involved, the affected muscles become shrunken and flabby. On the other hand, minute focal involvements may produce no appreciable loss of muscle mass, since adjacent unaffected fibers undergo compensatory hypertrophy. Within the affected area, the histologic changes consist of reduction in the size of myofibers accompanied by an apparent increase in the number of sarcolemmal nuclei. With denervation, the atrophic fibers are grouped together (Fig. 21–8). The cross-striations are preserved for a long time after the shrinkage of myofibers. In later stages, the myofibers show degenerative changes with loss of striations and accumulation of lipofuscin pigment. Eventually, the myofibers are reduced to hollow tubes enclosed by sarcolemma. There is apparent increase in endomysial and perimysial connective tissue,

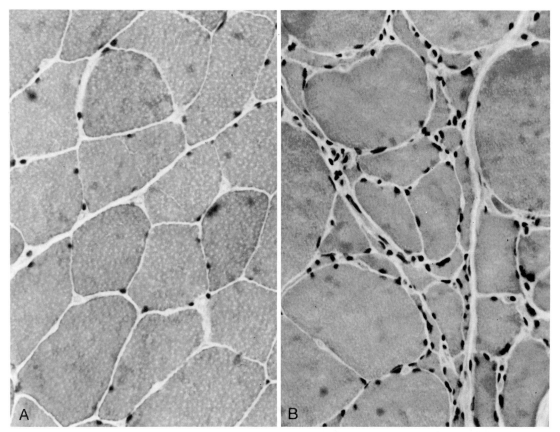

**Figure 21–8.** Normal and atrophic muscle (denervation atrophy). *A,* Fibers in the normal muscle are polygonal in shape and regular in diameter. Myofiber nuclei are located peripherally, at the sarcolemma. The amount of interstitial connective tissue is minimal. *B,* Atrophic fibers, interspersed with preserved fibers, are angulated and show a tendency to cluster (group atrophy). Myofiber nuclei retain their peripheral location, but they appear more numerous owing to a decrease in the amount of sacroplasm in atrophic fibers. (Courtesy of Dr. Charles L. White, Department of Pathology, Southwestern Medical School, Dallas, Texas.)

which accumulates scattered fat cells. Finally, sarcolemmal tubes disintegrate and are removed by macrophages.

## MUSCULAR DYSTROPHY

This term refers to *a group of genetically determined myopathies characterized by progressive atrophy or degeneration of increasing numbers of individual muscle cells.*[20] The histologic changes in the various types of muscular dystrophies are basically the same. However, the distribution of the affected muscles is quite distinctive. This, along with the mode of inheritance, forms the basis of the classification discussed below. Muscular dystrophies must be distinguished from *congenital myopathies, which are characterized by fairly specific distinctive morphologic changes.*[21] The pathogenesis of muscular dystrophies remains unknown. There is no lack of theories, but supporting evidence is scanty. Some evidence suggests the existence of a generalized

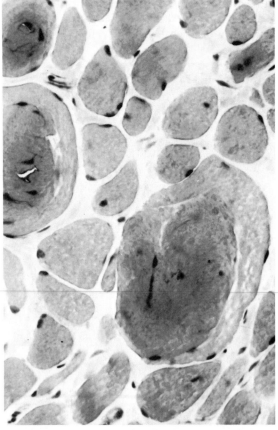

Figure 21–9. Muscular dystrophy. Numerous rounded atrophic fibers coexist with hypertrophied fibers. A few fibers show fragmentation (degenerative change). Several contain nuclei that have migrated toward the center of their fibers (regenerative change). Between muscle fibers there is significant fibrosis of the endomysium. Compare with normal and atrophic muscle in Figure 21–8. (Courtesy of Dr. Charles L. White, Department of Pathology, Southwestern Medical School, Dallas, Texas.)

membrane defect, which also involves cells other than myofibers.[22]

The involved muscles are shrunken, pale, and flabby. With the light microscope, individual muscle cells can be seen to be randomly affected, so that myocytes in various stages of degeneration may lie adjacent to abnormally large ones (Fig. 21–9). The coexistence of degenerative and regenerative changes in adjacent myocytes is in contrast with the grouped atrophy that characterizes denervation of the muscle. Degenerative changes include focal vacuolation, hyalinization, fragmentation of the cytoplasm, and shrinkage from the investing sarcolemmal sheath. Eventually, necrosis and phagocytosis of the fibers occurs. Dead fibers are replaced by fibrous and fatty tissue, which may cause the muscles to appear deceptively large (pseudohypertrophy). Regenerative changes include cytoplasmic basophilia, internal migration of sarcolemmal nuclei, and fiber splitting.

The muscular dystrophies are traditionally subdivided according to the patterns of initial muscle involvement, which in turn correlates fairly well with the type of genetic transmission. Despite such differences, however, it should be remembered that the histologic changes are very similar in all forms. The four major patterns in their order of prevalence are as follows:

1. Duchenne (pseudohypertrophic) muscular dystrophy: X-linked recessive
2. Myotonic dystrophy: autosomal dominant
3. Limb-girdle muscular dystrophy: autosomal recessive
4. Facioscapulohumeral muscular dystrophy: autosomal dominant

Only the two most common forms will be briefly described here. *Duchenne muscular dystrophy* is transmitted as an X-linked recessive trait and therefore affects males almost exclusively. The onset of muscle weakness occurs soon after birth, involving initially the pelvic girdle and later the shoulder girdle. A characteristic feature is enlargement or "pseudohypertrophy" of the calf muscles. Complete paralysis and death usually ensue within the first two decades of life. The diagnosis can usually be made by family history and clinical features and can be confirmed by biopsy and electromyography. Since the muscle fibers are richly endowed with several enzymes such as creatine kinase (CK), glutamic-oxaloacetic transaminase (GOT), cytidine triphosphate (CTP), and lactate dehydrogenase (LDH), the serum levels for these substances are elevated.

*Myotonic dystrophy,* in contrast to the Duchenne's type, usually sets in during early adulthood and is slowly progressive. Cranial muscles are frequently affected, and the involvement of the limbs usually begins with weakness of the distal muscles of hands and feet. An unusual feature of myotonic dystrophy is the impaired relaxation (tonic contraction) of the limb muscles. Unlike the case in other forms of muscular dystrophy, extraskeletal manifestations such as cataracts and testicular atrophy are also noted.

## MYOSITIS

Inflammation of the muscles may be encountered in a variety of clinical settings. Direct invasion by bacteria, virus, parasites, and fungi may occur in the course of systemic infections, or, less commonly, the muscle involvement may be primary (e.g., trichinosis, p. 720). Bacterial toxins, such as those produced by *Clostridium perfringens*, may injure muscle cells in the absence of direct bacterial invasion. Inflammatory myositis may also be encountered in many of the so-called connective tissue diseases, most of which are believed to be immunologic in origin. One such immunologic disorder that affects muscles predominantly, polymyositis-dermatomyositis, was discussed earlier in Chapter 5.

## MYASTHENIA GRAVIS

Myasthenia gravis is a relapsing, remitting neuromuscular disorder characterized by weakness and pronounced fatigability of the skeletal muscles. The disease may occur at any age, but the peak age of onset is 20 years; a second, smaller peak occurs in late adult life, at which time males are predominantly affected. In the younger age group females outnumber males by 3 to 1. There is a significant correlation between this age distribution and the occurrence of thymic lesions. Older males are likely to have thymic tumors, whereas young females tend to have thymic hyperplasia, as will be discussed later in greater detail.

**PATHOGENESIS.** Myasthenia gravis results from defective neuromuscular transmission across the motor end-plates of skeletal muscles. You may recall that skeletal contraction is triggered by interactions between acetylcholine released from the nerve terminals and acetylcholine receptors present on the motor end-plate. *In myasthenia gravis there is a severe reduction in acetylcholine receptors due to an autoimmune reaction directed against the receptor proteins.*[23] IgG antibodies against the acetylcholine receptors are found in the serum of over 85% of these patients.[24] These antibodies and C3 have been localized at the postsynaptic membranes of the neuromuscular junction. The antireceptor antibodies act by several mechanisms, the most important of which is the accelerated degradation of receptor proteins, leading to reduction in receptor concentration (Fig. 21–10). Complement-mediated lysis of the postsynaptic membranes and direct interference with the transmission of impulses also occur.

Despite the compelling evidence for the role of acetylcholine receptor antibodies in myasthenia

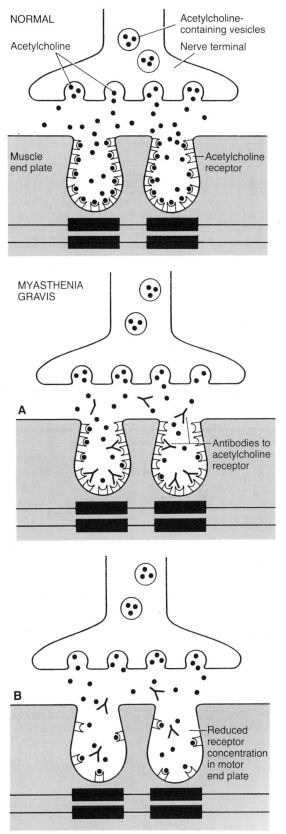

**Figure 21–10.** Normal neuromuscular junction (*top*) and the changes induced by the anti-acetylcholine-receptor antibody found in myasthenia gravis (*A* and *B*).

gravis, there is no good correlation between the titer of these antibodies and the degree of clinical weakness, suggesting that factors other than antibodies may also be involved. These factors could include a T cell–mediated attack on the receptors, but firm evidence is lacking.

About 75% of the patients with myasthenia gravis have thymic abnormalities. Ten to 15% (usually older males) have thymic tumors, whereas the others (younger females) have thymic hyperplasia. The hyperplastic thymus shows germinal centers that contain B cells, which can be shown to be active in secreting acetylcholine receptor antibodies. The presence of profound changes within the thymus adds strength to the hypothesis that immunologic aberrations are central to the pathogenesis of myasthenia gravis. Several other disorders of presumed autoimmune origin, such as pernicious anemia, rheumatoid arthritis, certain thyroid diseases, and systemic lupus erythematosus, all occur more commonly in patients with myasthenia gravis than in the general population. As in most other autoimmune diseases, genetic susceptibility may be important (p. 151). For example, there is an increased frequency of HLA-B8 in young females with myasthenia gravis. It is possible that environmental factors may trigger the autoimmune reactions in individuals who are genetically susceptible to loss of self-tolerance.[25]

In most cases, the muscles appear entirely normal, both grossly and by the light microscope. Subtle alterations can be seen in the motor end-plate under the electron microscope. Occasionally, small interstitial accumulations of lymphocytes are found. The thymus usually shows hyperplasia with the abnormal development of germinal follicles within the medulla. In addition, thymic tumors, usually of the epithelial type, may be present. (Reference should be made to page 700 for a description of thymic hyperplasia and the thymomas.)

**CLINICAL COURSE.** Myasthenia gravis manifests itself by slow to rapidly mounting fatigue of skeletal muscles. The muscles most severely involved are those in most active use: the extraocular muscles and those of the face, tongue, and extremities. In severely affected patients there is involvement of the respiratory muscles, which may lead to asphyxia. Usually the disease follows a long chronic course, interspersed with periods of spontaneous remission. The prognosis is highly variable and is not predictable in any one patient. Patients with myasthenia gravis respond dramatically to such anticholinesterase drugs as neostigmine. Indeed, lack of response should cast doubt on the diagnosis. However, acetylcholinesterase inhibitors do not completely reverse the symptoms, nor do they affect the course of the disease. Hence, treatment with immunosuppressive drugs such as steroids is often necessary. Thymectomy is beneficial in a large percentage of patients. Plasmapheresis has also been used to remove circulating acetylcholine-receptor antibodies.

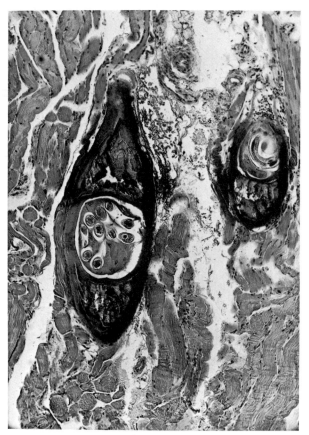

Figure 21–11. Trichinosis. Encysted parasites can be seen in striated muscle. The cyst on the right shows a coiled worm cut longitudinally. On the left, the parasite has been cut in numerous cross sections.

## TRICHINOSIS

This common disorder is caused by infection with the larvae of *Trichinella spiralis*. Some degree of infection, often subclinical, has been reported in about 4% of autopsies in the United States. Humans contract the disease by eating poorly cooked infected meat, usually pork. The larvae, encysted in the muscle cells of the meat, are released within the stomach and mature to adult worms within the duodenum. Here the female worm penetrates partially through the wall of the duodenum and her newly deposited larvae thus gain access to the bloodstream. They circulate throughout the pulmonic and systemic systems, ultimately emerging from capillaries to invade their preferred sites. The striated muscles provide the most suitable environment for their survival. The heaviest concentrations are usually found in the diaphragm and in the gluteus, pectoral, deltoid, gastrocnemius, and intercostal muscles. The brain and the heart also are frequently involved. However, no tissue or organ is exempt.

In the striated muscles the larvae penetrate the fibers and become enclosed in a membrane produced by the muscle cell.[26] The muscle cell is not killed. After several years of apparently peaceful coexistence, the larva and its host cell die, thus evoking an inflammatory reaction characterized principally by lymphocytes and eosinophils (Fig. 21–11). Fibrosis and calcification of the cysts ensue, yielding multiple minute radiodensities readily seen in the muscles on x-ray examination. In the heart, penetration of the fibers results in their death, and this evokes a widespread interstitial myocarditis. Encystment does not take place. Invasion of the central nervous system is usually reflected by a diffuse mononuclear infiltration in the leptomeninges and by the development of focal gliosis in and about the small capillaries of the brain substance.

The clinical manifestations of trichinosis depend on the size of the infection and on the stage of the involvement.[27] In most cases, the disease is mild or subclinical. With severe infection, the stage of invasion of the intestinal mucosa is usually marked by vomiting and diarrhea. During the hematogenous dissemination and muscular invasion, fever and widespread aches and pains appear. Muscle aches may persist. Often, invasion of the lungs evokes cough and dyspnea. Involvement of the central nervous system leads to headaches, disorientation, delirium, and other neurologic impairments. Heart failure may ensue when the myocardial injury is severe. The mortality rate is, however, low.

After the third week of the disease, the results of precipitin, complement fixation, and flocculation tests are positive except in overwhelming disease. The diagnosis may be established by muscle biopsy. In addition, it is strongly supported by the presence of a peripheral eosinophilia, which may constitute up to 70% of the circulating white cell count.

The exposure to live parasites can be easily avoided. Trichinae are killed by cooking at 60°C. for 30 minutes per pound of meat or by freezing of the meat at −15°C for 20 days.

# TUMORS

## DESMOID TUMOR

This refers to a curious fibrous proliferation that arises from the aponeuroses of muscles. Although histologically it appears quite benign and only rarely, if ever, does it metastasize, this lesion may be locally invasive. In this respect desmoid tumors resemble low-grade fibrosarcomas and may be considered to lie somewhere between hyperplastic and truly neoplastic proliferations. About 70% of desmoids occur in young women, frequently after pregnancy, and these usually affect the musculature of the anterior abdominal wall. However, men may also develop desmoids, and nearly any muscle of the body may be involved.

Desmoids appear grossly as firm, gray-white, poorly demarcated masses varying in size from small nodules 1 to 2 cm in diameter to large masses up to 15 cm in diameter. Microscopically, they resemble a somewhat cellular fibroma, with abundant collagenous fibrous tissue. The fibrocytes, which are uniform and innocent-appearing, insinuate themselves between muscle groups and individual muscle cells, frequently destroying the trapped myocytes.

The clinical presentation is of a slowly enlarging subcutaneous mass, sometimes but not usually producing pain.

## RHABDOMYOSARCOMA

These are highly malignant, but fortunately rare, tumors of striated muscle. Three distinct histologic and clinical patterns are recognized: (1) adult pleomorphic, (2) alveolar, and (3) embryonal. Although the adult pattern is least common, it will be described first, since it is more likely to contain the specific features indicating its origin from striated muscles. *Desmin, a muscle-specific intermediate filament, can be demonstrated by the immunoperoxidase technique in all variants.*[28]

**Adult pleomorphic rhabdomyosarcomas** occur in either sex, usually in individuals between the ages of 30 and 60 years. The lower extremities are most often involved. The tumor mass grows extremely rapidly and may be as large as 25 cm in diameter when the patient comes to medical attention. Grossly, these tumors are deeply situated within muscles and are composed of soft, gray-red, fish-flesh tissue, with areas of necrosis and hemorrhage. Since the tumors are typically quite pleomorphic, the light microscope may show a variety of cell types—sometimes racket-shaped cells with single, long protoplasmic processes; occasionally ovoid giant cells with peripheral vacuoles separated by thin strands of cytoplasm (**spider-web cells**); but most often sheets of varying-sized, totally undifferentiated cells. With luck, persistent searching will usually disclose characteristic striated cells that resemble normal myocytes. **With the identification of such cells or the intracellular localization of desmin, the diagnosis of rhabdomyosarcoma can be made with certainty.**

**Alveolar rhabdomyosarcomas** occur mainly in individuals who are 10 to 25 years old, and these tumors usually develop in a lower or upper extremity but occasionally involve the trunk. Grossly, these tumors may be similar in appearance to the adult rhabdomyosarcoma, although they rarely achieve such massive dimensions. Microscopically, the tumor cells are quite undifferentiated and round or oval. They typically are arranged in small nests or rosettes separated by an interlacing fibrous stroma. This stroma creates some resemblance to the alveolar pattern of the lung—with the neoplastic cells filling the "alveolar" spaces—hence the name. Intermingled with these are occasional multinucleate giant cells with deeply eosinophilic cytoplasm and, rarely, cells with cross striations.

**Embryonal rhabdomyosarcomas** occur most commonly in children and involve various sites such as the genitourinary tract, biliary passages, and the orbit. Very few involve the extremities. Those of the vagina are often termed **sarcoma botryoides** and were mentioned briefly on page 636. The term "botryoid" (grape-like) refers to the gross appearance of these cancers, which grow as large, pedunculated, multilobate masses resembling a cluster of grapes. The predominant cell type within these tumors is an undifferentiated, small, round or spindle-shaped cell that has a large hyperchromatic central nucleus and scant cytoplasm. An abundant loose myxoid stroma may be present. With careful searching, racket-shaped cells and elongated ribbon-like cells with cross-striations can be found.

Rhabdomyosarcomas in general are very aggressive tumors. Widespread dissemination tends to occur early, especially in the pleomorphic and alveolar variants. Their five-year survival rate is 10 to 30%. The embryonal type is less aggressive, and the localized lesions have a cure rate of up to 80%.

## References

1. Tannenbaum, H.: Osteopenia in rheumatology practice: Pathogenesis and therapy. Semin. Arthritis Rheum. 13:337, 1984.
2. Aloia, J. F., et al.: Risk factors for postmenopausal osteoporosis. Am. J. Med. 78:95, 1985.
3. Riggs, B. L., and Melton, L. J.: Involutional osteoporosis. N. Engl. J. Med. 314:1673, 1986.
4. Meier, D., et al.: Marked disparity between trabecular and cortical bone loss with age in healthy men. Ann. Intern. Med. 101:605, 1984.
5. Ettiger, B., et al.: Long-term estrogen replacement therapy prevents bone loss and fractures. Ann. Intern. Med. 102:319, 1985.
6. Mills, B. G., et al.: Evidence for both respiratory syncytial virus and measles virus antigens in the osteoclasts of patients with Paget's disease of bone. Clin. Orthop. 183:303, 1984.
7. Strewler, G. J.: Paget's disease of bone. West J. Med. 140:763, 1984.
8. Grabias, S. L., Campbell, C. J.: Fibrous dysplasia. Orthop. Clin. North Am. 8:771, 1977.
9. Goorin, A. M., et al.: Osteosarcoma: Fifteen years later. N. Engl. J. Med. 313:1637, 1985.
10. Dahlin, D. C., and Unni, K. K.: Osteosarcoma of bone and its important recognizable varieties. Am. J. Surg. Pathol. 1:61, 1977.
11. Burmester, C. R., et al.: Delineation of four cell types comprising the giant cell tumor of bone. J. Clin. Invest. 71:1633, 1983.
12. Schajowicz, F.: Current trends in the diagnosis and treatment of malignant bone tumors. Clin. Orthop. 180:220, 1983.
13. Navas-Palacios, J. J., et al.: On the histogenesis of Ewing's sarcoma: An ultrastructural, immuohistochemical, and cytochemical study. Cancer 53:1882, 1984.
14. Goldenberg, D. L., and Reed, J. I.: Bacterial arthritis. N. Engl. J. Med. 312:764, 1985.
15. Malawista, S. E., and Steere, A. C.: Lyme disease: Infectious in origin, rheumatic in expression. Adv. Intern. Med. 31:147, 1986.
16. Moffat, C. M., et al.: Cellular immune findings in Lyme disease. Am. J. Med. 77:625, 1984.
17. Bland, J. H., and Cooper, S. M.: Osteoarthritis: A review of the cell biology involved and evidence for reversibility. Management rationally related to known genesis and pathophysiology. Semin. Arthritis Rheum. 14:106, 1984.
18. Howell, D. S.: Pathogenesis of osteoarthritis. Am. J. Med. 80(Suppl. 4B):24, 1986.
19. Hamerman, D., and Klagsburn, M.: Osteoarthritis. Emerging evidence for cell interaction in the breakdown and remodeling of cartilage. Am. J. Med. 78:495, 1985.
20. Gardner-Medwin, D.: Clinical features and classification of muscular dystrophies. Br. Med. Bull. 36:109, 1980.
21. Dubowitz, V. (ed.): The congenital myopathies. In Dubowitz, V. (ed.): Muscle Disorders in Childhood. Philadelphia, W. B. Saunders Co., 1978, p. 70.
22. Pickard, N. A., et al.: Systemic membrane defect in proximal muscular dystrophies, N. Engl. J. Med. 299:136, 1978.
23. Seybold, M. E.: Myasthenia Gravis. A clinical and basic science review. J.A.M.A. 250:2516, 1983.
24. Vincent, A.: Acetylcholine receptors and myasthenia gravis. Clin. Endocrinol. Metab. 12:57, 1983.
25. Stefansson, K., et al.: Sharing of antigenic determinants between the nicotinic acetylcholine receptor and proteins in Escherichia coli, Proteus vulgaris and Klebsiella pneumoniae. Possible role in the pathogenesis of myasthenia gravis. N. Engl. J. Med. 312:221, 1985.
26. Despommier, D.: Adaptive changes in muscle fibers infected with Trichinella spiralis. Am. J. Pathol. 78:447, 1975.
27. Most, H.: Trichinosis, preventable yet still with us. N. Engl. J. Med. 298:1178, 1978.
28. Altmannsberger, M., et al.: Desmin is a specific marker for rhabdomyosarcomas of human and rat origin. Am. J. Pathol. 118:85, 1985.

# 22

# The Nervous System

JAMES H. MORRIS, M.A., D.Phil., B.M., B.Ch.*

To even the least introspective it is readily apparent that the brain is an organ of great complexity of organization and subtlety of operation. To an extent this complexity and subtlety are reflected in the pathologic disorders of the brain, and this can make neuropathology appear very intimidating to the be-

ginner. However, most of the ways that neuropathology differs from the pathology of the rest of the body are only a reflection of the differences between the brain and the other organs. Once these differences are understood—and they are quite easy to appreciate—much of the difficulty of neuropathology disappears. The most important of these differences are discussed below.

1. It is well known that different parts of the brain

---

*Pathologist, Brigham and Women's Hospital; Assistant Professor of Pathology, Harvard Medical School, Boston, Massachusetts perform different functions. This *localization of function* is the single most important difference between the brain and the rest of the body, and it has a number of consequences.

    a. The most important pathologic consequence of this localization of function is that a small focal lesion in the brain can produce a selective, and severe, deficit in a single function—for example, speech. The brain has, therefore, an *inherent vulnerability to small focal lesions* that is not seen in other organs such as the liver or the lung, in which one part of the organ performs much the same function as any other part and quite a large fraction of the organ can be destroyed without fatally compromising any particular function.

    b. Localization also accounts for the fact that *the same types of focal lesions, such as tumors, occurring in different parts of the nervous system (e.g., the frontal lobe or the spinal cord), will produce quite different manifestations.*

    c. In a different sense, localization is also important in pathologic diagnosis. Like other organs, *the brain has only a limited repertoire of pathologic responses, and the same type of pathologic change (e.g., neurofibrillary tangle formation) occurs in more than one disease.* Diagnosis then rests on the localization, or distribution, of tangles in the brain.

2. Although most diseases of the brain have their counterparts in other organs, *there are some disorders, namely, diseases of neurons and myelin, that are peculiar to the nervous system.* They are much less frequent than the diseases with systemic counterparts (e.g., infections, infarcts, and hemorrhages).

3. *The brain has a number of anatomic and physiologic features that very much affect the way that disease is expressed.* Many of these special features are double-edged swords, conferring protection against one form of attack while rendering the brain more vulnerable to another. The most important are the *skull*, which protects against trauma but makes possible raised intracranial pressure and herniation; the *cerebrospinal fluid*, which also protects against trauma but, conversely, is the medium for the development of hydrocephalus and for the dissemination of microorganisms and tumors; and the *absence of lymphatic drainage*, which makes the brain particularly sensitive to edema.

# NEURONS AND GLIAL CELLS—BASIC REACTIONS

The brain substance is composed of neurons embedded in a specialized supporting framework of glial cells—astrocytes, oligodendrocytes, ependymal cells, and the so-called microglia.

## Neurons

The typical neuron is the cortical pyramidal cell that has a large nucleus with watery chromatin and a prominent nucleolus. The cytoplasm contains clumps of rough-surfaced endoplasmic reticulum that stains strongly with basic dyes such as hematoxylin and is called *Nissl substance.* From this cell body, multiple dendrites and an axon emerge to make contact with other neurons at *synapses* and endow the brain with its unique conduction properties. Neurons, like people, come in a wide variety of shapes and sizes, ranging from the small granular cells of the cerebellar cortex to the large Betz cells of the motor cortex.

Neurons undergo a variety of different types of degeneration, many of which are associated with specific diseases or types of pathologic process, and these will be described with their diseases.

## Astrocytes

Normal astrocytes have an oval nucleus with finely dispersed chromatin and, as revealed by special stains, cytoplasmic processes extending through the tissue or attached to the walls of cerebral blood vessels by "end feet." They occur in two morphologic forms, *protoplasmic astrocytes,* which have more processes and are present in gray matter, and *fibrous astrocytes,* which are mostly in the white matter. In normal brain tissue, astrocytes act to insulate the electrically active processes from each other and stabilize the ionic constituents of the extracellular space. They also play a role in the maintenance of the blood-brain barrier.

In damaged brain tissue, astrocytes act rather like the fibroblasts in the rest of the body. When there is severe destruction, they produce a dense feltwork of cellular processes forming a *glial "scar."* An important difference between gliosis and fibrosis is that astrocytes do not produce an extracellular fibrous protein equivalent to collagen, so that glial scars are composed entirely of cellular processes. Early reactive astrocytes develop conspicuous pink cytoplasm, and the nucleus, which in this activated state may have a nucleolus, is often displaced to one side of the cytoplasm. In this state they are often called *gemistocytic* (stuffed) *astrocytes.* As the process resolves, astrocytes lose their cytoplasm but retain their processes and are then called *fibrillary astrocytes.* When there is prolonged stimulus to astrocytic reaction, *Rosenthal fibers* may form. These are elongated, irregular, densely eosinophilic structures in the astrocyte processes. They are found in some slowly growing tumors, notably pilocytic astrocytomas, and sometimes around chronic irritative lesions such as cavernous angiomas. *Corpora amylacea* are small, spherical inclusions in astrocyte processes that tend to accumulate with age under the pia and around blood vessels. They are composed of polyglucosans, which are nondegradable carbohydrates. They do not have a specific pathologic significance.

## Oligodendrocytes

As is implied by their name, these cells have fewer processes than astrocytes. Typically, they have a small, dark, lymphocyte-sized nucleus around which there is often a clear halo that is, although regularly present, an artifact of fixation. They are found in both gray and white matter, and, in the former, they often form small clusters around neurons, where they are called *satellite cells*. Their function is to produce the myelin that surrounds the axons in the central nervous system. Unlike the Schwann cells of the peripheral nervous system, in which there is only one Schwann cell per myelin internode, oligodendrocytes may produce myelin for several internodes of different axons.

*Myelin* is composed of oligodendrocyte cell membrane that is spirally wound around the axons. The membrane is modified by the addition of proteins such as myelin basic protein and myelin-associated glycoprotein. Removal of or damage to the myelin, such as occurs in the *demyelinating diseases* and the *leukodystrophies*, may either slow the conduction of the nerve impulse or stop it altogether.

## Ependymal Cells

The cerebral ventricles are lined by a single layer of ciliated cuboidal cells called ependymal cells. They do not play a prominent part in most reactions, but focal loss of these cells is followed by a compensatory proliferation of subependymal astrocytes, which produces small nodules on the walls of the ventricles, an appearance called *granular ependymitis*. These nodules are not etiologically specific but are seen in neurosyphilis as well as other disorders. Ependymal cells may also be the principal target of some pathologic processes, notably cytomegalovirus infection.

## Microglia

In spite of their name, these cells are the central nervous system's representative of the mononuclear-phagocyte system. In normal brain tissue they are very inconspicuous. Routine stains show only scattered, small, dark, elongated nuclei, though a few cytoplasmic processes are revealed by special stains. When they are stimulated by cerebral damage, their nuclei enlarge and become even more elongated, in which form they are called *rod cells*. More severe tissue damage results in the appearance of foamy macrophages (*gitter cells*) in the brain, most of which come from the bloodstream. There is still some dispute over whether microglia can turn into foamy macrophages.

# COMMON PATHOPHYSIOLOGIC COMPLICATIONS

*Raised intracranial pressure, cerebral herniation, cerebral edema*, and *hydrocephalus* are pathophysiologic complications that occur in a number of different disease processes. They are also interrelated; cerebral edema and hydrocephalus are both causes of raised intracranial pressure and may also produce cerebral herniation.

## RAISED INTRACRANIAL PRESSURE AND CEREBRAL HERNIATION

As has already been mentioned, the brain is enclosed in a rigid skull that, while it affords protection against injury, of necessity also restricts expansion of the intracranial contents. Small expansions can be accommodated by shifts of cerebrospinal fluid (CSF) and reduction in venous volume, but any further increase in intracranial volume will cause a rise in intracranial pressure. The principal detrimental effect of this rise in pressure is a reduction in cerebral arterial perfusion pressure and, therefore, cerebral blood flow. Small rises in intracranial pressure are compensated for by rises in the arterial blood pressure, but at higher levels of intracranial pressure (persistent elevation above 20 mm Hg) there is a progressive fall in cerebral perfusion pressure and blood flow and an increasing cerebral ischemia.

There are many causes of raised intracranial pressure, of which focal space-occupying lesions such as hemorrhages, tumors, and abscesses are obvious examples, but more diffuse processes such as edema, hydrocephalus, and meningitis also elevate intracranial pressure.

Clinically, the first symptom of raised intracranial pressure is usually headache, which typically is worst in the early morning. If intracranial pressure is raised for more than a week or two, papilledema of the head of the optic nerve and retinal hemorrhages may develop secondary to compression of the venous drainage, with consequent congestion of the retinal vasculature. With increasing severity, there may be dizziness, vomiting, and drowsiness progressing to coma. If the cause of the raised pressure cannot be eradicated or controlled, death will occur; raised intracranial pressure is often, in fact, the immediate cause of death in patients with fatal neurological disease.

*Cerebral herniation* is one of the most ominous developments in patients with focal space-occupying lesions or diffuse brain swelling. The skull cavity is partly divided into compartments by dural folds. These are the *falx cerebri*, which separates the cerebral hemispheres, and the *tentorium cerebelli*, separating the cerebellar hemispheres from the occipital poles of the cerebral hemispheres. Focal enlargement of any one compartment will tend to displace brain into adjacent compartments. This is called *herniation*.

There are three important types of herniation (Fig. 22–1). (1) *Subfalcine* (cingulate) herniation occurs when the cingulate gyrus herniates under the falx. (2) In *uncinate* (uncal, transtentorial) herniation, the

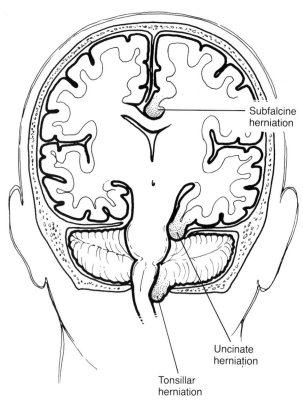

Figure 22–1. Herniations of the brain: subfalcine (cingulate), uncinate (uncal, transtentorial), and tonsillar. (Adapted from Fishman, R. A.: Brain edema. N. Engl. J. Med. 293:706, 1975. Adapted, with permission, from The New England Journal of Medicine.)

uncus of the temporal lobe is displaced medially and downwards through the incisura of the tentorium. This displacement also stretches the oculomotor (third cranial) nerve, causing a characteristic pupillary dilatation on the same side as the lesion. (3) *Tonsillar herniation* is displacement of the cerebellar tonsils through the foramen magnum. This compresses the medulla and its respiratory center which, if not relieved, will cause respiratory irregularities and eventually apnea and death.

In addition to the local compression of the herniated tissue, there are some secondary consequences of herniation. Downward displacement of the brain stem in uncinate herniation may rupture blood vessels in the mesencephalon and produce *Duret hemorrhages*. Kinking of arteries over the sharp edge of the dural partitions can cause distal infarction in the territory of the anterior cerebral artery in subfalcine herniation and of the posterior cerebral artery in uncinate herniation.

## CEREBRAL EDEMA

Because the brain is enclosed within the skull and therefore sensitive to quite small volume changes, it is severely affected by cerebral edema, which not only exacerbates the local effects of lesions but also causes raised intracranial pressure. This basic structural sensitivity of the brain to the volume effects of edema is exaggerated by the *absence of lymphatics*. The task of volume regulation is further complicated by the requirement for stability of the ionic composition of the extracellular fluid. Volume control in the brain is largely achieved at the *blood-brain barrier*, which regulates both the movement of molecules and bulk fluid flow.[1] The barrier is located at the capillary endothelium, which has tight junctions between the cells and a much smaller number of pinocytotic vesicles than are found in usual capillary endothelial cells.

There are two common types of cerebral edema. *Vasogenic edema* occurs because of bulk leakage of fluid across damaged or incompetent cerebral capillaries. *It is extracellular in location and is seen in white matter;* the gray matter is conspicuously spared. The edema may be general or focal, but is characteristically seen around mass lesions and is typically most apparent around lesions that exhibit marked capillary proliferation, such as metastatic implants and abscesses. This is probably because the newly formed capillaries do not have a properly functioning blood-brain barrier.

*Cytotoxic edema is an intracellular accumulation of excess fluid, and it affects gray matter more than white.* It results from processes such as ischemia or toxic exposure that impair the function of the cell membrane or ion pump, destroy the osmotic equilibrium of the cell, and lead to the ingress of excess water and other molecules into the cell. It is not infrequent for both types of edema to occur together in, for example, ischemic encephalopathy.

## HYDROCEPHALUS

Hydrocephalus means simply an increase in the volume of cerebrospinal fluid. Two general types occur.

*Hydrocephalus with normal CSF pressure* (compensatory hydrocephalus, hydrocephalus ex vacuo). In this type the volume of CSF is increased because the volume of the brain is decreased. Focal loss of brain substance, such as occurs in infarcts, is compensated for by local expansions of the ventricles or subarachnoid space, whereas diffuse atrophy, as occurs in Alzheimer's disease, is reflected in a general enlargement of the cerebral ventricles and widening of the cortical sulci.

*Hydrocephalus with raised CSF pressure.* This type of hydrocephalus can occur only because of the circulation pattern of the CSF. Cerebrospinal fluid is produced by the choroid plexus in the cerebral ventricles. From the lateral ventricles, the fluid flows through the foramina of Monro into the third ventricle and from there via the aqueduct of Sylvius into the fourth ventricle before it emerges into the sub-

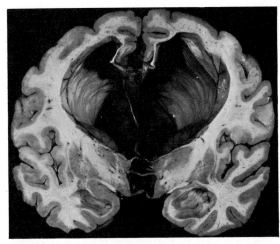

Figure 22–2. Hydrocephalus of moderate degree. This was associated with an Arnold-Chiari malformation. The basal ganglia have been displaced downward and laterally, and the overlying corpus callosum has been thinned.

arachnoid space around the medulla through the foramina of Luschka and Magendie. The CSF passes around the brain stem and over the cerebral hemispheres, and is absorbed into the venous circulation through the arachnoid granulations adjacent to the venous sinuses. The existence of this pattern of circulation creates the possibility of its obstruction and subsequent accumulation of CSF proximal to the site of the obstruction. This would raise the intraventricular (and intracranial) pressure and result in the *enlargement of the cerebral ventricles, the hallmark of this form of hydrocephalus.*

When the obstruction occurs early in life before fusion of the cranial sutures, the head enlarges and the worst sequelae of progressively rising intracranial pressure are avoided, or at least delayed. After fusion of the cranial sutures, rising intracranial pressure quickly necessitates that the obstruction be either removed or bypassed by a shunt.

If hydrocephalus occurs secondary to an obstruction within the ventricular system, it is often referred to as *noncommunicating,* whereas obstruction in the subarachnoid space outside the brain causes a *communicating* hydrocephalus. There are a large number of causes of hydrocephalus. Common causes are *tumors,* particularly around the aqueduct and fourth ventricle, and *infections* that may either cause an aqueductal stenosis or *postmeningitic fibrotic adhesions* in the subarachnoid space. The *Arnold-Chiari malformation,* in which the cerebellar tonsils descend into the upper cervical spinal canal and occlude the foramina of Luschka and Magendie, is an example of a *malformation* resulting in hydrocephalus (Fig. 22–2).

Pathologically, the raised CSF pressure in the ventricles may result in increased fluid accumulating in the periventricular white matter, a condition sometimes called *interstitial edema.* Microscopically, there

will often be breaks in the continuity of the ependymal lining of the ventricles and subependymal gliosis, together with attenuation of the periventricular white matter.

Clinically, the symptoms are very much dependent upon the cause of the hydrocephalus and the age of the patient. The CT scan has transformed the clinical evaluation and management of these patients.

## INFECTIONS

The nervous system is susceptible to a large number of infectious agents of all classes, including bacteria,[2] fungi, viruses, and, rarely, higher organisms (e.g., amebae). Because the clinical patterns of disease and causative agents differ, these infections are best divided into (1) infections of the meninges and CSF (meningitis) and (2) infections of the brain parenchyma (encephalitis).

Most infections reach the brain through the blood. Some agents, most notably herpes simplex virus and rabies, invade peripheral nerves and then ascend through them into the brain or sensory ganglia. Trauma to the brain may also be followed by infection, and sometimes, though fortunately only very occasionally, infection is introduced into the nervous system by medical procedures, most usually lumbar puncture. Involvement of one compartment in the CNS may, and often does, spill over into another. The inflammatory infiltrate in most infections of the brain (encephalitis) spills over into the CSF, and, conversely, a meningitis may invade the brain and produce a meningoencephalitis. Analogously, infections in the mastoid and frontal air sinuses or in the middle ear can eventually erode through the intervening bone and then involve either the meninges or penetrate the brain itself.

The three major categories of meningitis to be discussed are pyogenic, lymphocytic, and chronic. Similarly, there are several categories of encephalitis; in general, those caused by bacteria and fungi are focal and necrotizing and may develop into abscesses if sufficiently prolonged. Viral infections tend to be more diffuse and, with the exception of herpes simplex, cause individual cell death rather than frank tissue necrosis. Space limitations permit discussion of only the most important examples of the many infections of the CNS.

### MENINGITIS

Meningitis, sometimes called *leptomeningitis,* is an infection of the arachnoid mater and the CSF in the underlying subarachnoid space. It can occur only because the brain is floating in its cushioning bath of CSF and is yet another example of the disadvantages attendant on some of the protective features of the brain. Infection, once it breaches the protective wall of the meninges, is spread rapidly over the surface of the brain by the CSF.

Severe or prolonged meningitis may extend into the underlying brain and produce a meningoencephalitis. Three basic types of meningitis occur: acute pyogenic meningitis, which is usually caused by bacteria[3]; acute lymphocytic meningitis, which is generally viral; and chronic meningitis, which may be bacterial, fungal, or, rarely, be caused by some other organism such as amoeba.

### Pyogenic Meningitis

The most frequent causes of these infections are *Escherichia coli* in the neonate and, particularly, the neonate with a neural tube defect; *Haemophilus influenzae* in infants and children; *Neisseria meningitidis* in adolescents and young adults (which is also the most frequent cause of epidemic meningitis, since it is a mouth commensal and can be transmitted through air); and the *pneumococcus*, particularly in the very young and old and in meningitis following trauma.

Acutely, the brain and spinal cord are swollen and congested. The subarachnoid space contains exudate (Fig. 22–3), which varies in location. In meningitis caused by *H. influenzae*, for example, the exudate is usually basal, but in pneumococcal meningitis it is more often located over the cerebral convexity, near the longitudinal sinus. From the areas of greatest accumulation, tracts of pus can be followed around the blood vessels. Even in those areas where there is no gross exudate, the leptomeninges are opaque and congested. When the process

is fulminant, and especially if it is prolonged, the inflammation may extend to the ependymal surface of the ventricles and produce a ventriculitis.

Microscopically, the subarachnoid space contains a neutrophilic exudation that has varying amounts of fibrin. At its most severe, the entire subarachnoid space is filled with polymorphs, whereas in less severely affected cases, only the tissue around the leptomeningeal blood vessels contains cells. In fulminant infections, the inflammatory cells infiltrate the walls of the leptomeningeal veins, producing a vasculitis that may result in venous occlusion and hemorrhagic infarction of the cortex and underlying white matter.

Clinically, patients have a fever, the general signs of infection, and, in addition, the symptoms and signs of meningeal irritation (i.e., headache, photophobia, irritability, clouding of consciousness, and a stiff neck). A spinal tap yields cloudy or frankly purulent CSF, under increased pressure, with up to 90,000 polymorphs/mm,[3] a raised protein level, and a strikingly *reduced sugar content*. In fulminant infections, bacteria may sometimes be visible on smear or be readily cultured for a few hours before polymorphs appear.

Untreated, the usual outcome of pyogenic meningitis was death. Recovery, when it did occur, was accompanied by fibrous arachnoid adhesions between the meninges and the brain that obliterated the subarachnoid space around the brain stem and occluded the foramina of Magendie and Luschka. The resulting hydrocephalus was often fatal. Even with modern antibiotic treatment, hydrocephalus may still be a sequel, particularly in pneumococcal meningitis.

A particular problem of contemporary medicine is meningitis in the immunosuppressed patient.[4] It is often caused by an unusual agent, pursues a particularly fulminant course, and has atypical CSF findings, all of which render the diagnosis more urgent and more difficult.

### Lymphocytic Meningitis

Viral meningitis presents in much the same way as bacterial meningitis, with the clinical signs and symptoms of meningeal irritation, but the course is generally less fulminant and the CSF findings are markedly different. There is a lymphocytic rather than neutrophilic pleocytosis; the protein elevation is only moderate, and the CSF sugar content is normal, in sharp contrast to the reduced sugar content of the CSF in bacterial meningitides. The acute viral meningitides are self-limiting, and only symptomatic treatment is necessary. There are none of the life-threatening secondary complications that occur in pyogenic meningitis. A large number of different viruses have been isolated from these cases, including mumps, ECHO viruses, Coxsackie, Epstein-Barr virus, and herpes simplex type II, but they are often difficult to identify, and so viruses can be documented in only two thirds of cases.

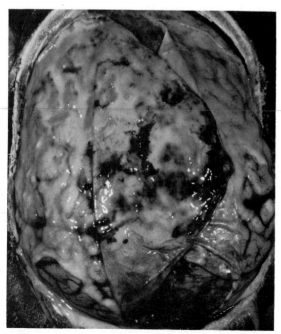

**Figure 22–3.** Pyogenic meningitis. A heavy layer of suppurative exudate is disclosed by folding back the dural covering.

## *Chronic Meningitis*

A number of agents produce a much more slowly evolving meningeal infection. The prototypic form of chronic meningitis is that produced by *Mycobacterium tuberculosis*, but all the relatively indolent infections in the meninges may produce similar changes.

In tuberculosis the meninges are filled with a gelatinous or fibrinous exudate in which focal densities may be visible macroscopically. These changes are usually most obvious around the base of the brain and may extend into the lateral sulcus. Microscopically, the meningeal exudate is composed of varying mixtures of chronic inflammatory cells including lymphocytes, plasma cells, macrophages, and fibroblasts. The local densities are tubercles, sometimes with caseous centers and giant cells. They are most frequently seen along the course of the cerebral vessels. In late cases there may be a dense fibrous arachnoiditis, most conspicuous around the base of the brain.

Clinically, tuberculous meningitis presents with relatively generalized neurologic complaints of headache and malaise, mental confusion, and vomiting. The CSF has only a moderate pleocytosis of up to about 1000 cells (the usual value is around 100), which are composed either entirely of mononuclear cells or a mixture of polymorphs and mononuclear cells. The protein level is elevated, often strikingly so, and the sugar level is typically moderately reduced but may be normal.

The most feared, and sometimes devastating, complications of tuberculous meningitis are consequences of the continuing chronic inflammatory reaction in the subarachnoid space. The arachnoid fibrosis already alluded to produces hydrocephalus. The inflammatory reaction around the vessels of the subarachnoid space may cause obliterative endarteritis. Affected vessels may be occluded to produce infarctions in the underlying brain. Spread of the infection into the parenchyma of the brain produces a meningoencephalitis.

Other organisms that produce meningitis with rather similar clinical and pathologic features include such bacteria as *Treponema pallidum* (syphilis) and species of *Brucella* and many of the fungi (e.g., Coccidioides and *Candida*).

Neurosyphilis may take one of three forms: (1) *Meningovascular neurosyphilis*, characterized by a mononuclear infiltration of the leptomeninges, particularly about the optic chiasm and brain stem, along with typical syphilitic endarteritis; (2) *paretic neurosyphilis*, characterized by atrophy of the entire brain due to loss of nerve cells, with perivascular cuffing and transformation of the microglia into rod cells; and (3) *tabes dorsalis (locomotor ataxia)*, characterized by atrophy of the posterior roots of the lumbar region, sometimes accompanied by optic nerve atrophy.

Cryptococcal meningitis differs from the general run of fungal meningitis mostly by virtue of its clinical and pathologic variability.[5] Pathologically, this organism sometimes elicits only a trivial inflammatory response, even in the presence of many organisms. Clinically, its course may be fulminant and fatal in as little as two weeks, or it may be indolent over months or even years. The CSF, particularly in the indolent cases, may have few cells but a notably high protein level (over 500 mg/dl). In most cases, the yeasts with their thick capsules can be seen in the CSF; they are most easily visualized by India ink preparations (p. 446). The most reliable diagnostic test, however, is the presence of cryptococcal antigen in the CSF.

## CEREBRAL ABSCESS

Abscesses may arise from direct implantation of organisms by trauma, by extension from nearby foci of infection (especially mastoiditis), or by hematogenous spread, particularly from a primary source in lung, heart, or bones. Cyanotic congenital heart disease is associated with a high incidence of cerebral abscesses. This is thought to be due to a right-to-left shunt and loss of pulmonary filtration of organisms. The microflora of intracranial abscesses is very varied but includes many anaerobic organisms, of which the anaerobic streptococci and *Bacteroides fragilis* are the most common. Other common organisms are aerobic streptococci and *Staphylococcus* species.

An abscess secondary to mastoiditis is usually preceded by an epidural extension from the infecting site, with spread into either the cerebellar hemisphere or the temporal lobe. During the stage of invasion there may be a "cellulitis" of brain substance, which then settles down into a nidus of organisms and necrotic tissue. Adhesions of the meninges then usually seal off the point of entry from the rest of the subarachnoid space. Gradually, an abscess expands, destroying and compressing contiguous tissues. As in somatic organs, a fibrous capsule surrounds brain abscesses. This is one of the very few instances in which there is fibrosis with collagen production in the brain. The fibroblasts that produce this collagen are derived from the walls of the blood vessels that proliferate around the edge of the necrotic brain. The new vessels are responsible for the pronounced vasogenic edema so characteristic around brain abscesses. Outside the fibrous capsule is a zone of conventional gliosis. The inflammatory reaction, both acute and chronic, that is associated with this advancing infection is reflected in the CSF by an increased pressure, and a raised white cell count and protein level, but the sugar content remains normal. No organisms will be present in the CSF unless the abscess has ruptured into a ventricle or the subarachnoid space.

*The patient with a brain abscess presents with general complaints relating to the raised intracranial pressure, caused by the mass effect, and focal complaints referable to the area of brain involved.* Abscesses are so destructive of tissue that a focal deficit is almost always present. Hemiparesis, convulsions in cerebral abscesses, and cerebellar incoordination in cerebellar abscesses are among the more dramatic signs. A systemic or local source of infection is usually detectable, but a small systemic focus may have ceased to be symptomatic by the time the patient presents with evidence of brain involvement.

Death may result from increased intracranial pressure and herniation. Rupture of the abscess may lead to ventriculitis, meningitis, or sinus thrombosis. With the use of surgery and antibiotics, the otherwise inevitable mortality can be reduced to less than 20%.

## VIRAL ENCEPHALITIS

Viral infection of the brain almost always reflects spread of the agent from some extracranial focus that may or may not be disease producing. Sometimes, as with *varicella-zoster virus* the primary infection is another recognized disease (for example, chicken pox), but it is often nonspecific, as in the gastroenteritis of *poliomyelitis*, or even unknown, as in *progressive multifocal leukoencephalopathy (PML)*, in which there is only serologic evidence of previous infection. *Rabies* is an exception in that at the site of the bite the virus is directly inoculated into the peripheral nerves, through which it ascends to the brain. Infection of the brain is almost invariably accompanied by some reaction in the meninges, so that there will be inflammatory cells, usually lymphocytes, in the CSF.

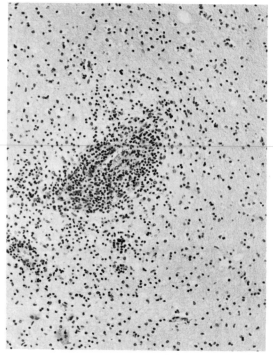

**Figure 22–4.** Microscopic detail of cerebral white matter in viral encephalitis. There is marked perivascular cuffing with lymphocytes, some of which have invaded the adjacent parenchyma.

The most characteristic histologic change in acute viral diseases is a mononuclear cell infiltrate (lymphocytes, plasma cells, and macrophages), generally located around blood vessels (Fig. 22–4). The presence of *glial nodules* and *neuronophagia* (individual neuron necrosis and phagocytosis) also suggest viral disease. A more direct expression of viral involvement is the presence of intranuclear *inclusion bodies* in some forms of viral infection. A well-known diagnostic inclusion is the intracytoplasmic *Negri body* of rabies.

A particularly striking feature of viral infections of the nervous system is the degree of tropism exhibited by some viruses.[6] Herpes zoster and poliomyelitis virus, for example, affect only specific subpopulations of neurons, the dorsal root ganglion cells and the anterior horn motor neurons, respectively. Other viruses affect whole classes of cells; the virus of PML infects primarily oligodendrocytes, and rabies virus attacks only neurons. Herpes simplex, although it infects all types of neural cells, is geographically restricted, affecting principally the temporal lobes. The basis for these different specificities is not clear, but they probably reflect surface receptor compatibility between the host cells and the infecting virus.

The capacity of some viruses for *latency* is important in viral diseases of the nervous system. Herpes simplex and varicella-zoster viruses can remain latent in their host cells in the nervous system, to be reactivated months or years after the initial infection.

Infections, overt or otherwise, do not make up the full gamut of viral effects on the nervous system. Systemic viral infections may occasionally be followed by an immune-mediated *perivenous encephalitis* or *polyneuritis* with no viral penetration of the nervous system. *Reye's syndrome*, a condition of unknown but possibly toxic origin, occurs most frequently after viral infection (usually influenza or chicken pox) and is associated with severe, often fatal brain edema. *Congenital malformations* can also be attributed to intrauterine viral infection, as occurs with rubella.

Virus infections of the brain can be divided into two general categories: (1) acute viral infections and (2) slow virus diseases.

### Acute Virus Infection

Acute viral infections of the brain have a wide spectrum of manifestations, ranging from a catastrophic acute necrotizing panencephalitis (e.g., neonatal herpes simplex encephalitis) to an infection that affects only specific subpopulations of neurons (e.g., polio).

**ARTHROPOD-BORNE ENCEPHALITIDES.** These are generalized encephalitides and are characterized by a panencephalitis without conspicuous localizing features. *All cause a perivascular, predominantly mononuclear reaction and a moderate CSF pleocytosis.* Most outbreaks of epidemic encephalitis are due to arthropod-borne viruses (arboviruses). The specific causative agents differ around the world. In the

Western Hemisphere, the most important ones are eastern and western equine, Venezuelan, St. Louis, and California encephalitis. Types found elsewhere include Japanese B (Far East), tick-borne (U.S.S.R. and Eastern Europe), and Murray Valley encephalitis (Australia and New Guinea). All have vertebrate hosts and mosquito vectors, except for the tick-borne. These viruses have many common properties, to the extent that some investigators wish to group them collectively as *encephaloviruses.*

*Eastern equine encephalitis* may serve as the example for all the arbovirus encephalitides. It was initially described in horses in 1933, and the first human cases were reported in 1939 when an outbreak in children followed an epidemic in horses. Serologic studies indicate that only about 5% of exposed persons develop encephalitis, but the mortality is 80%. Some survivors recover completely, but others, especially young children, are left with serious residual disability.

**Eastern equine encephalitis is a meningoencephalitis characterized by perivascular inflammatory cells, many focal areas of necrosis, and selective neuronal necrosis with neuronophagia.** In severe cases there may be a vasculitis and vascular necrosis. The location of the most severe damage varies; some cases have a predominantly cortical involvement, whereas in others the basal ganglia bear the brunt. In both eastern and western equine encephalitis, large numbers of polymorphs appear in the brain and CSF early in the disease. Later the polymorphs are replaced by mononuclear leukocytes. However, the level of CSF sugar is not decreased even when the cell count is exclusively polymorphonuclear.

The other arbovirus encephalitides differ in epidemiology and prognosis, but pathologically their appearance is very similar except for variations in severity and a tendency for there to be fewer polymorphs. There are no reliable morphologic distinguishing features.

In the arbovirus encephalitides, the brain is the principal site of significant infection, but *there are other viral diseases in which encephalitis is an occasional, and sometimes very severe, complication; these include measles, rubella, and chicken pox.* Most of these cases are probably examples of allergic perivenous encephalomyelitis, but in some cases (e.g., Epstein-Barr virus and mumps) the fact that virus can be recovered from the CSF is suggestive of direct neurotropic infection.

**HERPES SIMPLEX.** *HSV I encephalitis* typically involves the inferior and medial regions of the temporal lobes and the orbital gyri of the frontal lobes. Hemorrhagic necrosis and mononuclear perivascular infiltrates are almost always present, and intranuclear inclusion bodies may be found in neurons and glial cells. This infection may occur in any age group but is most often seen in children and young adults. Most cases are fatal, but some patients survive with severe dementia and, because of the temporal lobe damage,

a striking memory loss. Others may make a complete recovery. Most cases of so-called *acute necrotizing encephalitis* are probably due to herpes simplex.

The emergence of an effective therapy for HSV I encephalitis (acyclovir) has generated a requirement for rapid diagnosis, which can be achieved by the immunofluorescent or electron-microscopic demonstration of virus in brain biopsy material. Treatment of this disease has reduced the mortality to about 30%, compared with 70% in controls.

HSV II also produces disease in the nervous system; it is responsible for most cases of *herpetic viral meningitis.* More ominously, it causes a generalized and very severe *encephalitis* in neonates. With the current prevalence and resistance to treatment of herpes genitalis, obstetrics practice is moving toward recommending caesarean section in cases of active herpes genitalis rather than submitting the baby to the risk of encephalitis engendered by delivery through an infected birth canal.

**ACQUIRED IMMUNODEFICIENCY SYNDROME (AIDS).** Recent work has made it clear that the HTLV-III virus of AIDS frequently affects the brain.[7] Although the full range of the effects on the nervous system has yet to be defined, a meningitis, a myelopathy, and a subacute encephalopathy with dementia have all been ascribed to the direct action of the virus. In addition, opportunistic infections with cytomegalovirus, the papovavirus of PML, toxoplasma, and mycobacteria, among others, occur in the brain secondary to the immunosuppression caused by the AIDS virus infection.[8] Frequent occurrence of primary lymphomas in the brain is yet another manifestation of the impaired immunity in AIDS (p. 177).

### Slow Virus Diseases

The so-called slow virus diseases have a long latent period. When they produce disease, it evolves at a much slower pace than normal infections, and clinically it does not look like an infection at all. Recent advances have made it appropriate to divide the diseases in this category into two groups: (1) slow virus diseases and (2) unconventional agent encephalopathies.

The two major diseases in the slow virus group are subacute sclerosing panencephalitis (SSPE) and progressive multifocal leukoencephalopathy (PML).

**SUBACUTE SCLEROSING PANENCEPHALITIS (SSPE).** This disease generally attacks children, although it can sometimes be seen in adolescents and young adults. It has always been preceded by an attack of measles, often unusually early in life; very occasionally, it occurs after immunization against measles. The onset of the disease is usually heralded by personality changes followed by the development of involuntary movements. The EEG exhibits characteristic bursts of high-voltage activity. In most cases the disease progresses relentlessly to death. Given the poor prognosis of this disease, it is gratifying that measles immunization and the subsequent reduction in the number of cases of measles have strikingly reduced the incidence of SSPE.

On gross examination, the brain may appear normal or be unusually firm. Sometimes it contains regions of granularity and focal destruction. Microscopically, in all cases there is a perivascular mononuclear cell infiltrate and cytoplasmic or nuclear inclusion bodies in neurons and oligodendroglia. **Neuronophagia and extensive neuronal loss are present in severely involved regions**. Dense fibrillary gliosis follows as the process becomes older. Electron microscopy shows that the inclusion bodies contain particles very similar to measles virus.

*SSPE is caused by measles virus, which is present in large quantities in the affected brain.* The virus produced is defective in that it lacks the so-called M protein, which is one of the coat proteins of the virus. It is not known why the M protein is not produced in the brain.

PROGRESSIVE MULTIFOCAL LEUKOENCEPHALOPATHY (PML). This viral infection of oligodendrocytes causes demyelination as its principal pathologic effect.[9] It was first described in 1959 and occurs in association with advanced hematologic malignancies, immunosuppressive therapy, immunodeficiency diseases (including AIDS), and chronic debilitating diseases (tuberculosis, sarcoidosis, rheumatoid arthritis). In most cases, the associated illnesses have been present for months or years before PML becomes clinically manifest. Given the nature of the associated conditions, most cases are in middle-aged patients, but the condition also occurs in children. It becomes clinically apparent by the development of protean but focal and relentlessly progressive neurologic symptoms and signs. CT scans show extensive, often multifocal areas of lucency in the hemispheric or cerebellar white matter, or both. Currently there is no established treatment for this disorder.

Focal areas of white matter have irregular margins; a sunken, gray, translucent appearance; and a soft texture. Microscopically, **there are numerous areas of demyelination, ranging in size from minute foci to huge confluent lesions affecting whole lobes**. The cerebrum, brain stem, cerebellum, and, rarely, spinal cord can all be involved. The appearance of the oligodendrocytes is diagnostic. Their nuclei are still spherical but are grossly enlarged and contain **inclusion bodies, which range from violet smudges to discrete homogeneous eosinophilic masses**. They are most frequently seen at the edges of the lesions. There are also characteristic bizarre giant astrocytes, with irregular, hyperchromatic, sometimes multiple nuclei. Reactive fibrillary astrocytes are scattered among the bizarre forms, but there is strikingly little inflammatory reaction. Axons transversing the lesions are conspicuously preserved. Electron microscopy shows that the enlarged oligodendrocyte nuclei contain numerous papovavirus-like particles, often in par-

acrystalline arrays. Isolated virus particles are sometimes seen in astrocyte nuclei.

*Almost all cases of this disease are caused by the papovavirus called JC* (initials of a patient and unrelated to Creutzfeldt-Jakob disease). About 65% of normal persons have specific antibodies to the JC virus by the age of 12, but it is not known whether the development of PML is the rekindling of old infection or a new infection in a particularly susceptible host.

### Encephalopathies from Unconventional Agents

A small group of diseases, including Creutzfeldt-Jakob disease and kuru in humans and scrapie in sheep, are transmissible by injection but have a transmitting agent that does not appear to have most of the characteristics of a conventional virus or any other infectious agent. It now appears that the agent in question is largely, and perhaps exclusively, composed of protein that has a mass of about 30 kD. The name *prion* (from *pro*teinaceous *in*fective agent) has been applied to the agent by one of the major investigating groups, but it has not, at the time of this writing, been unequivocally established that there is no nucleic acid incorporated in the infectious material. The exact nature of this material, particularly whether it is the true infectious agent, is currently under study.

CREUTZFELDT-JAKOB DISEASE (TRANSMISSIBLE AGENT DEMENTIA, SUBACUTE SPONGIFORM ENCEPHALOPATHY). All these synonyms refer to a rare but well-characterized disease that presents clinically as a rapidly progressive dementia.[10] Despite the demonstrated experimental transmissibility of the causative agent, the disease is sporadic in occurrence, with a worldwide incidence of about one per million, and there is no discernible pattern of exposure in the patient population. The natural mode of transmission in humans is wholly obscure, although in a few cases, iatrogenic transmission by medical procedures (e.g., corneal transplantation) has occurred.

Morphologically, **the diagnostic feature is the presence of spongiform change ("bubbles and holes") in the cortex and, sometimes, the basal ganglia**. In the later stages there is also gross neuronal loss and an accompanying marked fibrillary gliosis. An inflammatory infiltrate is notably absent. By electron microscopy the "holes" appear as intracytoplasmic membrane-bound vacuoles in neuronal and glial processes. The progress of the disease is usually so rapid that, despite the degree of neuronal loss, there is little if any gross atrophy of the brain.

In the typical clinical presentation, abnormalities of personality and visual or spatial coordination are generally the first signs of illness. This is rapidly followed by a progressive severe dementia with myoclonus. The CSF is normal except for an occasional mild elevation of protein. The disease is uniformly fatal, with an average duration of seven months, although longer survival for three years or more occasionally occurs. All treatment has so far been unavailing.

## OTHER INFECTIONS

Protozoal diseases such as malaria, toxoplasmosis, amebiasis, and trypanosomiasis; rickettsial infections (typhus, Rocky Mountain spotted fever); and metazoal diseases such as echinococcosis and cysticercosis may also involve the CNS. Of these, cerebral toxoplasmosis merits a brief additional mention because, in its acquired form in adults, it occurs only in the immunosuppressed population, is particularly common in AIDS, and is treatable. Pathologically, it is a rapidly progressive, multifocal, necrotizing, and often hemorrhagic encephalitis.[11] The organisms are present in characteristic pseudocysts and free in the tissue, and they are usually most easily seen at the margins of the necrotic areas.

In this brief summary of infections there has been a considerable bias toward diseases encountered in Western European and North American practice. However, outside these privileged areas, cerebral malaria, cysticercosis, and tuberculosis are probably the most common infections of the nervous system.

# VASCULAR DISEASE

Vascular disease of the brain, in spite of a recent and gratifying reduction in its incidence, remains a very important cause of neurologic morbidity and mortality, with personal and social consequences extending far beyond the acute medical phase of the illness. It is hoped that the continued treatment of hypertension and progress in understanding the causes of atherosclerosis will further control these all too common disorders.

Cerebrovascular disease is most easily thought of in three general categories: (1) *General reductions in blood flow without vascular occlusion—ischemic encephalopathy and boundary zone infarcts.* (2) *Local cessation of blood flow caused by vascular occlusion—thrombotic and embolic infarcts, and venous obstruction.* (3) *Hemorrhages—within the brain (intracerebral hemorrhages), in the subarachnoid space (subarachnoid hemorrhages), or in both areas.*

## ISCHEMIC ENCEPHALOPATHY

The brain has a remarkably constant level of metabolic activity, and autoregulation of the cerebral circulation normally ensures the maintenance of cerebral perfusion pressure, and hence blood flow, over a wide range of systemic blood pressure and intra-

cerebral pressure. In normal persons, blood flow to the brain is adequate down to a systolic blood pressure of about 50 mm Hg.

Reductions in pressure below this level induce increasing tissue ischemia and subsequent ischemic encephalopathy.[12] In the brain, the cells most vulnerable to ischemia are the neurons, and they suffer first reversible and then irreversible damage. **For obscure reasons, some types of neurons, notably the pyramidal cells of the hippocampus and the Purkinje cells of the cerebellum, are more susceptible than others**, and consequently they are often the first to be lost.

The changes seen in the brain depend upon the duration and intensity of the ischemia and on the length of survival. When the insult has been slight, the nerve cells will recover function and no anatomic change occurs. In patients who survive only a few minutes or hours, no changes are seen regardless of the severity of the insult. The first demonstrable change is seen after survival for 12 to 24 hours. **All forms of ischemia initially result in either swelling or shrinkage of neurons.** Shortly thereafter, affected neurons may develop **ischemic cell change**, characterized by strikingly eosinophilic cytoplasm and a small pyknotic nucleus (red neurons) (Fig. 22–5). In the cortex, the process is usually widespread but not completely uniform; clusters of damaged cells may be found next to unaffected cells, even in the same cortical lamina. Subsequently, the nerve cells die and disappear, to be replaced by fibrillary gliosis. Frank cortical necrosis followed by gliosis occurs in areas of greater

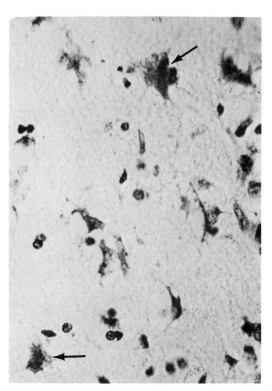

Figure 22–5. Shrunken and angular neurons (*arrows*) in the cerebral cortex have been caused by ischemia.

destruction, so that **laminar necrosis** interrupts the normal continuity of the cerebral cortex. In long-term survivors, the degree of cortical atrophy is proportional to the amount of cortical destruction. In generalized reductions of cerebral perfusion, the most severe ischemia is suffered by tissue supplied by the most distal branches of the arteries. This may be severe enough to result in wedge-shaped areas of tissue necrosis in the junctional zones between the major arterial territories, called **border-zone or watershed infarcts**. In the cerebral hemispheres, the border zone between the territories for the anterior and middle cerebral arteries seems to be most at risk. Damage to this region produces a linear parasagittal infarction, usually with some expansion over the lateral occipital gyri; the precise geometry of the infarct is governed by the degree of ischemia and the extent of narrowing of local vessels in the affected region. Border-zone infarcts are almost invariably seen in the context of a generalized severe ischemic encephalopathy.

The clinical expression of ischemic encephalopathy depends on the severity and duration of the period of ischemia. In mild cases, there may be only a transient postischemic confusional state and subsequent complete recovery, whereas more severely affected patients will be comatose, with loss of most cortical functions. Prolonged ischemia, which for the brain may be as little as four minutes, results, of course, in cerebral death, from which there is no appeal.

## CEREBRAL INFARCTION

Cerebral infarction occurs as a result of vascular occlusion; *the issue of whether infarction will or will not occur, and its size and shape, are determined by which vessel is occluded and the pattern and degree of anastomotic connections among the cerebral arteries.* In the case of the large internal carotid and vertebral arteries, the circle of Willis may provide a total functional anastomosis. The middle-sized intracranial arteries, such as the middle and anterior cerebral, have a partial anastomosis of their distal branches, so that, although a quite severe stenosis in one artery can be tolerated, a complete occlusion always causes an infarct that is smaller than the territory supplied by the obstructed vessel. In the small parenchymal arteries, such as the lenticulostriate and cortical penetrating arteries, there is little or no arterial anastomosis, and occlusion of these vessels always results in an infarct.

Clinically, the symptoms generated by vascular occlusion are called "strokes." "*Stroke*" is one of those old-fashioned clinical terms that is frequently used but is pathologically imprecise. *It implies the usually sudden onset of a focal neurologic syndrome,* such as a hemiparesis (weakness of the limbs on one side of the body) secondary to some sort of vascular event. This event may be either an occlusion, pro-

ducing a focal infarct, or a hemorrhage, which also causes local destruction of tissue. Other types of disease processes that cause local destruction (for example, tumors) may also occasionally present with a focal syndrome of rapid onset, thereby mimicking a "stroke."

Cerebral vascular occlusions can be divided into thrombotic or embolic. **The vast majority of thrombotic occlusions are atherosclerotic** and occur either in the internal carotid artery at the carotid bifurcation in the neck or in the vertebrobasilar system. The consequences of carotid occlusion are variable and depend to a large extent on the functioning of the circle of Willis. If this system of arterial anastomoses at the base of the brain is functioning normally, then occlusion of the carotid artery may cause no symptoms, as indeed occurs in many patients. In less favorable circumstances, when the anastomotic capacity of the circle of Willis is reduced by atherosclerotic narrowings or there is an abnormal pattern of cerebral circulation, there will be an infarction that can range in size from a small distal infarction in the territory of the middle cerebral artery to a catastrophic infarct of a whole hemisphere.

The posterior circulation is not afforded the same degree of anastomotic protection, and atherosclerotic occlusion of the basilar artery is invariably a seriously incapacitating and usually fatal event. Occlusion of a vertebral artery may, however, be asymptomatic.

Before total occlusion occurs, ephemeral focal neurologic symptoms and signs, called **transient ischemic attacks**, often point to significant atherosclerotic cerebrovascular disease.

Although atherosclerosis is the most frequent cause of thrombotic occlusion of a cerebral artery, other rarer causes exist—notably, the various arteritides. They usually cause occlusions in arteries smaller than those obstructed by atherosclerosis.

**Embolic occlusions** have a much wider range of origins. Common sources are atrial and ventricular mural thrombi; valvular vegetations, either infective or nonbacterial; and atherosclerotic debris from various sites, including, of course, the carotid and vertebrobasilar systems.

Emboli have a marked tendency to impact in the territory of the middle cerebral artery, probably for hemodynamic reasons, and they are usually small enough to affect only a part of the arborization of this artery (Fig. 22–6). As might be expected, very small emboli tend to affect the most distal branches of the artery, and many embolic infarcts occur in the boundary zone between the territories of the middle and anterior cerebral arteries. If small emboli are numerous, they may radiologically and pathologically simulate the boundary-zone infarcts seen in severe ischemic encephalopathy (p. 733).

By their very nature, some types of emboli tend to break up or completely lyse, allowing reflow of blood into vessels already damaged by ischemia. Not surprisingly, these damaged vessels tend to leak blood, thereby converting an anemic (bland) infarct into a hemorrhagic one.

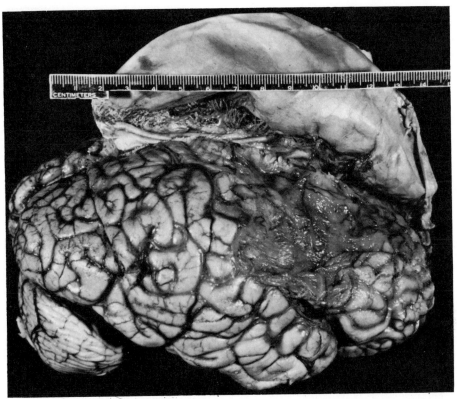

Figure 22–6. An old hemorrhagic infarct involving the superior lip of the sylvian fissure in the territory of the middle cerebral artery. The gyral pattern has been lost, the infarcted area has a yellow-brown discoloration, and there is gliotic scarring.

The hemorrhage is petechial in character and restricted to the infarcted cortex, unless the patient has received anticoagulants, in which case the hemorrhage may be massive and associated with an acute worsening of the patient's clinical state. In this situation it may be difficult pathologically to distinguish between a hemorrhagic infarct and a lobar hemorrhage.

**No matter what their cause, cerebral infarcts have a similar pattern of pathologic evolution.** Grossly, ischemic (bland) infarcts are not detectable with any certainty until six to 12 hours after their occurrence. The earliest visible change is a slight discoloration and softening of the affected area, so that the structure of the gray matter becomes blurred and the white matter loses its normal fine-grained appearance. **Within 48 to 72 hours necrosis is well established and there is softening and disintegration of the ischemic area and pronounced circumlesional swelling**, which may in lesions of sufficient size produce brain herniations. As resolution proceeds, there is liquefaction, resulting in cyst formation in larger lesions. These cysts are traversed by trabeculations of blood vessels and surrounded by firm glial tissue. The leptomeninges, when involved, become thickened and opaque and may form the outer wall of the cyst.

The first histologic change, seen after about six to 12 hours, is a diffuse reduction in the staining intensity of the tissue. In usual chromatic stains, the first discrete change is swelling of the nerve cell bodies and disarrangement and disorganization of the cytoplasm and nuclear chromatin. In addition, but probably following the initial swelling of the cells, large numbers of red neurons (p. 733) suffering from ischemic damage are present. As shown by special stains, there is fragmentation of the axons and early disintegration of the myelin sheaths. There is also loss of oligodendrocytes and astrocytes.

At about 48 hours the blood vessels stand out prominently and some neutrophils seep into the tissue. Occasionally, this response is so intense as to simulate a septic infarct, but usually it is replaced at 72 to 96 hours by the aggregation of macrophages around blood vessels. At this stage the macrophages are the dominant reactive cells, attaining their maximum number at about two weeks. After this they gradually disappear but even years later may still be found in the interstices of old infarcts. Astrocytosis becomes prominent during the second week and, eventually, as the final resolution of the infarct, it results in fibrillary gliosis, which replaces the necrotic region or encloses the cyst. The time required for an infarct to resolve ranges from weeks to many months, depending on its size. Hemorrhage within the infarct does not seem to affect the processes of infarct resolution, except that histologically, many of the macrophages contain hemosiderin.

**Lacunes** (little lakes) are small infarcts ranging from a few to 15 mm in diameter; they are most commonly found in the deep portions of the brain, especially the putamen, thalamus, internal capsule, basis pontis, and hemispheric white matter. Their occurrence is particularly associated with systemic arterial hypertension, and they are thought to result from the occlusion of deep arterioles either by emboli or hypertensive hyalinization of these arterioles.[13] Pigmented macrophages can be found in some lacunes, suggesting that a hemorrhagic component may have been present or that they may have been minute hemorrhages.

## INTRACRANIAL HEMORRHAGE

Spontaneous (nontraumatic) intracerebral hemorrhage falls into three basic categories: (1) intraparenchymal hemorrhage, (2) subarachnoid hemorrhage, and (3) mixed hemorrhage.

### Intraparenchymal Hemorrhage

Most intraparenchymal hemorrhages result from rupture of one of the small intraparenchymal arteries. Their occurrence is particularly associated with a prior history of hypertension and, it is thought, the formation of microaneurysms called *Charcot-Bouchard* aneurysms that burst and cause the bleeding. Rupture destroys the aneurysms and leads to hemorrhage into the immediately adjacent brain tissue. Studies of hypertensive patients without hemorrhage have shown that the occurrence of these microaneu-

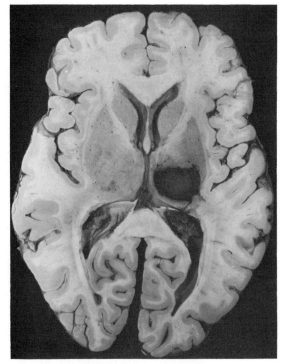

Figure 22–7. An intraparenchymal hemorrhage involving the basal ganglia and the posterior limb of the internal capsule.

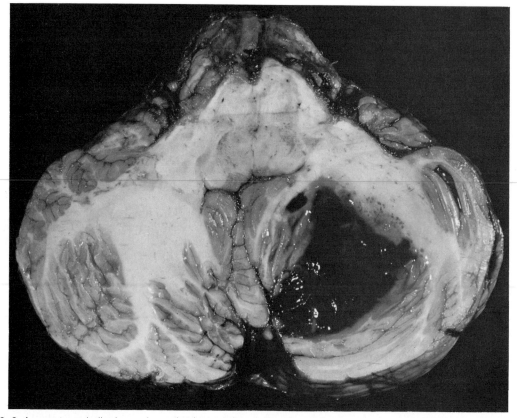

Figure 22–8. A recent cerebellar hemorrhage that has produced distortion of the vermis and compression of the fourth ventricle.

rysms in the arteries of the brain increases with age and with length of history of hypertension.

The aneurysms, and therefore the hemorrhages, occur most frequently in the basal ganglia (Fig. 22–7), the pons and cerebellar hemispheres (Fig. 22–8), and less frequently in the hemispheric white matter. Bleeding in this last location is often called a lobar hemorrhage.

The advent of the CT scan has led to some revision in our ideas about the natural history of intracerebral hemorrhages. Hemorrhages were thought to be usually large and frequently fatal, but CT has revealed that there are also a number of smaller hemorrhages that present as an occlusive stroke and, prior to the advent of CT, would not have been classed as hemorrhages. Cerebral hemorrhage is therefore not as invariably catastrophic as was previously thought. This is not to say that it is benign! Overall, there is an initial mortality of about 40%; most of these patients have extension of the hemorrhage into the cerebral ventricles. In those who survive, there is a relatively good prognosis for recovery of function, perhaps because hemorrhages tend to separate tissue planes rather than destroy the tissue, so that resolution of the mass of the hematoma may be accompanied by restitution of function. Generally, recurrent hemorrhage is rare, in contrast to the situation in subarachnoid hemorrhage, in which rebleeding is a major risk.

Gross inspection of the brain of a patient with, for example, a hemorrhage in the basal ganglia often shows obvious expansion of the affected hemisphere and flattening of the gyri. There will frequently be uncinate herniation (p. 725) and displacement of the midbrain to the side opposite the hemorrhage. If the hemorrhage has erupted into the ventricles, a blood clot may be present in the subarachnoid space and is often present around the foramina of Luschka and Magendie, where the ventricles communicate with the subarachnoid space.

The cut surface of the brain typically shows the blood clot expanding and separating the tissues of the basal ganglia. The parenchyma immediately adjacent to the clot is usually edematous and often discolored by degradation products of blood pigment, especially if the hemorrhage is some days old. **The mass effect of the blood clot causes distortion of the cerebral ventricles**; the ipsilateral one is usually compressed, but there may also be acute hydrocephalus if the aqueduct of Sylvius or either of the foramina of Monro is occluded by the ventricular distortion. Sometimes the hemorrhage ruptures into a ventricle and fills it. Resolution of a hemorrhage begins with the appearance of macrophages that, over a period of months, remove the clot and leave a slit-like cavity surrounded by a zone of fibrillary gliosis that contains scattered hemosiderin-laden macrophages.

Since in about 80% of cases there is a history of hypertension, vascular changes are also found in other parts of the brain. The most frequent is arteriolar sclerosis, with thickening and hyalinization of the walls of the arterioles seen most conspicuously in the deep white matter of the hemispheres. In the basal ganglia there is often arterial thickening, focal atherosclerosis, and expansion of the Virchow-Robin spaces with perivascular gliosis. Atherosclerosis of the larger arteries is also often severe but is not a necessary acompaniment to hypertensive hemorrhage.

Supratentorial hemorrhages tend to present as progressive hemiplegias. In the posterior fossa, cerebellar hematomas produce symptoms such as intractable vomiting. Whatever the location of the hemorrhage, if there is substantial bleeding and mass effect, the signs of raised intracranial pressure, coma, and the syndromes of herniation rapidly come to dominate the clinical picture.

### Subarachnoid Hemorrhage

Bleeding into the subarachnoid space usually results from rupture of either an aneurysm or, much less frequently, an arteriovenous malformation. *Aneurysms are divided into berry (congenital), arteriosclerotic, and mycotic, with berry aneurysms being the commonest.*

*Berry aneurysms* occur at bifurcations of cerebral arteries; the most common sites are at (1) the junction of the carotid and posterior communicating arteries, (2) the anterior communicating artery connecting the two anterior cerebral arteries, and (3) the major division of the middle cerebral artery in the Sylvian fissure. In 20 to 30% of cases they are multiple. Together these three sites account for at least 85% of ruptured aneurysms (Fig. 22–9); almost all the remainder are in the posterior circulation. Although often called congenital aneurysms, *they are not present at birth and develop at sites of medial weakness at arterial bifurcations.* The arterial wall bulges out

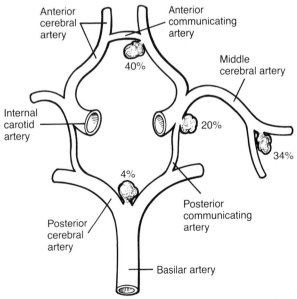

Figure 22–9. Common sites of berry aneurysms in the circle of Willis.

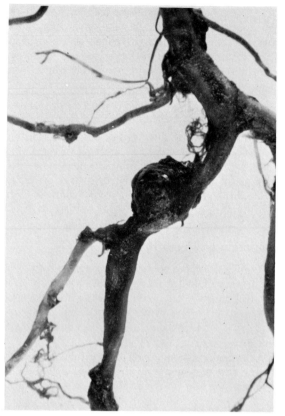

Figure 22–10. A berry aneurysm of the middle cerebral artery. The vessels have been dissected away from the brain.

reaching a ventricle and producing as much intraparenchymal as subarachnoid bleeding. This occurs in between 15 and 40% of patients and is particularly common in those who die within the first week after rupture. Alternatively, the blood may leak straight into the subarachnoid space and produce the more typical clinical presentation of a subarachnoid hemorrhage.

Patients usually complain of a sudden, severe, occipital headache and may rapidly lose consciousness. In most cases, they improve and are awake again within minutes. Arteriography and CT scan are helpful in determining the location of the aneurysm. About 25 to 50% of patients die with the first rupture. Rebleeding is common in those who survive, although it is impossible to predict in which patient this will occur; when it does, the prognosis is much more grave. Other complications include infarction, hydrocephalus, herniation, and brain stem hemorrhage.

Four to nine days after rupture, some patients develop additional neurologic deficits due to arterial vasospasm. About 40% of patients with ruptured aneurysms have arterial spasm that can be demonstrated arteriographically, but not all become symptomatic. Postmortem examination of patients dying with vasospasm frequently discloses infarcts in the territories supplied by the affected vessels. Experimentally, platelet products and red cell lysates cause constriction in cerebral vessels, but whether these play a role clinically is unknown.

### Mixed Intraparenchymal and Subarachnoid Hemorrhage (Vascular Malformations)

Arteriovenous malformations (AVMs) comprise about 1% of intracranial tumors. When they rupture, they bleed into both the brain and subarachnoid space in about two thirds of the cases, into only the subarachnoid space in about 25% of cases, and solely into the CNS in the remainder. They consist of tangles of abnormal vessels of varying sizes, many of which have a structure intermediate between arteries and veins. Ninety per cent of AVMs are in the cerebral hemispheres; about half are predominantly located on the surface of the brain, and the other half are more deeply situated. The abnormal vessels within the brain substance are separated by gliotic tissue in which there is either recent hemorrhage or evidence of old bleeding, in the form of hemosiderin-laden macrophages. Irregular, often grossly enlarged feeding arteries supply the vascular tangle, and veins that drain the malformation can usually be found.

Bleeding from AVMs is clinically most frequent between the ages of 10 and 30; after 60 it is rare. Males are affected twice as often as females. Subarachnoid and intracerebral hemorrhage associated with seizures is the most common clinical presentation. The most frequent site of bleeding is in the region of the middle cerebral artery.

through the muscular defect at this point to form a thin-walled sac composed only of fibrous tissue, in which there may be additional local degeneration and calcification (Fig. 22–10). Laminated blood clot and fibrin may be deposited on this attenuated wall. Rupture of aneurysms is frequently associated with acute rises in intracranial pressure, such as may be caused by straining at stool or lifting heavy weights.

Although acute elevation of blood pressure is often implicated in subarachnoid hemorrhage, there is no established association between chronic hypertension and either the development or the rupture of berry aneurysms. Conditions particularly associated with berry aneurysms include fibromuscular dysplasia, polycystic kidney disease, and cerebral arteriovenous malformations, but most are sporadic. There is clear evidence that aneurysms enlarge with time, and the likelihood of rupture rises when the diameter of the aneurysm is greater than 10 mm. However, not every aneurysm bursts, and small ones are a not infrequent incidental finding on carotid angiography and at autopsy.

The commonest site of rupture in an aneurysm is the thin-walled fundus, with consequences that depend on its orientation. If the fundus is pointing toward or applied to the surface of the brain, the escaping blood at high pressure may tunnel its way into the brain, sometimes

# TRAUMA

Cerebral trauma is most frequent in young males, who may then survive with varying degrees of incapacity for many years. It is estimated that in the United States there are more than 400,000 persons with major persisting handicap following head injury. Thus, as with cerebrovascular disease, trauma is an area of neuropathology with high costs to society as well as to the individual.

The most important anatomic feature that influences the effects of trauma on the brain is the skull. Although it protects against moderate forces, in more severe trauma it can turn into a weapon against the brain.

Injuries affecting the brain fall into three groups: (1) epidural hematomas, (2) subdural hematomas, and (3) parenchymal injuries.

## EPIDURAL HEMATOMA

*Epidural hematomas* develop after rupture of one of the meningeal arteries, usually the middle meningeal, that run between the dura and the skull. Since the dura is, in part, the periosteum of the skull and is therefore firmly attached to it, a skull fracture is usually present (Fig. 22–11A). Because they are a product of *arterial* bleeding, epidural hematomas accumulate quickly and cause a rapid and progressive rise in intracranial pressure, which usually develops within minutes to a few hours of the trauma. *Typically, patients recover from the initial trauma, the*

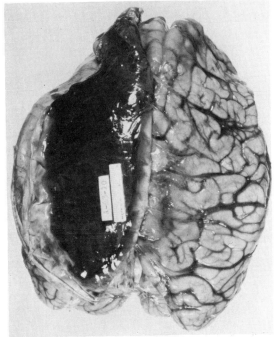

Figure 22–12. A relatively recent subdural hematoma, revealed by folding back the covering dura mater.

*so-called lucid interval, only to slip back into a progressively deepening coma.* Epidural hematomas are surgical emergencies which, if not immediately drained, will produce in rapid succession uncinate herniation, tonsillar herniation, medullary compression, respiratory paralysis, and death.

## SUBDURAL HEMATOMA

In contrast to epidural hematomas, which are the result of arterial bleeding, most subdural hematomas occur after rupture of some of the bridging veins that connect the venous system of the brain with the large venous sinuses that are enclosed within the dura. Since the brain in its bath of CSF can move, whereas the venous sinuses are fixed, the displacements of the brain that occur in trauma can tear some of these delicate veins at the point where they penetrate the dura, with subsequent bleeding into the subdural space (Fig. 22–11B). Subdural hematomas occur most frequently over the convexities of the hemispheres, where the freedom of movement of the brain is greatest (Fig. 22–12) and are relatively infrequent in locations such as the posterior fossa, where little movement is possible. They may be either acute or chronic.

*Acute subdural hematomas* are usually associated with obvious trauma and frequently with a laceration or contusion of the brain. *In contrast to the case with epidural hematomas, the onset of symptoms is generally delayed and is manifested clinically by fluc-*

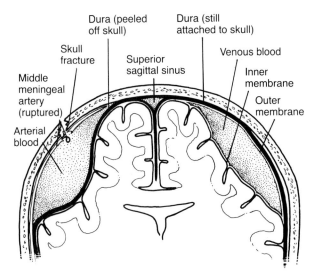

**A. Epidural hematoma**          **B. Subdural hematoma**

Figure 22–11. *A,* Epidural hematoma, in which rupture of a meningeal artery, usually associated with a skull fracture, leads to accumulation of arterial blood between the dura and the skull. *B,* In a subdural hematoma, damage to bridging veins between the brain and the superior sagittal sinus leads to the accumulation of blood between the dura and the brain.

*tuating levels of consciousness.* The outcome of an acute subdural hematoma depends not only on the effectiveness of surgical treatment but also on whether the adjacent brain is injured.

*Chronic subdural hematomas* are much less obviously symptomatic. Older persons and alcoholics are frequent victims. In such patients, there is usually some atrophy of the brain and consequently an increased range of movement of the brain within the skull cavity. This increased freedom of movement translates into an increased risk of rupture of the bridging veins, and in these patients subdural hematomas, often bilateral, may develop slowly after insignificant or even unnoticed trauma. The symptoms such as confusion, inattention, and progressive obtundation are often vague in nature and insidious in onset, although more rarely seizures or a progressive hemiparesis may occur. A source of clinical difficulty is that these protean symptoms may either mimic or be masked by concomitant disease, such as cerebrovascular disease or dementia. The CT scan has greatly simplified this diagnostic problem.

*Histologically, these hematomas consist of accumulations of blood encased by an outer membrane underlying the dura and an inner membrane that separates the blood from the adjacent arachnoid. Both subdural membranes are composed of granulation tissue derived from the dura.* Electron microscopy shows that the vascular channels within the membranes have incompletely endothelialized walls. This makes them very susceptible to rebleeding with only minimal trauma, resulting in progressive enlargement of the hematoma. Treatment consists of surgical drainage, but rebleeding from the membranes sometimes necessitates a craniotomy for their removal.

## PARENCHYMAL INJURIES

Trauma to brain itself can be grouped under five headings: (1) concussion, (2) contusions and lacerations, (3) diffuse axonal injury, (4) pure traumatic intracerebral hemorrhage, and (5) complications, which may be early or late.

*Concussion* is a transient loss of consciousness following head trauma. The duration of unconsciousness is usually short but may last for some hours. There is usually complete recovery. There is no established explanation for its occurrence, but one hypothesis is that torsion of the midbrain may temporarily disrupt the activating action of the reticular formation and may cause ensuing loss of consciousness.

*Contusions and lacerations* of the brain are traumatic lesions analogous to those of other soft tissues (p. 274).

**Contusions** occur when blunt trauma crushes or bruises brain tissue without rupturing the pia. The most common sites of contusions are either directly related to the trauma, in which case they may be at the site of impact (**coup lesions**) or at a point opposite (**contrecoup lesions**), where the brain in motion strikes against the inner surface of the skull, or at irregularities of the skull (e.g., the wing of the sphenoid and the orbital ridges, which produce contusions at the frontal and temporal poles and on the orbitofrontal gyri). The occipital poles are rarely damaged by this mechanism. Contusions usually damage only the crowns of the gyri, leaving the depths of the sulci intact. Histologically, acute contusions show foci of hemorrhagic necrosis. Later, macrophages remove dead tissue, and the area gradually resolves into an irregular, yellow-brown crater with a floor of glial tissue that is often covered by leptomeningeal fibrosis. Because of their color, these old contusions are referred to as "plaques jaunes." **Lacerations** are tears produced by severe blunt trauma, sometimes with an associated fracture followed by hemorrhage and necrosis. Resolution of lacerations is similar to that of contusions, except that it results in an irregular, yellow-brown, gliotic scar that involves not only cortex but also the deep underlying structures.

*Diffuse axonal injury* occurs in a group of patients who have severe neurologic impairment but do not have massive grossly visible brain damage.[14] Characteristically, these patients are deeply comatose from the moment of injury and recover only to the point of a persistent vegetative state. Microscopic examination of the brain shows widespread, diffuse damage to white matter in the form of *ruptured axons.* Older cases show microglial reaction, myelin degeneration, and sometimes microcavitation. There is some dispute over the pathogenesis of this lesion, but the most likely explanation is that shearing forces during the acceleration and deceleration of the brain cause actual physical rupture of axons.

*Pure traumatic intracerebral hemorrhages* are contained within the brain and do not extend to the surface. They are often multiple, involving the frontal and temporal lobes and the deep structures, and may be accompanied by contusions, lacerations, or acute axonal injury. It is not fully understood why they occur, but they probably result from direct rupture of intracerebral vessels at the time of trauma.

*Complications of trauma* may develop in patients who survive the initial insult. Posttraumatic *brain edema* may occur, especially in children; *herniation, brain stem compression,* and *Duret hemorrhage* (p. 726) may follow. Less frequently, skull fractures may provide a pathway for *infection,* especially from the ear or nose; *hydrocephalus* may develop secondary to blood or infection in the ventricular system, aqueduct, or subarachnoid space. In concluding this discussion of the more acute complications of trauma, it must be mentioned that there are a few patients in whom death may follow shortly after trauma when there is no apparent physical disruption of tissue. How and why death occurs in these cases is unknown.

*Delayed sequelae of trauma* include *posttraumatic epilepsy,* which usually occurs in patients who have sustained a cortical contusion or laceration, and *delayed intracerebral hemorrhage*, the so-called spät apoplexy, for totally obscure reasons.

# TUMORS

A somewhat simplified classification of tumors affecting the nervous system is given in Table 22–1. For operational purposes it is most convenient to divide tumors into three groups: (1) primary intracranial tumors of CNS parenchymal cells, (2) primary intracranial tumors that originate within the skull cavity but are not derived from the brain parenchyma itself, and (3) metastatic tumors.

In the *primary parenchymal tumors*, each type of cell in the nervous system gives rise to its own particular type or types of tumor, and there are some additional mixed, primitive, and mesenchymal tumors. The *primary nonparenchymal tumors*, as distinct from primary brain tumors, derive mostly either from the meninges or from adjacent structures such as the pituitary and pineal.[15]

**Table 22–1. TUMORS OF THE NERVOUS SYSTEM\***

**Primary Parenchymal Tumors**
  *Tumors of Neuroglia*
    Astrocytes
      *Astrocytoma*
      *Anaplastic astrocytoma*
      *Glioblastoma multiforme*
    *Pilocytic astrocytoma*
    Oligodendrocytes
      *Oligodendroglioma*
    Ependymal cells
      *Ependymoma* and its homologues

  *Tumors of Neurons*
    Neuroblastoma
    Ganglion cell tumors
      Ganglioneuroma
      Ganglioma

  *Tumors of Primitive Cells*
    *Medulloblastoma*

  *Tumors of Mesenchymal Cells*
    Lymphoma, primary and secondary
    Hemangioblastoma
    Vascular malformations

**Primary Nonparenchymal Tumors**
  *Meningeal Tumors*
    *Meningioma*
    Hemangiopericytoma
    Hemangioblastoma
    Meningeal sarcoma

  *Pineal Tumors (Non-neuroectodermal)*

  *Pituitary Tumors (Adenohypophyseal)*

  *Malformative Tumors*
    Craniopharyngioma
    Dermoid cyst
    Epidermoid

**Metastatic Tumors**

\*Tumors in light italics are discussed in the text.

An important feature of both primary categories is the discordance between the histologic appearance and the biologic consequences. Because some parts of the brain perform functions vital to life (e.g., the floor of the fourth ventricle, which controls respiration), there are some tumors, notably ependymomas, that are histologically benign or only trivially invasive but cannot be removed because of their location. They shorten the life of the patient and are "biologically malignant" although histologically benign.

## PRIMARY INTRACRANIAL TUMORS

Parenchymal brain tumors in general, and astrocytomas in particular, have a marked propensity for infiltrative growth into the interstices of the adjacent normal brain tissue. Thus they often do not have grossly or microscopically definable margins. Consequently, curative resection of such tumors is difficult and often impossible, even if the neurologic damage that would ensue were deemed to be acceptable. *Only rarely do they metastasize to the rest of the body, even the most anaplastic and histologically malignant. In the exceptional instance when this occurs, it is most frequently from a glioblastoma or medulloblastoma.* Surgical procedures that breach the dura or shunting operations have occasionally been associated with subsequent systemic dissemination of tumor. Although metastasis outside the nervous system is very infrequent, dissemination via the CSF within the nervous system may occur, and with some tumors, such as medulloblastomas, this is almost the rule rather than the exception.

*Some types of brain tumor have a predilection for specific sites within the brain. Medulloblastomas, for example, are confined to the cerebellum, and pilocytic astrocytomas are found predominantly in the cerebellum and hypothalamic area. There are also age preferences; medulloblastomas are the most frequent in the first decade of life, whereas hemispheric anaplastic astrocytomas and glioblastomas tend to occur in middle-aged and older patients, respectively.* Clinically, the most frequently encountered and important primary parenchymal tumors are astrocytomas, oligodendrogliomas, ependymomas, and medulloblastomas.

### Astrocytoma

Collectively, the astrocytomas are the most frequent type of primary parenchymal brain tumor, and most examples fall into one of three clinicopathologic groups: (1) astrocytomas, including glioblastoma multiforme, (2) brain stem glioma, and (3) pilocytic astrocytoma.

Astrocytomas in the cerebral hemispheres fall into three categories of increasing pathologic malignancy and rapidity of clinical progression. They are called *astrocytoma, anaplastic astrocytoma,* and *glioblastoma multiforme*, with astrocytomas being the least aggressive (though by no means benign) and glioblastomas the most.[16] Together they make up 80 to 90% of all the glial tumors arising in adults. They occur most frequently in middle age, with anaplastic astrocytomas having a peak incidence in the sixth decade and glioblastomas about ten years later.

The term "glioblastoma" requires a little clarification. In principle, this should be the term for the most anaplastic form of any glial tumor; in practice, it has come to be used for the most malignant variety of astrocytoma. It is also important to recognize that *astrocytic tumors have a marked tendency to become more anaplastic with time, so that a tumor initially diagnosed as an astrocytoma may, and frequently does, prove on later biopsy to be a glioblastoma.* A major practical difficulty in the interpretation of biopsies from these tumors is that in a single neoplasm different areas may have quite different histologic appearances, so that a small biopsy may incorrectly evaluate the full neoplastic potential of the tumor.

**Astrocytomas** are usually poorly defined, gray-white, infiltrative tumors that expand and distort the underlying brain. They are solid and, depending on their fibrillary content, may be firm or soft and gelatinous (Fig. 22–13). They range from a few centimeters in diameter to enormous lesions that replace the major part of a cerebral hemisphere and extend through the commissures into the opposite hemisphere.

Histologically, they may be composed of rather uniform populations of astrocytes that are given names such as protoplasmic, fibrillary, and gemistiocytic, but more usually they contain a mixture of astrocytic forms, many of which do not fall into one of the named types. Between the cells there is usually a highly characteristic fibrillary background of astrocytic processes of varying density and caliber.

**Anaplastic astrocytomas** are not grossly distinguishable from astrocytomas. Microscopically, they have typical anaplastic features such as hypercellularity, nuclear and cytoplasmic pleomorphism, and nuclear hyperchromatism. The presence in an astrocytoma of either vascular endothelial proliferation or a mitotic rate of greater than 1 per 10 high-power fields suggests this diagnosis.

Grossly, a **glioblastoma multiforme** can be distinguished from the other astrocytomas by its variegated appearance, hence the designation "multiforme." Some regions may be white and firm, others yellow and soft, and foci of necrosis, cysts, and hemorrhages are often seen (Fig. 22–14). **Microscopically, they are distinguished from anaplastic astrocytomas by the presence of necrosis**. As with anaplastic astrocytomas, vascular endothelial proliferation and mitoses are frequently seen (Fig. 22–15). In spite of the presence of these anaplastic features, areas of astrocytoma will usually be present intermixed with the more malignant regions. Both anaplastic astrocytomas and glioblastomas are occasionally disseminated throughout the neuraxis via the CSF.

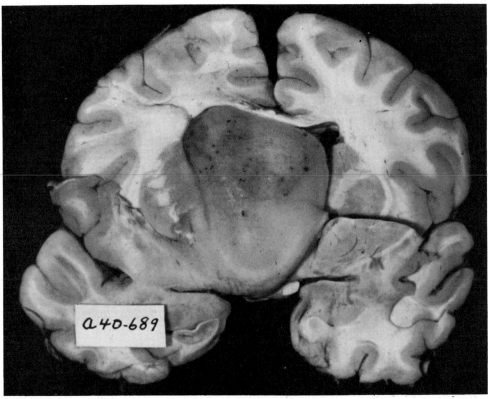

**Figure 22–13.** A large astrocytoma arising near the midline. Both lateral ventricles have been almost completely obliterated, and there is some distortion of the adjacent basal ganglia.

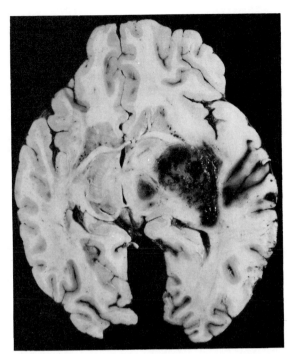

Figure 22–14. A glioblastoma multiforme showing hemorrhage into an area of cystic softening. The tumor and the surrounding edema have produced marked expansion of the affected hemisphere and a shift of the midline.

ever, patients usually enter a period of more rapid clinical deterioration that is generally correlated with the development of anaplastic features and more rapid growth in the tumor. The prognosis in patients with glioblastoma is grave indeed. With current treatment comprising palliative resection, where feasible, together with radiotherapy and steroids, mean survival is only between eight and 10 months; fewer than 10% of patients are alive after two years. Survival is substantially shorter in older patients. In anaplastic astrocytomas, the survival is more variable, but still dismal.

*Brain stem gliomas* mostly occur in the first two decades of life and make up about 20% of the primary brain tumors in this age group. Histologically, they resemble the astrocytomas in the hemispheres and, at autopsy, about 50% prove to be glioblastomas. With current radiotherapy, the five-year survival rate for the composite group is between 25 and 40%.

*Pilocytic astrocytomas* are distinguished from other astrocytomas by a distinctive pathologic appearance and *their almost invariably benign biologic behavior.* Typically, they occur in children and young adults and are usually located in the cerebellum, but they are also found in the floor and walls of the third ventricle, the optic chiasm and nerves, and, occasionally, in the cerebral hemispheres.

Grossly, they often manifest as a mural nodule in the wall of a cyst but, if solid, may be well circumscribed or apparently infiltrative. Microscopically, they are only moderately hypercellular and are composed of pilocytic astrocytes, which are bipolar cells with thin, hair-like processes. Rosenthal fibers (p. 724) and microcysts are also

Clinically, astrocytic neoplasms present with general or local signs and symptoms, or both, their nature depending largely on the location of the tumor. The symptoms may remain static or progress only slowly for a number of years. Eventually, how-

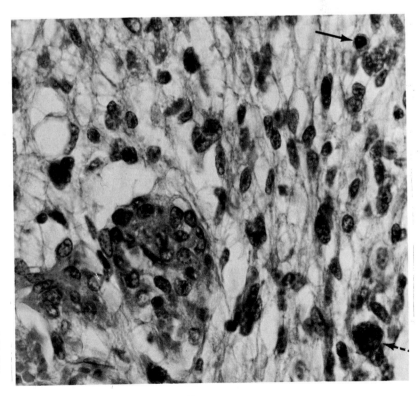

Figure 22–15. Microscopic detail of a glioblastoma multiforme. A mitotic figure (*solid arrow*), a giant cell (*dashed arrow*), and a cluster of hyperplastic endothelial cells are present.

characteristic. Vascular endothelial proliferation is often seen, but in this tumor, unlike the case in other astrocytomas, it does not imply an unfavorable prognosis, and other features of anaplasia are almost never seen.

These tumors are extremely slow growing and have the best prognosis of all brain tumors; patients have survived more than 40 years after incomplete resection.

## Oligodendroglioma

These tumors comprise about 5% of gliomas. They are most frequent in middle life and are found mostly in the cerebral hemispheres.

Grossly, they are well circumscribed, gelatinous gray masses, often with cysts, focal hemorrhages, and calcifications. **The calcification is often a valuable radiologic diagnostic clue**. As with other gliomas, there is occasionally extension of tumor into the subarachnoid space and dissemination through the CSF. Microscopically, **the tumor is composed of sheets of regular cells with spherical nuclei that contain finely granular chromatin** and are surrounded by a clear cytoplasmic halo that, although regularly present, is an artifact of fixation. Typically, a delicate vascular network of anastomosing capillaries separates the tumor cells into clusters. The calcifications range from microscopic foci to massive depositions. As many as 50% of these tumors contain foci of astrocytoma that, if anaplastic, determine the prognosis.

Clinically, these tumors have a very variable prognosis, and regrettably the pathologic characteristics of the tumor cells do *not* provide a good guide to the prognosis.

## Ependymoma

Ependymomas are derived from the single layer of epithelium that lines the ventricles and extends down the center of the spinal cord as the remnant of the central canal. Although they may occur at any age and anywhere in this epithelium, they are particularly likely to occur in the first two decades of life and in the fourth ventricle; they constitute between 5 and 10% of primary brain tumors of this age group. In middle life, the spinal cord is their most likely site of occurrence and, in this site, they comprise a large fraction of the intraparenchymal neoplasms.

Grossly, in the fourth ventricle they are typically **solid or papillary masses erupting from the floor of the ventricle and, although often well demarcated from the adjacent brain, their proximity to the vital medullary and pontine nuclei usually makes complete removal impossible**. With intraspinal tumors this sharp separation makes total removal, and therefore cure, sometimes possible. Microscopically, they are composed of elongated cells with rather regular round to oval nuclei that have abundant granular chromatin. Between the cells there is a fine fibrillary background, which may be very dense. The principal diagnostic features are **ependymal canals** and **rosettes**, in which the tumor cells form epithelial rings and surfaces that closely resemble ependyma, and perivascular **ependymal pseudorosettes**, in which there is a dense array of long, delicate ependymal processes inserted into the wall of the blood vessel, leaving a prominent nucleus-free halo around the vessel. Most tumors are well differentiated, but occasionally they are more anaplastic and may even resemble glioblastomas.

## Medulloblastoma

Medulloblastomas occur in the cerebellum and are overwhelmingly tumors of the first two decades of life.

Grossly, they are gray-white expansile lesions that sometimes appear to be quite well demarcated. In young children they are typically located in the vermis, but in older patients they are more often found laterally in the hemispheres. **Dissemination through the CSF with extensive ependymal and subarachnoid growth often occurs**. Microscopically, medulloblastomas are very cellular tumors with small but moderately pleomorphic nuclei containing variable densities of chromatin and very little, if any, visible cytoplasm. Some do not exhibit any form of differentiation, but in a few neuronal differentiation occurs, whereas other tumors show glial (spongioblastic) differentiation in the form of spindle cells, with delicate processes containing the specific glial fibrillary acidic protein. Occasionally, both types of differentiation are present in the same tumor. Usually, but not invariably, there are many mitoses in these rapidly growing tumors.

Clinically, patients tend to present with either hydrocephalus or progressive cerebellar signs (such as motor incoordination or unsteadiness of gait), or both. Because of the high frequency of CSF dissemination, treatment is by radiotherapy to the entire neuraxis. Currently, about 50% survival at 10 years is achieved.

## Meningioma

Meningiomas develop from the meningothelial cells of the arachnoid and are thus outside the brain. They comprise about 20% of all primary tumors of the brain and meninges. *Their commonest sites of occurrence are in the front half of the cranial cavity and include the hemispheric convexity, the falx, the lesser wing of the sphenoid bone, and the olfactory groove.* Other rarer but clinically important locations are the choroid plexus inside the cerebral ventricles, the cerebellopontine angle, the foramen magnum, and the spinal cord. Although usually solitary, multiple tumors may occur and are particularly likely in von Recklinghausen's neurofibromatosis. Meningiomas are generally tumors of middle and later life and are more frequent in women (3:2 ratio of women to men). Some tumors have estrogen receptors and grow rapidly during pregnancy.

Grossly, meningiomas are usually irregular, bosselated masses that are firmly attached to the dura and indent the surface of the brain but rarely invade it. Growth occasionally occurs in a plate-like fashion, producing the so-called **meningioma en plaque**. Hyperostosis of the overlying bone is frequently seen and occasionally superficial invasion of it. They are usually firm, solid tumors, often with a whorl-like pattern on their cut surfaces.

Microscopically, there are three major histologic types: **syncytial, fibroblastic**, and **transitional**. They form a spectrum rather than three completely separable entities. **Syncytial** meningiomas tend to recapitulate the normal appearance of meningothelial cells, with prominent cellular whorls and nodules (Fig. 22–16). The cell borders are indistinct, and electron microscopy reveals a complex interdigitation of the cell membranes, with desmosomes and gap junctions. **Fibroblastic** meningiomas have spindle-shaped bipolar cells arranged in interwoven bands and swaths. Their nuclei tend to be more elongated and have denser chromatin, and so the cells look like fibroblasts. **Transitional** meningiomas express intermediate characteristics and often contain **psammoma bodies**, which are roughly spherical, laminated, calcified structures. Psammoma bodies are also often found in small numbers in both syncytial and fibroblastic meningiomas.

Other histologic configurations such as microcystic variants are occasionally seen, as are various forms of degenerative change, such as xanthomatous degeneration and bone or, more rarely, cartilage formation. To an extent these descriptions are of academic interest in that none of these histologic variants have prognostic significance; all the variants are slow growing and histologically benign. Malignant meningiomas do occasionally occur, either as rather ordinary looking tumors with a high mitotic rate or as more frankly sarcomatous lesions that resemble fibrosarcomas.

## METASTATIC TUMORS

About 25 to 30% of tumors in the brain are metastatic implants. They are most frequent in older people, and the vast majority are carcinomas. About 80% arise in the lung, breast, skin (melanoma), kidney, and gastrointestinal tract, in order of frequency. Some tumors, such as choriocarcinomas, are quite rare but have a high likelihood of metastasizing to the brain; others, notably prostatic cancers and squamous cell carcinomas of the head and neck, almost never do, even when disseminated to adjacent bone.

Solitary metastases are unusual. Typically, there are multiple, well-circumscribed, roughly spherical masses of varying size that are usually located at the junction of the gray and white matter and are surrounded by zones of edematous white matter. Necrosis, cyst formation, and hemorrhage are frequent. Carcinomatous meningitis, with large numbers of tumor nodules studding the surface of the brain, cord, and intradural nerve roots, is an occasional complication that is particularly associated with small cell carcinomas and adenocarcinomas of the lung and carcinoma of the breast. Microscopically, most metastases recapitulate their primary tumors. Occasionally, small cell carcinomas of the lung may histologically resemble primary gliomas. The sharp demarcation between metastatic tumor and the surrounding reactive brain tissue, however, aids in distinguishing them from the usually infiltrative primary brain tumors.

The symptoms and signs are those of any intracranial mass. Occasionally, and particularly with carcinoma of the lung, they may even induce the presenting symptoms and be the unexpected diagnostic outcome of a biopsy of an ostensibly primary tumor. In general, treatment is symptomatic and palliative. Carcinoma of the kidney is an occasional exception to the rule that even apparently solitary metastases are not candidates for surgical resection.

## DEGENERATIVE DISEASES

Unlike most other categories of disease such as infections or trauma that share an etiological origin, the degenerative diseases are unified only by some general clinicopathologic features. Currently, almost all are of obscure origin, and there is no compelling reason to suppose that they have the same, or even a similar, type of etiology.

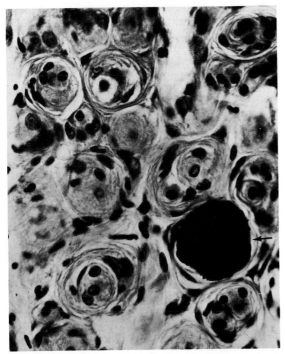

Figure 22–16. Microscopic detail of a meningioma, showing numerous concentric whorls and a large psammoma body (*arrow*).

*The two major common features of degenerative diseases are: (1) They are diseases of neurons and selectively affect one or more functional systems of neurons while they leave others intact. For example, in Parkinson's disease there is selective degeneration of the striatonigral dopaminergic system. (2) They are marked generally by symmetrical and progressive involvement of the CNS.*

In other ways these diseases differ among themselves quite sharply: some have a clear pattern of heritability, others are sporadic; some exhibit intracellular abnormalities of greater or lesser specificity, whereas in others the pathological process is atrophy and loss of the affected neurons without specific features.

Degenerative diseases that affect similar regions of the brain tend to produce clinical syndromes with many similarities, so that, for example, diseases of the cortex and basal ganglia tend to manifest as dementias and extrapyramidal movement disorders, respectively. Thus a diagnosis can often only be made by correlation of the clinical and pathologic findings.

For ease of description it is most convenient to group these diseases according to the part or parts of the brain that are principally affected, and an abbreviated list is given below. No etiologic connections among the diseases in each group are implied. Only a few of the more important entities (in *italics*) will be discussed.

| Diseases affecting the cortex | 1. *Alzheimer's disease*<br>2. *Pick's disease* |
| Diseases of the basal ganglia and mesencephalon | 1. *Huntington's disease*<br>2. *Idiopathic Parkinson's disease*<br>3. Postencephalitic Parkinson's disease<br>4. Striatonigral degeneration<br>5. Progressive supranuclear palsy<br>6. Shy-Drager syndrome |
| Spinocerebellar degenerations | 1. Olivopontocerebellar degeneration<br>2. Friedreich's ataxia<br>3. Ataxia-telangiectasia |
| Motor neuron diseases | 1. *Motor neuron disease (amyotrophic lateral sclerosis complex)*<br>2. Werdnig-Hoffmann disease<br>3. Kugelberg-Welander syndrome |

The major degenerative diseases with a large cortical component are *Alzheimer's disease* and *Pick's disease*, and their principal clinical manifestation is *dementia*. There are many other causes of dementia, including cerebrovascular disease, encephalitis, hydrocephalus, Creutzfeldt-Jakob disease, and metabolic diseases.

## ALZHEIMER'S DISEASE

Historically, the term *Alzheimer's disease* was used if the onset of the disease was before age 65, and *senile dementia* was used if the onset was later. However, currently Alzheimer's disease refers to dementia associated with the characteristic pathologic changes described below, regardless of the age of onset. Symptoms are rare before 50 years, and the usual initial complaints are of subtle impairment of higher intellectual functions or increased emotional lability. Later, progressive disorientation, memory loss, and language disorders indicate a more severe cortical dysfunction that eventually develops into a profound, mute, immobile dementia over the course of five to 10 years. Death is usually from an intercurrent infection exacerbated by inanition and dehydration. Most cases are sporadic, although some are familial. CT scans in advanced cases show the marked sulcal widening and ventricular enlargement of brain atrophy.

On gross examination of the brain there is widening of the cerebral sulci, usually most pronounced in the frontal and temporal regions (Fig. 22–17). Cut sections show compensatory ventricular enlargement secondary to tissue loss (hydrocephalus ex vacuo). The significant microscopic features of Alzheimer's disease are **neurofibrillary tangles, senile plaques, granulovacuolar degeneration**, and **Hirano bodies. Neurofibrillary tangles** are bundles of fibrils in the cytoplasm of a neuron that displace or encircle the nucleus. They are mildly basophilic in hematoxylin-eosin stains but are strongly stained by silver methods. Ultrastructurally, they are composed mostly of paired, helically wound filaments and have a diameter of 7 to 9 nm and a periodicity of about 80 nm. Neurofibrillary tangles are very insoluble and may remain

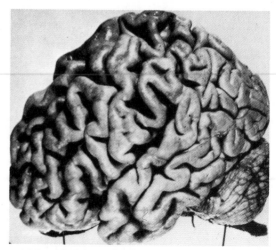

Figure 22–17. Alzheimer's disease. Cerebral atrophy is demonstrated by narrowed gyri and sulcal widening that is particularly marked in the frontal and superior temporal lobes. (Courtesy of Dr. Robert D. Terry.)

visible and stainable as "ghost tangles" for long periods after the death of the neuron. Their precise composition has not yet been elucidated. Although found in Alzheimer's disease, **neurofibrillary tangles are not specific to this condition**, since they are also found sometimes in other parts of the brain in other conditions such as Down's syndrome. They probably represent the end point of a number of different cellular pathophysiologic processes.

Early **senile plaques** are focal extracellular structures (20 to 150 μm in diameter) of dilated, tortuous, presynaptic axon terminals (and probably dendrites) that are found almost exclusively in the cerebral cortex. Microglial cells are often seen at the periphery of the plaques, as is, sometimes, astrocytosis. Later in their evolution they develop a central extracellular core of amyloid. **The plaques appear as irregular formations of silver-positive fibers and particulate material that surrounds, but is separated from, the central silver-positive amyloid core by a clear halo.** The electron microscope shows that the axonal terminals contain paired helical filaments similar to those seen in neurofibrillary tangles, together with degenerating lysosomes and mitochondria.

**Granulovacuolar degeneration** appears as small (5 μm in diameter), clear, intraneuronal cytoplasmic vacuoles, each of which contains an argyrophilic granule. The constituents of the granule are unknown, as is the pathophysiologic significance of this form of degeneration. This latter qualification also applies to **Hirano bodies**, seen in proximal dendrites as glassy eosinophilic inclusions. Ultrastructurally, they consist of regular arrays of beaded filaments, which biochemical analysis shows to be mostly actin filaments.

All of these structures can be seen in patients who do not have any known disease, and it is their number and distribution rather than their mere presence that allow the diagnosis of Alzheimer's disease to be made.[17] In Alzheimer's disease Hirano bodies are numerous, and granulovacuolar degeneration is present in more than 10% of the neurons of the hippocampus. Plaques and tangles are found extensively in the amygdala and most of the cerebral cortex, and tangles are present in the basal forebrain nuclei (basal nucleus of Meynert).[18]

The basic pathogenetic defect in Alzheimer's disease is unknown. The number of neurofibrillary tangles and senile plaques can be roughly correlated with the degree of dementia, but the mechanisms underlying their formation are obscure. The most consistent biochemical abnormalities in Alzheimer's disease are deficiencies in acetylcholine and associated enzymes choline acetyltransferase and acetylcholinesterase in the cerebral cortex, amygdala, and hippocampus. The major cortical and hippocampal cholinergic inputs from the basal forebrain nuclei (including the basal nucleus of Meynert) are severely depleted of cells in Alzheimer's disease, and some of the remaining cells exhibit neurofibrillary tangles or granulovacuolar change, or both.

## PICK'S DISEASE

Pick's disease occurs far less frequently than Alzheimer's disease, is often not distinguishable on clinical grounds from it, and leads to a similarly profound dementia. As with Alzheimer's disease, there are also occasional familial cases.

Typically, there is marked, although sometimes asymmetric, atrophy of the frontal and temporal lobes, with sparing of the posterior two thirds of the superior temporal gyrus and only very rare involvement of either the parietal or the occipital lobes. This pattern of atrophy is usually sufficient to distinguish Pick's disease, sometimes also called lobar atrophy, from Alzheimer's disease. The atrophy can be very severe, reducing the gyri to a thin wafer—the so-called knife blade atrophy or walnut brain. Microscopically, the atrophic cortex reveals neuronal loss that is most marked in the outer cortical layers and that may superficially resemble laminar necrosis (p. 734). Surviving neurons may contain **Pick bodies**, cytoplasmic, round to oval, filamentous inclusions that are only weakly eosinophilic but stain strongly with silver. Ultrastructurally, they are composed of neurofilaments, paired helical filaments, and vesiculated endoplasmic reticulum. In severe cases, in addition to the cortical damage, there is also marked subcortical degeneration of white matter.

## HUNTINGTON'S DISEASE

This disease usually first appears in persons between 20 and 50 years of age and is characterized by extrapyramidal or choreiform movements combined with a progressive dementia. It is inherited as an autosomal dominant, with the interesting but unexplained feature that those who inherit the disease from their fathers tend to manifest it much earlier in life than those who inherit from their mothers. *This combination of autosomal dominant inheritance with symptomatic onset that is often delayed until middle life turns this disease into a medical sword of Damocles over the heads of the children of affected persons.* For these offspring, an already difficult personal situation is exacerbated by the dilemma as to whether they themselves should have children and perhaps pass on the disease. The recent discovery that a genetic defect in these patients is located on chromosome 4 may lead to the removal of this sword, for although the precise mutant gene has not yet been identified, its localization to a chromosome offers the hope of antenatal diagnosis.[20]

On gross examination the brain is small (less than 1000 gm) and shows striking atrophy of the caudate nucleus and, less dramatically, of the putamen. The globus pallidus may be secondarily atrophied, and the lateral and third ventricles are enlarged. Atrophy of the frontal lobes, occasionally of the parietal lobes, and (more rarely) of the entire cortex may be present.

Microscopically, there is severe loss of neurons, particularly in the dorsal part of the striatum (with relative preservation of the nucleus accumbens in the inferior striatum) and also in the globus pallidus.[19] In the striatum, both the small and large neurons are affected, but loss of the small neurons generally seems to precede that of the larger. There is also a pronounced fibrillary gliosis that seems out of proportion to the usual reaction to neuronal loss.

Clinically, delusions, paranoia, neurosis, dementia, and abnormal eye movements are seen, and a hypothalamic component is suggested by abnormalities in glucose metabolism, aberrant levels of growth hormone, and altered prolactin release in some patients. The disease is relentlessly progressive, with an average course of 15 years, terminating in death. The neurochemical aspects of this disease are complex—some neurotransmitters such as GABA, acetylcholine, and substance P are decreased in concentration, whereas others are either unchanged or even, as with somatostatin, increased. It is not clear which of these changes is primary or secondary.

## PARKINSONISM

Parkinsonism is the name given to a disturbance of motor function characterized by expressionless facies, stooped posture, slowness of voluntary movement, festinating gait (progressively shortened, accelerated steps), rigidity, and sometimes, characteristic tremor. It is named after James Parkinson, who described idiopathic parkinsonism in 1817, but *this type of motor disturbance is seen in a number of different disease states that have in common damage to the striatonigral dopaminergic system.* It may also be produced by drugs, particularly dopamine antagonists, and by toxins.

### Idiopathic Parkinson's Disease (Paralysis Agitans)

This is a progressive disorder appearing spontaneously between 50 and 80 years of age.

Grossly, the substantia nigra and locus ceruleus are depigmented and, microscopically, there is loss of the melanin-containing neurons in these regions. **Lewy bodies** may be present in some of the remaining neurons. These are intracytoplasmic eosinophilic, round to elongated inclusions that have a dense core surrounded by a lighter rim. They are composed of filaments that are densely packed in the core but quite loose at the rim.

**Histologically, there is degeneration of the dopaminergic nigrostriatal pathway, with loss of cell bodies from the substantia nigra, degeneration of their axons and synapses in the striatum, and, consequently, a reduction in striatal dopamine content.**

Neurochemically, the severity of the parkinsonian syndrome is proportional to the dopamine deficiency, a deficiency that can, at least in part, be corrected by replacement therapy with L-dopa (the immediate precursor of dopamine). Treatment does not, however, reverse the morphologic changes or arrest the progress of the disease.

## MOTOR NEURON DISEASE (AMYOTROPHIC LATERAL SCLEROSIS COMPLEX)

Nowhere is the term "system degeneration" more appropriately applied than with this complex of clinical variants. *All are marked by degeneration of the pyramidal motor system, with its two levels of motor neurons in series.* The *upper motor neuron* is found in the motor cortex, and its axon traverses the internal capsule, brain stem, and corticospinal tract to end at a synapse on the *lower motor neuron* in a cranial motor nucleus or the anterior horn of the spinal cord.

Clinically, four variants are recognized. The most frequent is *amyotrophic lateral sclerosis*, in which patients show evidence of both lower motor neuron impairment (muscular atrophy and weakness) and upper motor neuron damage (hyperreflexia and a positive Babinski reflex). In *progressive bulbar palsy* there is predominant involvement of cranial nerves and brain stem, in *progressive muscular atrophy* there is principally lower motor neuron dysfunction, and in *primary lateral sclerosis* only the upper motor neurons are affected.

The pathologic changes are principally loss of motor neurons and their axons, with very little gliotic reaction. The distribution of the cell loss very much reflects the clinical symptoms and signs.[20]

Most cases of motor neuron disease are sporadic, although a few familial cases have been reported. Males are more often affected than females, the onset is typically in late middle age, and there is a progressive and inevitably fatal course over two to six years. Progressive bulbar palsy tends to run a shorter course, probably because of earlier involvement of the respiratory and pharyngeal musculature.

The etiology and pathogenesis of motor neuron disease are unknown. A high prevalence of HLA-A2, -A3, and -A28 haplotypes has been described. Needless to say, many possible etiologies have been explored, but without reward.

## DEMYELINATING DISEASES

The major pathologic process in the demyelinating diseases is loss of the myelin sheath that surrounds and insulates the axon. The axons themselves are relatively preserved. *Demyelination results either from damage to the oligodendrocytes that produce the myelin or a direct, usually immunologic or toxic assault on the myelin itself.* The demyelinating diseases, like the degenerative diseases, are a group of conditions bound together by a common pathologic process rather than an etiologic association. However, unlike the degenerative diseases, advances in understanding have allowed the transfer of many disorders previously included in the demyelinating diseases to more explicit etiologic categories. The most important diseases still remaining in this category are *multiple sclerosis* and its variants, and the *acute disseminated encephalomyelitides.* The *leukodystrophies* (inborn errors of metabolism), *progressive multifocal leukoencephalopathy* (slow virus disease), and *central pontine myelinolysis* (toxic metabolic disorder) are examples of diseases in which the principal pathologic process is demyelination but that are now more appropriately included in other etiologic categories.

## MULTIPLE SCLEROSIS (MS)

Since multiple sclerosis was first described by Charcot in 1868, it has been the subject of exhaustive but inconclusive study. The onset is between 20 and 40 years of age in about two thirds of the cases and is rare in individuals under 15 or over 50 years. The natural history of the disease is as varied as the number and distribution of the "plaques" of demyelination in the brain. *A relapsing and remitting course over many years is by far the most frequent pattern, but some patients have only a few brief episodes of mild disability, whereas others have a relentless downhill course to death in weeks or months.* Common early manifestations are paresthesias, retrobulbar neuritis, mild sensory or motor symptoms in a limb, or cerebellar incoordination. Intellectual deterioration is not usually an early feature. As the disease progresses, remissions become less complete. Although not all patients become totally disabled, the end stage is often that of unsteadiness of gait, incontinence, and paralysis due to widespread cerebral and spinal cord demyelination. There is no effective treatment, though ACTH and sometimes other immunosuppressive agents are often administered during relapses with some benefit.

The external appearance of the brain and spinal cord is usually normal. On cut section, **multiple, irregularly shaped, sharp-edged areas of demyelination called "plaques" are seen** (Fig. 22–18). Their appearance varies with their age; they are initially slightly pink and swollen but later become gray, sunken, and opalescent. Less frequently plaques have a diffuse rather than a sharp border, and they may be only faintly visible (shadow plaques). They occur in gray and white matter, range from barely visible to many centimeters in diameter, and

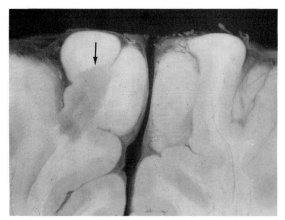

Figure 22–18. A plaque of multiple sclerosis in the subcortical white matter of a cerebral gyrus.

may be sparsely scattered or involve a large fraction of the brain and spinal cord. Although they have a predilection for the angles of the ventricles, they may occur anywhere in the CNS, but often they are bilaterally distributed in a relatively symmetrical fashion.

Microscopically, the earliest loss of myelin is seen around small veins and venules (perivenous demyelination). Mononuclear cells and lymphocytes are present around these vessels (Fig. 22–19). **As the demyelina-**

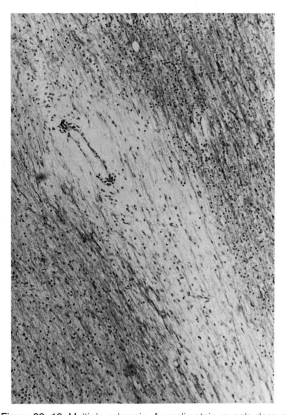

Figure 22–19. Multiple sclerosis. A myelin stain reveals demyelination adjacent to a small vessel in the white matter.

**tion progresses, the perivenular foci expand to form the macroscopically visible plaques**. In actively enlarging plaques, there is a lymphocytic inflammatory infiltrate at the border between the demyelinated and normal areas. Within the plaque, there is loss of oligodendrocytes but a pronounced reactive astrocytosis and numerous neutral lipid–laden macrophages. The axons traversing the plaque are conspicuously spared. Old inactive plaques have sharply defined edges, profound myelin loss, almost total absence of oligodendrocytes, and scattered fibrillary astrocytes. Although axons are relatively preserved, some loss is often detectable.

There is a great deal of interesting but ultimately inconclusive evidence about the cause of MS. A number of tantalizing epidemiologic observations have been made. There is a slight excess of females in the patient population, a higher incidence of disease in first-degree relatives of patients, and an excess of HLA-A3, -B7, and -DW2 antigens in northern European and white American patients. The disease is much more prevalent in the temperate latitudes in both the Northern and Southern Hemispheres and is most frequent in populations of European origin—there is a notably low incidence of MS in Oriental, African, and American Indian peoples. Migration studies have indicated that persons who move from regions of high incidence to lower-risk tropical climes (and conversely) tend to retain the risk of their birthplace if they move after the age of 15 years but adopt the risk of their new home if they migrate as children.

In isolated communities there is evidence of epidemic outbreaks of MS, notably in the Faroe Islands.[21] In this locale the outbreak began when British troops were present during the Second World War but persisted long after the withdrawal of the occupation forces, although it now seems to have died out. These findings suggest exposure to an environmental agent that can predispose to the later development of multiple sclerosis. Much effort has been devoted to the search for a viral association, but so far no really convincing candidate viru  has emerged.

As has been described, the demyelination in MS is marked by a prominent lymphocytic invasion into the lesions. Both T4 (helper) and T8 (suppressor) cells are present, and at least in some patients acute declines in the suppressor cell population in the blood accompany exacerbations of clinical symptoms. Although these findings suggest a role for the immune system in the process of demyelination, its precise contribution remains elusive. The immunoglobulin oligoclonal bands that are found in the CSF of patients with MS are probably epiphenomena, resulting from the trapping of activated B lymphocytes within the CSF, and although helpful diagnostically, they are not etiologically significant.

It is clear that the evidence concerning the pathogenesis of MS, although both confusing and incomplete, is suggestive of a role for infective and immune mechanisms, perhaps operating at different times in the life of the patient.

## PERIVENOUS ENCEPHALOMYELITIS

The term "perivenous encephalomyelitis" is applied to disorders associated with perivenous and perivenular demyelination accompanied by a pronounced mononuclear cell infiltration. *They usually follow a viral infection, vaccination, or a vague respiratory illness and are characterized by a monophasic, rapid, and relentless course that frequently terminates in death.* The two major disorders in this category are *acute disseminated encephalomyelitis* and *acute hemorrhagic leukoencephalitis.*

# NUTRITIONAL, ENVIRONMENTAL, AND METABOLIC DISORDERS

## NUTRITIONAL DISEASES

The major vitamin deficiencies that affect the adult nervous system involve *thiamine* and *cobalamin.*

### Thiamine Deficiency

A deficiency of thiamine has many systemic effects (p. 244) but in addition may result in the Wernicke-Korsakoff syndrome, a peripheral neuropathy, or both conditions. Clinically, these complications are most often but not exclusively encountered in alcoholics but are not a direct toxic effect of the alcohol itself. *Wernicke's encephalopathy* is an acute syndrome with confusion, eye movement abnormalities, and cerebellar signs that rapidly progress to coma but are completely reversible with thiamine if it is administered in time. *Korsakoff's psychosis* is a chronic memory disorder that causes an inability to form new memories or retrieve old ones. Both states are characterized by lesions in the mammillary bodies and the walls of the third ventricle (and sometimes other locations), in which there is prominent dilatation of small vessels and hyperplasia of endothelial cells in the affected regions. It is probable that the principal effect of the deficiency is on the vessels rather than the nervous system itself.

### Cobalamin Deficiency

An inadequacy of vitamin $B_{12}$ (cobalamin), if prolonged, results in pernicious anemia (p. 366) and its *subacute combined degeneration of the cord,* marked by a characteristic vacuolation and degeneration of both axons and myelin in the dorsal columns and lateral white columns of the spinal cord. The gray matter is entirely unaffected.

## ENVIRONMENTAL DISEASES

The central and peripheral nervous systems are the target of a very large number of environmental agents, so large indeed that not even a basic outline can be given here. Among the major categories of neurotoxic substances are *metals*, examples of which are lead, mercury, and arsenic; a wide variety of *industrial chemicals*, including aromatic hydrocarbon solvents, organophosphates, methyl alcohol, and carbon disulfide; and a range of *naturally occurring toxins* such as botulinum toxin and the chick-pea toxin that causes lathyrism.

Therapeutic agents are an additional important and expanding category of neurotoxins; some of the many types of adverse effects are *peripheral neuropathies* (vinca alkaloids, isoniazid), *tardive dyskinesias* (neuroleptics), and *convulsions* (metronidazole). Many neurotoxic effects have occurred after antitumor treatment. *Ionizing radiation*, as it does in other organs, can cause a vasculopathy leading to tissue ischemia and infarction. *Radiation/chemotherapy leukoencephalopathy* is particularly associated with the combination of radiation and intrathecal or high-dose intravenous methotrexate, and it consists of irregularly shaped, necrotic lesions in the white matter. Even saline solution can have neurotoxic effects. *Central pontine myelinolysis* is associated with the over-rapid correction of a low serum sodium, a therapeutic maneuver made possible by the availability of hypertonic saline solutions.[22] The demyelination can be extensive enough to involve the whole of the basis pontis and may cause complete paralysis.

*Ethyl alcohol* is a widely used, and abused, neurotoxin. Acutely, it causes a CNS depression that can be fatal. With chronic administration, in addition to the Wernicke-Korsakoff syndrome and a peripheral neuropathy that are associated with thiamine deficiency, there is also a cerebellar vermis degeneration that may be a direct toxic effect of the alcohol (p. 267).

## METABOLIC ENCEPHALOPATHY

The blood-brain barrier protects the CNS neurons from all but large or prolonged changes in the levels of electrolytes and metabolites in the blood. When deviations from the norm produce disturbances in cerebral function, it is referred to as a *metabolic encephalopathy*. Frequently encountered causes include diabetes, in which *exogenous insulin-induced hypoglycemia* produces an acute confusional state that can be rapidly reversed by the administration of glucose. *Hyperglycemic coma* is more complicated, with additional changes in pH, electrolytes, and osmotic pressure all contributing to a cerebral disequilibrium that can persist for several days after the

serum levels have been restored to normal. This persistence of dysfunction presumably reflects the time required to reestablish intracellular biochemical normality. Other frequent causes of a more chronic metabolic encephalopathy are uremia (p. 458), hypercalcemia (p. 26), and hepatic failure. Despite the sometimes profound disturbance in cerebral function, there is often little or no morphologic change, a finding that reflects the predominantly biochemical nature of the cerebral disorder.

### Hepatic Encephalopathy

Patients with hepatic failure exhibit a characteristic clinical picture that includes a peculiar flapping tremor of the extremities, called *asterixis*, and a disturbance in consciousness that progresses to coma and even death in severe cases.[23] The course of the encephalopathy parallels that of the hepatic failure. A similar encephalopathy can be produced, and marginally compensated patients precipitated into encephalopathy, by portacaval shunting. Although the severity of the encephalopathy is generally correlated with the raised blood ammonia level seen in hepatic failure, it is probably not a simple toxic effect of the hyperammonemia.

Pathologically, *the only consistent abnormality is a proliferation of protoplasmic astrocytes that have enlarged, watery, deformed nuclei, each containing a "glycogen dot" (Alzheimer II astrocytes).* They are found predominantly in gray matter and are especially prominent in the lenticular nucleus, thalamus, red nucleus, substantia nigra, and the deeper layers of the cerebral cortex. Nuclei that are similar but without the "glycogen dot" can be seen in patients with many of the other metabolic encephalopathies.

Severe and long-standing hepatic encephalopathy can lead to a cerebral degeneration morphologically similar to that seen in Wilson's disease.

# INBORN ERRORS OF METABOLISM

The variety and range of effects of the inborn errors of metabolism on the nervous system are legion. Many of these diseases have effects both inside and outside the nervous system; it is the balance of these effects that determines whether they present clinically as diseases of the nervous system or as systemic diseases. For example, in *Wilson's disease* some patients present with hepatic failure with little nervous system involvement, whereas others present with choreoathetosis and dementia, diseases of the brain. In *phenylketonuria* (p. 108), although the inborn error affects all tissues, the clinical manifestations are overwhelmingly in the nervous system. In this section only the neurologic features of *Wilson's disease* and the *leukodystrophies* will be considered.

## WILSON'S DISEASE

This autosomal recessive disorder of copper metabolism was discussed on page 110. It generally presents clinically with a rather characteristic combination of progressive choreoathetoid or parkinsonian motor symptoms coupled with evidence of liver disease.

In accordance with the predominantly extrapyramidal nature of the neurologic complaints, the most severe lesions in the brain are seen in the basal ganglia. There is a variable degree of brownish discoloration and atrophy of the caudate and lentiform nuclei with, in severe cases, cavitation in the putamen. Microscopically, the changes are more widely distributed but are again most obvious in the basal ganglia; the putamen is the most severely affected area. The major histologic features are large numbers of Alzheimer II astrocytes (p. 751), neuronal loss, and in some cases large multinucleate (Alzheimer I) astrocytes and Opalski cells, which are large cells of uncertain origin that have foamy cytoplasm and small, dense nuclei. The cavitation of the putamen, when it occurs, seems to result from the confluence of areas of severe degeneration of nerve cells and astrocytes.

## LEUKODYSTROPHIES

These are diseases of white matter in which the inborn error is known, or presumed, to be in the pathways of myelin metabolism. In all the leukodystrophies in which the biochemical defect has been identified, it is a deficiency of a lysosomal degradative enzyme. *Pathologically, the principal process is demyelination, but there may also be some neuronal storage.* From their biochemical origin it might be expected that all leukodystrophies would become manifest in early childhood as symmetrical disorders of myelination, affecting the entire neuraxis. In many cases (e.g., the childhood form of metachromatic leukodystrophy) this is so, but in other conditions (e.g., adrenoleukodystrophy) there is marked phenotypic variation in spite of the apparent uniformity of the biochemical defect.

The major leukodystrophies are *metachromatic leukodystrophy*, in which a deficiency of arylsulphatase A leads to the accumulation of galactosyl sulphatides; *globoid cell leukodystrophy* (Krabbe's disease), in which galactocerebroside accumulates because of a lack of galactocerebroside β-galactosidase; and the *adrenoleukodystrophy/adrenomyeloneuropathy* complex, in which the enzyme deficiency is not known but there is defective handling of long-chain fatty acids that leads to a raised C26:C20 fatty acid ratio in many tissues.[24]

## THE PERIPHERAL NERVOUS SYSTEM (PNS)

Unlike the brain, in which there is effectively no regeneration, both *degeneration* and *regeneration* can occur in the PNS. There are three basic degenerative processes, *Wallerian degeneration*, *axonal degeneration*, and *segmental demyelination*.[25]

*Wallerian degeneration* follows peripheral transection of the axon. Proximal to the site of transection there is degeneration back to the nearest node of Ranvier and, if the transection is sufficiently proximal, there will be chromatolysis in the cell body of the transected axon. Distal to the transection there is degeneration of the axon and its myelin sheath, both of which are digested by the Schwann cells, which proliferate to accomplish this task.

*Axonal degeneration* occurs when neuronal dysfunction renders the neuron unable to maintain its axon, which therefore starts to degenerate. The degeneration begins at the distal, or peripheral, end of the axon and proceeds back toward the cell body, a process called "dying back." There is often chromatolysis of the cell body. Schwann cell proliferation occurs in the region of active axonal degeneration, though it is less pronounced than that seen in Wallerian degeneration.

If the neuronal dysfunction can be halted or reversed, regeneration and some recovery of nerve function can occur.

*Regeneration* occurs by the outgrowth of multiple sprouts from the distal ends of the surviving segments of the axons. If there is no obstruction to their growth, the regenerating axons grow back down the nerve trunk at a rate of about 1 mm per day in association with the Schwann cells, which remain after digesting the degenerated axon. If, as is frequently the case in Wallerian degeneration secondary to a traumatic injury, there is hematoma or fibrous scar preventing the regenerating sprouts from entering the distal stump of the nerve, the obstructed regenerating axons then form a tangled, often painful mass of intertwined nerve fibers called an *amputation*, or *traumatic neuroma*.

*Segmental demyelination* is analogous to demyelination in the brain and is the selective loss of individual myelin internodes with preservation of the underlying axon (Fig. 22–20). After an episode of demyelination, remyelination can be accomplished by the remaining Schwann cells, which proliferate. Repeated episodes of demyelination and remyelination can occur and generate concentric arrangements of alternating Schwann cell processes and collagen, called "onion bulbs," which are found in the hypertrophic neuropathies.

### PERIPHERAL NEUROPATHY

Both diffuse demyelination and axonal degeneration tend to affect the longest axons first and produce

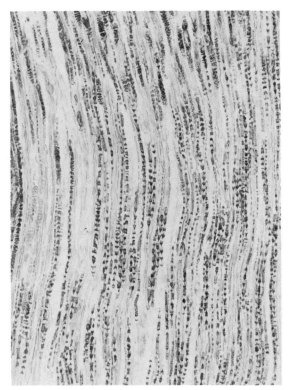

**Figure 22–20.** Demyelinating neuropathy. A myelin stain reveals focal loss of myelin in a peripheral nerve.

a syndrome called a *polyneuropathy*. Polyneuropathies are typically symmetrical and present with distal signs and symptoms in the limbs, such as motor weakness and loss of deep tendon reflexes or a "glove and stocking" sensory loss. If the autonomic system is affected, there may be postural hypotension, constipation, and impotence. When there is muscle weakness, axonal degeneration will be accompanied by muscle fasciculation and wasting; in demyelination, where there is conduction failure but no denervation, these are not present. Clinically, different etiologic agents preferentially tend to affect axons of different diameters or to affect sensory, motor, and autonomic axons to different degrees. The balance of symptoms and signs will reflect the axons principally involved. Neuropathies may also be mild or severe; they may be acute, subacute, or chronic in time course and may have relapses and remissions.

While many etiologic agents produce generalized damage, there are also pathologic processes that are focal (e.g., vasculitis) and affect only individual nerves, producing a *mononeuropathy* or, if more than one nerve is affected, a *mononeuropathy multiplex*. When they are widespread, even pathologically focal processes may present, usually asymmetrically, as a *polyneuropathy*.

Most clinical classifications of peripheral neuropathies are based on the type of clinical syndrome that develops. A simplified version of a widely used one is given in Table 22–2, which includes an indication

## Table 22–2. PRINCIPAL NEUROPATHIC SYNDROMES*

**Acute Ascending Motor Paralysis with Variable Sensory Disturbance**—*Acute demyelinating neuropathies*
  Acute idiopathic polyneuropathy (Landry-Guillain-Barré syndrome)
  Infectious mononucleosis with polyneuropathy
  Hepatitis and polyneuropathy
  Diphtheritic polyneuropathy
  Toxic polyneuropathies (e.g., triorthocresyl phosphate)

**Subacute Sensorimotor Polyneuropathy**
  (1) Symmetric—*Mostly axonal neuropathies*
       Alcoholic polyneuropathy and beriberi
       Arsenic polyneuropathy
       Lead polyneuropathy
       Vinca alkaloids and other intoxications
  (2) Asymmetric—*Axonal neuropathies with focal and/or diffuse pathology*
       Polyarteritis nodosa and other arteritides
       Sarcoidosis

**Chronic Sensorimotor Polyneuropathy**
  (1) Acquired—*Axonal neuropathies with focal and/or diffuse pathology*
       Carcinomatous
       Paraproteinemias (demyelinating)
       Uremia
       Diabetes
       Connective tissue diseases
       Amyloidosis
       Leprosy
  (2) Inherited—*Mostly chronic demyelination with hypertrophic changes*
       Peroneal muscular atrophy (Charcot-Marie-Tooth disease)
       Hypertrophic polyneuropathy (Dejerine-Sottas disease)
       Refsum's disease

**Chronic Relapsing Polyneuropathy**—*Mixed pathology*
  *Idiopathic polyneuropathy*
  *Porphyria*
  *Beriberi and intoxications*

**Mono or Multiple Neuropathy**—*Focal axonal or demyelinating pathology*
  Pressure palsies
  Traumatic palsies
  Serum neuritis
  Zoster
  Tumor invasion with neuropathy
  Leprosy

*Adapted from Adams, R. D., and Asbury, A. K.: Diseases of the peripheral nervous system. *In* Petersdorf, R. G., et al. (eds.): Harrison's Principles of Internal Medicine. 10th ed. New York, McGraw-Hill Book Co., 1983, p. 2158. Reprinted from Robbins, S. C., Cotran, R. S., and Kumar, V.: Pathologic Basis of Disease. 3rd ed. Philadelphia, W. B. Saunders, 1984, p. 1431. Reproduced with permission.

in each clinical category of the predominant pathologic process encountered.

In most clinical series, between 25 and 70% of peripheral neuropathies remain undiagnosed in etiologic terms. Intensive evaluation of a series of such cases has shown that at least 40% were probably hereditary and 20% were inflammatory or demyelinating, but that a significant number remained undiagnosed.[26] In this section only two examples of peripheral neuropathy will be discussed.

## Acute Idiopathic Polyneuropathy (Landry-Guillain-Barré Syndrome)

This acute demyelinating neuropathy has been associated with a bewildering variety of antecedent events. About 40% of the cases are associated with a "viral prodrome," with mycoplasma infection in about 5% of the cases, with allergic phenomena in 10%, and with a wide variety of other associations, including surgery, in 25%; the residual 20% of cases have no known antecedent event. It presents as a rapidly progressive motor neuropathy that has variable sensory features. In severe cases, the muscular weakness may be so profound and proceed so far proximally as to produce potentially fatal respiratory paralysis and facial diplegia. The CSF often, but not invariably, reveals a strikingly raised protein level and a normal or only slightly raised cell count.

Pathologically, focal inflammatory lesions marked by demyelination and an accumulation of lymphocytes and macrophages are scattered throughout the peripheral nerves, although there is some predilection for the proximal nerve trunks. Ultrastructurally, the earliest visible change is splitting of the myelin lamellae. Later, the myelin is apparently stripped off the axon and digested by macrophages, leaving the Schwann cells intact. This demyelination occurs without, apparently, the direct participation of the lymphocytes.

## Diabetic Neuropathy

Peripheral neuropathy frequently develops in diabetes and is often one of its most troublesome complications. One of its outstanding clinical features is its seemingly capricious occurrence—sometimes it is not present even after 40 years of poorly controlled juvenile onset diabetes, whereas in other cases it may even antedate measurable hyperglycemia. However, most cases occur late in the course of the disease. Clinically, *it is a distal, symmetric, predominantly sensory polyneuropathy, and, pathologically, it is principally an axonopathy* but with features suggesting the presence of a demyelinating component.

## PERIPHERAL NERVE TUMORS

### Schwannomas (Neurilemmomas) and Neurofibromas

Despite their usually quite distinct clinical presentations and histological features, both these tumors are derived from Schwann cells.

Grossly, both types of tumor have a white to gray color and a firm texture, but schwannomas are typically solitary, circumscribed, and encapsulated lesions that are **eccentrically located on proximal nerves or spinal nerve roots**. By contrast, neurofibromas are more often multiple and usually but not invariably unencapsulated; they appear as **fusiform enlargements of distal nerves**. Many are subcutaneous. Microscopically, **schwannomas are distinguished by the presence of areas of high and low cellularity called Antoni A and B tissue, respectively**. In the Antoni A tissue there may be foci of palisaded nuclei called **Verocay bodies**. Blood vessels in schwannomas often have **hyaline thickening**, around which there may be pseudopalisading of the tumor nuclei. **Neurofibromas have none of these features and usually consist of a loose pattern of interlacing bands of delicate spindle cells with elongated, slender, and sometimes wavy nuclei**. In both types of tumor there may be quite marked nuclear pleomorphism and irregularity, and even occasional giant cells, but these are not necessarily ominous findings. Myxoid or xanthomatous degeneration may also be seen. **In schwannomas, no nerve fibers are present in the body of the tumor, although the residual nerve of origin of the tumor may be seen compressed to one side. In neurofibromas, nerve fibers are found scattered throughout the tumor mass, as though it had arisen by expansion of the entire nerve fascicle**. This distinction has practical significance, as the compression of the nerve to one side in a schwannoma may permit its removal without requiring transection of the nerve, a course of action not possible with neurofibromas, in which the entire nerve is involved in the tumor process.

Malignant transformation may occur in both types of tumor, but it is much less frequent in schwannomas. It is characterized by hypercellularity, pleomorphism, mitoses, and blood vessel proliferation, so that the tumor resembles a fibrosarcoma. **Most cases of malignant neurofibroma are encountered in patients with von Recklinghausen's neurofibromatosis** (p. 106).

Except in von Recklinghausen's disease,[27] these are usually tumors of adults, presenting most frequently in the fifth and sixth decades. The most serious symptoms are those produced by schwannomas on the cranial and spinal nerve roots. Patients with acoustic (VIII nerve) schwannomas typically present with complaints of deafness and tinnitus, associated, if the tumor is large enough, with pressure palsies of the adjacent fifth and seventh cranial nerves or evidence of brain stem compression and hydrocephalus. Those with spinal root neurilemmomas may present with signs of slowly progressive cord compression or a cauda equina syndrome. With more distal tumors on nerve trunks there may be local complaints in the territory of the affected nerve, and, finally, there are the ubiquitous subcutaneous "lumps and bumps," which, if of neural origin, usually prove to be neurofibromas.

## References

1. Bradbury, M. W. B.: The structure and function of the blood-brain barrier. Fed. Proc. 43:186, 1984.
2. Harriman, D. G. F.: Bacterial infections of the central nervous system. *In* Blackwood, W., and Corsellis, J. A. N. (eds.): Greenfield's Neuropathology. 4th ed. London, Arnold Ltd., 1984, pp. 236–259.

3. Carpenter, R. R., and Petersdorf, R. G.: The clinical spectrum of bacterial meningitis. Am. J. Med. 33:262, 1962.

4. Hooper, D. C., et al.: Central nervous system infection in the chronically immunosuppressed. Medicine 61:166, 1982.

5. Myerowitz, R. L.: The Pathology of Opportunistic Infections. New York, Raven Press, 1983, p. 145.

6. Johnson, R. T.: Selective vulnerability of neural cells to viral infections. Brain 103:447, 1980.

7. Ho, D. D., et al.: Isolation of HTLV-III from cerebrospinal fluid and neural tissues from patients with neurologic syndromes related to the acquired immunodeficiency syndrome. N. Engl. J. Med. 313:1493, 1985.

8. Snider, W. D., et al.: Neurological complications of acquired immune deficiency syndrome: Analysis of 50 patients. Ann. Neurol. 14:403, 1983.

9. Walker, D. L.: Progressive multifocal leukoencephalopathy and opportunistic viral infection of the central nervous system. In Vinken, P. J., and Bruyn, G. W. (eds.): Handbook of Clinical Neurology. Vol. 34. Infection of the Nervous System, Part II. Amsterdam, North-Holland Publishing Co., 1978, pp. 307–329.

10. Manuelidis, E. E.: Creutzfeldt-Jakob Disease. J. Neuropathol. Exp. Neurol. 44:1, 1985.

11. Bradford, A. N., et al.: Cerebral toxoplasmosis complicating the acquired immune deficiency syndrome. Clinical and neuropathological findings in 27 patients. Ann. Neurol. 19:224, 1986.

12. Garcia, J. H., and Conger, K. A.: Ischaemic brain injuries: Structural and biochemical effects. In Grenvik, A. K., and Safar, P. (eds.): Brain Failure and Resuscitation. London, Churchill Livingstone, 1981, pp. 35–54.

13. Fisher, C. M.: Lacunar strokes and infarcts: A review. Neurology (N.Y.) 32:871, 1982.

14. Hume-Adams, J., et al.: Diffuse axonal injury due to non-missile head injury in humans: An analysis of 45 cases. Ann. Neurol. 12:557, 1982.

15. Russell, D. S., and Rubenstein, L. J.: Pathology of Tumors of the Nervous System. 4th ed. London, Arnold Ltd., 1977.

16. Burger, P. C., and Vogel, F. S.: Surgical Pathology of the Nervous System and Its Coverings. 2nd ed. New York, John Wiley & Sons, 1982, pp. 223–458.

17. Tomlinson, B. E., et al.: Observations on the brains of demented old people. J. Neurol. Sci. 11:205, 1970.

18. Whitehouse, P. J., et al.: Alzheimer's disease and senile dementia: Loss of neurones in the basal forebrain. Science 215:1237, 1982.

19. Martin, J. D.: Huntington's disease: New approaches to an old problem. Neurology (Clev.) 34:1059, 1984.

20. Martin, J. B., and Gusella, J. F.: Huntington's disease. Pathogenesis and management. N. Engl. J. Med. 315:1267, 1986.

21. Kurtzke, J. F., and Hyllested, K.: Multiple sclerosis in the Faroe Islands: II. Clinical update, transmission and the nature of M.S. Neurology 36:307, 1986.

22. Norenberg, M. D., et al.: Association between rise in serum sodium and central pontine myelinolysis. Ann. Neurol. 11:128, 1982.

23. Fraser, C. L., and Arieff, A. I.: Hepatic encephalopathy. N. Engl. J. Med. 313:865, 1985.

24. Kolodney, E. H., and Cable, W. J. L.: Inborn errors of metabolism. Ann. Neurol. 11:221, 1982.

25. Asbury, A. K., and Johnson, P. C.: Pathology of Peripheral Nerve. Philadelphia, W. B. Saunders Co., 1978.

26. Dyck, P. J., et al.: Intensive evaluation of referred unclassified neuropathies yields improved diagnosis. Ann. Neurol. 10:222, 1981.

27. Riccardi, V. M.: von Recklinghausen's neurofibromatosis. N. Engl. J. Med. 305:1617, 1981.

# Index

Note: Numbers in *italics* refer to figures; numbers followed by t refer to tables.